NUTRITION

FOR HEALTH, FITNESS & SPORT

Melvin H. Williams

Old Dominion University

J. David Branch

Old Dominion University

Eric S. Rawson

Bloomsburg University

McGraw Hill Education

NUTRITION FOR HEALTH, FITNESS AND SPORT: ELEVENTH EDITION

Published by McGraw-Hill Education, 2 Penn Plaza, New York, NY 10121. Copyright © 2017 by McGraw-Hill Education. All rights reserved. Printed in the United States of America. Previous editions © 2013, 2010, and 2007. No part of this publication may be reproduced or distributed in any form or by any means, or stored in a database or retrieval system, without the prior written consent of McGraw-Hill Education, including, but not limited to, in any network or other electronic storage or transmission, or broadcast for distance learning.

Some ancillaries, including electronic and print components, may not be available to customers outside the United States.

This book is printed on acid-free paper.

1 2 3 4 5 6 7 8 9 0 RMN/RMN 1 0 9 8 7 6

ISBN 978-0-07-802135-0
MHID 0-07-802135-9

Senior Vice President, Products & Markets: *Kurt L. Strand*
Vice President, General Manager, Products & Markets: *Marty Lange*
Vice President, Content Production & Technology Services: *Kimberly Meriwether David*
Managing Director: *Michael Hackett*
Brand Manager: *Marija Magner*
Director, Product Development: *Rose Koos*
Product Developer: *Mandy Clark*
Marketing Manager: *Kristine Rellihan*
Director, Content Design & Delivery: *Linda Avenarius*
Program Manager: *Faye M. Herrig*
Content Project Manager: *Jessica Portz, Brent Dela Cruz*
Buyer: *Laura Fuller*
Cover Image: *Upper left: © Terry Vine/Blend Images LLC; (clockwise) © 2009 Jupiter Images Corporation; © Trinette Reed/Blend Images LLC; Koji Aoki/Aflo/Getty Images; Comstock/Jupiter Images*
Compositor: *SPi Global*
Typeface: *10/12 STIXMathJax Main*
Printer: *R. R. Donnelley*

All credits appearing on page or at the end of the book are considered to be an extension of the copyright page.

Library of Congress Cataloging-in-Publication Data

Names: Williams, Melvin H. | Rawson, Eric S. | Branch, J. David, 1956-
Title: Nutrition for health, fitness, and sport / Melvin H. Williams, Old
    Dominion University, Eric S. Rawson, Bloomsburg University, J. David
    Branch, Old Dominion University.
Description: Eleventh edition. | New York, NY : McGraw-Hill, [2017] |
    Includes index.
Identifiers: LCCN 2015038385 | ISBN 9780078021350 (alk. paper)
Subjects: LCSH: Nutrition. | Physical fitness. | Sports—Physiological
    aspects.
Classification: LCC QP141 .W514 2017 | DDC 613.2—dc23 LC record available at
    http://lccn.loc.gov/2015038385

The Internet addresses listed in the text were accurate at the time of publication. The inclusion of a website does not indicate an endorsement by the authors or McGraw-Hill Education, and McGraw-Hill Education does not guarantee the accuracy of the information presented at these sites.

www.mhhe.com

To Jeanne,
Sara, Nik, Katy, Lucy, and Jake May
Serena, Jeff, Daniel, and David Newsom
—Melvin H. Williams

To Carol, David, Anne Randolph, Ellie,
Gracie, and the rest of my family
—J.David Branch

To Debbie, Christopher, Matthew,
and Erica
—Eric S. Rawson

and

To our teachers, colleagues,
and students
Mel, David and Eric

Brief Contents

Contents

CHAPTER THREE

Human Energy 90

Protein: The Tissue Builder 223

Vitamins: The Organic Regulators 277

CHAPTER EIGHT

Minerals: The Inorganic Regulators 327

CHAPTER NINE

Water, Electrolytes, and Temperature Regulation 370

CHAPTER TWELVE

Weight Gaining through Proper Nutrition and Exercise 539

Food Drugs and Related Supplements 565

Preface

According to the World Health Organization, better health is the key to human happiness and well-being. Many factors influence one's health status, including some provided by various government and health agencies, such as safe living environments and access to proper health care. However, in general, one's personal health over the course of a lifetime is dependent more on personal lifestyle choices, two of the most important being proper exercise and healthy eating.

In the twenty-first century, our love affair with fitness and sports continues to grow. Worldwide, although physical inactivity is still very prevalent in developed nations, more of us are joining fitness facilities or initiating fitness programs, such as bicycling, running, swimming, walking, and weight training. Improvement in health and fitness is one of the major reasons that more and more people initiate an exercise program, but many may also become more interested in sports competition, such as age-group road racing; running and walking race competitions have become increasingly popular, and every weekend numerous road races can be found within a short drive. Research has shown that adults who become physically active also may become more interested in other aspects of their lifestyles—particularly nutrition—that may affect their health in a positive way. Indeed, according to all major health organizations, proper exercise and a healthful diet are two of the most important lifestyle behaviors to help prevent chronic disease.

Nutrition is the study of foods and their effects upon health, development, and performance. Over the years, nutrition research has made a significant contribution to our knowledge of essential nutrient needs. During the first part of the twentieth century, most nutrition research focused on identification of essential nutrients and amounts needed to prevent nutrient-deficiency diseases, such as scurvy from inadequate vitamin C. As nutrition science evolved, medical researchers focused on the effects of foods and their specific constituents as a means to help prevent the major chronic diseases, such as heart disease and cancer, that are epidemic in developed countries. *Nutriceutical* is a relatively new term used to characterize the drug, or medical, effects of a particular nutrient. Recent research findings continue to indicate that our diet is one of the most important determinants of our health status. Although individual nutrients are still being evaluated for possible health benefits, research is also focusing on dietary patterns, or the totality of the diet, and resultant health benefits. However, we should note that research relative to the effects of diet, including specific nutrients, on health is complex and dietary recommendations may change with new research findings. For example, as shall be noted later in the text, the guidelines regarding dietary intake of cholesterol have been modified after being in effect for more than 50 years.

Other than the health benefits of exercise and fitness, many physically active individuals also are finding the joy of athletic competition, participating in local sports events such as golf tournaments, tennis matches, triathlons, and road races. Individuals who compete athletically are always looking for a means to improve performance, be it a new piece of equipment or an improved training method. In this regard, proper nutrition may be a very important factor in improving sports performance. Various sports governing agencies indicate today's athletes need accurate sports nutrition information to maximize sports performance. Although the effect of diet on sports and exercise performance was studied only sporadically prior to 1970, subsequently numerous sports scientists and sports nutritionists have studied the performance-enhancing effects of nutrition, such as diet composition and dietary supplements. Results of these studies have provided nutritional guidance to enhance performance in specific athletic endeavors. In the United States, many universities and professional sports teams, such as those in Major League Baseball and the National Football League, employ registered dietitians as well as culinary chefs to provide dietary guidance to their athletes.

With the completion of the Human Genome Project, gene therapies are being developed for the medical treatment of various health problems. Moreover, some contend that genetic manipulations may be used to enhance sports performance. For example, gene doping to increase insulin-like growth factor, which can stimulate muscle growth, may be applied to sport.

Our personal genetic code plays an important role in determining our health status and our sports abilities, and futurists speculate that one day each of us will carry our own genetic chip that will enable us to tailor food selection and exercise programs to optimize our health and sports performance. Such may be the case, but for the time being we must depend on available scientific evidence to provide us with prudent guidelines.

Each year thousands of published studies and reviews analyze the effects of nutrition on health or exercise and sports performance. The major purpose of this text is to evaluate these scientific data and present prudent recommendations for individuals who want to modify their diet for optimal health or exercise/sports performance.

Textbook Overview

This book uses a question-answer approach, which is convenient when you may have occasional short periods to study, such as riding a bus or during a lunch break. In addition, the questions are arranged in a logical sequence, the answer to one question often leading into the question that follows. Where appropriate, cross-referencing within the text is used to expand the discussion. No deep scientific background is needed for the chemical aspects of nutrition and energy expenditure, as these have been simplified. Instructors who use this book as a course text may add details of biochemistry as they feel necessary.

Chapter 1 introduces you to the general effects of exercise and nutrition on health-related and sports-related fitness, including the importance of well-controlled scientific research. Chapter 2 provides a broad overview of sound guidelines relative to nutrition for optimal health and physical performance. Chapter 3 focuses on energy and energy pathways in the body, the key to all exercise and sports activities.

Chapters 4 through 9 deal with the six basic nutrients—carbohydrate, fat, protein, vitamins, minerals, and water—with emphasis on the health and performance implications for the physically active individual. Chapters 10 through 12 review concepts of body composition and weight control, with suggestions on how to gain or lose body weight through diet and exercise, as well as the implications of such changes for health and athletic performance. Chapter 13 covers several drug foods, such as alcohol and caffeine, and other related dietary supplements regarding their effects on health and exercise performance. Several appendixes complement the text, providing data on caloric expenditure during exercise; detailed metabolic pathways for carbohydrate, fat, and protein; methods to determine body composition; nutritional value of fast foods; and other information pertinent to physically active individuals.

New to the Eleventh Edition

The first edition of this textbook, titled *Nutrition for Fitness and Sport*, was published in 1983. I am joined in this eleventh edition by two professors who are actively involved in the disciplines of exercise physiology and sports nutrition, and who have used this text over the years to teach their university classes. J. David Branch is an associate professor in the Department of Human Movement Sciences at Old Dominion University in Virginia. His e-mail address is dbranch@odu.edu. Eric Rawson is a professor in the Department of Exercise Science at Bloomsburg University in Pennsylvania. His e-mail address is erawson@bloomu.edu. Dr. Branch revised chapters 6, 9, 10, 11, 12, and 13; Dr. Rawson revised chapters 4, 5, and 6; and I revised chapters 1, 2, 3, and 8.

The content throughout each chapter of the book has been updated, where merited, based on contemporary research findings regarding the effects of nutritional practices on health, fitness, and sports performance. Many sections throughout the text were completely rewritten in attempts to improve presentation and clarity, such as the use of bullet points to summarize key points. More than 700 new references, including clinical studies, reviews, and meta-analyses, have been added to the text. Major changes include incorporation of the new *Dietary Guidelines for Americans*. The MyPlate model is designed to be more user friendly for the American population and is discussed in several chapters. New information from authoritative position statements dealing with exercise and nutrition issues has been incorporated into various chapters where relevant. These position statements have been developed by such prominent groups as the Academy of Nutrition and Dietetics, the American College of Sports Medicine, the American Academy of Pediatrics, the American Heart Association, the American College of Cardiology, the European College of Sport Science, the European Food Safety Authority, and Sports Dietitians Australia. Additionally, numerous Websites have been listed to help students explore various exercise and nutrition issues in more depth.

Chapter 1—Introduction to Nutrition for Health, Fitness, and Sports Performance
- New information on the use of various applications for health promotion
- Increased discussion of the use of various exercise gadgets, such as fitness bands and fitness watches, to help document daily amounts of physical activity and other aspects of lifestyle
- Update on the role of exercise to enhance health
- Introduction of high-intensity interval training (HIIT) and its possible application to exercise for health
- Introduction of the Compendium of Physical Activities, which is used in various chapters referring to energy expenditure during physical activities
- Increased use of reputable Websites to provide more detailed information on exercise and diet for health
- Discussion of new position stands, as related to a healthy diet by the Academy of Nutrition and Dietetics, the new name for the American Dietetic Association
- Introduction to the *2015 Dietary Guidelines for Americans*, the most recent report of the 2015 Dietary Guidelines Advisory Committee
- New application exercise for diet appraisal using several Website-based diet analyses by the Academy of Nutrition and Dietetics and other health profession groups
- Over 40 new references added and numerous dated citations deleted

Chapter 2—Healthful Nutrition for Fitness and Sport: The Consumer Athlete
- Updated discussion of dietary guidelines, including the debate over research with saturated fatty acids and the proposed new guidelines for cholesterol
- Introduction to the Academy of Nutrition and Dietetics position stand on the total diet approach to healthy eating
- Discussion of several smartphone applications (apps) to help you eat a healthier diet
- More details on how to use the MyPlate program to plan a healthier diet

- How to become an ambassador for ChooseMyPlate and healthy eating on your college campus
- Presentation of the Harvard Medical School modified MyPlate to present more specific recommendations for healthy eating
- Discussion of the proposed new food labels designed to make food shopping easier to select healthier foods
- An update on the controversy concerning use of GMO foods
- Use of various Websites to stay current, such as fruits and vegetables that fall into those with the lowest and highest pesticide content
- Over 40 new references, most of them reviews and meta-analyses

Chapter 3—Human Energy
- Enhanced discussion of techniques to measure energy expenditure, including the use of various commercial apps
- Presentation of more details on the use of the MET system to measure energy expenditure
- Presentation of a link to calculate your daily energy expenditure via five methods
- Over 30 new references

Chapter 4—Carbohydrates: The Main Energy Food
- Updated information on the role of the glycemic index in the risk of cardiovascular disease
- New data on the effectiveness of carbohydrate mouthrinse on endurance exercise performance
- New information on the effects of carbohydrate supplementation on exercise performance
- Updated information on the role of carbohydrate ingestion and resistance training
- New data on the effects of cycling carbohydrate intake on training adaptations and performance
- Update on approved sugar substitutes and artificial sweeteners and the effects on performance and weight gain
- Latest data on the effects of dietary fiber on morbidity and mortality
- Over 20 new references

Chapter 5—Fat: An Important Energy Source during Exercise
- Update on the effect of saturated fat on health
- New data on the effects of conjugated linoleic acid supplementation on body composition
- Update on the effects of omega fatty acid consumption on disease
- New data on avocado intake and cardiovascular health
- New research on the effects of dietary medium-chain triglycerides on weight loss and body composition
- Update on the effects of ketogenic diets on satiety and appetite
- Updated information on low-carbohydrate diets and weight loss
- Discussion of the potential effects of high-fat diets in endurance athletes
- Update on fasting and endurance exercise performance
- Over 20 new references

Chapter 6—Protein: The Tissue Builder
- Updated data on the effects of protein supplements on muscle mass, strength, and power
- New information on the effects of protein supplements on muscle damage, soreness, and recovery

- New data on the effects of protein plus carbohydrate ingestion on acute and repeated endurance exercise performance
- The latest protein intake recommendations on postexercise and before-sleep protein supplementation
- Update on the importance of dietary protein in satiety and weight loss
- Newest data on the safety of high protein intakes
- New data on creatine supplementation and muscle strength
- Latest information on beta-alanine supplementation
- Updated information on the effectiveness of HMB supplementation
- Update on the role of beetroot/nitrate ingestion on endurance exercise performance
- Over 20 new references

Chapter 7—Vitamins: The Organic Regulators
- New data on deficiency prevalence rates for folate and vitamins B_6, D, B_{12}, A, C, and E
- New information on vitamin D status, deficiency, and supplementation in athletes
- New information on vitamin E status and exercise performance
- New information on the effects of certain medications on vitamin B_{12} deficiency
- New information on pantothenic acid and choline supplementation and performance
- Link to current comments from the American College of Sports Medicine regarding vitamin/mineral supplementation and exercise
- New information on the role of antioxidant supplementation in the older athlete
- New reviews on the ergogenic effects of coenzyme Q_{10} and quercetin
- New studies of the role of vitamin B supplementation on homocysteine levels and primary and secondary stroke prevention
- New information on vitamin supplementation and the management of age-related macular degeneration and cataracts
- New information on the roles of antioxidant vitamins and vitamin D in mental health
- Over 50 new references

Chapter 8—Minerals: The Inorganic Regulators
- New information on who may be at risk for calcium deficiency.
- New data on research involving the ergogenic aspects of phosphate salt supplementation, including new studies and reviews
- New information on all trace minerals, including iron, zinc, copper, chromium, and others
- New section on manganese as a trace mineral
- New discussion of the metal hypothesis of Alzheimer's disease, which suggests some minerals may be protective but others may increase the risk
- Over 100 new references

Chapter 9—Water, Electrolytes, and Temperature Regulation
- Extensive revision to introduction and other parts of the text
- Several revised or new figures
- Updated information on U.S. and global sodium intake.

- Updated discussion of theoretical mechanisms of heat-related central nervous fatigue
- Updated information on glycerol's status as a WADA banned substance
- Updated U.S. and global prevalence rates for hypertension
- Updated information on evolving guidelines for dietary sodium intake
- Over 70 new references

Chapter 10—Body Weight and Composition for Health and Sport
- Several revised or new figures
- Updated global prevalence rates for obesity
- New photograph of bioelectrical impedance procedure for body-composition assessment
- Inclusion of BMI categories representing apparent chronic energy deficiency
- Inclusion of body fat categories by gender and age, modified from *American College of Sports Medicine's Guidelines for Exercise Testing and Prescription*, 9th edition, and The Cooper Institute, Dallas, Texas
- Updated discussion of brown adipose tissue
- Updated discussion of non-exercise activity thermogenesis (NEAT)
- Updated discussion of genetic contributions to obesity from genome-wide association studies (GRAS)
- Discussion of socioeconomic factors contributing to energy balance, such as more fast-food restaurants and unhealthy food choices in low-income areas
- New information on Calories consumed as sugar-sweetened beverages
- Expanded discussion of stress, environmental, viral exposure, and epigenetic factors and the built environment as contributors to obesity
- Discussion of the role of disruptions of normal intestinal bacteria in obesity
- Discussion of models other than the set-point theory as theoretical regulators of energy balance
- Expanded discussion of "screen-based" behaviors in impacting energy expenditure (sedentary activity) and intake (advertisements for energy-dense foods) in children and adults
- Expanded discussion of the health impacts of obesity to include increased risk for Alzheimer's disease and other dementia
- Updated information on prescription weight-loss drugs approved by the U.S. Food and Drug Administration
- Updated information reflecting the four clinical eating disorders currently described in the American Psychiatric Association's *Diagnostic and Statistical Manual of Mental Disorders—V*
- Discussion of the controversy surrounding replacing the term "female athlete triad" with "relative energy deficiency in sport (RED-S)"
- Over 140 new references

Chapter 11—Weight Management and Loss through Proper Nutrition and Exercise
- New information on a gastric stimulation device approved by the U.S. Food and Drug Administration

- New and revised figures throughout the chapter
- Incorporation of the Compendium of Physical Activities, which lists MET intensity values of many leisure and recreational activities as well as activities of daily living
- Discussion of the conversion of MET values into caloric expenditure to complement appendix B
- Incorporating the energy expenditure based on MET values from the Compendium with Physical Activity Levels and Coefficients in the National Academy of Sciences Estimated Energy Requirement formulas
- Inclusion of a web link to 171 small steps to a healthier diet and increased physical activity
- Inclusion of the proposed requirement by the U.S. Food and Drug Administration to include "added sugars" on Nutrition Facts labeling
- Inclusion of selected Websites listing caloric and nutritive value of fast-food restaurant foods to complement appendix E
- Inclusion of the current list of risk factors and signs/symptom of possible disease according to the American College of Sports Medicine
- Discussion of high-intensity interval training (HIIT) as a physical activity component of weight loss and weight maintenance
- Expanded discussion and figure for the "fat burning" myth in the selection of exercise intensity for fat loss and weight loss
- Recent studies comparing the efficacy of commercial weight-loss programs
- Over 90 new references

Chapter 12—Weight Gaining through Proper Nutrition and Exercise
- Updated *Healthy People 2020* information on the prevalence of resistance training among U.S. adults
- Added information on the importance of the branch-chain amino acid leucine in muscle growth
- New research on the effects of resistance training in the older adult
- New research on the efficacy of creatine supplementation combined with resistance training in the older adult
- Additional information on regulatory factors and cell signaling pathways in adaptations to resistance training
- New research on nutrient timing to facilitate postexercise muscle growth
- Revised sample weekly resistance training record sheet
- New research on the potential efficacy of higher protein intake in maintaining lean mass and reducing fat mass
- Over 20 new references

Chapter 13—Food Drugs and Related Supplements
- Revised figures throughout the chapter
- Updated World Health Organization data on the global effects of alcohol abuse on health and mortality
- Information on potential interactions between alcohol and prescribed pharmacological agents, especially in older adults
- Information on a potential role of coffee in decreasing alcoholic cirrhosis
- A link to recent alcohol-impaired traffic safety data

- Updated data on the health, academic, and psychological effects of alcohol in high school and college students
- Updated information from studies by the World Cancer Research Fund (WCRF)/ American Institute of Cancer Research (AICR) and the International Agency for Research of Cancer (IARC) on the link between alcohol and breast and other cancers
- Discussion of American Psychiatric Association's *Diagnostic and Statistical Manual of Mental Disorders—V* alcohol use disorder (AUD) diagnosis
- Links to online screening questionnaires for possible alcohol use disorder
- New information on the association of alcohol and Alzheimer's disease, mental health, and cognitive function
- Updated information on the role of alcohol and other ingredients in alcoholic drinks (e.g., polyphenols) on lipid metabolism, vascular function
- Research on the role of genetic variants in alcohol dehydrogenase in cardiovascular disease risk
- Updated data on the prevalence of coffee/caffeine use in the United States
- Updated information on the prevalence of energy drink use and concerns about the use of such products that also contain alcohol
- Updated research on the role of coffee/caffeine consumption and blood pressure and cardio-metabolic health
- Updated research on the role of coffee/caffeine in mental health, cognitive function, and multiple sclerosis
- Updated information on caffeine use in pregnancy and in infant health
- Updated information in recent discovery of amphetamine isomers in over-the-counter dietary supplements
- Updated status of pseudoephedrine (in addition to ephedrine, ephedra, and ma huang) as substances that are prohibited for use in competition by the WADA
- Updated information on U.S. Food and Drug Administration–mandated warnings about testosterone replacement therapy and increased risk for heart attacks and strokes
- Updated Centers for Disease Control and Prevention data on the prevalence of steroid use by teenagers
- Updated information on the efficacy of various herbals in improving body composition or performance
- Updated Australian Institute of Sports Classification System of Nutritional Supplements
- Over 110 new references

Appendices
- Updated several appendices, including those dealing with energy expenditure during exercise and the nutrient composition of products sold in fast-food restaurants

Enhanced Pedagogy

Each chapter contains several features to help enhance the learning process. **Chapter Learning Objectives** are presented at the beginning of each chapter, highlighting the key points and serving as a studying guide. **Key Terms** also are listed at the beginning of each chapter, along with the page number on which they are first highlighted and defined. Although some terms may appear in the text before they are defined, a thorough glossary includes the key terms as well as other terms warranting definition. **Key Concepts** provide a summary of essential information presented throughout each chapter. Students are encouraged to participate in several practical activities to help reinforce learning. **Check for Yourself** includes individual activities, such as checking food labels at the supermarket or measuring one's own body fat percentage. The **Application Exercise** at the end of each chapter may require more extensive involvement, such as a case study in weight control involving yourself or a survey of an athletic team. Students may wish to peruse all application exercises at the beginning of the course, as some may take several weeks or months to complete.

The reference lists have been completely updated for this edition, with the inclusion of more than 700 new references, and provide the scientific basis for the new concepts or additional support for those concepts previously developed. These references provide greater in-depth reading materials for the interested student. Although the content of this book is based on appropriate scientific studies, a reference-citation style is not used, that is, each statement is not referenced by a bibliographic source. However, names of authors may be used to highlight a reference source where deemed appropriate.

This book is designed primarily to serve as a college text in professional preparation programs in health and physical education, exercise science, athletic training, sports medicine, and sports nutrition. It is also directed to the physically active individual interested in the nutritional aspects of physical and athletic performance.

Those who desire to initiate a physical training program may also find the nutritional information useful, as well as the guidelines for initiating a training program. This book may serve as a handy reference for coaches, trainers, and athletes. With the tremendous expansion of youth sports programs, parents may find the information valuable relative to the nutritional requirements of their active children.

In summary, the major purpose of this book is to help provide a sound knowledge base relative to the role that nutrition, complemented by exercise, may play in the enhancement of both health and sports performance. We hope that the information provided in this text will help the reader develop a more healthful and performance-enhancing diet. Bon appetit!

Acknowledgments

This book would not be possible without the many medical/health scientists and exercise/sports scientists throughout the world who, through their numerous studies and research, have provided the scientific data that underlie its development. We are fortunate to have developed a friendship with many of you, and we extend our sincere appreciation to all of you.

We would like to acknowledge deep gratitude to Mandy Clark, Product Developer at McGraw-Hill, for her dedicated support throughout the revision process. Mandy was always available to address queries regarding various facets of the production process, and her responses were very prompt. We would also like to thank Anna Hoppmann, Digital Asset Librarian, for her assistance in navigating the photo database of McGraw-Hill, and Jessica Portz, our project manager. Our deep gratitude to Marija Magner, Brand Manager.

Melvin H. Williams
Norfolk, Virginia
J. David Branch
Norfolk, Virgina
Eric S. Rawson
Bloomsburg, Pennsylvania

Instructor Resources

Available at www.mhhe.com/williams11e are a number of instructor and student resources to accompany the text. For students, these include a BMI calculator, animations, daily food log, and more. For instructors, resources include PPT lecture outlines, image PowerPoint files, and more.

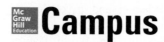 **McGraw—Hill Create**™ is a self—service website that allows you to create customized course materials using McGraw—Hill Education's comprehensive, cross—disciplinary content and digital products.

Campus MH Campus® integrates all of your digital products from McGraw—Hill Education with your school LMS for quick and easy access to best—in—class content and learning tools.

LEARNSMART PREP® Fueled by LearnSmart—the most widely used and intelligent adaptive learning resource—LearnSmart Prep® is designed to get students ready for a forthcoming course by quickly and effectively addressing prerequisite knowledge gaps that may cause problems down the road.

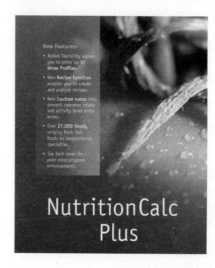

Inspire behavior change. NutritionCalc Plus is an online suite of powerful dietary self—assessment tools that help students track their food intake and activity and analyze their diet and health goals. Students and instructors can trust the reliability of the ESHA database while interacting with a robust selection of reports.

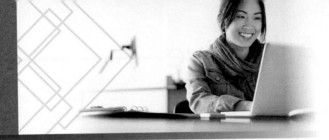

McGraw-Hill Connect®
Learn Without Limits

Connect is a teaching and learning platform that is proven to deliver better results for students and instructors.

Connect empowers students by continually adapting to deliver precisely what they need, when they need it, and how they need it, so your class time is more engaging and effective.

Course outcomes improve with Connect.

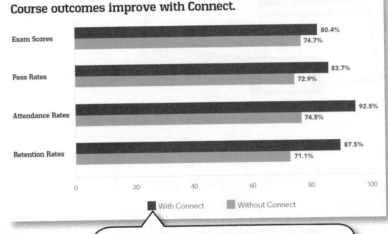

Using **Connect** improves passing rates by **10.8%** and retention by **16.4%**.

88% of instructors who use **Connect** require it; instructor satisfaction **increases** by 38% when **Connect** is required.

Analytics

Connect Insight®

Connect Insight is Connect's new one-of-a-kind visual analytics dashboard—now available for both instructors and students—that provides at-a-glance information regarding student performance, which is immediately actionable. By presenting assignment, assessment, and topical performance results together with a time metric that is easily visible for aggregate or individual results, Connect Insight gives the user the ability to take a just-in-time approach to teaching and learning, which was never before available. Connect Insight presents data that empowers students and helps instructors improve class performance in a way that is efficient and effective.

Connect helps students achieve better grades

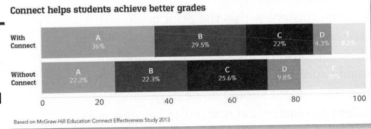

Based on McGraw-Hill Education Connect Effectiveness Study 2013

Students can view their results for any **Connect** course.

Mobile

Connect's new, intuitive mobile interface gives students and instructors flexible and convenient, anytime–anywhere access to all components of the Connect platform.

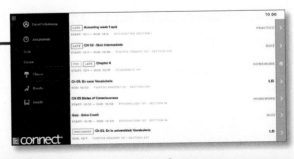

Adaptive

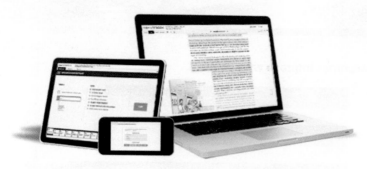

THE FIRST AND ONLY **ADAPTIVE READING EXPERIENCE** DESIGNED TO TRANSFORM THE WAY STUDENTS READ

More students earn **A's** and **B's** when they use McGraw-Hill Education **Adaptive** products.

SmartBook®

Proven to help students improve grades and study more efficiently, SmartBook contains the same content within the print book, but actively tailors that content to the needs of the individual. SmartBook's adaptive technology provides precise, personalized instruction on what the student should do next, guiding the student to master and remember key concepts, targeting gaps in knowledge and offering customized feedback, and driving the student toward comprehension and retention of the subject matter. Available on smartphones and tablets, SmartBook puts learning at the student's fingertips—anywhere, anytime.

Over **4 billion questions** have been answered, making McGraw-Hill Education products more intelligent, reliable, and precise.

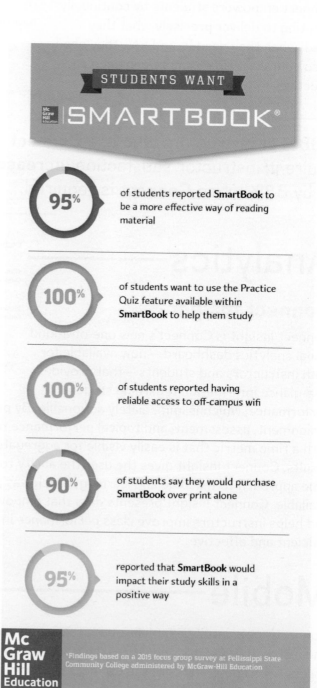

STUDENTS WANT

SMARTBOOK®

95% of students reported **SmartBook** to be a more effective way of reading material

100% of students want to use the Practice Quiz feature available within **SmartBook** to help them study

100% of students reported having reliable access to off-campus wifi

90% of students say they would purchase **SmartBook** over print alone

95% reported that **SmartBook** would impact their study skills in a positive way

Mc Graw Hill Education

*Findings based on a 2015 focus group survey at Pellissippi State Community College administered by McGraw-Hill Education

Introduction to Nutrition for Health, Fitness, and Sports Performance

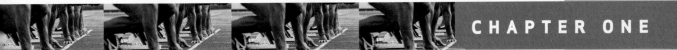

CHAPTER ONE

LEARNING OBJECTIVES

After studying this chapter, you should be able to:

1. Explain the role of both genetics and environment, particularly nutrition and exercise, in the determination of optimal health and successful sport performance.

2. List each of the components of health-related fitness and then identify the potential health benefits of an exercise program designed to enhance both aerobic and musculoskeletal fitness.

3. Define sports-related fitness and compare it to health-related fitness, noting similarities and differences.

4. List the seven principles of exercise training and explain the importance of each.

5. List the 12 guidelines underlying the Prudent Healthy Diet and discuss, in general, the importance of proper nutrition to optimal health.

6. Understand the importance of proper nutrition, including the role of dietary supplements as ergogenic aids, to sports performance.

7. Define nutritional quackery and understand the various strategies you can use to determine whether claims regarding a dietary supplement are valid.

8. Explain what types of research have been used to evaluate the relationship between nutrition and health or sport performance, and evaluate the pros and cons of each type.

There are two major focal points of this book. One is the role that nutrition, complemented by physical activity and exercise, may play in the enhancement of one's health status. The other is the role that nutrition may play in the enhancement of fitness and sports performance. Many individuals today are physically active, and athletic competition spans all ages. Healthful nutrition is important throughout the life span of the physically active individual because suboptimal health status may impair training and competitive performance. In general, as we shall see, the diet that is optimal for health is also optimal for exercise and sports performance.

Nutrition, fitness, and health. Health care in most developed countries has improved tremendously over the past century. Although some rather rare diseases, such as Ebola, are a cause for concern, primarily because of the dedicated work of medical researchers we no longer fear the scourge of major acute infectious diseases such as polio, smallpox, or tuberculosis. However, we have become increasingly concerned with the treatment and prevention of chronic diseases. The World Health Organization (WHO) indicates that chronic diseases are now the major cause of death and disability worldwide. According to the U.S. Department of Health and Human Services (HHS), unhealthy eating and physical inactivity are leading causes of death in the United States. Given with rank in parentheses, they include (1) diseases of the heart, (2) cancer, (3) stroke, (4) chronic lung diseases, (6) diabetes, (8) Alzheimer's disease, and (9) chronic kidney diseases. These diseases cause more than 85 percent of all deaths, and this figure is destined to rise as the U.S. population becomes increasingly older, particularly during the first quarter of this century when the baby boomers of the 1940s and 1950s reach their senior years.

The two primary factors that influence one's health status are genetics and lifestyle. According to Simopoulos, all diseases have a genetic predisposition. The Human Genome Project, which deciphered the DNA code of our 80,000 to 100,000 genes, has identified various genes associated with many chronic diseases, such as breast and prostate cancer. Genetically, females whose mothers had breast cancer are at increased risk for breast cancer, while males whose fathers had prostate cancer are at increased risk for prostate cancer.

Completion of the Human Genome Project is believed to be one of the most significant medical advances of all time. Although multiple genes are involved in the etiology of most chronic diseases and research regarding the application of the findings of the Human Genome Project to improve health is still in its initial stages, the future looks bright. For individuals with genetic profiles predisposing them to a specific chronic disease, such as cancer, genetic therapy eventually may provide an effective treatment or cure.

Although genetic influences may play an important role predisposing an individual to a chronic disease, so, too, does lifestyle. The CDC notes that although chronic diseases are among the most common and costly health problems, they are also among the most preventable by adopting a healthy lifestyle. Over the years, scientists in the field of epidemiology have identified a number of lifestyle factors considered to be health risks; these lifestyle factors are known as risk factors. A **risk factor** is a lifestyle behavior that has been associated with a particular disease, such as cigarette smoking being linked to lung cancer.

A major risk factor is being overweight or obese, a condition which affects almost two-thirds of Americans and is increasing worldwide. The Department of Health and Human Services recently listed the leading lifestyle-related causes of premature death in the United States. The combination of an unhealthy diet and physical inactivity, which may contribute to being overweight or obese, was ranked as the leading cause, followed by tobacco use and alcohol abuse.

In a recent review, Hall noted that our genes harbor many secrets to a long and healthy life but also noted that genes alone are unlikely to explain all the secrets of longevity. The role of a healthful diet and exercise are intertwined with your genetic profile. What you eat and how you exercise may influence your genes. **Epigenetics** is a relatively new field of research involving the role of the **epigenome,** a structure located just outside the genome that may activate or deactivate DNA and subsequent genetic and cellular activity. Cloud noted that various factors in our environment, such as substances in the foods we eat, may interact with the epigenome and thus modify cell functions—either in a positive or negative manner. Exercise, as noted later, also stimulates release of substances from muscle cells that may affect the epigenome. Cloud notes that comparable to the Human Genome Project, a Human Epigenome Project is under way, and epigenetics may eventually lead to many beneficial health-related applications. For example, if personal genetic code indicates that your genetic profile predisposes you to certain forms of cancer, and if your genetic profile indicates that you will respond favorably to specific nutritional or exercise interventions, then a preventive diet and an exercise plan may be individualized for you. Genomics represents the study of genetic material in body cells, and the terms *nutrigenomics* and *exercisenomics* have been coined to identify the study of the genetic aspects of nutrition and exercise, respectively, as related to health benefits. *Sportomics* involves study of the metabolic response of the athlete in an actual sport environment, not in a laboratory.

Treatment of chronic diseases is very expensive. Foreseeing a financial health-care crisis associated with an increasing prevalence of such diseases during the first half of this century, most private and public health professionals have advocated health promotion and disease prevention as the best approach to address this potential major health problem. Martinez-Perez and others note that with more than 1 billion smart phones around the world, the use of various applications for health promotion has great potential. The HHS, beginning in the 1980s, has published a series of reports designed to increase the nation's health; the latest version is entitled *Healthy People 2020: National Health Promotion/Disease Prevention Objectives.* Physical activity/fitness and overweight/obesity are two of the major focus areas. These reports emphasize that lifestyle behaviors that promote health and reduce the risk of chronic diseases are basically under the control of the individual. The role of diet and

exercise in health promotion has become a worldwide priority, as documented in the WHO report *Global Strategy on Diet, Physical Activity and Health.* The guidelines presented in these reports underlie the recommendations presented in this book. For both reports, see web addresses below.

As we shall see, proper exercise and proper nutrition, both individually and combined, may reduce many of the risk factors associated with the development of chronic diseases. These healthful benefits will be addressed at appropriate points throughout the book.

Nutrition, fitness, and sport. *Sport* is now most commonly defined as a competitive athletic activity requiring skill or physical prowess, for example, baseball, basketball, soccer, football, track, wrestling, tennis, and golf. As with health status, athletic ability and subsequent success in sport are based primarily upon genetics and epigenetics. In a review of epigenetics in sport, Ehlert and others note that natural genetic endowment with characteristics important to a specific sport must be maximized through epigenetic modifications by appropriate type and amount of training.

To be successful at high levels of competition, athletes must possess the appropriate biomechanical, physiological, and psychological genetic characteristics associated with success in a given sport. International-class athletes have such genetic traits. In recent reviews, Tucker and others highlighted the genetic basis for elite running performance while Eynon and others discussed the role of genes for elite power and sprint performance. Moreover, Wolfarth and others have

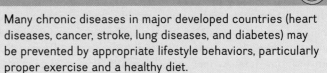

assembled a human gene map for performance and health-related fitness.

To be successful at high levels of competition, athletes must also develop their genetic characteristics maximally through proper biomechanical, physiological, and psychological coaching and training. Whatever the future holds for genetic enhancement of athletic performance, specialized exercise training will still be the key to maximizing genetic potential for a given sport activity. Training programs at the elite level have become more intense and individualized, sometimes based on genetic predispositions. Modern scientific training results in significant performance gains, and world records continue to improve. David Epstein, in his book *The Sports Gene,* provides a fascinating account of the role both genes and the training environment play relative to elite sport performance.

Proper nutrition also is an important component in the total training program of the athlete. Certain nutrient deficiencies can seriously impair performance, whereas supplementation of other nutrients may help delay fatigue and improve performance. Over the past 50 years, research has provided us with many answers about the role of nutrition in athletic performance, but unfortunately some findings have been misinterpreted or exaggerated so that a number of misconceptions still exist.

The purpose of this chapter is to provide a broad overview of the role that exercise and nutrition may play relative to health, fitness, and sport, and how prudent recommendations may be determined. More detailed information regarding specific relationships of nutritional practices to health and sports performance is provided in subsequent chapters.

www.health.gov/healthypeople Check for the full report of *Healthy People 2020.*

www.who.int/dietphysicalactivity/en/ Check for the World Health Organization report on diet and physical activity for health.

www.ncbi.nlm.nih.gov/genome/guide/human/ For the interested reader, this site accesses the human genome map and the National Institutes of Health Epigenetics Roadmap.

Key Concepts

▶ Many chronic diseases in major developed countries (heart diseases, cancer, stroke, lung diseases, and diabetes) may be prevented by appropriate lifestyle behaviors, particularly proper exercise and a healthy diet.

▶ The two primary determinants of health status are genetics and lifestyle.

Health-Related Fitness: Exercise and Nutrition

Physical fitness may be defined, in general terms, as a set of abilities individuals possess to perform specific types of physical activity. The development of physical fitness is an important concern of many professional health organizations, including the Society of Health and Physical Educators (SHAPE), which has classified fitness components into two different categories. In general, these two categories may be referred to as health-related fitness and sports-related fitness. Both types of fitness may be influenced by nutrition and exercise.

Exercise and Health-Related Fitness

What is health-related fitness?

As mentioned previously, one's health status or wellness is influenced strongly by hereditarian predisposition and lifestyle behaviors, particularly appropriate physical activity and a high-quality diet. As we shall see in various sections of this book, one of the key factors in preventing the development of chronic disease is maintaining a healthful body weight.

Proper physical activity may certainly improve one's health status by helping to prevent excessive weight gain, but it may also enhance other facets of health-related fitness as well. **Health-related fitness** includes not only a healthy body weight and composition but also cardiovascular-respiratory fitness, adequate muscular strength and muscular endurance, and sufficient flexibility (figure 1.1). As one ages, other measures used as markers of health-related fitness include blood pressure, bone strength, postural control and balance, and various indicators of lipid and carbohydrate metabolism.

Several health professional organizations, such as the American College of Sports Medicine (ACSM) and American Heart Association (AHA), have indicated that various forms of physical activity may be used to enhance health. In general, **physical activity** involves any bodily movement caused by muscular contraction that results in the expenditure of energy. For purposes of studying its effects on health, some epidemiologists classify physical activity as either unstructured or structured.

Unstructured physical activity, also known as leisure-time activity, includes many of the usual activities of daily living, such as leisurely walking and cycling, climbing stairs, dancing, gardening and yard work, various domestic and occupational activities, and games and other childhood pursuits. These unstructured activities are not normally planned to be exercise. However, as will be noted in chapter 11, these so-called nonexercise activities may play an important role in body weight control.

Structured physical activity, as the name implies, is a planned program of physical activities usually designed to improve physical fitness, including health-related fitness. For the purpose of this book, we shall refer to structured physical activity as **exercise,** particularly some form of planned moderate or vigorous exercise, such as brisk, not leisurely, walking.

What are the basic principles of exercise training?

Exercise training programs may be designed to provide specific types of health-related fitness benefits and/or enhance specific types of sports-related fitness. However, no matter what the purpose, several general principles are used in developing an appropriate exercise training program.

Principle of Overload Overload is the basic principle of exercise training, and it represents the intensity, duration, and frequency of exercise. For example, a running program for cardiovascular-respiratory fitness could involve training at an intensity of 70 percent of maximal heart rate, a duration of 30 minutes, and a frequency of 5 times per week. The adaptations the body makes are based primarily on the specific exercise overload. The terms *moderate* exercise and *vigorous* exercise are often used to quantify exercise intensity and are discussed later in this chapter and in more detail in chapter 11.

Principle of Progression Progression is an extension of the overload principle. As your body adapts to the original overload, the overload must be increased if further beneficial adaptations are desired. For example, you may start lifting a weight of 20 pounds, increase the weight to 25 pounds as you get stronger, and so forth. The overloads are progressively increased until the final health-related or sports-related goal is achieved or exercise limits are reached.

Principle of Specificity Specificity of training represents the specific adaptations the body will make in response to the type of exercise and overload. For example, running and weight lifting impose different demands on muscle energy systems, so the body adapts accordingly. Both types of exercise may provide substantial, yet different, health benefits. Exercise training programs may be designed specifically for certain health or sports-performance benefits.

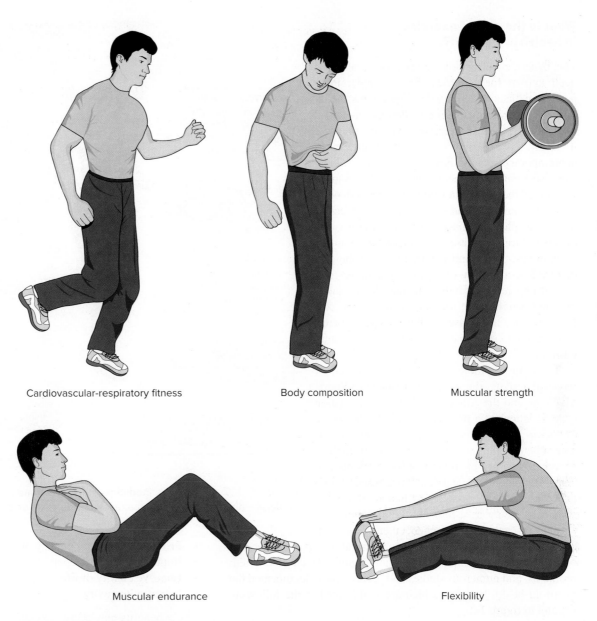

FIGURE 1.1 Health-related fitness components. The most important physical fitness components related to personal health include cardiovascular-respiratory fitness, body composition, muscular strength, muscular endurance, and flexibility.

Cardiovascular-respiratory fitness

Body composition

Muscular strength

Muscular endurance

Flexibility

Principle of Recuperation   Recuperation is an important principle of exercise training. Also known as the principle of recovery, it represents the time in which the body rests after exercise. This principle may apply within a specific exercise period, such as including rest periods when doing multiple sets during a weight-lifting workout. It may also apply to rest periods between bouts of exercise, such as a day of recovery between two long cardiovascular workouts.

Principle of Individuality   Individuality reflects the effect exercise training will have on each individual, as determined by genetic characteristics. The health benefits one receives from a specific exercise training program may vary tremendously among individuals. For example, although most individuals with high blood pressure may experience a reduction during a cardiovascular-respiratory fitness training program, some may not.

Principle of Reversibility   Reversibility is also referred to as the principle of disuse, or the concept of *use it or lose it*. Without the

use of exercise, the body will begin to lose the adaptations it has made over the course of the exercise program. Individuals who suffer a lapse in their exercise program, such as a week or so, may lose only a small amount of health-related fitness gains. However, a total relapse to a previous sedentary lifestyle can reverse all health-related fitness gains.

Principle of Overuse   Overuse represents an excessive amount of exercise that may induce some adverse, rather than beneficial, health effects. Overuse may be a problem during the beginning stages of an exercise program if one becomes overenthusiastic and exceeds her capacity, such as developing shin splints by running too far. Overuse may also occur in elite athletes who become overtrained, as discussed in chapter 3.

Specific exercise programs for healthy body weight and composition, cardiovascular-respiratory fitness, and muscular strength and muscular endurance are detailed in chapters 11 and 12, and several of these principles are discussed in more detail.

What is the role of exercise in health promotion?

The beneficial effect of exercise on health has been known for centuries. For example, Plato noted that "lack of activity destroys the good condition of every human being while movement and methodical physical exercise save and preserve it." Plato's observation is even more relevant in contemporary society. Frank Booth, a prominent exercise scientist at the University of Missouri, has coined the term **Sedentary Death Syndrome,** or **SeDS,** and he and his colleagues recently noted that physical inactivity is a primary cause of most chronic diseases, the major killers in the modern era. Slentz and others discussed the cost of physical inactivity over time. The *short-term* cost of physical inactivity is metabolic deterioration and weight gain; the *intermediate-term* cost is an increase in disease, such as type 2 diabetes, whereas the *long-term* cost is increased premature mortality.

To help promote the health benefits of physical activity, the American College of Sports Medicine and the American Medical Association (AMA) launched a program, entitled *Exercise Is Medicine^TM*, designed to encourage physicians and other health-care professionals to include exercise as part of the treatment for every patient. Clinical, epidemiological, and basic research evidence clearly supports the inclusion of regular physical activity as a tool for the prevention of chronic disease and the enhancement of overall health. Booth and others note that physical activity/exercise has been studied as a primary prevention against 35 chronic health problems, and numerous studies and reviews have documented the manifold health benefits, which are highlighted in the following list and in figure 1.2.

- Control body weight
- Reduce risk of metabolic syndrome
- Reduce risk of high blood pressure
- Reduce risk of type 2 diabetes
- Enhance blood lipid profile
- Reduce risk of heart disease
- Promote recovery from heart disease
- Reduce risk of stroke
- Reduce risk of breast cancer
- Reduce risk of colon cancer
- Improve self-image
- Reduce risk of mental depression
- Enhance cognitive functions in the elderly
- Reduce risk of falls in the elderly
- Delay onset and severity of Alzheimer's disease
- Strengthen bones and muscles
- Reduce arthritis pain
- Improve immune functions

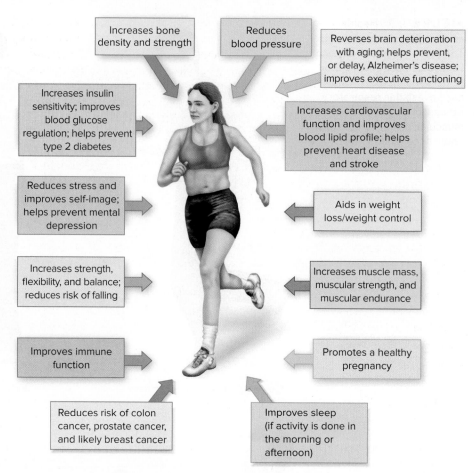

FIGURE 1.2 Exercise is medicine. Here are some of the benefits of regular moderate physical activity and exercise. See text for discussion.

- Promote healthy pregnancy of mother and fetus
- Improve quality of sleep
- Improve quality of life
- Increase longevity

These benefits may accrue to males and females of all races across all age spans. You are never too young or too old to reap some of these health benefits of exercise.

In essence, physically active individuals enjoy a higher quality of life, a *joie de vivre,* because they are less likely to suffer the disabling symptoms often associated with chronic diseases, such as loss of ambulation experienced by some stroke victims. As noted in the next section, physical activity may also increase the quantity of life. As quoted by Greider, James Fries, an emeritus professor who studies healthy aging at the Stanford University School of Medicine's Center on Longevity, said, "If you had to pick one thing, one single thing that came closest to the fountain of youth, it would have to be exercise."

How does exercise enhance health?

Recent news reports made headlines around the world, such as one entitled *Exercise Benefits: Rivals Drugs for Stroke, Heart Disease Treatment.* The question is, How?

The specific mechanisms whereby exercise may help to prevent the development of various chronic diseases are not completely understood but are involved with changes in gene expression that modify cell structure and function. Physical inactivity is a major risk factor for chronic diseases. As noted previously, Booth and Neufer indicated physical inactivity causes genes to misexpress proteins, producing the metabolic dysfunctions that result in overt clinical disease if continued long enough. In contrast, exercise may cause the expression of genes with favorable health effects.

Most body cells can produce and secrete small proteins known as **cytokines,** which are similar to hormones and can affect tissues throughout the body. Cytokines enter various body tissues, influencing gene expression that may induce adaptations either favorable or unfavorable to health (figure 1.3). Two types of cytokines are of interest to us. Muscle cells produce various cytokines called *myokines* (referred to as *exerkines* when produced during exercise), whereas fat (adipose) cells produce cytokines called *adipokines.* Muscle cells also produce *heat shock proteins (HSPs),* which may have beneficial health effects. The following represent several important cytokines produced in muscle and fat cells:

Muscle Cells	Fat Cells
Interleukin-6 (IL-6)	Tumor Necrosis Factor-alpha (TNF-α)
Brain-Derived Neurotropic Factor (BDNF)	Adiponectin

Overall, Brandt and Pederson theorize that exercise-induced cytokine effects on genes reduce many of the traditional risk factors associated with development of chronic diseases; Geiger and others note similar effects for HSPs. In particular, McAtee notes that one of the common causes of various chronic diseases is an inflammatory environment created by the presence of excess fat, particularly within blood vessels. Local inflammation is thought to promote the development of heart disease, cancer, diabetes, and dementia. According to Nimmo and others, exercise produces an anti-inflammatory cytokine that may help cool inflammation and reduce such health risks. They note that the most marked improvements in the inflammatory profile are conferred with exercise performed at higher intensities, with combined aerobic and resistance exercise training potentially providing the greatest benefit.

Cytokines and heat shock proteins may prevent chronic diseases in other ways as well, such as increasing the number of glucose receptors in muscle cells, improving insulin sensitivity, and helping to regulate blood glucose and prevent type 2 diabetes.

There are also other health-promoting mechanisms of exercise. One of the most significant contributors to health problems with aging is sarcopenia, or loss of muscle tissue. In their review, Landi and others conclude that regular exercise is the only strategy found to consistently prevent frailty and improve sarcopenia and physical function in older adults. The following are some other examples:

- Loss of excess body fat may reduce production of cytokines that may impair health.
- Loss of excess body fat may reduce estrogen levels, reducing risk of breast cancer.
- Reduction of abdominal obesity may decrease blood pressure and serum lipid levels.
- Increased mechanical stress on bone with high-impact exercise may stimulate increases in bone density.
- Production of some cytokines, such as BDNF, may enhance neurogenesis and brain functions.

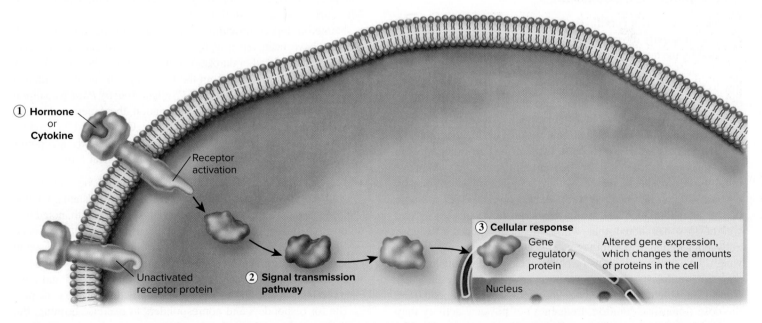

FIGURE 1.3 Exercise may induce adaptations that have favorable health effects in various body tissues. One suggested mechanism is the effect that various hormones or cytokines, which are produced during exercise, may have on gene regulation in body cells. (*1*) The hormone or cytokine binds to a cell receptor that activates a signal within the cell, (*2*) the signal is transmitted along a specific pathway, (*3*) the signal may alter gene expression and induce changes within the cell. Cell signals may also affect enzymes or other cell structures that may induce beneficial health effects.

Some healthful adaptations may occur with a single bout of exercise. Nimmo and others reported that single bouts of exercise have a potent anti-inflammatory influence, while others have noted that a single exercise session can acutely improve the blood lipid profile, reduce blood pressure, and improve insulin sensitivity, all beneficial responses. However, such adaptations will regress unless exercise becomes habitual. Thus, to maximize health benefits, exercise should be done most days of the week because many of its benefits stem from the most recent exercise sessions. The role that exercise may play in the prevention of some chronic diseases, such as heart disease and diabetes, and associated risk factors, such as obesity, are discussed throughout this book where relevant.

Do most of us exercise enough?

In general, NO. Surveys reveal that most adult Americans and Canadians have little or no physical activity in their daily lives. For example, the *Healthy People 2020* report from the United States Department of Health and Human Services indicates that more than 80 percent of adults do not meet the guidelines for both aerobic and muscle-strengthening activities. Similarly, a recent study by Song and others indicated more than 80 percent of adolescents do not do enough aerobic physical activity to meet the guidelines for youth. Harvey and others reported the majority of older adults are sedentary, many sitting for prolonged periods. Thus, one of the major goals of *Healthy People 2020* is to decrease the amount of physical inactivity, such as television viewing, and increase the amount of physical activity in both adults and youth.

How much physical activity is enough for health benefits?

In general, there is a curvilinear relationship between the amount of physical activity (dose) and related health benefits (response), as depicted by the dose-response graph in figure 1.4. A sedentary lifestyle has no health benefits, but health benefits increase rapidly with low to moderate levels of weekly activity. Beyond moderate levels of weekly physical activity, the increase in health benefits will continue to increase gradually and then plateau. Excessive exercise may actually begin to have adverse effects on some health conditions.

However, as noted by Bouchard, there may be other specific dose–response curves. Some health conditions may improve rapidly with low to moderate weekly levels of physical activity, whereas others may necessitate increased levels. As an example of the latter, the ACSM Position Stand on physical activity and weight loss has noted that while moderate-intensity exercise between 150 and 250 minutes weekly will provide only modest weight loss, greater amounts of physical activity, averaging more than 250 minutes weekly, have been associated with clinically significant weight loss. Dependent on the desired health outcome, the dose (intensity, duration, frequency) of physical activity may vary accordingly, as will type of physical activity. To reap the health benefits of exercise, most health professionals recommend a comprehensive program of physical activity, including aerobic exercise and resistance training. Flexibility and balance exercises become increasingly important for older adults. In general, the

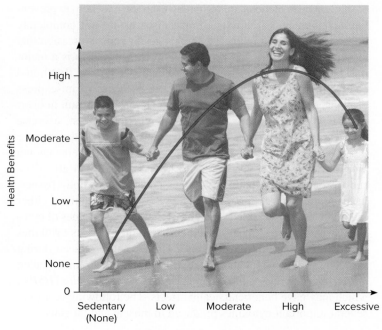

FIGURE 1.4 Significant health benefits may occur at low to moderate levels of physical activity with diminishing returns at higher levels. Excessive amounts or intensity of exercise, depending on the individual, may predispose to various types of health problems. See text for discussion.

following recommendations for adults have been formatted into a MyActivity Pyramid, a graphic depicting exercise guidelines. The latest version, developed by Stephen Ball at the University of Missouri, is presented in figure 1.5.

Numerous reports providing exercise recommendations for health benefits have been released by various professional and governmental health-related organizations, including the *Physical Activity Guidelines for Americans* from the U.S. Department of Health and Human Services and the *National Physical Activity Plan,* a coalition report from the American Heart Association, the American College of Sports Medicine, the Centers for Disease Control and Prevention, and many other such organizations. Here are some of the key points to help you reap the many health benefits of physical activity.

- *Individualization.* Exercise programs should be individualized based on physical fitness level and health status. Claude Bouchard, an expert in genetics, exercise, and health, noted that due to genes, physical activity may benefit some, but not others. For example, although most sedentary individuals will respond favorably to an aerobic exercise training program, such as an improved insulin sensitivity, others will not respond and have no change in insulin sensitivity. Currently, there is no gene profile for responders and nonresponders to exercise training, but that may change in the future so that specific exercise programs may be designed for individuals.
- *Leisure-time activity.* A key component of a fitness plan is simply to reduce the amount of daily sedentary activity. One important modification to your daily lifestyle is to sit less and

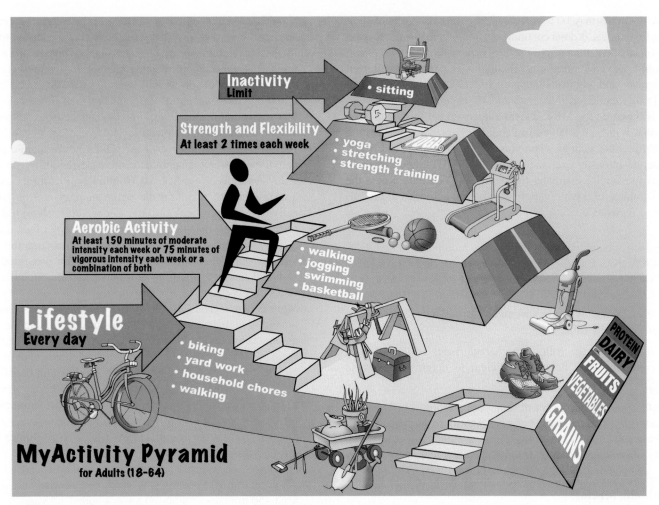

FIGURE 1.5 One version of a physical activity pyramid. See text for more specific information regarding exercise intensity and duration for adults and older adults.

Courtesy of Dr. Stephen D. Ball. Department of Nutrition and Exercise Physiology, University of Missouri, Columbia, MO.

move more. Here are some examples to help build light physical activity into your daily schedule:

- If you sit all day at work, take a short break every hour and walk around for several minutes.
- Take a walk after lunch and dinner.
- Walk to the store instead of driving.
- Stand instead of sit when you can.
- Get up and move during commercial breaks when watching television.
- Take the stairs instead of the elevator.
- Walk your dog instead of letting him out into the backyard (your dog needs exercise too).

Accumulating more daily unstructured physical activity may be very helpful in maintaining a healthy body weight. Additionally, leisurely walking may be adequate physical activity for elderly individuals with compromised health status or very low fitness levels.

- *Aerobic exercise.* For important health benefits, both adults and older adults should engage in moderate-intensity aerobic (endurance) exercise, such as brisk walking, for a minimum

of 150 minutes every week, or about 30 minutes for 5 days. Alternatively, both may engage in vigorous-intensity exercise, such as jogging or running, for 75 minutes every week. Gibala and others noted the term **high-intensity interval training (HIIT)** should be used to describe protocols in which the training stimulus is "near maximal" or the target intensity is between 80 and 100 percent of maximal heart rate. They also suggest *sprint interval training (SIT)* be used for protocols that involve supramaximal efforts, in which target intensities correspond to workloads greater than what is required to elicit 100 percent of maximal oxygen uptake (VO_2 max). These supramaximal exercise tasks may be accomplished in much less time as compared to moderate-intensity exercise, and Kilpatrick and others indicate 75 minutes weekly of such exercise could provide significant health benefits. Additionally, adults may engage in an equivalent mix of moderate- and vigorous-intensity exercise over the course of the week.

Children and adolescents should do 60 minutes of moderate to vigorous physical activity daily. Short bursts of vigorous activity in games are included. Exergames, interactive video games that promote physical activity, may hold promise to promote aerobic physical activity in youth.

Health benefits may be achieved whether the daily minute allotment for exercise is done continuously, or as three 10-minute *exercise snacks* done throughout the day, such as three brisk walks. Aerobic exercise programs, including the determination of moderate- and vigorous-intensity exercise and discussion of HIIT, are detailed in chapters 3 and 11. In brief, exercise intensity is based on the MET, a term associated with the metabolic rate that will be explained in detail in chapter 3. Your resting metabolic rate, such as when you are sitting quietly, is 1 MET. Moderate-intensity exercise is about 3–6 METs, and vigorous-intensity exercise is greater than 6 METs. You may access the MET values for a wide variety of physical activities at the following Website.

https://sites.google.com/site/compendiumofphysicalactivities/. Click on Activity Categories, such as bicycling, and the METs value will be provided for a wide variety of bicycling activities.

- Some examples of moderate- and vigorous-intensity exercise are presented in Table 1.1.

For the present, the following characteristics of the *talk test* while exercising may be may sufficient to determine exercise intensity.

Light: You can carry on a normal conversation.
Moderate: You can talk, but not sing but a few notes before taking a breath.
Vigorous: You cannot say more than a few words.

- *Resistance exercise.* Resistance exercise also conveys significant health benefits.

    Both adults and older adults should engage in muscle-strengthening activities on 2 or more days a week that work all major muscle groups (legs, hips, back, abdomen, chest, shoulders, and arms). Children and adolescents should do the same at least 3 days a week. The recommendation includes about 8 to 10 exercises that stress these major muscle groups. Individuals should perform about 8 to 12 repetitions of each exercise at least twice a week on nonconsecutive days. Older adults may lift lighter weights or use less resistance, but do more repetitions. Resistance exercises may include use of weights or other resistance modes or weight-bearing activities such as stair climbing, push-ups, pull-ups, and various other calisthenics that stress major muscle groups. Resistance exercise programs will be discussed in chapter 12.

- *Flexibility and balance exercise.* Older adults should perform activities that help maintain or increase flexibility on at least 2 days each week for at least 10 minutes. Flexibility exercises are designed to maintain the range of joint motion for daily activities and physical activity. Older adults should also perform exercises that help maintain or improve balance about 3 times a week. Such exercises may help reduce the risk of injury from falls. Appropriate exercises are presented in the National Institute of Aging program, Go4Life, included in the following Websites.

- *More is better.* The *Physical Activity Guidelines for Americans* notes that more exercise time, particularly increasing the weekly amount of moderate-intensity aerobic activity to 300 minutes or vigorous-intensity aerobic activity to 150 minutes, or an equivalent combination of the two, equals more health benefits. The *Guidelines* also note that going beyond this 300 or 150 minutes a week will provide even more health benefits. Some support for this viewpoint was provided in a recent *Consumer Reports on Health* article. In a summary of an analysis of studies involving 655,000 adults, 75 minutes a week of moderate physical activity, such as brisk walking, was linked to an additional 1.8 years of life expectancy, whereas people who were active at least 450 minutes (7.5 hours) a week added 4.5 years.

    For those who have the time and energy, exceeding the recommended amounts of physical activity may provide additional health benefits. In particular, as noted previously, more exercise may be an important consideration to promote weight loss and prevent weight gain, a major factor in promoting health.

If you are interested in starting an exercise program, you may preview chapter 3 for a discussion of energy expenditure during exercise. The Compendium of Physical Activities and the concept of the MET as a measure of exercise intensity is introduced. You may also preview chapter 11 to design an aerobics exercise program for cardiovascular-respiratory fitness and proper weight control, and chapter 12 to design a resistance training program for muscular strength and endurance. Additionally, the following excellent Websites provide detailed guidelines for physical activity as indicated.

TABLE 1.1	Some examples of moderate-intensity and vigorous-intensity exercise
Moderate-Intensity Exercise	**Vigorous-Intensity Exercise**
Leisurely bicycling, 5–8 mph	Bicycling, 12 mph and faster
Walking, leisurely, 2 mph	Walking, 4.5 mph and faster
Dancing, slow ballroom	Dancing, aerobic, with 6- to 8-inch step
Jogging, slow on a mini-tramp	Jogging/running, 4 mph and faster
Swimming, slow leisurely	Swimming, fast crawl, 50 yards/minute
Tennis, doubles	Tennis, singles
Golf, walking, carrying clubs	Basketball, competitive game
Pilates, general	Exergaming, vigorous effort

www.health.gov/paguidelines Provides detail on the Physical Activity Guidelines for children, adults, and older adults.
http://go4life.nia.nih.gov/ The National Institute of Aging provides a comprehensive exercise program for senior citizens.
www.shapeamerica.org/standards/guidelines/paguidelines.cfm The Society for Health and Physical Educators provides physical activity guidelines for children.

Am I exercising enough?

Several approaches may be used to answer this question. One approach is to keep a record of all your physical activity for a week, such as how many minutes you walk; engage in some type of aerobic physical activity such as swimming, cycling, or jogging; or perform resistance exercise such as lifting weights. Chapter 11 contains a form you can use, modifying it as you see fit, to record your daily physical activities. Tallying your totals for the week and comparing them to the previously mentioned recommendations for aerobic and resistance exercise will give you a good idea as to whether you are meeting current recommendations. Another method, which provides a more detailed analysis, is to use the program at *www.ChooseMyPlate.gov.* Click on Interactive Tools, then Food Tracker to assess your physical activity.

The most recent method involves the use of exercise gadgets that can monitor and record your daily levels of physical activity. Such gadgets started with the basic pedometer, but according to a recent *Consumer Reports* review, currently there are numerous gadgets you can wear on your wrist or put in your pocket that will effortlessly synchronize with your smartphone and provide you data on heart rate, blood pressure, energy (Calories) expended, and other health-related variables.

Consumer Reports suggests the *Fitbit One* may be worth your money. It counts steps, calculates Calories expended, and tells you how close you are to meeting your daily health goals. Other *Fitbit* models log foods you eat and track caloric intake. Highly recommended for iPhone users is *Moves,* a free app that records your running, cycling, swimming, exercise time in the gym, and much more, including periods of physical inactivity.

Numerous other fitness apps are available. About the time this book went to press, Hongu and others indicated more than 13,600 mobile phone health apps were currently available on the market. You can Google the terms *Fitness Apps* and *Free Fitness Apps* and peruse those available. These fitness apps not only record your physical activity; many also are designed to help promote regular physical activity and related health behaviors.

Can too much exercise be harmful to my health?

In general, the health benefits far outweigh the risks of exercise. Although individuals training for sport may need to undergo prolonged, intense exercise training, such is not the case for those seeking health benefits of exercise. Given our current state of knowledge, adhering to the guidelines presented above, preferably at the upper time and day limits, should be safe and provide optimal health benefits associated with physical activity. However, exercise, particularly when excessive and in individuals with preexisting health problems, may increase health risks. Training for and participating in various sports may also predispose one to various health problems.

- *Orthopedic problems.* Too much exercise may lead to orthopedic problems, such as stress fractures in the lower leg in those who run, particularly in those with poor biomechanics. Injuries to tendons and bones are common in some sports. However, recovery from such orthopedic problems occurs with proper rest.
- *Impaired immune functions.* Couto and others noted that while moderate physical activity may enhance immune function, prolonged, high-intensity exercise temporarily impairs immune competence, which may be associated with an increased incidence of upper respiratory tract infections. Moreover, according to a recent review by Nijs and others, individuals with chronic fatigue syndrome, discussed in chapter 3, may have an altered immune response to exercise and other reports link it to excessive exercise.
- *Exercise-induced asthma.* Couto and others indicate some endurance athletes, such as runners and cross-country skiers, particularly when exercising in cold weather, may be more prone to exercise-induced asthma. Excessive lung ventilation may dry the airways with subsequent release of inflammatory mediators that cause contraction of the airways, making breathing more difficult. In severe cases, exercise-induced asthma may be fatal.
- *Exercise addiction.* Exercise is known to release various brain chemicals, including endorphins, which may elicit euphoric feelings such as the *runners high.* However, Weinstein and Weinstein note that exercise addiction may also have an obsessive-compulsive dimension and may be linked to other psychiatric disorders, such as substance abuse and eating disorders.
- *Osteoporosis.* When coupled with inadequate dietary energy intake, exercise that leads to excessive weight loss may contribute to the menstrual irregularities in female athletes that may exacerbate loss of bone mass, or osteoporosis. Known as the female athlete triad, this topic is discussed in chapters 8 and 10.
- *Heat illness and kidney failure.* Exercising in the heat may cause heat stroke or other heat illnesses with serious consequences, such as kidney failure and death, as discussed in chapter 9.
- *Brain damage.* As noted previously, exercise exerts multiple beneficial effects on the brain, such as improved psychological health and reduced risk of mental decline with aging. McKee and others document the multiple benefits but also note that participation in some sports may be associated with mild traumatic brain injury (mTBI) and, rarely, catastrophic traumatic injury and death. Repetitive mTBIs, such as concussions, can lead to neurodegeneration, or chronic traumatic encephalopathy (CTE). CTE has been reported most frequently in American football players and boxers but is also associated with other sports such as ice hockey, soccer, rugby, and baseball.

- *Heart attacks and sudden death.* Varró and Baczkó note that although sudden death among young athletes is very rare, it is still two to three times more frequent than in the age-matched control population and attracts significant media attention.

  Sudden death in older athletic individuals may be associated with coronary heart disease, discussed in detail in chapter 5. In brief, atherosclerosis in the heart's blood vessels may limit oxygen supply to the heart muscle, triggering what is known as an ischemic heart attack. In his review, Williams cautions heart attack survivors to use caution with exercise, noting moderate levels may be beneficial but higher levels may attenuate the benefits. He notes that for heart attack survivors, more exercise is better, up to a point.

- *Accidents.* Given the nature of physical activity, particularly competitive sports, accidental injuries occur, and some may be fatal, such as a concussion causing serious head injury. Use safety gear as appropriate for your physical activity, such as helmets for bicycling, rollerblading, and skiing, as well as other protective sportswear as appropriate for any given activity. Adhere to safety protocols for various activities, such as cycling in traffic. About 700 cyclists are killed annually in the United States in collisions with automobiles. In recent years, reports indicate increasing emergency room visits by those who walk and talk on their cell phones and experience an accident, either by falls or being hit by motor vehicles.

It is important to emphasize that although a properly planned exercise program may be safe and confer multiple health benefits to most individuals, exercise may be hazardous to some. The most common concern is a heart attack. Individuals who have any concerns about their overall health, particularly those over age 35, should have a medical screening to detect risk factors for heart disease, such as high blood pressure, before increasing their level of physical activity. Such a medical screening might include an exercise stress test during which your heart rate and blood pressure are monitored for abnormal responses. Although exercise may be a temporary risk, it conveys lasting protection. The best protection for the heart is to exercise frequently, mainly because regular exercise helps prevent heart disease, as well as many other diseases, in the first place. Additional details are provided in subsequent chapters.

Key Concepts

▶ Health-related fitness includes a healthy body weight, cardiovascular-respiratory fitness, adequate muscular strength and muscular endurance, and sufficient flexibility.

▶ Overload is the key principle underlying the adaptations to exercise that may provide a wide array of health benefits. The intensity, duration, and frequency of exercise represent the means to impose an overload on body systems that enable healthful adaptations.

▶ Physical inactivity may be dangerous to your health. Some contend "Sitting is the new smoking." Exercise, as a form of physical activity, is becoming increasingly important as a

means to achieve health benefits, by preventing the development of many chronic diseases.

▶ Physical activity need not be strenuous to achieve health benefits, but additional benefits may be gained through more vigorous and greater amounts of physical activity.

▶ In general, more exercise is better, up to a point. Excessive exercise may cause some minor and major health problems in some individuals. You should be aware of personal health issues or other factors that may be related to exercise-associated health risks.

Check for Yourself

▶ As a prelude to activities presented in later chapters, make a detailed record of all your physical activities for a full 24-hour day, from the moment you arise in the morning until you go to bed at night, and include sleep time.

Nutrition and Health-Related Fitness

What is nutrition?

Nutrition usually is defined as the science of food, involving the sum total of the processes involved in the intake and utilization of food substances by living organisms, including ingestion, digestion, absorption, transport, and metabolism of nutrients found in food. This definition stresses the biochemical or physiological functions of the food we eat, particularly in relation to health and disease. Additionally, the Academy of Nutrition and Dietetics notes that nutrition may be interpreted in a broader sense and be affected by a variety of psychological, sociological, and economic factors.

From a standpoint of health and sport performance, it is the biochemical and physiological role or function of food that is important. However, economic factors, particularly with some college students, may influence healthful food selection. For example, healthier foods such as fresh fruits and vegetables, even though they require minimal processing, are more expensive than highly processed food laden with highly refined grains, sugar, and fat, three inexpensive ingredients. Calculations derived from a recent visit to a local discount food supermarket indicated that this is what $1 will buy:

- 600 Calories of a top brand of potato chips
- 750 Calories of store-brand cola
- 40 Calories of fresh asparagus
- 50 Calories of fresh strawberries

The primary purpose of the food we eat is to provide us with a variety of nutrients. A **nutrient** is a specific substance found in food that performs one or more physiological or biochemical functions in the body. There are six major classes of essential nutrients found in foods: carbohydrates, fats, proteins, vitamins, minerals, and water. However, as noted in chapter 2, food contains substances other than essential nutrients that may affect body functions.

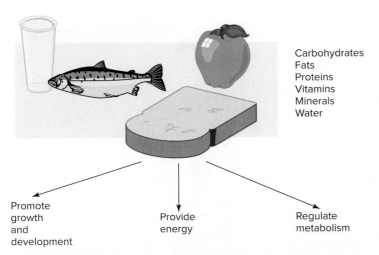

Carbohydrates
Fats
Proteins
Vitamins
Minerals
Water

Promote growth and development

Provide energy

Regulate metabolism

FIGURE 1.6 Three major functions of essential nutrients in food. Many nutrients have only one key role (e.g., glucose provides energy), whereas others have multiple roles (e.g., protein is necessary for growth and development and regulation of metabolism, and it may be used as a source of energy).

As illustrated in figure 1.6, the essential nutrients perform three basic functions. First, they provide energy for human metabolism (see chapter 3). Carbohydrates and fats are the prime sources of energy. Protein may also provide energy, but this is not its major function. Vitamins, minerals, and water are not energy sources. Second, all nutrients are used to promote growth and development by building and repairing body tissue. Protein is the major building material for muscles, other soft tissues, and enzymes, while certain minerals such as calcium and phosphorus make up the skeletal framework. Third, all nutrients are used to help regulate and maintain the diverse physiological processes of human metabolism.

In order for our bodies to function effectively, we need more than 40 specific essential nutrients, and we need these nutrients in various amounts as recommended by nutrition scientists. Dietary Reference Intakes (DRI) represent the current recommendations in the United States and include the Recommended Dietary Allowances (RDA). These recommendations are detailed in chapter 2. Nutrient deficiencies or excesses may cause various health problems, some very serious.

Although nutrients are important for our health, it is also important to note that we do not eat nutrients; we eat food.

What is the role of nutrition in health promotion?

As noted previously, your health is dependent upon the interaction of your genes and your environment, and the food you eat is part of your personal environment.

> *Let food be your medicine and medicine be your food.*

This statement by Hippocrates, made over two thousand years ago, is becoming increasingly meaningful as the preventative and therapeutic health values of food relative to the development of chronic diseases are being unraveled. Nutrients and other substances in foods, similar to the aforementioned cytokines produced in muscle and fat cells, may influence gene expression, some having positive and others negative effects on our health. For example, adequate amounts of certain vitamins and minerals may help prevent damage to DNA, the functional component of your genes, while excessive alcohol may lead to DNA damage.

Most chronic diseases have a genetic basis; if one of your parents has had coronary heart disease or cancer, you have an increased probability of contracting that disease. Such diseases may go through three stages: initiation, promotion, and progression. Your genetic predisposition may lead to the initiation stage of the disease, but factors in your environment that influence your epigenome may promote its development and eventual progression. In this regard, some nutrients are believed to be **promoters** that lead to progression of the disease, while other nutrients are believed to be **antipromoters** that deter the initiation process from progressing to a serious health problem.

What you eat plays an important role in the development or progression of a variety of chronic diseases. For example, the Centers for Disease Control and Prevention indicates that good nutrition lowers people's risk for many chronic diseases, including heart disease, stroke, some types of cancer, diabetes, and osteoporosis (see figure 1.7). The National Cancer Institute estimates that one-third of all cancers are linked in some way to diet, ranking just behind tobacco smoking as one of the major causes of cancer. Schwingshackl and Hoffman recently noted that high adherence to a healthy diet, such as the Mediterranean diet, is associated with a significant reduction in the risk of overall cancer mortality, particularly colorectal, prostate, and aerodigestive cancer.

As noted previously, *exercise is medicine.* In a like manner, *food is medicine* may also be an appropriate phrase, not only attributable to the quote from Hippocrates but also based on modern medicine as well. The types and amount of carbohydrate, fat, and protein that we eat; the amount and type of other substances such as vitamins, minerals, and phytochemicals found in our foods; the source of our food; and the method of food preparation are all factors that may influence the epigenome and subsequent gene expression or other metabolic functions that may affect our health status. The following are some of the proposed effects of various nutrients and appropriate energy intake that may help promote good health:

- Inactivate carcinogens or kill bacteria that damage DNA
- Help repair DNA
- Increase insulin sensitivity
- Relax blood vessels and improve blood flow
- Reduce blood pressure
- Optimize serum lipid levels
- Reduce inflammation
- Inhibit blood clotting
- Enhance immune system functions
- Prevent damaging oxidative processes
- Dilute harmful chemicals in the intestines
- Promote more frequent bowel movements
- Curb appetite to help reduce body fat

The beneficial, or harmful, effects of specific nutrients and various dietary practices on mechanisms underlying the development of chronic diseases will be discussed as appropriate in later sections of this book.

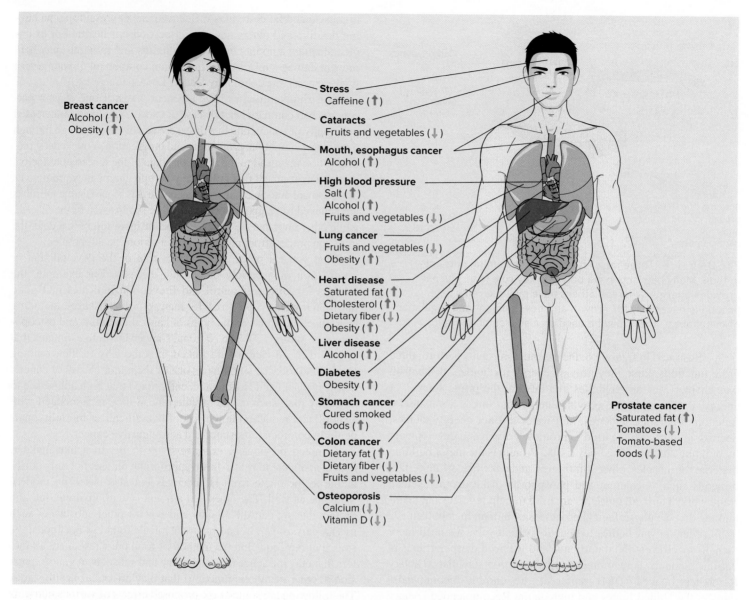

Breast cancer
Alcohol (↑)
Obesity (↑)

Stress
Caffeine (↑)

Cataracts
Fruits and vegetables (↓)

Mouth, esophagus cancer
Alcohol (↑)

High blood pressure
Salt (↑)
Alcohol (↑)
Fruits and vegetables (↓)

Lung cancer
Fruits and vegetables (↓)
Obesity (↑)

Heart disease
Saturated fat (↑)
Cholesterol (↑)
Dietary fiber (↓)
Obesity (↑)

Liver disease
Alcohol (↑)

Diabetes
Obesity (↑)

Stomach cancer
Cured smoked
foods (↑)

Colon cancer
Dietary fat (↑)
Dietary fiber (↓)
Fruits and vegetables (↓)

Osteoporosis
Calcium (↓)
Vitamin D (↓)

Prostate cancer
Saturated fat (↑)
Tomatoes (↓)
Tomato-based
foods (↓)

FIGURE 1.7 Some possible health problems associated with poor dietary habits. An upward arrow (↑) indicates excessive intake, while a downward arrow (↓) indicates low intake or deficiency.

Do we eat right?

Surveys indicate that most people are aware of the role of nutrition in health and want to eat better for healthful purposes, but they do not translate their desires into appropriate action. Poor eating habits span all age groups. According to the recent *Dietary Guidelines for Americans* report, on average Americans of all ages consume too few vegetables, fruits, high-fiber whole grains, low-fat milk products, and seafood and they eat too much added sugars, solid fats, refined grains, and sodium. The *Dietary Guidelines* recommend that solid fats and sugars (SoFAS) should constitute only 15 percent of Calories in the American diet, but they account for 35 percent of daily caloric intake for most Americans. In a study of more than 16,000 Americans, Krebs-Smith and others concluded that nearly the entire U.S. population consumes a diet that is not on par with recommendations. In particular, many Americans, Canadians, and

others throughout the world are consuming too many Calories, one of the leading causes of the global obesity problem.

To relate these nutrition findings to health in simplistic terms, most Americans eat more food (Calories) than they need, due in part to the increase in food portion sizes in recent years, and eat less of the food that they need more. The major nutrition goal of *Healthy People 2020* is to get more Americans to change their faulty dietary habits. Some advances are being made in the battle against unhealthy eating and obesity. For example, some food manufacturers have reduced the amount of fat and salt in their products. Some fast-food restaurants are offering healthier alternatives, such as oatmeal with fruit for breakfast. The National School Lunch Program has promoted a program to incorporate more fresh fruit and vegetables into daily school lunches. Although these are worthwhile endeavors, many more are needed before we can state that "We are eating right."

What are some general guidelines for healthy eating?

Because the prevention of chronic diseases is of critical importance, thousands of studies have been and are being conducted to discover the intricacies of how various nutrients may affect our health. Particular interest is focused on nutrient function within cells at the molecular level, the interactions between various nutrients, and the identification of other protective factors in certain foods. All of the answers are not in, but sufficient evidence is available to provide us with some useful, prudent guidelines for healthful eating practices.

Over the past two decades, in response to the need for healthier diets, a variety of public and private health organizations analyzed the research relating diet to health and developed some basic guidelines for the general public. The details underlying these recommendations may be found in several voluminous governmental reports, most recently the totally revamped eighth edition of *Nutrition and Your Health: Dietary Guidelines for Americans,* released by the U.S. Departments of Agriculture and Health and Human Services in 2015 and *Healthy People 2020.* These reports serve as the basis for dietary guidelines in ChooseMyPlate. Additionally, governmental health agencies in other countries, such as Britain, Canada, Germany, Japan, and Mexico, have developed dietary guidelines for health promotion in their countries, as has the WHO on a global basis. Several health organizations have promoted diets to help prevent specific diseases. The American Heart Association released a set of dietary guidelines to help prevent heart disease, the American Cancer Society released a similar set to help prevent cancer, and the American Diabetes Association did likewise for prevention of diabetes. In its recent position statement, headed by Freeland-Graves, the Academy of Nutrition and Dietetics supported the position that the total diet or overall pattern of food eaten is the most important focus of healthy eating. Classification of specific foods as good or bad is overly simplistic and can foster unhealthy eating behaviors. The Academy noted that all foods can fit within the total diet approach if consumed in moderation with appropriate portion size and combined with physical activity. Healthy eating messages should emphasize a balance of food and beverages within energy needs, rather than any one food or meal.

The dietary guidelines promoted by these government and professional health organizations have much in common and are related to some of the diet plans we will discuss in subsequent chapters, notably the Mediterranean diet and the DASH diet. For example, Sofi's review indicated that the Mediterranean diet has been consistently shown to be associated with favorable health outcomes and a better quality of life. Details are presented in a new book by Barry Sears, *The Mediterranean Zone: Unleash the Power of the World's Healthiest Diet for Superior Weight Loss, Health, and Longevity.*

Although we do have considerable research to support dietary recommendations to promote health, the research is incomplete. Moreover, inconsistencies in research findings, such as the health effects of saturated fat, discussed later in this chapter, may affect recommendations. Thus, the following recommendations may be considered to be prudent, and throughout this book we will refer to

these recommendations as a **Prudent Healthy Diet.** These recommendations are in accordance with the *total diet* approach of the Academy of Nutrition and Dietetics and the various governmental and professional health organizations noted above. Each specific dietary recommendation may convey some health benefit, so the more of these dietary guidelines you adopt, the greater should be your overall health benefits.

1. Balance the food you eat with physical activity to maintain or improve your body weight. Consume only moderate food portions. Be physically active every day.
2. Eat a nutritionally adequate diet consisting of a wide variety of nutrient-rich foods. Eat more whole foods in their natural form. Eat fewer highly processed foods.
3. Eat a diet rich in plant foods. Choose plenty of fruits and vegetables, whole-grain products, and legumes, which are rich in healthy carbohydrates, phytochemicals, and fiber.
4. Choose a diet moderate in total fat but low in saturated and *trans* fat and cholesterol.
5. Choose beverages and foods that moderate or reduce your intake of sugars, particularly added sugars.
6. Choose and prepare foods with less salt and sodium.
7. Maintain protein intake at a moderate yet adequate level, obtaining much of your daily protein from plant sources, complemented with smaller amounts of fish, skinless poultry, and lean meat.
8. Choose a diet adequate in calcium and iron.
9. Practice food safety, including proper food storage, preservation, and preparation.
10. Consider the possible benefits and risks of food additives and dietary supplements.
11. If you drink alcoholic beverages, do so in moderation. Pregnant women should not drink any alcohol.
12. Enjoy your food. Eat what you like, but balance it within your overall healthful diet.

An expanded discussion of these guidelines along with practical recommendations to help you implement them is presented in chapter 2. Additional details on how each specific recommendation may affect your health status, including specific considerations for women, children, and the elderly, are presented in appropriate chapters throughout this book. The following Websites present detailed information on healthy dietary guidelines:

---

www.dietaryguidelines.gov The *Dietary Guidelines for Americans 2015* focus on the total diet and how to integrate all of the recommendations into practical terms, encouraging personal choice but result in an eating pattern that is nutrient dense and Calorie balanced.

www.ChooseMyPlate.gov ChooseMyPlate offers personalized eating plans and interactive tools to help you plan your food choices based on *Dietary Guidelines for Americans.* Click on SuperTracker, a series of applications including Daily Food Plans for planning a healthy diet.

Am I eating right?

As part of this course, you may be required to document your actual food intake for several days and then conduct a computerized dietary analysis to determine your nutrient intake. Many computerized dietary analysis programs assess the quality of your diet from a health perspective and make recommendations for improvement where necessary.

For the time being, you may wish to take the brief diet quizzes in the Application Exercise at the end of this chapter to provide you with a general analysis of your current eating habits. Moreover, you may also analyze your diet at the ChooseMyPlate Website. Although more detailed information on healthy eating is presented in subsequent chapters, these application exercises may help you obtain some useful preliminary information on the overall healthfulness of your current diet.

Are there additional health benefits when both exercise and diet habits are improved?

A poor diet and physical inactivity are individual major risk factors for the development of chronic diseases. Collectively, however, they may pose additional risks, particularly prediabetes, a condition preceding type 2 diabetes, and for the two most deadly chronic diseases—heart disease and cancer. Recent research also indicates certain that dietary factors may complement exercise for enhanced brain function. Thus, combining a recommended exercise program with a healthy diet may have additive effects on one's health.

Prediabetes Several factors, such as excess body weight, impaired fasting blood glucose, and glucose intolerance, may be associated with prediabetes and predispose one to type 2 diabetes. In their recent review, Aguiar and others concluded that prevention interventions that include diet and both aerobic and resistance exercise training are modestly effective in reducing risk factors associated with prediabetes in adults, which help in the prevention of type 2 diabetes.

Heart Disease Lloyd-Jones and others, discussing the American Heart Association's Strategic Impact Goal through 2020 and beyond, reported that ideal cardiovascular health is associated with physical activity at goal levels and pursuit of a diet consistent with current guideline recommendations. As indicated in table 1.2, which highlights risk factors for heart disease, the key lifestyle behaviors that may be effective in favorably modifying heart disease risk factors are proper nutrition and exercise. Moreover, several of the risk factors for heart disease are diseases themselves, such as diabetes, obesity, and high blood pressure, all of which may benefit from the combination of proper nutrition and exercise.

TABLE 1.2 Modifiable risk factors associated with coronary heart disease

Risk Factors	Classification	Positive Health Lifestyle Modification
High blood pressure	Major	Proper nutrition, aerobic exercise
High blood lipids	Major	Proper nutrition, aerobic exercise
Smoking	Major	Stop smoking
Sedentary lifestyle	Major	Aerobic exercise
ECG abnormalities	Major	Proper nutrition, aerobic exercise
Obesity	Major	Low-calorie diet, aerobic exercise
Diabetes	Major	Proper nutrition, weight loss, aerobic exercise
Stressful lifestyle	Contributory	Stress management
Dietary intake	Contributory	Proper nutrition

Cancer In its recent extensive worldwide report on the means to prevent cancer, the American Institute of Cancer Research highlighted the three most important means to prevent a wide variety of cancers, and all are related to exercise and nutrition:

- Choose mostly plant foods, limit red meat, and avoid processed meat.
- Be physically active every day in any way for 30 minutes or more.
- Aim to be a healthy weight throughout life as much as possible.

Brain Health Meeusen noted that exercise and nutrition clearly are both powerful means to positively influence the brain and may influence brain health through several mechanisms that create new neurons (neurogenesis). In their review, Gomez-Pinilla and Hillman cite recent studies indicating that exercise collaborates with other aspects of lifestyle to influence cognition. In particular, select dietary factors share brain-enhancement mechanisms similar to exercise, and in some cases can complement the action of exercise. They conclude exercise and diet appear to be an effective strategy to counteract neurological and cognitive disorders.

Prevention of chronic diseases is a high priority for most governmental and professional health organizations, and they have developed appropriate healthy lifestyle behaviors to maximize prevention efforts. Most such healthy lifestyle behaviors include exercise and healthful eating. The possible complementary effect of exercise and nutrition on chronic diseases will be presented in later chapters as appropriate. In particular, as will be discussed in chapter 10, the most significant adverse health effect resulting from the combination of a poor, hypercaloric diet and physical inactivity is obesity, which may be involved in the etiology of numerous chronic health diseases.

However, although appropriate lifestyle behaviors, such as exercise, a healthful diet, and maintaining a healthy body weight, may help prevent the development of chronic diseases, individuals with a strong genetic predisposition to various risk factors, such as high serum cholesterol levels and high blood pressure, or those who are nonresponders to exercise or diet changes, may need medication to reduce these to a level compatible with protective effects.

www.fitness.gov/ The President's Council on Fitness, Sports, & Nutrition provides guidelines for children and adults to Be Active and Eat Healthy.

www.choosemyplate.gov/downloads/SuperTrackerHS LessonPlans1.pdf For teachers, this site presents lesson plans for promoting healthy nutrition among high school students using SuperTracker.

Key Concepts

▶ The primary purpose of the food we eat is to provide us with nutrients essential for the numerous physiological and biochemical functions that support life.

▶ Dietary guidelines developed by major professional health organizations are comparable, and collectively help prevent major chronic diseases such as heart disease, cancer, diabetes, high blood pressure, and obesity.

▶ Poor eating habits span all ages. The *Dietary Guidelines for Americans* and the *Healthy People 2020* report note that poor nutrition is a major health problem in the United States.

▶ Basic guidelines for a Prudent Healthy Diet include maintenance of a proper body weight and consumption of a wide variety of natural foods rich in nutrients associated with health benefits. The more healthful dietary guidelines that you adopt, the greater will be your overall health benefits.

▶ Although both proper exercise and sound nutrition habits may confer health benefits separately, health benefits may be maximized when both healthy exercise and nutrition lifestyles are adopted.

Check for Yourself

▶ As a prelude to activities presented in later chapters, make a detailed record of everything you eat for a full day, from breakfast until your late snack at night.

Sports-Related Fitness: Exercise and Nutrition

As with health, genetic endowment plays an important underlying role in the development of success in sport. In his book *The Sports Gene,* senior writer for *Sports Illustrated* and former college runner David Epstein notes that nature and nurture are both essential ingredients for superior performance in a given sport. Nature is in the genes, the hardware, whereas nurture is in the environment, the

software. Nurture involves not only exposure to the sport at a specific time but expert training as well. But Ahmetov and Rogozkin indicate that optimal responses to training are also dependent on possession of appropriate genes. Genes explain why some individuals benefit while others do not from the same sport training program. Elite athletes are not only born with the right genes for a given sport but must also have the right genes to benefit from proper training. Moreover, Joyner and Coyle note that complex motivational and sociological factors also play important roles in who does or does not become a sport champion. For example, one is more likely to be successful in ice hockey if born in Canada rather than Brazil, but the Brazilian child may be more successful in soccer.

What is sports-related fitness?

One of the key factors determining success in sport is the ability to maximize your genetic potential with appropriate physical and mental training to prepare both mind and body for intense competition. In this regard, athletes develop **sports-related fitness,** that is, fitness components such as strength, power, speed, endurance, and neuromuscular motor skills specific to their sport.

The principles of exercise training introduced earlier, such as overload and specificity, are as applicable to sports-related fitness as they are to health-related fitness. However, training for sports performance is more intense, prolonged, and frequent than training for health, and training is specific to the energy demands and skills associated with each sport. We will discuss energy expenditure for sports performance in chapter 3, but here are some examples of sport events with varying rates of energy expenditure or energy needs:

- Explosive, power sports
  – Olympic weight lifting
- Very high-intensity sports
  – 100-meter dash
- High-intensity, short duration sports
  – 5,000-meter run (3.1 miles)
- Intermittent high-intensity sports
  – Soccer
- Endurance sports
  – Marathon running (26.2 miles; 42.2 kilometers)
- Low-endurance, precision skill sports
  – Golf
- Weight-control and body-image sports
  – Bodybuilding

Training of elite athletes at the United States Olympic Training Center (USOTC) focuses on three attributes:

- Physical power
- Mental strength
- Mechanical edge

Coaches and scientists work with athletes to maximize physical power production for their specific sport, to optimize mental strength in accordance with the psychological demands of the sport, and to provide the best mechanical edge by improving specific fitness and sport skills, sportswear, and sports equipment. Jay Kearney, former senior sports scientist at the USOTC, has noted that sports science and technology provide elite competitors with the tiny margins needed to win in world-class competition (figure 1.8).

Athletes at all levels of competition, whether an elite international competitor, a college wrestler, a high school baseball player, a seniors age-group distance runner, or a youth league soccer player, can best improve their sports-related fitness and performance by intense training appropriate for their age, physical and mental development, and sport. For example, in a review as to how we should spend our time and money to improve cycling performance, Jeukendrup and Martin indicated that, of the many ways possible, training is the first and most effective means. To paraphrase Theodore Roosevelt, "Do the best with what you got." However, sports and exercise scientists have investigated a number of means to improve athletic performance beyond that attributable to training, and one of the most extensively investigated areas has been the effect of nutrition.

What is sports nutrition?

At high levels of athletic competition, athletes generally receive excellent coaching to enhance their biomechanical skills (mechanical edge), sharpen their psychological focus (mental strength), and maximize the physiological functions (physical power) essential for optimal performance. Clyde Williams, a renowned sport scientist from England, notes that, in addition to specialized training, from earliest times certain foods were regarded as essential preparation for sports competition, including the Olympics in ancient Greece.

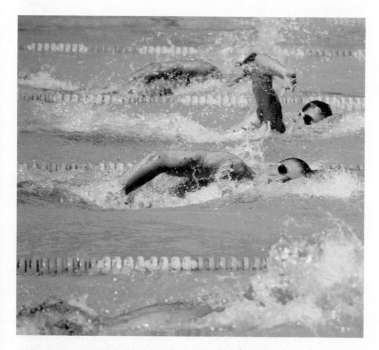

FIGURE 1.8 Elite athletes are exposed to state-of-the-art physiological, psychological, and biomechanical training that may provide an advantage measured in milliseconds, which could mean the difference between the gold and silver medal in world-class competition.

As we shall see, there are various dietary factors that may influence biomechanical, psychological, and physiological considerations in sport. For example, losing excess body fat will enhance biomechanical efficiency; consuming carbohydrates during exercise may maintain normal blood sugar levels for the brain and prevent psychological fatigue; and providing adequate dietary iron may ensure optimal oxygen delivery to the muscles. All these sports nutrition factors may favorably affect athletic performance.

Sports nutrition involves the application of nutritional principles to enhance athletic performance. Louise Burke, an internationally renowned sports nutritionist from Australia, defined sports nutrition as the application of eating strategies with several major objectives:

- To promote good health
- To promote adaptations to training
- To recover quickly after each training session
- To perform optimally during competition

Sports nutritionists may meet these objectives in various ways, such as developing meal plans for training, recovery, and competition; providing appropriate information about healthy diets; discussing the efficacy, safety, and permissibility of sports supplements; counseling individual athletes with special diets, such as vegetarians; and monitoring athletes for weight loss and eating disorders.

Although investigators have studied the interactions between nutrition and various forms of sport or exercise for more than a hundred years, it is only within the past several decades that extensive research has been undertaken regarding specific recommendations for athletes.

Is sports nutrition a profession?

Sports nutrition is recognized as an important factor for optimal athletic performance. Sports nutrition is sometimes referred to as *exercise nutrition* when coupled with exercise designed for health-related fitness, as discussed in the previous section, but that term is less frequently used. Several factors indicate that sports nutrition has become a profession and is a viable career opportunity.

Professional Associations Several professional associations, such as the Sports and Cardiovascular Nutritionists (SCAN) subsection of the Academy of Nutrition and Dietetics, Professionals in Nutrition for Exercise and Sport (PINES), the Collegiate & Professional Sports Dietitians Association (CPSDA), and the International Society of Sports Nutrition (ISSN), are involved in the application of nutrition to sport, health, and wellness.

Certification Programs Several professional and sports-governing organizations have developed a recognized course of study or certification program to promote the development of professionals who can provide athletes with sound information about nutrition. For example, the Academy of Nutrition and Dietetics has established a program for certification as a Specialist in Sports Dietetics (CSSD), while the International Olympic Committee offers a diploma in sports nutrition.

Research Productivity Numerous exercise-science/nutrition research laboratories at major universities are dedicated to sports nutrition research. Almost every scientific journal in sport/exercise science, and even in general nutrition, appears to contain at least one study or review in each issue that is related to sports nutrition. Several journals, such as the *International Journal of Sport Nutrition and Exercise Metabolism*, focus almost exclusively on sports nutrition.

International Meetings Numerous international meetings have focused on sports nutrition, some meetings highlighting nutritional principles for a specific sport, such as soccer or track and field, while others may focus on a specific sport supplement, such as creatine.

Consensus Statements and Position Stands Several international sports-governing organizations have developed consensus statements on nutrition for their specific sport. For example, the International Swimming Federation (Fédération Internationale de Natation, FINA) recently published a consensus statement on nutrition for the aquatic sports, which is designed to provide sound nutrition information for aquatic athletes worldwide. A more generalized position stand entitled "Nutrition and Athletic Performance" was issued jointly by the American Dietetic Association (now the Academy of Nutrition and Dietetics), Dietitians of Canada, and the American College of Sports Medicine.

National Sports Nutrition Programs Many countries have developed sports nutrition programs for international competition, such as the Olympic Games. Burke and others reported on such programs for the London Olympic Games.

Career Opportunities Sports nutritionists are employed by professional sport teams and athletic departments of major universities to design optimal nutritional programs for their athletes. Some dietitians market themselves as full-time or part-time sports nutritionists within their communities. Many are members of CPSDA.

Sports nutrition as we know it today has a relatively short history, but it appears to be an important aspect in the total preparation of the athlete.

---

www.acsm.org You may access the position stand entitled "Nutrition and Athletic Performance" by clicking on Access Public Information and then Position Stands.

www.scandpg.org/sports-nutrition/be-a-board-certified-sports-dietitian-cssd/ Check this SCAN site to see what is necessary to become a Certified Specialist in Sports Dietetics.

www.sportsoracle.com Check this PINES site to see what is needed to become a member and the requirements for the IOC Diploma in Sports Nutrition.

www.sportsrd.org Check this CPSDA site for information on membership.

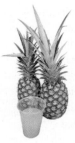

Are athletes today receiving adequate nutrition?

Numerous survey studies regarding dietary intake of athletes have been conducted over the course of the past two decades and, in general, present mixed results. Based on recommended dietary practices for athletes, the following is a brief summarization of the findings.

- Many athletes do not consume adequate amounts of energy, particularly carbohydrate.
- Many athletes consume more dietary fat than recommended, particularly saturated fat.
- Intake of micronutrients, such as vitamins and minerals, varies. Some athletes exceed current recommended intakes, while others have inadequate intakes.
- Athletes involved in weight-control sports who may restrict energy intake may be at high risk for micronutrient deficiencies. Iron and calcium deficiencies may be common in female athletes.
- Many athletes, including youth athletes, take dietary supplements, not only vitamins and minerals to help prevent deficiencies but also supplements designed to enhance performance.

This brief review indicates that some athletic groups are not receiving the recommended allowances for a variety of essential nutrients or may not be meeting certain recommended standards. It should be noted, however, that these surveys have analyzed the diets of the athletes only in reference to a standard, such as the RDA, and many studies have not analyzed the actual nutrient or biochemical status (such as by a blood test) of the athlete or the effects that the dietary deficiency exerted on exercise performance capacity or sport performance. The RDA for vitamins and minerals incorporates a safety factor, so an individual with a dietary intake of essential nutrients below the RDA may not necessarily suffer a true nutrient deficiency. If, however, the athlete does develop a nutrient deficiency, then athletic performance may deteriorate and health may be impaired. Examples discussed in later chapters include impaired aerobic endurance capacity associated with iron deficiency and premature decreases in bone density with calcium deficiency.

Why are some athletes malnourished?

Studies over the course of the past two decades have indicated a variety of factors that may contribute to poor dietary habits in many athletes, including the following:

- Athletes may not possess sufficient knowledge to make appropriate food choices.
- Christine Rosenbloom, a distinguished sports nutritionist, and her colleagues indicate that athletes have misconceptions about the roles of specific nutrients in sport performance, and if they choose foods based on these misconceptions then sports performance may suffer.
- Athletes may not be getting sound sports nutrition information. Jacobson and others reported that although some college varsity

athletes received nutrition information from reliable sources, such as dietitians and athletic trainers, considerable nutrition information was obtained from less reliable sources such as magazines and coaches with an inadequate education in sports nutrition.

- Finances and time may limit preparation of healthier meals, particularly with college athletes. Healthy meal preparation may take a back seat to time needed for sport practice and class and study time.

However, the future looks bright. SCAN and the CPSDA have partnered with the NCAA Sports Science Institute to publish nutrition information monthly on its Website. Along with increased emphasis on sports nutrition education for collegiate strength and conditioning coaches, such endeavors may help improve nutrition among collegiate athletes. Various education programs also are being developed for professional and youth sports by various groups, such as, respectively, the National Football League and the President's Council on Fitness, Sports, & Nutrition. Such programs should help. For example, Valliant and others reported a nutrition education program was useful in improving dietary intake and nutrition knowledge of female athletes.

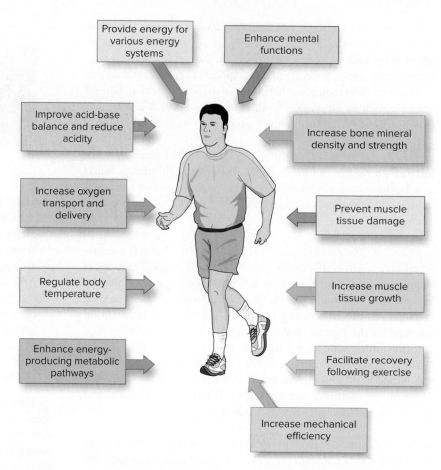

How does nutrition affect athletic performance?

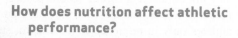

The nutrients in the foods we eat can affect exercise and sports performance in accordance with the three major functions of nutrients. First, nutrients may provide energy for the different energy-producing systems discussed in chapter 3. Second, nutrients also help regulate metabolic processes important to energy production and temperature regulation during exercise. Third, nutrients support the growth and development of specific body tissues and organs as they adapt to exercise training; figure 1.9 highlights some of the roles diet and nutrients play during exercise. A well-planned sport-specific diet will help optimize sports performance, but a poor diet plan may lead to impaired performance.

Malnutrition represents unbalanced nutrition and may exist as either undernutrition or overnutrition, that is, an individual does not receive an adequate intake (*undernutrition*) or consumes excessive amounts of single or multiple nutrients (*overnutrition*). Either condition can hamper athletic performance. An inadequate intake of certain nutrients may impair athletic performance due to an insufficient energy supply, an inability to regulate exercise metabolism at an optimal level, or a decreased synthesis of key body tissues or enzymes. In contrast, excessive intake of some nutrients may also impair athletic performance, and even the health of the athlete, by disrupting normal physiological processes or leading to undesirable changes in body composition.

FIGURE 1.9 Nutrients in the foods we eat and dietary strategies may influence exercise or sport performance in a variety of ways. They may provide energy for the various human energy systems, may help regulate various metabolic processes important to exercise, and may promote the growth and development of various body tissues and organs important for energy production during exercise.

What should athletes eat to help optimize sport performance?

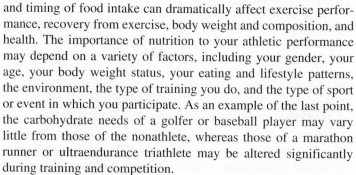

Melinda Manore, an expert in sports nutrition, noted that there is no doubt that the type, amount, composition, and timing of food intake can dramatically affect exercise performance, recovery from exercise, body weight and composition, and health. The importance of nutrition to your athletic performance may depend on a variety of factors, including your gender, your age, your body weight status, your eating and lifestyle patterns, the environment, the type of training you do, and the type of sport or event in which you participate. As an example of the last point, the carbohydrate needs of a golfer or baseball player may vary little from those of the nonathlete, whereas those of a marathon runner or ultraendurance triathlete may be altered significantly during training and competition.

The opinions offered by researchers in the area of exercise and nutrition relative to optimal nutrition for the athlete run the gamut. At one end, certain investigators note that the daily food requirement of athletes is quite similar to the nutritionally balanced diet for everyone else, and therefore no special recommendations are needed. At the other extreme, some, such as sports supplement companies, state that it is almost impossible to obtain all the nutrients the athlete requires from the normal daily intake of food, and for that reason nutrient supplementation is absolutely necessary. Other reviewers advocate a compromise between these two extremes, recognizing the importance of a nutritionally balanced diet but also stressing the importance of increased consumption of specific nutrients or dietary supplements for athletes in certain situations.

The review of the scientific literature presented in this book supports the latter point of view. In general, athletes who consume enough Calories to meet their energy needs and who meet the requirements for essential nutrients should be obtaining adequate nutrition. The dietary guidelines for better health, as discussed previously and expanded upon in chapter 2, are the same for optimal physical performance. The key to sound nutrition for the athletic individual is to eat a wide variety of healthful foods.

Although a healthy diet is the foundation of a dietary plan for athletes, modifications may be important for training and competition in various sports. For example, adequate carbohydrate is important as an energy source for aerobic endurance athletes, adequate protein may help optimize muscle development in strength/power athletes, and adequate iron may help ensure adequate oxygen delivery in female athletes. Some basic guidelines regarding eating for training and for competition are presented in chapter 2, whereas details regarding the use of specific nutrients, such as carbohydrate and protein, are presented in the chapter highlighting that nutrient.

Some athletes believe that there are *super* foods or diets that provide a competitive advantage in sports. Numerous *sports supplements* are marketed to athletes with this premise in mind and have been the subject of considerable research by sports nutrition scientists. The following section discusses the general role of such supplements in the enhancement of sports performance, while more details on specific sports supplements are presented in the chapter highlighting that nutrient. Chapter 13 also details the role of herbals and other sports supplements.

Key Concepts

▶ Success in sports is primarily dependent on genetic endowment and proper training, but nutrition can also be an important contributing factor.

▶ The major objectives of sports nutrition are to promote good health and adaptations to training, to recover quickly after each training session, and to perform optimally during competition.

▶ Studies reveal that although athletes desire to eat a diet that may enhance sports performance, their knowledge of nutrition is often inadequate, and some are not meeting the dietary recommendations of sports nutritionists.

▶ In general, the diet that is optimal for health is optimal for sports performance. However, athletes involved in certain sports may benefit from specific dietary modifications.

Ergogenic Aids and Sports Performance: Beyond Training

Since time immemorial, athletes have attempted to use a wide variety of techniques or substances to enhance sports performance beyond the effects that could be obtained through training. In sport and exercise science terminology, such techniques or substances are referred to as **ergogenic aids.**

What is an ergogenic aid?

As mentioned previously, the two key factors important to athletic success are genetic endowment and state of training. At certain levels of competition, the contestants generally have similar genetic athletic abilities and have been exposed to similar training methods, and thus they are fairly evenly matched. Given the emphasis placed on winning, many athletes training for competition are always searching for the ultimate method or ingredient to provide that extra winning edge. Indeed, some suggest that two of the key factors leading to better athletic records in recent years are improved diet and ergogenic aids.

The word *ergogenic* is derived from the Greek words *ergo* (meaning work) and *gen* (meaning production of) and is usually defined as *to increase potential for work output.* In sports, various ergogenic aids, or ergogenics, have been used for their theoretical ability to improve sports performance by enhancing physical power, mental strength, or mechanical edge. There are several different classifications of ergogenic aids, grouped according to the general nature of their application to sport. The first two classifications below are often referred to as *performance-enhancing techniques,* whereas the last three classifications involve taking some substance into the body and are known as *performance-enhancing substances.* We have listed several major categories with an example of one theoretical ergogenic aid for each.

Mechanical Aids Mechanical, or biomechanical, aids are designed to increase energy efficiency, to provide a mechanical edge. Lightweight racing shoes may be used by a runner in place of heavier ones so that less energy is needed to move the legs and the economy of running increases.

Psychological Aids Psychological aids are designed to enhance psychological processes during sport performance, to increase mental strength. Hypnosis, through posthypnotic suggestion, may help remove psychological barriers that limit physiological performance capacity.

Physiological Aids Physiological aids are designed to augment natural physiological processes to increase physical power. Blood doping, or the infusion of blood into an athlete, may increase oxygen transport capacity and thus increase aerobic endurance. However, its use is illegal.

Pharmacological Aids Pharmacological aids are drugs designed to influence physiological or psychological processes to increase physical power, mental strength, or mechanical edge. Anabolic steroids, whose use is prohibited in sports, are still used by some athletes to help increase muscle mass, strength, and power.

Nutritional Aids Nutritional aids are nutrients designed to influence physiological or psychological processes to increase physical power, mental strength, or mechanical edge. Protein supplements may be used by strength-trained athletes in attempts to increase muscle mass because protein is the major dietary constituent of muscle.

Athletes often use multiple sources of ergogenic aids in attempts to gain a competitive edge. Check the following *New York Times* link for a detailed listing of drugs and supplements used by a professional athlete.

www.nytimes.com/interactive/2014/01/13/sports/baseball/alex-rodriguez-alleged-drug-regimen.html

Why are nutritional ergogenics so popular?

Probably the most used ergogenic aids are dietary supplements. Dietary supplements marketed to physically active individuals are commonly known as sports nutrition supplements, or simply **sports supplements.** Companies market their products as "Supplements for the Competitive Athlete," and the overall sports supplement business is brisk. One business journal categorizes sports nutrition supplements into three categories:

- Sports supplements, including powders, pills, and ready-to-drink products
- Nutrition bars and gels
- Sports and energy drinks and shots

Collectively, annual sales approximate $20 billion.

Sports supplements are popular worldwide. Sports supplements are used by all types of athletes: male and female, young and old, professional and amateur. Reports indicate that 90 percent or more of elite, international-class athletes consume dietary supplements. Other surveys document significant use among high school and collegiate athletes, military personnel in elite groups such as SEALS, and fitness club members.

Sports supplements are popular for several reasons. Athletes have believed that certain foods may possess magical qualities, so it is no wonder that a wide array of nutrients or special preparations have been used since time immemorial in attempts to run faster, jump higher, or throw farther. Shrewd advertising and marketing strategies promote this belief, enticing many athletes and physically active individuals to try sports supplements. Many of these products may be endorsed by professional athletes, giving the product an aura of respectability. Specific supplements also may be recommended by coaches and fellow athletes. Additionally, as drug testing in sports gets increasingly sophisticated, leading to greater detection of pharmacological ergogenics, many athletes may resort to sports supplements, believing them to be natural, safe, and legal. However, as noted later, this may not be the case.

Are nutritional ergogenics effective?

There are a number of theoretical nutritional ergogenic aids in each of the six major classifications of nutrients, and athletes have been known to take supplements of almost every nutrient in attempts to improve performance. Here are a few examples:

Carbohydrate. Special metabolites of carbohydrate have been developed to facilitate absorption, storage, and utilization of carbohydrate during exercise.

Fats. Special fatty acids have been used in attempts to provide an alternative fuel to carbohydrate.

Protein. Special amino acids derived from protein have been developed and advertised to be more potent than anabolic steroids in stimulating muscle growth and strength development.

Vitamins. Special vitamin mixtures and even "nonvitamin vitamins," such as vitamin B_{15}, have been ascribed ergogenic qualities ranging from increases in strength to improved vision for sport.

Minerals. Special mineral supplements, such as chromium, vanadium, and boron, have been advertised to promote muscle anabolism.

Water. Special oxygenated waters have been developed specifically for aerobic endurance athletes, theoretically designed to increase oxygen delivery.

In addition to essential nutrients derived from foods, there are literally hundreds of nonessential substances or compounds that are classified as dietary supplements and targeted to athletes as potent ergogenics, such as creatine, L-carnitine, coenzyme Q_{10}, inosine, octacosonal, and ginseng. Moreover, many products contain multiple ingredients, each purported to enhance sports performance. For example, one of the "energy" drinks on the market includes carbohydrates, amino acids, vitamins, minerals, metabolites, herbs, and caffeine.

Supplementation with essential nutrients above and beyond the RDA is not necessary for the vast majority of well-nourished athletes. In general, consumption of specific nutrients above the RDA has not been shown to exert any ergogenic effect on human physical or athletic performance. In one review, Deldicque and Francaux indicated that the bulk of sports supplements sold on the market are labeled with various performance-enhancement claims without any scientific evidence. However, there are some exceptions. As noted in chapters 4 through 10, there may be some justification for nutrient supplementation or dietary modification in certain athletes under specific conditions, particularly in cases where nutrient deficiencies may occur. Some specific dietary supplements and food drugs may also possess ergogenic potential under certain circumstances.

The effectiveness of almost all of the popular nutritional ergogenics, including the essential nutrients, the nonessential nutrients, the food drugs caffeine and alcohol, the steroid precursor androstenedione, and other agents, will be covered in this book. A summary is presented in chapter 13.

Are nutritional ergogenics safe?

The majority of over-the-counter dietary supplements, particularly those containing essential nutrients, appear to be safe for the general population when taken in recommended dosages. However, in a *Sports Illustrated* article entitled "What You Don't Know Might Kill You," Epstein and Dohrmann indicated that sports supplements may be dangerous. Some dietary supplements, including sports supplements, may contain ingredients that pose serious health risks in several ways.

The FDA has noted that some sports supplements contain chemicals that have been linked to numerous serious illnesses and even death, particularly when taken in excess. For example, Navarro and Seeff noted that although perceived as safe, many different herbal and dietary supplements have been reported to cause liver injury, but the exact component that is responsible for injury is difficult to discern. In the United States, products used for bodybuilding and weight loss are the most commonly implicated.

Supplements that are mislabeled and contain unlisted substances pose a serious health threat. Some companies are unscrupulous and surreptitiously may add chemicals, such as stimulants or steroids, to help make the product more effective, but which also may have adverse health effects. Another potential problem is that some, particularly younger, athletes may have the mentality that "if one is good, then ten is better" and thus may overdose, increasing the potential health risk of a potentially harmful ingredient.

Fortunately, in the United States, the government is working to require that all ingredients be listed on dietary supplement labels, and hopefully appropriate warnings of any potential health risks will be provided as new laws take effect. Currently, some companies are voluntarily adding warnings in their advertisements and product labels.

Throughout this text, possible health risks associated with nutritional ergogenics are discussed when such information is available.

Are nutritional ergogenics legal?

The use of pharmaceutical agents to enhance performance in sport has been prohibited by the governing bodies of most organized sports. The use of drugs in sports is known as **doping,** and the World Anti-Doping Agency (WADA) has promulgated an extensive list of drugs and doping techniques that have been prohibited.

At present, all essential nutrients are not classified as drugs and are considered to be legal for use in conjunction with athletic competition. Most other food substances and constituents sold as dietary supplements are also legal. However, some dietary supplements are prohibited, such as androstenedione, because they are classified as anabolic steroids, which are prohibited drugs. Nevertheless, such supplements may still be obtained via Internet sales. Other dietary supplements may contain substances that are prohibited; for example, Chinese ephedra and some forms of ginseng may contain ephedrine, a stimulant prohibited in competition. Various athletic governing associations have addressed the issue of sports supplements. For example, the National Football League (NFL), partnering with the NSF Certified for Sports program, has developed strict requirements for the manufacturing of dietary supplements approved for use by its players. The National Collegiate Athletic Association (NCAA) places supplements for student athletes into three categories:

- Permissible—may be provided by the university. Supplements include vitamins, minerals, sports drinks, energy bars, and similar products.

- Impermissible—may not be provided by the university but may be purchased by the student athlete. These supplements are mainly high-protein products, such as those rich in whey protein.
- Banned—mainly drugs, such as those banned by WADA, including stimulants and anabolic agents. Some prescription drugs may also be banned unless under guidance of a physician.

Ron Maughan, an international expert in sports nutrition, noted that contamination of sports supplements that may cause an athlete to fail a doping test is widespread. Some studies of sports supplements targeted for muscle building and marketed on the Internet have reported that up to 25 percent were contaminated with prohibited substances and note that many athletes, including Olympic champions, who have claimed they have not taken drugs, but only dietary supplements, have tested positive for doping.

It is hoped that, with pending legislation, all ingredients will be listed in correct amounts on dietary supplement labels. In the meantime, athletes should consult with appropriate authorities before using any sports nutrition supplements marketed as performance enhancers.

Some organizations, such as NSF International, have created programs such as NSF Certified for Sport®, designed to minimize the risk of contaminated sports supplements. Another such group is Informed-Sport. Both groups have Websites (www.nsfsport.com; www.informed-sport.com). Nevertheless, WADA notes that the use of nutritional or dietary supplements is completely at the athlete's own risk, even if the supplements are labeled as "approved" or "verified."

Where can I find more detailed information on sports supplements?

Although details on various sports supplements are presented in later chapters, space limitations prevent detailed accounts of each supplement. The following resources may provide detailed information regarding efficacy and safety of numerous supplements, including sports supplements.

This United States Department of Agriculture website provides numerous links to ergogenic aids and dietary supplements marketed to athletes, and you can search for specific supplements. You may access this information at www.nutrition.gov/dietary-supplements/dietary-supplements-athletes.

The Australian Institute of Sport provides a comprehensive coverage of sports supplements in four categories based on scientific evidence:

A–supported for use in specific sports situations
B–deserving of additional research
C–have little meaningful proof of beneficial effects
D–banned or high risk of containing substances that could lead to a positive doping test

The site also contains a section, A–Z Factsheets, that contains more detailed coverage of some supplements. You may access this information at www.ausport.gov.au/ais/nutrition/supplements.

Additionally, over the course of several years the *British Journal of Sports Medicine* published a series of reviews semimonthly entitled *A–Z of Nutritional Supplements,* with each review focusing on specific supplements. A total of 48 reviews were authored by leading sports scientists. Unfortunately, no abstracts are presented with the listing on the National Library of Medicine Website, nor is the identification of the supplements reviewed.

Key Concepts

▶ Probably the most prevalent ergogenic aids used to increase sports performance are those classified as nutritional, for theoretical nutritional aids may be found in all six classes of nutrients.

▶ Although most sports supplements are safe and legal, most are not effective ergogenic aids, and some are unsafe or illegal. Before using a sports supplement, athletes should try to determine if it is effective, if it is safe, and if it is legal.

Check for Yourself

▶ Go to a health food store, peruse the multiple dietary supplements available, and ask the clerk for advice on a supplement to help you enhance your sports performance, such as increasing your muscle mass or losing body fat. Write down the advice and check out advertisements on the Internet. Then, research the supplements on the Websites noted above and compare the findings.

Nutritional Quackery in Health and Sports

Increasing numbers of dietary supplements are being marketed to the general population as health enhancers and to athletes as performance enhancers. Unfortunately, many of the products that advertise extravagant claims of enhanced health or performance are promoted by unscrupulous entrepreneurs, have no legitimate basis, and may be regarded as quackery.

What is nutritional quackery?

According to the Food and Drug Administration (FDA), **quackery,** as the term is used today, refers not only to the fake practitioner but also to the worthless product and the deceitful promotion of that product. Untrue or misleading claims that are deliberately or fraudulently made for any product, including food products, constitute quackery. The Academy of Nutrition and Dietetics (AND), formerly the American Dietetic Association (ADA), in its position statement on food and nutrition misinformation authored by Wansink, notes that such misinformation can have harmful effects on the health and economic status of consumers.

Knowledge relative to all facets of life, the science of nutrition included, has increased phenomenally in recent years. Thousands of studies have been conducted, revealing facts to help unravel some of the mysteries of human nutrition. The AND indicates that consumers are taking greater responsibility for self-care and are eager to receive food and nutrition information. However, that creates opportunities for nutrition *mis*information, health fraud, and

quackery to flourish. The AND further notes that the media are consumers' leading source of nutrition information but that news reports of nutrition research often provide inadequate depth for consumers to make wise decisions. Certain individuals may capitalize on these research findings for personal financial gain. For example, isolated nutritional facts may be distorted or the results of a single study will be used to market a specific nutritional product. Health hustlers will use this information to capitalize on people's fears and hopes, be it the fear that the nutritional quality of our food is being lessened by modern processing methods or the hope of improved athletic performance capacity.

Health quackery is big business. Reports suggest that Americans spend almost $27 billion annually on questionable health practices. A substantial percentage of this amount is spent on unnecessary nutritional products. Authorities in this area have noted that the amount of misinformation about nutrition is overwhelming, and it is circulated widely, particularly by those who may profit from it. Although we may still think of quacks as sleazy individuals selling patent medicine from a covered wagon, the truth is quite different. Nutritional quacks today are super salespeople, using questionable scientific information to give their products a sense of authenticity and credibility and using sophisticated advertising and marketing techniques.

As noted previously, there are some bona fide health benefits associated with the foods we eat, but, as shall be noted in chapter 2, federal legislation establishes strict guidelines regarding the placement of health claims on food labels for most of the packaged foods that we buy. Such may not be the case, however, with dietary supplements.

Before the passage of the 1994 Dietary Supplements Health and Education Act (DSHEA), many extravagant health claims were made by some unscrupulous companies in the food supplement industry. As an example, the deceptive label of one secret formula noted that it would help you lose excess body fat while sleeping, a false claim. Although the DSHEA was designed to eradicate such fraudulent health claims, dietary supplements today appear to have more leeway than packaged foods to imply health benefits. Technically, labels on dietary supplements are not permitted to display scientifically unsupported claims. However, companies are allowed to make general health claims like "boosts the immune system" if, for example, the product contains a nutrient, such as zinc, that has been deemed important in some way to immune functions in the body. Although companies may not claim that the product prevents diseases associated with impaired immune functions, such as the common cold, cancer, or AIDS, the consumer may erroneously make such an assumption.

Many companies now use a disclaimer for general health claims on their labels, noting "These statements have not been evaluated by the Food and Drug Administration" and "This product is not intended to diagnose, treat, cure, or prevent any disease." Companies may also circumvent government regulations by using *freedom of the press.* They may provide information in the form of a reprint of an article, a brochure with highlighted research, or other printed materials that are distributed in connection with the sale of the product. Many dietary supplement companies also have developed infomercials for television or home pages on the

Internet to provide comparable biased advertising information to potential consumers.

Although these advertising strategies may contain fraudulent information, the federal agencies that monitor such practices are understaffed and cannot litigate every case of misleading or dishonest advertising. Thus, unsuspecting consumers may be lured into buying an expensive health-food supplement that has no scientific support of its effectiveness. To help remedy this problem, a Dietary Supplement Safety Act was proposed in the Senate in 2010, but a popular senator recently withdrew his support and the legislation has not been passed at the time this book went to press.

Nutritional quackery is widespread, as documented in the position stand on food and nutrition misinformation by the AND. Years ago J. V. Durnin, an international authority on nutrition and exercise, stated that there is still no sphere of nutrition in which faddism, misconceptions, ignorance, and quackery are more obvious than in athletics, a situation that continues today.

Why is nutritional quackery so prevalent in athletics?

As with nutritional quackery in general, hope and fear are the motivating factors underlying the use of nutritional supplements by athletes. They hope that a special nutrient concoction will provide them with a slight competitive edge, and they fear losing if they do not do everything possible to win.

Various factors within the athletic environment help nurture these hopes and fears, but the most significant factor contributing to nutritional quackery in sports is direct advertising, as caricatured by the fabricated advertisement in figure 1.10. If you scan through various magazines targeting bodybuilders or endurance athletes, you will see dozens of advertisements suggesting enhancement of strength, endurance, and sports performance. Such advertisements often use endorsements by star athletes. However, in most cases, there is little or no research supporting the purported ergogenic effects of the advertised supplement.

Additionally, many sports magazines will run articles on the ergogenic benefits of a particular nutrient and in close proximity to the article place an advertisement for a product that contains that nutrient. Freedom of speech guaranteed by the First Amendment permits the author of the article to make sensational and deceptive claims about the nutrient. However, freedom of speech does not extend to advertising, so fraudulent or deceptive claims may be grounds for prosecution by the FDA or the Federal Trade Commission (FTC). Thus, by cleverly positioning the article and the advertisement, the promoter can make the desired claims about the value of the product and yet avoid any illegality. Classic examples of this technique may be found with protein and amino acid supplement advertising in magazines for bodybuilders. Moreover, many advertisements now appear in a format designed to look like a scientific review, though in actuality they are deceptive advertisements for sports supplements. Check the top of the page of such articles and you will find *Advertisement* in small print.

Most of these advertised products are economic frauds. The prices are exorbitant in comparison to the same amount of nutrients that may be obtained in ordinary foods. Besides being an economic fraud, these products are an intellectual fraud, for there is very little scientific evidence to support their claims. Simple basic facts about the physiological functions of the nutrients in these products are distorted, magnified, and advertised in such a way as to make one believe that they will increase athletic performance. Unfortunately, in the area of nutrition and sport, it is very easy to distort the truth and appeal to the psychological emotions of the athlete. Epstein and Dohrmann recently documented the shadowy behaviors in the multibillion-dollar sports-supplement industry, suggesting that sports supplements may be comparable to snake oil for sale. The supplements are usually manufactured by a third party and sold to many different companies, which market them under their personal brand and slick advertising.

How do I recognize nutritional quackery in health and sports?

It is often difficult to differentiate between quackery and reputable nutritional information, but the following may be used as guidelines in evaluating the claims made for a nutritional supplement or nutritional practice advertised or recommended to athletes and others. If the answer to any of these questions is yes, then one should be skeptical of such supplements and investigate their value before investing any money.

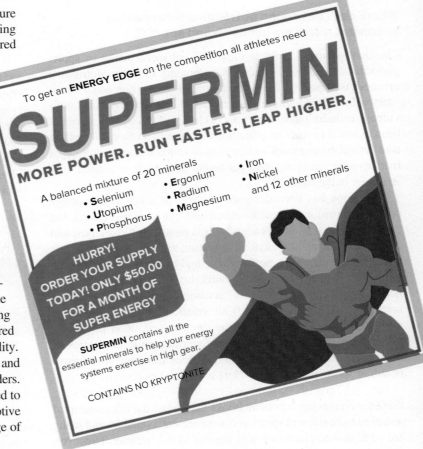

FIGURE 1.10 Simulated nutritional supplement advertisement aimed at athletes.

1. Does the product promise quick improvement in health or physical performance?
2. Does it contain some secret or magical ingredient or formula?
3. Is it advertised mainly by use of anecdotes, case histories, or testimonials?
4. Are currently popular personalities or star athletes featured in its advertisements?
5. Does it take a simple truth about a nutrient and exaggerate that truth in terms of health or physical performance?
6. Does it question the integrity of the scientific or medical establishment?
7. Is it advertised in a health or sports magazine whose publishers also sell nutritional aids?
8. Does the person who recommends it also sell the product?
9. Does it use the results of a single study or dated and poorly controlled research to support its claims?
10. Is it expensive, especially when compared to the cost of equivalent nutrients that may be obtained from ordinary foods?
11. Is it a recent discovery not available from any other source?
12. Is its claim too good to be true? Does it promise the impossible?

For additional tips on identifying nutrition quacks, check www.dietitian.com/quack.html.

Where can I get sound nutritional information to combat quackery in health and sports?

The best means to evaluate claims of enhanced health or sports performance made by dietary supplements or other nutritional practices is to possess a good background in nutrition and a familiarity with related high-quality research. Unfortunately, most individuals, including most athletes, coaches, and physicians, have not been exposed to such an educational program, so they must either take formal course work in nutrition or sports nutrition, develop a reading program in nutrition for health and sport, or consult with an expert in the field.

This book has been designed to serve as a text for a college course in nutrition for health-related and sports-related fitness, but it may also be read independently. It is an attempt to analyze and interpret the available scientific literature as to how nutrition may affect health and sports performance and to provide some simple guidelines for physically active individuals to help improve their health or athletic performance. It should provide the essential science-based (evidence-based) information you need to plan an effective nutritional program, either for yourself, other physically active individuals, or athletes, and to evaluate the usefulness of many nutritional supplements or practices designed to improve health or sports performance. Here are some key resources.

Books Numerous reputable books that detail the relationship of nutrition to health and sports performance are available, and many are cited in the reference list at the end of this chapter. However, some books, such as diet books based on an author's personal experiences, may not contain reputable information. A good guide is to check the author's credentials.

Government, Health Professional, Consumer, and Commercial Organizations and Related Websites Accurate information relating nutrition to health is published by governmental agencies such as the FDA and USDA; health professional groups such as the Academy of Nutrition and Dietetics, Dietitians of Canada, American College of Sports Medicine, and American Medical Association; consumer groups such as Consumers Union and Center for Science in the Public Interest; and some commercial groups such as the National Dairy Council and the PepsiCo's Gatorade Sports Science Institute. As noted previously, the Australian Institute of Sport provides detailed, accurate information on a wide variety of sports supplements. Excellent materials relative to nutrition may be obtained free or at small cost from some of these organizations.

www.hsph.harvard.edu/nutritionsource Excellent Website for nutrition information from the Harvard School of Public Health.
www.gssiweb.com Website for the Gatorade Sports Science Institute, providing detailed reviews on various topics in sports nutrition.
www.healthfinder.gov U.S. Department of Health and Human Services Website for information on various health topics, including nutrition.
http://medlineplus.gov National Library of Medicine, a comprehensive health-information retrieval Website.

Scientific Journals Many scientific journals publish reputable findings about nutrition, exercise, and health. These technical journals may not be readily available in public libraries but may be found in university and medical libraries. Examples of such publications include *Medicine & Science in Sports & Exercise, The Journal of the Academy of Nutrition and Dietetics, American Journal of Clinical Nutrition, Sports Medicine,* and *International Journal of Sport Nutrition and Exercise Metabolism.*

www.pubmed.gov National Library of Medicine Website provides abstracts of original research studies and excellent reviews and meta-analyses published in scientific medical journals. Free full-text articles are provided for some journals.

Popular Magazines Articles in popular health and sports magazines may or may not be accurate. The credentials of the author, if listed, should be a good guide to an article's authenticity. A Ph.D. listed after the author's name may not guarantee accuracy of the content of the article. Be wary of publications emanating from organizations or publishers that also sell nutritional supplements.

Consultants Nutritional consultants are another source of information. Such consultants should have a solid background in nutrition, particularly sports nutrition if they are to advise athletes. The consultant should be a registered dietitian (RD) or possess appropriate professional certification, such as the Certified Nutrition

Specialist (CNS). He or she should be a member of a reputable organization of nutritionists, such as the Academy of Nutrition and Dietetics, which can be contacted at its Website address to provide you with the name of a local dietitian. Other recognized nutritional organizations include the American Society for Nutrition, the American College of Nutrition, and the Dietitians of Canada. Qualified nutritionists are able to provide you with nutritional advice to help you meet your health goals.

> *www.eatright.org* Contact the Academy of Nutrition and Dietetics for the names of local dietitians, as well as other sources of sound nutrition information.

As noted previously, the Academy of Nutrition and Dietetics Commission on Dietetic Registration, working with members of Sports, Cardiovascular and Wellness Nutritionists (SCAN), has developed a certification program for registered dietitians (RD) who work in sports to achieve the status of Certified Specialist in Sports Dietetics (CSSD). A qualified sports nutritionist will be able to assess your nutritional status, including variables such as body composition, dietary analysis, and eating and lifestyle patterns, and relate these nutritional factors to the physiological and related nutritional demands of your sport or exercise program, providing you with a plan to help you reach your performance goals.

> *www.scandpg.org/search-rd* Use this Website to find a sports nutritionist. Click on your state to find one closest to you. Those with the CSSD designation have earned the designation as a Certified Specialist in Sports Dietetics.

Be wary of individuals who do not possess professional degrees or appropriate certification, such as "experts" in nutrition or fitness. Many states do not have regulations restricting the use of various terms, such as *nutritionist* or *fitness professional*. Although these individuals may have some practical experience with helping people change their diets and initiate exercise programs, they normally do not have the depth of knowledge required in some cases. For proper nutritional advice, be certain to ask for proof of certification from recognized nutrition professional groups as cited previously. For fitness professionals, check for certification by such groups as the American College of Sports Medicine (ACSM), the American Council on Exercise (ACE), or the National Strength and Conditioning Association (NSCA).

Cautions on Using the Internet The U.S. Department of Health and Human Services has recommended caution in using the Internet to find health information. Along with others, here are some of its major points:

- No one regulates information on the Internet. Thus, anyone can set up a home page and claim anything.
- Some official-sounding Websites, such as Wikipedia, permit anyone to enter or modify the information presented.
- Search engines, such as Google and Yahoo, host paid advertisements which usually have priority listing and may contain biased information.

- Compare the information you find on the Internet with other resources, such as medical journals and textbooks.
- Check the author's or organization's credentials. Unfortunately, there are many so-called nutritionists and other health professionals making false claims on the Internet.
- Be wary of Websites advertising and selling products that claim to improve your health.
- Be cautious when using information found on bulletin boards or during chat sessions with others.
- Don't believe everything you read.

Several Websites listed previously provide reputable information. Although some commercial (.com) and organization (.org) Websites provide trustworthy information and may be cited in this text, others may not be as reputable, as they may be sponsored by unethical supplement companies. In general, education (.edu) and government (.gov) Websites provide trustworthy information. The Websites cited in this text are deemed to be reliable.

For those who would like to view a National Library of Medicine tutorial on evaluating Internet health information, check the following website.

> *www.nlm.nih.gov/medlineplus/webeval/.*

Key Concepts

▶ Nutritional quackery is widespread as related to the purported benefits of specific dietary supplements, particularly so with dietary supplements marketed to physically active individuals.

▶ There are a number of guidelines to help identify quackery and false claims regarding dietary supplements, but one of the critical points to consider is if the claim simply appears to be too good to be true.

▶ The best means to counteract nutritional quackery is to possess a good background in nutrition. Reputable sources of information are available to help provide contemporary viewpoints on the efficacy, safety, and legality of various dietary supplements for health or sport.

Research and Prudent Recommendations

By now you should realize that nutrition and exercise may influence health and sports performance. But how do we know what effect a nutrient, food, or dietary supplement we consume or exercise program we undertake will have on *our* health or performance? To find answers to specific questions, we should rely on the findings derived from scientific research, which is the heart of *evidence-based* medicine. As sophisticated sciences, nutrition and exercise science have a relatively short history. Not too long ago, nutrition scientists were concerned primarily with identifying the major constituents of the foods we eat and their general functions in the human body, while those investigating exercise concentrated more on its application to enhance sports performance. Over time, however, numerous scientists have turned their attention to the possible health benefits of certain foods and various forms of exercise, and, in the case of sports scientists, the possible applications to athletic performance. These scientists are not only attempting to determine the general effects of diet and exercise on health and performance but also investigating the effects of specific nutrients at the molecular and genetic levels to determine possible mechanisms of action to improve health or performance in sport.

Because this book makes a number of nutritional (and some exercise) *evidence-based* recommendations relative to sports and health, it is important to review briefly the nature and limitations of nutritional and exercise research with humans. For the purpose of this discussion, our emphasis will be on nutritional research, although the same research considerations apply to exercise as well.

What types of research provide valid information?

Several research techniques have been used to explore the effect of nutrition on health or athletic performance. The two major general categories have been epidemiological research and experimental research.

Epidemiological research, also known as *observational research,* involves studying large populations to find relationships between two or more variables, such as dietary fat and heart disease. However, the treatment of interest, such as dietary fat, is not assigned to the subjects. Their normal diet and its relationship to the development of heart disease is the main variable of interest. There are various forms of epidemiological research. One general form uses retrospective techniques. In this case, individuals who have a certain disease are identified and compared with a group of their peers, called a *cohort,* who do not have the disease. Researchers then trace the history of both groups through interviewing techniques to identify dietary practices that may have increased the risk for developing the disease. Another general form of epidemiological research uses prospective techniques. In this case, individuals who are free of a specific disease are identified and then followed for years, during which time their diets are scrutinized. As some individuals develop the disease and others do not, the investigators then attempt to determine what dietary behaviors may increase the risk for the disease.

Epidemiological research helps scientists identify important relationships between nutritional practices and health. For example, years ago several epidemiological studies reported that individuals who consumed a diet high in fat were more likely to develop heart disease. One should note that such epidemiological research does not prove a cause-and-effect relationship. Although these studies did note a deleterious association between a diet high in fat and heart disease, they did not actually prove that fat consumption (possible cause) leads to heart disease (possible effect), but only that some form of relationship between the two existed. However, in some cases, the relationship between a lifestyle behavior and a disease is so strong that causality is inferred. In this regard, epidemiologists often calculate and report relative risks (RR) or odds ratios (OR), which are probability estimates of getting some disease by practicing some unhealthful behavior. An RR of 1.0 is normal probability, so if a study reports an RR of 2.5 for developing heart disease in individuals who consumed a diet rich in saturated fatty acids, such diets may increase one's risk 2.5 times normal. Conversely, if a study reports an RR of 0.5 for developing heart disease by consuming a purely vegetarian diet, such diets may cut heart disease risk in half. Epidemiological research is useful in identifying relationships between variables and generating hypotheses and is often a precursor to experimental research, but it does not prove a cause-and-effect relationship.

Experimental research is essential to establishing a cause-and-effect relationship (figure 1.11). In human nutrition research, experimental studies are often referred to as *randomized clinical trials (RCTs)* or *intervention studies,* usually involving a treatment group and a control, or placebo, group. RCTs may involve

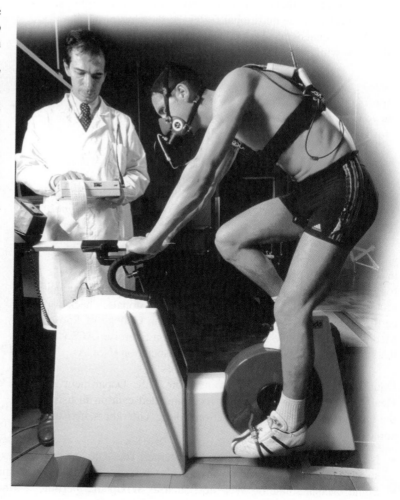

FIGURE 1.11 Well-controlled experimental research serves as the basis underlying recommendations for the use of nutritional strategies to enhance health status or sports performance.

studying a smaller group of subjects under tightly controlled conditions for a short time frame or larger population groups living freely over a long time frame. In RCTs, an independent variable (cause) is manipulated so that changes in a dependent variable (effect) can be studied. If we continue with the example of fat and heart disease, a large (and expensive) clinical intervention study could be designed to see whether a low-fat diet could help prevent heart disease. Two groups of subjects would be matched on several risk factors associated with the development of heart disease, and over a certain time, say ten years, one group would receive a low-fat diet (treatment, or cause) while the other would continue to consume their normal high-fat diet (control or placebo). At the end of the experiment, the differences in the incidence of heart disease (effect) between the two groups would be evaluated to determine whether or not the low-fat diet was an effective preventive strategy. Bouchard presents an excellent, detailed overview of the quality of different research-based sources of evidence, noting that RCTs with large populations represent one of the richest sources of data. If the results of an RCT showed that consumption of a low-fat diet had no effect upon the incidence rate of heart disease, should you continue to consume a high-fat diet? The answer to this question, as we shall see later, is "not necessarily." The type of fat may be an important consideration.

Most of the research designed to explore the effect of nutrition on sports performance is experimental in nature, and of a much shorter duration than studies investigating the relationship of nutrition and health. Additionally, most sports nutrition studies are conducted in a laboratory with tight control of extraneous variables. Very few studies have actually investigated the effect of nutritional strategies on actual competitive sports performance. Nevertheless, although most of our information about the beneficial effects of various nutritional strategies on sports performance is derived from laboratory-based research, many of these studies use laboratory protocols designed to mimic the physiological demands of a specific sport. In later chapters, as we discuss the effects of various nutritional strategies or dietary supplements on sports performance, we will often refer to studies that have problems with their experimental methodology, but we will also note studies that were well controlled. Following are some major questions you should ask when evaluating the experimental methodology of a study to see if it has been well designed. We shall use research investigating creatine supplementation as a means to increase muscular strength and power as an example.

1. Is there a legitimate reason for creatine supplementation? Theoretically, creatine may add to the stores of creatine phosphate in the muscle, an important energy source.
2. Were appropriate subjects used? As creatine phosphate may theoretically benefit power performance, trained strength athletes would be ideal subjects. However, if the purpose of the study was to evaluate the effect of creatine to prevent sarcopenia, then older subjects would be appropriate subjects.
3. Are the performance tests valid? Validated tests should be used to collect data on the dependent variable, in this case valid strength and power tests.

4. Was a placebo control used? A placebo similar in appearance and taste to creatine should be used in the control trial. Ideally, a control trial in which no substance is consumed should also be incorporated into the study. Beedie and others found that inert substances could induce a positive (placebo) effect or even a negative (nocebo) effect on performance, depending on the respective perception of the subject.
5. Were the subjects randomly assigned to treatments? Subjects should be randomly assigned to separate groups, either the treatment (creatine) or the control (placebo) group. In a repeated-measures design, in which all subjects take both the creatine and the placebo in different trials, the order of administration of the creatine and placebo is counterbalanced, which is known as a *crossover design*. In general, a repeated-measures design is preferable because each subject serves as his or her own control.
6. Was the study double-blind? Neither the investigators nor the subjects should know which groups received the treatment or the placebo until the conclusion of the study.
7. Were extraneous factors controlled? Investigators should try to control other factors that may influence power, such as physical training, diet, and activity prior to testing.
8. Were the data analyzed properly? Appropriate statistical techniques should be used to reduce the risk of statistical error. Using a reasonable number of subjects also helps to minimize statistical error.

Most experienced contemporary investigators generally use similar sophisticated research designs to generate meaningful data, and their studies appear in peer-reviewed journals. A peer-reviewed journal uses a process whereby each manuscript submitted undergoes a review and critique by several experts who recommend for or against publication. However, some researchers do not apply such strict research protocols as noted above, a fact that, if overlooked by reviewers, may result in publication of a faulty study.

Why do we often hear contradictory advice about the effects of nutrition on health or physical performance?

It is very difficult to conduct nutritional research about health and athletic performance with human subjects. For example, many diseases such as cancer and heart disease are caused by the interaction of multiple risk factors and may take many years to develop. It is not an easy task to control all of these risk factors in freely living human beings so that one independent variable, such as dietary fat, can be isolated to study its effect on the development of heart disease over 10 or 20 years. In a similar manner, numerous physiological, psychological, and biomechanical factors also influence athletic performance on any given day. Why can't athletes match their personal records day after day, such as the world-record 43.18-second 400-meter dash performance by Michael Johnson? Because their physiology and psychology vary from day to day and even within the day.

Although well-designed studies in peer-reviewed scientific journals serve as the basis for making an informed decision as to whether or not to use a particular nutritional strategy or dietary supplement to enhance health or sports performance, it is important to realize that the results from a single study with humans do not prove anything. For example, Ioannidis noted that even the most highly cited RCTs, particularly small ones with a limited number of subjects, may be challenged and refuted over time. Although most investigators attempt to control extraneous factors that may interfere with the interpretation of the results of their study, there may be some unknown factor that leads to an erroneous conclusion. For example, investigators studying the effect of creatine supplementation need to control dietary intake prior to testing. If not, consumption by some subjects of beverages containing caffeine, an effective ergogenic aid, could confound the results. Consequently, for this and other reasons, the results of single studies, whether epidemiological or experimental should be taken with a grain of salt—figuratively speaking, of course.

The Center for Science in the Public Interest published an article entitled "Behind the Headlines," noting that headlines often neglect to consider important limitations to the study. In this regard, Wellman and others indicated that, unfortunately, all too often the media make bold headlines based on the findings of an individual study, and often these headlines inadvertently exaggerate the findings of the study and their importance to health or physical performance. For example, a newspaper headline might blare "Coffee drinking causes heart disease" after a study is published indicating that coffee drinking could increase blood cholesterol levels slightly. The study did *not* show that coffee drinking caused heart disease, but only that it may have adversely affected one of its risk factors. A year or so later one may read headlines that report "Coffee drinking does not cause heart disease" because a more recent individual study did not find an association between coffee use and serum cholesterol levels. Is it no wonder consumers are often confused about nutrition and its effects on health or sports performance? Wellman and others note that nutrition scientists should be more involved in helping the media accurately convey diet and health messages.

For the purpose of improving public understanding, the National Cancer Institute provided some guidelines for journalists and others in the communications business for reporting health-related nutrition research. Key points included the following:

- The quality and credibility of the study. Was it well designed and published in a high-quality journal?
- Peer-reviewed study or presentation at a meeting. Was it presented at a meeting, which normally does not require a review by other scientists?
- Comparison of findings to other studies. Was the study compared to other studies reporting contrasting findings?
- Funding sources. Was it funded by a company that could benefit financially from the results?
- Putting findings in context, such as risk/benefit trade-offs. Are the health risks meaningful? An increased health risk from one in a million to three in a million, if reported as a three-fold

increase, may appear to be more unhealthful than it really is. Although these guidelines were presented almost 20 years ago, their use by the media does not appear to have increased appreciably.

What is the basis for the dietary recommendations presented in this book?

Scientists consider each single study as only one piece of the puzzle in attempting to find the truth. To evaluate the effects of nutritional strategies or dietary supplements on health or sports performance, individual studies should be repeated by other scientists and, if possible, a consensus developed. Reviews and meta-analyses provide a stronger foundation than the results of an individual study.

In reviews, an investigator analyzes most or all of the research on a particular topic and usually offers a summarization and conclusion. However, the conclusion may be influenced by the studies reviewed or by the reviewer's orientation. There have been instances in which different reviewers evaluated the same studies and came up with diametrically opposed conclusions.

Meta-analysis, a review process that involves a statistical analysis of previously published studies, may actually provide a quantification and the strongest evidence available relative to the effect of nutritional strategies or dietary supplements on health or sports performance. According to Binns and others, the meta-analysis is the gold standard for evidence-based clinical practice guidelines.

The value of reviews and meta-analyses is based on the quantity and quality of studies reviewed. If the number of studies is limited and they are not well controlled, or if improper procedures are used in analyzing and comparing the findings of each study, the conclusions may be inaccurate. For example, Hart and Dey noted that three meta-analyses of the use of Echinacea for the prevention of colds had somewhat different conclusions, as selection criteria for studies used in the analysis varied. Nevertheless, well-designed reviews and, in particular, meta-analyses provide us with valuable data to make prudent decisions. In particular, position statements and position stands of various groups, such as the American College of Sports Medicine and the Academy of Nutrition and Dietetics, are developed using an *evidence-based* approach, which includes an evaluation of the quality of the studies reviewed. Such groups normally use only RCTs to support their position on specific topics. A number of such position statements are cited throughout this text where relevant.

Within the lifetime of many students, a tremendous amount of both epidemiological and experimental research has been concerned with the effect nutrition may have upon health and athletic performance. Based on evolving research findings, dietary recommendations change over time. For example, in a 25th anniversary issue spanning the years 1977 to 2002, *Environmental Nutrition* compared 10 different dietary recommendations based on current research and that available 25 years ago. Here is 1 of the 10: Then, in the 1970s, dietary fat was at the root of most illnesses, including heart disease and cancer, and there was no distinction between different types of fat. However, in 2002, dietary fat was in good favor if consumed in moderation and if unsaturated fats, particularly monounsaturated fats, were substituted for saturated fats, which were considered to be unhealthy fat contributing to development of chronic diseases, particularly heart disease. But a dozen years later, in 2014, newspaper headlines around the world claimed "Butter Is Back," based on a meta-analysis of 76 studies. Chowdhury and others concluded that the available research evidence does not clearly support current dietary guidelines, particularly to consume a diet low in saturated fat, as a means to help prevent heart disease. Nevertheless, as noted above, even meta-analyses may be flawed, resulting in erroneous conclusions. Numerous scientists criticized this meta-analysis, indicating the authors misinterpreted some research and failed to include other studies; some even suggested the authors retract it. More details are presented in chapter 5. Stay tuned.

Comparable to the science of other human behaviors, the science of human exercise and nutrition is not, as many may believe, exact. Although in many cases we still do not have absolute proof that a particular nutritional practice will produce the desired effect, we do have sufficient information to make a recommendation that is prudent, meaning that it is likely to do some good and cause no harm. Thus, the recommendations offered in this text should be considered prudent; they are based upon a careful analysis and evaluation of the available scientific literature, primarily comprehensive reviews and meta-analyses of the pertinent research by various scientists or public and private health or sports organizations. Most such organizations use RCTs as the basis for their guidelines, while some recognize possible limitations of RCTs in making specific nutrition recommendations and incorporate the totality of evidence, including epidemiological findings. In cases where the research data are limited, recommendations may be based on several individual studies if they have been well designed.

www.nel.gov The USDA Nutrition Evidence Library collaborates with leading scientists using state-of-the-art methodology to review, evaluate, and synthesize research to answer important diet-related questions.

How does all this relate to me?

Remember that we all possess biological individuality and thus might react differently to a particular nutritional or exercise intervention. For example, relative to health, most of us have little or no reaction to an increase in dietary salt, but some individuals are very sensitive to salt intake and will experience a significant rise in blood pressure with increased dietary salt. Relative to athletic performance, Mann and others note there are high responders and low responders to the same standardized exercise training program, some individuals improving markedly but others less so. Such individual reactions have been noted in some research studies and are discussed where relevant in the following chapters. With advances in genetic technology, diets and

exercise training may one day be individualized to conform to our genetically determined favorable responses to particular dietary strategies. However, to our knowledge, individualized diets and exercise training for health or sports performance based on one's genetic profile have not yet been developed. For example, Sales and others note that the science of nutrigenomics seeks to explain the interactions between genes and nutrients in order to customize diets according to each individual's genotype, which may help prevent some chronic diseases. Moreover, in a major review of the genomics of elite sporting performance, Wang and others noted that progress has been made, such as identifying single genes with sprint or endurance performance, but they note that only after a lengthy and costly process will the true potential of genetic testing in sport be determined.

Thus, recommendations offered in this text should not be regarded as medical advice. Individuals should consult a physician or another appropriate health professional for advice on taking any dietary supplement for health purposes. Additionally, although information presented in this book may help athletes make informed decisions regarding the use of nutritional strategies as a means to improve sports performance, athletes should confer with an appropriate health professional before using sports supplements or nutritional ergogenics.

Key Concepts

► Epidemiological research helps to identify relationships between nutritional practice and health or sports performance and may be helpful in developing hypotheses for experimental research. However, experimental studies such as randomized controlled trials are needed to establish a cause-effect relationship. Such experimental studies should adhere to appropriate research design protocols.
► Prudent nutritional recommendations for enhancement of health or athletic performance are based on reputable evidence-based research.

Check for Yourself

► Obtain a scientific article from your library that involves the use of a dietary supplement to improve some facet of sports performance. To get a list of studies, you may go to www.pubmed.gov, and type in the name of the supplement and the term "exercise" in the search column, or simply scan some sports medicine journals in your library. Compare the methodology to the recommended criteria presented on page 29.
► As a student scientist, periodically check your local paper for articles that are based on a recent study about nutrition or exercise and health. Find the research study on which the newspaper article is based and compare the findings. Can you find any examples of exaggeration in the newspaper article?

APPLICATION EXERCISES

Rating Your Diet

Several instruments, varying in detail, may help you evaluate your diet based on healthy eating guidelines. Try one or more of the following to see if your diet may need to be improved and, if so, how.

The Academy of Nutrition and Dietetics has developed a short quiz to rate your diet to see if you are eating right. Click on the following link to take the quiz: www.eatright.org/nnm/games/quiz/index.html.

Use the following link to take a more detailed Healthy Eating Quiz, which is designed to assess your current dietary practices and compare them to healthy eating recommendations. Although the quiz was developed in Australia, it is applicable to American diets. http://healthyeatingquiz.com.au.

For increased detail, analyze your diet at the ChooseMyPlate Website. Under SuperTracker and Other Tools, click on Supertracker and then Create a Profile. You can then use Food Tracker to enter your daily food intake for comparison to

recommended goals for improved health. You may also use *Physical Activity Tracker* to assess your daily exercise routine. These programs may be used throughout this course. www.choosemyplate.gov."

Numerous other instruments are available to provide you with an analysis of your diet. Some may be applicable for specific countries. Simply Google the term *Healthy Eating Quiz* to access some of those available.

Review Questions—Multiple Choice

1. Which of the following would not be regarded as unstructured physical activity, sometimes referred to as activities of daily living?
   a. gardening
   b. housework
   c. jogging
   d. leisurely walking
   e. driving the car

2. Which basic principle of exercise training is associated with the concept that cardiovascular-respiratory training will enhance adaptations primarily in the heart, whereas resistance training will enhance adaptations primarily in the skeletal muscles?
   a. overuse
   b. overload
   c. specificity
   d. progression
   e. reversibility

3. Increased levels of both aerobic and musculoskeletal fitness through physical activity may produce numerous health benefits. Which of the following is least likely to occur from a combined aerobic and resistance exercise training program?
   a. prevention of heart disease
   b. building of bone density
   c. prevention of weight gain

   d. prevention of type 1 diabetes
   e. improvement of life expectancy

4. Which of the following is not a recommended dietary guideline associated with the Prudent Healthy Diet?
   a. Maintain a healthy body weight.
   b. Eat a variety of wholesome, natural foods.
   c. Choose a diet with plenty of simple, refined carbohydrates.
   d. Abstain from alcohol if you are pregnant.
   e. Choose a diet rich in plant foods.

5. Poor nutrition may contribute to the development of numerous chronic diseases. For example, obesity, high blood pressure, diabetes, and heart disease are most associated with which of the following nutritional problems?
   a. diets rich in vitamins and minerals
   b. diets rich in dietary fiber
   c. diets rich in fat and Calories
   d. diets rich in complex carbohydrates
   e. diets rich in plant proteins

6. Which group of athletes is most likely to suffer from nutritional inadequacies?
   a. male baseball players
   b. female gymnasts
   c. male tennis players
   d. female basketball players
   e. male football players

7. Based on recent recommendations of the American College of Sports Medicine and the American Heart Association relative to exercise and health benefits for adults, which of the following statements is false?
   a. Moderate-intensity aerobic exercise should be done for a minimum of 30 minutes daily on 5 days each week.
   b. Vigorous-intensity exercise may be done for a minimum of 20 minutes on 3 days each week.
   c. Each daily exercise bout of aerobic exercise may be done continuously or in smaller segments, such as 3 10-minute bouts.
   d. In general, more is better, as exceeding the minimum recommended amounts of exercise may provide additional health benefits.
   e. Resistance exercise, including exercises for the major muscle groups in the body, is recommended at least 5, and preferably 7, days per week.

8. Which of the following statements regarding ergogenic aids is false?
   a. They are designed to enhance sports performance.
   b. Use of any aid that enhances sports performance is illegal and is grounds for disqualification.

c. Although most nutritional ergogenics are safe, some dietary supplements pose significant health risks.

d. Endorsement of a nutritional ergogenic by a professional athlete does not necessarily mean that it is effective as advertised.

e. Some nutritional supplements marketed as ergogenics may contain prohibited drugs.

9. In an experimental study to evaluate the effect of creatine supplementation on muscular power for sport, which of the following would not be considered acceptable for the research methodology to be followed in the conduct of the study?

a. Use well-trained power sport athletes.

b. Use a double-blind protocol.

c. Use a placebo control group.

d. Use a sport-related performance task.

e. Use caffeine as the placebo.

10. A meta-analysis is

a. an ergogenic aid for mathematicians.

b. a technique to evaluate the presence of drug metabolites in athletes.

c. a statistical evaluation of a collection of studies in order to derive a conclusion.

d. an evaluation of the daily metabolic rate.

e. an analytical technique to evaluate biomechanics in athletes.

Answers to multiple choice questions:
1. c; 2. c; 3. d; 4. c; 5. c; 6. b; 7. e; 8. b; 9. e; 10. c

Review Questions—Essay

1. Describe the possible mechanisms whereby exercise may enhance health status, and list at least eight of the potential health benefits of a regular, comprehensive exercise program.

2. Name and describe the various principles of exercise.

3. Define the term *sports nutrition* and explain how appropriate eating strategies may enhance sports performance.

4. List at least five guideline questions one may use to evaluate advertised claims for nutritional supplements.

5. Differentiate between epidemiological research and experimental research, discussing the protocols used in each and the pros and cons of each.

References

Books

American Institute of Cancer Research. 2007. *Food, Nutrition, Physical Activity, and the Prevention of Cancer: A Global Perspective.* Washington, DC: AICR.

Antonio, J., and Stout, J. 2001. *Sports Supplements.* Philadelphia: Lippincott Williams & Wilkins.

Bahrke, M., and Yesalis, C. 2002. *Performance-Enhancing Substances in Sport and Exercise.* Champaign, IL: Human Kinetics.

Benardot, D. 2006. *Advanced Sport Nutrition.* Champaign, IL: Human Kinetics.

Burke, L. 2007. *Practical Sports Nutrition.* Champaign, IL: Human Kinetics.

Clark, N. 2008. *Nancy Clark's Sports Nutrition Guidebook: Eating to Fuel Your Active Lifestyle.* Champaign, IL: Human Kinetics.

Department of Health and Human Services, Office of Disease Prevention and Health Promotion. 2015. *Dietary Guidelines for Americans, 2015.* Washington, DC: U.S. Government Printing Office.

Dunford, M. 2010. *Fundamentals of Sport and Exercise Nutrition.* Champaign, IL: Human Kinetics.

Dunford, M. 2006. *Sports Nutrition: A Practice Manual for Professionals.* Chicago: SCAN and the American Dietetic Association.

Duyff, R. 2006. *The American Dietetic Association's Complete Food and Nutrition Guide.* New York: Wiley.

Epstein, D. 2013. *The Sports Gene: Inside the Science of Extraordinary Athletic Performance.* New York: Penguin Group.

Ivy, J., and Portman, R. 2004. *Nutrient Timing: The Future of Sports Nutrition.* North Bergen, NJ: Basic Health Publications.

Jeukendrup, A., and Gleeson, M. 2010. *Sport Nutrition.* Champaign, IL: Human Kinetics.

Kreider, R. B., et al. (eds.) 2009. *Exercise & Sport Nutrition: Principles, Promises, Science & Recommendations.* Santa Barbara: Fitness Technologies Press.

Manore, M., et al. 2009. *Sport Nutrition for Health and Performance.* Champaign, IL: Human Kinetics.

Maughan, R. J. 2000. *Nutrition in Sport.* Oxford: Blackwell Science.

McArdle, W. D., et al. 2009. *Sports and Exercise Nutrition.* Baltimore: Lippincott Williams & Wilkins.

Mooren, F., and Völker, K. 2005. *Molecular and Cellular Exercise Physiology.* Champaign, IL: Human Kinetics.

National Academy of Sciences. 2006. *Dietary Reference Intakes: The Essential Guide to Nutrient Requirements.* Washington, DC: National Academies Press.

Ross, C., et al. 2014. *Modern Nutrition in Health and Disease.* Philadelphia: Lippincott Williams & Wilkins.

Sears, B. 2014. *The Mediterranean Zone: Unleash the Power of the World's Healthiest Diet for Superior Weight Loss, Health, and Longevity.* New York: Zink Ink, Random House.

Seaver, B., and Newby, P. 2013. *National Geographic Foods for Health.* Washington, DC: National Geographic Society.

United States Anti-Doping Agency. 2005. *Optimal Dietary Intake.* Colorado Springs, CO: USADA.

U.S. Department of Health and Human Services. 2010. *Healthy People 2020.* Washington, DC: U.S. Government Printing Office.

Wardlaw, G., and Hampf, J. 2007. *Perspectives in Nutrition.* New York: McGraw-Hill.

Wolinsky, I., and Driskell, J. 2008. *Sports Nutrition: Energy Metabolism and Exercise.* Boca Raton, FL: CRC Press.

Reviews and Specific Studies

Aguiar, E., et al. 2014. Efficacy of interventions that include diet, aerobic and resistance training components for type 2 diabetes prevention: A systematic review with meta-analysis. *International Journal of Behavior Nutrition and Physical Activity* 11:2. doi: 10.1186/1479-5868-11-2.

Ahmetov, I., and Rogozkin, V. 2009. Genes, athlete status and training—An overview. *Medicine and Sport Science* 54:43–71.

American Cancer Society. 2002. Nutrition and Physical Activity Guidelines Advisory Committee. American Cancer Society guidelines on nutrition and physical activity for cancer prevention: Reducing the risk of cancer with healthy food choices and physical activity. *CA: A Cancer Journal for Clinicians* 52:92–119.

American College of Sports Medicine. 2009. Position of the American Dietetic Association, Dietitians of Canada, and the American College of Sports Medicine: Nutrition and athletic performance. *Medicine & Science in Sports & Exercise* 41:709–31.

American College of Sports Medicine and American Heart Association. 2007. Exercise and acute cardiovascular events: Placing the risks into perspective. *Medicine & Science in Sports & Exercise* 39:886–97.

American Diabetes Association. 2003. Evidence-based nutrition principles and recommendations for the treatment and prevention of diabetes and related complications. *Diabetes Care* 26:S51–61.

American Dietetic Association. 2000. *10 Tips to Healthy Eating.* Chicago: The American Dietetic Association.

American Heart Association Nutrition Committee. 2006. Diet and lifestyle recommendations revision 2006: A scientific statement from the American Heart Association Nutrition Committee. *Circulation* 114:82–96.

Angevaren, M., et al. 2008. Physical activity and enhanced fitness to improve cognitive function in older people without known cognitive impairment. *Cochrane Database of Systematic Reviews* April 16; (2): CD005381.

Beedie, C., et al. 2007. Positive and negative placebo effects resulting from the deceptive administration of an ergogenic aid. *International Journal of Sport Nutrition & Exercise Metabolism* 17:259–69.

Binns, C., et al. 2008. Tea or coffee? A case study on evidence for dietary advice. *Public Health Nutrition* 11:1132–41.

Blair, S., et al. 2004. The evolution of physical activity recommendations: How much is enough? *American Journal of Clinical Nutrition* 79:919S–20S.

Booth, F., and Chakravarthy, M. 2002. Cost and consequences of sedentary living: New battleground for an old enemy. *President's Council on Physical Fitness and Sports Research Digest* 3 (13):1–8.

Booth, F., and Lees, S. 2007. Fundamental questions about genes, inactivity, and chronic diseases. *Physiological Genomics* 28:146–57.

Booth, F., et al. 2012. Lack of exercise is a major cause of chronic diseases. *Comprehensive Physiology* 2:1143–211.

Booth, F. W., and Neufer, P. D. 2006. Exercise genomics and proteomics. In *ACSM's Advanced Exercise Physiology,* ed. C. M. Tipton. Philadelphia: Lippincott Williams & Wilkins.

Bouchard, C., et al. 2000. Genomic scan for maximal oxygen uptake and its response to training in the HERITAGE family study. *Journal of Applied Physiology* 88:551–59.

Bouchard, C. 2001. Physical activity and health: Introduction to the dose-response symposium. *Medicine & Science in Sports & Exercise* 33:S347–50.

Brandt, C., and Pedersen, B. 2010. The role of exercise-induced myokines in muscle homeostasis and the defense against chronic diseases. *Journal of Biomedicine & Biotechnology* 520258.

Burke, L. 1999. Nutrition for sport: Getting the most out of training. *Australian Family Physician* 28:561–7.

Burke, L. 2001. Nutritional practices of male and female endurance cyclists. *Sports Medicine* 31:521–32.

Burke, L., et al. 2013. National Nutritional Programs for the 2012 London Olympic Games: a systematic approach by three different countries. *Nestle Nutrition Institute Workshop Series* 76:103–20.

Carmichael, M. 2007. Stronger, faster, smarter. *Newsweek* 156 (13):38–47.

Center for Science in the Public Interest. 2006. Behind the headlines. *Nutrition Action Health Letter* 33 (3):3–7.

Chowdhury, R., et al. 2014. Association of dietary, circulating, and supplement fatty acids with coronary risk: A systematic review and meta-analysis. *Annals of Internal Medicine* 160:398–406.

Cloud, J. 2010. Why genes aren't destiny. *Time* 175 (2):49–53.

Colberg, S., et al. 2010. Exercise and type 2 diabetes: American College of Sports Medicine and the American Diabetes Association: Joint Position Statement. Exercise and type 2 diabetes. *Medicine & Science in Sports & Exercise* 42:2282–303.

Consumer Reports. 2014. Get-healthy gadgets that really work. *Consumer Reports on Health* 26 (9):8.

Consumer Reports. 2013. More exercise, longer life. *Consumer Reports on Health* 25 (2):3.

Consumers Union. 2007. Simple steps may slow aging. *Consumer Reports on Health* 19 (4):1, 4–5.

Cordain, L., et al. 2005. Origins and evolution of the Western diet: Healthy implications for the 21st century. *American Journal of Clinical Nutrition* 81:341–54.

Couto, M., et al. 2013. Exercise and airway injury in athletes. *Acta Medica Portuguesa* 26:56–60.

Deldicque, L., and Francaux, M. 2008. Functional food for exercise performance: Fact or foe? *Current Opinion in Clinical Nutrition & Metabolic Care* 11:774–81.

Donnelly, J., et al. 2009. American College of Sports Medicine Position Stand. Appropriate physical activity intervention strategies for weight loss and prevention of weight regain for adults. *Medicine & Science in Sports & Exercise* 41:459–71.

Durnin, J.V. 1967. The influence of nutrition. *Canadian Medical Association Journal* 96:715–20.

Ehlert, T., et al. 2013. Epigenetics in sports. *Sports Medicine* 43:93–110.

Environmental Nutrition Editors. 2002. Celebrating 25 years of *Environmental Nutrition:* What we believed then, what we think we know now. *Environmental Nutrition* 25(1):8.

Epstein, D., and Dohrmann, G. 2010. What you don't know might kill you. *Sports Illustrated* 110 (20):54–63.

Epstein, D., and Dohrmann, G. 2013. The strongest stuff. *Sports Illustrated* 118 (4):58–66.

Erdman, K. 2006. Influence of performance level on dietary supplementation in elite

Canadian athletes. Medicine & Science in Sports & Exercise 38:348–56.

Eynon, N., et al. 2013. Genes for elite power and sprint performance: ACTN3 leads the way. *Sports Medicine* 43:803–17.

Fédération Internationale de Football Association (FIFA). 2006. *Nutrition for Football* [pamphlet]. Altstätten, Switzerland: Druck und Medun, AG.

Febbraio, M., and Pedersen, B. 2005. Contraction-induced myokine production and release: Is skeletal muscle an endocrine organ? *Exercise and Sport Sciences Reviews* 33:114–19.

Freeland-Graves, J., et al. 2013. Position of the Academy of Nutrition and Dietetics: Total diet approach to healthy eating. *Journal of the Academy of Nutrition and Dietetics.* 113:307–17.

Friedenreich, C., and Orenstein, M. 2002. Physical activity and cancer prevention: Etiologic evidence and biological mechanisms. *Journal of Nutrition* 132:3456S–64S.

Geiger, P., et al. 2011. Heat shock proteins are important mediators of skeletal muscle insulin sensitivity. *Exercise and Sport Sciences Reviews* 39:34–42.

Gibala, M., et al. 2014. Physiological and health-related adaptations to low-volume interval training: Influences of nutrition and sex. *Sports Medicine* 44: Supplement 2, 127–37.

Gomez-Pinilla, F., and Hillman C. 2013. The influence of exercise on cognitive abilities. *Comprehensive Physiology* 3:403–28.

Greider, K. 2011. The real fountain of youth: Exercise. *AARP Bulletin.* 12(1):10.

Gremeaux, V., et al. 2012. Exercise and longevity. *Maturitas* 73:312–17.

Hall, S. On Beyond 100. *National Geographic.* 223 (5):28–49.

Hart, A., and Dey, P. 2009. Echinacea for prevention of the common cold: An illustrative overview of how information from different systematic reviews is summarised on the internet. *Preventive Medicine* 49:78–82.

Harvey, J., et al. 2013. Prevalence of sedentary behavior in older adults: A systematic review. *International Journal of Environmental Research and Public Health.* 10:6645–61.

Haskell, W., et al. 2007. Physical activity and public health: Updated recommendation for adults from the American College of Sports Medicine and the American Heart Association. *Medicine & Science in Sports & Exercise* 39:1423–34.

Higgins, J., et al. 2013. Sudden cardiac death in young athletes: Preparticipation screening for underlying cardiovascular abnormalities and approaches to prevention. *The Physician and Sportsmedicine* 41(1):81–93.

Hinton, P., et al. 2004. Nutrient intakes and dietary behaviors of male and female collegiate athletes. *International Journal of Sport Nutrition and Exercise Metabolism* 14:389–405.

Hongu, N., et al. 2014. Mobile technologies for promoting health and physical activity *ACSM's Health & Fitness Journal* 18 (4):8–15.

Ioannidis, J. 2005. Contradicted and initially stronger effects in highly cited clinical research. *Journal of the American Medical Association* 294:218–28.

Jacobson, B., et al. 2001. Nutrition practices and knowledge of college varsity athletes: A follow-up. *Journal of Strength and Conditioning Research* 15:63–68.

Jeukendrup, A., and Martin, J. 2001. Improving cycling performance: How should we spend our time and money. *Sports Medicine* 31:559–69.

Jonnalagadda, S., et al. 2000. Assessment of under-reporting of energy intake of elite female gymnasts. *International Journal of Sport Nutrition and Exercise Metabolism* 10:315–25.

Joyner, M., and Coyle, E. 2008. Endurance exercise performance: The physiology of champions. *Journal of Physiology* 586:35–44.

Kearney, J. 1996. Training the Olympic athlete. *Scientific American* 274 (June):52–63.

Kilpatrick, M., et al. 2014. High-intensity interval training. A review of physiological and psychological responses. *ACSM's Health & Fitness Journal* 18 (5):11–16.

Krebs-Smith, S., et al. 2010. Americans do not meet federal dietary recommendations. *Journal of Nutrition* 140:1832–8.

Kristiansen, M., et al. 2005. Dietary supplement use by varsity athletes at a Canadian University. *International Journal of Sport Nutrition and Exercise Metabolism* 15: 195–210.

Kushi, L., et al. 2006. American Cancer Society Guidelines on Nutrition and Physical Activity for cancer prevention: Reducing the risk of cancer with healthy food choices and physical activity. *CA Cancer Journal for Clinicians* 56:254–81.

Landi, F., et al. 2014. Exercise as a remedy for sarcopenia. *Current Opinion in Clinical Nutrition and Metabolic Care.* 17:25–31.

LeLorier, J., et al. 1997. Discrepancies between meta-analyses and subsequent large, randomized, controlled trials. *New England Journal of Medicine* 337:559–61.

Liebman, B. 2007. Staying sharp. *Nutrition Action Health Letter* 34 (5):1, 3–7.

Lloyd-Jones, D., et al. 2010. Defining and setting national goals for cardiovascular health promotion and disease reduction: The American Heart Association's strategic Impact Goal through 2020 and beyond. *Circulation* 121:586–613.

Mann, T., et al. 2014. High responders and low responders: Factors associated with individual variation in response to standardized training. *Sports Medicine* 44:1113–24.

Manore, M. 2004. Nutrition and physical activity: Fueling the active individual. *President's Council on Physical Fitness and Sports Research Digest* 5(1):1–8.

Martínez-Pérez, B., et al. 2013. Mobile health applications for the most prevalent conditions by the World Health Organization: Review and analysis. *Journal of Medical Internet Research* (June 14); 15(6):e120

Maughan, R., et al. 2004. Dietary supplements. *Journal of Sports Sciences* 22:95–113.

Maruti, S., et al. 2008. A prospective study of age-specific physical activity and premenopausal breast cancer. *Journal of the National Cancer Institute* 100:728–37.

McAtee, C. 2013. Fitness, nutrition and the molecular basis of chronic disease. *Biotechnology & Genetic Engineering Reviews* 29:1–23.

McKee, A., et al. 2014. The neuropathology of sport. *Acta Neuropathologica* 127:29–51.

Meadows, M. 2005. Genomics and personalized medicine. *FDA Consumer* 39(6):12–17.

Meeusen, R. 2013. Exercise, nutrition & the brain. *Sports Science Exchange* 26 (112):1–6.

Mooren, F., et al. 2005. Inter- and intracellular signaling. In *Molecular and Cellular Exercise Physiology,* eds. F. Mooren and K. Völker. Champaign, IL: Human Kinetics.

Morrison, L., et al. 2004. Prevalent use of dietary supplements among people who exercise at a commercial gym. *International Journal of Sport Nutrition & Exercise Metabolism* 14:481–92.

National Cancer Institute. 1998. Commentary: Improving Public Understanding: Guidelines for communicating emerging science on nutrition, food safety, and health. *Journal of National Cancer Institute* 90 (3):194–99.

National Institutes of Health. 2006. National Institutes of Health State-of-the-Science conference statement: Multivitamin/

mineral supplements and chronic disease prevention. *Annals of Internal Medicine* 145:364–71.

Navarro, V., and Seeff, L. 2013. Liver injury induced by herbal complementary and alternative medicine. *Clinical Liver Disease* 17:715–35.

Nieman, D. 2000. Is infection risk linked to exercise workload? *Medicine & Science in Sports & Exercise* 32:S406–11.

Nijs, J., et al. 2014. Altered immune response to exercise in patients with chronic fatigue syndrome/myalgic encephalomyelitis: A systematic literature review. *Exercise Immunology Review* 20:94–116.

Nimmo, M., et al. 2013. The effect of physical activity on mediators of inflammation. *Diabetes, Obesity and Metabolism* 15: Supplement 3, 51–60.

Østergård, T., et al. 2007. The effect of exercise, training, and inactivity on insulin sensitivity in diabetics and their relatives: What is new? *Applied Physiology, Nutrition, and Metabolism* 32:541–48.

Peplonska, B., et al. 2008. Adulthood lifetime physical activity and breast cancer. *Epidemiology* 19:226–36.

Rankinen, T., et al. 2010. Advances in exercise, fitness, and performance genomics. *Medicine & Science in Sports & Exercise* 42:835–846.

Rogers, C., et al. 2008. Physical activity and cancer prevention: Pathways and targets for intervention. *Sports Medicine* 38:271–96.

Rosenbloom, C. 2002. Nutrition knowledge of collegiate athletes in a Division I National Collegiate Athletic Association institution. *Journal of the American Dietetic Association* 102:418–20.

Sales, N., et al. 2014. Nutrigenomics: Definitions and advances of this new science. *Journal of Nutrition and Metabolism* 2014:202759. doi: 10.1155/2014/202759. Epub 2014 Mar 25.

Simopoulos, A. 2010. Nutrigenetics/nutrigenomics. *Annual Review Public Health* 21:53–68.

Schwingshackl, L. and Hoffmann, G. 2014. Adherence to Mediterranean diet and risk of cancer: A systematic review and meta-analysis of observational studies. *International Journal of Cancer* 135:1884–97.

Slentz, C., et al. 2007. Modest exercise prevents the progressive disease associated with physical inactivity. *Exercise and Sport Sciences Reviews* 35:18–23.

Smith, J., et al. 2014. The health benefits of muscular fitness for children and adolescents: A systematic review and meta-analysis. *Sports Medicine* May 1. [Epub ahead of print]

Sofi, F., et al. 2010. Effectiveness of the Mediterranean diet: Can it help delay or prevent Alzheimer's disease? *Journal of Alzheimers Disease.* 20:795–801.

Song, M., et al 2013. Meeting the 2008 physical activity guidelines for Americans among U.S. youth. *American Journal of Preventive Medicine* 44:216–22.

Stewart, L., et al. 2007. The influence of exercise training on inflammatory cytokines and C-reactive protein. *Medicine & Science in Sports & Exercise* 39:1714–19.

Tucker, R., et al. 2013. The genetic basis for elite running performance. *British Journal of Sports Medicine* 47:545–49.

Valliant, M., et al. 2012. Nutrition education by a registered dietitian improves dietary intake and nutrition knowledge of a NCAA female volleyball team. *Nutrients* 4:506–16.

Varró, A., and Baczkó, I. 2010. Possible mechanisms of sudden cardiac death in top athletes: A basic cardiac electrophysiological point of view. *Pflugers Archiv* 460:31–40.

Vuori, I. 2001. Health benefits of physical activity with special reference to

interaction with diet. *Public Health Nutrition* 4:517–28.

Wansink, B. 2006. Position of the American Dietetic Association: Food and nutrition misinformation. *Journal of the American Dietetic Association* 106:601–7.

Wang, G., et al. 2013. Genomics of elite sporting performance: What little we know and necessary advances. *Advances in genetics* 84:123–49.

Weissgerber, T., et al. 2006. Exercise in the prevention and treatment of maternal-fetal disease: A review of the literature. *Applied Physiology, Nutrition and Metabolism* 31:661–74.

Wellman, N., et al. 1999. Do we facilitate the scientific process and the development of dietary guidance when findings from single studies are publicized? An American Society for Nutritional Sciences controversy session report. *American Journal of Clinical Nutrition* 70:802–5.

Williams, C. 1998. Diet and sports performance. In *Oxford Textbook of Sports Medicine,* eds. M. Harries et al. Oxford: Oxford University Press.

Williams, M. 2014. Sports nutrition. In *Modern Nutrition in Health and Disease,* eds. A. C. Ross, et al. Baltimore: Williams & Wilkins.

Williams, M., and Branch, J. D. 2000. Ergogenic aids for improved performance. In *Exercise and Sport Science,* eds. W. E. Garrett and D. T. Kirkendall. Philadelphia: Lippincott Williams & Wilkins.

Williams, P. T. 2014. Increased cardiovascular disease mortality associated with excessive exercise in heart attack survivors. *Mayo Clinic Proceedings* 89:1187–94.

Wolfarth, B., et al. 2014. Advances in exercise, fitness, and performance genomics in 2013. *Medicine & Science in Sports & Exercise* 46:851–59.

Healthful Nutrition for Fitness and Sport: The Consumer Athlete

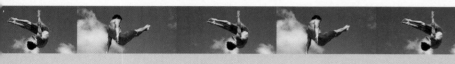

CHAPTER TWO

LEARNING OBJECTIVES

After studying this chapter, you should be able to:

1. List the six major classes of nutrients that are essential for human nutrition and identify specific nutrients within each class.

2. Explain the development of the DRI and explain the meaning of its various components, including the RDA, AI, AMDR, UL, EAR, and EER.

3. Discuss the concept of the balanced diet as applied to the MyPlate food guide.

4. Explain the concept of nutrient density and provide an example.

5. Outline the 12 guidelines for healthy eating and provide several examples for each as to how food might be selected or prepared in order to adhere to these guidelines.

6. Describe the various classes of vegetarians, what foods they may consume in their diets, and the potential health benefits.

7. List the nutrients that must be included on a food label and explain how reading food labels may help one consume a healthier diet.

8. Identify the various types of dietary supplements and discuss, in general, the potential benefits and risks associated with taking dietary supplements.

9. Describe how commercial and home food processing may enhance or impair the quality of food we eat.

10. Differentiate among food intolerance, food allergy, and food poisoning regarding causes and consequences of each.

11. Understand how dietary practices as related to training and competition may help optimize sports performance.

What you eat can have a significant effect on your health. Hippocrates, the Greek physician known as the father of medicine, recognized the value of nutrition and the power of food to enhance health when he declared that you should let food be your medicine and medicine be your food. As noted in chapter 1, the foods we eat contain various nutrients to sustain life by providing energy, promoting growth and development, and regulating metabolic processes. Basically, healthful nutrition is designed to optimize these life-sustaining properties of nutrients and other substances found in food.

Although the Paleolithic (Paleo) diet has been promoted in recent years, Gibbons notes that the hunter/gatherer diet was not all meat and marrow; fossil research suggests humans may have been eating grains and tubers for at least 100,000 years, suggesting Neanderthals were omnivores, not total carnivores. A natural diet of animal and plant foods provided the nutrients necessary to sustain the lives of our hunter/gatherer ancestors. Through trial and error in selecting and consuming various foods, our ancient ancestors were able to obtain the numerous specific nutrients essential to life.

As science evolved, human food consumption patterns gradually changed. For example, food scientists identified specific nutrients, foods rich in such nutrients, and the amounts of each necessary to life. Food hazards, such as bacteria, were also uncovered and methods to combat them were developed. Foods could be packaged, refrigerated, and shipped thousands of miles. Overall, modern developments in the food industry have improved food quality and safety. For example, provision of a wide variety of foods has helped to eradicate most nutrient-deficiency diseases in industrialized nations. However, some current practices in the food industry are a cause for concern. For example, increased availability of a wide variety of high-fat, high-sugar, high-Calorie, low-fiber foods appears to have increased the possibility of the development of various chronic diseases.

The three keys to a healthful diet are *balance, variety,* and *moderation.* In general, a healthful diet is simply one that provides a balanced proportion of foods from different food groups, a variety of foods from within the different food groups, and moderation in the consumption of any food. Such a diet should provide us with the nutrients we need to sustain life and, as noted later, food scientists have determined the amounts of each we need.

In past years, nutrition research focused on the determination of how specific nutrients in our diet, such as saturated fat, affect our health, primarily as related to the development of chronic diseases. Although such research continues to be important, in recent years an increased focus has involved the health effects of the overall diet and whole foods within such diets, and such diets have been promoted by governmental health agencies and professional health organizations. For example, the United States Department of Agriculture, in its *Dietary Guidelines for Americans, 2015,* focuses on food and beverages to promote health. In its recent position statement, authored by Freeland-Graves and Nitzke, the Academy of Nutrition and Dietetics advocated a *total diet* approach to healthy eating, while *Consumer Reports,* in an article entitled "Eat Your Way to Good Health," cited five total diet plans that could promote good health, including the Dietary Approaches to Stop Hypertension (DASH) and Mediterranean diets.

In general, a common core of these dietary recommendations underlies the Prudent Healthy Diet, a dozen guidelines used in this text to promote healthful eating. Although the basic guidelines underlying the Prudent Healthy Diet are rather simple, selecting the appropriate foods in modern society may be somewhat confusing. Fortunately, nutrition labels should provide the knowledgeable consumer with sufficient information to make intelligent choices and select high-quality foods. Food safety is also another consumer concern, and appropriate food selection and preparation practices may help minimize most of the health risks associated with certain foods.

The Prudent Healthy Diet also serves as the basic diet for those interested in optimal physical performance, although it may be modified somewhat for specific types of athletic endeavors, as shall be noted as appropriate throughout the book.

Several smartphone applications (apps) to help you eat a healthier diet are presented in this chapter and throughout the book. Many such apps are available, and new versions continue to be developed.

Essential Nutrients and Recommended Nutrient Intakes

"You are what you eat" is a popular phrase that contains some truth, particularly in its implications for both health and athletic performance. The foods you eat contain a wide variety of nutrients, both essential and nonessential, as well as other substances that may affect your body functions. These nutrients are synthesized by plants from water, carbon dioxide, and various elements in the soil, and they also become concentrated in animals that consume plant foods. Various nutrients may also be added to foods in the manufacturing process. Careful selection of wholesome, natural foods will provide you with the proper amounts of nutrients to optimize energy sources, to build and repair tissues, and to regulate body processes. However, as we shall see in later chapters, poor food selection with an unbalanced intake of some nutrients may contribute to the development of significant health problems and impair sports performance.

What are essential nutrients?

As noted in chapter 1, six classes of nutrients are considered necessary in human nutrition: carbohydrates, fats, proteins, vitamins, minerals, and water. Within most of these general classes (notably protein, vitamins, and minerals) are a number of specific nutrients necessary for life. For example, more than a dozen vitamins are needed for optimal physiological functioning.

In relation to nutrition, the term **essential nutrients** describes nutrients that the body needs but cannot produce at all or cannot produce in adequate quantities. Thus, in general, essential nutrients must be obtained from the food we eat. Essential nutrients also are known as *indispensable nutrients*.

Table 2.1 lists the specific nutrients currently known to be essential or probably essential to humans. Some of the nutrients listed have been shown to be essential for various animals and are theorized to be essential for humans. Curing a nutrient-deficiency disease by a specific nutrient has been the key factor underlying the determination of nutrient essentiality. However, the concept of nutrient essentiality has evolved to include substances that may help prevent the development of chronic diseases. Most recently, the essentiality of choline was included with the B vitamin group, and the list is likely to expand in the future as research reveals health benefits of various plant substances.

Some foods, such as whole wheat bread, may contain all six general classes of nutrients, whereas others, such as table sugar, contain only one nutrient class. However, whole wheat bread cannot be considered a complete food because it does not contain a proper balance of all essential nutrients.

The human body requires substantial amounts of some nutrients, particularly those that may provide energy and support growth and development of the body tissues, namely carbohydrate, fat, protein, water, and several minerals and electrolytes. These nutrients are referred to as **macronutrients** because the daily requirement usually is greater than a few grams. Most nutrients that help to regulate metabolic processes, particularly vitamins and minerals, are needed in much smaller amounts (usually measured in milligrams or micrograms) and are referred to as **micronutrients**,

TABLE 2.1	Nutrients essential or probably essential to humans	
Carbohydrates		
Fiber		
Sugars and starches		
Fats (essential fatty acids)		
Linoleic fatty acid		
Alpha-linolenic fatty acid		
Protein (essential amino acids)		
Histidine	Phenylalanine and tyrosine	
Isoleucine	Threonine	
Leucine	Tryptophan	
Lysine	Valine	
Methionine and cysteine		
Vitamins		
Water soluble	*Fat soluble*	
B_1 (thiamin)	A (retinol)	
B_2 (riboflavin)	D (calciferol)	
Niacin	E (tocopherol)	
B_6 (pyridoxine)	K	
Pantothenic acid		
Folacin		
B_{12} (cyanocobalamin)		
Biotin		
Choline*		
C (ascorbic acid)		
Minerals		
Major	*Trace/Ultratrace*	
Calcium	Boron	Manganese
Chloride	Chromium	Molybdenum
Magnesium	Cobalt	Nickel
Phosphorus	Copper	Selenium
Potassium	Fluorine	Silicon
Sodium	Iodine	Vanadium
Sulfur	Iron	Zinc
Water		

*Technically not classified as a vitamin (see chapter 7).

although as noted in chapter 8, minerals may be classified by other terminology according to the daily requirement.

Essential nutrients are necessary for human life. An inadequate intake may lead to disturbed body metabolism, certain disease states, or death. Conversely, an excess of certain nutrients may also disrupt normal metabolism and may even be lethal (see figure 2.1).

What are nonessential nutrients?

Those nutrients found in food but that also may be formed in the body are known as **nonessential nutrients**, or dispensable nutrients. A good example of a nonessential nutrient is creatine. Although we may obtain creatine from food, the body can also manufacture

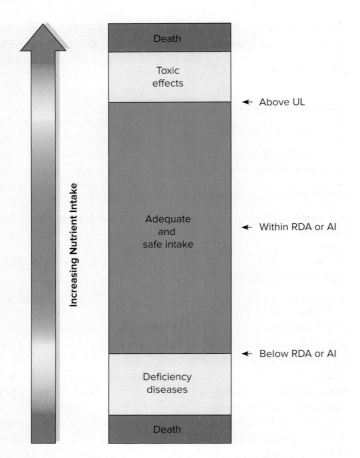

FIGURE 2.1 One model of the possible relationship between nutrient intake and health status. An inadequate intake may lead to nutrient-deficiency diseases, while excessive amounts may cause various toxic reactions. Both deficiencies and excesses may be fatal if carried to extremes. Nutrient intakes within the Recommended Dietary Allowance (RDA) or Adequate Intake (AI) levels are normally adequate and safe, while those below these levels may lead to deficiency diseases. Nutrient intakes above the Tolerable Upper Intake Level (UL) may lead to toxic reactions.

TABLE 2.2	Examples of nonessential nutrients and other substances found in foods
Nonessential nutrients	
Carnitine	
Creatine	
Glycerol	
Drugs	
Caffeine	
Ephedrine	
Phytochemicals	
Phenols	
Plant sterols	
Terpenes	
Extracts	
Bee pollen	
Ginseng	
Yohimbe	
Antinutrients	
Phytates	
Tannins	

creatine from several amino acids when necessary. Thus, we need not consume creatine *per se* but must consume adequate amounts of the amino acids from which creatine is made. As we shall see later, creatine combined with phosphate is a very important nutrient for energy production during very high intensity exercise.

Other than nonessential nutrients, foods contain nonessential substances that may be involved in various metabolic processes in the body. These substances, sometimes referred to as *non-nutrients,* include those found naturally in foods and those added either intentionally or inadvertently during the various phases of food production and preparation. Classes of these substances include phytochemicals, extracts, herbals, food additives, drugs, and even antinutrients (substances that may adversely affect nutrient status). Many of these nonessential nutrients and other substances are marketed as a means to enhance health or sports performance. Table 2.2 provides some examples that will be covered later in this text. Nielsen discusses the issue of whether some nonessential nutrients, particularly various phytochemicals found in plants, may eventually be classified as essential nutrients if they are found to provide significant health benefits.

How are recommended dietary intakes determined?

As noted in table 2.1, humans have an essential requirement for more than 40 specific nutrients. A number of countries, as well as the Food and Agriculture and World Health Organizations (FAO/WHO), have estimated the amount of each nutrient that individuals should consume in their diets. In the United States, the recommended amounts of certain of these nutrients have been established by the Food and Nutrition Board, Institute of Medicine, of the National Academy of Sciences. The first set of recommendations, **Recommended Dietary Allowances (RDA),** was published in 1941 and revised periodically over the years. In general, scientists with considerable knowledge of a specific nutrient met to evaluate the totality of scientific data concerning the need for that nutrient in the diet. Based on their analysis, specific dietary intake recommendations were made.

In the past the Recommended Dietary Allowances were developed to prevent deficiency diseases. For example, the RDA for vitamin C was set to prevent scurvy. However, more recently scientists have discovered that higher amounts of some nutrients may confer some health benefits in specific population groups, such as prevention of birth defects by adequate folic acid intake in the early stages of pregnancy and the prevention of various chronic diseases by sufficient intake of nutrients found in fruits and vegetables. Conversely, scientists have also noted that overconsumption of some nutrients may increase health risks.

Expert scientists still meet to evaluate the available scientific data that serve as the basis for dietary recommendations, but the basis for such recommendations has been expanded beyond the objective of simply preventing deficiency diseases. The current philosophy relative to the development of recommendations for dietary intake focuses on a continuum of nutrient intake. Several points along this continuum for a specific nutrient may be (1) the amount that prevents a nutrient-deficiency disease, (2) the amount that may reduce the risk of a specific health problem or chronic diseases, and (3) the amount that may increase health risks.

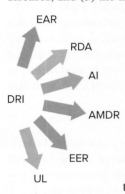

Based on this concept, the Food and Nutrition Board, working with Health Canada, developed new standards for nutrient intake, the **Dietary Reference Intakes (DRI)**, for Americans and Canadians. The most recent DRI were developed for vitamin D and calcium in 2010. The *DRI* is an umbrella term, consisting of various reference intakes, that replaces and expands on the Recommended Dietary Allowances. The DRI consists of the following.

The Recommended Dietary Allowance (RDA)   The RDA represents the average daily dietary intake that is sufficient to meet the nutrient requirement of nearly all (97 percent to 98 percent) healthy individuals in a group. The RDA is to be used as a goal for the individual. You may use the RDA to evaluate your intake of a specific nutrient. The *RDA* term is used throughout this book as the means to express nutritional adequacy.

The Adequate Intake (AI)   The AI is a recommended daily intake level based on observed or experimentally determined approximations of nutrient intake by a group of healthy people. When an RDA cannot be set because extensive scientific data are not available, an AI may be established because the limited data available may provide grounds for a reasonable judgment. You may also use the AI to evaluate your intake of a specific nutrient, but remember that it is not as well established as the RDA. The *AI* term is used throughout this book as appropriate.

The Acceptable Macronutrient Distribution Range (AMDR)   The AMDR is defined as a range of intakes for a particular energy source that is associated with reduced risk of chronic disease while providing adequate intakes of essential nutrients. The AMDR is expressed as a percentage of total energy intake and has both an upper and a lower level. Individuals consuming below or above this range are at more risk for inappropriate intake of essential nutrients and development of chronic diseases. AMDRs have been set for carbohydrate, fat, and protein.

The Tolerable Upper Intake Level (UL)   The UL is the highest level of daily nutrient intake that is likely to pose no risks of adverse health effects to most individuals in the general population. The UL is given to assist in advising individuals what levels of intake may result in adverse effects if habitually exceeded.

The UL is not intended to be a recommended dietary intake; you should consider it as a maximum for your daily intake of a specific nutrient on a long-term basis. The UL is cited throughout this book when data are available.

The Estimated Average Requirement (EAR)   The EAR represents a nutrient intake value that is estimated to meet the requirement of half the healthy individuals in a group. Conversely, half of the individuals consuming the EAR will not meet their nutrient needs. The EAR is used to establish the RDA. Depending on the data available, the RDA is some multiple of the EAR, mathematically calculated to provide adequate amounts to 97 percent to 98 percent of the general population. When sufficient scientific data are not available to calculate an EAR, then an AI may be provided.

The Estimated Energy Requirement (EER)   The EER is an estimate of the amount of energy needed to sustain requirements for daily physical activity. The EER is covered in detail in chapter 3.

Figure 2.1 highlights several of these terms in relation to nutritional deficiency, adequacy, and excess. These terms, and others, are described in detail in the National Academy of Sciences series on Dietary Reference Intakes.

Currently, DRI have been established for all classes of essential nutrients, including carbohydrate, fat, protein and amino acids, vitamins, minerals, and water. The new DRI also, for the first time, provide recommendations for those 70 years and older. Tables containing the current DRI may be found on the inside of the front and back covers of this text. The current DRI will be updated, with inclusion of additional substances such as phytochemicals, as future research data merits.

http://fnic.nal.usda.gov/dietary-guidance/dietary-reference-intakes/dri-tables   You may access the DRI, including RDA, AI, AMDR, and UL for all age groups. Click on Dietary Reference Intakes: Recommended intakes for individuals. *www.nap.edu/catalog/11537.html.*   For those who are interested, the entire Dietary Reference Intakes book may be read online or downloaded free of cost.

An interactive Website has also been developed to provide your personal DRI.

http://fnic.nal.usda.gov/fnic/interactiveDRI/   By entering your age, gender, height, weight, and daily physical activity level, you can use this Website to obtain your personal DRI for vitamins, minerals, and macronutrients. Your body mass index (BMI) and daily caloric needs will also be provided.

The DRI have been developed for several purposes, one of the most important being the assessment of dietary intake and planning diets for individuals and groups. In this context, the DRI for specific nutrients will be provided in the appropriate chapter. However, another term, *Daily Value (DV),* is used with food labels and may be useful in helping you plan your dietary intake. The DV is discussed later in this chapter.

These standards are designed to ensure adequate nutrition for most individuals in the population. They may also be used to plan diets for individuals with special needs. If individuals in a population consume foods in amounts adequate to meet these standards, there will be very little likelihood of nutritional inadequacy or impairment of health. An individual does not necessarily have a deficient diet if the recommendation for a given nutrient is not received daily. The daily recommendation for any nutrient should average over a five- to eight-day period, so one may be deficient in iron consumption one day but compensate for this one-day deficiency during the remainder of the week. Thus, comparison of our nutrient intake to these standards over a sufficient period may be useful in estimating our risk for deficiency. However, one should realize that only a clinical and biochemical evaluation can reveal an individual's nutritional status in regard to any specific nutrient.

Although the RDA are useful because they state approximately how much of all the essential nutrients we need, they are not designed to inform us as to which specific foods we may need to consume to obtain these nutrients. Other dietary guidelines have been developed to help us select foods that will provide us with the RDA for all essential nutrients.

Key Concepts

▶ Balance, variety, and moderation are the three keys to a healthful diet.
▶ The principal purposes of the nutrients we eat are to provide energy, build and repair body tissues, and regulate metabolic processes in the body.
▶ More than 40 specific nutrients are essential to life processes. They may be obtained in the diet through consumption of the six major nutrient classes: carbohydrates, fats, proteins, vitamins, minerals, and water.
▶ The Dietary Reference Intakes (DRI) provide us with a set of standards for our nutritional needs and have been developed with the goal of promoting optimal health.

Check for Yourself

▶ Use the interactive Website listed previously to determine your personal DRI for vitamins, minerals, and macronutrients.

The Balanced Diet and Nutrient Density

One of the major concepts advanced by nutritionists over the years to teach proper nutrition is that of the balanced diet, one containing a variety of foods that provide us with the wide variety of nutrients essential to life. Early food guides, in the 1940s, had little focus on healthful nutrition, mainly because the role of nutrition in chronic disease prevention was not a major research focus. However, as such research developed in the 1950s, food guides began to evolve and promoted healthier eating practices. In accordance with this concept the Academy of Nutrition and Dietetics, in its recent position statement on the total diet approach to healthy eating, indicated the diet should focus on variety, moderation, and proportionality in the context of a healthy lifestyle, today's concept of a balanced diet.

What is a balanced diet?

As noted previously, the human body needs more than 40 different nutrients to function properly. The concept of the balanced diet is that by eating a wide variety of foods in moderation you will obtain all the nutrients you need to support growth and development of all tissues, regulate metabolic processes, and provide adequate energy for proper weight control (see figure 2.2). You should obtain the RDA or AI for all essential nutrients and adequate food energy to achieve a healthy body weight.

Although everyone's diet requires the essential nutrients and adequate energy, the proportions differ at different stages of the life cycle. The infant has needs differing from those of his grandfather, and the pregnant or lactating woman has needs differing from those of her adolescent daughter. There also are differences between the needs of males and females, particularly in regard to the iron content of the diet. Moreover, individual variations in lifestyle may impose different nutrient requirements. A long-distance runner in training for a marathon has some distinct nutritional needs compared to a sedentary colleague. The individual trying to lose weight needs to balance Calorie losses with nutrient adequacy. The diabetic individual needs strict nutritional counseling for a balanced diet. Thus, a number of different conditions may influence nutrient needs and the concept of a balanced diet.

The food supply in the United States is extremely varied, and most individuals who consume a wide variety of foods do receive an adequate supply of nutrients. However, there appears

 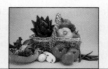 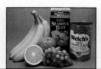

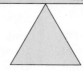

| Milk, yogurt, cheese | Vegetables | Fruits | Bread, cereal, rice, pasta | Meat, poultry, fish, dry beans, eggs, nuts | Fats, oils, sweets |

FIGURE 2.2 The key to sound nutrition is a balanced diet that is high in nutrients and adequate in Calories. For balance, select a wide variety of foods from among and within the food groups in the MyPlate food guide or the Exchange Lists (appendix D).

to be some concern that many Americans are not receiving optimal nutrition because they consume excessive amounts of highly processed foods. This may be true, as improper food processing may lead to depletion of key nutrients and the addition of high-Calorie and low-nutrient ingredients, such as sugar. For example, the World Health Organization recommends consuming no more than 5 percent of daily caloric intake from sugar, but one report indicates the typical American gets 16 percent of his or her total daily Calories from added sugars.

An unbalanced diet is due not to the unavailability of proper foods but rather to our choice of foods. To improve our nutritional habits we need to learn to select our foods more wisely.

What foods should I eat to obtain the nutrients I need?

Although the RDA, AI, and AMDR provide us with information relative to the nutrients we need, they don't guide us in appropriate food selection. Thus, over the years a number of educational approaches have been used to convey the concept of a balanced diet to help individuals select foods that will provide sufficient amounts of all essential nutrients. In essence, foods with similar nutrient content were grouped into categories.

In the past, foods were grouped into the Basic Seven or the Basic Four Food Groups, but today there is some consensus that six general categories of foods may be used to represent the grouping of various nutrients. Although different terminology may be used with various food guides, the six categories are (1) dairy, (2) protein foods, (3) grains, (4) vegetables, (5) fruits, and (6) oils and empty Calories. Table 2.3 lists some of the major nutrients found in each of these six food categories.

One concept of balance focuses on the macronutrients, from which we derive our food energy. Although an RDA for protein had previously been established, the National Academy of Sciences has since released DRI for carbohydrate, fat, and protein as a guide to provide adequate energy but also to help minimize the risk of chronic disease. For adults, the AMDR should be composed of approximately 45–65 percent of carbohydrate, 20–35 percent of fat, and 10–35 percent of protein. Similar percentages are recommended for children, except that younger children need a slightly higher percentage of fat. Carbohydrates are found primarily in the Grains, Vegetable, and Fruit groups but also in beans and sweets listed in other categories. Protein and fats are both found primarily in the Protein foods group and the Dairy group, while solid fats and added sugars are major components of the Oils and Empty Calories group.

Two contemporary food guides using a six-level classification system are MyPlate and the Food Exchange system.

What is the MyPlate food guide?

The most recent government food guide designed to provide sound nutritional advice for daily food selection is MyPlate (figure 2.3), developed by the United States Department of Agriculture (USDA). The USDA originally published guidance on food selection in the 1900s. In the 1940s, the Basic Seven food guide program was published, which was changed to the Four Food Groups program in 1956. The 1979 Hassle-Free daily food guide featured the basic four food groups but also suggested moderate intake of a fifth group consisting of fats, sweets, and alcohol. In 1984, the Food Wheel was published, which featured the five groups that formed the basis of the Food Guide Pyramid, which existed from 1992 to 2011. In addition to the food groups included, it graphically illustrated how variety, moderation, and proportion were important for healthy eating. MyPyramid evolved to include physical activity and the slogan "steps to a healthier you." The most recent food guide is MyPlate, which represents the 2015 Dietary Guidelines for Americans. Health Canada has developed a similar program, Eating Well with Canada's Food Guide, as have many other countries.

www.health.gov/dietaryguidelines/2015.asp Use to access the full documentation of the development of the 2015 Dietary Guidelines for Americans.

MyPlate is a comprehensive program including many features to help promote health through proper nutrition and physical activity. Numerous features of the ChooseMyPlate Website can be found under the menus on the top and bottom of the page on your computer screen, including the following.

- Food groups: detailed information on fruits, vegetables, and the other food groups
- MyPlate Videos: videos on cooking and other topics
- Healthy Eating on a Budget: hints for grocery shopping and cooking
- SuperTracker: analyze your current eating and physical activity habits

TABLE 2.3	Major nutrients found in the five food groups and the oils and empty Calories categories described in the MyPlate food guide				
Dairy group	**Protein foods group**	**Grains group**	**Vegetable group**	**Fruit group**	**Oils and Empty Calories***
Calcium	Protein	B vitamins	Vitamins A, (carotene)	Vitamin A (carotene)	Vitamin A
Protein	B Vitamins	Iron	Vitamin C	Vitamin C	Vitamin D
Riboflavin	Iron	Fiber	Iron	Potassium	Vitamin E
Vitamin A, D	Potassium		Potassium	Fiber	
	Zinc		Fiber		

*Mainly contains Calories. Fat-soluble vitamins found in some foods.

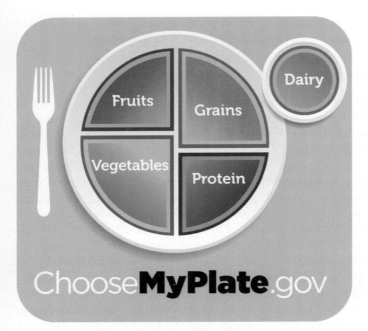

FIGURE 2.3 The food guide for the *2015 Dietary Guidelines for Americans* is MyPlate. The guide consists of five food groups, plus oils and empty Calories, and offers tips on how to balance Calories, which foods to increase in the diet, and which foods to reduce. Physical activity is an important part of the MyPlate program. Personalized diet and physical activity programs are available through the ChooseMyPlate.gov Website.

Source: U.S. Department of Agriculture, U.S. Department of Health and Human Services.

TABLE 2.4 Serving sizes for the MyPlate food guide

MyPlate food group	Serving size
Dairy	1 cup milk or yogurt 1 1/2 ounces natural cheese 2 ounces processed cheese
Protein	1 ounce cooked lean meat, poultry, or fish 1/4 cup cooked dry beans 1 egg 1 tablespoon peanut butter
Grains	1 slice of bread 1 ounce ready-to-eat cereal 1/2 cup cooked cereal, rice, or pasta
Vegetable	1 cup raw, leafy vegetables 1/2 cup other vegetables, cooked or chopped raw 1 cup vegetable juice
Fruit	1 medium apple, banana, or orange 1 cup chopped, cooked, or canned fruit 1 cup fruit juice 1/2 cup dried fruit
Oils and empty Calories (not an official food group)	1 teaspoon

- 10 Tips Nutrition Education Series: tips to help you eat healthier
- Healthy menus and recipes: includes tips from the White House chefs
- Daily food plans: personalize your daily meals
- Audiences: dietary information for preschoolers, pregnant women, dieters, and others
- Educational materials: handouts, videos, and lesson plans for teachers and health professionals
- Additional information: resources to obtain more details on various aspects of healthful nutrition

MyPlate is designed to be simple, yet motivational, with the intent to help individuals make healthier lifestyle choices relative to diet and exercise. Serving sizes for each food group are presented in table 2.4, while key points for healthful eating and physical activity are presented in figure 2.4. One of the key points of MyPlate is to make changes in your diet and physical activity levels gradually, or in small steps one at a time.

The beauty of MyPlate, as the name implies, is its design to individualize dietary recommendations. Here is what you can do when you access the MyPlate Website:

- Click on the text in the *SuperTracker* box, and then click on Create Profile.
- You are asked to input your age, gender, height, weight, and activity level.
- You will be provided with a dietary plan based on your predicted daily caloric expenditure.

- To modify your personalized plan, you can select one or more of five goals (Weight Management; Physical Activity; Calories; Food Groups; Nutrients) to modify your daily caloric recommendation.
- You can sign up for My Coach Center to send you messages in support of achieving your goal(s).
- You can use Food Tracker to record your daily food intake and compare to your goals.
- You can use Physical Activity Tracker to record your daily levels of activity and progress toward your weekly goals.
- You may use Food-a-Pedia to get quick access to nutrition information for over 8,000 foods, and you can choose and compare two foods.
- You can generate a variety of reports, such as your average intake of food groups and Calories for any period of time, your average intake of various nutrients such as calcium, your weekly physical activities compared to Physical Activity Guidelines for Americans, and a graph charting your history of food intake and physical activity.

The MyPlate Website contains an impressive amount of useful information to help individuals. In particular, the SuperTracker program helps you initiate changes to your diet and level of physical activity, all with the goal of enhancing your personal health.

www.ChooseMyPlate.gov Provides an impressive amount of valuable information regarding diet and exercise, personalized for you with the *SuperTracker* program.

GRAINS Make half your grains whole	VEGETABLES Vary your veggies	FRUITS Focus on fruits	DAIRY Get your calcium-rich foods	PROTEIN Go lean with protein
Eat at least 3 oz. of whole-grain cereals, breads, crackers, rice, or pasta every day 1 oz. is about 1 slice of bread, about 1 cup of breakfast cereal, or ½ cup of cooked rice, cereal, or pasta	Eat more dark-green veggies like broccoli, spinach, and other dark leafy greens Eat more orange vegetables like carrots and sweet potatoes Eat more dry beans and peas like pinto beans, kidney beans, and lentils	Eat a variety of fruit Choose fresh, frozen, canned, or dried fruit Go easy on fruit juices	Go low-fat or fat-free when you choose milk, yogurt, and other milk products If you don't or can't consume milk, choose lactose-free products or other calcium sources such as fortified foods and beverages	Choose low-fat or lean meats and poultry Bake it, broil it, or grill it Vary your protein routine — choose more fish, beans, peas, nuts, and seeds

For a 2,000-Calorie diet, you need the amounts below from each food group. To find the amounts that are right for you, go to ChooseMyPlate.gov.

Eat 6 oz. every day	Eat 2½ cups every day	Eat 2 cups every day	Get 3 cups every day; for kids aged 2 to 8, it's 2	Eat 5½ oz. every day

Find your balance between food and physical activity

- Be sure to stay within your daily Calorie needs.
- Be physically active for at least 30 minutes most days of the week.
- About 60 minutes a day of physical activity may be needed to prevent weight gain.
- For sustaining weight loss, at least 60 to 90 minutes a day of physical activity may be required.
- Children and teenagers should be physically active for 60 minutes every day, or most days.

Know the limits on fats, sugars, and salt (sodium)

- Make most of your fat sources from fish, nuts, and vegetable oils.
- Limit solid fats like butter, stick margarine, shortening, and lard, as well as foods that contain these.
- Check the Nutrition Facts label to keep saturated fats, *trans* fats, and sodium low.
- Choose food and beverages low in added sugars. Added sugars contribute Calories with few, if any, nutrients.

FIGURE 2.4 MyPlate provides guidelines for healthful eating and physical activity.
Source: United States Department of Agriculture; ChooseMyPlate.gov.

www.healthcanada.org Click on Food and Nutrition and then Nutrition and Healthy Eating to access *Canada's Food Guide.* *www.choosemyplate.gov/Ambassadors/ambassadorlist. aspx.* College students interested in promoting healthy eating on campus may become ChooseMyPlate ambassadors. Contact the Website for more information.

Contrary to popular belief, you can eat healthy on a budget. Some techniques include the following:

- Choose seasonal fruits and vegetables.
- Capitalize on store specials on fresh chicken, fish, and low-fat meat. Buy quantities, repackage into smaller portions, and freeze for future use.
- Purchase whole-grain cereals, rice, and similar products in bulk at warehouse stores.
- Buy bags of frozen fruits and vegetables, which are cheaper and do not spoil.

The following Website provides some detailed information in accordance with MyPlate goals for eating healthy on a budget.

www.eggnutritioncenter.org/wp-content/uploads/2014/01/ Meeting-MyPlate-Goals-on-a-Budget.pdf

What is the Food Exchange System?

A food guide similar to MyPlate is the **Food Exchange System**, a grouping of foods developed by the American Dietetic Association, American Diabetes Association, and other professional and governmental health organizations. Foods in each of the six exchanges contain similar amounts of Calories, carbohydrate, fat, and protein. As with the MyPlate food guide, eating a wide variety of foods from the various food exchanges will help guarantee that you receive the RDA for essential nutrients. The basic content of the six primary food exchanges is presented in table 2.5. There are several differences between the food groups in MyPlate and the Food Exchange Lists. First, the milk exchange list has three levels based on fat content. Second, cheese is found in the meat and meat substitutes exchange list. Third, the meat and meat substitutes exchange list has four levels based on fat content. Fourth, the starch exchange list includes starchy vegetables. Fifth, nuts and seeds are found in the fat exchange list. A detailed list of common foods in the various exchanges may be found in appendix D. The Food Exchange System was developed for diabetics and for weight control, but it also can be used as the basis for a healthy diet. Because it may be an effective means to judge the caloric content of foods during a weight-management program, it will be covered in greater detail in chapter 11.

TABLE 2.5 Carbohydrate, fat, protein, and Calories in the six Food Exchanges (typical serving sizes)

Food Exchange	Carbohydrate	Fat	Protein	Calories
Milk (1 cup)				
Skim/very low fat	12	0–3	8	90
Low fat	12	5	8	120
Whole	12	8	8	150
Meat and meat substitutes (1 ounce)				
Very lean*	0	0–1	7	35
Lean	0	3	7	55
Medium fat	0	5	7	75
High fat	0	8	7	100
Starch (1 ounce; 1/2 cup)	15	0–1	3	80
Fruit (1 medium; 1/2 cup)	15	0	0	60
Vegetable (1/2 cup)	5	0	2	25
Fat (1 teaspoon)	0	5	0	45

Carbohydrate, fat, and protein in grams (g)
    1 g carbohydrate = 4 Calories
           1 g fat = 9 Calories
      1 g protein = 4 Calories

*Legumes (beans) are meat substitutes but per ounce have more carbohydrate (7~ grams) and less protein (~2 grams) than very lean meat, fish, or poultry.

---

www.uaex.edu/publications/pdf/FSHED-86.pdf Provides examples of foods found in each food group of the Food Exchange System.

What is the key-nutrient concept for obtaining a balanced diet?

As already noted, humans require many diverse nutrients, including 20 amino acids, 13 vitamins, and more than 15 minerals. To plan our daily diet to include all of these nutrients would be mind-boggling, so simplified approaches to diet planning have been developed.

The nutritional composition of foods varies tremendously. If you wish, you may evaluate the nutrient content of your favorite foods on the MyPlate Website, or for a more detailed evaluation go to the USDA Website.

http://ndb.nal.usda.gov/ndb/ Provides a detailed analysis of the nutrient content, over 60 individual nutrients, of various foods.

This site analyzes for nearly 120 nutrients and food components. If you examine a food-composition table, you will quickly see that no two foods are exactly alike in nutrient composition. However, certain foods are similar enough in nutrient content to be grouped accordingly. This fact is the basis for approaching nutrition education by way of the MyPlate food guide and the Food Exchange Lists. In essence, foods are grouped or listed according to approximate caloric content and nutrients in which they are rich.

Eight nutrients are central to human nutrition: protein, thiamin, riboflavin, niacin, vitamins A and C, iron, and calcium (figure 2.5). When found naturally in plant and animal sources, these nutrients are usually accompanied by other essential nutrients. The central

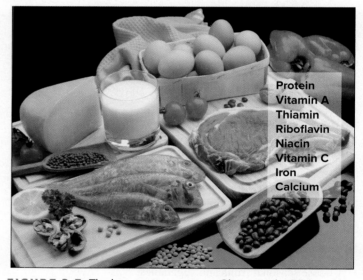

Protein
Vitamin A
Thiamin
Riboflavin
Niacin
Vitamin C
Iron
Calcium

FIGURE 2.5 The key-nutrient concept. Obtaining the RDA or AI for these eight key nutrients from a balanced diet of wholesome, natural foods among the six Food Exchanges will most likely support your daily needs for all other essential nutrients.

theme of the **key-nutrient concept** is simply that if these eight key nutrients are adequate in your diet, you will probably receive an ample supply of *all* nutrients essential to humans. It is important to note that for the key-nutrient concept to work, you must obtain the nutrients from a wide variety of minimally processed whole foods. For example, highly processed foods to which some vitamins have been added will not contain all of the trace elements, such as chromium, that were removed during processing.

TABLE 2.6   Eight key nutrients and significant food sources from plants and animals

Nutrient	RDA or AI		Plant source	Animal source	Food group/ Food Exchange
	M	F			
Protein	58 g	46 g	Dried beans and peas, nuts	Meat, poultry, fish, cheese, milk	Meat, milk
Vitamin A	0.9 mg	0.7 mg	Dark-green leafy vegetables, orange-yellow vegetables, margarine	Butter, fortified milk, liver	Vegetable, fat, meat
Vitamin C	90 mg	75 mg	Citrus fruits, broccoli, potatoes, strawberries, tomatoes, cabbage, dark-green leafy vegetables	Liver	Fruit, vegetable
Thiamin (vitamin B_1)	1.2 mg	1.1 mg	Breads, cereals, pasta, nuts	Pork, ham	Grain (starch), meat
Riboflavin (vitamin B_2)	1.3 mg	1.1 mg	Breads, cereals, pasta	Milk, cheese, liver	Grain (starch), milk
Niacin	16 mg	14 mg	Breads, cereals, pasta, nuts	Meat, fish, poultry	Grain (starch), meat
Iron	8 mg	18 mg	Dried peas and beans, spinach, asparagus, dried fruits	Meat, liver	Meat, grain (starch)
Calcium	1,000 mg	1,000 mg	Turnip greens, okra, broccoli, spinach, kale	Milk, cheese, sardines, salmon	Milk, meat (fish), vegetable

Recommended Dietary Allowance (RDA) or Adequate Intake (AI) for males (M) and females (F) age 19–50.

Table 2.6 presents the eight key nutrients and some significant plant and animal sources. You can see that the food groups and Food Exchanges can be a useful guide to securing these eight key nutrients. Keep in mind, however, that there is some variation in the proportion of the nutrients, not only between the food groups but also within each food group. For example, the grain food group does contain some protein, but it is not as good a source as the meat or milk group. Within the fruit group, oranges are an excellent source of vitamin C, but peaches are not, although peaches are high in vitamin A. If you select a wide range of foods within each group, the nutrient intake should be balanced over time. Table 2.7 presents a daily diet based upon the Food Exchanges. An example of a low-Calorie diet plan based upon the Food Exchanges is presented in chapter 11, together with methods for planning a diet based upon a specific number of Calories.

What is the concept of nutrient density?

As mentioned before, the nutrient content of foods varies considerably, and the differences between food groups are more distinct than the differences between foods in the same group. **Nutrient density** is an important concept relative to the proportions of essential nutrients such as protein, vitamins, and minerals that are found in specific foods. In essence, a food with high nutrient density possesses a significant amount of a specific nutrient or nutrients per serving compared to its caloric content. We refer to these as *quality Calories*.

Let's look at an extreme example between two different food groups. Consider the nutrient differences between 6 ounces of baked yellowfin tuna (meat and meat substitute exchange) and six strips of fried bacon (fat exchange), each containing about 220 Calories. The tuna fish would provide a young adult female with 100 percent of her requirement for two key nutrients (protein and niacin) along with substantial amounts of several other vitamins, and minerals, but very little fat. The bacon would contain less than 25 percent of the protein requirement and about 10 percent of the niacin requirement, with greater amounts of total and saturated fat. Hence, the tuna fish has greater nutrient density and considerably greater nutritional value. Another example is presented in figure 2.6, which compares the nutrient density of milk and sweetened cola.

Let's also look at a comparison of two foods within the same group, the meat and meat substitute exchange. Consider the following nutritional data for 3 ounces of fresh yellowfin tuna and 3 ounces of raw Eastern oysters:

	Calories	Protein	Iron
3 oz. yellowfin tuna	93	22 g	0.65 mg
3 oz. Eastern oysters	43	5 g	3.87 mg

Per serving, both of these seafood choices are relatively low in Calories and good sources of protein and iron. Although the tuna contains more than twice the Calories as oysters per serving, it also contains more than 4 times the amount of protein. And although the tuna is a relatively good source of iron, the oysters contain nearly 6 times as much iron per serving and more than 12 times as much based on Calories. These examples illustrate the

TABLE 2.7   Example of a daily menu based on the Food Exchanges

Exchange	Food selections		Exchange	Food selections
Breakfast			*Dinner*	
Meat	Canadian bacon		Meat substitute	Baked beans
Starch	English muffin, whole wheat		Starch	Rice or pasta
Milk	Skim milk			Bagel
Fruit	Orange juice		Milk	Yogurt
Fat	Low-fat margarine, *trans* fat free		Fruit	Sliced peaches (in yogurt)
			Vegetable	Mixed salad
Lunch			Fat	Low-fat salad dressing
Meat	Tuna fish (water pack)		*Snacks*	
Starch	Whole wheat bread			
Milk	Skim milk		Fruit	Banana
Fruit	Apple			
Vegetable	Lettuce and tomato			
Fat	Low-fat mayonnaise			

Note: This table presents some common examples of foods within each of the six Food Exchanges. As discussed in the text, however, you should select food wisely among exchanges and within each exchange. For example, to avoid excessive amounts of Calories and saturated fats, you should select skim milk, lean meats such as skinless turkey and chicken, water-packed tuna fish, low-fat yogurt, and low-fat, soft tub margarine.

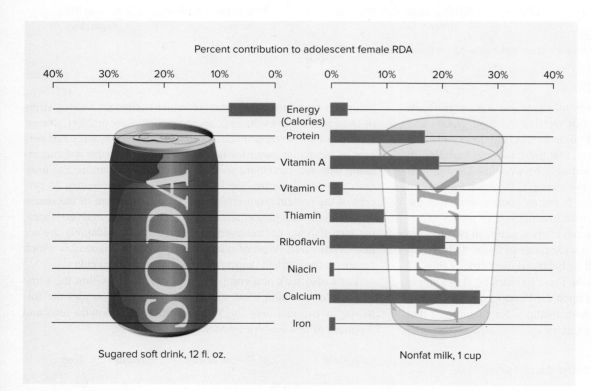

Sugared soft drink, 12 fl. oz.
Nonfat milk, 1 cup

FIGURE 2.6 Comparison of the nutrient density of a sugared soft drink with that of nonfat milk. Both contribute fluid to the diet. However, choosing a glass of nonfat milk makes a significantly greater contribution to nutrient intake in comparison with a sugared soft drink. An easy way to determine nutrient density is to see how many of the nutrient bars in the graph are longer than the energy (Calories) bar. The soft drink has no longer nutrient bars. Nonfat milk has longer nutrient bars for protein, vitamin A, thiamin, riboflavin, and calcium. Including many nutrient-dense foods in your diet aids in meeting nutrient needs.

need to consume a wide variety of foods among food groups and within each food group to satisfy your nutrient needs.

Several groups offer tools to help increase dietary nutrient density. Yale University's Griffin Prevention Research Center developed an Overall Nutritional Quality Index (ONQI), which rates individual foods on a scale from 1 to 100 based on nutrient content and effects on health concerns. For example, broccoli scores 100, while soda scores 1. The ONQI serves as the basis for the NuVal™ Nutritional Scoring System to rate foods in some supermarkets.

www.nuval.com   Go to the NuVal™ site to obtain the ONQI score for a wide variety of foods found in some local supermarkets. You may use your zip code to search for supermarkets that use the NuVal™ scoring system.

Will using the MyPlate food guide or the Food Exchange System guarantee me optimal nutrition?

If you use the key-nutrient and nutrient density concepts, MyPlate or the Food Exchange System may be an effective means to obtain optimal nutrition and help sustain a healthful body weight. However, although the MyPlate food guide and the Food Exchange System represent a significant improvement over previous food guides to help ensure proper nutrition, both have some flaws if foods are not selected carefully. For example, individuals who predominantly choose the high-fat and high-sugar foods from among the food lists may be more susceptible to the development of chronic health problems.

Although the MyPlate figure by itself does not indicate which foods may be healthful or unhealthful, the accompanying guidelines do. For example, the guidelines presented in figure 2.4 provide suggestions for selecting healthier foods and limiting less healthful foods. More detailed information concerning healthful food selection is presented on the MyPlate Website. Some modifications of MyPlate, such as the Harvard Healthy Eating Plate, as well as other healthy eating plans, such as the Mediterranean and DASH diets, focus on healthy food selection. Basically, most healthy eating plans attempt to reduce the consumption of or modify the type of fat, to increase the consumption of whole-grain products, and to increase the consumption of plant products, particularly beans and other legumes, fruits, and vegetables.

www.health.harvard.edu/plate/healthy-eating-plate **The Harvard Medical School modified MyPlate to present more specific recommendations for healthy eating.**

In a recent position statement, the Academy of Nutrition and Dietetics (AND) indicated that the dietary patterns of MyPlate support the total diet approach to healthy eating. The AND position focuses on the message that healthful eating should emphasize the total diet, or overall pattern of food eaten, rather than any one food or meal, and that if consumed in moderation all foods can fit into a healthful diet. In concert with this AND viewpoint, and reflecting healthful recommendations in MyPlate, the major guidelines for healthier food choices are presented in the following section.

▶ The MyPlate food guide and the related Food Exchange System—meat, milk, starch, fruit, vegetable, and fat—should be viewed as an educational approach to help individuals obtain proper nutrition. Foods of similar nutrient value are found in each of the six exchanges.

▶ There are eight key nutrients (protein, vitamin A, thiamin, riboflavin, niacin, vitamin C, calcium, and iron) that, if adequate in the diet and obtained from wholesome foods, should provide an ample supply of all nutrients essential to human nutrition.

▶ Some foods contain a greater proportion of these key essential nutrients than other foods and thus have a greater nutrient density or nutritional value.

Healthful Dietary Guidelines

In past centuries most morbidity and mortality in industrialized nations were caused by nutrient-deficiency diseases and infectious diseases, but advances in nutritional and medical science have almost eliminated most of the adverse health consequences associated with these diseases. Today, most morbidity and mortality are associated with chronic diseases (e.g., coronary heart disease, stroke, cancer, diabetes, osteoporosis, obesity), and most dietary guidelines for healthful nutrition are targeted to prevent these chronic diseases.

Nutrition scientists are using both epidemiological and experimental research in attempts to determine what types of diet, specific foods, and specific nutrients or food constituents may either cause or prevent the development of chronic diseases. Such research, coupled with the application of nutrigenomics, may provide each of us with individualized diets for optimal health.

What is the basis underlying the development of healthful dietary guidelines?

In general, healthful dietary guidelines are based on appropriate research. Over the years, epidemiologists have attempted to determine the relationship between diet and the development of chronic diseases. In early research, the focus was simply on the overall diet and its relationship to disease, such as comparing the typical American diet to the Mediterranean (Greece, Italy, Spain) or Japanese diet. If a significant relationship was found between the diets of two nations, for example, more heart disease among Americans compared to those consuming the Mediterranean diet, scientists then attempted to determine what specific foods, particularly which macronutrients (carbohydrate, fat, and protein) in those foods, may have been related to either an increased or a decreased risk for heart disease. In more recent years, scientists have been investigating the roles of specific nutrients or food constituents and their potential to prevent or deter chronic diseases.

Based on the evaluation of current research findings, nutritional scientists believe that the development of most chronic diseases may be associated with either deficiencies or excesses of various nutrients or food constituents in the diet. Most Americans eat more food than they need and eat less of the food they need more.

In general, many Americans eat too many Calories; consume too much fat, saturated fat, refined sugars and starches, and salt and sodium; and drink too much alcohol. Such dietary practices may predispose them to several chronic diseases, including obesity, heart disease, hypertension, and cancer.

Conversely, possibly because they rely more on highly processed foods, many Americans do not consume a diet rich in whole-grain products, legumes, fruits, and vegetables, foods that are rich in dietary fiber and other healthful nutrients, including phytonutrients. Some may not obtain adequate amounts of calcium and iron. These dietary practices may lead to such chronic diseases as cancer, osteoporosis, and anemia.

To help prevent chronic diseases, over the years numerous governmental and professional health organizations have developed general dietary guidelines for good health. Some of these guidelines have been criticized, possibly because they were not based on the best science. Most of the early research relating diet to disease was epidemiological in nature, which may have led to some erroneous dietary recommendations. However, experimental studies involving randomized controlled trials (RCTs) have predominated in recent years and, as noted by Woolf, rigorous procedures involving evidence-based approaches are currently used to develop dietary guidelines to promote health. Nevertheless, as noted in chapter 1, some dietary recommendations based on research, even using meta-analysis of numerous studies, may be the subject of debate.

Although there is no absolute proof that dietary changes will enhance the health status of every member of the population, scientists involved in the development of healthful dietary guidelines believe that they are *prudent* recommendations for most individuals and are based on the available scientific evidence.

What are the recommended dietary guidelines for reducing the risk of chronic disease?

In chapter 1 we introduced the concept of the Prudent Healthy Diet, a dozen guidelines to healthier eating. These prudent dietary recommendations represent a synthesis of various recent reports from governmental, educational, and professional health organizations, including the following:

- Academy of Nutrition and Dietetics
- American Cancer Society
- American Diabetes Association
- American Heart Association
- American Institute of Cancer Research
- Harvard School of Public Health
- United States Department of Agriculture
- United States Department of Health and Human Services

These recommendations are also in accord with *Dietary Guidelines for Americans, 2015*. The guidelines are not considered to be static and may be modified somewhat as we gain more knowledge through research. In particular, healthful dietary recommendations may be individualized in the future when the full impact of nutrigenomics is realized.

Taken together, these recommendations may be helpful in preventing most chronic diseases, including cardiovascular diseases and cancer. The rationale as to how these dozen healthful dietary recommendations may promote good health is presented in later chapters where appropriate. These guidelines do, however, come with several caveats.

Remember, diet is only one factor that may influence the development of chronic diseases. As noted by the American Heart Association Nutrition Committee, other positive lifestyle behaviors, such as exercise and avoiding tobacco use, are also important.

Most dietary guidelines have been developed for Americans over age 2, but some organizations, such as the American Heart Association, have developed separate dietary guidelines for children. Children and adolescents need energy to support growth and development, so it is important that adequate Calories be provided if dietary fat is restricted. Several of the guidelines presented in this section have special implications for children.

Healthy diets today have an increased focus on whole foods rather than specific nutrients such as carbohydrate, fat, and protein. Although we need nutrients, we eat food. Many of the diets designed to promote health are food based. The foods in healthy diets contain specific nutrients we need but also contain numerous phytonutrients, and evidence suggests the combined effect of nutrients and phytonutrients in the overall diet may be responsible for its beneficial health effects. *Consumer Reports* highlights five diet plans that could be used to promote health, including the Mediterranean and DASH diets, both of which are recommended in the U.S. Dietary Guidelines.

The Mediterranean diet has been the focus of increased research, and results suggest significant health benefits. In a recent detailed review, Gotsis and others cited increasing evidence suggesting that the Mediterranean diet could increase secretion of anti-inflammatory cytokines and antioxidant activity, which could counter diseases associated with chronic inflammation, including metabolic syndrome, atherosclerosis, cancer, diabetes, obesity, pulmonary diseases, and cognition disorders. Relative to the last example, Swaminathan and Jicha indicate the Mediterranean diet may protect against Alzheimer's disease. Gostis and others noted that these health benefits involve the impact of a holistic dietary approach rather than single nutrients. Some contend there is no such thing as an official Mediterranean diet, but it has certain characteristics. The Prudent Healthy Diet is based on these characteristics as well as other guidelines for healthful eating.

The benefits that may accrue from adhering to only a few healthful eating recommendations may be negated if most dietary guidelines are ignored. To maximize your health benefits, adopt as many of these healthful dietary guidelines as possible. In general, your diet should focus on healthy carbohydrates, healthy fats, and healthy protein. Some examples are presented in table 2.8.

The Healthy Prudent Diet

1. *Balance the food you eat with physical activity to maintain or achieve a healthy body weight.* Consume only moderate food portions. Be physically active every day. Preventing obesity helps to reduce the risk of numerous chronic diseases, such as heart disease and cancer. To avoid becoming overweight, you should consume only as many Calories as you expend daily. Relative to diet, an appropriate phrase is "Don't eat more of anything without eating less of something else." Methods of regulating your body weight are presented in detail in chapter 11. An appropriate exercise program and adherence to the concept of nutrient density, which includes a number of the following recommendations, could serve as the basis for a sound weight-control program.

2. *Eat a nutritionally adequate diet consisting of a wide variety of nutrient-rich foods.* Build a healthy base. Eating a wide variety of natural foods from within (and among) the MyPlate food groups or the Food Exchange Lists will assure you of obtaining a balanced and adequate intake of all essential nutrients. Stress foods that are nutrient dense, particularly those that are rich in the key nutrients.

   However, keep the concept of variety in perspective. Research has shown that the more food choices we have, the more likely we are to eat more. Our supermarket society, with more than 50,000 food products in the typical store, provides us with so many choices that it is very easy to overeat and become overweight. Thus, although consuming a wide variety of foods is a good strategy to get the nutrients we need, we must keep in mind the first point, to maintain or achieve a healthy body weight. MyPlate provides guidance for healthy food selection at the supermarket, even on a budget. Simply type *Grocery* in the search box on its Website.

Each year various health professional groups have created lists of so-called superfoods based on various criteria, primarily nutrient-dense foods with potential health benefits. The lists vary somewhat, but the following have been listed as superfoods in recent years.

- Fruit–guava, watermelon, kiwi
- Vegetables–kale, spinach, collard greens, asparagus
- Leanest meat–turkey breast, no skin; chicken breast, no skin
- Beans–soybeans, pinto beans, chickpeas
- Grains–quinoa, amaranth, buckwheat groats, brown rice
- Nuts–walnuts, almonds, pecans
- Seafood–Alaska wild salmon; Pacific sardines
- Oils–olive oil

3. *Choose a plant-rich diet with plenty of fruits and vegetables, whole-grain products, and legumes, foods that are rich in complex carbohydrates, phytonutrients, and fiber* (see figure 2.7). In general, healthy carbohydrates are the ones that nature makes and are found naturally in whole fruits, whole vegetables, and whole grains. About 45–65 percent or more of your daily Calories should come from carbohydrates, about 35–55 percent from complex carbohydrates, and the other 10 percent or less from simple, naturally occurring carbohydrates. To accomplish this, you need to eat more whole-grain breads, cereal, rice, and pasta; more legumes such as beans and peas; more fruits and vegetables; and fewer refined grain products, such as white bread, rice, and pasta.

   Numerous epidemiological studies have shown that diets rich in plant foods confer significant health benefits, which are attributable mainly to the complex mixture of phytonutrients and dietary fibers. The health benefits of phytonutrients and dietary fiber are discussed, respectively, in the next section, on vegetarianism, and in chapter 4.

   Health professionals recommend that 50 percent or more of our total grain intake should be whole grains, but currently Americans consume less than 15 percent. A study

TABLE 2.8	Examples of healthy carbohydrates, healthy fats, and healthy proteins that should constitute the majority of the daily caloric intake		
Healthy carbohydrates	*Healthy* fats	*Healthy* proteins	
Whole wheat or grain	Plant oils	Very lean meat, fish, poultry	
Bread	Olive oil	Egg whites or substitutes	
Cereal	Canola oil	Legumes, beans	
Rice	Unsalted nuts and seeds	Vegetables	
Pasta	Pecans, walnuts, almonds	Meat substitutes	
Fruits	Fish and seafood oil	Unsalted nuts and seeds	
Vegetables	Avocados and olives	Pecans, walnuts, almonds	

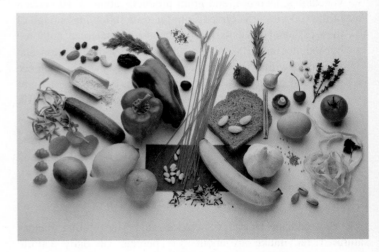

FIGURE 2.7 Include in your diet foods high in plant starch and fiber. Eat more fruits, vegetables, legumes, and whole-grain products.

of more than 13,000 adults by O'Neil and colleagues showed that, on average, Americans consumed less than one serving of whole grains per day and that those who consumed the most whole grains had better diet quality and nutrient intakes. When buying cereal, bread, rice, and other grain products, ensure that they contain whole grains, preferably stating 100 percent whole grain on the food label. Whole-grain products are rich in dietary fiber and phytonutrients as well as several key nutrients. Select whole wheat bread in which you can see the grain; whole-grain cereals such as Cheerios, Wheaties, and Quaker Oatmeal; and whole-grain pasta. Consume 3- to 4- ounce equivalents, or more, of whole-grain products per day, and check food labels that list grams of fiber per serving.

In particular, eat a wide variety of fruits and vegetables, including legumes. Two recent meta-analyses, led by Fulton and Wang, concluded that increased fruit and vegetable consumption is associated with reduced risk of major diseases, particularly cardiovascular diseases, as well as increased longevity. The slogan "Eat your colors every day to stay healthy and fit" refers to the health benefits associated with eating fruits and vegetables of different colors and the associated phytonutrients that appear to protect you against heart disease, strokes, and several forms of cancer. Eat at least five servings of fruits and vegetables daily, but this is a minimum. Another slogan, "Fruits & veggies—more matters," reflects the importance of consuming more than the minimum. Grill vegetables and bake fruits to add flavor. Eat larger portions. For example, 1/2 cup of cooked vegetables is a standard serving size, so a full cup represents two servings.

4. *Choose a diet moderate in total fat but low in saturated and trans fats.* There is no specific requirement for fat in the diet. However, a need exists for essential fatty acids (linoleic and alpha-linolenic fatty acids) and vitamins that are components of fat. Since almost all foods contain some fat, sufficient amounts of the essential fatty acids and related vitamins are found in the average diet. Even on a vegetarian diet of fruits, vegetables, legumes, and grain products, about 5–10 percent of the Calories are derived from fat, thus supplying enough of these essential nutrients. In a recent position statement authored by Vannice and Rasmussen, the Academy of Nutrition and Dietetics, within the context of the rapidly evolving science relative to dietary fats and human health, made some recommendations. In general, the Academy recommended the following, which it considered a prudent approach:

- 20–35 percent of Calories from fat
- Increased consumption of omega-3 polyunsaturated fatty acids
- Limited intake of saturated fats
- Limited intake of *trans* fat.

The American Heart Association suggests limiting dietary saturated fat intake to about 5-6 percent of daily caloric intake.

The following practical suggestions will help you meet the recommended dietary goal.

a. Choose plant oils or other healthy fats. In general, most dietary fat should come from sources of monounsaturated and polyunsaturated fatty acids, such as fish, nuts, seeds, and vegetable oils, particularly olive and canola oils.

b. Eat less meat with a high-fat content. Avoid hot dogs, luncheon meats, sausage, and bacon. Trim off excess fat before cooking. Eat only limited amounts of meat, mostly lean red meat and white meat, such as turkey and chicken, which have less fat. Remove the skin from poultry. Eat no more than 3–6 ounces of animal meat per day.

c. Eat more fish. Many fish, such as sardines, salmon, tuna, and mackerel, are rich in omega-3 fatty acids. White fish, such as flounder, is very low in fat Calories. However, as noted in chapter 5, children and some women should limit intake of or avoid fish that may be polluted with mercury.

d. Eat cholesterol-rich foods, such as eggs, in moderation. Eckel and others, in a recent joint American Heart Association/ American College of Cardiology report, indicated there is little evidence that lowering dietary cholesterol will reduce blood cholesterol. Previously, the American Heart Association recommended consuming 300 milligrams or less of cholesterol per day. Egg yolks are rich in cholesterol, containing about 220–250 milligrams, but research by Rong and others indicated consuming one egg daily has no effect on the risk of heart disease and stroke, two diseases associated with high blood serum cholesterol. A recent study by Katz and others also found that even in individuals with heart disease, consuming two eggs daily had no adverse effect on several cardiovascular disease risk factors. If you want to cut Calories, egg whites have none of the fat of yolks and are excellent sources of high-quality protein.

As this book went to press, the Dietary Guidelines Advisory Committee was considering the removal of restrictions on dietary cholesterol intake, which have been part of United States nutrition guidelines since the early 1960s. Many countries do not limit dietary cholesterol intake in their nutrition guidelines, and such a viewpoint is being considered in the United States.

e. Eat fewer dairy products that are high in fat. Switch from whole milk to low-fat or skim milk. Eat other dairy products made from skim or nonfat milk, such as yogurt and cottage cheese. Most cheeses, except low-fat cottage cheese, are high in fat and Calories, but some fat-free cheeses are now available.

f. Eat less butter, which is high in saturated fats, by substituting soft margarine made from liquid oils that are monounsaturated or polyunsaturated, such as corn oil. Eat butter and margarine sparingly. Some fat-free and other healthier margarines are also available.

g. Avoid foods that contain *trans* fats, considered by many health professionals to be the worst type of fat you can eat. Many food manufacturers have removed *trans* fats from their products, but some remain, particularly some canned and packaged foods. You can check the ingredient list on food labels to look for hydrogenated or partially hydrogenated oils, the source of *trans* fats.

h. Limit your consumption of fast foods. Although fast-food chains generally serve grade A foods, many of their products are high in fat. The average fast-food sandwich contains approximately 50 percent of its Calories in fat. Appendix E lists a number of websites that provide a breakdown of the fat Calories in products served by popular fast-food restaurants. Some fast-food restaurants do serve nutrient-dense foods. Wise choices, such as baked fish, grilled skinless chicken, lean meat, baked potatoes, and salads, can provide healthy nutrition. But avoid high-fat sauces. For example, the mayonnaise serving on a Burger King TENDERGRILL® chicken sandwich adds 90 Calories, or about 10 grams of fat, which accounts for about 20 percent of the total Calories of the sandwich.

i. Use food labels to help you select foods low in total fat, saturated fat, *trans* fat, and fat Calories, all of which are listed on the food label for most products. In the ingredients list, look for the terms presented on the right-hand side of figure 2.8, all of which contain fat.

j. Broil, bake, or microwave your foods. Limit frying. If you must use oil in your cooking or food preparation, try to use monounsaturated oils such as olive, canola, or peanut oil. For other health reasons, as noted later, avoid charring foods when grilling or broiling.

k. If you reduce intake of dietary fats, do not replace them with sugar or refined carbohydrates.

5. *Choose beverages and foods to moderate your intake of added sugars and highly refined carbohydrates.* In general, unhealthy carbohydrates include added sugars and highly refined white flour or rice found in such foods as bread, cereal, pasta, crackers, and pastry. Sugar is somewhat addictive because it may stimulate the same pleasure centers of the brain that respond to drugs, such as cocaine, and thus may be consumed in excess. In some aspects, refined carbohydrates may have effects comparable to sugar in human physiology. In an article entitled "Sugar Love (A Not So Sweet Story)," Cohen indicates that although the World Health Organization recommends consuming no more than 6 teaspoons of sugar per day, one report noted the typical American eats and drinks over 22 teaspoons daily, including sucrose, high-fructose corn syrup, and other sweeteners. On average, Americans get 16 percent of their total Calories from added sugars. The major sources of added sugars in the diet (with the highest sources listed first) are soda, energy and sports drinks, grain-based desserts, sugar-sweetened fruit drinks, dairy-based desserts, and candy.

Excessive intake of added sugar is associated with high blood triglyceride levels and high blood pressure, risk factors for heart disease. Added sugars may also increase the caloric content of food without an increase in nutritional value, so they may contribute to weight gain with an increased risk of obesity and type-2 diabetes.

Thus, moderation in sugar intake is recommended. As noted above, the World Health Organization, along with other health organizations, recommends an intake approximating 5 percent of daily caloric intake. For someone on a 2000-Calorie diet, that amount approximates about 6 teaspoons.

To meet this goal you should reduce your intake of common table sugar and products high in refined sugar, such as nondiet soft drinks, as noted, the largest source of added sugars in the American diet. Sugar is one of the major additives in processed foods, so check the labels. If sugar is listed first, it is the main ingredient. Also look for terms such as *high-fructose corn syrup, dextrose, fructose, malt sugar,* and even *fruit juice concentrate,* which are also primarily refined sugars (figure 2.7). Food labels list the total amount of sugar per serving.

Use naturally occurring sugars to satisfy your sweet tooth. Most fruits have a high sugar content but also contain vitamins, minerals, and fiber.

6. *Choose and prepare foods with less salt and sodium.* Restrict sodium intake to less than 1,500 milligrams daily, which is the equivalent of 3,750 milligrams, or 3.75 grams, of table salt. This lower amount will provide sufficient sodium for normal physiological functioning.

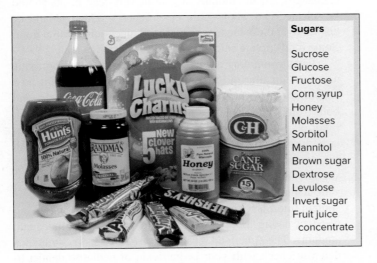

Sugars

Sucrose
Glucose
Fructose
Corn syrup
Honey
Molasses
Sorbitol
Mannitol
Brown sugar
Dextrose
Levulose
Invert sugar
Fruit juice concentrate

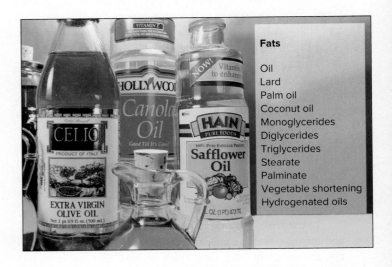

Fats

Oil
Lard
Palm oil
Coconut oil
Monoglycerides
Diglycerides
Triglycerides
Stearate
Palminate
Vegetable shortening
Hydrogenated oils

FIGURE 2.8 Nutritional labeling as a guide to sugar and fat in processed foods. Refined sugar and fats may appear in processed foods in a variety of forms. Check for these terms on nutrition labels.

Sodium is found naturally in a wide variety of foods, so it is not difficult to get an adequate supply. Several key suggestions may help you reduce the sodium content in your diet.

a. Get rid of your salt shaker. One teaspoon of salt is 2,000 mg of sodium; the average well-salted meal contains about 3,000 to 4,000 mg. Put less salt on your food both in your cooking pot and on your table.

b. Reduce the consumption of obviously high-salt foods such as most pretzels and potato chips, pickles, and other such snacks. For a healthy snack, eat some unsalted nuts, such as almonds and walnuts. They are rich in protein and healthy fats.

c. Check food labels for sodium content. Salt is a major additive in many processed foods, and food labels list the sodium content per serving.

d. Eat more fresh fruits and vegetables, which are very low in sodium. Fruits, both fresh and bottled or canned, have less than 8 mg of sodium per serving. Fresh and frozen vegetables may have 35 mg or less but if bottled or canned may contain up to 460 mg.

e. Use fresh herbs, spices that do not contain sodium, or lite salt as seasoning alternatives.

The DASH (Dietary Approaches to Stop Hypertension) diet, discussed in chapter 9, is low sodium.

7. *Maintain protein intake at a moderate yet adequate level, obtaining much of your daily protein from plant sources complemented with smaller amounts of fish, skinless poultry, and lean meats.* The recommended dietary intake is 0.8 gram of protein per kilogram body weight, which averages out to about 50 to 60 grams per day for the average adult male and somewhat less for the average adult female, or about 10 percent of daily Calories, which is about 100 Calories on a 2,000-Calorie diet. The current recommendation of the National Academy of Sciences is to obtain 10–35 percent of daily Calories from protein. Since the average daily American intake of protein is about 100 grams, we appear to be staying within the guidelines. A healthy breakfast is a good way to get a jumpstart on daily protein intake. A bowl of high-protein cereal, such as Post Grape Nuts, in a bowl of milk with a quarter cup of almonds on top, along with an egg, will provide about 30 grams of protein.

Most of the protein Americans eat is found in the meat from various animals. Meat is an excellent source of complete protein and, compared to plant foods, is a better source of dietary iron and other minerals such as zinc and copper. Three to six ounces of lean meat, fish, or poultry, together with two glasses of skim milk, will provide the average individual with the daily RDA for protein, totaling about 40–60 grams of high-quality protein. Combining this animal protein intake with plant foods high in protein, such as whole-grain products, soy-protein meat substitutes, beans and peas, and vegetables, will substantially increase your protein intake and more than meet your needs.

In particular, soy-protein products, such as tofu, tempeh, and miso, as well as commercial products such as soy burgers, are excellent meat substitutes because they are complete proteins. The possible health benefits of soy are highlighted in chapter 6.

For health promotion, the general recommendation is to eat less meat, particularly less red meat. Red meat may contain more fat, particularly saturated fat, and may contain other compounds that may interfere with cholesterol metabolism. Processed red meats may contain cancer-causing compounds and, as noted later in this chapter, cooking meats at high temperatures may produce carcinogenic compounds. In her recent review on reasons medical experts advise us to eat less red meat, Liebman indicates high red-meat intake is associated with various chronic diseases, including heart disease, stroke, diabetes, and colorectal cancer, all contributing to premature death.

Most Americans enjoy eating meat. It is the centerpiece of most meals. However, for health reasons, it is recommended that we change our eating habits. Instead of red meat, we are advised to eat more seafood, such as tuna, salmon, and shrimp, as well as more white poultry meat, such as turkey and chicken breast. If red meat must be part of your diet, some suggestions are to consume small amounts only several times weekly and to choose USDA Extra Lean cuts, such as eye of round steak. When selecting ground beef, look for the lowest percentage of fat, such as 93 percent fat free. Other healthier meat alternatives include buffalo, ostrich, and venison, which are very low in total and saturated fat yet rich in protein and iron. Another healthful recommendation is to use meat as a condiment, such as by adding small amounts to help add flavor to stir-fried vegetable dishes. Using such strategies, you can, so to speak, *have your meat and eat it too.*

8. *Choose a diet adequate in calcium and iron.* Adequate calcium and iron are particularly important for women and children. Skim or low-fat milk and other low-fat dairy products are excellent sources of calcium. For example, one glass of skim milk provides nearly one-third the RDA for calcium. Milk substitutes, such as soy, almond, coconut, and rice milk, may have similar or lower Calories and comparable amounts of calcium but may contain much lower amounts of protein. Certain vegetables, such as broccoli, are also good sources of calcium. Iron is found in good supply in the meat and starch exchanges. Small amounts of lean or very-lean meats should be selected and whole-grain or enriched products should be chosen over those made with bleached, unenriched white flour. Some foods rich in calcium and iron are listed in table 2.9.

Diets containing a wide variety of foods should provide adequate amounts of other minerals. Potassium intake is now considered important enough to appear on food labels, and both fruits and vegetables are good sources of this mineral. Fluoride, a salt of fluorine, is an important nutrient, particularly during childhood when the primary and secondary teeth are developing, for fluoride helps prevent tooth decay by strengthening the tooth enamel. Fluoride may also help prevent dental caries in adults. Most community water systems contain fluoride, either naturally or artificially, so drinking tap water or eating food cooked in water will provide adequate amounts. The American Academy of Pediatrics recommends that you check with your pediatrician or pediatric dentist to find out if any additional fluoride supplements are necessary, or whether your child is already receiving the right amount. In

TABLE 2.9	Foods rich in calcium and iron
Mineral	**Food source**
Calcium	All dairy products: milk, cheese, ice milk, yogurt; egg yolk; dried peas and beans; dark-green leafy vegetables such as beet greens, spinach, and broccoli; cauliflower
Iron	Organ meats such as liver; meat, fish, and poultry; shellfish, especially clams and oysters; dried beans and peas; whole-grain products such as breads and cereals; dark-green leafy vegetables such as spinach and broccoli; dried fruits such as figs, raisins, apricots, and dates

addition, comparable to potassium, vitamin D is considered a very important vitamin. It may be found in dairy products, particularly milk, as well as vitamin D–fortified products; adequate sunshine also promotes vitamin D synthesis in the body.

Although adequate amounts of calcium and iron, as well as other minerals, are important for optimal health, excessive intakes may cause health problems, as noted in chapter 8.

9. *Practice food safety, including proper food preservation and preparation.* Although food safety is a key responsibility of food producers, government agencies, and food distributors, we, the consumers, also play a key role. Using recommended protocols during food preservation and preparation may help prevent food poisoning and decrease the formation of potential risk factors for chronic disease.

To prevent food poisoning, the Academy of Nutrition and Dietetics recommends a four-step protocol.

- Wash to keep bacteria at bay. Wash hands, surfaces, cutting boards, cooking utensils, dishes, and produce.
- Separate. When shopping for, storing, and preparing foods, prevent cross-contamination of harmful bacteria from juices of some foods, such as meat and chicken, to other ready-to-eat foods, such as fruit and vegetables.
- Cook. Use a food thermometer for cooking foods to the safe minimum temperatures to kill harmful bacteria.
- Refrigerate. Refrigerate foods quickly to a temperature of 40°F or below to slow the growth of bacteria that could cause food poisoning.

Some methods of food preparation, such as excessive use of heating techniques, like grilling, baking, and frying, may produce carcinogenic compounds. More detailed information on this topic, as well as food safety in general, is presented later in this chapter.

10. *Consider the benefits and risks of food additives and dietary supplements.* More than 3,000 food additives are used in the United States. Additives are used by food manufacturers to enhance their products for a variety of reasons, such as color, texture, and nutrient density. The use of any additive in food must be tested for safety and approved by the Food and Drug Administration. Eating fresh, natural foods is one of the best approaches to avoiding additives. However, nutrients such as vitamins and minerals are often used as food additives to increase the nutritional quality of a food product, which may benefit some individuals. Food additives are covered in more detail later in this chapter.

As noted in chapters 7 and 8, dietary supplements of most vitamins and minerals are not necessary for individuals consuming a balanced diet. If you adhere to the recommendations listed here, you are not likely to need any supplementation at all, for the consumption of natural, whole, nutrient-dense foods should guarantee adequate vitamin and mineral nutrition. If you feel a supplement is needed, the ingredients should not exceed 100 percent of the daily RDA for any vitamin or mineral. Many one-a-day vitamin-mineral supplements do adhere to this standard.

As noted later in the section on dietary supplements, many health professionals, such as the Academy of Nutrition and Dietetics, may recommend dietary supplements for certain segments of the population. For example, the American Heart Association recommends patients with high triglyceride (blood fats) levels or documented heart disease may be advised to consume omega-3 fatty acids, which in some cases may be obtained from supplements. As shall be noted in chapter 7, some health professionals believe it may be prudent for most individuals to take a daily multivitamin.

Conversely, excess supplementation with some vitamins and minerals, as well as other dietary supplements, may elicit some serious adverse health effects.

The possible health benefits of dietary supplements, as well as possible adverse effects, are discussed in later chapters where appropriate.

11. *If you drink alcoholic beverages, do so in moderation.* The current available scientific evidence does not suggest that light to moderate daily alcohol consumption will cause any health problems to the healthy, nonpregnant adult. A drink is defined as one 12-ounce bottle of beer, one 4-ounce glass of wine, or 1.5 ounces of 80-proof distilled spirits. Current guidelines for moderate alcohol intake recommend no more than two drinks per day for males and one for females. However, even small amounts may pose health problems to some individuals. Alcohol intake is associated with breast cancer. Castor and Castro note that although the suggested acceptable dose for prevention of breast cancer is one drink per day, women at risk may wish to abstain from alcohol consumption, as it is one of the avoidable causes of breast cancer. Certainly, excessive alcohol consumption is one of the most serious health problems in our society today. An expanded discussion is presented in chapter 13.

12. *Enjoy your food. Eat what you like, but balance it within your overall healthful diet.* It is important to note that you can eat whatever you want with the Prudent Healthy Diet. There are no unhealthy foods, only unhealthy diets. The dietary advice regarding moderate intake of certain foods, such as high-fat meats and ice cream, does not mean that they have to be eliminated from the diet, only that their intake should be limited

and balanced with other nutrient-dense foods in the total diet. Portion control is an important concept to limit caloric intake. It is balance, variety, and moderation in the overall diet that is important, not any single food.

Fast foods can fit into a healthy diet. All fast-food restaurants have healthy foods on their menu, but in a review of America's best and worst fast foods, *Consumer Reports* reported that if you want more healthful choices, the top three restaurants are Subway, Jason's Deli, and Panera. Others listed included Baja Fresh Mexican Grill, Au Bon Pain, and Chipotle Mexican Grill.

However, many fast-food restaurants continue to serve what *Consumer Reports* calls *foods to fear,* including monster burgers with over 1,300 Calories, more than half the daily caloric needs for many individuals. Appendix E provides a list of popular fast-food restaurants with Websites to obtain nutritional information on their products.

In this context, it is important to note that although healthful eating may confer numerous health benefits, some may take it to extremes that may become counterproductive. In his book *Health Food Junkies: Overcoming the Obsession with Healthful Eating,* Bratman indicates that taking the quest for a healthful diet to excess can become a disease in its own right.

Enjoy eating; it is one of life's pleasures. To make healthier foods such as chicken, fish, and vegetables taste better, season them with spices. Spices not only enhance the flavor of some foods but also contain various phytonutrients that may have beneficial health effects. Some suggestions include the following:

- Basil: use on tomatoes, green salads, and strawberries
- Oregano: use on ground beef and vegetable casserole
- Turmeric: use on chicken, eggs, and fish
- Cayenne: use on chicken, beef, fish, and vegetables and in pasta sauce
- Nutmeg: use on oatmeal, rice, yogurt, vegetables, and fruit

The Healthy Prudent Diet Your health depends on a variety of factors such as heredity and certain aspects of your environment. Adherence to these 12 simple guidelines will not guarantee you good health; however, the available data indicate that these dietary practices have the potential to keep you healthy or even to improve upon your current health status.

The sooner in life one develops healthy eating habits, the better. Research has shown that preadolescent children can modify their lifestyle by eating healthier foods and engaging in exercise. The National Institute of Health has launched a national public education program entitled *We Can! Ways to Enhance Children's Activity & Nutrition.*

www.nhlbi.nih.gov/health/educational/wecan/ http://www .letsmove.gov/eat-healthy Several national programs entitled We Can! And Let's Move! present ways to enhance children's participation in physical activity and encourage healthy eating.

A Dietary Guidelines Alliance, with representatives from several leading health, government, and food industry organizations, has proposed five simple messages to motivate you into positively changing your eating and physical activity routines:

- Be realistic. Make small changes over time in what you eat and the level of activity you do. Small steps work better than giant leaps.
- Be adventurous. Expand your tastes to enjoy a variety of foods.
- Be flexible. Balance what you eat and the physical activity you do over several days. No need to worry about just one meal or one day.
- Be sensible. Enjoy all foods; just don't overdo it.
- Be active. Start moving, even in small steps. Walk the dog; don't just watch the dog walk.

Although it may not appear obvious, the general nature of the Prudent Healthy Diet is a shift toward vegetarianism, so it may be important to address the nature of this dietary regimen.

Key Concept

▶ Here are 12 recommendations for healthier nutrition.
 1. Maintain or improve a healthy weight.
 2. Consume a wide variety of natural, whole, nutrient-rich foods.
 3. Choose a plant-rich diet with plenty of whole-grain products, legumes, fruits, and vegetables.
 4. Choose a diet moderate in total fat and low in saturated and *trans* fats.
 5. Choose a diet moderate in sugars.
 6. Choose a diet with less salt and sodium.
 7. Eat protein at a moderate yet adequate level.
 8. Choose a diet adequate in calcium and iron.
 9. Practice food safety.
 10. Consider the benefits and risks of food additives and dietary supplements.
 11. Drink alcoholic beverages in moderation, if at all.
 12. Enjoy your food!

Check for Yourself

▶ Think about your dietary habits and then determine how many of the 12 healthful dietary guidelines you follow.

Vegetarianism

Many individuals have been changing their diets to improve their health. One of the major changes has been a shift toward a vegetarian-type diet.

What types of foods does a vegetarian eat?

There are a variety of ways to be a vegetarian. A strict vegetarian, known also as a **vegan**, eats no animal products at all. Most nutrients are obtained from fruits, vegetables, breads, cereals, legumes, nuts, and seeds. **Ovovegetarians** include eggs in their diet, while lactovegetarians include foods in the milk group such as cheese and other dairy products. An **ovolactovegetarian** eats both eggs and milk products. These latter classifications are not strict vegetarians, because eggs and milk products are derived from animals.

Others may call themselves **flexitarians,** because they occasionally may eat meat, fish, or poultry. Flexitarians are also known as **semivegetarians.** Those who eat fish, but not poultry, are known as **pescovegetarians.** In practice, then, vegetarians range on a continuum from those who eat nothing but plant foods to those who eat a typical American diet.

As a general guide, table 2.10 presents the amounts of food that should help meet daily nutrient requirements for the vegan. The amounts may be increased to provide additional Calories. Foods rich in iron, calcium, zinc, and riboflavin should be included daily.

Use of fortified foods or supplements can be helpful in meeting recommendations for individual nutrients. Other classes of vegetarians may obtain nutrients from cow milk, eggs, cheese, yogurt, and in the case of semivegetarians, from fish or poultry.

What are some of the nutritional concerns with a vegetarian diet?

In its position statement, the Academy of Nutrition and Dietetics (AND) noted that planned vegetarian diets are healthful, nutritionally adequate, and provide health benefits in the prevention and treatment of certain diseases. However, if foods are not selected carefully, the vegetarian may suffer nutritional deficiencies involving Calories, vitamins, minerals, and protein.

TABLE 2.10   Daily food guidelines for a vegetarian (vegan) diet

Grains and starchy vegetables

Servings: 8–11 or more daily
Note: Use whole wheat or other whole grains. Products made of oats, rice, rye, corn, and whole wheat are good sources of protein, B vitamins, and iron, more so if they are fortified products. Fortified cereals may provide adequate vitamin B_{12}.
Food examples:

Barley	Macaroni, enriched
Bran flakes	Oatmeal
Bread, whole wheat	Potatoes
Buckwheat pancakes	Rice, brown
Corn	Rye wafers
Corn muffins	Spaghetti, enriched
Farina, cooked	Sweet potatoes
Fortified cereals	Wheat, shredded

Legumes

Servings: 3 or more daily
Note: Good sources of protein, niacin, iron, and Calories.
Food examples:

Great northern beans	Soybeans
Navy beans	Tofu
Red kidney beans	Split peas
Pinto beans	Chickpeas
Lima beans	Lentils

Nuts and seeds

Servings: 3 or more daily
Note: Good sources of Calories, protein, niacin, and iron. May be excellent snack foods.
Food examples:

Almonds	Pecans
Brazil nuts	Walnuts
Cashew nuts	Sesame seeds
Peanuts	Sunflower seeds
Peanut butter	Pumpkin seeds

Fruits

Servings: 4 or more daily
Note: Fruits are generally good sources of vitamins and minerals. At least one fruit should come from the citrus group and one from the high-iron group. Select fruits of different colors.
Food examples:

Regular	*Citrus*	*High iron*
Apples	Oranges	Dried apricots
Bananas	Orange juice	Dried prunes
Grapes	Grapefruit	Dried dates
Peaches	Grapefruit juice	Dried figs
Pears	Lemon juice	Dried peaches
Pineapple		Raisins
		Prune juice

Vegetables

Servings: 4–6 or more daily
Note: Vegetables are good sources of vitamins and minerals. At least one serving should come from the dark-green or deep-yellow vegetables. Select other color vegetables as well.
Food examples:

Regular	*Dark-green or deep-yellow*
Artichokes	Beet greens
Asparagus	Broccoli
Beans, green	Carrots
Cabbage	Collard greens
Cauliflower	Kale
Cucumbers	Lettuce
Eggplant	Spinach
Radishes	Squash
Tomatoes	

Milk products (calcium-rich foods)

Servings: 3 or more daily
Note: Good source of protein and calcium, if fortified.
Food examples:
Non-dairy soy milk
Non-dairy rice milk

Sweets and vegetable oils may be added to increase caloric intake.

Vegetarian diets, particularly vegan diets, should be well-planned, especially for children. The AND states that vegetarian diets are appropriate for all stages of the life cycle. Although vegetarian diets can be adequate for children, the lack of food variety and too much reliance on vegetarian convenience foods, which may not possess the nutritional quality of unprocessed plant foods, can be a concern.

Calories   Caloric deficiency is one of the lesser concerns of a vegetarian diet. However, because plant products are generally low in caloric content, a vegetarian may be on a diet with insufficient Calories for proper body weight maintenance. This may be particularly true for children, who need energy for growth and development, and for the active individual who may be expending more than 1,000 Calories per day through exercise. The solution is to eat greater quantities of the foods that constitute the diet, and to include some of the higher-Calorie foods like nuts, beans, corn, green peas, potatoes, sweet potatoes, avocados, orange juice, raisins, dates, figs, whole wheat bread, and pasta products. These foods may be used in main meals and as snacks.

On the other hand, the low caloric content of vegetarian diets may be a desirable attribute for some, as it may be useful in weight-reduction programs or helpful in maintenance of proper body weight. However, Martins and others have voiced concern that some individuals may adopt a vegetarian dietary style in an attempt to mask their dieting behavior from others. Adopting a vegetarian-type diet may be a very useful strategy for weight control, but may be detrimental if associated with eating disorders, a topic discussed in chapter 10.

Vitamins   Strict vegetarians may incur a vitamin B_{12} deficiency because this vitamin is not found in plant foods. In a recent review, Pawlak and others indicated that vegetarians, especially vegans, have a relatively high rate of vitamin B_{12} deficiency. Vitamin B_{12} is found in many animal products such as meat, eggs, fish, and dairy products, so the addition of these foods to the diet will help prevent a deficiency state. An ovolactovegetarian should have no problem getting the required amounts. A vegan will need a source of B_{12}, such as fortified soy milk, fortified breakfast cereal, or a B_{12} supplement. If not exposed to sunlight, vegans will also need dietary supplements of vitamin D, which is not found in plant foods.

Minerals   Mineral deficiencies of iron, calcium, and zinc may occur. During the digestion process, some plant foods form compounds known as phytates and oxalates that can bind these minerals so that they cannot be absorbed into the body. Avoidance of unleavened bread helps reduce this effect, as does thorough cooking of legumes such as beans. In general, research has revealed that a balanced intake of grains, legumes, and vegetables will not significantly impair mineral absorption. Foods rich in iron, calcium, and zinc should also be included in the vegetarian diet.

Iron-rich plant foods include nuts, beans, split peas, dates, prune juice, raisins, green leafy vegetables, and many iron-enriched grain products. Special attention should be given to dietary practices that promote absorption of iron and zinc from plant foods. For example, consuming foods rich in vitamin C will increase the absorption of dietary iron from plant sources. Semivegetarians may obtain high-quality iron in fish and poultry.

Calcium-rich plant foods include many green vegetables such as broccoli, cabbage, mustard greens, and spinach. Dairy products added to the diet supply very significant amounts of calcium, as do calcium-fortified soy milk or fruit juices. According to the AND the calcium intake of some vegan vegetarians is below recommended levels, while calcium intake in ovolacto vegetarians is similar to that of nonvegetarians. Craig notes that increased bone fracture risk in vegans may be a consequence of low calcium intake.

Zinc-rich plant foods include whole wheat bread, peas, corn, and carrots. Egg yolk and seafood also add substantial zinc to the diet.

Iodine deficiency may occur with strict vegetarian diets, particularly when plant foods grown in iodine-depleted soils are ingested. In such cases, use of iodized salt will prevent iodine deficiency.

Protein   The major concern of the vegetarian is to obtain adequate amounts of the right type of protein, particularly in the case of young children. Generally speaking, obtaining sufficient protein on a vegetarian diet is not difficult. Consuming enough Calories to maintain an optimal body weight will provide adequate amounts of protein.

As will be noted in chapter 6, proteins are classified as either complete or incomplete. A protein is complete if it contains all of the essential amino acids that the human body cannot manufacture. Animal products generally contain complete proteins, whereas plant proteins are incomplete. Certain vegetable products may also provide good sources of protein. Grain products such as wheat, rice, and corn, as well as beans (particularly soybeans), peas, and nuts, have a substantial protein content. However, most vegetable products lack one or more essential amino acids in sufficient quantity. They are incomplete proteins and, eaten individually, are generally not adequate for maintaining proper human nutrition. But, if certain plant foods are eaten together, they may supply all the essential amino acids necessary for human nutrition and may be as good as animal protein (see figure 2.9).

The strict vegetarian must receive nutrients from breads and cereals, nuts and seeds, legumes, fruits, and vegetables. To receive a balanced distribution of the essential amino acids, the vegan must eat plant foods that possess **complementary proteins**. In essence, a vegetable product that is low in a particular amino acid is eaten with a food that is high in that same amino acid. For example, grains and cereals, which are low in lysine, are complemented by legumes, which have adequate amounts of lysine. The low level of methionine in the legumes is offset by its high concentration in the grain products. These types of food combinations are practiced throughout the world. Traditionally, many Hispanic peoples have eaten beans and corn; many Asians, soybeans and rice. Through the proper selection of foods that contain complementary proteins, the vegan can get an adequate intake of the essential amino acids. Because all amino acids must be present for tissue formation, a deficiency of one or two essential amino acids will limit the proper development of protein structures in the body.

In their position statement regarding vegetarian diets, the AND noted that complementary proteins should be consumed over the

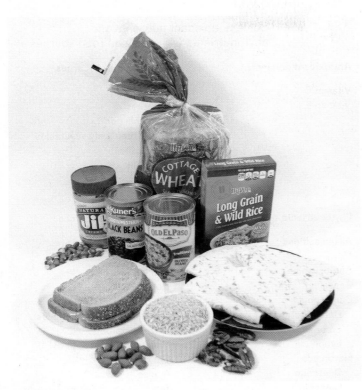

FIGURE 2.9 It is important for the vegetarian to eat protein foods that complement each other (e.g., nuts and bread, rice and beans) so that all the essential amino acids are obtained in the diet.

course of the day, indicating that because endogenous sources of amino acids are available, it is not necessary that complementation of amino acids occur at the same meal.

Table 2.11 provides some examples of food combinations that achieve protein complementarity. Milk is included because it is a common means of enhancing the quality of plant protein for lactovegetarians, but eggs could also be substituted by ovovegetarians where appropriate. The two most common plant foods that vegans combine to achieve protein complementarity are grains and legumes. Grains such as wheat, corn, rice, and oats are combined with legumes such as soybeans, peanuts, navy beans, kidney beans, lima beans, black-eyed peas, and chickpeas.

Is a vegetarian diet more healthful than a nonvegetarian diet?

Numerous epidemiological studies have suggested that a vegetarian diet, when compared to the typical nonvegetarian Western diet, is associated with reduced risk for numerous chronic diseases and health problems, including obesity, hypertension, blood sugar and lipid control, heart disease, stroke, and some types of cancer. As noted previously in The Healthy Prudent Diet, two recent meta-analyses reported increased fruit and vegetable consumption is associated with reduced risk of major diseases, particularly cardiovascular diseases, as well as increased longevity. However, some critics note that many vegetarians, such as Seventh-Day Adventists, may lead lifestyles conducive to longevity, such as being more highly educated, less likely to smoke, exercise more,

and are thinner. Nevertheless, the vegetarian diet is based on nutritional concepts that may reduce health risks, including the following.

Nutrient Density   Vegetarian diets contain substantial amounts of nutrient-dense foods, particularly vegetables. For example, one 54-Calorie cup of cooked broccoli contains the following:

- 4 grams of protein
- 5 grams of dietary fiber
- 10 or more vitamins and minerals
- 170 percent of the Daily Value for vitamin C
- 50 percent of the Daily Value for vitamin A, as carotenoids
- 42 percent of the Daily Value for folate
- 30 percent of the Daily Value for potassium
- 6 percent of the Daily Value for calcium and iron

Low Fat   The total fat and saturated fat content in a vegetarian diet is usually low because the small amounts of fats found in plant foods are generally polyunsaturated. This may account for the finding that vegetarians generally have lower blood triglycerides and cholesterol than meat eaters, and these lower levels may be important to the prevention of coronary heart disease.

High Fiber   Plant foods possess a high content of fiber, which may help reduce levels of serum cholesterol and help in the prevention of heart disease. Diets rich in fiber may also prevent certain disorders in the gastrointestinal tract. Moreover, increased fiber intake may help maintain normal blood glucose levels and a healthy body weight, two factors involved in the prevention of diabetes. More details on the health benefits of fiber are presented in chapter 4.

TABLE 2.11   Combining foods for protein complementarity
Milk and grains
Pasta with milk or cheese
Rice and milk pudding
Cereal with milk
Macaroni and cheese
Cheese sandwich
Cheese on nachos*
Milk and legumes
Creamed bean soups*
Cheese on refried beans*
Grains and legumes
Rice and bean casserole
Wheat bread and baked beans
Corn tortillas and refried beans*
Pea soup and toast
Peanut-butter sandwich

*Low-fat, low-sodium versions should be selected to minimize excessive saturated fat and sodium intake.

Low Calorie If the proper foods are selected, the vegetarian diet supplies more than an adequate amount of nutrients and is rather low in caloric content. Plant foods can be high in nutrient density, providing bulk in the diet without the added Calories of fat. Hence, the vegetarian diet can be an effective dietary regimen for losing excess body weight. However, vegetarians who consume excess amounts of high-Calorie foods, such as cheese, whole milk, and processed vegetarian products containing added sugars and fat, may be at risk for excess weight gain.

High Vitamin and Phytonutrient Content Plant foods are rich in antioxidant vitamins, particularly vitamin C and beta-carotene, a precursor to vitamin A. Polyunsaturated plant oils provide substantial amounts of vitamin E. Selenium, an antioxidant mineral, is found in other plant foods.

Other than nutrients, plants also contain numerous phytonutrients (plant chemicals), such as phenols, plant sterols, and terpenes, which are not considered essential nutrients but may still influence various metabolic processes in the body. Collectively, these antioxidant nutrients and phytonutrients are referred to as **nutraceuticals**, parts of food that may provide a medical or health benefit. As suggested in a position statement by the Academy of Nutrition and Dietetics, foods containing such phytonutrients may be classified as functional foods, a topic covered in the next section of this chapter. Table 2.12 provides a list of some antioxidant nutrients and phytochemicals and their common plant sources.

Although the exact mechanisms whereby antioxidant nutrients and phytonutrients may help prevent chronic diseases such as cancer or heart disease have not been identified, several hypotheses are being studied. Potential health benefits of antioxidants and phytonutrients may be related to one or more of their possible roles in human metabolism:

- Affect enzyme activity
- Detoxify carcinogenic compounds
- Block cell receptors for natural hormones
- Prevent formation of excess oxygen-free radicals
- Alter cell membrane structure and integrity
- Suppress DNA and protein synthesis

Some of these actions may favorably affect health, as in the following two examples. Antioxidants, such as carotenoids, may block the oxidation of certain forms of serum cholesterol, reducing their potential to cause atherosclerosis and possible heart disease. Also, phytochemicals known as phytoestrogens may compete with natural forms of estrogen in the body for estrogen receptors in various tissues, blocking estrogen's natural proliferative activity and possibly suppressing cancer development.

Most nutrition scientists indicate that many of these nutrients and phytonutrients share the same food sources, so the protective

www.ars-grin.gov/duke/plants.html Obtain a list of all the vitamins and other phytonutrients found in your favorite food or plant, like strawberries.

TABLE 2.12 Some antioxidant nutrients and phytonutrients with common food sources

Antioxidant nutrients	Common plant sources
Vitamin C	Citrus fruits
Vitamin E	Potatoes
	Strawberries
	Dark-green leafy vegetables
	Margarine
	Vegetable oils
	Wheat germ
	Whole grains

Phytonutrients	Common plant sources
Allium sulfides	Garlic
	Onions
Anthocyanins	Blueberries
Capsaicin	Hot peppers
Carotenoids	Carrots
Beta-carotene	Dark-green leafy vegetables
Lycopene	Sweet potatoes
Lutein	Tomatoes
Flavonoids	Citrus fruits
Quercetin	Apples
Catechin	Tea
Indoles	Cruciferous vegetables
	Broccoli
	Brussels sprouts
	Cabbage
	Cauliflower
	Kale
Isoflavones	Soybeans
Phytoestrogens	Peanuts
Genistein	Soy milk
Isothiocyanates	Cruciferous vegetables
Sulforaphane	Brocoli
	Brussels sprouts
	Cabbage
	Cauliflower
	Kale
Phenolic acids	Carrots
	Citrus fruits
	Tomatoes
	Whole grains
Polyphenols	Grapes
Resveratrol	Red wines
	Grapes
Saponins	Beans
	Legumes
Terpenes	Cherries
Limonene	Citrus fruits

health effect associated with a plant-rich diet may not be attributed to a single food constituent, but may be due to the collective effect of multiple nutraceuticals. Thus, health professionals currently recommend that consuming natural plant foods, rather than supplements, is the best way to obtain these purported nutraceuticals.

TABLE 2.13 Food colors of various fruits and vegetables

Red	Yellow/orange	Green	Blue/purple	White/brown
Cherries	Apricots	Artichokes	Blackberries	Bananas
Cranberries	Cantaloupe	Avocados	Blueberries	Cauliflower
Raspberries	Corn	Collards	Dried plums	Garlic
Red cabbage	Carrots	Cucumbers	Eggplant	Jicama
Red grapes	Lemons	Green grapes	Plums	Onions
Strawberries	Mangos	Kiwi fruit	Purple cabbage	Pears
Tomatoes	Oranges	Lettuce	Purple grapes	Potatoes
Watermelon	Pineapple	Spinach	Raisins	Turnips

To help ensure that you obtain a wide variety of healthful phytochemicals in your diet, eating foods of many different colors is one strategy recommended by health professionals. *Eat Your Colors* is a popular phrase, and the title of a book highlighting related health benefits. Table 2.13 lists the key colors and some examples of foods found within each color group. In brief, the following highlights one of the main health effects for one food of each color:

> Red—Tomatoes and tomato products contain lycopene, which may help prevent prostate cancer.
> Blue/purple—Blueberries contain anthocyanins, which may help lower blood pressure and risk of heart disease.
> Yellow/orange—Carrots contain carotenoids, which may reduce risk of heart disease.
> Green—Broccoli contains sulforaphane, which may help prevent cancer.
> White/brown—Onions contain allicin, which may help lower cholesterol and risk of heart disease.

In summary, although a vegetarian diet is more healthful than a typical high-fat diet, it should be emphasized that the nonvegetarian who eats a vegetarian-type diet and who carefully selects foods from the meat and milk group, including limited amounts of lean red meat, may attain the same health benefits as the vegetarian.

How can I become a vegetarian?

People become vegetarians for a number of reasons, including weight control, improved health, religion, love for all animals, protecting the environment, and taste preferences. Choosing to adopt a vegetarian diet is up to the individual and may represent a significant change in dietary habits. Anyone desiring to make an abrupt change to a vegetarian diet should do some serious reading on the matter beforehand. Once you have done some reading on vegetarianism, there may be several ways to gradually phase yourself into a vegetarian diet.

- You may become a part-time vegetarian simply by eating less red meat. For example, you may have several meatless meals each day by skipping the ham or sausage at breakfast and having a big salad for lunch. Eventually, you may move toward having several meatless days per week, possibly incorporating meat analogues such as meatless chicken, meatless smoked turkey, or tasty veggie burgers in your meals.
- You may become a semivegetarian, substituting white meat such as chicken and turkey breast, with its generally lower fat content, for red meat. You may become a pescovegetarian, eating fish as your main animal food.
- You may wish to become an ovolactovegetarian, eating eggs and dairy products. These excellent sources of complete protein can be blended with many vegetable products or eaten separately.
- You may use the above methods as forerunners to a strict vegan diet, gradually phasing out animal products altogether as you learn to select and prepare vegetable foods to obtain protein complementarity and adequate intake of essential nutrients.

The following simple suggestions may help you incorporate more fruits, vegetables, and whole grains in your diet.

- Keep 100-percent fruit juices available, but limit those which provide few nutrients, such as apple and white grape juice.
- Buy only bread products that list whole wheat as the first ingredient on the food label.
- Buy large bags of frozen fruits, such as blueberries and raspberries, at club warehouses. Top breakfast cereals with a serving or two.
- Keep a variety of raw fruits handy for snacks, such as bananas, grapes, apples, and oranges.
- Keep a bowl of raw vegetables in the refrigerator, such as small carrots, cut-up celery, broccoli, cauliflower, and radishes, along with a tasty low-Calorie dip, for handy snacks.
- Use frozen vegetables for quick stir-fry meals.
- Add vegetables, such as onions, tomatoes, lettuce, spinach, and peppers, to your sandwiches.
- Load up on fresh vegetables at the supermarket salad bar, putting meal-sized portions in small containers to take for lunch during the week.
- Add cut-up vegetables to canned beans, soups, or omelets to increase their nutrient value.
- Use your microwave to cook sweet potatoes and baked potatoes, and to steam vegetables with a little water.
- Bake fruits for dessert.

The scope of this book does not permit a discussion of food preparation. A number of excellent cookbooks for vegetarian meals are available at local bookstores, the titles of which may be obtained from a local dietitian or local branch of the American Heart Association. These cookbooks provide the vegetarian with a variety of appetizing recipes that not only incorporate complementary proteins with a balance of vitamins and minerals, but also make vegetarianism a gastronomical delight. An excellent example is the *Vegetarian Times Complete Cookbook.*

http://vegetariannutrition.net/ The Academy of Nutrition and Dietetics practice group on vegetarian diets provides useful information on all aspects of vegetarianism, including a step-by-step approach to becoming a vegan, vegetarian diets, recipes, meal planning, and resources to cookbooks and useful Websites.

Will a vegetarian diet affect physical performance potential?

As noted previously, a diet that follows vegetarian principles is considered to be more healthful than the typical American diet today. But will such a diet have any significant impact upon physical performance? In a review of nutritional considerations for vegetarian athletes, Barr and Rideout noted that well-controlled long-term studies assessing the effects of vegetarian diets on athletes have not been conducted. Nevertheless, based on their review and the reviews of Venderley and Campbell and Fuhrman and Ferrari, the following observations can be made.

- Well-planned, appropriately supplemented vegetarian diets appear to effectively support athletic performance. Including fortified foods, such as soy milk and whole-grain cereals, may help provide adequate amounts of some vitamins and minerals that may be low in vegetarian diets.
- Plant and animal protein sources appear to provide equivalent support to athletic training and performance provided protein intakes are adequate to meet needs for total nitrogen and the essential amino acids.
- Vegetarian athletes (particularly women) are at increased risk for non-anemic iron deficiency, which may limit endurance performance.
- Vegetarian diets are low in creatine, and thus vegetarian athletes may have lower muscle creatine concentrations than meat-eating athletes. Lower creatine levels may impair very high intensity exercise. Details are presented in chapter 6.
- Vegetarian diets may be high in healthful carbohydrates and be effective for weight control, which could be to the advantage of some athletes, particularly endurance runners. However, if used improperly as a strategy for weight control, vegetarian diets could lead to eating disorders and impaired performance and health, a topic discussed in chapter 10.

As shall be noted later in this text, the amino acid leucine appears to be critical to promote muscle protein synthesis, and increased muscle mass, when consumed during resistance training programs. Whey protein, from milk, contains substantial amounts of leucine, while soy protein contains slightly lower amounts. In one study, Tang and others found that although both whey and soy protein supplementation increased muscle protein synthesis, whey protein was about 30 percent more effective, possibly due to its slightly greater leucine content. Such a finding may be of interest to individuals attempting to maximize muscle mass for sport competition.

Some world-class athletes have been vegetarians, and on occasion their diets have been cited as a reason for their success. On the other hand, there are a far greater number of world-class athletes who eat a balanced diet including animal products. Both types of diet may supply the nutrients necessary for the physically active individual if foods are selected properly.

However, as noted previously, if you want to shift toward a vegetarian diet, you would need to do some careful reading beforehand and then initiate the process gradually. During the process, you should listen to your body—a common phrase among many athletes today. If you are active, how do you feel during your workouts? Do you have more or less stamina? Are you gaining or losing weight? Is your physical performance getting better or worse? The answers to these questions, together with other body reactions, may offer you some feedback as to whether the dietary change is beneficial.

Remember, there is nothing magical about a vegetarian diet that will increase your physical performance capacity. It can be a healthful way to obtain the nutrients your physically active body needs, but so too is a well-balanced diet containing animal products.

Key Concepts

▶ Vegetarians must be careful in selecting foods in order to obtain a balanced mixture of amino acids and adequate amounts of B_{12}, calcium, iron, and zinc.
▶ Vegetarian diets are based on healthful nutritional concepts that may help reduce chronic disease, particularly cardiovascular disease, but nonvegetarian diets may confer similar health and sport performance benefits if limited animal foods are carefully chosen.

Check for Yourself

▶ If you are not a vegetarian, eat a vegetarian diet for a day or two to see if it may fit into your lifestyle.

Consumer Nutrition— Food Labels and Health Claims

Guidelines for a healthful diet will not be effective unless people change their behavior to buy and eat healthier foods. A model often used to explain the development of a set of behaviors involves a sequence of (1) acquisition of knowledge, (2) formation of an attitude or set of values, and (3) development of a particular behavior. In this sequence, knowledge is the first step that may enhance the development of proper health behaviors. Knowing how to interpret food labels may guide you in developing a nutritious, safe, and healthful diet.

What nutrition information do food labels provide?

Food manufacturers view labels as a device for persuading you to buy their product instead of a competitor's product. Just walk down the cereal aisle next time you visit the supermarket and notice the bewildering number of choices. As manufactured food products multiplied over the years, and as competition for your food dollar intensified, food companies began to manipulate their labels to enhance sales. Unfortunately, many of these practices were deceptive, and the consumer had a difficult time determining the nutritional quality of many processed foods. Thus, Congress passed a law designed to establish a set of standards to help Americans base their food choices on sound nutritional information.

This set of standards resulted in **nutritional labeling**, whereby major nutrients found in a food product must be listed on the label. It is not the total solution to the problem of poor food selection existing among many Americans, but combined with an educational program to increase nutritional awareness, it may effectively improve the nutritional health of our nation.

Initial food labeling legislation was passed in 1973, but it contained numerous flaws. Because of pressure from a variety of consumer interest groups, a major overhaul of the nutritional labeling program was signed into law as the Nutrition Labeling and Education Act in 1990, and it was in full effect in 1994. Under this law, nutrition labeling is mandatory for almost all foods regulated by the Food and Drug Administration (FDA). However, there are some exceptions. Food produced by very small businesses; food served in restaurants, hospital cafeterias, and airplanes; ready-to-eat food prepared primarily on site; and several other categories are exempt from these regulations. Other modifications may be used for young children. Additionally, providing nutrition information is currently voluntary for many raw foods such as fresh fruits, vegetables, meat, and fish, but may become mandatory in the future.

The food label illustrated in figure 2.10 is called *Nutrition Facts,* and it is designed to provide information on the nutrients that are of major concern for consumers. This food label was in effect when this book went to press. However, under the Food Labeling Modernization Act the FDA has proposed many changes to the food label, which may be in effect in the next few years. Currently, food labels must contain the following information:

List of ingredients
    Ingredients will be listed in descending order by weight.
Serving size
    Serving size has been standardized.
Servings per container
Amount per serving of the following:
    Total Calories
    Calories from fat
Total fat
    Saturated fat
    Trans fat
Cholesterol
Sodium
Total carbohydrate
    Dietary fiber
    Sugars

Protein
Vitamin A
Vitamin C
Calcium
Iron

    The following are optional:

Calories from saturated fat	Phosphorus
Polyunsaturated fat	Magnesium
Monounsaturated fat	Zinc
Potassium	Selenium
Soluble fiber	Copper
Insoluble fiber	Manganese
Sugar alcohols	Molybdenum
Other carbohydrates	Iodine
Vitamins D, E, K	Potassium
All B vitamins	Chloride

How can I use this information to select a healthier diet?

The **Daily Value (DV)**, which is based on dietary standards discussed earlier in this chapter, represents how much of a specific nutrient you should obtain in your daily diet. DVs have been established for macronutrients and micronutrients that may affect our health. In essence, a food label indicates how much of a given nutrient is present in that product, and for some nutrients, what percentage of the DV is provided by one serving.

The DVs cover the macronutrients that are sources of energy, consisting of carbohydrate (including fiber), fat, and protein. The DVs for the energy-producing nutrients are based on the number of Calories consumed daily. On the food label, the percent of the DV that a single serving of a food contains is based on a 2,000-Calorie diet, which has been selected because it is believed to have the greatest public health benefit for the nation. However, the DV may be higher or lower depending on your Calorie needs. Values for

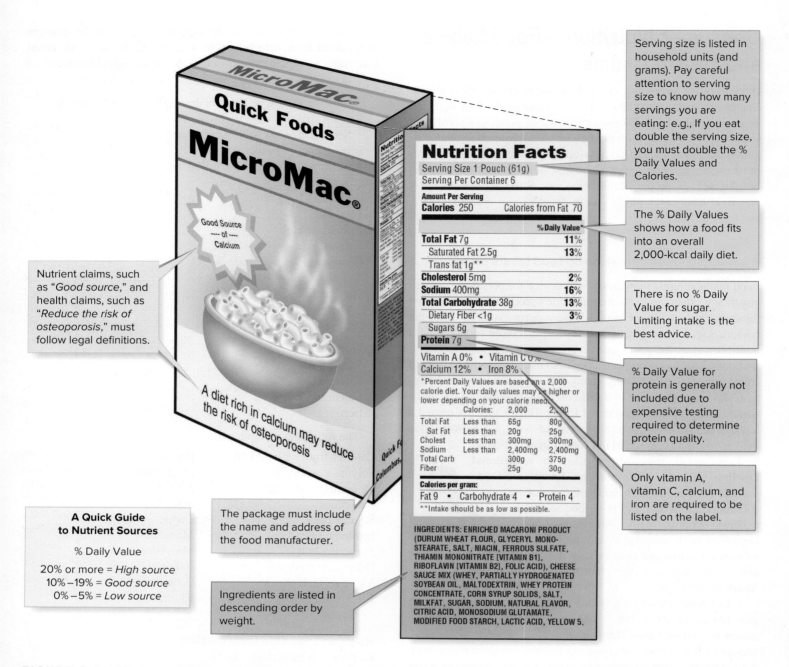

Nutrient claims, such as *"Good source,"* and **health claims,** such as *"Reduce the risk of osteoporosis,"* must follow legal definitions.

Serving size is listed in household units (and grams). Pay careful attention to serving size to know how many servings you are eating: e.g., If you eat double the serving size, you must double the % Daily Values and Calories.

The **% Daily Values** shows how a food fits into an overall 2,000-kcal daily diet.

There is **no % Daily Value for sugar.** Limiting intake is the best advice.

% Daily Value for protein is generally not included due to expensive testing required to determine protein quality.

Only **vitamin A, vitamin C, calcium, and iron** are required to be listed on the label.

A Quick Guide to Nutrient Sources

% Daily Value

20% or more = *High source*
10%–19% = *Good source*
0%–5% = *Low source*

The package must include the name and address of the **food manufacturer.**

Ingredients are listed in descending order by weight.

Nutrition Facts

Serving Size 1 Pouch (61g)
Serving Per Container 6

Amount Per Serving

Calories 250   Calories from Fat 70

	% Daily Value*
Total Fat 7g	**11%**
Saturated Fat 2.5g	**13%**
Trans fat 1g**	
Cholesterol 5mg	**2%**
Sodium 400mg	**16%**
Total Carbohydrate 38g	**13%**
Dietary Fiber <1g	**3%**
Sugars 6g	
Protein 7g	

Vitamin A 0% • Vitamin C 0%
Calcium 12% • Iron 8%

*Percent Daily Values are based on a 2,000 calorie diet. Your daily values may be higher or lower depending on your calorie needs.

		Calories:	2,000	2,500
Total Fat	Less than		65g	80g
Sat Fat	Less than		20g	25g
Cholest	Less than		300mg	300mg
Sodium	Less than		2,400mg	2,400mg
Total Carb			300g	375g
Fiber			25g	30g

Calories per gram:
Fat 9 • Carbohydrate 4 • Protein 4

**Intake should be as low as possible.

INGREDIENTS: ENRICHED MACARONI PRODUCT (DURUM WHEAT FLOUR, GLYCERYL MONO-STEARATE, SALT, NIACIN, FERROUS SULFATE, THIAMIN MONONITRATE [VITAMIN B1], RIBOFLAVIN [VITAMIN B2], FOLIC ACID), CHEESE SAUCE MIX (WHEY, PARTIALLY HYDROGENATED SOYBEAN OIL, MALTODEXTRIN, WHEY PROTEIN CONCENTRATE, CORN SYRUP SOLIDS, SALT, MILKFAT, SUGAR, SODIUM, NATURAL FLAVOR, CITRIC ACID, MONOSODIUM GLUTAMATE, MODIFIED FOOD STARCH, LACTIC ACID, YELLOW 5.

FIGURE 2.10 The Nutrition Facts panel on a current food label. This nutrition information is required on virtually all processed food products. The % Daily Value listed on the label is the percentage of the generally accepted amount of a nutrient needed daily that is present in one serving of the product. See text for additional discussion.

some of the macronutrients are also provided for a 2,500-Calorie diet on the food label.

The DVs are based on certain minimum and maximum allowances, including the following for a 2,000-Calorie diet:

Total fat: Maximum of 30 percent of Calories, or less than 65 grams.
Saturated fat: Maximum of 10 percent of Calories, or less than 20 grams.
Carbohydrate: Minimum of 60 percent of Calories, or more than 300 grams.

Protein: Based on 10 percent of Calories. Applicable only to adults and children over age 4; 50 grams for a 2,000-Calorie diet.
Fiber: Based on 12.5 grams of fiber per 1,000 Calories.
Cholesterol: Less than 300 milligrams.
Sodium: Less than 2,400 milligrams.

The DVs for vitamins and minerals, based on previously established RDA, are presented in table 2.14. The list includes those whose listing is mandatory and some selected others. Although the RDA for several nutrients has changed with recent DRI updates, the DVs are still based on 1968 standards of the RDA.

TABLE 2.14 DVs for protein, dietary fiber, and some vitamins and minerals on food labels

Mandatory listing	
Protein	56 grams
Vitamin A	5,000 IU; 1 milligram
Vitamin C	60 milligrams
Calcium	1,000 milligrams
Iron	18 milligrams
Dietary fiber	25 grams

Optional listing	
Thiamin	1.5 milligrams
Riboflavin	1.7 milligrams
Niacin	20 milligrams
Vitamin D	400 IU
Vitamin E	30 IU
Vitamin B_6	2 milligrams
Folic acid	400 micrograms
Vitamin B_{12}	6 micrograms
Zinc	15 milligrams
Copper	2 milligrams
Magnesium	400 milligrams
Potassium	3,500 milligrams

Some important points to consider in reading a food label are as follows:

1. The DV for a nutrient represents the percentage contribution one serving of the food makes to the daily diet for that nutrient based on current recommendations for healthful diets. A lower DV is desirable for total fat, saturated fat, cholesterol, and sodium; a DV of 5 percent or less is a good indicator. There is no DV for *trans* fat; only the number of grams is listed, and intake should be as low as possible, preferably 0 grams. A higher DV is desirable for dietary fiber, iron, calcium, vitamins A and C, and other vitamins and minerals that may be listed, with 10 percent or more representing a good source.

2. To calculate the percentage of fat Calories in one serving, divide the value for Calories from fat by the total Calories and multiply by 100. For example, if one serving contains 70 Calories from fat and the total number of Calories is 120, the food consists of 58 percent fat Calories (70/120 × 100). It should be noted that this percentage is not the same as the DV percentage for fat, which is based on your total daily diet, not an individual serving of the food product.

3. Related to carbohydrates, sugars include both natural and added sugars. There is no DV for sugar, but the fewer grams, the better. Dietary fiber is the total amount of fiber per serving. The term *Other Carbohydrates* may be listed, which represents carbohydrates other than sugar and dietary fiber.

4. Be aware of serving size tricks. A serving size for a cola drink may be 8 ounces (100 Calories), so a 20-ounce bottle of soda is 2.5 servings (250 Calories). However, most people drink it all at one time, thinking it is only one serving and may consume more than twice the Calories as expected. Recommended changes are to provide nutrition information for a single serving as well as for the entire package; so for a 20-ounce bottle of soda, you will get the nutrition breakdown for 8 ounces as well as for the entire 20 ounces.

5. Check the ingredient list. Although in small type, it may provide very useful information. As noted, the list of ingredients is in order by weight. As noted, *trans* fat may be listed as 0 on the label, but the product contains some *trans* fat if hydrogenated or partially hydrogenated oils are in the ingredient list. Some additional information is presented later in this chapter in the discussion of food additives.

Labels also must disclose certain ingredients, such as sulfites, certain food dyes, and eight food allergens, so food-sensitive consumers may avoid foods that may cause allergic responses. Others may be added as deemed necessary. Food allergies are discussed later in this chapter.

In the past, many terms used on food labels, such as "lean" and "light," had no definite meaning. However, currently most terms used have specific definitions. A summary of these terms is presented in table 2.15. Additionally, milk labels are based on fat content, expressed as percent or grams of fat, as follows: fat-free, skim, or nonfat milk (0 grams); low-fat or light milk (1% or 2.5 grams); reduced fat milk (2% or 5 grams); and whole milk (3.5% or 8 grams).

In a survey, Rothman and others reported that many Americans, even well-educated individuals with good literacy and math skills, do not know how to interpret food labels. However, other studies have shown that individuals with high blood pressure have used food labels to reduce their consumption of sodium, a dietary risk factor for some. Take time to learn to read food labels; it's a smart thing to do.

As noted later in this chapter, some smart phone apps may be very useful when grocery shopping. Simply scanning the bar code on the food label may provide significant information relative to the health benefits or concerns with the product.

What are the proposed changes to the current food label?

As noted, numerous changes have been suggested to help make the food label friendlier to the consumer. As this book went to press, proposed changes were under discussion and the food industry would have two years to put the new rules in effect once approved. Here are some of the key proposed changes.

- Change the serving size requirements on packaged foods, including drinks that individuals normally consume at one time. Serving sizes have changed over the years. Based on a serving size of 8 ounces, a 20-ounce bottle of soda currently may list 2.5 servings, and 100 Calories per serving. However, most individuals consume the entire bottle, so the new requirement would list only one serving, and 250 Calories.
- Make Calories and serving sizes more prominent, increasing the type size and using bold print. This emphasis is considered

Sugar
- **Sugar free:** less than 0.5 g per serving
- **No added sugar; without added sugar; no sugar added:**
  - No sugars were added during processing or packing, including ingredients that contain sugars (for example, fruit juices, applesauce, or jam).
  - Processing does not increase the sugar content above the amount naturally present in the ingredients. (A functionally insignificant increase in sugars is acceptable for processes used for purposes other than increasing sugar content.)
  - The food that it resembles and for which it substitutes normally contains added sugars.
  - If the food doesn't meet the requirements for a low- or reduced-Calorie food, the product bears a statement that the food is not low Calorie or Calorie reduced and directs consumers' attention to the Nutrition Facts panel for further information on sugars and Calorie content.
- **Reduced sugar:** at least 25% less sugar per serving than reference food

Calories
- **Calorie free:** fewer than 5 kcal per serving
- **Low Calorie:** 40 kcal or less per serving and, if the serving is 30 g or less or 2 tbsp or less, per 50 g of the food
- **Reduced or fewer Calories:** least 25% fewer kcal per serving than reference food

Fiber
- **High fiber:** 5 g or more per serving. (Foods making high-fiber claims must meet the definition for low fat, or the level of total fat must appear next to the high-fiber claim.)
- **Good source of fiber:** 2.5 to 4.9 g per serving
- **More or added fiber:** at least 2.5 g more per serving than reference food

Fat
- **Fat free:** less than 0.5 g of fat per serving
- **Saturated fat free:** less than 0.5 g per serving, and the level of *trans* fatty acids does not exceed 0.5 g per serving
- **Low fat:** 3 g or less per serving and, if the serving is 30 g or less or 2 tbsp or less, per 50 g of the food. 2% milk can no longer be labeled low-fat, as it exceeds 3 g per serving. *Reduced fat* is the term used instead

- **Low saturated fat:** 1 g or less per serving and not more than 15% of kcal from saturated fatty acids
- **Reduced or less fat:** at least 25% less per serving than reference food
- **Reduced or less saturated fat:** at least 25% less per serving than reference food

Cholesterol
- **Cholesterol free:** less than 2 mg of cholesterol and 2 g or less of saturated fat per serving
- **Low cholesterol:** 20 mg or less cholesterol and 2 g or less of saturated fat per serving and, if the serving is 30 g or less or 2 tbsp or less, per 50 g of the food
- **Reduced or less cholesterol:** at least 25% less cholesterol and 2 g or less of saturated fat per serving than reference food

Sodium
- **Sodium free:** less than 5 mg per serving.
- **Very low sodium:** 35 mg or less per serving and, if the serving is 30 g or less or 2 tbsp or less, per 50 g of the food
- **Low sodium:** 140 mg or less per serving and, if the serving is 30 g or less or 2 tbsp or less, per 50 g of the food
- **Light in sodium:** at least 50% less per serving than reference food
- **Reduced or less sodium:** at least 25% less per serving than reference food

Other Terms
- **Fortified or enriched:** Vitamins and/or minerals have been added to the product in amounts in excess of at least 10% of that normally present in the usual product. *Enriched* generally refers to replacing nutrients lost in processing, whereas *fortified* refers to adding nutrients not originally present in the specific food.
- **Healthy:** An individual food that is low fat and low saturated fat and has no more than 360 to 480 mg of sodium or 60 mg of cholesterol per serving can be labeled "healthy" if it provides at least 10% of the Daily Value for vitamin A, vitamin C, protein, calcium, iron, or fiber.
- **Light or lite:** The descriptor *light* or *lite* can mean two things: first, that a nutritionally altered product contains one-third fewer kcal or half the fat of reference food (if the food derives 50% or more of its kcal from fat, the reduction must be 50% of the fat) and, second, that the sodium content of a low-Calorie, low-fat food has been reduced by 50%. In addition, "light in sodium" may be used for foods in which the sodium content

has been reduced by at least 50%. The term *light* may still be used to describe such properties as texture and color, as long as the label explains the intent—for example, "light brown sugar" and "light and fluffy."
- **Diet:** A food may be labeled with terms such as *diet, dietetic, artificially sweetened,* or *sweetened with nonnutritive sweetener* only if the claim is not false or misleading. The food can also be labeled *low Calorie* or *reduced Calorie.*
- **Good source:** *Good source* means that a serving of the food contains 10 to 19% of the Daily Value for a particular nutrient. If 5% or less, it is a **low source.**
- **High:** *High* means that a serving of the food contains 20% or more of the Daily Value for a particular nutrient.
- **Organic:** Federal standards for organic

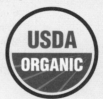

foods allow claims when much of the ingredients do not use chemical fertilizers or pesticides, genetic engineering, sewage sludge, antibiotics, or irradiation in their production. At least 95% of ingredients (by weight) must meet these guidelines to be labeled "organic" on the front of the package. If the front label instead says "made with organic ingredients," only 70% of the ingredients must be organic. For livestock, the animals need to be allowed to graze outdoors and be fed organic feed as well. They also cannot be exposed to large amounts of antibiotics or growth hormones.
- **Natural:** The food must be free of food colors, synthetic flavors, or any other synthetic substance.

Milk
- **Fat-free, skim, or nonfat:** Contains 0 grams of fat
- **Low-fat or light:** Contains 1% or 2.5 grams of fat
- **Reduced fat:** Contains 2% or 5 grams of fat
- **Whole:** Contains 3.5% or 8 grams of fat

The following terms apply only to meat and poultry products regulated by USDA.
- **Extra lean:** less than 5 g of fat, 2 g of saturated fat, and 95 mg of cholesterol per serving (or 100 g of an individual food)
- **Lean:** less than 10 g of fat, 4.5 g of saturated fat, and 95 mg of cholesterol per serving (or 100 g of an individual food)

Many definitions are from FDA's *Dictionary of Terms*, as established in conjunction with the 1990 Nutrition Education and Labeling Act (NELA).

important because obesity and its adverse impact on health is an important health concern.

- Shift the Percent Daily Value to the left of the label. Placing it in a more prominent position helps inform the shopper of the nutrient value of the product.
- Update the DV for several nutrients, such as sodium, vitamin D, and dietary fiber, based on more current research.
- Include potassium and Vitamin D on the label because the FDA has determined they are nutrients of importance to public health. Calcium and iron would remain, but the listing of vitamins A and C would be voluntary. Include actual amount and percent of DV for each nutrient listed.
- Include *Added Sugars* indented under the current Sugar listing to help consumers understand how much sugar is naturally occurring and how much has been added to the product.
- Place *Percent Daily Value* in a more prominent location and provide a better explanation of its intent.

> *http://www.fda.gov* Type Food Label in the search box to access numerous links to use the food label for healthy eating and to review the proposed changes. A good link is How to Understand and Use the Nutrition Facts Label.

What health claims are allowed on food products?

Food manufacturers want your business. Given the public's growing awareness of the relationship between nutrition and health, many food labels now list various health claims or use terminology to entice you to buy their product. For example, one snack product has a label claiming it is made with 5 grams of whole grain, but it is mostly sugar and white flower. And consumers do view a food product as healthier if it carries a health claim or uses *health* terminology.

The FDA permits food manufacturers to make specific health claims on food labels only if the food meets certain minimum standards. These health claims are permitted because the FDA believes there may be significant scientific agreement supporting a relationship between consumption of a specific nutrient and possible prevention of a certain chronic disease. However, there are several requirements, such as not stating the degree of risk reduction, using only terms such as "may" or "might" in reference to reducing health risks, and indicating that other foods may provide similar benefits. Figure 2.11 provides an example.

The FDA approves the use of health claims on food labels based on the underlying research, usually only approving the claim if it is supported by significant scientific evidence. See table 2.16. Currently, there are 12 FDA-approved, qualified health claims, while 4 are authorized based on statements from federal scientific agencies. The following are the approved health claims for various food nutrients and the health problems they may help prevent; the 4 with an asterisk are the agency-approved health claims:

- Calcium and vitamin D and osteoporosis
- Dietary fat and cancer
- Dietary saturated fat and cholesterol and risk of coronary heart disease

- Dietary noncariogenic carbohydrate sweeteners and dental caries
- Fiber-containing grain products, fruits, and vegetables and cancer
- Folate and neural-tube defects (spina bifida)
- Fruits and vegetables and cancer
- Fruits, vegetables, and grain products that contain fiber, particularly soluble fiber, and risk of coronary heart disease
- Plant sterol/stanol esters and risk of coronary heart disease
- Sodium and hypertension
- Soluble fiber from certain foods and risk of coronary heart disease
- Soy protein and risk of coronary heart disease
- Whole-grain foods and risk of heart disease and certain cancers*
- Whole-grain foods with moderate fat content and risk of heart disease*
- Potassium and the risk of high blood pressure and stroke*
- Fluoridated water and reduced risk of dental caries*

> *www.fda.gov* Access the FDA Website and type Appendix C: Health Claims in the search box to access details of all approved health claims for foods.

Appropriate food labeling may help us select healthier foods, and the forthcoming changes hopefully will do so. A simple, yet effective, approach is needed. Some countries, such as Sweden and Great Britain, have a national system that uses traffic light symbols (Red = High; Yellow = Medium; Green = Low) to instantly highlight the contents of less healthy ingredients, such as fat, saturated fat, sugars, and sodium. This traffic light system, or the NuVal™ scoring system discussed earlier, may be a useful approach to help us select healthier foods.

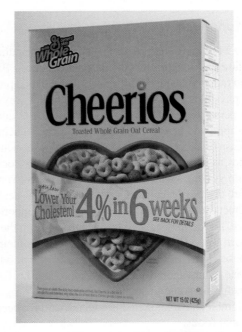

FIGURE 2.11 An example of a Nutrition Facts food label with an approved health claim.

TABLE 2.16 Qualified health claims. FDA-approved model health claims for foods that have significant scientific evidence supporting the claim

Calcium and vitamin D and osteoporosis: Regular exercise and a healthy diet with enough calcium helps teen and young adult white and Asian women maintain good bone health and may reduce their high risk of osteoporosis later in life.

Dietary fat and cancer: Development of cancer depends on many factors. A diet low in total fat may reduce the risk of some cancers.

Dietary saturated fat and cholesterol and risk of coronary heart disease: Development of heart disease depends upon many factors, but its risk may be reduced by diets low in saturated fat and cholesterol and healthy lifestyles.

Dietary noncariogenic carbohydrate sweeteners and dental caries: Frequent eating of foods high in sugars and starches as between-meal snacks can promote tooth decay. The sugar alcohol used to sweeten this food may reduce the risk of dental caries.

Fiber-containing grain products, fruits, and vegetables and cancer: Low fat diets rich in fiber-containing grain products, fruits, and vegetables may reduce the risk of some types of cancer, a disease associated with many factors.

Folate and neural-tube defects (spina bifida): Healthful diets with adequate folate may reduce a woman's risk of having a child with a brain or spinal cord birth defect.

Fruits and vegetables and cancer: Low-fat diets rich in fruits and vegetables (foods that are low in fat and may contain dietary fiber, vitamin A, and vitamin C) may reduce the risk of some types of cancer, a disease associated with many factors.

Fruits, vegetables, and grain products that contain fiber, particularly soluble fiber, and risk of coronary heart disease: Diets low in saturated fat and cholesterol and rich in fruits, vegetables, and grain products that contain some types of dietary fiber, particularly soluble fiber, may reduce the risk of heart disease, a disease associated with many factors.

Sodium and hypertension: Diets low in sodium may reduce the risk of high blood pressure, a disease associated with many factors.

Soluble fiber from certain foods and risk of coronary heart disease: Soluble fiber from foods such as oats and barley, as part of a diet low in saturated fat and cholesterol, may reduce the risk of heart disease. A serving of this food supplies 0.75 gram of the soluble fiber from oats necessary per day to have this effect.

Soy protein and risk of coronary heart disease: Diets low in saturated fat and cholesterol that include 25 grams of soy protein a day may reduce the risk of heart disease. One serving of this food provides 8 grams of soy protein.

Plant sterol/stanol esters and risk of coronary heart disease: Foods containing at least 0.65 g per serving of *plant sterol* esters eaten twice a day with meals for a daily total intake of at least 1.3 g (or 1.7 g per serving of *plant stanol* esters for a total daily intake of at least 3.4 g) as part of a diet low in saturated fat and cholesterol may reduce the risk of heart disease. A serving of this food supplies 0.75 gram of vegetable oil sterol (stanol) esters.

Source: U.S. Food and Drug Administration. Health Claims That Meet Significant Scientific Agreement.

Note: Given changing opinions on dietary cholesterol, some health claims may be modified in the future.

What are functional foods?

In 1994, the FDA permitted dietary supplement manufacturers to make structure and function claims on their products. Basically, a structure and function claim simply means that the food product may affect body physiology in some way, usually in some way beneficial to health or performance. These claims may not be as authoritative as the FDA-approved claims cited above (such as reducing the risk of heart disease or cancer), but these claims may use such terminology as "helps to maintain healthy cholesterol levels" or "supports your immune system," which the consumer may interpret as preventing heart disease or cancer. Technically, these health claims must be correct, but they need not have as much supportive scientific evidence, nor do they have to have approval from the FDA.

Based partly on such health claims, dietary supplement sales have skyrocketed in the past 20 years, and the food industry jumped on the bandwagon. In recent years, numerous food manufacturers, including some giants such as Kellogg, Tropicana, and Procter & Gamble, have marketed products that have been referred to as functional foods.

In its recent position statement authored by Crowe and Francis, the Academy of Nutrition and Dietetics indicated that all food is essentially functional, such as providing energy, promoting growth and development, and regulating body metabolism. However, the Academy indicates increasing scientific evidence suggests that some food components, not considered nutrients in the traditional sense, may provide positive health benefits. Foods containing these food components, including natural, fortified, and enriched products, are called **functional foods**. In this regard, many of the foods listed in Tables 2.12 and 2.13 may be classified as functional foods. Other foods, including fish such as salmon and various Greek yogurts, also may fit this category.

The Academy further notes that functional food research holds many promises for improving the quality of life for consumers. Indeed, Claus indicates that by using modern genomic technology, individual metabolic profiles may be used to develop personalized functional foods for enhanced health. However, the Academy notes there remain some complexities in defining functional foods and their application to promote health. One major complexity is the fact there is no legal or governmental definition of functional food. Thus, the food industry may use health claims to market their products.

Fortification with nutrients or nutraceuticals is a current technique to make functional foods. In a sense, functional foods have been around for nearly a century, as salt was fortified with iodine, and milk was fortified with vitamins A and D, to help prevent nutrient deficiencies. More recently, calcium-fortified juices and multivitamin/mineral–fortified cereals are breakfast mainstays designed, in part, to help us obtain adequate amounts of specific nutrients. Some of these products may be worthwhile, for they may be in accord with the principles underlying FDA approval of food health claims. For example, calcium-fortified orange juice may be an excellent source of calcium for someone who does not drink milk. Cereals fortified with psyllium may be an excellent source of soluble dietary fiber. On the other hand, a sugar drink with added vitamins is a different story, as it is simply a vitamin pill with added sugar.

Some functional foods are designed to satisfy the criteria for qualified health claims on food labels. Many other products marketed as functional foods are simply dietary supplements in disguise, and use structure and function claims to suggest health benefits. Such products include soups with St. John's wort, snack foods with kava kava, cereals with ginkgo biloba, and energy drinks with caffeine.

In the next section we discuss dietary supplements and health claims. However, in the meantime, remember that fruits, vegetables, whole grains, and other plant foods are the optimal functional foods. Their health benefits have been well established.

Key Concepts

► Information provided through nutritional labeling on most food products may serve as a useful guide in finding foods that have a high nutrient density and are healthy choices.

► The Daily Value (DV) on a food label represents the percentage of a nutrient, such as saturated fat or carbohydrate, provided in a single serving that is recommended for an individual who consumes 2,000 Calories daily.

► Terms used on food labels, such as *fat free*, must meet specific standards. In this case, use of *fat free* indicates that a serving of the food contains less than 0.5 gram of fat.

► Health claims may be placed on food labels only if they are supported by adequate scientific data and have been approved by the Food and Drug Administration (FDA).

► Some functional foods may provide some health benefits, adhering to qualified health claims. Other products marketed as functional foods may use structure and function claims, which do not have the scientific support of qualified health claims.

Check for Yourself

► Go to a supermarket and compare food labels for various products. In particular, compare the caloric content of some fat-free products with their non–fat-free counterparts to see the Calorie reduction, if there is any.

Consumer Nutrition—Dietary Supplements and Health

Nutrition scientists indicate that foods, particularly fruits and vegetables, contain numerous nutrients or other food substances, such as vitamins, minerals, and phytonutrients, that may have pharmaceutical properties when taken in appropriate dosages. The potential health benefits of specific nutrients and phytonutrients will be covered in the following chapters as appropriate. The purpose of this section is to provide a broad overview of possible health effects of such supplements when marketed as dietary supplements.

What are dietary supplements?

The dietary supplement industry is a multibillion-dollar business. According to Dickinson and MacKay, numerous surveys indicate that somewhere between 50 percent and 75 percent of American adults use dietary supplements—mostly vitamins and minerals but also other substances marketed for potential health benefits (figure 2.12). Americans have been using such supplements since the 1940s, when they were regulated as either food or drugs. However, in 1994, the United States passed the Dietary Supplements Health and Education Act (DSHEA), which defined a **dietary supplement** as a food product, added to the total diet, that contains at least one of the following ingredients:

- Vitamin
- Mineral
- Herb or botanical

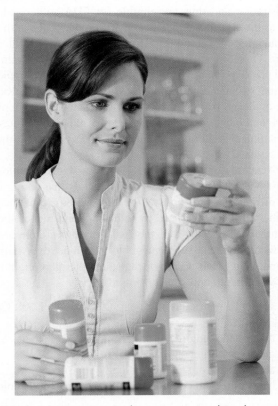

FIGURE 2.12 Dietary supplements are marketed as a means of enhancing both health and physical performance.

- Amino acid
- Metabolite
- Constituent
- Extract
- Combination of any of these ingredients

It is important to note that the DSHEA stipulates that a dietary supplement cannot be represented as a conventional food or as the sole item of a meal or diet.

As noted by this definition, dietary supplements may contain essential nutrients such as essential vitamins, minerals, and amino acids, but also other nonessential substances such as ginseng, ginkgo, yohimbe, ma huang, and other herbal products. The technical definition of a supplement is something added, particularly to correct a deficiency. Theoretically, then, dietary supplements should be used to correct a deficiency of a specific nutrient, such as vitamin C. However, numerous dietary supplements contain substances other than essential nutrients and are marketed not to correct a deficiency but rather to increase the total dietary intake of some food or plant substance that allegedly may enhance one's health status. Like foods, dietary supplements must carry labels, or *supplement facts;* an example is presented in figure 7.5 on page 316.

Will dietary supplements improve my health?

Dietary supplements are usually advertised to the general public as a means to improve some facet of their health and are usually under governmental regulation. In the United States, dietary supplements are regulated under food law by the Food and Drug Administration and thus are eligible for FDA-authorized health claims, as discussed previously. Dietary supplement health claims in Canada are governed by Health Canada's Natural Health Products Directorate. In some countries, such as Germany, a medical prescription is needed to obtain some dietary supplements containing strong herbal products. Dickinson and MacKay note that the evidence from numerous surveys shows that supplement users are making a greater effort to seek health and wellness. Can dietary supplements improve your health? Possibly, but there are several caveats.

The Academy of Nutrition and Dietetics states that most people don't need supplements and recommends that eating a wide variety of nutrient-rich foods is the best way for most people to obtain the nutrients they need to be healthy and reduce their risk of chronic disease. However, the Academy notes there are some people who may need supplements to help meet their nutritional needs, indicating your doctor or registered dietitian might recommend a vitamin/mineral supplement when

- You are on a restrictive diet, eating less than 1,600 Calories per day.
- You are an older adult (50+).
- You are a vegetarian or vegan.
- You are pregnant or a woman of child-bearing age.
- You have a medical condition that limits your food choices.

Consumers should be aware of exceeding recommended upper limits of some vitamins and minerals. Some prudent

recommendations for vitamin and mineral supplementation will be presented in chapters 7 and 8.

In general, as shall be noted in chapter 6, individual amino acid supplements may not enhance health if adequate protein is consumed in the diet. However, research is ongoing with several amino acids.

Of the other classes of nonvitamin, nonmineral dietary supplements (herb or botanical, metabolite, constituent, extract, or combinations), numerous products are marketed for their purported health benefits. In a recent survey of college students from five universities, Harris and others found that college students appear more likely to use dietary supplements than the general population and many use multiple types of supplements weekly. Although we have no specific requirement for these substances, as they are not essential for normal physiological function, some may affect physiological functions in the body associated with health benefits. Using a broad interpretation of the FDA health claim regulations for dietary supplements, some supplement companies advertise their supplements as "miracle products" that can produce "magical results" in a short period of time.

Under current federal law, any dietary supplement can be marketed without advance testing. The only restriction is that the label cannot claim that the product will treat, prevent, or cure a disease. However, as noted previously, the label may make vague claims, referred to as structure/function claims, such as "enhances energy" or "supports testosterone production." Unfortunately, for most of these dietary supplements there are few research data to support their claims. Most advertisements are based on theory alone, testimonials or anecdotal information, or the exaggeration or misinterpretation of research findings relative to the health effects of specific nutrients or other food constituents. Many labels carry a notice stating *This statement has not been evaluated by the FDA,* a disclaimer regarding the health claim. Moreover, although advertisers may not make unsubstantiated health claims, the 1994 DSHEA stipulates that the burden of proving the claims false rests with the government. Currently, under the DSHEA, the FDA must show in court that an unreasonable risk is posed by consumption of a dietary supplement.

Various governmental and other agencies have developed guidelines for the supplement industry to help the consumer have confidence in the composition, labeling, and safety of dietary supplement products. The FDA has established current good manufacturing practice requirements, noting that manufacturers are required to evaluate the identity, purity, quality, strength, and composition of dietary supplements. The Federal Trade Commission has indicated that marketers of dietary supplements must have above-board scientific evidence to support any health claims. Additionally, U.S. Pharmacopeia, a respected nonprofit medical agency, launched a certification program for dietary supplements. If the dietary supplement contains what the label indicates, then it may carry the USP seal of approval. However, the USP seal does not mean the product is effective or even that it is safe to use, just that it contains what the label promises.

It should be noted that some of these types of dietary supplements, such as herbals and food extracts, have been the subject of research to evaluate their health effects. Such effects will be discussed in later chapters as appropriate.

Again, to reiterate the point, dietary supplements may exert some beneficial healthful effects in certain cases, but as Thomas points out, for most of us the substances found in most dietary supplements are readily available in familiar and attractive packages called fruits, vegetables, legumes, fish, and other healthy foods. Although the Prudent Healthy Diet is the optimal means to obtain the nutrients we need, dietary supplements may be recommended under certain circumstances. When deemed to be prudent behavior, such recommendations will be provided at specific points in this text.

Can dietary supplements harm my health?

In his review of dietary supplements, Thomas noted that although they may be beneficial to some individuals, their use may be harmful in some ways. Some of his key points, and others, are

1. Nutrition is only one factor that influences health, well-being, and resistance to disease. Individuals who rely on dietary supplements to guarantee their health may disregard other very important lifestyle behaviors, such as appropriate exercise and a healthy diet.
2. Dietary supplements may provide a false sense of security to some individuals who may use them as substitutes for a healthful diet, believing they are eating healthfully and not attempting to eat right.
3. Taking supplements of single nutrients in large doses may have detrimental effects on nutritional status and health. Although large doses of some vitamins or minerals may be taken to prevent some conditions, excesses may lead to other health problems.
4. Individuals who use dietary supplements as an alternative form of medicine may avoid seeking effective medical treatment.
5. Dietary supplements vary tremendously in quality, including best-selling store brands marketed by national retailers, such as GNC and Walgreens. Numerous independent analyses of specific dietary supplements, such as those by ConsumerLab.com, reveal that some may contain less than that listed, sometimes even none of the main ingredient. Some products contain substances not listed on the label. This may pose a health risk.
6. Numerous case studies have shown that the use of various dietary supplements may impair health, and may even be fatal.

www.ConsumerLab.com Check the content analysis of various brands of popular dietary supplements. Fee charged for some reports.

Although most dietary supplements are safe, some may induce adverse health effects. In a recent analysis of dangerous supplements, *Consumer Reports* reported that of the more than 50,000 dietary supplement products in the Natural Medicines Comprehensive Database, close to 12 percent have been linked to safety concerns or problems with product quality. They cite 12 supplements, mostly herbals, that should be avoided, including bitter orange, chaparral, comfrey, germanium, kava, and yohimbe.

Where appropriate, the effectiveness and safety of various dietary supplements will be discussed in later sections of this book, but some general safeguards recommended by consumer health organizations to protect your health represent sound advice.

- Before trying a dietary supplement to treat a health problem, try changing your diet or lifestyle first.
- Check with your doctor before taking any dietary supplement, particularly herbal preparations. This is especially important for pregnant and nursing women, children, and individuals taking prescribed drugs whose effects may be impaired by herbal interactions.
- Buy standardized products. Most dietary supplements in the United States should be standardized according to federal regulations. Supplement Facts labels should provide information comparable to the Nutrition Facts food label.
- Use only single-ingredient dietary supplements. Use of combination supplements may make it difficult to determine the cause of any side effects.
- Be alert to both the positive and negative effects of the supplement. Try to keep an objective record of the effects.
- Stop taking the supplement immediately if you experience any health-related problems. Contact your physician and local health authorities to report the problem. This may help establish a database for the safety of dietary supplements.

The following Websites provide detailed information on various aspects of dietary supplements.

www.dsld.nlm.nih.gov/dsld/ The National Institutes of Health database of dietary supplements contains thousands of supplements. Use the search box to obtain product information.

http://ods.od.nih.gov/factsheets/list-all/ The Office of Dietary Supplements provides detailed information, including safety, for most common supplements.

www.fda.gov/Food/DietarySupplements/ Use the search box to find reports on the safety and effectiveness of specific dietary supplements

www.ConsumerLab.com Check the content analysis of various brands of popular dietary supplements. Fee charged for some reports.

https://myds.nih.gov Use this site to obtain an app, MyDS (My Dietary Supplements) to assess information about supplements you use. You can share this information with your doctor.

Consumer Nutrition—Food Quality and Safety

We all have the basic assumption that the food we eat is safe and of high quality. Several federal agencies, such as the USDA and FDA, effectively regulate food quality and safety. The FDA Food Safety Modernization Act (FSMA) was effective in 2011, helping ensure that our food supply is safe by enacting measures to prevent contamination. In general, our assumption of food safety is correct. However, foods are not necessarily risk free or high quality. One newspaper headline, titled *Food Frights,* noted that the FDA is one busy agency, recalling numerous products annually for suspected bacteria, contamination, and mislabeling. Many factors may influence food quality and safety in the development of a food product. For example, from the time a plant seed is created until the final food product hits our kitchen table, the food may have been treated with plant chemicals, loaded with additives, contaminated with bacteria, or prepared improperly, all of which may affect food quality and safety. Food safety is an important consideration in healthful eating, and thus has been included in the 2015 *Dietary Guidelines for Americans.* The purpose of this section is to discuss several of the major factors and concerns influencing food quality and safety in developed nations.

www.foodsafety.gov Represents the gateway to food safety information presented by the FDA.

Is current food biotechnology effective and safe?

Food biotechnology has been around for thousands of years, as farmers used plant breeding techniques to enhance desired traits, such as the ability of plants to produce higher yields or to resist pests and diseases. Today, genetic engineering, which involves the insertion of favorable genes into plants or animals, is a key feature of food biotechnology. Genetically engineered foods are also known as genetically modified (GM) foods and genetically modified organisms (GMO). GM foods have their proponents as well as opponents, as highlighted in reviews by Bawa and Anilakumar, Moses and Brookes, and Kramkowska and others.

Proponents of GM foods indicate that GM foods offer dramatic promise for meeting some areas of greatest challenge for the 21st century, citing various potential benefits from such products, including the following:

• Enable production of greater quantities of food or prevention of food spoilage by making plants less vulnerable to insects, viruses, drought, or frost, which may help meet the needs of the world's growing population without damaging the environment

• Enhance food quality by increasing the nutrient content, such as more beta-carotene, a precursor of vitamin A, in rice, preventing millions of deaths annually caused by vitamin A deficiency. An increase in the growth rate and size of fish, such as salmon, can help produce a source of high-quality, healthful protein.

Contrarily, in addition to possible philosophical and religious concerns associated with "messing with Mother Nature," opponents of GM foods indicate they have been marketed without adequate research and cite potential risks, including the following.

• Cause plant pests to develop increased resistance to the GM crops that were supposed to combat them. Such effects could have adverse effects on the environment.

• Lead to the synthesis of various proteins that may cause allergies or other health problems, with possible long-term adverse health effects, particularly in young children

In the United States, GM foods are regulated by three federal agencies, including the FDA. Commercial GM food crops include soybeans, corn, canola, Hawaiian papaya, zucchini, and yellow squash. Most recently, a GM potato that eliminates the formation of a possible carcinogen during frying has been approved by the FDA. Since 1992 the FDA has determined that GM foods must meet the same rigorous standards for safety as those created through traditional means and is not aware of any information that GM foods differ from conventional foods in quality, safety, or any other characteristic.

Although most of us are probably unaware of the fact, we have eaten GM products. About 70 percent of foods in a typical supermarket contain at least one GM ingredient, typically from corn or soybeans. Are they safe for us to eat? The available scientific evidence suggests *yes.* In a recent review of 24 studies involving GM plant diets, Snell and others concluded the results show that GM plants are nutritionally equivalent to their non-GM counterparts, can be safely used in food and feed, and do not suggest any health hazards.

Nevertheless, some may wish to avoid consuming GM products. Currently, GM foods need not be identified on food labels in the United States unless the food is significantly different in nutrient content from its conventional counterpart, unless a known food allergen has been introduced, or unless the food is to be exported, the last because GM foods must be identified on food labels in the European Union.

One way to avoid GM products is to buy certified organic products, discussed later in this chapter, because they cannot intentionally include GM ingredients. Also, some food manufacturers may produce non-GM products and include various non-GM seals on the food label. In a recent survey conducted by *Consumer Reports,* 92 percent of responders think that GM foods should be labeled before they are sold.

www.nongmoproject.org/find-non-gmo/search-participating-products/ This Website of the NON GMO Project lists various food manufacturers that produce non-GM products, including listings of such products.

Do pesticides in food present significant health risks?

Modern production techniques are designed to increase both the quantity and quality of plant and animal food and yet maintain appropriate safety standards. One potential problem is bacterial contamination, discussed later, and another is the potential health risks of pesticides.

As noted previously, plants contain substances called phytochemicals, (phytonutrients) which may contribute to various health benefits associated with a diet high in fruits, vegetables, and other wholesome plant foods. Ames and Gold note that 99.99 percent of the pesticides we eat are naturally present in plants. Many of these phytochemicals also help the plant survive, primarily by acting as herbicides or pesticides to prevent damage from naturally occurring weeds and insects. Nevertheless, more than two thousand insects, weeds, or plant diseases damage nearly one-third of our nation's farm crop each year. To help minimize crop damage from these pests, agriculturalists have developed synthetic herbicides and pesticides to augment plants' natural defenses.

Synthetic herbicides and pesticides can enter the body via absorption through the skin, inhalation into the lungs, or ingestion when found in food and water. Although synthetic herbicides and pesticides may effectively control weeds and pests harmful to plants, they appear to function differently in the human body than do natural plant phytochemicals. Prolonged exposure to synthetic chemicals may cause various health problems, including respiratory diseases, nervous system disorders, genetic defects and miscarriages in pregnant women, cancer, and death. On the one hand, we need to control those pests destructive to our food supply, but on the other hand, the health of the public should not be harmed by the chemicals being used. This is the dilemma concerning the use of pesticides and similar chemicals.

Most of the serious diseases from pesticide use have been associated with occupational exposure, such as in farm workers and crop-dusting pilots, who may be exposed to high concentrations on a daily basis, or in people who live near sprayed areas. For example, Ye and others reported strong evidence for an association between occupational pesticide exposure and asthma, especially in agricultural occupations. However, direct exposure to even small amounts of household insect spray has been known to alter brain function, causing irritability, insomnia, and reduced concentration. The prudent individual should avoid direct contact with these substances as much as possible, for even thorough washing with soap and water has little effect upon the absorption through the skin of some insect sprays.

Ames and Gold note that 99.99 percent of the pesticides we eat are naturally present in plants, but synthetic pesticides may also be on the food we eat and in the water we drink. The FDA and state government agencies conduct spot surveys to analyze the pesticide content of produce for sale. In a report that analyzed data on more than 200 known carcinogens in foods, the National Research Council of the National Academy of Sciences concluded that both synthetic and naturally occurring pesticides are consumed at such low levels that they pose little threat to human health. Moreover, in its comprehensive, worldwide review, the American Institute for Cancer Research found no convincing evidence that eating foods containing trace amounts of chemicals, such as pesticides and herbicides, and drugs used on farm animals, changes our risk for cancer.

However, there is increasing concern that children may be exposed to higher levels of pesticides because children are smaller and normally consume greater amounts of fruits and vegetables per unit of body weight. Recent reviews suggest children may experience various health problems associated with exposure to pesticides. Doust and others indicated that exposure to pesticides may be associated with asthma, more so in children than adults. Muñoz-Quezada and others noted that all but 1 of 27 studies with early childhood exposures to pesticides showed some negative effects of pesticides on neurobehavioral development, such as cognitive, behavioral, and motor deficits, while the American Academy of Pediatrics reported that epidemiological evidence demonstrates associations between early life exposure to pesticides and pediatric cancers, decreased cognitive function, and behavioral problems. The impact of pesticides on the developing brain and nervous system is a major concern, and health professionals recommend that baby foods contain no pesticides.

Government agencies are attempting to reduce pesticide residues in the food we eat, and more farmers are turning to pesticide-free farming, producing more organic foods certified to be free of any pesticide residue. Genetically engineered plants may also reduce the need for pesticides. According to Needham and others, these efforts are working, as the level of environmental chemicals in humans is decreasing.

Based on current knowledge, the following points appear to be sound advice to help reduce, though they may not completely eliminate, the pesticide content in the foods we eat.

1. Avoid direct skin contact or breathing exposure to pesticides.
2. Food preparation may reduce pesticide residues. Wash produce thoroughly; some, but not all, pesticides on fruits and vegetables are water soluble. Washing may be particularly helpful to remove pesticide residues from apples, bananas, corn, grapes, lettuce, peaches, and tomatoes. Peeling some fruits and vegetables also helps. Peeling is effective for apples, carrots, cucumbers, grapes, oranges, peaches, and potatoes. Remove outer leaves of produce. Cooking may also help, particularly with broccoli, green beans, potatoes, and tomatoes.
3. Eat less animal fat and seafood from contaminated waters. Pesticides may concentrate in animal fat. In particular, farmed fish such as Atlantic salmon may contain high concentrations of several contaminants.
4. Buy fruits and vegetables locally and in season. Farmers are less likely to use pesticides if the food is to be sold locally.

5. Eat a wide variety of foods. A food that contains pesticides will then contribute only a small amount as part of your overall diet.

6. Buy certified organic foods, because they contain fewer pesticide residues than conventionally grown alternatives. The Environmental Working Group annually ranks fruits and vegetables based on pesticide content. Table 2.17 presents the most current listing. If you want the fewest pesticides in your diet, you might consider choosing organic alternatives for the *dirty* dozen.

www.ewg.org/foodnews/list.php Consult the Environmental Working Group Website to find the ranking of fruits and vegetables relative to pesticide content.

www.epa.gov/pesticides/health/human.htm For more information relative to the effects of pesticides on human health, consult the Website of the Environmental Protection Agency.

Are organic foods safer and healthier choices?

The USDA has established rules regarding certified **organic foods**. One stipulation is prohibition of certain synthetic pesticides and fertilizers in plant production. Additionally, the use of antibiotics and growth hormones in animal production is prohibited, as is the use of irradiation and genetically modified organisms. Moreover, no food additives may be used with organic foods.

Foods whose ingredients are all organic may be labeled as 100 percent organic, while those containing at least 95 percent organic ingredients may carry the USDA organic label (see table 2.15), while foods with the notation "Made With Organic Ingredients" must contain at least 70 percent organic ingredients

TABLE 2.17	The environmental working group ranks fruits and vegetables on pesticide content. The lower the rank, the higher the pesticide content. Out of 51 fruits and vegetables, this list contains the most recent ranking of the 10 based on lowest (clean) and highest (dirty) pesticide content. If you want the fewest pesticides in your diet, you might consider choosing organic alternatives of those with the lowest pesticide content.

Lowest Pesticide Content (Clean)		Highest Pesticide Content (Dirty)	
51	Avocados	1	Apples
50	Sweet corn	2	Strawberries
49	Pineapples	3	Grapes
48	Cabbage	4	Celery
47	Sweet peas—frozen	5	Peaches
46	Onions	6	Spinach
45	Asparagus	7	Sweet bell peppers
44	Mangoes	8	Nectarines—imported
43	Papayas	9	Cucumbers
42	Kiwi	10	Cherry tomatoes

but cannot use the organic label. Are such foods safer or healthier? Let's look at several proposed differences between organic and conventional food products.

Pesticides Most studies report lower levels of pesticides in organic foods. For example, Barański and others conducted a meta-analysis of 343 studies and reported that organic crops, on average, have a lower incidence of pesticide residues than the non-organic crops. However, Magkos and others note that although organic foods may contain less pesticide residues than conventionally grown foods, the significance of this difference is questionable, inasmuch as actual levels of contamination in both types of food are generally well below acceptable limits. This is especially so with the *clean* fruits and vegetables mentioned above. Most health professionals agree that you should not cut back on fruits and vegetables, because the associated health benefits discussed previously far outweigh potential risks from pesticides.

Bacteria Bacteria levels in organic foods are comparable to those in conventional foods. The Center for Science in the Public Interest indicated that organic fruits or vegetables are no less likely to be contaminated with bacteria, such as *E. coli,* than conventional ones. The Consumers Union also noted that chickens labeled as *organic* were more likely to harbor salmonella bacteria than were conventionally produced broilers. However, the Centers for Disease Control and Prevention indicated that there is no evidence that foodborne diseases, such as food poisoning, are a greater or lesser risk with organic foods. As discussed later in this chapter, food poisoning may have serious health consequences.

Nutritional Value Marketing of organic foods may be problematic. The Consumers Union notes that as more companies enter the organic market, government standards come under attack. Today we have numerous organic products in the marketplace, some of which have been termed *organic junk foods,* such as peanut butter cookies, sweetened cereals, potato chips, and soda, which may contain significant amounts of sugar and fat; although organic, such foods may not be healthful.

Overall, in a systematic review, Dangour and others determined that evidence is lacking for health effects resulting from the consumption of organic foods. However, Dangour, as well as Williams, notes that we need higher-quality research than that currently available.

Beyond health considerations, many promote buying organic as a means to help protect the environment. Organic farming practices may reduce pollution of our waters, while organic animal farming may be more humane.

Does commercial food processing affect food quality and safety?

Numerous federal, state, and local government agencies are involved in the process of ensuring the safety of the food we eat. Such agencies monitor production of food on farms, preparation in food establishments such as restaurants, and processing in plants of the commercial food industry. Ideally, relative to the last, commercial food processing would make food more healthy, safe, delicious, attractive, and stable. In many cases it does. In a scientific statement by the Academy of Nutrition and Dietetics (AND), Weaver and others note that both fresh and processed foods make up vital parts of the food supply. Processed food contributes to both food security (ensuring that sufficient food is available) and nutrition security (ensuring that food quality meets human nutrient needs), and nutrient-dense processed foods may help meet food guidance recommendations for healthy diets. Dwyer and others note that fortification of foods during processing is an important public health objective, indicating that many individuals in the United States would not achieve recommended micronutrient intakes without fortification of the food supply.

Commercial food processing may provide other benefits. For example, some frozen foods may have higher concentrations of nutrients than their fresh counterparts because they are usually "flash-frozen" soon after picking. Processed tomatoes, such as spaghetti sauce, may increase the bioavailability of phytonutrients, such as lycopene, by breaking cell walls. Although some commercial processing techniques may reduce the quantity of some nutrients, enrichment with vitamins and minerals will help restore such losses.

The AND statement indicates the food industry is part of the process to improve the diets of Americans by providing a nutritious food supply that is safe, enjoyable, affordable, and sustainable. However, certain commercial food-processing practices may be detrimental to our health in several ways. Potential health risks of several food-processing practices, such as the intentional inclusion of food additives and the unintentional inclusion of bacteria, are discussed later in this chapter. The major problem with some forms of commercial food-processing techniques is adding the wrong stuff and taking away the good stuff, possibly converting a healthful food into a potentially harmful one. The major feature of the Prudent Healthy Diet is the consumption of wholesome, natural, low-fat foods. But most of us do consume a wide variety of packaged foods, some of which may be highly processed and may be of questionable nutritional value. There has been increasing concern over the years that the nutritional quality of our food has been declining because many of our foods are overprocessed.

The following are some concerns with highly processed foods.

- They contain too much refined sugar, which has no nutritional value except Calories.
- They contain too much extracted oils, which has no nutritional value except Calories.
- They contain white flour, overprocessed wheat with less nutrient value.
- They contain more salt and sodium, which may pose a health risk to some.
- Fruits and vegetables are artificially ripened, with lower quantities of vitamins and minerals.
- Synthetic products, such as artificial orange juice and imitation ice cream, do not possess the same nutrient values as their natural counterparts.
- Indiscriminate fortification of foods could result in excess amounts of micronutrients, which could pose some health problems.

Wise food selection can help avoid some of these concerns. In its scientific statement, the Academy of Nutrition and Dietetics indicates the key to meeting healthful dietary guidelines is to select nutrient-dense foods, either processed or not. However, this may be somewhat tricky in today's food marketplace. Careful reading of food labels may be the key.

Does home food processing affect food quality and safety?

Somewhat like commercial food processing, you process food at home. You may wash, cut, blend, freeze, and cook a variety of foods at home in preparation for a meal, and home food processing, like commercial food processing, may lead to loss of some nutrients, particularly several water-soluble vitamins. You can minimize nutrient losses and preserve the healthful quality of foods by following these procedures at home:

- Keep most fruits and vegetables chilled in the refrigerator to prevent enzymic destruction of nutrients. For similar reasons, keep frozen foods in the freezer until ready for preparation to eat. To help preserve perishable foods, set an appropriate temperature for your refrigerator ($\leq 40°$) and freezer ($\leq 0°$).
- After cutting, wrap most fruits and vegetables tightly to prevent exposure to air, which may accelerate oxidation and spoiling, and store them in the refrigerator.
- Buy milk in cardboard or opaque plastic containers to prevent light from destroying riboflavin, a B vitamin. For similar reasons, keep most grain products stored in opaque containers or dark cupboards.
- Steam or microwave vegetables in very little water to prevent the loss of water-soluble vitamins and some minerals. Microwaving is very effective in preserving the nutrient value of food. Use microwave-safe dishes or glass cookware. Do not use plastic wrap, plastic containers, or Styrofoam because chemicals can leach into the food when heated. Cover food with a paper towel instead.
- Avoid cooking with high temperatures and prolonged cooking of foods, particularly in hot water, which may increase nutrient losses such as of water-soluble vitamins.
- Avoid using high-temperature methods when cooking certain foods. Research suggests some cooking protocols may induce the formation of carcinogens in some foods. Although Virk-Baker and others noted more high-quality research is needed to ascertain a link between such cooking protocols and increased risk of cancer, caution is advisable.
  - Cooking some foods at high temperatures, about 250° Fahrenheit or higher, may induce the formation of acrylamide, a possible carcinogen, from the interaction of an amino acid and some sugars in food, such as potatoes. French fries may contain acrylamide, but a genetically modified potato has recently been developed that reduces the amount of acrylamide produced when the potato is fried.
  - Grilling or broiling meat, including beef, pork, poultry, and fish, with an open flame may cause the formation of heterocyclic amines (HCAs), possible mutagens/carcinogens, from the interaction of amino acids and creatine.

Cooking meats at lower temperatures, such as oven roasting, baking, steaming, and boiling, as well as marinating meats or use of a microwave to partially cook meat before grilling may help reduce the formation of HCAs.

Using these techniques, nutrient losses incurred with home food processing are minimal, and an adequate nutrient intake will be obtained if you consume a wide variety of foods.

What is food poisoning?

The major health problem associated with home food processing is the presence of foodborne bacteria. Food bacteria are of two types. One type causes food spoilage, which probably won't make you sick, while the other type doesn't spoil food but can make you sick.

Food poisoning is caused primarily by consuming foods or fluids contaminated with certain bacteria, particularly Salmonella, Escherichia, Staphylococcus, Clostridium, Campylobacter, and Listeria. Torgerson and others noted that foodborne diseases are a global problem and a major cause of morbidity and mortality in humans. Staphylococcus and Escherichia (*E. coli*) are the most commonly reported bacterial causes of food poisoning in the United States. The FDA recently indicated that one in six Americans suffers from a foodborne illness each year, including several thousand deaths.

Bacteria that cause food poisoning are found mainly in animal foods. The Consumers Union reported that 83 percent of whole chicken broilers bought nationwide, even premium and organic broilers, harbored Campylobacter or Salmonella. Bacteria are also common in produce. The contamination of fresh spinach with the bacterium *E. coli* led to one of the largest and deadliest outbreaks of foodborne illness in recent years. The most common sources of food poisoning are

- Raw and undercooked meat and poultry
- Raw or undercooked eggs
- Raw or undercooked shellfish
- Contaminated produce
- Improperly canned foods

The most common symptoms of food poisoning include nausea, vomiting, and diarrhea, which normally clear up in a day or two. However, individuals should seek medical help in cases involving headache, stiff neck, and fever occurring together; bloody diarrhea; diarrhea lasting longer than three days; fever that lasts more than 24 hours; or sensations of weakness, numbness, and tingling in the arms and legs. Some cases of food poisoning may lead to lifelong health problems and may be fatal if not treated properly.

Most cases of food poisoning occur at home and may be associated with inappropriate commercial food processing. Although governmental health agencies attempt to control the spread of bacteria to food through appropriate regulations governing the food industry, the Consumers Union noted that occasional outbreaks occur because of food contamination during industrial processing, such as ground meat contamination with *Escherichia coli* (*E. coli*). *E. coli* can lead to kidney failure. Millions of Americans experience a significant foodborne illness each year, with several thousand fatalities.

Food poisoning may be prevented by improving both commercial and home food processing. One commercial procedure is **irradiation**, a process whereby food products are subjected to powerful gamma rays from ionizing radiation, such as radioactive cobalt-60. Although food irradiation has been used since the 1990s to reduce food bacteria, the Centers for Disease Control and Prevention (CDC) recently noted that irradiation holds great potential for preventing many important foodborne diseases that are transmitted through meat, poultry, fresh produce, and other foods. The CDC further noted that an overwhelming body of scientific evidence demonstrates that irradiation does not harm the nutritional value of food, nor does it make the food unsafe to eat, and is a logical means to help reduce the burden of foodborne disease in the United States. Irradiation may also reduce the need for many food preservatives. The FDA has approved irradiation for poultry, beef, pork, and lamb. Irradiated food products must have a label containing a statement that they have been treated and the international symbol of irradiation known as a *radura,* which is depicted in figure 2.13. The position of the Academy of Nutrition and Dietetics, developed by Wood and Bruhn, is that food irradiation enhances the safety and quality of the food supply and helps protect consumers from foodborne illness.

If you prefer to not purchase irradiated meats, at the minimum the following guidelines should be helpful in preventing the spread of bacteria in food prepared at home. Even if you buy irradiated foods, which may reduce the possibility of bacterial contamination, these guidelines are still recommended.

1. Wash hands thoroughly and often before and during food preparations.
2. Treat all raw meat, poultry, fish, seafood, and eggs as if they were contaminated. When shopping, place meat in separate bags, and store them that way in the refrigerator. Rinsing raw meat is more likely to contaminate the kitchen than decontaminate the food. Handle raw meat in just one part of the kitchen, on a cutting board used only for such food. Prevent juices from getting on other foods.
3. Eating raw fruits and vegetables is healthy. However, produce is often coated with wax, which can trap potentially dangerous bacteria. Wash all fruits and vegetables thoroughly with running water, even if you are going to peel them with a knife. The knife can transfer bacteria to the fruit as you recut it. Peel only a thin layer because many vitamins and minerals

FIGURE 2.13 The radura, the international symbol of irradiation.
U.S. Environmental Protection Agency

are found just under the skin. Wash the fruit once it is peeled to help remove any bacteria transferred by the peeler. Organic fruits and vegetables normally are not waxed, but they may be. Check with your grocer.

4. Thoroughly clean with hot, soapy water all utensils used in food preparation. Microwaving your sponges and other food preparation utensils for about 30 to 60 seconds may help kill bacteria.

5. Use a clean preparation surface. After preparing poultry or other animal foods, clean the preparation surface thoroughly before using it to prepare other foods. When using the same surface, prepare animal foods last.

6. Do not use canned foods that are extensively dented or bulging.

7. Cook all meat, poultry, seafood, and eggs thoroughly according to directions. Use a meat thermometer inserted deep into the meat, especially with ground meat, because bacteria may get from the surface to the interior. Heat meat to the desired temperature, usually noted on the meat package. Guidelines include heating beef, pork, lamb, and veal to 160° and poultry to 170°–180°. However, do not overcook or char meats, as this process may produce carcinogens.

8. Do not eat raw shellfish.

9. Store heated foods promptly in the refrigerator or freezer. Reheat foods thoroughly.

10. Use leftovers within a few days. When in doubt, throw it out.

Are food additives safe?

Do you ever read the list of ingredients on the labels of highly processed food products? If not, check one out soon. My guess is you will not know what half the ingredients are or why they are there (unless the reason is listed). A box of long grain & wild rice with herb seasoning, thought to be totally natural, had the main ingredients of enriched parboiled long grain rice, wild rice, and dehydrated vegetables (onion, parsley, spinach, garlic, celery) as the herb seasoning—along with hydrolyzed vegetable protein, salt, sugar, monosodium glutamate, autolyzed yeast, sodium silicoaluminate, disodium inosinate, disodium guanylate, and sodium sulfite. The rice was delicious, but were all the additives necessary?

The Food and Drug Administration classifies a **food additive** as any substance added directly to food. There are more than 40 different purposes for the additives in the foods we eat, but the 4 most common are to add flavor, to enhance color, to improve texture, and to preserve the food. For example, vanilla extract may be added to ice cream to impart a vanilla flavor, vitamin C (ascorbic acid) may be added to fruits and vegetables to prevent discoloration, emulsifiers may be added to help blend oil evenly throughout a product, and sodium propionate may be used to prolong shelf life. Nutrients may also be added to increase the quality of the product, a process called *fortification.*

To earn FDA approval, additives must be **generally recognized as safe (GRAS)**. The Office of Food Additive Safety of the FDA has determined an acceptable daily intake (ADI) for some, but not all, food additives. The ADI represents the amount of food additive that an individual may consume daily without any adverse effect, and includes a 100-fold safety factor. Additives may be added only to specific foods for specific purposes, and in general

must improve the quality of the food without posing any hazards to humans. Only the minimum amount necessary to achieve the desired purpose may be added.

Although we realize that absolute safety does not exist in anything we do, including eating, we do have a right to expect that the food we purchase is generally safe for consumption. The government and food manufacturers must take utmost care to ensure that food additives do not create any appreciable health risks. On the other hand, we as consumers also have a responsibility to select foods necessary for good nutrition. Food product labeling has helped us in this regard, for we now can tell what ingredients we are eating, although we may not always know why they are there.

The general consensus is that most additives used in processed foods are safe. However, there are some concerns. Neltner and others recently reported that the approval process for a GRAS additive appeared to be flawed. They noted that over a 15-year period, individuals or groups determining whether a food additive was GRAS had financial conflicts of interest, raising concerns about the integrity of the process and whether it ensures the safety of the food supply. Moreover, Wilson and Bahna note that although adverse reactions to additives seem to be rare, they are likely to be underdiagnosed in part due to low index of suspicion. Some research has shown that certain additives, such as food dyes, may cause allergic reactions or cause some children to become measurably more hyperactive and distractible. When such adverse effects are documented, as has happened in past years, the FDA has removed such additives from the GRAS list. More details on specific food additives may be found on the FDA Website.

http://www.nutrition.gov/whats-food/food-additives **The FDA provides detailed information on a wide variety of food additives.**

Based on such findings, consumer interest groups such as the Center for Science in the Public Interest (CSPI) have concerns about the safety of many additives. The CSPI places additives in five categories ranging from Safe to Avoid. You can check the many food additives in each of the five categories on the CSPI Website.

www.cspinet.org/reports/chemcuisine.htm **Check the CSPI Website, Chemical Cuisine, regarding its evaluation of the safety of various food additives. The safety rating categories are Safe, Cut Back, Caution, Certain People Should Avoid, and Avoid. The Website provides details on each additive listed.**

However, there remains some debate relative to the safety of various additives. For example, the CSPI has placed aspartame, a popular artificial sweetener, in its Avoid category and reportedly was to formally call on the FDA to ban it, citing three Italian animal studies indicating aspartame may cause cancer. Conversely, most major reviews, including a report by the FDA, have reported no significant health risks associated with aspartame.

Health professional organizations reiterate the point that natural foods, such as fruits, vegetables, and lean animal protein foods, contain little to no additives and are the best approach to reduce such intake if a concern. Moreover, avoiding or minimizing intake of additives such as sugar, corn syrup, and partially hydrogenated vegetable oil, all products with few nutrients and excess Calories, may be one of the best ways to avoid development of chronic diseases.

Why do some people experience adverse reactions to some foods?

Although most food we eat is safe and causes no acute health problems, some individuals may experience mild to severe reactions, or possibly death, from eating certain foods. These reactions may be attributed to food intolerance or food allergy.

Food intolerance, the most common problem, is a general term for any adverse reaction to a food or food component that does not involve the immune system. The body cannot properly digest a portion of the food because it lacks the appropriate enzyme, resulting in gastrointestinal distress such as bloating, abdominal pain, nausea, and diarrhea. Lactose and gluten intolerance are relatively common.

- Lactose intolerance is a problem for many African-Americans because they lack lactase, the enzyme needed to digest lactose (milk sugar).
- Gluten intolerance, or gluten sensitivity, is caused by gluten, a protein found in wheat, barley, and rye. Gluten may irritate the lining of the intestine, and symptoms may vary, including bloating and irritable stomach as well as fatigue and depression.

Both conditions will be discussed in chapter 4.

Food allergy, also known as food hypersensitivity, involves an adverse immune response to an otherwise harmless food substance. Many foods contain allergens, usually proteins, that may stimulate the immune system to manufacture antibodies (immunoglobulin E, or IgE) specific to that food. When individuals who have inherited a food allergy are first exposed to that food, their immune system produces millions of IgE antibodies. These antibodies reside in some white blood cells and mast cells in the body, particularly in the skin, respiratory tract, and gastrointestinal tract, the parts of the body that come into contact with air and the food we eat. These cells also contain substances, such as histamine, that are released when the antibodies are exposed again to the offending food allergen.

Histamine and other chemicals cause the allergic reaction, which may involve the skin (swelling, hives, itchy skin and eyes), gastrointestinal tract (nausea, vomiting, abdominal cramps, diarrhea), or respiratory tract (runny nose, sneezing, coughing). In severe cases, an allergic response may involve anaphylactic shock and death by respiratory failure. According to a recent review by Sicherer and Sampson, food allergy likely affects nearly 5 percent of adults and 8 percent of children, whereas Syed and others indicate it affects up to 10 percent of the population, but both research groups indicate an increased prevalence.

More than 700 food allergens have been identified. Although allergens may be found in many foods, 90 percent of the offenders are proteins found in several common foods. The FDA mandates clear labeling and source of ingredients derived from commonly allergenic sources. Labels are required to state clearly whether the food contains one of the eight "major food allergens" listed:

- Milk
- Fish
- Tree nuts
- Wheat
- Eggs
- Crustacean shellfish
- Peanuts
- Soybeans

Some additives also may cause allergic responses, particularly sulfites used as preservatives.

For individuals who know which food substances may trigger an allergic response, food labels may be helpful in determining the allergen's presence. Food manufacturers are placing notices on food labels for "Food Allergic Consumers" to check the ingredient list and note that the product may have been manufactured in a factory that makes other products containing allergenic foods.

If you experience problems when you consume certain foods, you may be able to make a self-diagnosis by simply avoiding that food and noting whether or not you experience a recurrence. But because there may be many causes of food-related illness, you should consult an allergist or other appropriate physician to determine whether you have either food intolerance or food allergy.

According to Syed and others, there is currently no accepted treatment for food allergy. Current management involves avoidance of the offending food and emergency preparedness, particularly for anaphylaxis. Some foods, such as milk and eggs, may be denatured via extensive heating, then incorporated into the diet of children. Additionally, Kostadinova and others indicate allergen-specific immunotherapy may be effective; use of tablets or injections may strengthen the immune response to the allergen.

If you want to complain to the FDA about food-related illnesses, adverse events after taking dietary supplements, products not labeled for allergens, or other problems with food products, you may use the Consumer Complaint System.

www.fda.gov/Safety/ReportaProblem/ConsumerComplaint Coordinators/ To complain to the FDA about various food-related health problems, this site provides a contact phone number for your state and information to include in your report.

Key Concepts

▶ In general, current food biotechnology techniques, such as genetically modified (GM) food, help provide a food supply that is high quality and safe. However, preventing the introduction of allergy-causing ingredients in GM foods is a concern.

▶ Pesticide residues in most foods are minimal, but some foods may contain more than others. The major concern is reducing pesticide intake in children, as some scientists believe neurological development may be impaired.

▶ Although organic foods may contain lesser amounts of pesticides than conventional foods, they may not contain fewer bacteria or higher nutrient density. The available research

- is insufficient to determine whether consumption of organic foods confers any health benefits.
- ▶ Commercial food processing can provide safe and healthful foods. However, excess sugar and fat added during commercial food processing may dilute health benefits.
- ▶ Proper food preparation practices may help preserve the nutrient quality and safety of foods prepared at home.
- ▶ Certain individuals may be intolerant to various foods or experience allergic responses to others and thus should take precautions to avoid such foods.

Check for Yourself

- ▶ Check the food label for several commercial food products you love most. Check the list of ingredients. Do you recognize any of the additives?

Healthful Nutrition: Recommendations for Better Physical Performance

Sports nutrition for the physically active person may be viewed from two aspects: nutrition for training and nutrition for competition. Of the three basic purposes of food—to provide energy, to regulate metabolic processes, and to support growth and development—the first two are of prime importance during athletic competition, while all three must be considered during the training period in preparation for competition.

Articles about nutrition for athletes in popular sports magazines, and food supplements advertised therein, give the impression that athletes have special nutritional requirements above those of non-athletes. In general, however, the diet that is optimal for health is also optimal for physical or sports performance. The Prudent Healthy Diet will provide adequate food energy and nutrients to meet the need of almost all athletes in training and competition.

Nevertheless, modifications to the Prudent Healthy Diet may help enhance performance for certain athletic endeavors, and subsequent chapters will focus on specific recommendations relative to the use of various nutrients and dietary supplements to enhance physical performance. The purpose of this section is to provide some general recommendations regarding use of the Prudent Healthy Diet by the athlete for training and competition.

However, it is very important for athletes to individualize their dietary practices. The nutrient needs and dietary practices of athletes may vary significantly, such as daily carbohydrate intake of a golfer as compared to that of a marathon runner. All athletes should keep track of what, how much, and when they eat and drink during training and competition and experiment with dietary strategies to find those that are optimal. Several prominent sports organizations have developed nutrition guides for athletes. The United States Olympic Committee published a comprehensive guide to sports nutrition entitled the *Athlete's Plate,* providing details on a wide variety of topics such as caution when traveling internationally. The United States Anti-Doping Agency also published a pamphlet, *TrueSport® Nutrition Guide,* with a focus on a healthy diet designed to provide optimal dietary intake for sport and for life.

http://coachrey.com/volleyball-blog/wp-content /uploads/2014/04/USOC-Nutrition-Guide.pdf The *Athlete's Plate,* a guide to sports nutrition for the athlete, has been developed by the United States Olympic Committee.

www.usada.org/resources/nutrition/ The United States Anti-Doping Agency provides information on carbohydrate, protein, vitamins, and other nutrients relative to health and sport performance. A PDF file may be used to print the pamphlet.

What should I eat during training?

Both sport scientists and coaches stress the importance of proper nutrition during training. Ron Maughan, an expert in exercise metabolism and sports nutrition, notes that the main role of nutrition for the athlete may be to support consistent intensive training. As noted in chapter 1, optimal training is the most important factor contributing to improved sport performance.

Because energy expenditure increases during a training period, the caloric intake needed to maintain body weight may increase considerably—an additional 500–1,000 Calories or more per day in certain activities. By selecting these additional Calories wisely from a wide variety of foods, you should obtain an adequate amount of all nutrients essential for the formation of new body tissues and proper functioning of the energy systems that work harder during exercise. A balanced intake of carbohydrate, fat, protein, vitamins, minerals, and water is all that is necessary. For endurance athletes, dietary carbohydrates should receive even greater emphasis.

However, there may be some circumstances during sport training that make particular attention to the diet important. For example, during the early phases of training, the body will begin to make adjustments in the energy systems so that they become more efficient. This is the so-called **chronic training effect**, and many of the body's adjustments incorporate specific nutrients. For example, one of the chronic effects of long-distance running is an increased hemoglobin content in the blood and increased myoglobin and cytochromes in the muscle cells; all three compounds require iron in order to be formed. Hence, the daily diet would have to contain adequate amounts of iron not only to meet normal needs but also to make effective body adjustments due to the chronic effects of training.

Nutrient timing, the intake of carbohydrate and protein just before or after an intense training session, has been advocated to promote recovery and anabolism for several decades. However, Aragon and Schoenfeld indicated recent research has challenged its applicability to the athlete. Nevertheless, if convenient, consuming a carbohydrate/protein combination shortly before or after strenuous exercise may be a recommended procedure for some athletes. More details are presented in chapters 4 and 6.

Breakfast may be especially important during training. A balanced breakfast provides a significant amount of Calories and other nutrients in the daily diet of the physically active person. A breakfast of skim milk, a poached egg, whole-grain toast, fortified high-fiber cereal, and orange juice will help provide a substantial part of the RDA for protein, calcium, iron, fiber, vitamin C, and other nutrients and is relatively high in complex carbohydrates. A balanced breakfast high in fiber with an average amount of protein also will help prevent the onset of mid-morning hunger. The fiber and protein may help maintain a feeling of satiety throughout the morning, whereas a breakfast of refined carbohydrates, such as doughnuts, may trigger an insulin response and produce hypoglycemia (low blood sugar) in the middle of the morning. The resultant hunger is typically satisfied by eating other refined carbohydrates, which will satisfy the hunger urge only until about lunchtime. A balanced breakfast having a high nutrient density is therefore preferable to a breakfast based on refined carbohydrate products. Nontraditional breakfast foods, such as pizza, may also provide a balanced meal for breakfast.

Moreover, for young athletes, Nicklas and others have noted that breakfast consumption is an important factor in their nutritional well-being, enhancing their academic performance, an important consideration for those aspiring to college scholarships. Although individual preferences should be taken into account, a balanced breakfast could provide a good source of some major nutrients to the individual who is involved in a physical conditioning program. For those on a tight time schedule, a bowl of ready-to-eat, fortified high-fiber, protein-rich cereal with skim milk and fruit may be an ideal choice. Nancy Clark, a nationally acclaimed sports nutritionist, notes that this breakfast is not only quick, easy, and convenient but also rich in carbohydrate, fiber, iron, calcium, and vitamins.

Proper nutrition should enhance the physiological responses to training, and thus enhance competitive sports performance. The nutrient needs of athletes in training will be highlighted throughout the remainder of this text where relevant.

When and what should I eat just prior to competition?

In competition an athlete will utilize specific body energy sources and systems, depending upon the intensity and duration of the exercise. The three human energy systems will be discussed in detail in chapter 3. Briefly, however, high-energy compounds stored in the muscle are utilized during very short, high-intensity exercise; carbohydrate stored in the muscle as glycogen may be used without oxygen for intense exercise lasting about 1 to 3 minutes; and

the oxidation of glycogen and fats becomes increasingly important in endurance activities lasting longer than 5 minutes. The release of energy in each of these three systems may require certain vitamins and minerals for optimal efficiency.

If an individual is well nourished, athletic competition normally will not impose any special demands for any of the six major classes of nutrients. Body energy stores of carbohydrate and fat are adequate to satisfy the energy demands of most activities lasting less than 1 hour. Protein is not generally considered a significant energy source during exercise. The vitamin and mineral content of the body will be sufficient to help regulate the increased levels of metabolic activity, and body-water supply will be adequate under normal environmental conditions.

However, content and timing of the precompetition intake may be critical. It is a well-established fact that the ingestion of food just prior to competition will not benefit physical performance in most athletic events, yet the pregame meal, so to speak, is one of the major topics of discussion among athletes. A number of special meals have been utilized throughout the years because of their alleged benefits to physical performance, and special products have been marketed as pre-event nutritional supplements. Although research has not substantiated the value of any one particular precompetition meal, some general guidelines have been developed from practical experience over the years.

There are several major goals of the precompetition meal that may be achieved through proper timing and composition. In general, the precompetition meal should do the following:

1. *Allow the stomach to be relatively empty at the start of competition.* In general, a solid meal should be eaten about 3 to 4 hours prior to competition. This should allow ample time for digestion to occur so that the stomach is relatively empty yet hunger sensations are minimized. However, pre-event emotional tension or anxiety may delay digestive time, as will a meal with a high-fat or high-protein content. Hence, the composition of the meal is critical. It should be high in carbohydrate, low in fat, and low to moderate in protein, providing for easy digestibility.

2. *Help to prevent or minimize gastrointestinal distress.* The composition of the precompetition meal should not contribute to any gastrointestinal distress, such as flatulence, increased acidity in the stomach, heartburn, or increased bulk that may stimulate the need for a bowel movement during competition. In general, foods to be avoided include gas formers such as beans, spicy foods that may elicit heartburn, and bulk foods such as bran products. High-sugar compounds may delay gastric emptying or create a reverse osmotic effect, possibly increasing the fluid content of the stomach, which may lead to a feeling of distress, cramps, or nausea. High-sugar loads, particularly fructose, may also lead to other forms of gastrointestinal distress, such as diarrhea. Individuals with known food intolerances, such as lactose intolerance, should use due caution. Through experience, you should learn what foods disagree with you during performance and, of course, avoid these prior to competition.

3. *Help avoid sensations of hunger, light-headedness, or fatigue.* A small amount of protein in a carbohydrate meal will help

delay the onset of hunger. Large amounts of concentrated sugars can cause a reactive drop in blood sugar in susceptible individuals, which may cause light-headedness and fatigue.

4. *Provide adequate energy supplies, primarily carbohydrate, in the blood and muscles.* A wide variety of foods may be selected for the precompetition meal. The meal should consist of foods that are high in complex carbohydrates with moderate to low amounts of protein. Examples of such foods are presented in later chapters as well as in appendix D, particularly those in the starch list. The foods should be agreeable to you. You should eat what you like within the guidelines presented above.

5. *Provide an adequate amount of body water.* Adequate fluid intake should be assured prior to an event, particularly if the event will be of long duration or conducted under hot environmental conditions. Diuretics such as alcohol, which increase the excretion of body water, should be avoided. Large amounts of protein increase the water output of the kidneys and thus should be avoided. Fluids may be taken up to 15 to 30 minutes prior to competition to help ensure adequate hydration.

Two examples of precompetition meals, each containing about 500–600 Calories with substantial amounts of carbohydrate, are presented in table 2.18.

One important last point: Meals other than the precompetition meal eaten on the same day should not be skipped. They should adhere to the basic principles set forth earlier in this chapter. Authored by Helen DeMarco, the American College of Sports Medicine published recommendations, as follows, on pre-event meals scheduled at different times of the day.

- Morning events: The night before, eat a high-carbohydrate meal. Early morning, eat a light breakfast or snack: cereal and nonfat milk, fresh fruit or juice, toast, bagel or English muffin, pancakes or waffles, nonfat or low-fat fruit yogurt, or a liquid pre-event meal
- Afternoon events: Eat a high-carbohydrate meal both the night before and for breakfast. Follow with a light lunch: salads with low-fat dressings, turkey sandwiches with small portions of turkey, fruits, juice, low-fat crackers, high-carbohydrate nutritional bars, pretzels, rice cakes.
- Evening events: Eat a high-carbohydrate breakfast and lunch, followed by a light meal or snack: pasta with marinara sauce, rice with vegetables, light-cheese pizza with vegetable toppings, noodle or rice soups with crackers, baked potato, frozen yogurt.

TABLE 2.18	Two examples of precompetition meals containing 500–600 Calories
Meal A	**Meal B**
Glass of orange juice	One cup low-fat yogurt
One bowl of oatmeal	One banana
Two pieces of toast with jelly	One toasted bagel
Sliced peaches with skim milk	One ounce of turkey breast
	One-half cup of raisins

Pre-event nutritional strategies will vary somewhat for athletes involved in prolonged exercise tasks, such as running a marathon. As noted by prominent Australian exercise scientist Mark Hargreaves, body stores of both carbohydrate and fluids should be optimized. To achieve this goal, athletes may engage in practices such as carbohydrate loading and water hyperhydration, which will be detailed in chapters 4 and 9.

The ACSM notes that no one food or group of foods works for everybody; individuals may need to experiment to find which foods and amount of food that work best. Food choices may vary based on the type of exercise, as well as the intensity and duration of the exercise. However, it is important to experiment with new foods during training rather than around competition.

What should I eat during competition?

There is no need to consume anything during most types of athletic competition with the possible exception of carbohydrate and water. Carbohydrate may provide additional supplies of the preferred energy source during prolonged, high-intensity intermittent and endurance exercise, while water intake may be critical for regulation of body temperature when exercising in warm environments. In ultradistance competition, a hypotonic salt solution also may be recommended. Appropriate details are presented in chapters 4 and 9.

What should I eat after competition?

In general, a balanced diet is all that is necessary to meet your nutrient needs and restore your nutritional status to normal following competition or daily, hard physical training. Carbohydrate and fat are the main nutrients used during exercise and can be replaced easily from foods among the Food Exchange Lists. The increased caloric intake that is needed to replace your energy expenditure also will help provide you with the additional small amounts of protein, vitamins, minerals, and electrolytes that may be necessary for effective recovery. Thirst will normally help replace water losses on a day-to-day basis; you can check this by recording your body weight each morning to see if it is back to normal.

As noted previously, nutrient timing may be an important consideration. Simple sugars eaten immediately after a hard workout may help restore muscle glycogen fairly rapidly. Consuming a small amount of high-quality protein may also be prudent. Specific guidelines are presented in chapters 4 and 6.

For those who must compete several times daily and eat between competitions, such as in tennis tournaments or swim meets, the principles relative to pregame meals may be relevant, with a focus on carbohydrate-rich foods or fluids and moderate protein intake.

Should athletes use commercial sports foods?

The sports nutrition industry is booming. Numerous products are marketed to athletes, including meal replacement powders, sports drinks, sports bars, sports gels, sports candy, and sports supplements. It is important to note that although many of these products may be convenient and appropriate for a pregame, post-training, or postcompetition meal, they do not contain all the healthful nutrients found in natural foods and thus should not be used on a long-term basis to replace the Prudent Healthy Diet.

Liquid Sports Meals **Liquid meals**, many of them designed specifically for athletes, usually contain high-quality sources of carbohydrate and protein, a low-to-moderate fat content, vitamins and minerals, and various other supplements. The food label will provide the amounts of each. They are very convenient for precompetition meals as well as for recovery nutrition after training or competition.

Liquid meals available include Nutrament, Ensure, Slim-Fast, Boost, Gatorade Nutrition Shake, and PowerBar ProteinPlus. Some liquid meals come premixed, while others come as powders. You can make your own liquid sports meal, or *smoothie,* from high-quality carbohydrate/protein powders, such as whey powder, nonfat dry milk powder, and/or other healthful sources of carbohydrate and protein, such as yogurt and fruits. The following formula will provide 1 quart of a tasty liquid meal:

½ cup water/ice cubes
½ cup nonfat dry milk powder
¼ cup glucose polymer
1 frozen banana
3 cups cold skim milk
1 teaspoon flavoring for palatability (cherry, vanilla)

A liquid meal may be assimilated more readily than a solid meal, and thus may be useful as a precompetition meal because it may be taken closer to competition—say, 2 to 3 hours before. Research has shown that there is no difference between a liquid and a solid meal relative to subsequent hunger, nausea, diarrhea, or physical performance.

Sports Bars Sports bars have become increasingly popular in recent years, and several dozen products are targeted to physically active individuals. **Sports bars** vary in composition. Some are high carbohydrate, some are high protein, and some have nearly equal mixtures of carbohydrate, protein, and fat. Many are vitamin and mineral fortified, and some are designed to serve as a meal replacement. Others contain drugs, such as caffeine. As with liquid meals, the food label on the sports bar will describe its contents. When compared to comparable energy sources from ordinary food, sports bars do not possess any magical qualities to enhance physical performance, but they possess some advantages similar to liquid meals, such as convenience. Because the major ingredient in many sports bars is carbohydrate, an expanded discussion is presented in chapter 4.

Sports Drinks Sports drinks are generally referred to as carbohydrate and electrolyte replacement fluids and may be consumed by athletes before, during, and after training and competition. Examples include Gatorade and Powerade. They are designed to provide carbohydrate, water, and electrolytes, and their role in sport is discussed in chapters 4 and 9.

Sports Gels and Candy Sports gels and candy normally provide carbohydrate but may contain other substances such as vitamins, minerals, and caffeine. Their primary purpose is to provide a source of easily digested carbohydrates for energy during exercise.

Sports Supplements As noted in chapter 1, numerous sports supplements are marketed to athletes, including various forms of carbohydrates, fats, and protein; many vitamins and minerals; several food drugs; and selected herbal or botanical products. Based on the available scientific data, the use of most sports supplements does not appear to be necessary for the well-nourished athlete during training. However, nutrient supplementation may be warranted in some cases. For example, in activities where excess body weight may handicap performance, a loss of some body fat may be helpful. During weight loss, vitamin-mineral supplements may be recommended to prevent a nutrient deficiency. Athletes may use sports supplements in attempts to enhance performance, and in their review Russell and Kingsley noted that the use of nutritional ergogenic aids in team sports such as soccer is now commonplace. Use of several sports supplements has been supported by research because they may enhance physical performance, may not pose any health risks, and may be legal. Research evaluating the effectiveness of purported sport ergogenics is presented throughout the book. Pertinent discussion topics include the following.

Chapter 4: Carbohydrate ergogenics
Chapter 5: Ergogenics that affect fat metabolism
Chapter 6: Amino acids, creatine, and other protein-related ergogenics
Chapter 7: Vitamins and other vitamin-related ergogenics
Chapter 8: Mineral ergogenics
Chapter 9: Glycerol
Chapter 13: Alcohol, caffeine, and other food-drug and herbal ergogenics

How can I eat more nutritiously while traveling for competition?

Athletes who must travel to compete are often faced with the problem of obtaining proper pre-event and postevent nutrition. After reading this chapter, you should be aware of how to select foods that are high in carbohydrate, low in fat, and moderate in protein. More guidelines are presented in chapters 4 through 6.

One possible solution is to pack your own food and fluids in a traveling bag or cooler. Foods from each of the Food Exchange Lists can be easily packed or kept on ice, such as skim milk; precooked low-fat meats; bagels and cereal; fruits, juices, and vegetables; sports drinks; and high-carbohydrate snacks, including whole wheat crackers and pretzels and low-fat cookies such as Fig Newtons and vanilla wafers. Small containers of condiments can also be easily transported in the cooler, along with proper eating utensils. Taking your own food means you can eat your pre-event or postevent meal as planned, and you may save money as well. Such an approach may be very effective for short, one-day trips and may be used to complement other meals on longer journeys. Some easily packed snack foods are presented in table 2.19.

TABLE 2.19　Easily packed snacks for traveling or brown bag lunches

Grains	Meats/Others	Vegetables
Bagels	Small can of baked beans	Sliced carrots
Pita bread	Cooked chicken or turkey, small 2-ounce commercial	Broccoli stalks
Muffins	packages, packed in airtight plastic bags	Cauliflower pieces
Fig Newtons	Small can of tuna fish, salmon, or sardines	Tomatoes
Vanilla wafers	Peanut butter	Canned vegetable juices
Whole wheat crackers and pretzels	Reduced-fat cheese slices	Cherry tomatoes
Graham crackers	String cheese	
Dry cereals	Hummus	
Wheat Chex	Turkey breast	
Grapenuts		
Plain popcorn		

Fruits	Milk	Nuts
Small cans of fruit in own juice	Small containers of skim or low-fat milk; chocolate milk;	Almonds
Small containers of fruit juice, aseptic	aseptic packaging if available	Walnuts
packages	Dried skim milk powder, to be reconstituted	
Oranges	Packaged yogurt	
Apples		
Other raw fruits		
Dried fruits		

While traveling, you have a variety of eating places from which to select your food, including full-service restaurants, restaurants with all-you-can-eat buffets, steakhouses and fishhouses, fast-food restaurants, pizza parlors, sub shops, supermarkets, convenience stores, and even vending machines. With a solid background on the nutritional principles presented in this chapter, you should be able to select healthful, high-carbohydrate and low-fat foods at any of these establishments but, of course, the variety of food choices will vary depending on the place you choose. Keep in mind that you can always ask to see if they will create a meal for you. For example, order a salad and ask to have extra vegetables and fish or chicken breast added, with the dressing on the side.

Although all fast foods can be part of a healthy diet when consumed in moderation, many are relatively high in fat content, and their intake should be restricted. However, many restaurants do provide a few healthier choices with individual sandwiches containing less than 30 percent of their Calories from fat, including grilled or broiled chicken, lean roast beef, and veggie burgers. In some cases, particularly with grilled, skinless chicken sandwiches, much of the fat content is in the sauce added to the sandwich, so ordering the sauce on the side allows you to control the amount added. Other sandwich shops, such as Au Bon Pain and Subway, may serve healthful sandwiches, but unwise selections in these stores may also contain substantial amounts of fat.

You can eat fast food and stay within the recommended nutrition guidelines for a healthy diet, but obtaining a healthful diet requires careful selection of foods. Fast-food restaurants provide materials detailing the nutrient content of each of their products. In some cases the materials may be obtained in the restaurant, and all have Websites detailing nutrient analysis of their products. See appendix E for appropriate Websites.

The following suggestions may be helpful if you are dining in a fast-food or budget-type restaurant, such as McDonald's, Wendy's, Arby's, Pizza Hut, Baja Fresh, Applebee's, or Ruby Tuesday. Many supermarkets also have takeout departments or salad bars from which to select lunch or dinner.

Breakfast selections

English muffins, unbuttered, with jelly
English muffins with Canadian bacon
Whole wheat pancakes with syrup
French toast
Bran muffins, fat-free or low-fat
Hot whole-grain cereal, oatmeal
Ready-to-eat fortified, high-fiber cereal
Skim or low-fat milk
Orange juice
Hot cocoa

Lunch or dinner selections

Any low-fat sandwiches, no mayonnaise or high-fat sauces
Grilled chicken breast sandwich, on whole-grain bun
Baked or broiled fish sandwich
Lean roast beef sandwich, on whole-grain bun
Single, plain hamburger, on whole-grain bun
Baked potato, with toppings on the side (add sparingly)
Pasta dishes, spaghetti, and macaroni, with low-fat sauces
Rice dishes
Lo mein noodles, not chow mein (fried noodles)
Soups, rice and noodle
Salsas, made with tomatoes
Chicken or seafood tostadas, made with cornmeal tortillas

Bean and rice dishes

All whole-grain and other breads

Salads, low-fat dressing

Salad bar, focus on vegetables and high-carbohydrate foods; avoid high-fat items

Pizza, thick crust, vegetable type with minimum cheese topping

Skim or low-fat milk; chocolate milk

Orange juice

Frozen yogurt, fat-free or low-fat

Sherbet

With any of these selections, it is always a good idea to order toppings, for example, mayonnaise, salad dressing, and so on, on the side so that you can control portions. When selecting sandwiches, ask for those that are either baked, broiled, or grilled.

Athletes who travel internationally for competition should use special caution, including the following:

- Drink only bottled water and other beverages.
- Avoid use of tap water.
- Eat only food that is fully cooked.
- Do not eat raw foods.
- Do not eat food from street vendors.

How do gender and age influence nutritional recommendations for enhanced physical performance?

The diet that is optimal for health is the optimal diet for physical performance. This is the key principle of sports nutrition and it applies to physically active males and females of all ages. However, as shall be noted at certain points in this text, specific nutrient needs may vary by gender and age, and various forms of exercise training may influence nutrient requirements as well.

Gender Seiler and others note that exercise performance is, in general, about 10 percent greater in males than females, mainly because males have greater levels of muscle mass and strength, anaerobic power and capacity, and maximal aerobic capacity, as well as lower levels of body fat. Nevertheless, most physiological adaptations to exercise are similar for males and females. Moreover, Maughan and Shirreffs, discussing nutrition and hydration needs of football (soccer) players, noted that the differences between males and females are smaller than differences between individuals, so principles developed for male players also apply to women. However, some physiological differences between males and females could influence nutritional requirements.

Adolescent and adult premenopausal females need more dietary iron than males. Female athletes, especially those participating in aerobic endurance sports such as distance running, must include iron-rich foods in their diet or risk incurring iron-deficiency anemia and impaired running ability.

Being smaller in size, women need fewer Calories than men, yet many may not consume adequate energy and may develop disordered eating practices as they attempt to lose body mass for competition purposes. Disordered eating is more prevalent in female athletes and may contribute to the development of premature osteoporosis due to calcium imbalance. A discussion of the topic, relative to energy deficiency in sport, which is also referred to as the female athlete triad, is presented in chapters 8 and 10.

http://reference.medscape.com/article/108994-overview#aw2aab6b3   This site provides some detailed information on the nutrition needs of the female athlete.

Age Youth sports competition is worldwide, ranging from community-based games to Olympic competition, and proper nutrition is important for these young athletes. Petrie and others have noted that child and adolescent athletes typically consume more food to meet their energy expenditure and thus are more likely to obtain an adequate supply of nutrients. However, Oded Bar-Or noted that while nutritional considerations are similar for all athletes irrespective of age, children have several physiological characteristics that may require specific nutritional considerations. For example, their relative protein needs may be greater to support growth, and their relative calcium needs may be greater for optimal bone development. Young athletes may experience greater thermal stress during exercise. Roberts indicates it may be unwise to allow children to exercise hard in high heat and humidity conditions, but also notes that there are few data to support this concern. Those who participate in weight-control sports involving excessive exercise and inadequate energy intake may be at risk for nutrient deficiencies and impaired growth and development. The American Academy of Pediatrics has developed a policy stand on promotion of healthy weight-control practices in young athletes.

http://kidshealth.org/kid/stay_healthy/food/sports.html
Eating for Sports provides some useful dietary information for young athletes, with sections designed for kids and for their parents.

Sport participation is also very popular at the other end of the age spectrum, and older athletes may also have special nutrient needs. In general, resting metabolism declines in older age, so caloric need may decrease. Older people also eat less, so they need to make wiser food choices, that is, foods with high nutrient density. Campbell and Geik noted that nutrition is a tool that the older athlete should use to enhance exercise performance and health. In particular, they noted that older athletes may need to focus on obtaining sufficient micronutrients, such as the B vitamins and vitamin D. Supplements may be recommended to obtain adequate vitamin B_{12} and calcium if not obtained from the diet, such as from fortified foods. Female athletes over age 50, because of decreased estrogen levels associated with menopause, need to focus on obtaining adequate calcium. However, they may need less dietary iron compared to their younger counterparts. Older individuals also need to ensure adequate fluid intake because of increased susceptibility to dehydration.

www.ideafit.com/fitness-library/nutrition-needs-of-senior-athletes   The IDEA Health & Fitness Association presents tips on how nutrition may help improve performance in physically active older adults.

The special nutrient requirements of females, the young, and the elderly, as they relate to physical activity, will be incorporated into the text where relevant. However, most of the nutritional principles underlying exercise and sports performance that are presented in this text apply to most physically active individuals.

www.eatright.org/Public/   The Academy of Nutrition and Dietetics provides detailed information on a wide array of sport nutrition topics. Click on Sports and Exercise.

What apps are available to help me in my quest to develop a diet plan to improve both my health and my sports performance?

There are hundreds, if not thousands, of software programs designed to promote health through diet and/or exercise. Such a program is known as an application, or app, and is most commonly used in conjunction with a smartphone. Two popular versions are the Apple and Android models. Many may be used free of charge, while others carry small fees.

Various apps may be mentioned throughout this text, but keep in mind that such apps constantly are being upgraded and newer models also may appear on the marketplace. Here are several that may help you plan a healthier diet. The comments are current as this book went to press.

- Nutrino—Enter your current weight and your goal weight, along with your food preferences, and a personalized diet will be developed for you. This app is available at the Apple Store and is free.

- Fooducate—Scan bar codes on food labels at the grocery, and view important nutrition information, both good and bad, about the product. It rates the product with a nutrient grade from A to D. Basic model is free but fee-based for advanced version.
- Healty Out—Search for healthy choices at local restaurants that match your preferences.

To find an app suitable for your goals, you can use a search engine such as Google, entering terms such as *Healthy Eating Apps* or *Fitness Apps* to find a wide variety of possibilities.

Key Concepts

▶ The precompetition meal should be easily digestible, high in carbohydrates, moderate in protein, and low in fat, and it should be consumed about 3–4 hours prior to competition. Athletes should determine what types of foods are compatible with their sport.

▶ Liquid meals and sports bars may be convenient as an occasional meal replacement, including use as a precompetition meal, but should be used only occasionally and not serve as a substitute for healthful whole foods.

▶ A healthful diet is the key to nutrition for male and female athletes at all age levels. However, female, young, and older athletes may have some specific nutritional needs in certain circumstances.

Check for Yourself

▶ Interview a coach or some athletes at your school about their meal strategies prior to competition. How do their strategies compare with general recommendations?

APPLICATION EXERCISE

In the Application Exercise in chapter 1, we recommended that you evaluate your normal daily diet with one or more of the dietary assessment instruments. Switch to a vegetarian diet, as close to a vegan diet as possible, for a day or two and use the same dietary assessment. Compare the results.

1. The guide to eating from the United States Department of Agriculture, MyPlate, has five food groups. Which of the following is *not* considered an official food group by the USDA?
   a. grains
   b. protein
   c. oils
   d. fruit
   e. dairy
   f. vegetables

2. Which of the following is not an acceptable definition for food labels with the listing "free"?
   a. fat free—less than 0.5 gram of total fat per serving
   b. cholesterol free—less than 2 milligrams per serving
   c. sugar free—less than 0.5 gram per serving
   d. Calorie free—less than 40 Calories per serving
   e. sodium free—less than 5 milligrams per serving

3. Approximately how many Calories are in a meal with two starch/bread exchanges, four lean meat exchanges, one fruit exchange, two vegetable exchanges, three fat exchanges, and one skim milk exchange?
   a. 450
   b. 540
   c. 670
   d. 715
   e. 780

4. Which of the following statements regarding consumer nutrition is false?
   a. Dietary supplements include vitamins, minerals, amino acids, herbals and botanicals, and various extracts and metabolites.

   b. Genetically modified foods may be designed to increase the content of a specific nutrient.
   c. Organic foods are healthier than conventional foods because they contain fewer bacteria and substantially more healthful nutrients.
   d. Various products in foods may cause food intolerance or food allergies in susceptible individuals.
   e. Food poisoning may be fatal.

5. Which of the following is not a key (indicator) nutrient as defined by the key-nutrient concept?
   a. iron
   b. calcium
   c. vitamin A
   d. protein
   e. vitamin D
   f. riboflavin
   g. niacin
   h. All are key nutrients.

6. The recommended dietary goals for healthy Americans suggest that the intake of saturated fat, as a percentage of daily Calories, be less than what percent?
   a. 10
   b. 20
   c. 30
   d. 40
   e. 50

7. Which key nutrient is not usually found in substantial amounts in the meat group?
   a. vitamin C
   b. iron
   c. protein
   d. niacin
   e. thiamin

8. A food label lists the amount of complex carbohydrates as 5 grams, the amount of simple sugars as 10 grams, the amount of protein as 5 grams, and the amount of fat as 10 grams. Which of the following is true?
   a. Simple sugars make up the majority of the Calories.
   b. Carbohydrate makes up the majority of the Calories.
   c. The amount of Calories from protein and carbohydrate is equal.
   d. The majority of the Calories is derived from fat.
   e. None of the above statements is true.

9. A vegetarian-type diet may be more healthful than the current typical American diet for all of the following reasons *except* which?
   a. higher in iron
   b. higher in fiber
   c. lower in saturated fats
   d. a higher polyunsaturated to saturated fat ratio
   e. lower in cholesterol

10. Which of the following is a recommendation for the precompetition meal for an endurance athlete who will be competing in warm environmental conditions?
    a. water
    b. sports drinks
    c. high carbohydrate content
    d. moderate protein content
    e. moderate salt content
    f. all of the above

Answers to multiple choice questions:
1. c; 2. d; 3. d; 4. c; 5. e; 6. a; 7. a; 8. d; 9. a; 10. f.

1. Name the eight key nutrients and identify a food source that is particularly rich in each nutrient. For example, lean meat is a rich source of iron.

2. Discuss the five categories of foods depicted in the MyPlate design in respect to the concepts of variety, proportionality, and moderation.

3. Compare and contrast the MyPlate food guide with the Food Exchange System. What similarities and differences do you note?

4. List and explain the potential health benefits of a vegan diet as compared to the typical American diet today.

5. Identify the nutrients that must be listed on food labels, how the DV is determined for each, and why you may want to have a high percent of the DV for some and a low percent for others.

Books

American Dietetic Association and American Diabetes Association. 1995. *Exchange Lists for Meal Planning.* Chicago: American Dietetic Association.

American Institute for Cancer Research. 2007. *Food, Nutrition, Physical Activity, and the Prevention of Cancer: A Global Perspective.* Washington, DC: AICR.

Bratman, S. 2000. *Health Food Junkies: Overcoming the Obsession with Healthful Eating.* New York: Bantam Doubleday.

Larson-Meyer, D. 2007. *Vegetarian Sports Nutrition.* Champaign, IL: Human Kinetics.

National Academy of Sciences. Institute of Medicine, Food and Nutrition Board. 2011. *Dietary Reference Intakes for Calcium and Vitamin D.* Washington, DC: National Academies Press.

National Academy of Sciences. Institute of Medicine, Food and Nutrition Board. 2004. *Dietary Reference Intakes for Water, Potassium, Sodium, Chloride, and Sulfate.* Washington, DC: National Academies Press.

National Academy of Sciences. Institute of Medicine, Food and Nutrition Board. 2002. *Dietary Reference Intakes for Vitamin A, Vitamin K, Arsenic, Boron, Chromium, Copper, Iodine, Iron, Manganese, Molybdenum, Nickel, Silicon, Vanadium, and Zinc.* Washington, DC: National Academies Press.

National Academy of Sciences. Institute of Medicine, Food and Nutrition Board. 2002. *Dietary Reference Intakes for Energy, Carbohydrates, Fiber, Fat, Protein and Amino Acids (Macronutrients).* Washington, DC: National Academies Press.

National Academy of Sciences. Institute of Medicine, Food and Nutrition Board. 2000. *Dietary Reference Intakes for Thiamin, Riboflavin, Niacin, Vitamin B6, Folate, Vitamin B12, Pantothenic Acid, Biotin, and Choline.* Washington, DC: National Academies Press.

National Academy of Sciences. Institute of Medicine, Food and Nutrition Board. 2000. *Dietary Reference Intakes for Vitamin C, Vitamin E, Selenium, and Carotenoids.* Washington, DC: National Academies Press.

National Academy of Sciences. Institute of Medicine, Food and Nutrition Board.

1999. *Dietary Reference Intakes for Calcium, Phosphorus, Magnesium, Vitamin D, and Fluoride.* Washington, DC: National Academies Press.

National Research Council. 1989. *Diet and Health: Implications for Reducing Chronic Disease Risk.* Washington, DC: National Academies Press.

Otten, J., et al. 2000. *Dietary Reference Intakes: The Essential Guide to Nutrient Requirements.* Washington, DC: National Academies Press.

Ross, C. et al. (Eds.). 2014. *Modern Nutrition in Health and Disease.* Philadelphia: Lippincott Williams & Wilkins.

U.S. Department of Agriculture and U.S. Department of Health and Human Services. 2015. *Nutrition and Your Health: Dietary Guidelines for Americans.* Washington, DC: U.S. Government Printing Office.

U.S. Department of Health and Human Services. 2010. *Healthy People 2020: National Health Promotion and Disease Prevention Objectives.* Washington, DC: U.S. Government Printing Office.

Reviews and Specific Studies

Allen, K., et al. 2006. Food allergy in childhood. *Medical Journal of Australia* 185:394–400.

American Academy of Pediatrics. 2005. Promotion of healthy weight-control practices in young athletes. *Pediatrics* 116:1557–64.

American Academy of Pediatrics, Council on Environmental Health. 2012. Pesticide exposure in children. *Pediatrics* 130:1757–63.

American Cancer Society 2001 Nutrition and Physical Activity Guidelines Advisory Committee. 2002. American Cancer Society guidelines on nutrition and physical activity for cancer prevention: Reducing the risk of cancer with healthy food choices and physical activity. *CA: A Cancer Journal for Clinicians* 52:92–119.

American Diabetes Association. 2003. Evidence-based nutrition principles and recommendations for the treatment and prevention of diabetes and related complications. *Diabetes Care* 26:S51–61.

American Dietetic Association. 2009. Position of the American Dietetic Association: Functional foods. *Journal of the American Dietetic Association* 109:735–46.

American Dietetic Association. 2009. Position of the American Dietetic Association: Vegetarian diets. *Journal of the American Dietetic Association* 109:1266–82.

American Dietetic Association. 2009. Position of the American Dietetic Association: Nutrient supplementation. *Journal of the American Dietetic Association* 109:2073–85.

American Dietetic Association. 2000. *10 Tips to Healthy Eating.* Chicago: ADA.

American Heart Association. 2006. Diet and lifestyle recommendations revision 2006: A scientific statement from the American Heart Association Nutrition Committee. *Circulation* 114:82–96.

American Heart Association. 2002. *Dietary Guidelines for Healthy Children.* Dallas: AHA.

Aragon, A., and Schoenfeld, B. 2013. Nutrient timing revisited: Is there a post-exercise anabolic window: Post-exercise nutrient timing. *Journal of the International Society of Sport Sciences* 10:5.

Barański, M., et al. 2014. Higher antioxidant and lower cadmium concentrations and lower incidence of pesticide residues in organically grown crops: A systematic literature review and meta-analyses. *British Journal of Nutrition* 112:794–81.

Bar-Or, O. 2001. Nutritional considerations for the child athlete. *Canadian Journal of Applied Physiology* 26:S186–91.

Barr, S., and Rideout, C. 2004. Nutritional considerations for vegetarian athletes. *Nutrition* 20:696–703.

Bawa, A., and Anilakumar, K. 2013. Genetically modified foods: Safety, risks and public concerns-a review. *Journal of Food Science and Technology* 50:1035–46.

Campbell, W., and Geik, R. 2004. Nutritional considerations for the older athlete. *Nutrition* 20:603–8.

Castro, G., and Castro, J. 2014. Alcohol drinking and mammary cancer: Pathogenesis and potential dietary preventive alternatives. *World Journal of Clinical Oncology* 5:713–29.

Center for Science in the Public Interest. 2008. Chemical cuisine: A guide to food additives. *Nutrition Action Health Letter* 35 (4):1–8.

Center for Science in the Public Interest. 2006. Eating green: The case for a plant-based diet. *Nutrition Action Health Letter* 33 (7):3–7.

Center for Science in the Public Interest. 2006. Fear of fresh. *Nutrition Action Health Letter* 33 (10):3–6.

Center for Science in the Public Interest. 2002. Genetically engineered foods: Are they safe? *Nutrition Action Health Letter* 28 (9):1–8.

Center for Science in the Public Interest. 1999. Chemical cuisine. *Nutrition Action Health Letter* 26 (2):4–9.

Clark, N. 1987. Breakfast of champions. *Physician and Sportsmedicine* 15(January):209–12.

Claus, S. P. 2014. Development of personalized functional foods needs metabolic profiling. *Current Opinion in Clinical Nutrition and Metabolic Care* 17:567–73.

Cohen, R. 2013. Sugar love (a not so sweet story). *National Geographic* 224 (2):78–97.

Consumer Reports. 2015. GMOs: Your right to know. *Consumer Reports* 80 (3): 7, 12–14.

Consumer Reports. 2014. America's best & worst fast food. *Consumer Reports* 79 (8):15–21.

Consumer Reports. 2013. Eat your way to good health. *Consumer Reports on Health* 25 (8):1, 4–5.

Consumer Reports. 2010. Dangerous supplements. *Consumer Reports* 75 (9):16–23.

Consumers Union. 2007. Dirty birds. *Consumer Reports* 72 (1):20–23.

Consumers Union. 2007. Functional—or dysfunctional—foods. *Consumer Reports on Health* 19 (2):8–9.

Consumers Union. 2007. Eat right, at any age. *Consumer Reports on Health* 19 (8):1, 4–5.

Consumers Union. 2006. Buy quality organic foods and save. *Consumer Reports* 71 (2):12–17.

Consumers Union. 2006. Diet and cancer: Can one size fit all? *Consumer Reports on Health* 18 (11):8–9.

Consumers Union. 2005. 'Super' foods: Do you really need them. *Consumer Reports on Health* 17 (6):1, 4–6.

Consumers Union. 2005. You are what they eat. *Consumer Reports* 70 (1):26–31.

Consumers Union. 2003. The truth about irradiated meat. *Consumer Reports* 68 (8):34–37.

Consumers Union. 2002. How safe is that burger? *Consumer Reports* 67 (11):29–35.

Craig, W. 2009. Health effects of vegan diets. *American Journal of Clinical Nutrition* 89:1627S–33S.

Crowe, K., and Francis, C. 2013. Position of the Academy of Nutrition and Dietetics:

Functional foods. *Journal of the Academy of Nutrition and Dietetics* 113:1096–103.

Dangour, A., et al. 2010. Nutrition-related health effects of organic foods: A systematic review. *American Journal of Clinical Nutrition* 92:203–10.

Dickinson, A., and MacKay, D. 2014. Health habits and other characteristics of dietary supplement users: A review. *Nutrition Journal* 13:14. doi:10.1186/1475-2891-13-14.

Doust, E., et al. 2014. Is pesticide exposure a cause of obstructive airways disease? *European Respiratory Review* 23:180–92.

Dwyer, J., et al. 2014. Fortification: New findings and implications. *Nutrition Reviews* 72:127–41.

Eckel, R. 2014. Association Task Force on Practice 2013 AHA/ACC guideline on lifestyle management to reduce cardiovascular risk. *Journal of the American College of Cardiology* 63(25 Pt B):2960–84.

Fairfield, K., and Fletcher, R. 2002. Vitamins for chronic disease prevention in adults. *Journal of the American Medical Association* 287:3116–26.

Fletcher, R., and Fairfield, K. 2002. Vitamins for chronic disease prevention in adults: Clinical applications. *Journal of the American Medical Association* 287:3127–29.

Freeland-Graves, J., and Nitzke, S. 2013. Position of the Academy of Nutrition and Dietetics: Total diet approach to healthy eating. *Journal of the Academy of Nutrition and Dietetics* 113:307–17.

Fuhrman, J., and Ferreri, D. 2010. Fueling the vegetarian (vegan) athlete. *Current Sports Medicine Reports* 9:233–41.

Fulton, S., et al. 2014. The effect of increasing fruit and vegetable consumption on overall diet: A systematic review and meta-analysis. *Critical Reviews in Food Science and Nutrition* (August 13).

Gibbons, A. 2014. The evolution of diet. *National Geographic* 226 (3):34–61.

Gotsis, E., et al. 2015. Health benefits of the Mediterranean diet: An update of research over the last 5 years. *Angiology* 66:307–18.

Hargreaves, M. 2001. Pre-exercise nutritional strategies: Effects on metabolism and performance. *Canadian Journal of Applied Physiology* 26:S64–70.

Hawley, J., et al. 2006. Promoting training adaptations through nutritional interventions. *Journal of Sports Sciences* 24:709–21.

International Food Information Council Foundation. 1999. Myths and facts

about food biotechnology. *Food Insight* (September/October):2–3.

Katz, D., et al. 2015. Effects of egg ingestion on endothelial function in adults with coronary heart disease: A randomized, controlled, crossover trial. *American Heart Journal* 169:162–9.

Kostadinova, A., et al. 2013. Immunotherapy—risk/benefit in food allergy. *Pediatric Allergy and Immunology* 24:633–44.

Kramkowska, M., et al. 2013. Benefits and risks associated with genetically modified food products. *Annals of Agriculture and Environmental Medicine* 20:413–9.

Lieberman, H. et al. 2015. Patterns of dietary supplement use among college students. *Clinical Nutrition* 34:976–85.

Liebman, B. 2013. Six reasons to eat less red meat. *Nutrition Action Health Letter* 40(5):3–7.

Magkos, F., et al. 2006. Organic food: Buying more safety or just peace of mind? A critical review of the literature. *Critical Reviews in Food Science & Nutrition* 46:23–56.

Martins, Y., et al. 1999. Restrained eating among vegetarians: Does a vegetarian eating style mask concerns about weight? *Appetite* 32:145–54.

Maughan, R. 2002. The athlete's diet: Nutritional goals and dietary strategies. *Proceedings of the Nutrition Society* 6:87–96.

Maughan, R., and Shirreffs, S. 2007. Nutrition and hydration concerns of the female football player. *British Journal of Sports Medicine* 41 (Supplement 1):60–63.

Meadows, M. 2007. How the FDA works to keep produce safe. *FDA Consumer* 41 (2):13–19.

Moses, V., and Brookes, G. 2013. The world of "GM-free." *GM Crops & Food* 4:135–42.

Mozaffarian, D., and Rimm, E. 2006. Fish intake, contaminants, and human health: Evaluating the risks and the benefits. *Journal of the American Medical Association* 296:1885–99.

Muñoz-Quezada, M., et al. 2013. Neurodevelopmental effects in children associated with exposure to organophosphate pesticides: A systematic review. *Neurotoxicology* 39:158–68.

Needham, L., et al. 2005. Concentrations of environmental chemicals associated with neurodevelopmental effects in U.S. population. *Neurotoxicology* 26:531–45.

Neltner, T., et al. 2013. Conflicts of interest in approvals of additives to food determined to be generally recognized as safe: Out of balance. *JAMA Internal Medicine* 173:2032–6.

Nicklas, T., et al. 1998. Nutrient contribution of breakfast, secular trends, and the role of ready-to-eat cereals: A review of data from the Bogalusa Heart Study. *American Journal of Clinical Nutrition* 67:757S–763S.

Nielsen, F. H. 2014. Should bioactive trace elements not recognized as essential, but with beneficial health effects, have intake recommendations. *Journal of Trace Elements in Medicine and Biology.* 28:406–8.

O'Neil, C., et al. 2010. Whole-grain consumption is associated with diet quality and nutrient intake in adults: The National Health and Nutrition Examination Survey, 1999–2004. *Journal of the American Dietetic Association* 110:1461–8.

Ortega, R. 2006. Importance of functional foods in the Mediterranean diet. *Public Health Nutrition* 9:1136–40.

Palupi, E., et al. 2012. Comparison of nutritional quality between conventional and organic dairy products: A meta-analysis. *Journal of the Science of Food and Agriculture* 92:2774–81.

Pawlak, R., et al. 2014. The prevalence of cobalamin deficiency among vegetarians assessed by serum vitamin B12: a review of literature. *European Journal of Clinical Nutrition* 68:541–48.

Petrie, H., et al. 2004. Nutritional concerns for the child and adolescent competitor. *Nutrition* 20:620–31.

Roberts, W. O. 2007. Can children and adolescents run marathons? *Sports Medicine* 37:299–301.

Rock, C. 2007. Multivitamin-multimineral supplements: Who uses them? *American Journal of Clinical Nutrition* 85:277S–79S.

Rong, Y., et al. 2013. Egg consumption and risk of coronary heart disease and stroke: Dose-response meta-analysis of prospective cohort studies. *BMJ* 346:e8539.

Rosenbloom, C., et al. 2006. Special populations: The female player and the youth player. *Journal of Sports Sciences* 24:783–93.

Rothman, R., et al. 2006. Patient understanding of food labels: The role of literacy and numeracy. *American Journal of Preventive Medicine* 31:391–98.

Russell, M., and Kingsley, M. 2014. The efficacy of acute nutritional interventions on soccer skill performance. *Sports Medicine* 44:957–70.

Schardt, D. 2007. Organic foods: Worth the price? *Nutrition Action Health Letter* 34 (6):3–8.

Seiler, S., et al. 2007 . The fall and rise of the gender difference in elite anaerobic performance, 1952–2006. Medicine and Science in Sports & Exercise 39:534–40.

Sicherer, S., and Sampson, H. 2013. Food allergy: Epidemiology, pathogenesis, diagnosis, and treatment. *Journal of Allergy and Clinical Immunology* 133:291–307.

Smith-Spangler, C., et al. 2012. Are organic foods safer or healthier than conventional alternatives? A systematic review. *Annals of Internal Medicine* 157:348–66.

Snell, C., et al. 2012. Assessment of the health impact of GM plant diets in long-term and multigenerational animal feeding trials: A literature review. *Food and Chemical Toxicology* 50:1134–48.

Swaminathan, A., and Jicha, G. 2014. Nutrition and prevention of Alzheimer's dementia. *Frontiers in Aging Neuroscience* 6:282; 10.3389/fnagi.2014.00282.

Syed, A., et al. 2013. Food allergy diagnosis and therapy: Where are we now? *Immunotherapy* 5:931–44.

Tang, J., et al. 2009. Ingestion of whey hydrolysate, casein, or soy protein isolate: Effects on mixed muscle protein synthesis at rest and following resistance exercise in young men. *Journal of Applied Physiology* 107:987–92.

Torgerson, P., et al. 2014. The global burden of foodborne parasitic diseases: An update. *Trends in Parasitology* 30:20–6.

Tufts University. 2008. Can you afford to eat right? *Health & Nutrition Letter* 26 (3):4–5.

Van Maele-Fabry, G., et al. 2006. Review and meta-analysis of risk estimates for prostate cancer in pesticide manufacturing workers. *Cancer Causes & Control* 17:353–73.

Vannice, G., Rasmussen, H. 2014. Position of the Academy of Nutrition and Dietetics: Dietary fatty acids for healthy adults. *Journal of the Academy of Nutrition and Dietetics* 114:136–53.

Venderley, A., and Campbell, W. 2006. Vegetarian diets: Nutritional considerations for athletes. *Sports Medicine* 36:293–305.

Virk-Baker, M., et al. 2014. Dietary acrylamide and human cancer: A systematic review of literature. *Nutrition and Cancer* 66:774–90.

Volek, J., et al. 2006. Nutritional aspects of women strength athletes. *British Journal of Sports Medicine* 40:742–48.

Wang, X., et al. 2014. Fruit and vegetable consumption and mortality from all causes, cardiovascular disease, and cancer: Systematic review and dose-response meta-analysis of prospective cohort studies. *BMJ* 349:g4490.

Weaver, C., et al. 2014. Processed foods: Contributions to nutrition. *American Journal of Clinical Nutrition* 99:1525–42.

Weiss, B., et al. 2004. Pesticides. *Pediatrics* 113:1030–36.

Willett, W. 2006. The Mediterranean diet: Science and practice. *Public Health & Nutrition* 9:105–10.

Williams, C. 2006. Nutrition to promote recovery from exercise. *Sports Science Exchange* 19 (1):1–6.

Williams, C. 2002. Nutritional quality of organic food: Shades of grey or shades of green? *Proceedings of the Nutrition Society* 61:19–24.

Williams, M. 2008. Nutrition for the school aged child athlete. In *The Young Athlete,* eds. H. Hebestreit and O. Bar-Or. Oxford: Blackwell.

Wood, O., and Bruhn, C. 2000. Position of the American Dietetic Association: Food irradiation. *Journal of the American Dietetic Association* 100:246–53.

Woolf, S. 2006. Weighing the evidence to formulate dietary guidelines. *Journal of the American College of Nutrition* 25:277S–84S.

Ye, M., et al. 2013. Occupational pesticide exposures and respiratory health. *International Journal of Environmental Research and Public Health* 10:6442–71.

Human Energy

CHAPTER THREE

LEARNING OBJECTIVES

After studying this chapter, you should be able to:

1. Understand the interrelationships among the various forms of chemical, thermal, and mechanical energy, and be able to perform mathematical conversions from one form of energy to another.

2. Identify the three major human energy systems, their major energy sources as stored in the body, and various nutrients needed to sustain them.

3. List the components of total daily energy expenditure (TDEE) and how each contributes to the total amount of caloric energy expended over a 24-hour period.

4. Describe the various factors that may influence resting energy expenditure (REE).

5. List and explain the various means whereby energy expenditure during exercise, or the thermic effect of exercise (TEE), may be measured, and be able to calculate conversions among the various methods.

6. Describe the three different muscle fiber types and the major characteristics of each in relation to energy production during exercise.

7. Explain the relationship between exercise intensity and energy expenditure and how the MET values in the Compendium of Physical Activities may be used to design an exercise program.

8. Understand the concept of the physical activity level (PAL) and how it relates to estimated energy expenditure (EER). Calculate your EER based on an estimate of your PAL and the physical activity coefficient (PA).

9. Describe the role of the three energy systems during exercise.

10. Explain the various causes of fatigue during exercise and discuss nutritional interventions that may help delay the onset of fatigue.

As noted in chapter 1, the body uses the food we eat to provide energy, to build and repair tissues, and to regulate metabolism. Of these three functions, the human body ranks energy production first and will use food for this purpose at the expense of the other two functions in time of need. Energy is the essence of life.

Through technological processes, humans have harnessed a variety of energy sources, such as wind, waterfalls, the sun, wood, and oil, to operate the machines invented to make life easier. However, humans cannot use any of these energy sources for their own metabolism but must rely on food sources found in nature. The food we eat must be converted into energy forms that the body can use. Thus, the human body is equipped with a number of metabolic systems to produce and regulate energy for its diverse needs, such as synthesis of tissues, movement of substances between tissues, and muscular contraction.

The underlying basis for the control of movement in all sports is human energy, and successful performance depends upon the ability of the athlete to produce the right amount of energy and to control its application to the specific demands of the sport. Sports differ in their energy demands. In some events, such as the 100-meter dash, success is dependent primarily on the ability to produce energy very rapidly. In others, such as the 26.2-mile marathon, energy need not be produced so rapidly but must be sustained at an optimal rate for a much longer period. In still other sports, such as golf, the athlete need not only produce energy at varying rates (compare the drive with the putt) but must carefully control the application of that energy. Thus, each sport imposes specific energy demands upon the athlete. Sports scientists have coined the term *sportomics* to evaluate the metabolic response of the athlete under varying conditions, such as weather changes.

A discussion of the role of nutrition as a means to help provide and control human energy is important from several standpoints. First, inadequate supplies of necessary energy nutrients as a source of fuel, such as muscle glycogen or blood glucose, may cause fatigue. Fatigue also may be caused by the inability of the energy systems to function optimally because of a deficiency of other nutrients, such as selected vitamins and minerals. In addition, the human body is capable of storing energy reserves in a variety of body forms, including body fat and muscle tissue. Excess body weight in the form of fat or decreased body weight due to losses of muscle tissue may adversely affect some types of athletic performance.

One purpose of this chapter is to review briefly the major human energy systems and how they are used in the body under conditions of exercise and rest. Following this, chapters 4 through 9 discuss the role of each of the major classes of nutrients as they relate to energy production in the human body, with the primary focus on prevention of fatigue caused by impaired energy production; chapter 13 details the effects of various food drugs and supplements on human energy systems. Another purpose of this chapter is to discuss the means by which humans store and expend energy. Chapters 10 through 12 focus on weight-control methods and expand on some of the concepts presented in this chapter.

Measures of Energy

What is energy?

For our purposes, **energy** represents the capacity to do work. **Work** is one form of energy, often called *mechanical* or *kinetic energy.* When we throw a ball or run a mile, we have done work; we have produced mechanical energy.

Energy exists in a variety of other forms in nature, such as the light energy of the sun, nuclear energy in uranium, electrical energy in lightning storms, heat energy in fires, and chemical energy in oil. The six forms of energy—mechanical, chemical, heat, electrical, light, and nuclear—are interchangeable according to various laws of thermodynamics. We take advantage of these laws every day. One such example is the use of the chemical energy in gasoline to produce mechanical energy—the movement of our cars.

In the human body, four of these types of energy are important. Our bodies possess stores of *chemical energy* that can be used to produce *electrical energy* for creation of electrical nerve impulses, to produce *heat energy* to help keep our body temperature at 37°C (98.6°F) even on cold days, and to produce *mechanical energy* through muscle shortening so that we may move about.

For earthlings, the sun is the ultimate source of energy. Solar energy is harnessed by plants, through photosynthesis, to produce either plant carbohydrates, fats, or proteins, all forms of stored chemical energy. When humans consume plant and animal foods, the carbohydrates, fats, and proteins undergo a series of metabolic changes and are utilized to develop body structure, to regulate body processes, or to provide a storage form of chemical energy (figure 3.1).

The optimal intake and output of energy is important to all individuals, but especially for the physically active person. To perform to capacity, body energy stores must be used in the most efficient manner possible.

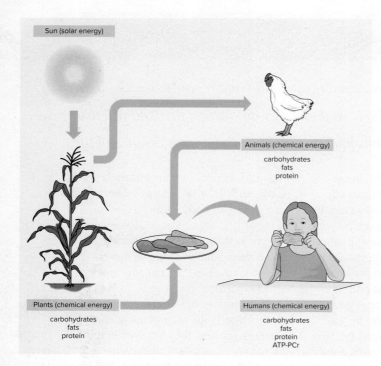

FIGURE 3.1 Through photosynthesis, plants utilize solar energy and convert it into chemical energy in the form of carbohydrates, fats, or proteins. Animals eat plants and convert the chemical energy into their own stores of chemical energy—primarily fat and protein. Humans ingest food from both plant and animal sources and convert the chemical energy for their own stores and use.

What terms are used to quantify work and power during exercise?

Energy has been defined as the ability to do work. According to the physicist's definition, work is simply the product of force times vertical distance, or in formula format, Work = Force × Distance. When we speak of how fast work is done, the term **power** is used. Power is simply work divided by time, or Power = Work/Time.

Two major measurement systems have been used in the past to express energy in terms of either work or power. The metric system has been in use by most of the world, while England, its colonies, and the United States have used the English system. In an attempt to provide some uniformity in measurement systems around the world, the International Unit System (*Systeme International d'Unites,* or SI) has been developed. Most of the world has adopted the SI, which is comparable to the metric system. Although legislation has been passed by Congress to convert the United States into the SI, and terms such as *gram, kilogram, milliliter, liter,* and *kilometer* are becoming more prevalent, it appears that it will take some time before this system becomes part of our everyday language.

The SI is used in most scientific journals today, but the other two systems appear in older journals. Terms that are used in each system are presented in table 3.1. For our purposes in this text, we shall use several English terms that are still in common usage in the United States, but if you read scientific literature, you should be able to convert values among the various systems if necessary. For example,

TABLE 3.1 Terms in the English, metric, and international systems

Unit	English system	Metric system	International system
Mass	slug	kilogram (kg)	kilogram (kg)
Distance	foot (ft)	meter (m)	meter (m)
Time	second (s)	second (s)	second (s)
Force	pound (lb)	newton (N)	newton (N)
Work	foot-pound (ft-lb)	kilogram-meter (kgm)	joule (J)
Power	horsepower (hp)	watt (W)	watt (W)

work may be expressed as either foot-pounds, kilogram-meters (kgm), joules, or watts. If you weigh 150 pounds and climb a 20-foot flight of stairs in 1 minute, you have done 3,000 foot-pounds of work, which maybe converted to the metric system and International system. One kgm is equal to 7.23 foot-pounds, so you would do about 415 kgm (3,000 foot pounds ÷ 7.23 foot pounds = 415 kgm). One **joule** is equal to about 0.102 kgm, so you have done about 4,062 joules of work (415 kgm ÷ 0.102 kgm = 4,062 joules). One watt is equal to one joule per second, so you have generated about 68 watts of power (4,062 joules ÷ 60 = 67.7 watts). Some basic interrelationships among the measurement systems are noted in table 3.2. Other equivalents may be found in appendix A.

How do we measure physical activity and energy expenditure?

For research purposes, exercise and nutrition scientists are interested in measuring work output and energy expenditure under two conditions. One condition involves specific techniques in controlled laboratory research, whereas the other condition involves normal daily activities, including actual sports performance. Other than researchers, many physically active individuals, for various reasons such as body weight control, want to know how much exercise they have done and how much energy they have expended.

Over the years numerous techniques have been used to quantify physical activity and energy expenditure. Given the worldwide increase in obesity and related diseases, such as diabetes, quantifying physical activity is very important, not only for medical scientists but also for the typical individual who exercises for its manifold health benefits. Recent research and reviews, such as those by Bort-Roig, *Consumer Reports,* and Psota and Chen, as well as Hills, Hongu, Lee, Liu, Montoye, and Schoeller and their colleagues, have documented various methods used and provided an analysis of their accuracy and usefulness, and they serve as the basis for the following discussion.

Hills and others indicate that it is important to appreciate that physical activity and energy expenditure are different constructs. Physical activity involves bodily movement, which increases energy expenditure above resting levels. In many cases, objective measures of physical activity may be used to predict energy expenditure. All of the following techniques have been used to

TABLE 3.2 Some interrelationships between work measurement systems

Weight	Distance	Work	Power
1 kilogram = 2.2 pounds	1 meter = 3.28 feet	1 kgm = 7.23 foot-pounds	1 watt = 1 joule per second
1 kilogram = 1,000 grams	1 meter = 1.09 yards	1 kgm = 9.8 joules	1 watt = 6.12 kgm per minute 1 watt = 0.0013 horsepower
454 grams = 1 pound	1 foot = 0.30 meter	1 foot-pound = 0.138 kgm	1 horsepower = 550 foot-pounds per second
1 pound = 16 ounces	1,000 meters = 1 kilometer	1 foot-pound = 1.35 joules	1 horsepower = 33,000 foot-pounds per minute
1 ounce = 28.4 grams	1 kilometer = 0.6215 mile	1 newton = 0.102 kg	1 horsepower = 745.8 watts
3.5 ounces = 100 grams	1 mile = 1.61 kilometers 1 inch = 2.54 centimeters 1 centimeter = 0.39 inch	1 joule = 1 newton meter 1 kilojoule = 1,000 joules 1 megajoule = 1,000,000 joules 1 joule = 0.102 kgm 1 joule = 0.736 foot-pound 1 kilojoule = 102 kgm	

collect data on physical activity and energy expenditure specifically for research purposes, but many may be useful for individuals interested in monitoring their personal exercise habits. A detailed discussion of such measurement techniques is beyond the scope of this text but, based on the research cited above, here are some highlights of the various methods.

Physical Activity Questionnaires The use of questionnaires was one of the first methods to assess physical activity and is still widely used. Although some researchers note that physical activity questionnaires may have potential as a source of rich descriptive data, most contend the data obtained are subjective, not objective, in nature and thus the validity of the data obtained is questionable. For example, Matthews and others note that attempts to quantify physical activity energy expenditure via questionnaires are known to contain substantial errors.

Heart Rate Monitoring Heart rate monitoring is an easy, effective means to monitor exercise intensity in aerobic exercise. In and by itself heart rate does not measure energy expenditure, but if calibrated with oxygen consumption in an exercise protocol, it may be used to assess energy expenditure in a given individual. The use of heart rate in planning an exercise program is presented in chapter 11.

Ergometers and Exercise Equipment When conducting research, exercise scientists need accurate measures of work output and energy expenditure. An **ergometer**, such as a cycle or arm ergometer, is designed to provide accurate measurement of work, including measures of power and total work output over specific periods of time. For example, bicycle ergometers provide work output in joules and watts, measures of work and power, respectively. However, ergometers do not evaluate energy expenditure, such as Calories expended.

Exercise machines, particularly cardio machines such as treadmills, stationary cycling devices, elliptical trainers, and step machines are examples of ergometers. Many commercial machines are configured to provide an estimate of exercise intensity, such as heart rate monitoring, as well as energy expenditure,

such as Calories expended. Some of these machines use computerized standard formulas to predict energy expenditure based on a *typical* individual, while others incorporate data input from the user, such as gender, age, body weight, fitness level, and heart rate. In general, the more personal data the machine uses, the more accurate will be the prediction of energy expenditure.

Calorimetry Our bodies produce heat at all times, even at rest. When we exercise, heat production increases rapidly, and in proportion to energy expenditure. **Calorimetry** is the measurement of heat production by the body. Figure 3.2 illustrates a bomb

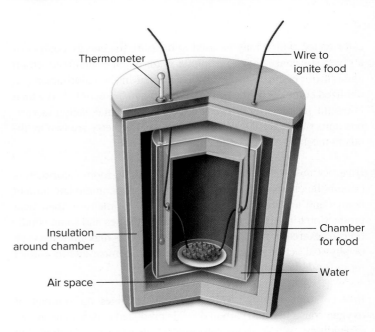

FIGURE 3.2 A bomb calorimeter. The food in the calorimeter is combusted via electrical ignition. The heat (Calories) given off by the food raises the temperature of the water, thereby providing data about the caloric content of specific foodstuffs.

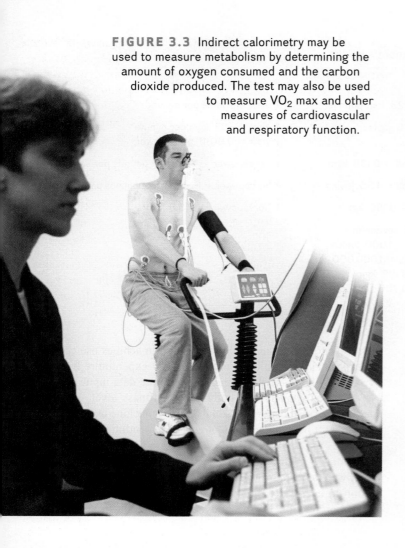

FIGURE 3.3 Indirect calorimetry may be used to measure metabolism by determining the amount of oxygen consumed and the carbon dioxide produced. The test may also be used to measure VO$_2$ max and other measures of cardiovascular and respiratory function.

calorimeter, which may be used to measure the energy content of a given substance. For example, a gram of fat contains a certain amount of chemical energy. When placed in the calorimeter and oxidized completely, the heat it gives off can be recorded. We then know the heat energy of one gram of fat and can equate it to various units of energy. Direct and indirect calorimetry are two methods to measure energy expenditure in humans.

Direct calorimetry Large, expensive whole-room calorimeters (metabolic chambers) are available that can accommodate human beings and a water-cooled gradient layer can measure their heat production directly under normal home activities and some conditions of exercise. The limited size of such units may limit the type of physical activity, but they are equipped comparable to a hotel room for daily living activities.

Indirect calorimetry This method determines the amount of oxygen consumed and carbon dioxide produced to calculate energy expenditure. Whole-room calorimeters also use this method, but it may also be used in other laboratory conditions (see figure 3.3). Moreover, lightweight portable oxygen analyzers are also available to record energy expenditure in freely moving individuals, including those involved in some sport activities. In essence, oxygen is

needed to metabolize carbohydrate, fat, and protein for energy production in the body, and if we can accurately measure the oxygen consumption (and carbon dioxide production) of an individual, we can get a pretty good measure of energy expenditure.

Doubly Labeled Water (DLW) Technique Scientists indicate that the DLW technique is the "gold standard" technique for measuring total daily energy expenditure in individuals in a free-living environment. It is safe, noninvasive, and convenient for users over the course of a week or more. In brief, the subject ingests water with stable isotopes of hydrogen and oxygen ($^2H_2^{18}O$), which emit no radiation. Analysis of urine and blood samples provides data on ^2H and ^{18}O excretion. The labeled oxygen is eliminated from the body as water and carbon dioxide, whereas the hydrogen is eliminated only as water, which may provide an estimate of carbon dioxide fluctuation that may be converted to energy expenditure. Despite the advantages of this technique, it does not provide information on the type, intensity, or duration of physical activity accounting for some of the total energy expenditure.

Physical Activity Level (PAL) As a measure of physical activity and energy expenditure, the Institute of Medicine has developed four physical activity level (PAL) categories based on the equivalent of walking various distances daily. This procedure is discussed in more detail later in this chapter and in chapter 11 for its role in body weight control.

Metabolic Equivalents (METs) The metabolic equivalent, or MET, of physical activity is based on the amount of oxygen consumed and thus may be converted into energy expenditure. Details on the MET are presented later in this chapter, and as discussed in chapter 11, may be a useful procedure when calculating energy expenditure during exercise for purposes of body weight control. Appendix B also provides some useful data.

Motion Sensors Motion sensors are electronic devices worn on various parts of the body and are designed to monitor body motion during physical activity. The pedometer and accelerometer are two commonly used devices. These devices generate electrical signals, the pedometer through the pendular motion of walking and the accelerometer when piezoelectric transmitters are stressed by acceleration forces.

The pedometer has been in use for many years. It is easy to use, is inexpensive, and measures step counts when walking or jogging throughout the day. Thus, it may be very useful in determining the PAL mentioned above, which is based on daily walking distance. However, pedometers cannot measure exercise intensity. Various models are available, but some may not be reliable. The Yamax Digi-Walker SW-200 has been highly recommended for its consistent accuracy in laboratory and field tests. By providing feedback to the user, pedometers may also be useful as a means to encourage individuals to do more exercise. Although the basic pedometer may serve its intended purpose, some consider it old-fashioned because it lacks the advanced features of more modern devices.

The accelerometer is relatively small, is usually worn at the waist, and can record data for days. It measures changes in acceleration in one to three planes, can be used to assess physical activity and energy expenditure, and can estimate exercise intensity. The tri-axial accelerometer can evaluate motion in all three planes (vertical, anterior-posterior, and medial-lateral) and is considered to provide a more detailed analysis of motion than pedometers or uni-axial accelerometers. Moreover, wearing multiple accelerometers, on the wrist, thigh, and ankle, significantly improves the prediction of energy expenditure as compared to a single accelerometer on the hip. However, scientists note accelerometers have some shortcomings, including the inability to record static exercise, unsuitability to quantify movement in some activities such as swimming and cycling, and inability to differentiate energy expenditure when walking on the level as compared to uphill. Nevertheless, comparable to pedometers accelerometers may be appropriate for many physically active individuals. Various companies manufacture accelerometers for personal use, and the ActiGraph is one reported to have high validity and reliability.

Combination Devices Combining the use of two or more techniques to quantify physical activity and energy expenditure may help improve accuracy as compared to a single measure. For example, Hills and others indicated that a potentially powerful approach to quantifying energy expenditure is the simultaneous use of accelerometry and heart rate monitoring; matching the accelerator data with the heart rate data could verify that the increase in heart rate was due to physical activity. Many such devices are currently available for individual use, including the following.

- Actiheart—combines data from an accelerometer and heart rate monitor
- Samsung Gear Fit—combines data from accelerometer, heart rate monitor, gyroscope, and pedometer

Hills and others note an increasing number of such sophisticated products are becoming available for personal use. For example, a Personal Calorie Monitor is an arm band containing a heat flow sensor, serving as your own personal calorimeter to calculate the Calories you are expending while doing various activities.

Smartphone Applications (Apps) for Physical Activity As mentioned in previous chapters, applications (apps) for exercise and nutrition are becoming increasingly popular. In a recent review, Hongu and others noted more than 13,600 mobile phone health apps currently exist on the market, and the list is increasing. Numerous wearable, wireless gadgets are available, including fashion designer clothing, jewelry, and watches, incorporating various technologies such as global positioning system (GPS) navigation, accelerometers, heart rate monitors, and cameras that can interact with your smartphone and provide a wealth of data on your physical activity. Bort-Roig noted that although Smartphone use is a relatively new field of study in physical activity research, the few studies that evaluated the validity of physical activity assessment found average-to-excellent levels of accuracy for different behaviors.

Numerous smartphone apps are available to assess one's level of physical activity. You can use Google to access information on *Fitness Apps* or *Free Fitness Apps* to evaluate their features and their reliability. *Consumer Reports* provides periodic analyses

of fitness applications, and in a recent review indicated the Fitbit One, which calculates Calories expended and progress toward your daily health goals, may be worth your money. When possible, select devices that can be tailored for individual characteristics, such as gender, age, and body weight.

All of these measures, from the questionnaire to the smartphone, may be useful as a means to measure and promote physical activity. Some, such as direct calorimetry and the DLW technique, are relatively expensive and used primarily for research purposes, but many, such as smartphone apps, are becoming increasingly available and effective with reasonable cost for use by the general population.

What is the most commonly used measure of energy?

Although there are a number of different ways to express energy, the most common term used in the past and still most prevalent and understood in the United States by most people is **Calorie**.

A calorie is a measure of heat. One gram calorie represents the amount of heat needed to raise the temperature of 1 gram of water 1 degree Celsius. A kilocalorie is equal to 1,000 small calories. It is the amount of heat needed to raise 1 kg of water (1 L) 1 degree Celsius. In human nutrition, because the gram calorie is so small, the kilocalorie is the main expression of energy. It is usually abbreviated as kcal, kc, or C, or capitalized as Calorie. Throughout this book, *Calorie* or *C* will refer to the kilocalorie.

According to the principles underlying the first law of thermodynamics, energy may be equated from one form to another. Thus, the Calorie, which represents thermal or heat energy, may be equated to other forms of energy. Relative to our discussion concerning physical work such as exercise and its interrelationships with nutrition, it is important to equate the Calorie with mechanical work and the chemical energy stored in the body. As will be explained later, most stored chemical energy must undergo some form of oxidation in order to release its energy content as work.

The following represents some equivalent energy values for the Calorie in terms of mechanical work and oxygen utilization. Some examples illustrating several of the interrelationships will be used in later chapters.

$$1 \text{ C} = 3{,}086 \text{ foot-pounds}$$
$$1 \text{ C} = 427 \text{ kgm}$$
$$1 \text{ C} = 4.2 \text{ kilojoules (kJ), or 4{,}200 joules}$$
$$1 \text{ C} = 200 \text{ ml oxygen (approximately)}$$

Although the Calorie is the most commonly used expression in the United States for energy, work, and heat, the **kilojoule** is the proper term in the SI and is used by the rest of the world. It is important for you to be able to convert from Calories into kilojoules, and vice versa. To convert Calories into kilojoules, multiply the number of Calories by 4.2 (4.186 to be exact); to convert kilojoules into Calories, divide the number of kilojoules by 4.2. Simply multiplying or dividing by 4 for each respective conversion will provide a ballpark estimate. In some cases, megajoules (MJ), a million joules, are used to express energy. One MJ equals about 240 Calories, or 4.2 MJ is the equivalent of about 1,000 Calories.

Through the use of a calorimeter, the energy contents of the basic nutrients have been determined. Energy may be derived from the three major foodstuffs—carbohydrate, fat, and protein—plus alcohol. The caloric value of each of these three nutrients may vary somewhat, depending on the particular structure of the different forms. For example, carbohydrate may exist in several forms—as glucose, sucrose, or starch—and the caloric value of each will differ slightly. In general, 1 gram of each of the three nutrients and alcohol, measured in a calorimeter, yields the following Calories:

$$1 \text{ gram carbohydrate} = 4.30 \text{ C}$$
$$1 \text{ gram fat} = 9.45 \text{ C}$$
$$1 \text{ gram protein} = 5.65 \text{ C}$$
$$1 \text{ gram alcohol} = 7.00 \text{ C}$$

Unfortunately, or fortunately if one is trying to lose weight, humans do not extract all of this energy from the food they eat. The human body is not as efficient as the calorimeter. For one, the body cannot completely absorb all the food eaten. Only about 97 percent of ingested carbohydrate, 95 percent of fat, and 92 percent of protein are absorbed. In addition, a good percentage of the protein is not completely oxidized in the body, with some of the nitrogen waste products being excreted in the urine. In summary, then, the caloric value of food is reduced somewhat in relation to the values given previously. Although the following values are not exactly precise, they are approximate enough to be used effectively in determining the caloric values of the foods we eat. Thus, the following caloric values are used throughout this text as a practical guide:

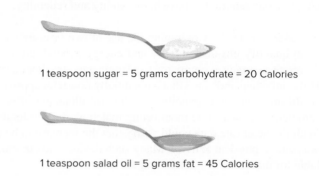

Carbohydrate
4 kcal per gram

Protein
4 kcal per gram

Energy sources for body functions

Alcohol
7 kcal per gram

Fat
9 kcal per gram

$$1 \text{ gram carbohydrate} = 4 \text{ C}$$
$$1 \text{ gram fat} = 9 \text{ C}$$
$$1 \text{ gram protein} = 4 \text{ C}$$
$$1 \text{ gram alcohol} = 7 \text{ C}$$

For our purposes, the Calories in food represent a form of potential energy to be used by our bodies to produce heat and work (figure 3.4). However, the fact that fat has about twice the amount of energy per gram as carbohydrate (figure 3.5) does not mean that it is a better energy source for the active individual, as we shall see in later chapters when we talk of the efficient utilization of body fuels.

1 teaspoon sugar = 5 grams carbohydrate = 20 Calories

1 teaspoon salad oil = 5 grams fat = 45 Calories

FIGURE 3.5 The Calorie as a measure of energy.

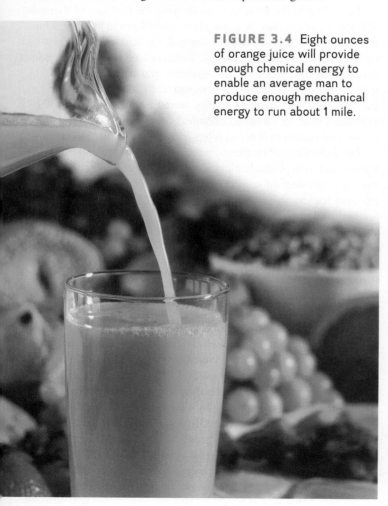

FIGURE 3.4 Eight ounces of orange juice will provide enough chemical energy to enable an average man to produce enough mechanical energy to run about 1 mile.

Key Concepts

▶ Energy represents the capacity to do work, and food is the source of energy for humans.
▶ Energy expenditure in humans may be estimated in a variety of ways, including both direct and indirect calorimetry, doubly labeled water, accelerometers, and pedometers. Smartphones may contain devices to measure physical activity and energy expenditure. Each of these techniques has advantages and disadvantages.
▶ The Calorie, or kilocalorie, is a measure of chemical energy stored in foods; this chemical energy can be transformed into heat and mechanical work energy in the body. A related measure is the kilojoule. One Calorie is equal to 4.2 kilojoules.
▶ Carbohydrates and fats are the primary energy nutrients, but protein may also be an energy source during rest and exercise. In the human body 1 gram of carbohydrate = 4 Calories, 1 gram of fat = 9 Calories, and 1 gram of protein = 4 Calories. Alcohol is also a source of energy; 1 gram = 7 Calories.

Check for Yourself

▶ Measure the height of a step on a flight of stairs or bleachers and convert it into feet (9 inches = 0.75 foot). Stepping in

Human Energy Systems

How is energy stored in the body?

The ultimate source of all energy on earth is the sun. Solar energy is harnessed by plants, which take carbon, hydrogen, oxygen, and nitrogen from their environment and manufacture either carbohydrate, fat, or protein. These plant foods contain not only the energy stored in carbohydrate, fat, and protein but also various vitamins and minerals the body needs to process them during energy production. When we consume these foods, our digestive processes break them down into simple compounds that are absorbed into the body and transported to various cells. One of the basic purposes of body cells is to transform the chemical energy of these simple compounds into forms that may be available for immediate use or other forms that may be available for future use.

Energy in the body is available for immediate use in the form of **adenosine triphosphate (ATP)**. It is a complex molecule constructed with high-energy bonds, which, when split by enzyme action, can release energy rapidly for a number of body processes, including muscle contraction. ATP is classified as a high-energy compound and is stored in the tissues in small amounts. It is important to note that ATP is the immediate source of energy for all body functions, and the other energy stores are used to replenish ATP at varying rates. Myburgh notes that muscle contraction is totally dependent on ATP, so the body has developed an intricate system to help replenish ATP as rapidly as needed.

Another related high-energy phosphate compound, **phosphocreatine (PCr)**, is also found in the tissues in small amounts. Although it cannot be used as an immediate source of energy, it can rapidly replenish ATP.

ATP also may be formed from either carbohydrate, fat, or protein after those nutrients have undergone some complex biochemical changes in the body. Figure 3.6 represents a basic schematic of how ATP is formed from each of these three nutrients.

Because ATP and PCr are found in very small amounts in the body and can be used up in a matter of seconds, it is important to have adequate energy stores as a backup system. Your body stores of carbohydrate, fat, and protein can provide you with ample amounts of ATP, enough to last for many weeks even on a starvation diet. The digestion and metabolism of carbohydrate, fat, and protein are discussed in their respective chapters, so it is unnecessary to present that full discussion here. However, you may wish to preview figure 3.12 to visualize the metabolic interrelationships among the three nutrients in the body. For those who desire more detailed schematics of energy pathways, appendix F provides some of the major metabolic pathways for carbohydrate, fat, and protein.

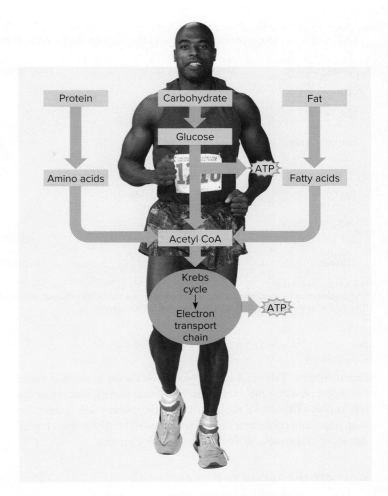

FIGURE 3.6 Simplified schematic of ATP formation from carbohydrate, fat, and protein. All three nutrients may be used to form ATP, but carbohydrate and fat are the major sources via the aerobic metabolism of the Krebs cycle. Carbohydrate may be used to produce small amounts of ATP under anaerobic conditions, thus providing humans with the ability to produce energy rapidly without oxygen for relatively short periods. For more details, see appendix F.

It is important to note that parts of each energy nutrient may be converted into the other two nutrients in the body under certain circumstances. For example, protein may be converted into carbohydrate during prolonged exercise, whereas excess dietary carbohydrate may be converted into fat in the body during rest.

Table 3.3 summarizes how much energy is stored in the human body as ATP, PCr, and various forms of carbohydrate, fat, and protein. The total amount of energy, represented by Calories, is approximate and may vary considerably between individuals depending on body size and composition, diet, and physical fitness level. Carbohydrate is stored in limited amounts as blood (serum) glucose, liver glycogen, and muscle glycogen. The largest amount of energy is stored in the body as fats. Fats are stored as triglycerides in both muscle tissue and adipose (fat) tissue; triglycerides and free fatty acids (FFA) in the blood are a limited supply. The protein of the body tissues, particularly muscle tissue, is a large reservoir of energy but is not used to any great extent under normal

Energy source	Major storage form	Total body Calories	Total body kilojoules	Distance covered**
ATP	Tissues	1	4.2	17.5 yards
PCr	Tissues	4	16.8	70 yards
Carbohydrate	Serum glucose	20	88	350 yards
	Liver glycogen	400	1,680	4 miles
	Muscle glycogen	1,500	6,300	15 miles
Fat	Serum-free fatty acids	7	29.2	123 yards
	Serum triglycerides	75	315	0.75 mile
	Muscle triglycerides	2,500	10,500	25 miles
	Adipose tissue triglycerides	80,000	336,000	800 miles
Protein	Muscle protein	30,000	126,000	300 miles

See text for discussion.
*These values may have extreme variations depending on the size of the individual, amount of body fat, physical fitness level, and diet.
**Running at an energy cost of 100 Calories per mile (1.6 kilometers).

circumstances. Table 3.3 also depicts how far an individual could run based on using the total of each of these energy sources as the sole supply. The role of each of these energy stores during exercise is an important consideration that is discussed briefly in this chapter and more extensively in their the following chapters.

What are the human energy systems?

Why does the human body store chemical energy in a variety of forms? If we look at human energy needs from an historical perspective, the answer becomes obvious. Sometimes humans needed to produce energy at a rapid rate, such as when sprinting to safety to avoid dangerous animals. Thus, a fast rate of energy production was an important human energy feature that helped ensure survival. At other times, our ancient ancestors may have been deprived of adequate food for long periods, and thus needed a storage capacity for chemical energy that would sustain life throughout these times of deprivation. Hence, the ability to store large amounts of energy was also important for survival. These two factors—rate of energy production and energy capacity—appear to be determining factors in the development of human energy systems.

One need only watch weekend television programming for several weeks to realize the diversity of sports popular throughout the world. Each of these sports imposes certain requirements on humans who want to be successful competitors. For some sports, such as weight lifting, the main requirement is brute strength, while for others such as tennis, quick reactions and hand/eye coordination are important. A major consideration in most sports is the rate of energy production, which can range from the explosive power needed by a shot-putter to the tremendous endurance capacity of an ultramarathoner. The physical performance demands of different sports require specific sources of energy.

As noted previously, the body stores energy in a variety of ways—in ATP, PCr, muscle glycogen, and so on. In order for this energy to be used to produce muscular contractions and movement, it must undergo certain biochemical reactions in the muscle. These biochemical reactions serve as a basis for classifying human energy expenditure by several energy, or power, systems.

In his 1979 text *Sports Physiology,* one of the first to discuss the application of human energy systems to sport, Edward L. Fox named three human energy systems—the ATP-PCr system, the lactic acid system, and the oxygen system. As noted below, other terminology may be used to describe the metabolic relationships to these three energy systems, but the original classification is still useful when discussing the application of human energy to sports performance.

ATP-PCr Energy System   The **ATP-PCr system** is also known as the *phosphagen system* because both adenosine triphosphate and phosphocreatine contain phosphates. ATP is the immediate source of energy for almost all body processes, including muscle contraction. This high-energy compound, stored in the muscles, rapidly releases energy when an electrical impulse arrives in the muscle. See figure 3.7 for a graphical representation of ATP breakdown. No matter what you do, scratch your nose or lift 100 pounds, ATP breakdown makes the movement possible. ATP must be present for the muscles to contract. The body has a limited supply of ATP and must replace it rapidly if muscular work is to continue. The main purpose of every other energy system, including PCr, is to help regenerate ATP to enable muscle contraction to continue at the optimal desired rate.

PCr, which is also a high-energy compound found in the muscle, can help form ATP rapidly as ATP is used. Energy released when PCr splits is used to form ATP from ADP and P. PCr is also in short supply (but more than ATP) and has to be replenished if used. PCr breakdown to help resynthesize ATP is illustrated in figure 3.8.

The ATP-PCr system is critical to energy production. Because these phosphagens are in short supply, any all-out exercise for 5 to 10 seconds could deplete the supply,

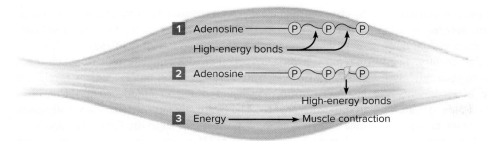

FIGURE 3.7 ATP, adenosine triphosphate. *(1)* ATP is stored in the muscle in limited amounts. *(2)* Splitting of a high-energy bond releases adenosine diphosphate (ADP), inorganic phosphate (P), and energy, which *(3)* can be used for many body processes, including muscular contraction. The ATP stores may be used maximally for fast, all-out bursts of power that last about 1 second. ATP must be replenished from other sources for muscle contraction to continue.

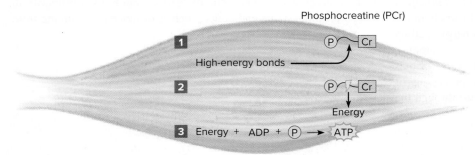

FIGURE 3.8 Phosphocreatine (PCr). *(1)* PCr is stored in the muscle in limited amounts. *(2)* Splitting of the high-energy bond releases energy, which *(3)* can be used to rapidly synthesize ATP from ADP and P. ATP and PCr are called phosphagens and together represent the ATP-PCr energy system. This system is utilized primarily for quick, maximal exercises lasting about 1 to 6 seconds or more, such as sprinting.

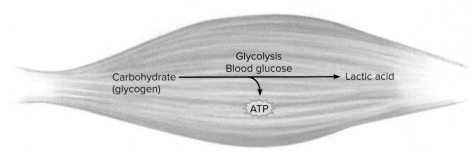

FIGURE 3.9 The lactic acid energy system. Muscle glycogen and glucose can break down without the utilization of oxygen. This process is called anaerobic glycolysis. (See appendix F, figure F.1, for more details.) ATP is produced rapidly, but lactic acid is the end product. Lactic acid may be a major cause of fatigue in the muscle. The lactic acid energy system is utilized primarily during exercise bouts of very high intensity, those conducted at maximal rates for about 30 to 120 seconds.

particularly PCr, in a given muscle. Hence, the phosphagens must be replaced, and this is the function of the other energy sources. Increasing the level of PCr in the muscle would provide a greater fuel reserve and possibly enhance the performance of brief, high-intensity exercise. Creatine supplementation, discussed in later chapters, is one way athletes are increasing muscle PCr in an effort to enhance performance. In summary, the value of the ATP-PCr system is its ability to provide energy rapidly, for example, in sport events such

as competitive weight lifting or sprinting 100 meters. *Anaerobic power* is a term often associated with the ATP-PCr energy system.

Lactic Acid Energy System The **lactic acid system** cannot be used directly as a source of energy for muscular contraction, but it can help replace ATP rapidly when necessary. If you are exercising at a high intensity level and need to replenish ATP rapidly, the next best source of energy besides PCr is glucose. Glucose may enter the muscle from the bloodstream or may be derived from the breakdown of glycogen stored in the muscle. The glucose molecule undergoes a series of reactions to eventually form ATP, a process called **glycolysis**. One of the major factors controlling the metabolic fate of glucose is the capacity of the **mitochondria**, which are cell organelles that *need oxygen* to process glucose to ATP. If the muscle cell mitochondria can process the available glucose, then adequate oxygen is assumed to be available. This is known as **aerobic glycolysis**. Conversely, if the rate of glycolysis surpasses the capacity of mitochondrial oxidation to meet the energy demands of the exercise task or to maintain a high level of aerobic glycolysis, then insufficient ATP is formed and lactic acid is a by-product of the process necessary to increase ATP production. This process has been referred to as anaerobic because of inadequate aerobic processing by the mitochondria, and the term **anaerobic glycolysis** has been used as a scientific term for the lactic acid energy system.

The lactic acid system is diagrammed in figure 3.9. It is used in sports events in which energy production is near maximal for 30–120 seconds, such as a 200- or 800-meter run. *Anaerobic capacity* is a term often associated with the lactic acid energy system.

The lactic acid system has the advantage of producing ATP rapidly. Its capacity is limited in comparison to aerobic glycolysis, for only about 5 percent of the total ATP production from muscle glycogen can be released. Moreover, the lactic acid produced as a by-product may be associated with the onset of fatigue, as discussed later in this chapter. In brief, a prevailing hypothesis suggests that anaerobic glycolysis releases hydrogen ions, increasing the acidity within the muscle cell and disturbing the normal cell environment. The processes of energy release and muscle contraction in the muscle cell are controlled by enzymes whose functions may be impaired by the increased acidity in the cell. However, it is important to note that the lactate present after loss of the hydrogen ion still has considerable energy content, which may be used by other tissues for energy or converted back into glucose in the liver.

Oxygen Energy System   The third system is the **oxygen system**. It is also known as the oxidative or aerobic system. *Aerobics* is a term used by Dr. Kenneth Cooper in 1968 to describe a system of exercising that created an exercise revolution in this country. In essence, aerobic exercises are designed to stress the oxygen system and provide benefits for the heart and lungs. Figure 3.10 represents the major physiological processes involved in the oxygen system. The oxygen system, like the lactic acid system, cannot be used directly as a source of energy for muscle contraction, but it does produce ATP in rather large quantities from other energy sources in the body. Muscle glycogen, liver glycogen, blood glucose, muscle triglycerides, blood FFA and triglycerides, adipose cell triglycerides, and body protein all may be ultimate sources of energy for ATP production and subsequent muscle contraction. To do this, glycogen, fats, and protein must be present within the muscle cell or must enter the muscle cell as glucose, FFA, or amino acids. Through a complex series of reactions, metabolic by-products of carbohydrate, fat, or protein combine with oxygen to produce energy, carbon dioxide, and water. These reactions occur in the energy powerhouse of the cell, the mitochondrion. The whole series of events of oxidative energy production primarily involves aerobic processing of carbohydrates and fats (and small amounts of protein) through the

Krebs cycle and the **electron transfer system**. The oxygen system is depicted in figure 3.11. The Krebs cycle and the electron transfer system represent a highly structured array of enzymes designed to remove hydrogen, carbon dioxide, and electrons from substrates such as glucose. At different steps in this process, energy is released and ATP is formed, with most of the ATP produced during the electron transfer process. The hydrogen and electrons eventually combine with oxygen to form water (see appendix F for more details).

Although the rate of ATP production is lower, the major advantage of the oxygen system over the other two energy systems is the production of large amounts of energy in the form of ATP. However, oxygen from the air we breathe must be delivered to the muscle cells deep in the body and enter the mitochondria to be used. This process may be adequate to handle mild and moderate levels of exercise but may not be able to meet the demand of very strenuous exercise. The oxygen system is used primarily in sports emphasizing endurance, such as distance runs ranging from

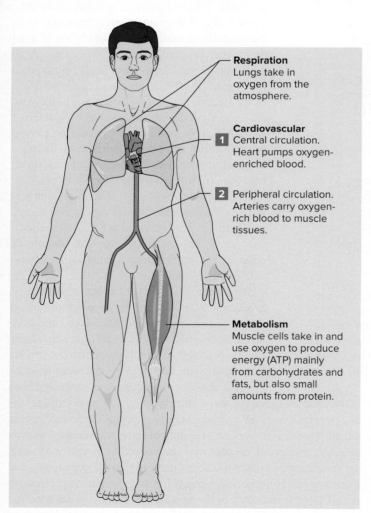

Respiration
Lungs take in oxygen from the atmosphere.

Cardiovascular
1 Central circulation. Heart pumps oxygen-enriched blood.

2 Peripheral circulation. Arteries carry oxygen-rich blood to muscle tissues.

Metabolism
Muscle cells take in and use oxygen to produce energy (ATP) mainly from carbohydrates and fats, but also small amounts from protein.

FIGURE 3.10 Physiological processes involved in oxygen uptake.

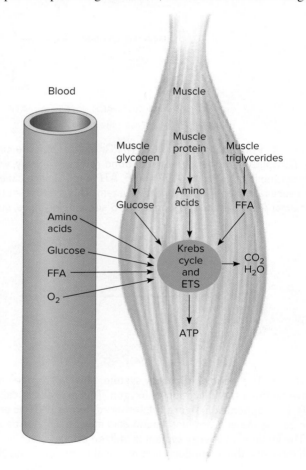

FIGURE 3.11 The oxygen energy system. The muscle stores of glycogen and triglycerides, along with blood supplies of glucose and free fatty acids (FFA), as well as small amounts of muscle protein and amino acids, undergo complex biochemical changes for entrance into the Krebs cycle and the associated electron transfer system (ETS). In this process, in which oxygen is the final acceptor to the electron, large amounts of ATP may be produced. The oxygen energy system is utilized primarily during endurance-type exercises, those lasting longer than 4 or 5 minutes. (See appendix F for more details.)

5 kilometers (3.1 miles) to the 26.2-mile marathon and beyond.

Hawley and Hopkins subdivided the oxygen energy system into two systems. The scientific terms for these two subdivisions are aerobic glycolysis, which uses carbohydrates (muscle glycogen and blood glucose) for energy production, and **aerobic lipolysis**, which uses fats (muscle triglycerides, blood FFA). As discussed in the next two chapters, carbohydrate is the more efficient fuel during high-intensity exercise, whereas fat becomes the predominant fuel used at lower levels of exercise intensity. Thus, aerobic glycolysis provides most of the energy in high-intensity aerobic running events such as 5 kilometers (3.1 miles), 10 kilometers (6.2 miles), and even races up to 2 hours, while aerobic lipolysis may contribute significant amounts of energy in more prolonged aerobic events, such as ultramarathons of 50 to 100 kilometers (31 to 62 miles). Aerobic glycolysis and aerobic lipolysis may respectively be referred to as *aerobic power* and *aerobic capacity*. Details relative to the role of these energy systems during exercise are presented in chapters 4 and 5. Figure 3.12 presents a simplified schematic reviewing the three human energy systems.

Summary The energy systems for exercise are discussed later in this chapter, but in brief, human energy systems for exercise may be classified as anaerobic or aerobic, and each may be subdivided into energy systems for power and capacity as follows:

- Anaerobic power—ATP-PCr energy system
- Anaerobic capacity—lactic acid energy system (anaerobic glycolysis)
- Aerobic power—aerobic glycolysis
- Aerobic capacity—aerobic lipolysis

As noted, protein may be used as an energy source during exercise and has been referred to as aerobic *proteolysis,* but its contributions are considered minor and it is not classified here as a separate energy system. Its contributions to energy production during exercise are covered in chapter 6.

What nutrients are necessary for operation of the human energy systems?

Although the energy for the formation of ATP is derived from the energy stores in carbohydrate, fat, and sometimes protein, this energy transformation and utilization would not occur without the participation of the other major nutrients—water, vitamins, and minerals. These three classes of nutrients function very closely with protein in the structure and function of numerous enzymes, many of which are active in the muscle-cell energy processes.

Water is used to help break up and transform some energy compounds by a process known as *hydrolysis.*

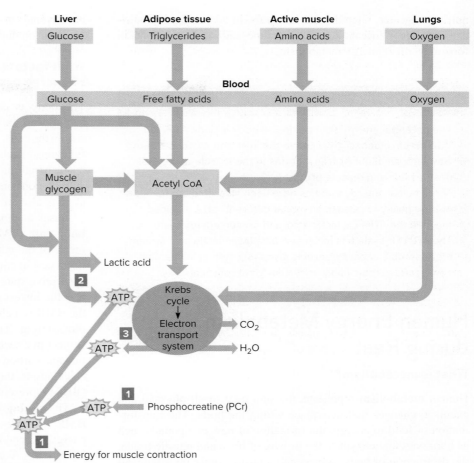

FIGURE 3.12 Simplified flow diagram of the three energy systems. The major nutrients and oxygen are transported to the cells for energy production. In the muscles, ATP is the immediate source of energy for muscle contraction. *(1)* The ATP-PCr system is represented by muscle stores of ATP and phosphocreatine (PCr); PCr can replenish ATP rapidly. *(2)* Glucose or muscle glycogen can produce ATP rapidly via the lactic acid system. *(3)* The oxygen system can produce large amounts of ATP via the aerobic processes in the Krebs cycle, primarily oxidation of carbohydrate and fatty acids. Numerous other energy pathways exist, and some are described in chapter 4 (carbohydrates), chapter 5 (fats), and chapter 6 (protein).

Several vitamins are needed for energy to be released from the cell sources. For example, niacin serves an important function in glycolysis, thiamin is needed to convert glycolytic end products to acetyl CoA for entrance into the Krebs cycle, and riboflavin is essential to forming ATP through the Krebs cycle and electron transfer system. A number of other B vitamins are also involved in facets of energy transformation within the cell.

Minerals, too, are essential for cellular energy processes. Iron is one of the more critical compounds. Aside from helping hemoglobin deliver oxygen to the muscle cell, it is also a component of myoglobin and the cytochrome part of the electron transfer system. It is needed for proper utilization of oxygen within the cell itself. Other minerals such as zinc, magnesium, potassium, sodium, and calcium are involved in a variety of ways, either as parts of active enzymes, in energy storage, or in the muscle-contraction process.

Proper utilization of body energy sources requires attention not only to the major energy nutrients but also to the regulatory nutrients—water, vitamins, and minerals. In addition, other nutrients and non-nutrients (such as creatine and caffeine) found in food may affect energy metabolism.

Human Energy Metabolism during Rest

What is metabolism?

Human **metabolism** represents the sum total of all physical and chemical changes that take place within the body. The transformation of food to energy, the formation of new compounds such as hormones and enzymes, the growth of bone and muscle tissue, the destruction of body tissues, and a host of other physiological processes are parts of the metabolic process.

Metabolism involves two fundamental processes, anabolism and catabolism. *Anabolism* is a building-up process, or constructive metabolism. Complex body components are synthesized from the basic nutrients. For the active individual, this may mean an increased muscle mass through weight training or an increased amount of cellular enzymes to better use oxygen following endurance-type training. Energy is needed for anabolism to occur. *Catabolism* is the tearing-down process. This involves the disintegration of body compounds into their simpler components. The breakdown of muscle glycogen to glucose and eventually CO_2, H_2O, and energy is an example of a catabolic process. The energy released from some catabolic processes is used to support the energy needs of anabolism.

Metabolism is life. It represents human energy. The metabolic rate reflects how rapidly the body is using its energy stores, and this rate can vary tremendously depending on a number of factors. For all practical purposes, the **total daily energy expenditure (TDEE)** may be accounted for by three factors:

• Energy for basal metabolism
• Energy for processing food intake
• Energy for physical activity

Basal energy expenditure accounts for the largest component of TDEE, whereas physical activity is the most variable. We shall examine basal energy expenditure and the effect of eating in this section, while the role of physical activity, or exercise, will be covered in the section "Human Energy Metabolism during Exercise."

What factors account for the amount of energy expended during rest?

The body is constantly using energy to build up and tear down substances within the cells. Certain automatic body functions, such as contraction of the heart, breathing, secretion of hormones, and the constant activity of the nervous system, also are consuming energy.

Basal metabolism, or the **basal metabolic rate (BMR)**, represents the energy requirements of the many different cellular and tissue processes that are necessary to continuing physiological activities in a resting, postabsorptive state throughout most of the day. Other than sleeping, it is the lowest rate of energy expenditure. The determination of the BMR is a clinical procedure conducted in a laboratory or hospital setting. The individual fasts for 12 hours. Then, with the subject in a reclining position, the individual's oxygen consumption and carbon dioxide production are measured. Through proper calculations, the BMR is determined. **Basal energy expenditure (BEE)** represents the BMR extrapolated over a 24-hour period.

The **resting metabolic rate (RMR)** is slightly higher than the BMR. It represents the BMR plus small amounts of additional energy expenditure associated with eating and previous muscular activity. According to the National Academy of Sciences, the BMR and RMR differ by less than 10 percent. Consequently, although there are some fine differences in the two terms, they are often used interchangeably. Additionally, the term **resting energy expenditure (REE)** is used to account for the energy processes at rest when extrapolated over 24 hours. In general, we shall use REE to also represent RMR.

Although some of the energy released during oxidative processes at rest supports physiological functions, such as pumping activity of the heart muscle, the majority of energy is released as heat, a thermal effect that keeps our body temperature at about 98.6° Fahrenheit (37° Celsius). Eating a meal and exercising are two other factors that induce a thermal effect.

White and Kearney note that BMR, and hence RMR, shows substantial variation between individuals, which may be a major factor in body weight control, a topic covered in chapter 10.

What effect does eating a meal have on the metabolic rate?

The significant elevation of the metabolic rate that occurs after ingestion of a meal was previously known as the *specific dynamic action of food* but is now often referred to as **dietary-induced thermogenesis (DIT)** or **thermic effect of food (TEF)**. This elevation is usually highest about 1 hour after a meal and lasts for about 4 hours, and it is due to the energy necessary to absorb, transport, store, and metabolize the food consumed. The greater the caloric content of the meal, the greater this TEF effect. Also, the type of food ingested may affect the magnitude of the TEF.

The TEF for protein approximates 20–30 percent, carbohydrate approximates 5–10 percent, and the effect of fat is minimal (0–5 percent). Crovetti and others noted that a very high protein meal (68% of Calories) elicited a greater TEF for 7 hours post-eating than did corresponding diets high in carbohydrate and fat. Even though the increased TEF amounts to only about 6 Calories more per hour, small daily changes in energy balance can lead to weight gain (e.g., 6 calories per hour for 7 hours × 365 days per year = 15,339 additional Calories per year). As shall be noted in chapter 11, there may be some advantage from incorporating more protein into the diet for weight-loss purposes.

The TEF is expressed as a percent of the energy content of the ingested meal. The normal increase in the BMR due to TEF from a mixed meal of carbohydrate, fat, and protein is about 5–10 percent. A TEF of 10 percent will account for 50 Calories of a 500-Calorie meal. The remaining 450 Calories are available for energy use by other body processes. The TEF effect accounts for approximately 5–10 percent of the total daily energy expenditure.

The role of TEF in obesity is somewhat controversial. Overfeeding may increase TEF, whereas underfeeding will decrease it. In a recent review, Westerterp indicated that alternating overfeeding and underfeeding may result in a positive energy balance, which may be one of the explanations for the increasing incidence of obesity in our current society. This topic is discussed in chapters 10 and 11 concerning diets for weight control.

How can I estimate my daily resting energy expenditure (REE)?

There are several ways to estimate your REE, but whichever method is used, the value obtained is an estimate and will have some error associated with it. To get a truly accurate value you would need a clinical evaluation, such as a standard BMR test. Accurate determination of REE is important for clinicians dealing with obesity patients, for such testing is needed to rule out hypometabolism. However, a number of formula estimates may give you an approximation of your daily REE.

Table 3.4 provides a simple method for calculating the REE of males and females of varying ages. Examples are provided in the table along with calculation of a 10 percent variability. Keep in mind that this is only an estimate of the daily REE, and additional energy would be expended during the day through the TEF effect and the effect of physical activity, as noted later.

A very simple, rough estimate of your REE is 1 Calorie per kilogram body weight per hour. Using this procedure, the estimated value for the male in table 3.4 is 1,680 Calories per day (1 × 70 kg × 24 hours) and for the female is 1,320 Calories (1 × 55 kg × 24 hours), values that are not substantially different from those calculated by the table procedure.

www.globalrph.com/harris-benedict-equation.htm Various Website calculators are available to estimate your REE. Enter your age, height, weight, and sedentary as the physical activity level to obtain your REE.

TABLE 3.4 Estimation of the daily resting energy expenditure (REE)

Age (years)	Equation
Males	
3–9	(22.7 × body weight*) + 495
10–17	(17.5 × body weight) + 651
18–29	(15.3 × body weight) + 679
30–60	(11.6 × body weight) + 879
>60	(13.5 × body weight) + 487

Example

154-lb male, age 20
154 lbs/2.2 = 70 kg
(15.3 × 70) + 679 = 1,750

Age (years)	Equation
Females	
3–9	(22.5 × body weight*) + 499
10–17	(12.2 × body weight) + 746
18–29	(14.7 × body weight) + 496
30–60	(8.7 × body weight) + 829
>60	(10.5 × body weight) + 596

Example

121-lb female, age 20
121 lbs/2.2 = 55 kg
(14.7 × 55) + 496 = 1,304

To get a range of values, simply add or subtract a normal 10 percent variation to the RMR estimate.

Male example: 10 percent of 1,750 = 175 Calories
Normal range = 1,575–1,925 Calories/day
Female example: 10 percent of 1,304 = 130 Calories
Normal range = 1,174–1,434 Calories/day

*Body weight is expressed in kilograms (kg).

What genetic factors affect my REE?

Your REE is directly related to the amount of metabolically active tissue you possess. At rest, tissues such as the heart, liver, kidneys, and other internal organs are more metabolically active than muscle tissue, but muscle tissue is more metabolically active than fat. Changes in the proportion of these tissues in your body will therefore cause changes in your REE.

Wu and others identified almost 2,400 genes significantly correlated with REE. Many factors influencing the REE, such as age, gender, natural hormonal activity, body size and surface area, and to a degree, body composition, are genetically determined. The effect of some of these factors on the REE is generally well known. Because infants have a large proportion of metabolically active tissue and are growing rapidly, their REE is extremely high. The REE declines through childhood, adolescence, and adulthood as full growth and maturation are achieved. Individuals with naturally greater muscle mass in comparison to body fat have a higher REE; the REE of women is about 10–15 percent lower than that of men, mainly because women have a higher proportion of fat to muscle tissue. Genetically lean individuals have a higher REE than do stocky individuals because their body surface area ratio is larger in proportion to their weight (body volume) and they lose more body heat through radiation. The role of genes in the etiology of obesity is discussed in detail in chapter 10.

How do dieting and body composition affect my REE?

Body composition may be changed so as to alter REE. Losing body weight, including both body fat and muscle tissue, generally lowers the total daily REE. The REE may be decreased significantly in obese individuals who go on a very low-Calorie diet of less than 800 Calories per day. The decrease in the REE, which is greater than would be due to weight loss alone, may be caused by lowered levels of thyroid hormones. In one study, the REE of obese subjects dropped 9.4 percent on a diet containing only 472 Calories per day. This topic is covered in more detail in chapters 10 and 11. The possibility of decreased REE in some athletes who maintain low body weight through exercise, such as female distance runners and male wrestlers, has been the subject of recent debate and will be covered in chapter 10 when we discuss body composition.

In contrast, maintaining normal body weight while reducing body fat and increasing muscle mass may raise the REE slightly because muscle tissue has a somewhat higher metabolic level than fat tissue or because the ratio of body surface area to body weight is increased. The decline in the REE that occurs with aging may be attributed partially to physical inactivity with a consequent loss of the more metabolically active muscle tissue and an accumulation of body fat. Methods to lose body fat and increase muscle mass are covered in chapters 11 and 12.

The type of body fat may also influence REE. White fat, or white adipose tissue, is metabolically different from brown fat, or brown adipose tissue. Park and others note that white fat is a major source of health problems associated with obesity, primarily via its role in promoting inflammation and metabolic dysfunction in the body. On the other hand, Lee and others note that brown fat plays a key role in energy homeostasis and, via its function to burn Calories to generate heat, may help protect against diet-induced obesity. The role of white and brown fat relative to obesity are discussed in chapter 10.

What environmental factors may also influence the REE?

Several lifestyle and environmental factors, including some foods we eat or drink, may influence our metabolism. For example, although caffeine is not a food, it is a common ingredient in some of the foods we may eat or drink. Caffeine is a stimulant and may elicit a significant rise in the REE. One study reported that the caffeine in two to three cups of regular coffee increased the REE 10–12 percent. Hot, spicy foods, such as hot peppers containing capsaicin, can also exert a modest stimulant effect on the metabolism.

Smoking cigarettes also raises the REE. Apparently the nicotine in tobacco stimulates the metabolism similarly to caffeine. This may be one of the reasons some individuals gain weight when they stop smoking. A long time ago cigarettes were advertised on major radio shows as a means to lose weight. Although some may still smoke cigarettes for weight-control purposes, such practices are strongly discouraged, given the many associated adverse health effects.

Climatic conditions, especially temperature changes, may also raise the REE. Exposure to the cold may stimulate the secretion of several hormones and muscular shivering, which may stimulate heat production up to 400 percent to help us stay warm. Exposure to warm or hot environments will increase energy expenditure through greater cardiovascular demands and the sweating response. Altitude exposure will also increase REE due to increased ventilation.

Many of these factors influencing the REE are important in themselves but may also be important considerations relative to weight-control programs and body temperature regulation. Thus, they are discussed further in later chapters.

As we shall see in the next section, the most important factor that can increase the metabolic rate is exercise.

What energy sources are used during rest?

The vast majority of the energy consumed during a resting situation is used to drive the automatic physiological processes in the body. Because the muscles expend little energy during rest, there is no need to produce ATP rapidly. Hence, the oxygen system is able to provide the necessary ATP for resting physiological processes.

The oxygen system can use carbohydrates, fats, and protein as energy sources. However, as noted in chapter 6, protein is not used as a major energy source under normal dietary conditions. Carbohydrates and fats, when combined with oxygen in the cells, are the major energy substrates during rest. Several factors may influence which of the two nutrients is predominantly used. In general, though, on a mixed diet of carbohydrate, protein, and fat, about 40 percent of the REE is derived from carbohydrate and about 60 percent comes from fat. However, eating a diet rich in carbohydrate or fat will increase the percent of the REE derived, respectively, from carbohydrate and fat. Also, when carbohydrate levels are low, such as after an overnight fast, the percentage of the REE derived from fat increases.

Key Concepts

▶ Human metabolism represents the sum total of all physiological processes in the body, and the metabolic rate reflects the speed at which the body utilizes energy.

▶ The basal metabolic rate (BMR) represents the energy requirements necessary to maintain physiological processes in a resting, postabsorptive state, while the resting metabolic rate (RMR) is a little higher due to the effects of prior eating and physical activity. The terms *BEE* and *REE* represent basal energy expenditure and resting energy expenditure, respectively, totaled over a 24-hour period.

- Eating a meal increases the metabolic rate as the digestive system absorbs, metabolizes, and stores the energy nutrients, a process termed the thermic effect of food (TEF). A meal will increase the RMR by about 5–10 percent, and some meals will elevate the RMR more than others.
- Various methods may be used to estimate daily resting energy expenditure (REE), but one simple means is to use the value of 1 Calorie per kilogram body weight per hour. For a 60-kilogram (132-pound) individual, this would represent 1,440 Calories over the course of 24 hours (60 × 1.0 × 24).
- A number of different factors may affect the REE, including body composition, drugs, climatic conditions, and prior exercise.
- Fats stored in the body serve as the main source of energy during rest.

Check for Yourself

- Using the formula in table 3.4, estimate your daily resting energy expenditure (REE) in Calories. Keep this record for later comparisons.

Human Energy Metabolism during Exercise

Exercise is a stressor to the body, and almost all body systems respond. If the exercise is continued daily, the body systems begin to adapt to the stress of exercise. As noted previously and as we shall see in later chapters, these adaptations may have significant health benefits. The two body systems most involved in exercise are the nervous system and the skeletal muscular system. The nervous system is needed to activate muscle contraction, but it is in the muscle cell itself that the energetics of exercise occur. Most other body systems are simply designed to serve the needs of the muscle cell during exercise.

How do my muscles influence the amount of energy I can produce during exercise?

Muscles constitute a significant percentage of our body weight, approximating 45 percent in the typical adult male and 35 percent in the typical adult female. However, in any given individual, these percentages may vary tremendously depending on various factors, such as type and intensity of physical activity. We shall discuss the potential health and sports performance benefits associated with modifying muscle mass in later chapters, but our focus here is on energy production for exercise.

The skeletal muscle cell, or muscle fiber, is a rather simple machine in design but extremely complex in function. It is a tube-like structure containing filaments that can slide by one another to shorten the total muscle. The shortening of the muscle moves bones, and hence work is accomplished, be it simply the raising of a barbell as in weight training or moving the whole body as in running. Like most other machines, the muscle cell has the capability of producing work at different rates, ranging from very low levels of energy expenditure during sleep to nearly a 90-fold increase during maximal, short-term anaerobic exercise.

The human body possesses several different types of skeletal muscle fibers, and their primary differences are in the ability to produce energy. Various types of proteins are found in muscle cells, and the production of energy is dependent on the specific type of proteins present. In general, three different types of skeletal muscle fiber types have been differentiated based on their rate of energy production, and table 3.5 presents various characteristics associated with each. For comprehensive details on muscle fiber types, see the review by Schiaffino and Reggiani.

Type I muscle fiber is also known as the *slow-twitch red fiber*, and as this name implies is used for slow muscle contractions, such as during rest and light aerobic physical activity. It is often

TABLE 3.5	Characteristics associated with the three types of skeletal muscle fibers		
Type	**I**	**IIa**	**IIb (IIx)**
Twitch speed	Slow	Faster	Fastest
Color	Red	Red	White
Size (diameter)	Small	Medium	Large
Fatigability	Slow	Moderate	Fast
Force production	Low	High	Highest
Oxidative processes	Highest	Moderate	Lowest
Mitochondria	Highest	Moderate	Low
Myoglobin	Highest	Moderate	Low
Blood flow	Highest	Moderate	Lowest
Triglyceride use	Highest	Moderate	Lowest
Glycogen use	Lowest	Moderate	Highest
Phosphocreatine levels	Lowest	Higher	Higher
Energy for sports	Aerobic capacity; aerobic power	Aerobic power; anaerobic capacity	Anaerobic power; anaerobic capacity

referred to as the *slow-oxidative (SO) fiber*. The characteristics associated with it, such as high mitochondria and myoglobin content, support its high oxidative capacity and resistance to fatigue. Use of the type I fiber is important during events associated with aerobic capacity and aerobic power.

The type IIa muscle fiber, also known as the *fast-twitch red fiber,* also possesses good aerobic capacity, but not as high as the type I fiber. However, it may also produce energy anaerobically via the lactic acid energy system. Hence, it is often referred to as the fast-oxidative glycolytic (FOG) fiber. It also has high ATP-PCr capacity. Use of the type IIa fiber is important during events associated with aerobic power and anaerobic capacity, but it fatigues sooner than the type I muscle fiber.

The type IIb (IIx) muscle fiber, also known as the *fast-twitch white fiber,* possesses poor aerobic capacity and is used primarily for anaerobic energy production. It is often referred to as the fast glycolytic (FG) fiber. Like the type IIa fiber, it also has high ATP-PCr capacity. Use of the type IIb muscle fiber is important during events associated with anaerobic power and anaerobic capacity, but it fatigues very rapidly.

Most muscles contain all three types of muscle fibers, and all fibers are used during exercise tasks of varying intensity. However, the use of one fiber type will usually predominate, dependent on the intensity of the exercise task and the associated human energy system. Physical training can improve the efficacy of each muscle fiber type, and the benefits that accrue to each depend on the type and extent of exercise training. Moreover, the distribution of muscle fiber types will vary among different individuals due to genetic predisposition, and such differences may influence the level of success in certain sport endeavors. Wilson and others indicate that type I muscle fibers are found in abundance in elite endurance athletes, while type IIa and IIb fibers are proportionally higher in elite strength and power athletes.

What effect does muscular exercise have on the metabolic rate?

As noted in the previous section, the REE is measured with the subject at rest in a reclining position. Any physical activity will raise metabolic activity above the REE and thus increase energy expenditure. Accounting for changes in physical activity over the day may provide a reasonable, although imprecise, estimate of the total daily energy expenditure. Very light activities such as sitting, standing, playing cards, cooking, and typing all increase energy output above the REE, but we normally do not think of them as exercise, as noted later in this chapter. For purposes of this discussion, the **exercise metabolic rate (EMR)** represents the increase in metabolism brought about by moderate or strenuous physical activity such as brisk walking, climbing stairs, cycling, dancing, running, and other such planned exercise activities. The EMR is known more appropriately as the **thermic effect of exercise (TEE)**.

The most important factor affecting the metabolic rate is the intensity or speed of the exercise. To move faster, your muscles must contract more rapidly, consuming proportionately more energy. Use of type I muscle fibers predominates during low-intensity exercise, and type II fibers are increasingly recruited with more intense exercise. The following represents approximate

energy expenditure in Calories per minute for increasing levels of exercise intensity for an average-sized adult male. However, for most of us, it would be impossible to sustain the higher levels of energy expenditure for long, less than a minute or so, and the highest level could be sustained for only a second or so.

Level of intensity	Caloric expenditure per minute
Resting metabolic rate	1.0
Sitting and writing	2.0
Walking at 2 mph	3.3
Walking at 3 mph	4.2
Running at 5 mph	9.4
Running at 10 mph	18.8
Running at 15 mph	29.3
Running at 20 mph	38.7
Maximal power weightlift	>90.0

Although the intensity of the exercise is the most important factor affecting the magnitude of the metabolic rate, there are some other important considerations. In some activities, the increase in energy expenditure is not directly proportional to speed, for the efficiency of movement will affect caloric expenditure. Very fast walking becomes more inefficient, so the individual burns more Calories per mile walking briskly compared to more leisurely walking. A beginning swimmer wastes a lot of energy, whereas one who is more accomplished may swim with less effort, saving Calories when swimming a given distance. Swimming and cycling at very high speeds exponentially increase water or air resistance, so caloric expenditure also increases exponentially. Moreover, the individual with a greater body weight will burn more Calories for any given amount of work in which the body has to be moved, as in walking, jogging, or running. It simply costs more total energy to move a heavier load.

How is energy expenditure of the three human energy systems measured during exercise?

As discussed earlier in this chapter, physical activity and energy expenditure can be measured in a variety of ways, such as with the use of ergometers and accelerometers. In this section, we discuss measurement techniques to quantify energy production from the three human energy systems.

Ward-Smith noted that due to accurate measurements of oxygen uptake and carbon dioxide output, the energy contributions from aerobic metabolism are readily quantifiable, whereas the energy contribution from anaerobic metabolism is far more difficult to determine.

ATP-PCr Energy System   Energy production from the ATP-PCr energy system has been measured by several procedures. One procedure involves a muscle biopsy with subsequent analysis for ATP and PCr levels to determine use following exercise, but the small muscle biopsy may not represent ATP-PCr use in other muscles.

ATP and PCr levels may also be determined by computerized imaging procedures, a noninvasive procedure, but the exercise task must be confined to specific movements due to the nature of the imaging equipment. Thus, Lange and Bury indicate that it is difficult to obtain precise physiological or biochemical data during common explosive-type exercise tests, such as short sprints.

Lactic Acid Energy System Laboratory techniques are also available to measure the role of the lactic acid system in exercise, primarily by measuring the concentration of lactic acid in the blood or in muscle tissues. One measure of exercise intensity is the so-called anaerobic threshold, or that point where the metabolism is believed to shift to a greater use of the lactic acid system. This point is often termed the **onset of blood lactic acid (OBLA)**, or *lactate threshold*. The anaerobic threshold may also be referred to as the **steady-state threshold**, indicating that endurance exercise may continue for prolonged periods if you exercise below this threshold value. Other procedures, such as the maximal accumulated oxygen deficit (MAOD), are used in attempts to quantify anaerobic energy expenditure, but Noordhof and others note that unlike aerobic capacity, anaerobic capacity cannot be easily quantified.

Oxygen Energy System Laboratory tests also are necessary to measure the contribution of the oxygen system during exercise, and this is the most commonly used technique for measuring exercise intensity (see figure 3.3). The most commonly used measurement is the **maximal oxygen uptake**, which represents the highest amount of oxygen that an individual may consume under exercise situations. In essence, the technique consists of monitoring the oxygen uptake of the individual while the exercise intensity is increased in stages. When oxygen uptake does not increase with an increase in workload, the maximal oxygen uptake has been reached. Maximal oxygen uptake is usually expressed as VO_2 **max**, which may be stated as liters per minute or milliliters per kilogram body weight per minute. An example is provided in figure 3.13. A commonly used technique to indicate exercise intensity is to report it as a certain percentage of an individual's VO_2 max, such as 50 or 75 percent. If blood samples are taken periodically to measure serum levels of lactic acid, the percent of VO_2 max at which the steady-state threshold occurs may be determined. Additionally, measurement of oxygen during recovery from exercise may be used to calculate the MAOD, as noted above, an indirect marker for anaerobic contributions to energy expenditure during exercise. Proper training may increase both VO_2 max and the steady-state threshold, as illustrated in figure 3.14.

How can I convert the various means of expressing exercise energy expenditure into something more useful to me, such as Calories per minute?

A number of research studies have been conducted to determine the energy expenditure of a wide variety of sports and other physical activities.

The energy costs have been reported in a variety of ways, including Calories, kilojoules (kJ), oxygen uptake, and **METS**.

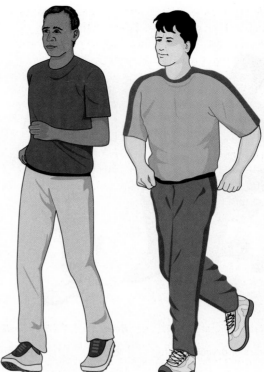

FIGURE 3.13 Maximal oxygen uptake (VO_2 max). The best way to express VO_2 max is in milliliters of oxygen per kilogram (kg) of body weight per minute (ml O_2/ kg/min). As noted in the figure, the leaner individual has a lower VO_2 max in liters but a higher VO_2 max when expressed relative to weight. In this case, the leaner individual has a higher degree of aerobic fitness, at least as measured by VO_2 max per unit body weight.

VO_2 max: liters/minute	3.6 L (3600 ml)	4.0 L (4000 ml)
kg body weight	60	80
VO_2 max: ml O_2/kg/minute	60	50

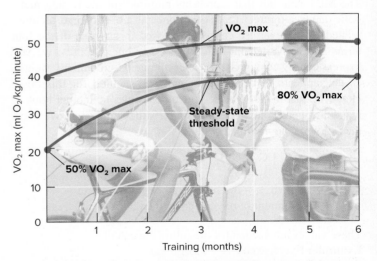

FIGURE 3.14 The effect of training upon VO_2 max and the steady-state threshold. Training increases both your VO_2 max and your steady-state threshold, which is the ability to work at a greater percentage of your VO_2 max without producing excessive lactic acid—a causative factor in fatigue. For example, before training the VO_2 max may be 40 ml while the steady-state threshold is only 20 ml (50% of VO_2 max). After training, VO_2 max may rise to 50 ml, but the steady-state threshold may rise to 40 ml (80% of the VO_2 max).

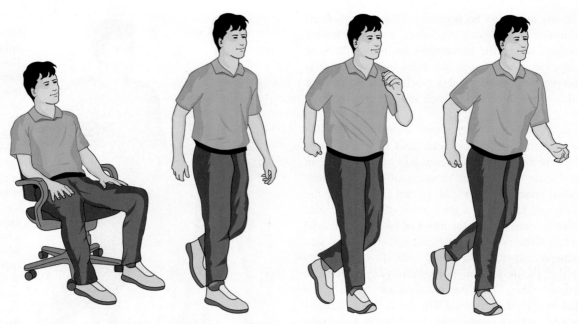

	Rest	Slow walk (2 mph)	Fast walk (5 mph)	Run (8 mph)
Liters of oxygen/minute	.25	.5−.75	1.5−1.75	2.5−3.0
Calories/minute	1.25	2.5−3.75	7.5−8.75	12.5−15.0
Kilojoules/minute	5	10−15	30−35	50−60
METS	1	2−3	6−7	10−12

FIGURE 3.15 Energy equivalents in oxygen consumption, Calories, Kilojoules, and METS. This figure depicts four means of expressing energy expenditure during four levels of activity. These approximate values are for an average male of 154 pounds (70 kg). If you weigh more or less, the values will increase or decrease accordingly.

The MET is a unit that represents multiples of the resting metabolic rate (see figure 3.15). These concepts are, of course, all interrelated, so an exercise can be expressed in any one of the four terms and converted into the others. For our purposes, we will express energy cost in Calories per minute based on body weight, as that appears to be the most practical method for this book. However, just in case you see the other values in another book or magazine, here is how you may simplify the conversion. We know the following approximate values:

$$1 \text{ C} = 4 \text{ kJ}$$
$$1 \text{ L O}_2 = 5 \text{ C}$$
$$1 \text{ MET} = 3.5 \text{ ml O}_2/\text{kg body weight/min}$$
(amount of oxygen consumed during rest)

These values are needed for the following calculations:

Example: Exercise cost = 20 kJ/minute
To get Calorie cost, divide kJ by the equivalent value for Calories.

$$20 \text{ kJ/min}/4 = 5 \text{ C/min}$$

Example: Exercise cost = 3 L of O_2/min
To get Calorie cost, multiply liters of O_2 × Calories per liter.

$$\text{Caloric cost} = 3 \times 5 = 15 \text{ C/min}$$

Example: Exercise cost = 25 ml O_2/kg body weight/min
You need body weight in kg, which is weight in pounds divided by 2.2. For this example 154 lbs = 70 kg. Determine total O_2 cost/min by multiplying body weight times O_2 cost/kg/min.

$$70 \times 25 = 1,750 \text{ ml O}_2$$

Convert ml into L: 1,750 ml = 1.75 L
Multiply liters O_2 × Calories per liter
Caloric cost = 1.75 × 5 = 8.75 C/min

Example: Exercise cost = 12 METS
You need body weight in kg—for this example, 70 kg.
Multiply total METS times O_2 equivalent of 1 MET.

$$12 \times 3.5 \text{ ml O}_2/\text{kg/min} = 42.0 \text{ ml O}_2/\text{kg/min}$$

Multiply body weight times this result
70 × 42 ml O_2/kg/min = 2,940 ml O_2/min
Convert ml into L: 2,940 ml O_2/min = 2.94 L O_2/min
Multiply liters O_2 × Calories per liter
Caloric cost = 2.94 × 5 = 14.70 C/min

We shall use this METS procedure later, using a simplified formula to calculate caloric expenditure:

$$\text{METS} \times 3.5 \text{ ml O}_2/\text{kg/min} \times \text{kg body weight} \div 200$$
$$12 \times 3.5 \times 70 \text{ kg} \div 200 = 14.70 \text{ C/min}$$

How can I tell what my metabolic rate is during exercise?

The human body is basically a muscle machine designed for movement. Almost all of the other body systems serve the muscular system. The nervous system causes the muscles to contract. The digestive system supplies nutrients. The cardiovascular system delivers these nutrients along with oxygen in cooperation with the respiratory system. The endocrine system secretes hormones that affect muscle nutrition. The excretory system removes waste products. When humans exercise, almost all body systems increase their activity to accommodate the increased energy demands of the muscle cell. In most types of sustained exercises, however, the major demand of the muscle cells is for oxygen.

As noted previously, the major technique for evaluating metabolic rate is to measure the oxygen consumption of an individual during exercise. Athletes may benefit from such physiological testing. Measurements of VO$_2$ max, maximal heart rate, and the anaerobic threshold may help in planning an optimal training program, and subsequent testing may illustrate training effects. Such testing is becoming increasingly available at various universities and comprehensive fitness/wellness centers, but very useful data, such as heart rate, may be obtained with use of the various gadgets and apps discussed previously.

Given the relationships among exercise intensity, oxygen consumption, and heart rate, the average individual may be able to get a relative approximation of the metabolic rate during exercise. A more or less linear relationship exists between exercise intensity and oxygen uptake. As the intensity level of work increases, so does the amount of oxygen consumed. The two systems primarily responsible for delivering the oxygen to the muscles are the cardiovascular and respiratory systems. There is also a fairly linear relationship between their responses and oxygen consumption. In general, maximal heart rate (HRmax) and VO$_2$ max coincide at the same exercise intensity level. A simplified schematic is presented in figure 3.16.

Because the heart rate (HR) generally is linearly related to oxygen consumption (the main expression of metabolic rate), and because it is easy to measure this physiological response during exercise either manually at the wrist or neck pulse or with a gadget that monitors heart rate, it may prove to be a practical guide to your metabolic rate. The higher your heart rate, the greater your metabolic rate. However, a number of factors may influence your specific heart rate response to exercise, such as the type of exercise (running vs. swimming), your level of physical fitness, your gender, your age, your skill efficiency, your percentage of body fat, and a number of environmental conditions. Thus, it is difficult to predict your exact metabolic rate from your exercise HR. As we shall see in chapter 11, however, the HR data during exercise may be used as a basis for establishing a personal fitness program for health and weight control.

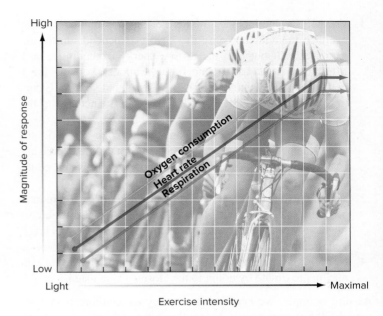

FIGURE 3.16 Relationships among oxygen consumption, heart rate, and respiration responses to increasing exercise rates. In general, as the intensity of exercise continues, there is a rise in oxygen consumption, which is accompanied by proportional increases in heart rate and respiration. VO$_2$ max and HRmax usually occur at the same exercise intensity.

How can I determine the energy cost of my exercise routine?

As noted previously in this chapter, there are a variety of ways to determine and express the energy cost of exercise. Unless we are conducting research, most of us are interested in the caloric cost of exercise, primarily for purposes of body weight control. Various devices and smartphone applications may provide us with a good estimate, but simply knowing the metabolic cost in Calories per minute for our usual physical activities may also be helpful. Bushman notes that the MET levels provided in the Compendium of Physical Activities can be a useful means to quantify the caloric expenditure of exercise.

Based on the MET level provided in the Compendium, appendix B provides an estimate of Calories expended per minute for individuals of varying body weights. You may use the following Website to find the MET level for a wide variety of physical activities.

https://sites.google.com/site/compendiumofphysicalactivities/
Click on Activity Categories and then select the appropriate activity, such as Walking. Scan the list to find the most appropriate type of walking you do to obtain the MET level.

Although the Compendium was not developed to determine the exact energy expenditure of physical activity for individuals, it may be a useful guide with the following considerations.

1. The MET value includes the REE. Thus, the total cost of the exercise includes not only the energy expended during the exercise itself but also the resting energy expenditure, or 1 MET, during the same time frame. Suppose you ran for 1 hour and expended a total of 800 Calories, but your REE during that hour was 1 MET, or 75 Calories. The net cost of the exercise was 725 Calories.

2. The MET values in the table are only for the time you are doing the activity. For example, if your total time exercising is 1 hour, but you take three 5-minute breaks for water, count only 45 minutes for the actual exercise task.

3. The MET values are not precise. Your energy expenditure may be more or less than the estimated amount. Actual caloric cost might vary somewhat because of such factors as your skill level, your training status, the environmental temperature, and others.

4. Not all body weights or MET levels could be listed, but you may approximate by going to the closest value listed.

As one example, we can find the energy expenditure of a 154-pound (70-kg) man who walked 4.0 miles in 1 hour, a very brisk pace on a level, firm surface. Consulting the Compendium, we find his MET value is 5.0. From appendix B, we find that approximately 6.1 Calories would be expended per minute. Selecting appropriate activities with individually appropriate MET levels is an important consideration in body weight control, as discussed in chapter 11.

What are the best types of activities to increase energy expenditure?

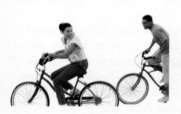

Activities that use the large muscle groups of the body and are performed continuously usually will expend the greatest amount of Calories. Intensity and duration are the two key determinants of total energy expenditure. Activities in which you may be able to exercise continuously at a fairly high intensity for a prolonged period will maximize your total caloric loss. Although this may encompass a wide variety of physical activities, popular modes include walking, running, swimming, bicycling, and aerobic dance. Walking and running are most popular because they are so practical to do. In essence, all you need is a good pair of shoes.

However, as noted in chapter 1, high-intensity interval training (HIIT) has become increasingly popular, particularly when time is an issue. A few general comments about some common modes of exercising would appear to be in order.

Walking Walking at a slow pace is more economical than walking at a faster pace or running. Kuo and others note that walking is a pendular motion, with the stance leg behaving as an inverted pendulum and the swing leg as a regular pendulum. Thus, the pendular motion of slow walking saves energy and reduces the metabolic cost. A good rule of thumb is that you expend about 1 Calorie per kilogram/body weight per mile walking at a speed of 2–3 miles per hour on a level, smooth surface.

However, walking faster may increase energy expenditure exponentially. The MET level for walking or jogging 5 mph is the same, 8.3 METS. At high walking speeds (above 5 mph), you may expend more energy than if you jogged at the same speed. Fast, vigorous walking, known as aerobic walking, can be an effective means to expend Calories. However, as with other exercise activities, it takes practice to become a fast walker.

Various terms, including the following, have been used to describe walking based on speed.

> Strolling–about 2 mph (30 minutes/mile)
> Leisurely walking–about 3 mph (20 minutes/mile)
> Aerobic or brisk walking–about 4 mph (15 minutes/mile)
> Power walking–about 5 mph (12 minutes/mile)
> Race walking, beginner–about 6 mph (10 minutes/mile)
> Race walking, elite–about 10 mph (6 minutes/mile)

Walking intensity can be increased in other ways. Climbing stairs, at home, at work, in an athletic stadium, or on step machines, is one means to make walking more vigorous. Carrying loads, such as backpacks or hand weights, is another. The Compendium of Physical Activities lists more than 60 modes of walking, with a range of 2 to 12 METS. Walking leisurely less than 2 miles per hour would be 2 METS, whereas climbing a hill while carrying a heavy load would approximate 12 METS. You may calculate the caloric cost of walking at various MET levels in appendix B.

For health purposes, walking may be as good as running, if you have the time. In a study comparing exercise and health benefits, Williams and Thompson noted that the more runners ran and the walkers walked, the better off they were in health benefits. If the amount of energy expended was the same between the two groups, then the health benefits were comparable. But the walkers need to spend about twice the amount of time as the runners to get the same benefits.

Running As a general rule, the caloric cost of running a given distance does not depend on the speed. It will take you a longer time to cover the distance at a slower running speed, but the total caloric cost will be similar to that expended at a faster speed. The MET levels for running at a pace of 4 mph, 8 mph, and 12 mph are, respectively, 6.0, 11.8, and 19, resulting is comparable calculated energy expenditures within a range of 108 to 116 Calories per mile for a 70-kilogram runner. The Compendium of Physical Activities lists more than 25 levels for running and jogging, ranging from 4.5 to 23 METS.

Swimming Because of water resistance, swimming takes more energy to cover a given distance than does either walking or running. Although the amount of energy expended depends somewhat on the type of swimming stroke used and the ability of the swimmer, swimming a given distance takes about four times as much energy as running. For example, swimming a quarter-mile is the energy equivalent of running a mile. Water aerobics and water running (doing aerobics or running in waist-deep, chest-deep, or deep water) may be effective exercise regimens that help prevent injuries due to impact. The MET values for swimming different strokes may be found in the Compendium of Physical Activities, listed under Water Activities.

Cycling Bicycling takes less energy to cover a given distance in comparison to running on a level surface. The energy cost of bicycling depends on a number of factors such as body weight, the type of bicycle, hills, and body position on the bike (assuming a streamlined position to reduce air resistance). Owing to rapidly increasing air resistance at higher speeds such as 20 mph, the energy cost of bicycling increases at a much faster rate at such speeds. A detailed method for calculating energy expenditure during bicycling is presented in the article by Hagberg and Pena. In general, cycling 1 mile is approximately the energy equivalent of running one-third the distance. The MET values for bicycling at different speeds and under different conditions are listed in the Compendium of Physical Activities.

Group Exercise Various types of group exercise classes have been popular for more than 30 years. These classes can include high- and low-impact aerobic dance, step aerobics, zumba, spin classes, and cardio-kickboxing. All of these classes vary in intensity based on participant effort but have been shown to burn up to about 10 Calories per minute. Though the energy expenditure of group exercise can be comparable to individual exercise tasks such as running or cycling, the greatest benefit of group exercise might be improved exercise adherence. Burke and colleagues examined 44 studies and showed that when exercisers were given the opportunity to interact with others, as when exercising in a group, adherence was better and the exercise program was more effective. The MET equivalents for various types of group exercise are listed in the Compendium of Physical Activities under the category Conditioning Exercise.

Home Aerobic Exercise Equipment Home exercise equipment may also provide a strenuous aerobic workout. Recent research suggests that for any given level of perceived effort, treadmill running burned the most Calories. Exercising on elliptical trainers, cross-country ski machines, rowing ergometers, and stair-climbing apparatus also expended significant amounts of Calories, more so than bicycling apparatus. Many modern pieces of exercise equipment are electronically equipped with small computers to calculate approximate energy cost as Calories per minute and total caloric cost of the exercise. However, as noted above, research shows that exercise adherence is better when there is contact with fellow exercisers, as in group exercise settings. Comparable to group exercise, the MET equivalents for various types of home exercises are listed in the Compendium of Physical Activities under the category Conditioning Exercise.

Resistance, or Weight, Training Resistance training, or weight training, may be an effective way to expend energy, but it is not as effective as aerobic types of exercise. For example, Bloomer compared energy expenditure during resistance training (free-weight squatting at 70% maximal) to aerobic training (cycling at 70 percent VO_2 max) for 30 minutes. Although the heart rates were the same for both types of exercise, the cycling protocol expended 441 Calories while the squatting protocol expended only 269 Calories, a 64 percent difference. Although this is a significant difference, Bloomer noted that the resistance exercise, if

performed 4–5 days a week, would meet the recommendations for energy expenditure as suggested by the ACSM. The MET equivalents for resistance-type exercises are listed in the Compendium of Physical Activities under the category Conditioning Exercise.

Sports activity One of the most enjoyable ways to increase energy expenditure is sports participation. As noted above, sports such as running, race walking, swimming, and bicycling provide opportunities to expend considerable amounts of energy, as do other sports such as soccer, basketball, handball, martial arts, singles tennis, and others. The MET equivalents of participation in a wide variety of sports are presented in the Compendium of Physical Activities.

Passive and Occupational Energy Expenditure Advances in technology have changed the way people accomplish their jobs. Specifically, people are spending more time sitting than ever, which has been implicated in decreased daily energy expenditure and as a contributing factor to the obesity epidemic. One-way people are increasing energy expenditure at work is to sit on a Physioball instead of a desk chair, or to abandon sitting entirely and simply do their job while standing at their desk or even walking slowly on a treadmill. In their review of 32 studies, Torbeyns and others concluded that active workstations could increase physical activity levels. One study reported an increased energy expenditure approximating 100 Calories per hour when using a "walk and work" treadmill. Now that sitting itself has been identified as an independent risk factor for mortality, researchers are focusing on how to increase passive energy expenditure to combat the decrease in occupational energy expenditure and to supplement daily energy expenditure to help maintain a healthy body weight.

Table 3.6 provides a classification of some common physical activities based on rate of energy expenditure. The implications of these types of exercises for weight-control programs are discussed in later chapters.

Does exercise affect my resting energy expenditure (REE)?

Exercise not only raises the metabolic rate during exercise but also, depending on the intensity and duration of the activity, will keep the REE elevated during the recovery period. The increase in body temperature and in the amounts of circulating hormones such as adrenaline (epinephrine) will continue to influence some cellular activity, and some other metabolic processes, such as circulation and respiration, will remain elevated for a limited time. This effect, which has been labeled the **metabolic aftereffects of exercise**, is calculated by monitoring the oxygen consumption for several hours during the recovery period after the exercise task. The amount of oxygen in excess of the pre-exercise REE, often called excess postexercise oxygen consumption (EPOC), reflects the additional caloric cost

TABLE 3.6	Classification of selective physical activities based on rate of energy expenditure*

Light, mild aerobic exercise (<5 Calories/min)

Archery
Badminton, social
Baseball
Bicycling (5 mph)
Bowling
Croquet
Dancing, slow ballroom
Golf (using power cart)
Horseback riding (walk)
Swimming (20–25 yards/min)
Tai Chi
Walking (2–3 mph)

Moderate aerobic exercise (5–10 Calories/min)

Badminton, competitive
Basketball, game
Bicycling (10 mph)
Dancing, aerobic
Racquetball
Rope skipping (60 rpm)
Running (5 mph)
Step aerobics (10 inches)
Skateboarding, moderate speed
Tennis, recreational singles
Volleyball, competitive
Walking (3.0–4.0 mph)

Moderately heavy to heavy aerobic exercise (>10 Calories/min)

Bicycling, mountain
Bicycling (15–20 mph)
Calisthenics, vigorous
Handball, competitive
In-line skating (10–15 mph)
Racquetball, competitive
Rope skipping (120–140 rpm)
Running (6–9 mph)
Swimming (50–70 yards/min)
Volleyball, competitive
Walking (5.0–6.0 mph)
Water jogging, vigorous

*Calories per minute based on a body weight of 70 kg, or 154 pounds. Those weighing more or less will expend more or fewer Calories, respectively, but the intensity level of the exercise will be the same. The actual amount of Calories expended may also depend on a number of other factors, depending on the activity. For example, bicycling into or with the wind will increase or decrease, respectively, the energy cost. See appendix B, the Compendium of Physical Activities, for more details.

of the exercise above and beyond that expended during the exercise task itself.

Recent research suggests that if the exercise task is sufficiently intense, the postexercise metabolic rate may remain elevated to burn additional Calories. Knab and others reported male subjects who cycled for 45 minutes at a high-intensity level approximating 75 percent of VO$_2$ max experienced an elevated EPOC for nearly 14 hours, totaling about 190 Calories. High-intensity interval training (HIIT), discussed in chapter 1, has also been promoted as a means to elevate EPOC. Skelly and others recently evaluated oxygen consumption over a 24-hour period after subjects performed either HIIT or continuous moderate-intensity training. The 20-minute HIIT exercise session consisted of ten 1-minute interval exercise bouts at 90 percent of maximal heart rate, with each interval interspersed with 1 minute of active recovery. The continuous moderate-intensity bout involved cycling at 70 percent of maximal heart rate for 45 minutes. Although the total oxygen cost during HIIT exercise was lower than during the continuous exercise, the total oxygen consumption over 24 hours was similar. For individuals who are aerobically fit but have limited time to exercise, for body weight-control purposes the HIIT protocol may be as effective as more prolonged moderate exercise. Resistance training may also increase the EPOC, but the increase is relatively small. For example, Haddock and Wilkin found that although a bout of resistance training increased the resting metabolic rate for 120 minutes afterwards, subjects expended only about 23 more Calories above the normal resting level for that time frame.

Although the metabolic aftereffects of exercise may be relatively modest, they may add up over time. Moreover, exercise may help mitigate the decrease in the REE often seen in individuals on very low-Calorie diets. This point is explored further in chapter 11.

Does exercise affect the thermic effect of food (TEF)?

Many studies have been conducted to investigate the effect of exercise on the thermic effect of food. Unfortunately, no clear answer has been found. Some studies have reported an increase in TEF when subjects exercise either before or after the meal, whereas others revealed little or no effects. Some research even suggests that exercise training decreases the TEF. In more recent studies, Warwick reported that prior low-intensity exercise had no effect on the TEF of a meal containing about 560 Calories. Binns and others found that exercising after consuming a high-protein meal increased TEF more so than exercising after fasting, but there were no differences in TEF when compared to a low-protein meal. As noted in chapter 11, the TEF associated with high-protein diets may play a role in body weight control.

Other studies have investigated differences between exercise-trained and untrained individuals relative to TEF, and although some preliminary research noted a decreased TEF in endurance-trained athletes, Tremblay and others also noted that it is still unclear if training causes any significant alterations in TEF. In any case, the increases or decreases noted in the TEF due to either exercise or exercise training were minor, averaging about 5–9 Calories for several hours.

How much energy should I consume daily?

The National Academy of Sciences, through the Institute of Medicine, has released its DRI for energy in conjunction with DRI for carbohydrate, fat, and protein, as noted in chapter 2. Because of possible problems in developing obesity, no RDA or UL were developed for energy. Instead, the Institute of Medicine uses the term **Estimated Energy Requirement (EER)**, which it defines as the dietary intake that is predicted to maintain energy balance in a healthy adult of a defined age, gender, weight, height, and level of physical activity consistent with good health. In essence, the EER estimates your REE based on age, gender, weight, and height, and then modifies this value depending on your daily level of physical activity, which we refer to in this book as the thermic effect of exercise (TEE).

Your total daily energy expenditure (TDEE) is the sum of your BEE, your TEF, and your TEE. Figure 3.17 provides some approximate values for the typical active individual, indicating that BEE accounts for 60–75 percent of the total daily energy expenditure, TEF represents 5–10 percent, and TEE explains 15–30 percent. These values are approximate and may vary tremendously, particularly TEE, which may range from near 0 percent in the totally sedentary individual to 50 percent or more in ultraendurance athletes.

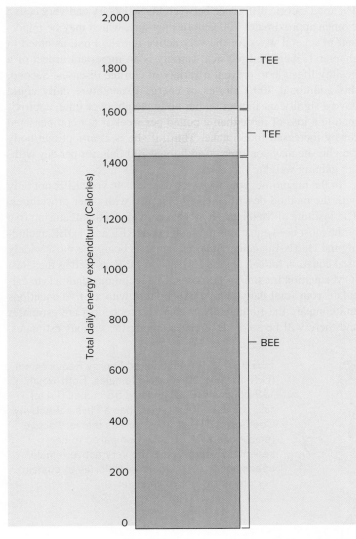

FIGURE 3.17 Total daily energy expenditure. Three major factors account for the total daily energy expenditure. Basal energy expenditure (BEE) accounts for 60–75 percent, the thermic effect of food (TEF) accounts for 5–10 percent, and 15–30 percent is accounted for by the thermic effect of exercise (TEE). However, all of these percentages are variable in different individuals, with exercise being the most modifiable component. In the figure, the BEE is 70 percent, the TEF is 10 percent, and the TEE is 20 percent.

To illustrate the effect that physical activity, or TEE, may have on your TDEE, the Institute of Medicine developed four **physical activity level (PAL)** categories, which are presented in table 3.7. The PAL describes the ratio of the TDEE divided by the BEE over a 24-hour period. The PAL (calculated as 2,000/1,400) in figure 3.17 is 1.43, or low active. The higher the ratio, the greater the amount of daily physical activity.

Sedentary Category   The energy expenditure in individuals in the Sedentary category represents their REE, including the TEF, plus various physical activities associated with independent living, such as walking from the house or work to the car, typing, and other forms of very light activity. Levine has coined the term **nonexercise activity thermogenesis (NEAT)** for these very light activities, which represent all the energy we expend daily that is not sleeping, eating, or sports-related exercise. NEAT includes such activities as playing the piano, dancing, housework, washing the car, and similar daily physical activities. We shall discuss the role of NEAT in weight control in chapter 10.

For the other three categories, the Institute of Medicine bases the PAL on the amount of daily physical activity that is the equivalent of walking at a rate of 3–4 miles per hour.

Low Active Category   An adult male who weighs 154 pounds (70 kg) and who, in addition to the normal daily activities of independent living, expended the physical activity equivalent of walking 2.2 miles per day would be in the Low Active category, with a PAL of 1.5.

Active Category   To be in the Active category with a PAL of 1.75, he would need to expend the physical activity energy equivalent of walking 7.0 miles per day.

Very Active Category   To be in this category, with a PAL of 2.2, he would need to expend the energy equivalent of 17 miles per day.

Keep in mind that you do not need to walk this many miles per day, but simply do a multitude of physical activities, such as climbing stairs, golfing, swimming, and jogging, that add up to this energy equivalent. Table 3.6 provides examples of physical activities ranging from light to heavy that may be used to total the required energy equivalents of walking.

TABLE 3.7   The Physical Activity Level Categories

Category	Physical Activity Level (PAL)	Physical Activity Coefficient (PA) Males/Females
Sedentary	≥ 1.0 − < 1.4	1.00/1.00
Low Active	≥ 1.4 − < 1.6	1.11/1.12
Active	≥ 1.6 − < 1.9	1.25/1.27
Very Active	≥ 1.9 − < 2.5	1.48/1.45

Note that walking at a speed of about 3-4 mph is considered to be moderate aerobic exercise, so equivalent amounts of the types of exercise in this category may serve as substitutes for actual walking. Light and heavy exercise activities may also be done in place of walking. Also note that the energy equivalent of moderate exercise is about 5-10 Calories per minute. Perusal of appendix B, in conjunction with the Compendium of Physical Activities, will provide you with a wide variety of activities that may cost about 5–10 Calories per minute and serve as substitutes for walking.

Based on a number of doubly labeled water studies, the Institute of Medicine developed equations, utilizing the Physical Activity Quotient (PA) described below, to determine the Estimated Energy Requirement (EER).

Males, 19 years and older:

$$EER = 662 - 9.53 \times age + [PA \times (15.91 \times Weight + 539.6 \times Height)]$$

Females, 19 years and older:

$$EER = 354 - 6.91 \times age + [PA \times (9.361 \times Weight + 726 \times Height)]$$

Age: In years.

Weight: In kilograms (kg). To convert weight in pounds into kilograms, multiply by 0.454.

Height: In meters (m). To convert height in inches into meters, multiply by 0.0254.

PA: PA is the physical activity coefficient, which is based on the PAL. Based on mathematical consideration to equate energy expenditure between the various PAL categories, the PA coefficient for the Sedentary category was set at 1.0 and the PA for the other categories adjusted accordingly. The PAs for the four PAL categories are presented for adult males and females in table 3.7.

Although there may be variances in this estimate of your EER, the estimate may provide you with a ballpark figure of your daily energy needs. Let's look at an example, as depicted in figure 3.18, of the difference that physical activity may have on the daily energy needs of a sedentary and very active adult female. Both are 20 years old, weigh 132 pounds (60 kg), and are 55 inches (1.4 m) tall.

Sedentary:

$$EER = 354 - 6.91 \times 20 + [1.0 \times (9.361 \times 60 + 726 \times 1.4)]$$
$$EER = 354 - 138.2 + [1.0 \times (561.66 + 1,016.4)]$$
$$EER = 215.8 + [1,578.06] = 1,794 \text{ Calories}$$

Very active:

$$EER = 354 - 6.91 \times 20 + [1.45 \times (9.361 \times 60 + 726 \times 1.4)]$$
$$EER = 354 - 138.2 + [1.45 \times (561.66 + 1,016.4)]$$
$$EER = 2,15.8 + [2,288.19] = 2,504 \text{ Calories}$$

The total caloric difference between the sedentary and very active women approximates 700 Calories per day, which may be important in several ways for the very active female. First, as noted in chapter 1, increased physical activity is an important aspect of a healthy lifestyle to prevent a variety of chronic diseases. Second, this additional 700 Calories of energy expenditure daily could have a significant impact on her body weight over time, approximating a loss of more than a pound per week if not compensated for by increased food intake. Third, if she is at an optimal body weight, she may consume an additional 700 Calories per day without gaining weight.

In the meantime, you may wish to calculate your EER not only with the method described above but also with other procedures. The Institute of Medicine (IOM) has provided a link featuring five of the most used equations to predict your REE and TDEE, including the Harris-Benedict equation, noted as being the most widely used equation for calculating BMR and TDEE, as well as the latest IOM equation for similar purposes. One recommendation is to calculate your total daily energy expenditure with all five equations and compare the findings. Note that all procedures are estimates and there will be some differences among the various estimates,

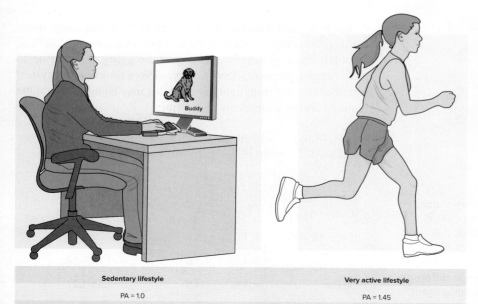

FIGURE 3.18 Estimated Energy Requirement (EER) for two 20-year-old females. Both weigh 132 pounds (60 kg) and are 55 inches (1.4 m) tall. The sedentary female has a Physical Activity Coefficient (PA) of 1.0, whereas the very active female has a PA of 1.45. Compared to her sedentary counterpart, the very active female needs about 700 additional Calories to sustain her physically active lifestyle.

Sedentary lifestyle	Very active lifestyle
PA = 1.0	PA = 1.45
EER = 1,794 Calories	EER = 2,504 Calories

but the data should provide some useful information regarding your daily energy expenditure. You may also compare the findings with your personal wearable gadget or smartphone app that estimates your daily energy expenditure.

> www.globalrph.com/estimated_energy_requirement. htm Use this Website to calculate your estimated EER with five different methods.

If you are interested in increasing your PAL, then your best bet is to incorporate more light, moderate, and moderately heavy to heavy physical activities into your daily lifestyle. Some additional guidelines for estimating your daily TDEE and EER, particularly in the design of a proper weight-control program, are presented in chapter 11.

Key Concepts

▶ The three major muscle fiber classifications are type I, type IIa, and type IIb. Type I, known as a slow-oxidative fiber, produces ATP aerobically. Type IIa, also known as a fast-oxidative glycolytic fiber, produces ATP both aerobically and anaerobically. Type IIb, also known as a fast glycolytic fiber, produces ATP anaerobically.

▶ The thermic effect of exercise (TEE), or exercise metabolic rate (EMR), provides us with the most practical means to increase energy expenditure.

▶ The metabolic rate during exercise is directly proportional to the intensity of the exercise, and the exercise heart rate may serve as a general indicator of the metabolic rate.

▶ Activities that use the large muscle groups of the body, such as running, swimming, bicycling, and aerobic dance, facilitate energy expenditure. Resistance training of sufficient intensity and duration may also help expend enough energy to satisfy exercise recommendations for caloric expenditure.

▶ The total daily energy expenditure (TDEE) is accounted for by BEE (60–75 percent), TEF (5–10 percent), and TEE (15–30 percent), although these percentages may vary considerably among individuals.

▶ The Estimated Energy Requirement (EER) is defined as the dietary intake that is predicted to maintain energy balance in a healthy adult of a defined age, gender, height, weight, and level of physical activity consistent with good health. Changing from a sedentary Physical Activity Level (PAL) to a very active PAL is a very effective means to increase TDEE and EER.

Check for Yourself

▶ Record the types and amounts (in minutes) of your daily physical activity. The application exercise on page 122 may be useful. Consult the Compendium of Physical Activities and Appendix B to determine your total amount of daily energy expenditure through physical activity and exercise. Compare your findings with the other website estimates of your TDEE.

Human Energy Systems and Fatigue during Exercise

In sport, energy expenditure can vary tremendously. For example, Asker Jeukendrup and his associates noted that in one sport, World Class Cycling, events may range in duration from 10 seconds to 3 weeks, involving race distances between 200-meters and 4,000 kilometers. Exercise intensity in a 200-meter event would be extremely high, and much lower during the prolonged event.

What energy systems are used during exercise?

The most important factor determining which energy system will be used is the intensity of the exercise, which is the rate, speed, or tempo at which you pursue a given activity. In general, the faster you do something, the higher your rate of energy expenditure and the more rapidly you must produce ATP for muscular contraction. Very rapid muscular movements are characterized by high rates of power production. If you were asked to run 100 meters as fast as you could, you would exert maximal speed for a short time. On the other hand, if you were asked to run 5 miles, you certainly would not run at the same speed as you would for the 100 meters. In the 100-meter run your energy expenditure would be very rapid, characterized by a high-power production. The 5-mile run would be characterized by low-power production, or endurance.

As noted previously in this chapter, the requirement of energy for exercise is related to a power-endurance continuum. On the power end, we have extremely high rates of energy expenditure that a sprinter might use; on the endurance end, we see lower rates that might be characteristic of a marathon runner. The closer we are to the power end of the continuum, the more rapidly we must produce ATP. As we move toward the endurance end, our rate of ATP production does not have to be as great, but we need the capacity to produce ATP for a longer time.

It should be noted from the outset that all three energy systems—ATP-PCr, lactic acid, and oxygen—are used in one way or another during most athletic activities. (Gastin provides an excellent overview.) However, one system may predominate, depending primarily on the intensity level of the activity. In this regard, the three human energy systems may be ranked according to several characteristics, which are displayed in table 3.8. You may recall that use of the ATP-PCr energy system is referred to as *anaerobic power,* and use of the lactic acid system is referred to as *anaerobic capacity,* whereas the terms *aerobic power* and *aerobic capacity* are used when the oxygen system uses, respectively, carbohydrate and fat as the main energy source.

Both the ATP-PCr and the lactic acid systems are able to produce ATP rapidly and are used in events characterized by high intensity levels that occur for short periods mainly because their capacity for total ATP production is limited. Because both of these systems may function without oxygen, they are called anaerobic. Relative to running performance, the ATP-PCr system predominates in short, powerful bursts of muscular activity such as the short dashes like the 100-meter dash, whereas the lactic acid

TABLE 3.8   Major characteristics of the human energy systems*

	ATP-PCr (Anaerobic power)	Lactic acid (Anaerobic capacity)	Oxygen (Aerobic power)	Oxygen (Aerobic capacity)
Main energy source	ATP; phosphocreatine	Carbohydrate	Carbohydrate	Fat
Intensity level	Highest	High	Lower	Lowest
Rate of ATP production	Highest	High	Lower	Lowest
Power production	Highest	High	Lower	Lowest
Capacity for total ATP production	Lowest	Low	High	Highest
Endurance capacity	Lowest	Low	High	Highest
Oxygen needed	No	No	Yes	Yes
Anaerobic/aerobic	Anaerobic	Anaerobic	Aerobic	Aerobic
Characteristic track event	100-meter dash	200–800 meters	5,000-meter (5-km) run	Ultradistance
Time factor	1–10 seconds	30–120 seconds	5 minutes or more	Hours

*Keep in mind that during most exercises, all three energy systems will be operating to one degree or another. However, one system may predominate, depending primarily on the intensity of the activity. See text for further explanation.

system begins to predominate during the longer sprints and middle distances such as 200, 400, and 800 meters. In any athletic event where maximal power production lasts about 1–10 seconds, the ATP-PCr system is the major energy source. The lactic acid system begins to predominate in events lasting 30–120 seconds, but studies have noted significant elevations in muscle lactic acid in maximal exercise even as brief as 10 seconds.

The oxygen system possesses a lower rate of ATP production than the other two systems, but its capacity for total ATP production is much greater. Although the intensity level of exercise while using the oxygen system is by necessity lower, this does not necessarily mean that an individual cannot perform at a relatively high speed for a long time. The oxygen system can be improved through a physical conditioning program so that ATP production may be able to meet the demands of relatively high-intensity exercise, as discussed previously and highlighted in figure 3.14. Endurance-type activities, such as those that last 5 minutes or more, are dependent primarily upon the oxygen system, but the oxygen system makes a very significant contribution even in events as short as 30–90 seconds, as documented by Spencer and Gastin.

In summary, we may simplify this discussion by categorizing the energy sources as either anaerobic or aerobic. Anaerobic sources include both the ATP-PCr and lactic acid systems, whereas the oxygen system is aerobic. Table 3.9 illustrates the approximate percentage contribution of anaerobic and aerobic energy sources, depending on the level of maximal intensity that can be sustained for a given time period. Thus, for a 100-meter dash covered in 10 seconds, 85 percent of the energy is derived from anaerobic sources. For an elite marathoner (26.2 miles) with times of approximately 125–130 minutes in international-level competition, the aerobic energy processes contribute 99 percent. Although Ward-Smith, using a mathematical approach to predict aerobic and anaerobic contributions during running, noted that these percentage values may be modified slightly for elite athletes, the concept is correct. For example, using track athletes as subjects, Spencer and Gastin found that the relative contribution of the aerobic energy system was 29 percent in the 200-meter run and increased progressively to 84 percent in the 1,500-meter run, noting that the contribution of the aerobic energy system during track running events is greater than traditionally thought. These values are somewhat higher than the aerobic percentage values presented in table 3.9 but support the concept. The key point is that the longer you exercise, the less your intensity has to be, and the more you rely on your oxygen system for energy production.

What energy sources are used during exercise?

The ATP-PCr system can use only adenosine triphosphate and phosphocreatine, but as noted previously, these energy sources are in short supply and must be replaced by the other two energy systems.

TABLE 3.9   Percentage contribution of anaerobic and aerobic energy sources during different time periods of maximal work*

Time	10 sec	1 min	2 min	4 min	10 min	30 min	60 min	120 min
Anaerobic	85	70	50	30	15	5	2	1
Aerobic	15	30	50	70	85	95	98	99

*Percentages are approximate and may vary between sedentary individuals and elite athletes.

The lactic acid system uses only carbohydrate, primarily the muscle glycogen stores. At high-intensity exercise levels that may be sustained for 1–2 minutes or less, such as exercising well above your VO₂ max, carbohydrate will supply more than 95 percent of the energy. However, the accumulation of lactic acid may be associated with the early onset of fatigue.

In contrast, the oxygen system can use a variety of energy sources, including protein, although carbohydrate and fat are the primary ones. The carbohydrate is found as muscle glycogen, liver glycogen, and blood glucose. The fats are stored primarily as triglycerides in the muscle and adipose cells, but small amounts are also present in the blood. As we shall see in this section and in chapters 4, 5, and 6, a number of different factors can influence which energy source is used by the oxygen system during exercise, but exercise intensity and duration are the two most important factors.

Under normal conditions, exercise intensity is the key factor determining whether carbohydrate or fat is used. Holloszy and others note that both absolute and relative (i.e., percent of VO₂ max) exercise intensities play important roles in the regulation of substrate metabolism. The absolute work rate determines the total quantity of fuel required, while relative exercise intensity plays a major role in determining the proportions of carbohydrate and fat oxidized by the working muscles.

Hoppeler and Weibel noted that as one does mild to moderate exercise, say up to 50 percent of one's VO₂ max, blood glucose and fat may provide much of the needed energy. However, the transfer of glucose and fat from the vascular system to the muscles becomes limited at about 50 percent of VO₂ max. Thus, as you start to exceed 50 percent of your VO₂ max, you begin to rely more on your intramuscular stores of glycogen and triglycerides. As you continue to increase your speed or intensity, you begin to rely more and more on carbohydrate as an energy source. Apparently the biochemical processes for fat metabolism are too slow to meet the increased need for faster production of ATP, and carbohydrate utilization increases. The major source of this carbohydrate is muscle glycogen.

The transition from use of fat to carbohydrate as the primary fuel source during increasing intensity of exercise has been referred to as the **crossover concept**, and although the technicalities of specific fuel contributions are the subject of debate, exercise scientists agree that at some specific point in the increase of exercise intensity an individual will begin to derive more energy from carbohydrate than fat (see figure 3.19). At high levels of energy expenditure, 70–80 percent of VO₂ max, carbohydrates may contribute more than 80 percent of the energy sources. Houston notes that elite marathoners burn about 19–20 Calories per minute and need about 4–5 grams of carbohydrate per minute. This speaks for the need of adequate muscle glycogen stores when this level of exercise is to be sustained for long periods, say in events lasting more than 60–90 minutes.

In events of long duration, when body stores of carbohydrate are nearly depleted, the primary energy source is fat. In the later stages of ultramarathoning events, fat may become the only fuel available, which may necessitate a slower pace because fat is a less efficient fuel. That is why Cermak and van Loon indicated

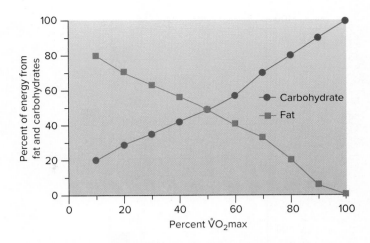

FIGURE 3.19 The crossover concept of carbohydrate and fat utilization during exercise. During low-intensity exercise (20 percent VO₂ max), the majority of energy production is derived from fat, but as exercise intensity increases, the use of carbohydrate for energy production increases and may be 80 percent or higher at very intense exercise. Highly trained endurance athletes will use less carbohydrate and more fat during submaximal exercise as compared to untrained individuals.

improving carbohydrate availability during prolonged exercise through carbohydrate ingestion has dominated the field of sports nutrition research. More detail on carbohydrate use during exercise is presented in chapter 4. Moreover, protein may become an important energy source in these circumstances; its role is detailed in chapter 6.

What is the "fat burning zone" during exercise?

As noted in chapter 11, the goal in weight-loss programs is to lose fat, not muscle. Various fitness-related Internet sites and the consoles of many pieces of cardiovascular exercise equipment instruct exercisers on how to train in the "fat burning zone" for weight loss, which as noted is most often low-intensity exercise, maybe only 40–50 percent of maximal heart rate. However, as shall be discussed in chapter 11, the best recommendation for most exercisers who want to achieve a healthy body weight and improve their fitness is to exercise at the highest intensity appropriate for their age, health, motivation, and current fitness level. Figure 3.20 illustrates this concept. At the top, about 80 percent of your total caloric expenditure will come from fat, and only 20 percent from carbohydrate, so based on these percentages you are exercising in the "fat burning zone" while walking at 2 mph. If you ran at a pace of 9 mph, the reverse would be true, with about 80 percent of your energy coming from carbohydrate and only 20 percent from fat.

However, one of the key concepts underlying exercise as a means for weight loss is to exercise as intensely as possible for a given time frame. Total caloric expenditure during exercise is the key to promote weight loss. At the bottom in figure 3.20, a typical average adult male walking for 30 minutes at a pace of 2 mph will burn about a total of 100 Calories, about 80 from fat and 20

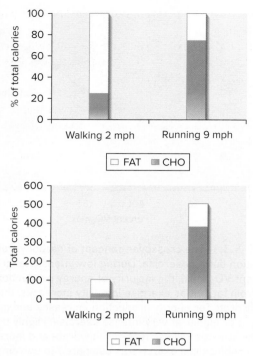

FIGURE 3.20 Top. Energy expenditure from fat and carbohydrate (CHO) during 30 minutes of low-intensity and high-intensity exercise expressed as a percentage of total Calories. **Bottom.** Energy expenditure from fat and carbohydrate (CHO) during 30 minutes of low-intensity and high-intensity exercise expressed in absolute total Calories. Although a greater percentage of fat is oxidized during low-intensity exercise, many more Calories are expended during high-intensity exercise.

from carbohydrate. Running at 9 mph for the same time frame will burn about 450 Calories, about 90 from fat and 360 from carbohydrate, more than four times the caloric expenditure in the same time frame and similar amounts of fat. Nevertheless, exercising in the "fat burning zone" may be very appropriate for some individuals, such as those beginning an exercise program, the elderly, and others. Additional details regarding exercise and weight loss are presented in chapter 11.

Other than exercise intensity and duration, a number of different factors are known to influence the availability and use of human energy sources during exercise. Gender, hormones, state of training, composition of the diet, time of eating prior to competition, nutritional status, nutrient intake during exercise, environmental temperature, and drugs are some of the more important considerations. For example, warm environmental temperatures may increase the use of carbohydrates, whereas fasting may facilitate the use of fats. These considerations will be incorporated into the following chapters where appropriate. For the interested reader, Hargreaves provides an excellent detailed review.

What is fatigue?

Fatigue is a very complex phenomenon. It may be chronic, or it may be acute. Both types may affect the athlete.

Chronic Fatigue **Chronic fatigue syndrome (CFS)**, or myalgic encephalomyelitis, is a medical condition characterized by numerous symptoms, the most prevalent being prolonged, incapacitating fatigue lasting at least six months. Moss-Morris and others note that the etiology of CFS is complex and unlikely to be understood through a single mechanism. Multiple factors may be involved, such as viral illnesses, sleep disturbances, immune system dysfunction, excessive mental stress, and prolonged overwork, factors which may be observed in athletes engaged in excessive physical training.

Chronic fatigue in the athlete may develop over time, usually in endurance athletes involved in prolonged, intense training that may involve conditions known as overreaching and overtraining. *Overreaching* is a condition of physical and mental stress that may impair physical performance, but it may be a planned phase of training in elite athletes followed by short-term recovery with return to previous or improved levels of performance. *Overtraining* is a term often used to characterize a syndrome in athletes involving prolonged periods of fatigue. However, Halson and Jeukendrup note that although some scientific and anecdotal evidence support its existence, there appear to be no clear markers for overtraining and more research is needed to establish its existence with certainty. Some contend that the term *overtraining* is misleading, and may actually be related to *underrecovery*, particularly involving inadequate nutrition.

Roy Shephard, the renowned Canadian sport scientist, indicated that overtraining and/or a negative energy balance may be related to the development of CFS in athletes. In such cases, training would be adversely affected and performance certainly would suffer. Given the debilitating effects on exercise and sports performance, scientists are attempting to identify the causes, prevention, and treatment of both overtraining and chronic fatigue syndrome. In a joint consensus statement, developed by Meeusen and others, the European College of Sport Science and the American College of Sports Medicine indicated that the etiology of the overtraining syndrome involves the exclusion of organic diseases or infections and factors such as dietary caloric restriction (negative energy balance) and insufficient carbohydrate and/or protein intake, iron deficiency, magnesium deficiency, allergies, and other possible initiating events or triggers. Treatment involves behavioral therapy and graded exercise, but recovery is a long process. Although chronic fatigue syndrome is a serious medical condition, its prevalence in the general population, including athletes, appears to be very low. In a recent meta-analysis, Johnston and others reported the incidence of CFS is low, less than 1 percent of the population with clinical assessment, but over 3 percent with self-diagnosis. CFS also affects children and adolescents. For more details on CFS, use the following Centers for Disease Control and Prevention Website.

www.cdc.gov/cfs/general/index.html

Acute Fatigue Acute mental or physical fatigue is experienced by most athletes at one time or another during maximal efforts. For purposes of the present discussion, **fatigue** will be defined as the inability to continue exercising at a desired level of intensity.

Relative to this definition, fatigue may be due to a failure of the rate of energy production in the human body to meet the demands of the exercise task. In simple terms, ATP production rates are unable to match ATP utilization rates.

As acute fatigue can adversely affect sports performance, it has been the subject of considerable research. In general, sports scientists classify the site of acute fatigue in the body as either central or peripheral (see figure 3.21). *Central fatigue* involves the brain or spinal cord of the central nervous system (CNS), while *peripheral fatigue* is associated primarily with the muscles and, under some conditions, other body organs such as the heart or lungs.

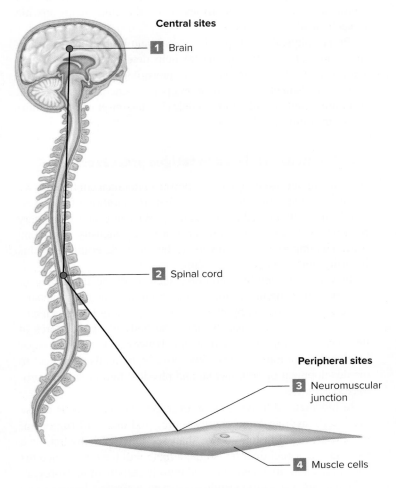

Central sites

1 Brain

2 Spinal cord

Peripheral sites

3 Neuromuscular junction

4 Muscle cells

FIGURE 3.21 Fatigue sites. The causes of fatigue are complex and may involve central sites such as the brain and spinal cord or peripheral sites in the muscles. Hypoglycemia, or low blood sugar, could adversely affect the functioning of the brain, while the acidity associated with the production of lactic acid could interfere with optimal energy production in the muscle cells.

What causes acute fatigue in athletes?

Robert Fitts, an expert on muscular fatigue during prolonged exercise, noted that the etiology of fatigue is not fully understood despite more than a century of research. He indicated that the mechanisms of muscle fatigue are complex and depend on the type of exercise, one's state of fitness, and the fiber type composition of the muscle.

Although the cause of acute exercise-induced fatigue has not been determined, numerous hypotheses exist, involving both peripheral and central fatigue.

Peripheral Fatigue Fatigue may develop in the muscle for various reasons, including depletion of energy sources or accumulation of fatigue-causing metabolites. For example, Hargreaves indicates that fatigue occurs when the compounds needed to produce ATP are depleted. Depletion of phosphocreatine could decrease the rapid replenishment of ATP in sprint-type events, such as the 200-meter track event. Depletion of muscle glycogen could impair marathon running performance. Relative to the accumulation of metabolites, Amenti and Verkerke indicate that some, such as hydrogen ions and inorganic phosphates, may accumulate within the muscle cell during intense exercise, disrupting biochemical equilibrium and causing fatigue. For example, Fitts indicates that hydrogen ion accumulation can decrease sensitivity of the myofibrils to calcium. Some potential factors involve the following:

Substrate Depletion	Metabolic By-Product Accumulation
ATP	Hydrogen ions
Phosphocreatine	ADP and inorganic phosphate
Muscle glycogen	Ammonia
Blood glucose	Reactive oxygen species

Central Fatigue In a recent review, Sidhu and others reported substantial evidence supporting the finding that fatigue during exercise is accompanied by changes within the central nervous system that may reduce muscle force production. For example, Noakes suggests that central fatigue may be associated with the depletion of critical neurochemicals or the accumulation of "toxic" concentrations of neurotransmitters at neural synapses, which could reduce neural impulses to the muscles. In this regard, Edgerton and Roy noted that elevated levels of serotonin, a neurotransmitter in the brain, are associated with fatigue, and exercise may increase levels of serotonin in the brain. In contrast, the neurotransmitter norepinephrine is a stimulant and may help prevent fatigue; its reduction may help induce fatigue. Relative to central fatigue, Noakes highlights the fact that the single variable that is always maximal at exhaustion during all forms of exercise is the rating of perceived exertion, a mental perception.

Peripheral and Central Fatigue Roelands and others have indicated the current focus on exercise fatigue research involves a complex interplay between peripheral and central limitations of performance. For example, both peripheral and central factors may be involved in setting the pace for a runner in a distance event. Changes within the muscle, such as increased acidity, provide feedback to the central nervous system. At the same time, anticipation by the central nervous system of forthcoming consequences, such as increased heat stress, provide feedforward input to the muscles. Both factors may be involved in setting of a race pace to help in the prevention of premature fatigue.

Dempsey and others note that most scientists agree that the *decision* to reduce power output during exercise clearly involves the higher areas of the central nervous system, but the real mystery is to identify those sources of input that trigger these decisions.

Some possible causes of fatigue are listed in table 3.10. Keep in mind that fatigue is complex and several of these factors may be involved simultaneously in the etiology of fatigue in certain sport-type events. For example, Houston indicates that fatigue in the 400-meter dash may involve depletion of PCr and muscle glycogen, but may also be associated with increases in hydrogen ion concentration.

TABLE 3.10	Some possible causes of fatigue during exercise
Increased formation of depressant neurotransmitters	
Increased serotonin levels	
Decreased levels of energy substrates	
Decrease in phosphocreatine levels	
Depletion of muscle glycogen	
Decrease in blood sugar levels	
Decrease in plasma branched-chain amino acids	
Increased levels of reactive oxygen and nitrogen species	
Impaired calcium recycling	
Decreased muscle contraction force	
Disturbed acid-base balance	
Increase in hydrogen ions due to excess lactic acid production	
Decreased oxygen transport	
Decreased blood volume due to dehydration	
Increased core body temperature resulting in hyperthermia	
Decreased cooling effect due to dehydration	
Disturbed electrolyte balance	
Increased or decreased concentration due to sweat losses and inadequate water replacement	

How can I delay the onset of fatigue?

The most important factor in the prevention of premature fatigue is proper training, including physiological, psychological, and biomechanical training.

Physiologically, athletes must train specifically on the energy system or systems that are inherent to their event. Under the guidance of sport physiologists and coaches, appropriate physiological training for each specific energy system may increase its energy stores, enzymatic activity, and metabolic efficiency, thus enhancing energy production. Physiological training enhances physical power.

Psychologically, athletes must train the mind to tolerate the stresses associated with their specific event. Sport psychologists may help provide the athlete with various mental strategies, such as inducing either a state of relaxation or arousal, whichever may be appropriate for their sport. Physiological training may also confer some psychological advantages, such as tolerating higher levels of pain associated with intense exercise. Psychological training enhances mental strength.

Biomechanically, athletes must maximize the mechanical skills associated with their sport. For any sport, sport biomechanists can analyze the athlete's skill level and recommend modifications in movement patterns or equipment to improve energy production or efficiency. In many cases, modification of the amount of body fat and muscle mass may provide the athlete with a biomechanical advantage. Biomechanical training helps provide a mechanical edge.

Proper physiological, psychological, and biomechanical training represents the best means to help deter premature fatigue. However, what you eat may affect physiological, psychological, and biomechanical aspects of sports performance. Thus, nutrition is an important consideration in delaying the onset of fatigue during sport training and competition.

How is nutrition related to fatigue processes?

As noted in our discussion of the power-endurance continuum, we can exercise at different intensities, but the duration of our exercise is inversely related to the intensity. We can exercise at a very high intensity for a short time or at a lower intensity for a long time. The importance of nutrition to fatigue is determined by this intensity-duration interrelationship.

In very mild aerobic activities, such as distance walking or low-speed running in a trained ultramarathoner, the body can sustain energy production by using fat as the primary fuel when carbohydrate levels diminish. Because the body has large stores of fat, energy supply is not a problem. However, low blood sugar levels, dehydration, and excessive loss of minerals may lead to the development of both mental and physical fatigue in very prolonged activities.

In moderate to heavy aerobic exercise, the body needs to use more carbohydrate as an energy source and thus will run out of muscle glycogen faster. As we shall see later, carbohydrate is a more efficient fuel than fat, so the athlete will have to reduce the pace of the activity when liver and muscle carbohydrate stores are depleted, such as during endurance-type activities lasting more than 90 minutes. Thus, energy supply may be critical. Low blood sugar, changes in blood constituents such as certain amino acids, and dehydration also may be important factors contributing to the development of mental or physical fatigue in this type of endeavor.

In very high-intensity exercise lasting only 1 or 2 minutes, the probable cause of fatigue is the disruption of cellular metabolism caused by the accumulation of hydrogen ions resulting from excess lactic acid production. There is some evidence to suggest that beta-alanine and sodium bicarbonate (discussed in chapters 6 and 13, respectively), which promote intracellular buffering, may help reduce the disruptive effect of lactic acid to some extent. Furthermore, a very low supply of muscle glycogen in fast-twitch muscle fibers may impair this type of performance.

In extremely intense exercise lasting only 5–10 seconds, a depletion of phosphocreatine (PCr) may be related to the inability to maintain a high force production. Supplementation with creatine monohydrate, discussed in chapter 6, has been shown to increase muscle PCr levels and many studies have reported improved performance in high-intensity exercise tasks.

In summary, a deficiency of almost every nutrient may be a causative factor in the development of fatigue. A poor diet can hasten the onset of fatigue. Proper nutrition is essential to assure the athlete that an adequate supply of nutrients is available in the diet, not only to provide the necessary energy, such as through carbohydrate and fat, but also to ensure optimal metabolism of the energy substrate via protein, vitamins, minerals, and water.

Moreover, as noted in chapter 2, an overall healthy diet is important for the physically active individual. For example, Gleeson indicated that prolonged exercise and heavy training may be associated with depressed immune function, which could lead to minor illnesses and possibly impair training. To help avoid immune system dysfunction, he recommends all athletes should eat a well-balanced diet sufficient to meet their energy, carbohydrate, protein, and micronutrient requirements. Guidelines are presented in chapter 2. The role of specific nutrients or dietary supplements relative to fatigue processes will be discussed in later sections of the book where appropriate. Table 3.11 provides some examples of how some nutrients or dietary supplements are thought to delay fatigue.

Key Concepts

▶ The ATP-PCr and lactic acid energy systems are used primarily during fast, anaerobic, power-type events, while the oxygen system is used primarily during aerobic, endurance-type events.

▶ Fats serve as the primary source of fuel during mild levels of aerobic exercise intensity, but carbohydrates begin to be the preferred fuel as exercise intensity increases.

▶ Fatigue may be classified as central (neural) or peripheral (muscular) fatigue. Fatigue may also be caused by a variety of factors, including the depletion of energy substrate or the accumulation of fatigue-causing metabolites.

▶ A sound training program and proper nutrition are important factors in the prevention of fatigue during exercise.

Check for Yourself

▶ Check the world records in running for 100 meters, 400 meters, 1,500 meters, and the marathon (42,200 meters). Calculate the average speed for each distance. Can you relate your findings to the human energy systems and their relationship to fatigue?

TABLE 3.11 Examples of some nutritional ergogenic aids and, theoretically, how they may influence physiological, psychological, or biomechanical processes to delay fatigue

Provide energy substrate

Carbohydrate: Energy substrate for aerobic glycolysis
Creatine: Substrate for formation of phosphocreatine (PCr)

Enhance energy-generating metabolic pathways

B vitamins: Coenzymes in aerobic and anaerobic glycolysis
Carnitine: Enzyme substrate to facilitate fat metabolism

Increase cardiovascular-respiratory function

Iron: Substrate for hemoglobin formation and oxygen transport
Nitrates: Promote utilization of oxygen for energy production

Increase size or number of energy-generating cells

Arginine and ornithine: Amino acids that stimulate production of human growth hormone, an anabolic hormone
Chromium: Mineral to potentiate activity of insulin, an anabolic hormone

Attenuate fatigue-related metabolic by-products

Beta-alanine: Amino acid that acts as an intracellular buffer and attenuates acidosis
Sodium bicarbonate: Buffer to reduce effects of lactic acid

Prevent catabolism of energy-generating cells

Antioxidants: Vitamins to prevent unwanted oxidation of cell membranes
HMB: By-product of amino acid metabolism to prevent protein degradation

Ameliorate psychological function

BCAA: Amino acids that favorably modify neurotransmitter production
Caffeine: Reduces the sensation of psychological effort during exercise

Improve mechanical efficiency

Ma huang: Stimulant to increase metabolism for fat loss
Hydroxycitrate (HCA): Supplement to increase fat oxidation for fat loss

Note: These examples as to how nutritional aids may delay fatigue are based on theoretical considerations. As shall be shown in respective chapters, supplementation with most of these nutritional ergogenic aids has not been shown to enhance exercise or sports performance.

	Distance logged Sunday	Distance logged Monday	Distance logged Tuesday	Distance logged Wednesday	Distance logged Thursday	Distance logged Friday	Distance logged Saturday
12:00–2:00 A.M.							
2:00–4:00 A.M.							
4:00–6:00 A.M.							
6:00–8:00 A.M.							
8:00–10:00 A.M.							
10:00–12:00 A.M.							
12:00–2:00 P.M.							
2:00–4:00 P.M.							
4:00–6:00 P.M.							
6:00–8:00 P.M.							
8:00–10:00 P.M.							
10:00–12:00 P.M.							

Borrow, rent, or buy a pedometer or an accelerometer and keep a record of your daily movement (recording the amount every 2 hours). This will provide you with an estimate of your daily physical activity involving movement and will be useful in determining your estimated energy requirement (EER) and maintaining an optimal body weight as discussed in chapter 11.

Review Questions—Multiple Choice

1. Which energy system would predominate in an all-out, high-intensity, 400-meter dash in track?
   a. ATP-PCr
   b. lactic acid
   c. oxygen–carbohydrate
   d. oxygen–fat
   e. oxygen–protein

2. If a 50-kilogram body-weight athlete was exercising at an oxygen consumption level of 2.45 liters (2,450 ml) per minute, approximately how many METS would she be attaining?
   a. 8
   b. 10
   c. 11
   d. 12
   e. 14
   f. insufficient data to calculate the answer

3. Which of the following classifications of physical activity is rated as light, mild aerobic exercise—because it is likely to burn less than 7 Calories per minute?
   a. competitive racquetball
   b. running at a speed of 7 miles per hour
   c. walking at a speed of 2.0 miles per hour
   d. competitive singles tennis
   e. bicycling at a speed of 15 miles per hour

4. Which of the following statements relative to the basal metabolic rate or resting metabolic rate is false?
   a. The BMR is high in infancy but declines throughout adolescence and adulthood.
   b. The BMR is higher in women than in men due to the generally higher levels of body fat in women.
   c. The resting metabolic rate is the equivalent of 1 MET.
   d. The resting metabolic rate is higher than the BMR.
   e. Dietary-induced thermogenesis raises the resting metabolic rate.

5. Which of the following is not likely to be a cause of fatigue?
   a. depletion of PCr in fast-twitch fibers in a 200-meter dash
   b. depletion of muscle glycogen in fast-twitch fibers in a 400-meter dash
   c. depletion of adipose cell fatty acids in a marathon
   d. depletion of muscle glycogen in a marathon
   e. accumulation of hydrogen ions in a 400-meter dash

6. Of the following statements concerning the interrelationships between various forms of energy, which one is false?
   a. A kilojoule is greater than a kilocalorie.
   b. A kilogram-meter is equal to 7.23 foot-pounds.
   c. A gram of fat has more Calories than a gram of carbohydrate.
   d. A gram of fat has more Calories than a gram of protein.
   e. A liter of oxygen can release more than 1 kilocalorie when metabolizing carbohydrate.

7. Approximately how many Calories will a 200-pound individual use while jogging a mile?
   a. 70
   b. 145
   c. 200
   d. 255
   e. 440

8. Which of the following statements relative to exercise and metabolic rate is false?
   a. The intensity of the exercise is the most important factor to increase the metabolic rate.

b. Increased efficiency for swimming a set distance will decrease the energy cost.

c. A heavier person will burn more Calories running a mile than a lighter person.

d. Oxygen consumption and heart rate are two ways to monitor the metabolic rate.

e. Walking a mile slowly and jogging a mile cost the same amount of Calories.

9. Which energy system has the greatest capacity for energy production (i.e., endurance?)
   a. ATP-PCr
   b. lactic acid

c. anaerobic glycolysis

d. oxygen

e. phosphagens

10. Which of the following is *not* needed to calculate the estimated energy requirement (EER)?
    a. body fat percentage
    b. age
    c. height
    d. weight
    e. physical activity level (PAL)

Answers to multiple choice questions: 1. b; 2. e; 3. c; 4. b; 5. c; 6. a; 7. b; 8. e; 9. d; 10. a

Review Questions—Essay

1. If an individual performed 5,000 foot-pounds of work in 1 minute, how many kilojoules of work were accomplished?

2. Name the sources of energy stored in the human body and discuss their role in the three human energy systems.

3. Differentiate among BMR, RMR, BEE, REE, TEF, TEE, EER, and TDEE as defined in this text.

4. Explain the role of the three energy systems during exercise and provide an example using track running events. Which muscle fiber types are the major source of energy production during these track events?

5. List the major causes of fatigue during exercise and indicate how various nutritional interventions may help prevent premature fatigue.

References

Books

Fox, E. L. 1979. *Sports Physiology.* Dubuque, IA: Wm. C. Brown.

Houston, M. 2006. *Biochemistry Primer for Exercise Science.* Champaign, IL: Human Kinetics.

McArdle, W., et al. 2015. *Exercise Physiology.* Baltimore: Wolters Kluwer.

National Academy of Sciences. 2005. *Dietary Reference Intakes for Energy, Carbohydrates, Fiber, Fat, Protein, and Amino Acids (Macronutrients).* Washington, DC: National Academies Press.

Reviews and Specific Studies

Ainsworth, B., et al. 2011. 2011 Compendium of Physical Activities: A second update of codes and MET values. *Medicine and Science in Sports and Exercise* 43:1575–81.

Binns, A., et al. 2015. Thermic effect of food, exercise, and total energy expenditure in active females. *Journal of Science and Medicine in Sport* 18:204–8.

Bloomer, R. 2005. Energy cost of moderate-duration resistance and aerobic exercise. *Journal of Strength and Conditioning Research* 19:878–82.

Bort-Roig, J. 2014. Measuring and influencing physical activity with smartphone technology: A systematic review. *Sports Medicine* 44:671–86.

Burke, S., et al. 2006. Group versus individual approach? A meta-analysis of the effectiveness of interventions to promote physical activity. *Sport & Exercise Psychology Review* 2:19–35.

Bushman, B. 2012. How can I use METS to quantify the amount of aerobic exercise? *ACSM's Health & Fitness Journal* 16 (2):5–7.

Cermak, N., and van Loon, L. 2013. The use of carbohydrates during exercise as an ergogenic aid. *Sports Medicine* 43:1139–55.

Consumer Reports. 2014. Get-healthy gadgets that really work. *Consumer Reports on Health* 26 (9):8.

Coyle, E. 2007. Physiological regulation of marathon performance. *Sports Medicine* 37:306–11.

Crovetti, R., et al. 1998. The influence of thermic effect of food on satiety. *European Journal of Clinical Nutrition* 52:482–88.

Dempsey, J., et al. 2008. Respiratory system determinants of peripheral fatigue and endurance performance. *Medicine & Science in Sports & Exercise* 40:457–61.

Edgerton, V., and Roy, R. 2006. The nervous system and movement. In *ACSM's Advanced Exercise Physiology,* ed. C. M. Tipton. Philadelphia: Lippincott Williams & Wilkins.

Fitts, R. 2006. The muscular system: Fatigue processes. In *ACSM's Advanced Exercise Physiology,* ed. C. M. Tipton. Philadelphia: Lippincott Williams & Wilkins.

Fitts, R. 2008. The cross-bridge cycle and skeletal muscle fatigue. *Journal of Applied Physiology* 104:551–58.

Gastin, P. 2001. Energy system interaction and relative contribution during maximal exercise. *Sports Medicine* 31:725–41.

Gleeson, M. 2013. Nutritional support to maintain proper immune status during intense training. *Nestle Nutrition Institute Workshop Series* 75:85–97.

Haddock, B., and Wilkin, L. 2006. Resistance training volume and post-exercise energy expenditure. *International Journal of Sports Medicine* 27: 143–48.

Hagberg, J., and Pena, N. 1989. Bicycling's exclusive calorie counter. *Bicycling* 30:100–103.

Halson, S., and Jeukendrup, A. 2004. Does overtraining exist? An analysis of overreaching and overtraining research. *Sports Medicine* 34:967–81.

Hargreaves, M. 2000. Skeletal muscle metabolism during exercise in humans. *Clinical & Experimental Pharmacology & Physiology* 27:225–28.

Hargreaves, M. 2005. Metabolic factors in fatigue. *Sports Science Exchange* 18 (3):1–6.

Hawley, J., and Hopkins, W. 1995. Aerobic glycolytic and aerobic lipolytic power systems. *Sports Medicine* 19:240–50.

Hills, A., et al. 2014. Assessment of physical activity and energy expenditure: An overview of objective measures. *Frontiers in Nutrition.* 1:5.

Holloszy, J., et al. 1998. The regulation of carbohydrate and fat metabolism during and after exercise. *Frontiers in Bioscience* 3:D1011–27.

Hongu, N., et al. 2014. Mobile technologies for promoting health and physical activity *ACSM's Health & Fitness Journal* 18 (4):8–15.

Hoppeler, H., and Weibel, E. 2000. Structural and functional limits for oxygen supply to muscle. *Acta Physiologica Scandinavica* 168:445–56.

Jeukendrup, A., et al. 2000. The bioenergetics of World Class Cycling. *Journal of Science & Medicine in Sport* 3:414–33.

Johnston, S., et al. 2013.The prevalence of chronic fatigue syndrome/myalgic encephalomyelitis: A meta-analysis. *Clinical Epidemiology* 5:105–10.

Knab, A., et al. 2011. A 45-minute vigorous exercise bout increases metabolic rate for 14 hours. *Medicine and Science in Sports and Exercise* 43:1643–8.

Kuo, A., et al. 2005. Energetic consequences of walking like an inverted pendulum: Step-to-step transitions. *Exercise & Sports Sciences Reviews* 33:88–97.

Lange, B., and Bury, T. 2001. Physiologic evaluation of explosive force in sports. *Revue Medicale de Liege* 56:233–38.

Lee, J.-M., et al. 2014. Validity and utility of consumer-based physical activity monitors. *ACSM's Health & Fitness Journal* 18 (4):16–21.

Lee, P., et al. 2013. Brown adipose tissue in adult humans: A metabolic renaissance. *Endocrine Reviews* 34:413–38.

Levine, J. 2004. Non-exercise activity thermogenesis. *Nutrition Reviews* 62:S82–S97.

Levine, J. 2005. Measurement of energy expenditure. *Public Health Nutrition* 8:1123–32.

Liu, S., et al. 2012. Computational methods for estimating energy expenditure in human physical activities. *Medicine & Science in Sports & Exercise* 44:2138–46.

Matthews, C., et al. 2012. Improving self-reports of active and sedentary behaviors in large epidemiologic studies. *Exercise and Sport Sciences Reviews* 40:118–26.

Meeusen, R., et al. 2013. Prevention, diagnosis, and treatment of the overtraining syndrome: Joint consensus statement of the European College of Sport Science and the American College of Sports Medicine. *Medicine & Science in Sports & Exercise* 45:186–205.

Montoye, A., et al. 2014. Use of a wireless network of accelerometers for improved measurement of human energy expenditure. *Electronics* 3:205–20.

Myburgh, K. 2004. Protecting muscle ATP: Positive roles for peripheral defense mechanisms. *Medicine & Science in Sports & Exercise* 37:16–19.

Noakes, T. 2011. Time to move beyond a brainless exercise physiology: The evidence for complex regulation of human exercise performance. *Applied Physiology Nutrition and Metabolism* 36:23–35.

Noakes, T. 2007. The central governor model of exercise regulation applies to the marathon. *Sports Medicine* 37:374–77.

Noordhof, D., et al. 2013. Determining anaerobic capacity in sporting activities. *International Journal of Sports Physiology and Performance* 8:475–82.

Park, Y., et al. 2014. Adipose tissue inflammation and metabolic dysfunction: Role of exercise. *Missouri Medicine* 111:65–72.

Psota, T., and Chen, K. 2013. Measuring energy expenditure in clinical populations: Rewards and challenges. *European Journal of Clinical Nutrition* 67:436–42.

Roelands, B., et al. 2013. Neurophysiological determinants of theoretical concepts and mechanisms involved in pacing. *Sports Medicine* 43:301–11.

Schiaffino, S., and Reggiani, C. 2011. Fiber types in mammalian skeletal muscles. *Physiological Reviews* 91:1447–531.

Schoeller, D., et al. 2013. Self-report-based estimates of energy intake offer an inadequate basis for scientific conclusions. *American Journal of Clinical Nutrition* 97:1413–15.

Shephard, R. 2001. Chronic fatigue syndrome: An update. *Sports Medicine* 31:167–94.

Sidhu, S., et al. 2013. Corticospinal responses to sustained locomotor exercises: Moving beyond single-joint studies of central fatigue. *Sports Medicine* 43:437–49.

Skelly, L., et al. 2014. High-intensity interval exercise induces 24-h energy expenditure similar to traditional endurance exercise despite reduced time commitment. *Applied Physiology, Nutrition, and Metabolism* 39:845–8.

Spencer, M., and Gastin, P. 2001. Energy system contribution during 200- to 1500-m running in highly trained athletes. *Medicine & Science in Sports & Exercise* 33:157–62.

Torbeyns, T., et al. 2014. Active workstations to fight sedentary behaviour. *Sports Medicine* 44:1261–73.

Tremblay, A., et al. 1985. The effects of exercise-training on energy balance and adipose tissue morphology and metabolism. *Sports Medicine* 2:223–33.

Tremblay, A., et al. 1990. Long-term exercise training with constant energy intake. 2: Effect of glucose metabolism and resting energy expenditure. *International Journal of Obesity* 14:75–81.

Ward-Smith, A. J. 1999. Aerobic and anaerobic energy conversion during high-intensity exercise. *Medicine & Science in Sports Exercise* 31:1855–60.

Warwick, P. M. 2007. Thermic and glycemic responses to bread and pasta meals with and without prior low-intensity exercise. *International Journal of Sport Nutrition and Exercise Metabolism* 17:1–13.

Westerterp, K. 2013. Metabolic adaptations to over--and underfeeding--Still a matter of debate? *European Journal of Clinical Nutrition* 67:443–5.

White, C., and Kearney, M. 2013. Determinants of inter-specific variation in basal metabolic rate. *Journal of Comparative Physiology* 183:1–26.

Williams, P., and Thompson, P. 2013. Walking versus running for hypertension, cholesterol, and diabetes mellitus risk reduction. *Arteriosclerosis, Thrombosis and Vascular Biology* 33:1085–91.

Wilson, J., et al. 2012. The effects of endurance, strength, and power training on muscle fiber type shifting. *Journal of Strength and Conditioning Research* 26:1724–29.

Wu, X., et al. 2010. Genes and biochemical pathways in human skeletal muscle affecting resting energy expenditure and fuel partitioning. *Journal of Applied Physiology* 110:746–55.

Carbohydrates: The Main Energy Food

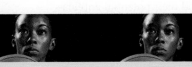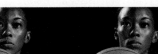

CHAPTER FOUR

LEARNING OBJECTIVES

After studying this chapter, you should be able to:

1. List the different types of dietary carbohydrates and identify foods typically rich in the different types.

2. Calculate the approximate number of Calories from carbohydrate that should be included in your daily diet.

3. Describe how dietary carbohydrate is absorbed, how it is distributed in the body, and what its major functions are in human metabolism.

4. Explain the role of carbohydrate in human energy systems during exercise.

5. Describe the various mechanisms whereby inadequate amounts of dietary carbohydrate may contribute to fatigue during exercise.

6. Understand the mechanisms whereby various dietary strategies involving carbohydrate intake (amount, type, and timing) before, during, and after exercise may help to optimize training for and competition in sport.

7. Identify athletes for whom carbohydrate loading may be appropriate and describe the full carbohydrate loading protocol, highlighting dietary intake and exercise training considerations.

8. Evaluate the efficacy of metabolic by-products of carbohydrate metabolism as ergogenic aids.

9. Identify carbohydrate-containing foods that are considered to be more healthful and explain why.

10. Describe the effects of chronic endurance exercise training on the subsequent use of carbohydrate as an energy source during exercise, including underlying mechanisms and potential health benefits.

One of the most important nutrients in your diet, from the standpoint of both health and athletic performance, is dietary carbohydrate.

Over the years the reputation of carbohydrate, particularly as a component of a weight-control diet, has seesawed between friend and foe. Most recently, some have dubbed carbohydrate as foe, alleging that high-carbohydrate diets are contributing to the epidemic of obesity within industrialized nations. Recently, interest in low-carbohydrate diets as a means to improve health and even endurance exercise performance have seen a resurgence. Although this is mostly supported through speculation or individual reports, some studies support low-carbohydrate diets as a means to decrease body mass or improve endurance exercise performance. Low-carbohydrate, high-fat diets are discussed in depth in the next chapter. In general, researchers and dietitians consider consumption of carbohydrate-rich foods to be one of the most important components of a healthful diet, but choosing good carbohydrates is key. The possible health benefits of a diet high in complex carbohydrates and fiber and low in added sugars were introduced in chapter 2 and are explained further in this chapter. The role of carbohydrate foods in a weight-control plan will be addressed in chapter 11 and, as we shall see, carbohydrates *per se* do not cause obesity, but excess Calories do.

As noted in chapter 3, the major role of carbohydrate in human nutrition is to provide energy, and scientists have long known that carbohydrate is one of the prime sources of energy during exercise. Of all the nutrients we consume, carbohydrate has received the most research attention in regard to a potential influence upon athletic performance, particularly in exercise tasks characterized by endurance, such as long-distance running, cycling, and triathloning. Such research is important to athletes who are concerned about optimal carbohydrate nutrition during training and competition. Indeed, continued research over the past quarter century has enabled sports nutritionists to provide more specific and useful responses to athletes' questions. For example, compared to the first edition of this book, published in 1983, readers of this edition will note several significant differences concerning dietary carbohydrate recommendations to athletes.

In this chapter, we explore the nature of dietary carbohydrates, their metabolic fates and interactions in the human body, their possible influence upon health status, and their potential application to physical performance, including the following: the adverse effects of low-carbohydrate diets; the value of carbohydrate intake before, during, and after exercise; the efficacy of different types of carbohydrates; the role of carbohydrate loading; and carbohydrate foods or compounds with alleged ergogenic properties. Although the role of sports drinks containing carbohydrate, such as Gatorade and PowerAde, is introduced in this chapter, additional detailed coverage of these beverages and their effect upon performance is presented in chapter 9: Water, Electrolytes, and Temperature Regulation.

Dietary Carbohydrates

What are the different types of dietary carbohydrates?

Carbohydrates represent one of the least expensive forms of Calories and hence are one of the major food supplies for the vast majority of the world's peoples. They are one of the three basic energy nutrients formed when the energy from the sun is harnessed in plants through the process of photosynthesis. Although the energy content of the various forms of carbohydrate varies slightly, each gram of carbohydrate contains approximately 4 Calories.

Carbohydrates are organic compounds that contain carbon, hydrogen, and oxygen in various combinations. A wide variety of forms exist in nature and in the human body, and novel manufactured carbohydrates, including sports drinks, have been developed for the food industry. In general terms, the major categories of importance to our discussion are simple carbohydrates, complex carbohydrates, and dietary fiber.

Simple carbohydrates, which are usually known as sugars, can be subdivided into two categories: disaccharides and monosaccharides. *Saccharide* means "sugar" or "sweet." The three major **monosaccharides** (single sugars) are **glucose, fructose**, and **galactose**. Glucose and fructose occur widely in nature, primarily in fruits, as free monosaccharides. Glucose is often called *dextrose* or *grape sugar,* while fructose is known as *levulose* or *fruit sugar.* Galactose is found in milk as part of lactose. Figure 4.1 presents two configurations illustrating the structure of monosaccharides.

The combination of two monosaccharides yields a **disaccharide**. The disaccharides (double sugars) include maltose (malt sugar), lactose (milk sugar), and sucrose (cane sugar or table sugar). Upon digestion these disaccharides yield the monosaccharides as follows.

Monosaccharides and disaccharides, such as glucose and sucrose, may be isolated from foods in purified forms known as *refined sugars.* Trisaccharides and higher saccharides also exist

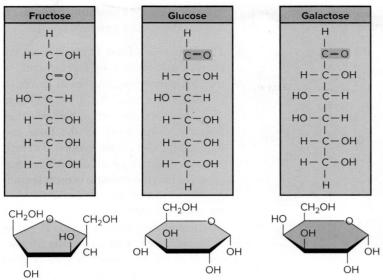

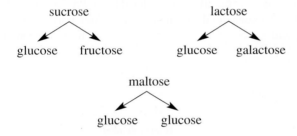

FIGURE 4.1 Chemical structure of the three monosaccharides is depicted in both the linear and ring configurations. Each corner in the ring structure contains a carbon atom, for a total of six carbons for each monosaccharide.

and may be found in commonly used sweeteners such as corn syrup. For example, high-fructose corn syrup, a common food additive, is a manufactured carbohydrate derived from the conversion of glucose in corn starch to fructose. Other food additives that are primarily sugar include honey, brown sugar, maple syrup, molasses, and fruit juice concentrate.

Complex carbohydrates, commonly known as *starches,* are generally formed when three or more glucose molecules combine. This combination is known as a **polysaccharide** when more than ten glucose molecules are combined and may contain thousands of linked glucose molecules. Starches, which exist in a variety of forms such as amylose, amylopectin, and resistant starch, are the storage form of carbohydrates. The vast majority of carbohydrates that exist in the plant world are in polysaccharide form. Of prime interest to us are the plant starches, through which we obtain a good proportion of our daily Calories along with a wide variety of nutrients, and the animal starch, glycogen, about which we shall hear more later in relation to energy for exercise. Additionally, **glucose polymers** are polysaccharides prepared commercially by controlled hydrolysis of starch. Maltodextrins are common glucose polymers used in sports drinks, which are discussed later.

Unfortunately, because of disagreements over the classification of various forms of carbohydrate, the term "complex carbohydrate" does not appear on the Nutrition Facts food label. You may obtain a rough estimate of the complex carbohydrate content by subtracting the grams of sugar from the grams of total carbohydrate. In some cases, the term "other carbohydrates" is used, which could include complex carbohydrates and other forms of carbohydrate as well.

Fiber is a complex carbohydrate. In its recent report on Dietary Reference Intakes, the National Academy of Sciences settled on three terms to define fiber. **Dietary fiber** consists of nondigestible carbohydrates and lignin that are intrinsic and intact in plants; this would include resistant starch. **Functional fiber** consists of isolated, nondigestible carbohydrates that have beneficial physiological effects in humans. **Total fiber** is the sum of dietary fiber and functional fiber. These nondigestible substances, which means that they are not digested and absorbed in the human small intestine, are usually a mixture of polysaccharides found in the plant wall or intracellular structures.

The National Academy of Sciences carefully defines both dietary and functional fiber, particularly as they may affect health. In essence, dietary fiber is consumed as part of intact foods (even if mechanically altered) containing other macronutrients, such as digestible carbohydrate and protein. For example, cereal brans derived from whole grains contain carbohydrate and protein, along with nondigestible fiber. Some examples of dietary fiber are cellulose, hemicellulose, lignin, pectin, and gums. When studying the health effects of dietary fiber, it is difficult to determine if health benefits are attributed to dietary fiber or to other potential healthful substances, such as certain phytochemicals, found in the food. The definition of dietary fiber includes the phytochemicals that come with it.

Functional fibers, in contrast, may be isolated or extracted from foods by chemical or other means, and may be manufactured synthetically. For example, various gums may be extracted from seeds and used as food ingredients for various purposes. Some examples of functional fiber are pectin, gums, and resistant starch. The specific fiber has to demonstrate a physiological effect in the body to be classified as a functional fiber, and this effect may be associated with a specific health benefit.

Total fiber is the sum of dietary fiber and functional fiber. A specific fiber may be classified as both dietary fiber and functional fiber. For example, cellulose can be classified as dietary fiber as a natural ingredient of an intact food, or it may be considered to be a functional fiber if extracted from a natural source and added to another food.

Previously, the various components of dietary and functional fiber have been classified on the basis of their solubility in water. Some fibers have been referred to as water soluble because they have been found to dissolve or swell in water and may be metabolized by bacteria in the large intestine. Others that do not possess these characteristics have been referred to as water-insoluble fibers. Common water-soluble fibers include gums, beta-glucans, and pectins. Common water-insoluble fibers include cellulose, hemicellulose, and lignin. Each of these types of fibers may confer specific health benefits, which will be discussed later in this chapter.

Sugar substitutes are designed to provide the sweetness of sugars, but with no or fewer Calories. A commonly used sugar substitute is sorbitol, a sugar alcohol. Health aspects of sugar substitutes are discussed later.

TABLE 4.1 Types of dietary carbohydrates***

Monosaccharides	Disaccharides	Polysaccharides	Other carbohydrates
Glucose	Sucrose	Plant starch	Sorbitol (sugar alcohol)
Fructose	Maltose	Amylose	Ribose (a five-carbon sugar)
Galactose	Lactose	Amylopectin	
		Resistant starch	
		Animal starch	
		Glycogen	

Dietary fiber	Functional fiber	Dietary/functional fiber**	
Hemicellulose	Polydextrin	Beta-glucans	
Resistant starch*	Psyllium	Cellulose	
	Resistant starch*	Gums	
		Pectins	

*Certain forms.
**Dietary fiber if found intact in food; functional fiber if extracted and added to foods.
***See text for food sources of the types of dietary carbohydrates.

A summary of the different types of carbohydrates is presented in table 4.1, and the effects of different forms of carbohydrate on physical performance or health are presented later in this chapter.

What are some common foods high in carbohydrate content?

Three of the six Food Exchanges are the primary contributors of carbohydrate in the diet; per serving, the starch exchange contains 15 grams, the fruit exchange 15 grams, and the vegetable exchange 5 grams. Some foods in the meat and milk groups also contain moderate to high amounts of carbohydrate. Dried beans and peas, because their protein content is comparable to that of meat, may be listed in the meat and meat substitute group. One-third cup of navy beans contains 15 grams of carbohydrate, which is nearly 70 percent of its energy content. A glass of skim milk contains 12 grams of carbohydrate, more than 50 percent of its energy content. Table 4.2 shows some foods in the different Food Exchanges that have high carbohydrate content. A more extensive listing is provided in appendix E. Complex-carbohydrate foods are accentuated, as they are highly recommended in the Prudent Healthy Diet.

Miscellaneous foods such as sodas, fruit ades, candy, pies, cake, and other processed sweets are high in carbohydrates.

TABLE 4.2 Foods high in carbohydrate content (grams per serving)[†]

Starch exchange (15 grams)	Fruit exchange (15 grams)	Vegetable exchange (5 grams)	Milk exchange (12 grams)	Meat exchange (15 grams)	Sports drinks/ gels/bars/chews (14–52 grams)	Miscellaneous (10–40 grams)
Whole grain	Apples	Asparagus	Ice milk	Kidney beans	Drinks:	Candy
Brown rice	Apricots	Broccoli	Rice milk	Navy beans	Gatorade	Cookies
Corn tortillas	Bananas	Carrots	Skim milk	Split peas	PowerAde	Fruit ades
Granola	Blueberries	Mushrooms	Soy milk	Lentils	Gels:	Soft drinks
Oatmeal	Cantaloupe	Radishes	Yogurt, fruit		ReLode	
Ready-to-eat cereal*	Cherries	Rutabaga			GU Energy Gel	
Rye crackers	Dried fruits	Squash, summer			Power Gel	
Whole wheat bread	Fruit juices	Tomatoes			Bars:	
Enriched	Oranges	Zucchini			Power Bar	
Bagels	Peaches				Clif Bar	
English muffins	Pineapple				Balance Bar	
Pasta	Plums				Chews:	
Ready-to-eat cereal*	Raspberries				GU Chomps	
White bread					Clif Shot Blocks	
White rice					Power Bar Blasts	
Starchy vegetables					Honey Stinger	
Corn					Energy Chews	
Green peas						
Potatoes						

*May be whole wheat or enriched, depending on the brand.
[†]Typical serving sizes: starch exchange (1 slice bread, ½ cup cereal); fruit exchange (1 medium; ½ cup); vegetable exchange (½ cup); milk exchange (1 cup; 8 fluid ounces); meat substitute exchange (½ cup). Check food labels, as grams of carbohydrate per serving, especially for cereals and sports products, may vary considerably.

Added sugars is the term applied to refined sugars that are added to foods during production. Reading food labels will provide you with the total amount of carbohydrate in grams, grams of sugar, and grams of fiber. The label will also provide you with the percentage of your recommended Daily Value for total carbohydrate and fiber, as explained on pages xxxxx.

As carbohydrates are the major fuel for most exercise tasks, several products have been marketed to athletes, particularly sports drinks, sports gels, and sports bars. Sports drinks, such as Gatorade and PowerAde, usually contain about 6–8 percent carbohydrates, or about 14–18 grams of carbohydrate per 8 fluid ounces. The carbohydrate source in each varies but usually contains a mixture of one of the following: glucose, fructose, sucrose, and glucose polymers. More details on sports drinks are presented in chapter 9. Sports gels, such as ReLode, GU, Power Gel, and Clif-Shot, contain forms of carbohydrates similar to those used in sports drinks, but in a more solid, gel form. They come in small squeeze containers (usually about 1 ounce) and contain roughly 20–30 grams of carbohydrate. Energy chews are a recent alternative for endurance athletes. They come in packets of three to ten chews containing 2.3–8 grams of carbohydrate per piece. Sports bars are also high in carbohydrate, usually with small amounts of protein and fats. The amount and type of carbohydrate per bar vary, the amount generally ranging between 20 to 45 grams. So-called energy drinks may contain substantial amounts of carbohydrate, often 30–50 or more grams in 8 ounces. Again, Nutrition Facts food labels on sports and "energy" drinks, sports gels, and sports bars provide information on the nutrient content, including amount of total carbohydrate, sugar, and fiber, as well as other ingredients such as caffeine, amino acids, vitamins, and minerals. By careful label reading and price comparisons, you may be able to get a better buy on some products. For example, sports bars are rather expensive, so purchasing lower-cost granola bars that contain similar nutrient value may provide some financial savings.

Foods high in dietary fiber include most vegetables and fruits, foods in the starch exchange made from whole grains, and dried beans and peas in the meat exchange. Wheat products are good sources of insoluble fiber, while oats, beans, dried peas, fruits, and vegetables are excellent sources of soluble fiber. Because of the purported health benefits of fiber, cereal manufacturers have released new products containing 13–14 grams of fiber per serving. Psyllium, rich in both soluble and insoluble fiber, is now added to several breakfast cereals. Table 4.3 presents the average fiber content in some common foods. Food labels also document fiber content per serving. Currently food labels document total fiber content per serving, but future labels may contain both dietary and functional fiber content.

How much carbohydrate do we need in the diet?

As we shall see, the human body can convert part of dietary protein and fat to carbohydrate. Thus, the National Academy of Sciences indicated that the lower limit of dietary carbohydrate compatible with life apparently is zero, provided that adequate amounts of protein and fat are consumed. Several populations around the world have subsisted on a diet with minimal amounts of carbohydrate without any apparent adverse effects. However, given that a very low-carbohydrate diet may be associated with various micronutrient deficiencies and health problems in Western societies, Dietary Reference Intakes (DRI) recently have been developed for carbohydrate and total fiber, and may be found in the DRI table for macronutrients in the front inside cover.

The RDA for carbohydrates is set at 130 grams per day for adults and children, which is based on the average minimum amount of glucose utilized by the brain. Fehm and others noted that although the brain constitutes only 2 percent of body mass, its metabolism accounts for 50 percent of total body glucose utilization. The Academy developed an Acceptable Macronutrient Distribution Range (AMDR), recommending that 45–65 percent of the daily energy intake be derived from carbohydrate. The AMDR for individuals has been set for carbohydrate based on scientific evidence suggesting such an intake may play a role in the prevention of increased risk of chronic diseases and may also ensure sufficient intakes of essential nutrients.

Most of us consume carbohydrate within this range and meet the RDA, as men consume an average 200–330 grams per day, while women average 180–230 grams per day. The Daily Value (DV) for carbohydrate on the food label is based on a recommendation of 60 percent of the caloric intake. The Daily Value (DV) for a 2,000-Calorie diet is 300 grams of carbohydrate, which represents 60 percent of the daily caloric intake ($4 \times 300 = 1,200$ carbohydrate Calories; $1,200/2,000 = 60$ percent).

The Academy also recommended that no more than 25 percent of total Calories come from added sugars. This standard was set based on evidence that individuals who exceed this level may not be obtaining adequate amounts of essential micronutrients that are not present in foods and beverages that contain added sugars. It should be stressed that the 25 percent is the maximal amount, not a recommended goal. In fact, the recommendation from most health professionals is to reduce this amount to approximately 10 percent. According to the *Dietary Guidelines for Americans* 2010, current estimates of sugar intake approximate 16 percent of daily energy intake.

The Academy recommends an Adequate Intake (AI) for total fiber as follows:

- Men
  - 38 grams up to age 50
  - 30 grams over age 50
- Women
  - 25 grams up to age 50
  - 21 grams over age 50

TABLE 4.3	Fiber content in some common foods[†]
Beans	7–9 grams per ½ cup, cooked
Vegetables	3–5 grams per ½ cup, cooked
Fruits	1–3 grams per piece
Breads and cereals*	1–3 grams per serving
Nuts and seeds	2–5 grams per ounce

*Fiber content may vary considerably in bran-type cereals, ranging up to 13–14 grams per serving. Select whole-grain products for higher fiber content.

[†]Check food labels for grams of fiber per serving.

The DV for a 2,000-Calorie diet is 25 grams of fiber, or 12.5 grams per 1,000 Calories. Thus, the DV is in accord with the AI for women but somewhat lower than the AI for men. The current average amount of total fiber intake is approximately 15 grams per day, so most individuals are not meeting this recommendation. An increased intake of complex carbohydrates would help meet this recommendation. Inadequate intake of dietary carbohydrate can have a negative impact on physical performance.

Sports nutritionists also recommend a high-carbohydrate diet for individuals engaged in athletic training programs. The general recommendation for most athletes parallels the recommended dietary goals noted above. For an athlete consuming 3,000 Calories per day, 55–60 percent from carbohydrate would be 1,650–1,800 Calories, or about 400–450 grams. Ron Maughan and Louise Burke, experts in sports nutrition, have described how carbohydrate intake varies considerably based on specific needs related to physical activity levels, sport, and individual goals. Thus, the amount of carbohydrate needed by an individual exercising to lose weight will be quite different from the amount needed by an individual in training to run a marathon. These considerations will be discussed later in this chapter and in chapter 11.

Many recent dietary surveys conducted with athletes, including endurance athletes, often reveal a carbohydrate intake significantly lower than these recommendations. Inadequate intake of dietary carbohydrate can have a negative impact on physical performance.

Key Concepts

▶ Dietary carbohydrates include monosaccharides and disaccharides (simple sugars) and polysaccharides (complex carbohydrates). Most foods in the starch, fruit, and vegetable exchanges contain a high percentage of carbohydrate, primarily complex carbohydrates.

▶ The RDA for carbohydrate is 130 grams daily, while the AMDR is 45–65 percent of energy intake. The AI for total fiber is 38 and 25 grams per day for young men and women, respectively, and somewhat lower for older men and women. However, the Daily Value (DV) for carbohydrate is 300 grams and for dietary fiber 25 grams, based on a 2,000-Calorie diet.

Check for Yourself

▶ Peruse food labels of some of your favorite foods and check carbohydrate. Pay particular attention to percent of Daily Value for total carbohydrates, sugars, and fiber. You can also go to www.ChooseMyPlate.gov. Click on Food Groups, then Grain Group, Vegetable Group, and Fruit Group to learn more about what foods are healthy choices for each of the food groups. The Food Gallery links may also help in determining serving sizes.

Metabolism and Function

The food we eat must be processed before the nutrients it contains may be used in the body for their various purposes. This process includes digestion, absorption, and excretion of nutrients, which is the responsibility of the gastrointestinal (GI) system, or alimentary canal, which extends from the mouth to the anus. Figure 4.2 presents the main organs involved in the GI system, some of their basic digestive functions, and the sites of nutrient absorption, which will be discussed in the following chapters.

Digestion is the process by which food is broken down mechanically and chemically in the digestive tract and converted into absorbable forms. Specific enzymes break down foods into smaller substances that may be absorbed. Specific enzymes of interest regarding carbohydrates, fats, and protein will be discussed where appropriate. Absorption of nutrients, as noted in figure 4.2, may occur in the stomach and large intestine, but the vast majority of nutrients are absorbed through the millions of villi lining the small intestine. Some substances are absorbed by diffusion, which may be passive or facilitated. In passive diffusion the substance simply diffuses across the cell membrane. Osmosis is the passive diffusion of water. In **facilitated diffusion**, a receptor in the cell membrane is needed to transport the substance from the intestine into the villi. No energy is required for diffusion, but other substances need energy supplied by the villi cells in order to be absorbed, a process known as **active transport**. Figure 4.3 presents a cross section of a villus and highlights some of the key nutrients and the associated process of absorption.

How are dietary carbohydrates digested and absorbed and what are some implications for sports performance?

Carbohydrates usually are ingested in the forms of polysaccharides (starches), disaccharides (sucrose, maltose, and lactose), and monosaccharides (glucose and fructose). In addition, special carbohydrate compounds, such as glucose polymers, have been developed for athletes. To be useful in the body, these carbohydrates must be digested, absorbed, and transported to appropriate cells for metabolism.

The digestion and absorption of dietary carbohydrates are highlighted in figure 4.4. The enzyme that digests complex carbohydrates is amylase, which is secreted by the salivary glands and pancreas. Saliva amylase initiates digestion of the polysaccharides to disaccharides, but most digestion is done in the small intestine by pancreatic amylase. Enzymes then digest the disaccharides to monosaccharides, which are absorbed by specific receptors in the villi.

The composition of the dietary carbohydrate may influence delivery into the body. For example, as noted later in this chapter, sports drinks may be designed to take advantage of the different monosaccharide receptors in the villi. Moreover, sports drinks containing carbohydrate and sodium may enhance water absorption via a co-transport mechanism, a topic that is discussed in chapter 9.

Optimal functioning of the GI tract following carbohydrate intake has been studied extensively because improper functioning may impair athletic performance. For example, although there is very little digestion of carbohydrate in the stomach, the rapidity with which carbohydrate leaves the stomach, and its impact upon the absorption of water, may be important considerations for athletes involved in prolonged exercise under warm environmental conditions.

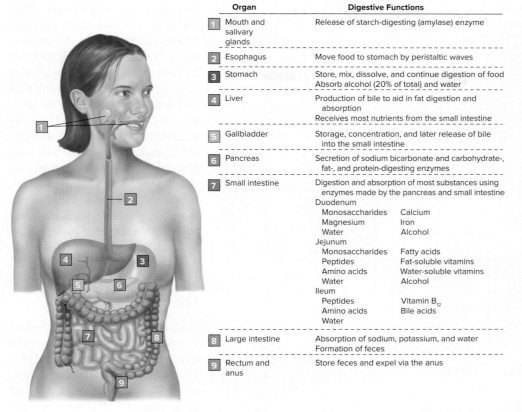

Organ		Digestive Functions
1	Mouth and salivary glands	Release of starch-digesting (amylase) enzyme
2	Esophagus	Move food to stomach by peristaltic waves
3	Stomach	Store, mix, dissolve, and continue digestion of food Absorb alcohol (20% of total) and water
4	Liver	Production of bile to aid in fat digestion and absorption Receives most nutrients from the small intestine
5	Gallbladder	Storage, concentration, and later release of bile into the small intestine
6	Pancreas	Secretion of sodium bicarbonate and carbohydrate-, fat-, and protein-digesting enzymes

7	Small intestine	Digestion and absorption of most substances using enzymes made by the pancreas and small intestine
		Duodenum
		  Monosaccharides Calcium
		  Magnesium Iron
		  Water Alcohol
		Jejunum
		  Monosaccharides Fatty acids
		  Peptides Fat-soluble vitamins
		  Amino acids Water-soluble vitamins
		  Water Alcohol
		Ileum
		  Peptides Vitamin B_{12}
		  Amino acids Bile acids
		  Water

8	Large intestine	Absorption of sodium, potassium, and water Formation of feces
9	Rectum and anus	Store feces and expel via the anus

FIGURE 4.2 The alimentary canal. The alimentary canal includes the mouth, the esophagus, the stomach, the small intestine (duodenum, jejunum, ileum), the large intestine (colon), the rectum, and the anal canal. Various glands and organs, including the salivary glands, the gallbladder, and the pancreas, secrete enzymes and other constituents into the digestive tract. Most blood draining from the intestines goes to the liver for processing. Note the general sites in the digestive tract where principal nutrients and other substances are absorbed (although there is some overlap in the exact site of absorption). Most absorption of nutrients occurs throughout the small intestine.

Certain dietary practices may predispose individuals to gastrointestinal distress, which will compromise exercise performance. High concentrations of simple sugars, particularly fructose, may exert a reverse osmotic effect in the intestines, drawing water from the circulatory system into the intestinal lumen. The resulting symptoms are referred to as the dumping syndrome and include weakness, sweating, and diarrhea. Lactose may present a problem to some athletes, and its possible effects are discussed later in the chapter.

What happens to the carbohydrate after it is absorbed into the body?

Of the three monosaccharides, glucose is of most importance to human physiology. Most dietary carbohydrates are broken down to glucose for absorption into the blood, while the majority of the absorbed fructose and galactose are converted to glucose by the liver. Glucose is the blood sugar.

The **glycemic index (GI)** represents a ranking system relative to the effect that consumption of 50 grams of a particular carbohydrate food has upon the blood glucose response over the course

of 2 hours. The normal baseline measure is 50 grams of glucose, and the resultant blood glucose response is scored as 100. In general, the following values are used to rank the glycemic index of foods:

- 70 or more—high GI foods
- 69–55—medium GI foods
- 55 or less—low GI foods

Many factors other than a food's carbohydrate content, such as the physical form (coarse or fine) and serving mode (raw or cooked), may influence the glycemic index of any given food. Moreover, the glycemic index for any given food may vary considerably between individuals, so although some general values of the glycemic index may be given, the effects of different foods should be tested individually in those who are concerned about their blood sugar levels. In general, foods containing high amounts of refined sugars have a high glycemic index because they lead to a rapid rise in the blood sugar, but some starchy foods also have a high glycemic index. In contrast, foods high in fiber, such as beans, generally have a low glycemic index. Interestingly, fructose has a low glycemic index, which is one of the reasons its use as the primary carbohydrate source in sports drinks had been advocated for endurance athletes. We shall discuss the role of fructose later in this chapter. Table 4.4 classifies some common foods according to their glycemic index.

The **glycemic load (GL)** also represents a ranking system relative to the effect that eating a carbohydrate food has on the blood glucose level, but GL also includes the portion size. While the glycemic index is based on 50 grams of a particular food, a typical serving size for that food may be 6–8 ounces (180–240 grams). The GL is calculated by the following formula:

$$GL = \frac{(\text{glycemic index}) \times (\text{grams of nonfiber carbohydrate in 1 serving})}{100}$$

The following values are used to rank the glycemic load of foods:

- 20 or more—high GL foods
- 19–11—medium GL foods
- 10 or less—low GL foods

The GL for some foods is presented in table 4.4.

The usefulness of glycemic index and glycemic load is the subject of debate. As reviewed by Mirrahimi and by Greenwood, glycemic index may play a role in reducing cardiovascular disease risk and diabetes, respectively. O'Reilly notes that research on glycemic

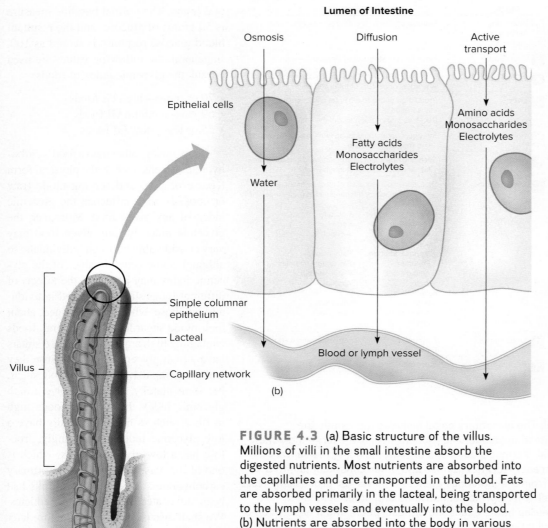

Lumen of Intestine

Osmosis   Diffusion   Active transport

Epithelial cells

Water

Fatty acids
Monosaccharides
Electrolytes

Amino acids
Monosaccharides
Electrolytes

Simple columnar epithelium

Lacteal

Blood or lymph vessel

Capillary network

(b)

Villus

Arteriole
Venule
Lymph vessel

(a)

FIGURE 4.3 (a) Basic structure of the villus. Millions of villi in the small intestine absorb the digested nutrients. Most nutrients are absorbed into the capillaries and are transported in the blood. Fats are absorbed primarily in the lacteal, being transported to the lymph vessels and eventually into the blood. (b) Nutrients are absorbed into the body in various ways. Water enters the cell by osmosis, most fatty acids by diffusion, and amino acids via active transport, a process that requires energy. Monosaccharides and electrolytes may use two pathways (i.e., diffusion and active transport).

to a given food may be very different from someone else's response. Moreover, individuals do not normally consume carbohydrate foods by themselves, but usually with other foods containing fat and protein such as a hamburger on a bun. The addition of fat and protein will usually reduce the glycemic index and glycemic load. The glycemic index and glycemic load can be used to help select more healthful carbohydrates. In general, the lower the glycemic index or glycemic load, the more healthful the source of carbohydrate, as discussed later in this chapter.

What is the metabolic fate of blood glucose?

Normal blood glucose levels (normoglycemia) range between 80 and 100 milligrams per deciliter of blood (80–100 mg/ml, or 80–100 milligram percent). The maintenance of a normal blood glucose level is very important for proper metabolism. Thus, the human body possesses a variety of mechanisms, primarily hormones, to help keep blood glucose levels under precise control. The rise in blood glucose, also known as *serum glucose,* stimulates the pancreas to secrete insulin into the blood. **Insulin** is a hormone that facilitates the uptake and utilization of glucose (facilitated diffusion) by various tissues in the body, most notably the muscles and adipose (fat) tissue. Cell membranes contain receptors to transport glucose into the cell. The primary receptors in muscle and fat cell membranes are known as GLUT-4 receptors, which are directly activated by insulin (see figure 4.5). Exercise also activates these receptors to transport blood glucose into the muscle cell, independently of the effect of insulin. Other hormones, discussed later in this chapter, are also involved in regulating blood glucose. With normal amounts of carbohydrate intake in a mixed meal, blood glucose levels remain normal.

However, foods with a high glycemic index may lead rapidly to high blood glucose levels, possibly **hyperglycemia** (>140 mg percent), which will cause an enhanced secretion of insulin from the pancreas. High serum levels of insulin will then lead to a rapid, and possibly excessive, transport of blood glucose into the tissues. This may lead in turn to **hypoglycemia** (<40–50 mg percent), or low blood glucose level. This insulin response and **reactive hypoglycemia** following carbohydrate intake may be an important consideration for some athletes and is discussed later.

index and exercise performance, discussed later in the chapter, is at an early stage but may have some benefit. However, Sacks and others recently demonstrated that when a large group of overweight adults were placed on a five-week high- or low-glycemic-index diet, the high-glycemic-index diet did not improve insulin sensitivity, systolic blood pressure, LDL-cholesterol, or HDL-cholesterol. The strength of this study is that food for the diets (all meals, snacks, and Calorie-containing beverages) were provided by the investigators for five-week diets. The authors suggested that selecting foods based on glycemic index may not improve cardiovascular risk factors or insulin resistance. As noted, one person's glycemic response

www.mendosa.com/gilists.htm   Check the glycemic index and the glycemic load for a wide variety of carbohydrate-containing foods.

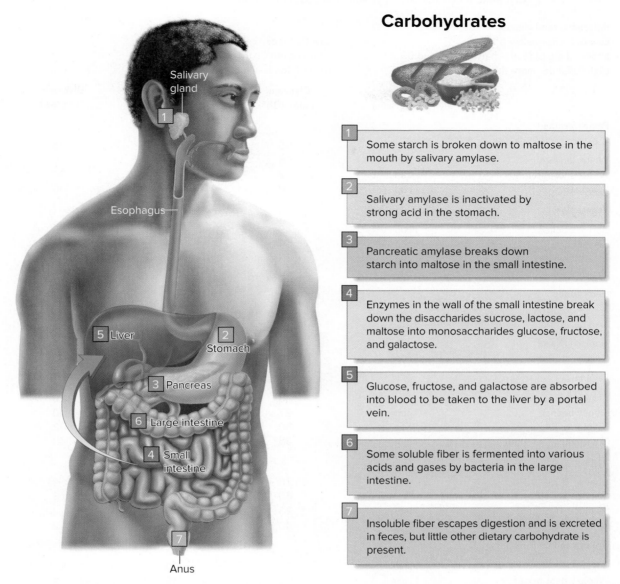

Carbohydrates

1. Some starch is broken down to maltose in the mouth by salivary amylase.

2. Salivary amylase is inactivated by strong acid in the stomach.

3. Pancreatic amylase breaks down starch into maltose in the small intestine.

4. Enzymes in the wall of the small intestine break down the disaccharides sucrose, lactose, and maltose into monosaccharides glucose, fructose, and galactose.

5. Glucose, fructose, and galactose are absorbed into blood to be taken to the liver by a portal vein.

6. Some soluble fiber is fermented into various acids and gases by bacteria in the large intestine.

7. Insoluble fiber escapes digestion and is excreted in feces, but little other dietary carbohydrate is present.

FIGURE 4.4 Carbohydrate digestion and absorption. Enzymes made by the mouth, pancreas, and small intestine participate in the process of digestion. Most carbohydrate digestion and absorption take place in the small intestine.

Foods with a low glycemic index, particularly soluble fiber forms, lead to a slower insulin response and a more stable blood glucose level. Consuming a diet based on the glycemic index has been studied as a possible means to enhance health, as well as sports performance, as noted later in this chapter.

The fate of blood glucose is dependent upon a multitude of factors, and exercise is one of the most important. The following points represent the major fates of blood glucose. Figure 4.6 schematically represents these fates.

1. Blood glucose may be used for energy, particularly by the brain and other parts of the nervous system that rely primarily on glucose for their metabolism. Hypoglycemia can impair the normal function of the brain. Although hypoglycemia as a clinical condition is quite rare in the general population, transitory hypoglycemia may occur in very prolonged endurance exercise.

2. Blood glucose may be converted to either liver or muscle glycogen. It is important to note that liver glycogen may later be reconverted to blood glucose. However, this does not occur to any appreciable extent with muscle glycogen. In essence, glucose is locked in the muscle once it enters, owing to the lack of a specific enzyme needed to change its form so that it can cross the cell membrane back into the bloodstream. Most of the muscle glycogen is converted to this locked form of glucose during the production of energy. Researchers discovered two forms of muscle glycogen, proglycogen and macroglycogen. Hargreaves indicates that the functional significance of these glycogen forms remains to be fully elucidated. Houston indicates that proglycogen seems to be preferentially used during muscle activity, while the macroglycogen may be more of a reserve supply of carbohydrate for prolonged exercise. In this text we shall use the term *glycogen* to represent both forms.

TABLE 4.4   Glycemic index (GI) and glycemic load (GL) of common foods

Reference food glucose = 100
Low GI foods—below 55
Intermediate GI foods—between 55 and 69
High GI foods—more than 70

Low GL foods—below 10
Intermediate GL foods—between 11 and 19
High GL foods—more than 20

	Serving size (grams)	Glycemic index (GI)*	Carbohydrate (grams)	Glycemic load (GL)
Pastas/grains				
Brown rice	1 cup	55	46	25
White, long grain	1 cup	56	45	25
White, short grain	1 cup	72	53	38
Spaghetti	1 cup	41	40	16
Vegetables				
Carrots, boiled	1 cup	49	16	8
Sweet corn	1 cup	55	39	21
Potato, baked	1 cup	85	57	48
New (red) potato, boiled	1 cup	62	29	18
Dairy foods				
Milk, whole	1 cup	27	11	3
Milk, skim	1 cup	32	12	4
Yogurt, low-fat	1 cup	33	17	6
Ice cream	1 cup	61	31	19
Legumes				
Baked beans	1 cup	48	54	26
Kidney beans	1 cup	27	38	10
Lentils	1 cup	30	40	12
Navy beans	1 cup	38	54	21
Sugars				
Honey	1 tsp	73	6	4
Sucrose	1 tsp	65	5	3
Fructose	1 tsp	23	5	1
Lactose	1 tsp	46	5	2
Breads and muffins				
Bagel	1 small	72	30	22
Whole wheat bread	1 slice	69	13	9
White bread	1 slice	70	10	7
Croissant	1 small	67	26	17
Fruits				
Apple	1 medium	38	22	8
Banana	1 medium	55	29	16
Grapefruit	1 medium	25	32	8
Orange	1 medium	44	15	7
Beverages				
Apple juice	1 cup	40	29	12
Orange juice	1 cup	46	26	13
Gatorade	1 cup	78	15	12
Coca-Cola	1 cup	63	26	16
Snack foods				
Potato chips	1 oz	54	15	8
Vanilla wafers	5 cookies	77	15	12
Chocolate	1 oz	49	18	9
Jelly beans	1 oz	80	26	21

*Based on a comparison to glucose.

Source: Foster-Powell, K. and others: International table of glycemic index and glycemic load. *American Journal of Clinical Nutrition* 76:5, 2002.

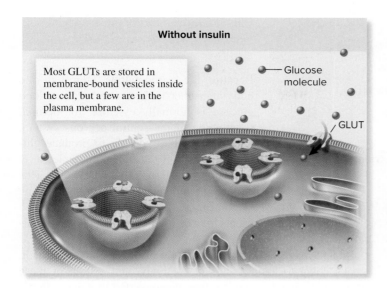
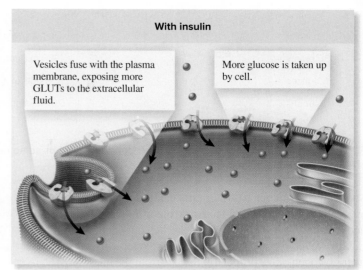

FIGURE 4.5 Insulin promotes the transport of glucose across plasma membranes. This is done by the recruitment of intracellular vesicles containing glucose transporter (GLUT) proteins to the plasma membrane, where they facilitate glucose diffusion into the cell.

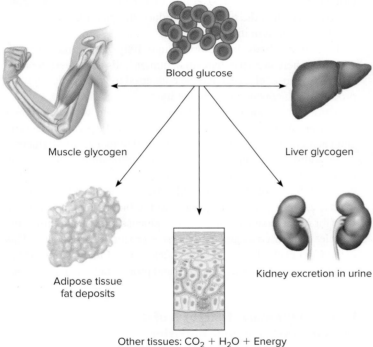

FIGURE 4.6 Fates of blood glucose. After assimilation into the blood, glucose may be stored in the liver or muscles as glycogen or be utilized as a source of energy by these and other tissues, particularly the nervous system. Excess glucose may be partially excreted by the kidneys, but major excesses are converted to fat and stored in the adipose tissues.

3. Blood glucose may be converted to and stored as fat in the adipose tissue. This situation occurs when the dietary carbohydrate, in combination with caloric intake of other nutrients, exceeds the energy demands of the body and the storage capacity of the liver and muscles for glycogen.

4. Some blood glucose also may be excreted in the urine if an excessive amount occurs in the blood because of rapid ingestion of simple sugars.

How much total energy do we store as carbohydrate?

A common method to express the concentration of carbohydrate stored in the body is in millimoles (mmol). A **millimole** is 1/1,000 of a mole, which is the term representing gram molecular weight. In essence, a mole represents the weight in grams of a particular substance such as glucose. The chemical formula for glucose is $C_6H_{12}O_6$, so it contains 6 parts of carbon and oxygen and 12 parts of hydrogen. The atomic weight of carbon is 12, hydrogen is 1, and oxygen 16. If you multiply the number of parts by the respective atomic weights of each of the elements for glucose [(6 × 12) + (12 × 1) + (6 × 16)], you get a total of 180. Thus, 1 mole of glucose is 180 grams, or about 6 ounces. One millimole is 1/1,000 of 180 grams, or 180 milligrams. (See figure 4.7.)

As an illustration, the normal glucose concentration is about 5 mmol per liter of blood, or 90 mg/100 ml (90 mg/dL). To calculate, 5 mmol × 180 mg = 900 mg/liter, which is the same as 90 mg/100 ml. The normal individual has about 5 liters of blood. Thus, this individual would have a total of 25 mmol of glucose in the blood, or a total of 4,500 milligrams (25 × 180), or 4.5 grams.

These calculations have been presented here because this is the means whereby concentrations of glucose, glycogen, and other nutrients are expressed in contemporary scientific literature. A knowledge of these mathematical relationships should help you interpret research more effectively. However, because we are using the Calorie as the measure of energy in this book, and because each gram of carbohydrate equals approximately 4 Calories, an estimate of the energy content of the major human energy sources of carbohydrate may be obtained.

For our purposes, the body has three major energy sources of carbohydrate: blood glucose, liver glycogen, and muscle glycogen.

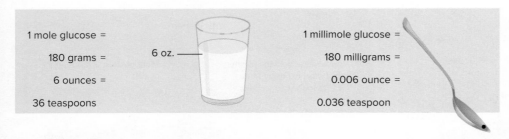

1 mole glucose =	6 oz.	1 millimole glucose =
180 grams =		180 milligrams =
6 ounces =		0.006 ounce =
36 teaspoons		0.036 teaspoon

FIGURE 4.7 The millimole concept. The concentration of some nutrients in the body is often expressed in millimoles. See text for explanation.

Some glucose (about 10–15 grams) is also found in the lymph and intercellular fluids. Initial stores of blood glucose are rather limited, totaling only about 5 grams, or the equivalent of 20 Calories (C). However, blood glucose stores may be replenished from either liver glycogen or absorption of glucose from the intestine. The liver has the greatest concentration of glycogen in the body. However, because its size is limited, the liver normally contains only about 75–100 g of glycogen, or 300–400 C. One hour of aerobic exercise uses more than half of the liver glycogen supply. It is also important to note that the liver glycogen content may be decreased by starvation or increased by a carbohydrate-rich diet. Fifteen hours or more of starvation will deplete the liver glycogen, whereas certain dietary patterns may nearly double the glycogen content of the liver, a condition that may be useful in certain tasks of physical performance.

The greatest amount of carbohydrate stored in the body is in the form of muscle glycogen. This is because the muscles compose such a large proportion of the body mass as contrasted to the liver. One would expect large differences in total muscle glycogen content between different individuals because of differences in body size. However, for an average-sized, untrained man with about 30 kg of his body weight consisting of muscle tissue, one could expect a total muscle glycogen content of approximately 360 g, or 1,440 C. This would represent a concentration of about 66 mmol, or 12 grams, per kg of muscle tissue. As with liver glycogen, the muscle glycogen stores also may be decreased or increased, with considerable effects on physical performance. For example, a trained endurance athlete may have twice the amount of stored muscle glycogen that an untrained, sedentary individual has.

If we calculate the body storage of carbohydrate as blood glucose, liver glycogen, and muscle glycogen, the total is only about 1,800–1,900 C, not an appreciable amount. One full day of starvation could reduce it considerably. Some normal ranges of carbohydrate stores are presented in table 4.5, although these normal ranges may be increased or decreased considerably by diet or exercise.

TABLE 4.5	Approximate carbohydrate stores in the body of a normal, sedentary adult	
Source	**Amount in grams**	**Equivalent amount in Calories**
Blood glucose	5	20
Liver glycogen	75–100	300–400
Muscle glycogen	300–400	1,200–1,600

Can the human body make carbohydrates from protein and fat?

Because the carbohydrate stores in the body are rather limited, and because blood glucose is normally essential for optimal functioning of the central nervous system, it is important to be able to produce glucose internally if the stores are depleted by starvation or a zero-carbohydrate diet. This process in the body is called **gluconeogenesis**, meaning the new formation of glucose. A number of different substrates from each of the three energy nutrients may be used and are depicted graphically in figure 4.8.

Protein may be a significant source of blood glucose. Protein breaks down to amino acids in the body, and certain of these amino acids, notably alanine, may be converted to glucose in the liver. This is referred to as the **glucose-alanine cycle**, which is explained further in chapter 6. A number of other amino acids also are gluconeogenic. Glucose is essential for the brain and several other tissues. If about 130 grams of carbohydrate are not consumed daily, then the body will produce the glucose it needs, primarily from protein in the body.

Fats in the body break down into fatty acids and glycerol. Although there is no mechanism in human cells to convert the fatty acids to glucose, glycerol may be converted to glucose through the process of gluconeogenesis in the liver.

Through gluconeogenesis, 1 gram of protein will yield about 0.56 gram of glucose. Triglycerides are about 10 percent glycerol, and each gram of glycerol may be converted to a gram of glucose.

In addition, certain by-products of carbohydrate metabolism, notably pyruvate and lactate, may be converted back to glucose in the liver. Some of the lactic acid produced in the muscle during intense exercise may be released into the blood and carried to the liver for reconversion to glucose. The glucose may then return to the muscles to be used as an energy source or stored as glycogen. This is the **Cori cycle**. Figure 4.9 illustrates some of the basic interrelationships among carbohydrate, fat, and protein in human nutrition.

What are the major functions of carbohydrate in human nutrition?

The major function of carbohydrate in human metabolism is to supply energy. Some body cells, such as the nerve cells in the brain and retina and the red blood cells, are normally totally dependent upon glucose for energy and require a constant source. Through a series of biochemical reactions in the body cells, glucose is oxidized, eventually producing water, carbon dioxide, and energy. Zierler notes that although carbohydrate is an excellent source of energy, it is not the major fuel when the body is at rest; fats are. Carbohydrate is the main fuel for certain tissues during rest, such as the brain, central nervous system, and red blood cells but provides only about 15–20 percent of muscle energy needs during rest. Thus, the body conserves its limited carbohydrate stores by using fats as the primary energy source during resting conditions.

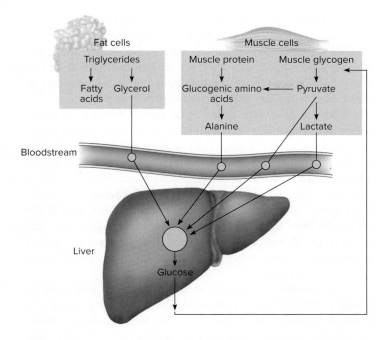

FIGURE 4.8 Gluconeogenesis. The liver is the major site for gluconeogenesis in the body. The breakdown products of fats, protein, and carbohydrate from other parts of the body may be transported to the liver by the blood for eventual reconversion into glucose. Glycerol, glucogenic amino acids, lactate, and pyruvate may be important sources for the new formation of glucose. The Cori cycle involves the transport of lactate to the liver and conversion to glucose, which may then be transported back to the muscle.

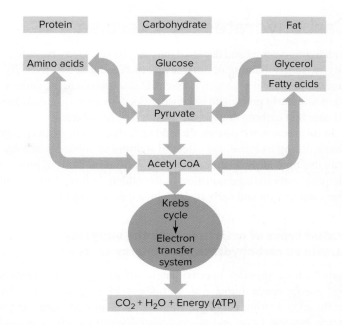

FIGURE 4.9 Interrelationships among carbohydrate, fat, and protein metabolism in humans. All three nutrients may be utilized for energy, although the major energy sources are carbohydrate and fat. Excess carbohydrate may be converted to fat; the carbohydrate structure also may be used to form protein, but nitrogen must be added. Fat cannot be used to generate carbohydrate to any large extent because acetyl CoA cannot be converted to pyruvate. The glycerol component of fat may form very small amounts of carbohydrate. Fats may serve as a basis for the formation of protein, but again, nitrogen must be added. Excess protein cannot be stored in the body but can be converted to either carbohydrate or fat.

As noted in chapter 3, carbohydrate can be used to produce energy either aerobically or anaerobically. Recall that in the lactic acid system, ATP is produced rapidly via anaerobic glycolysis, but for this system to continue functioning, the end product of glycolysis, pyruvic acid or pyruvate, must be converted into lactic acid. In the oxygen system, aerobic glycolysis predominates and pyruvic acid is converted into acetyl CoA, which enters into the Krebs cycle and electron transfer system for complete oxidation and the production of relatively large amounts of ATP. For the same amount of carbohydrate, anaerobic metabolism yields only 2 ATP, whereas aerobic metabolism yields 36 to 38 ATP. See appendix G, figures G.1 to G.3, for more detail.

Carbohydrates have some functions in the body other than energy production. Monosaccharides can be used to form other, smaller carbohydrate molecules such as trioses and pentoses. These substances may combine with other nutrients and form body chemicals essential to life, such as glycolipids or glycoproteins. Glycoproteins are very important components of cell membranes, serving as receptors to help regulate cell function. Ribose is a key pentose (5-carbon sugar) that is a part of a number of indispensable compounds in the body. One of those compounds is RNA, or ribonucleic acid, which plays an important part in anabolic processes in the cells.

Key Concepts

▶ Most ingested carbohydrates are initially converted into blood glucose and used for energy or stored as liver and muscle glycogen, but excess carbohydrates may be converted into fat.

▶ The glycemic index (GI) is a measure of the rate of digestion and absorption of 50 grams of a carbohydrate food and the resultant effect on the blood glucose level. The glycemic load (GL) is similar but is based on the typical serving size for carbohydrate foods. Different numerical rankings are used for the GI and GL.

▶ The three sources of carbohydrate in the body of an average adult male are blood glucose (5 grams; 20 Calories), liver glycogen (75–100 grams; 300–400 Calories), and muscle glycogen (350–400 grams; 1,400–1,600 Calories).

▶ The liver is the main organ that can produce glucose from certain by-products of protein and fat, a process known as gluconeogenesis.

▶ The major function of carbohydrates in human metabolism is to supply energy; blood glucose is essential for optimal functioning of the nervous system, whereas muscle glycogen is essential for both anaerobic capacity and aerobic power exercise.

Carbohydrates for Exercise

Both hypoglycemia and depleted muscle glycogen may precipitate fatigue, so maintaining optimal levels of blood glucose, liver glycogen, and muscle glycogen is essential in various athletic endeavors, particularly prolonged exercise tasks. Some sports authorities indicate that carbohydrate is the master fuel for athletes.

In this section we discuss the role of carbohydrate as an energy source during exercise, the effect of training to enhance carbohydrate use for energy when needed, and various methods to provide adequate carbohydrate nutrition to the athlete before, during, and after competition and carbohydrate intake during training.

In what types of activities does the body rely heavily on carbohydrate as an energy source?

Carbohydrate supplies approximately 40 percent of the body's total energy needs during rest, with about 15–20 percent used by the muscles. During very light exercise fat is an important energy source, but van Loon and others found that muscle glycogen and plasma glucose oxidation rates increased with every increment in exercise intensity. When exercise becomes more intense, such as when a person is working at 65–85 percent of capacity, carbohydrate becomes the preferred energy source; this is the crossover concept discussed in chapter 3. At maximal or supramaximal exercise levels, carbohydrate is used almost exclusively. Thus, carbohydrate may be the prime energy source for high-intensity anaerobic events lasting for less than 1 minute and high-intensity aerobic events lasting more than an hour or two.

As Holloszy and others summarized, carbohydrate use, then, is associated with the intensity level of the exercise. The more intense the exercise, the greater the percentage contribution of carbohydrate. Of course, the more intense the exercise, the sooner exhaustion occurs. A fairly well-conditioned person may be able to exercise for many hours at 40–50 percent of VO_2 max, for 1 to 2 hours or so at 70–80 percent of VO_2 max, but only for minutes at maximal or supramaximal levels of VO_2 max. As noted by Hargreaves, the fatigue that occurs in very high-intensity exercise of short duration, such as a 400-meter run, may be associated with the accumulation of hydrogen ions, a by-product of lactic acid production. In contrast, the fatigue associated with more prolonged exercise may be connected with depleted supplies of liver and muscle glycogen, both of which may be affected by dietary practices and exercise intensity and duration.

Carbohydrate intake is most important for prolonged endurance events lasting more than 90–120 minutes. Data from such endurance tasks as the Tour de France, the bicycle Race Across America, and the Ironman Triathlon, illustrate the importance of dietary carbohydrate in sustaining high energy output for prolonged periods. Most of the athletes in these events consumed high-caloric diets rich in carbohydrates both before and during competition. A classic example is the ultradistance runner from Greece, Yannis Kouros, who won the Sydney to Melbourne race in Australia, a distance of approximately 600 miles, in 5 days and 5 hours, or about 114 miles of running per day. He consumed up to 13,400 Calories per day, with up to 98 percent being derived from carbohydrates. Cyclists in major multiday races consume more than 800 grams of carbohydrate daily. Data obtained from exercise tasks of lesser magnitude, such as marathons (26.2 miles; 42.2 kilometers) and ultramarathons (50 kilometers and longer), also provide evidence for the importance of carbohydrate as the prime energy fuel, as evidenced in the review by Peters.

Carbohydrate is also an essential energy fuel for prolonged sports involving many intermittent bouts of high-intensity exercise, such as soccer, rugby, field hockey, ice hockey, and tennis. For example, Bangsbo noted that although soccer players are engaged in low-intensity exercise for about 70 percent of the time, there may be 150–250 bouts of brief, intense actions during a game. Athletes in these sports repeatedly use muscle glycogen stored in their fast-twitch muscle fibers, which may lead to a selective depletion in these fibers. Bangsbo identified muscle glycogen as the most important substrate for energy production in sports such as soccer.

Environmental conditions may also increase carbohydrate use during exercise. Carbohydrate oxidation, particularly muscle glycogen, is increased during exercise in the heat. Sawka and Young indicated that the increased glycogen utilization is probably mediated by elevated epinephrine and muscle hyperthermia. They also note that lactate uptake and oxidation by the liver are impaired during exercise heat stress. However, heat acclimatization helps reduce muscle glycogen use and lactate accumulation. Mazzeo and Fulco indicate that exercising at high altitude increases blood glucose compared to sea level, possibly because hypoxia may induce translocation of glucose transporters to the cell membrane, which may facilitate glucose entry and utilization in the muscle cell. Braun indicates that under conditions of low oxygen availability, glucose utilization will provide more ATP per unit of oxygen available.

Why is carbohydrate an important energy source for exercise?

Carbohydrate is the most important energy food for exercise. Besides being the only food that can be used for anaerobic energy production in the lactic acid system, it is also the most efficient fuel for the oxygen system. If we look at the caloric value of carbohydrate (1 gram = 4 C) and fat (1 gram = 9 C), we might think that fat is a better source of energy. Indeed, this is so if we just look at Calories per gram. However, more oxygen is needed to metabolize the fat, and if we look at how many Calories we get from 1 liter of oxygen, we will find that carbohydrate yields about 5.05 Calories and fat gives only 4.69. Thus, carbohydrate appears to be a more efficient fuel than fat, by about 7 percent. Houston notes an even greater benefit if we look at ATP production. You get more ATP from glucose than you do from a fatty acid. For each unit of oxygen consumed, glucose produces 2.7 ATP, whereas palmitic fatty acid produces 2.3 ATP, a 17 percent difference. The metabolic pathways for carbohydrate are also more efficient than those for fat. In essence, during aerobic glycolysis, carbohydrate is able to produce ATP for muscle contraction up to three times more rapidly than fat and even faster during anaerobic glycolysis.

The primary carbohydrate source of energy for physical performance is muscle glycogen, specifically the glycogen in the muscles that are active. Elite marathon runners may use about 4–5 grams of carbohydrate per minute. As the muscle glycogen is being used during exercise, blood glucose enters the muscles and the energy pathways. In turn, the liver will release some of its glucose to help maintain or elevate blood glucose levels and prevent hypoglycemia. Coyle noted that during moderate exercise, muscle glycogen and liver glycogen contribute equally to carbohydrate oxidation. At higher intensities, muscle glycogen use increases.

Thus, all body stores of carbohydrate—blood glucose, liver glycogen, and muscle glycogen—are important for energy production during various forms of exercise. Proper physical training is essential to optimize carbohydrate utilization during exercise, as is proper carbohydrate nutrition.

What effect does endurance training have on carbohydrate metabolism?

Because carbohydrate is a primary fuel for exercise, as you initiate an endurance exercise program, a major proportion of your energy will be derived from your muscle glycogen stores. A single bout of exercise can activate the genes that produce GLUT-4 receptors, which can exert an insulin-type effect by facilitating the transport of blood glucose into the muscle both during and immediately following the exercise bout.

As you continue your endurance exercise program, such as running or bicycling, the physical activity serves as a metabolic stressor to the body, and various tissues begin to adapt to better accommodate the exercise stress. Houston reported that as few as five days of training can exert favorable effects, such as decreasing the production of lactic acid for a standardized exercise task. These adaptations have implications for physical performance and the fuels used. Figure 4.10 schematically represents some of these changes at the cellular level. The following have been noted to occur in both males and females, young and old, after several months of endurance training:

1. You will increase your VO_2 max.
2. Of equal or greater importance, you will be able to work at a greater percentage of your VO_2 max without fatigue.
3. Endurance-trained muscles may use less glucose at low-intensity exercise but have the capacity to use more during intense, maximal exercise.
4. Endurance-trained muscle has an increased maximal capacity to utilize carbohydrates. As muscle cell mitochondria density increases, the enzymes that metabolize carbohydrate in the muscle cells will increase, especially oxidative enzymes associated with the Krebs cycle.
5. As we shall see in chapter 5, training also enhances the use of fat during exercise. By doing so, there is less reliance on carbohydrate oxidation during submaximal exercise.
6. More glycogen is stored in the muscle. Synthesis of muscle glycogen may be twofold faster in trained versus untrained individuals.

What do all these changes mean? You may be able to run a 10-kilometer (6.2-mile) road race at a 7-minute-per-mile pace instead of 8 minutes. You can cruise in high gear for longer periods because you have increased your ability to produce energy from carbohydrates. Also, by reducing your reliance on carbohydrates at lower running speeds, you may compete in more prolonged races, such as marathons, without becoming hypoglycemic.

How is hypoglycemia related to the development of fatigue?

As noted previously, blood glucose is in very short supply, so as it is being used during exercise it must be replenished from liver glycogen stores. A depletion of liver glycogen may lead to hypoglycemia during high-intensity aerobic exercise because gluconeogenesis normally cannot keep pace with glucose utilization by the muscles.

Hypoglycemia is known to impair the functioning of the central nervous system and is often accompanied by acute feelings of dizziness, muscular weakness, and fatigue. The normal blood glucose level usually ranges from 80 to 100 mg of glucose per 100 ml of blood (4.4–5.5 mmol per liter). As this level gets progressively lower, hypoglycemic symptoms may develop. The point usually used to identify hypoglycemia during research studies with exercise is 45 mg per 100 ml, or 2.5 mmol per liter, although some investigators have used higher levels.

Because hypoglycemia may disrupt functioning of the central nervous system (brain and spinal cord), the body attempts to maintain an optimal blood glucose level. Zierler noted that exercise increases muscle glucose uptake, in part due to increased cell membrane GLUT-4 receptors. Exercise may also increase the sensitivity to insulin, so more glucose is transported into the muscle for the same level of insulin. Thus, insulin levels normally drop during exercise so as to help maintain normal serum glucose. Other hormones—epinephrine (adrenaline), glucagon, and cortisol—also help maintain, and even increase, blood glucose levels during exercise.

Epinephrine is secreted from the adrenal gland during exercise, particularly intense exercise, and stimulates the liver to release glucose; it also accelerates the use of glycogen in the muscle. However, during the early phases of exercise, liver glucose output may exceed muscle glucose uptake, which may result in hyperglycemia. Glucagon and cortisol levels generally increase during the stress of exercise, cortisol particularly during prolonged exercise. **Glucagon** is released from the pancreas and generally increases the rate of gluconeogenesis in the liver. Kjaer noted that liver gluconeogenesis may contribute substantially during prolonged aerobic exercise when liver glycogen levels decline and gluconeogenic substrate becomes more abundant. **Cortisol** is secreted from the adrenal gland and facilitates the breakdown and release of amino acids from muscle tissue to provide some substrate to the liver for gluconeogenesis. Blood glucose normally increases during the initial stages of exercise and is normally well maintained by these hormonal mechanisms. A summary of hormonal actions in the regulation of blood glucose is presented in table 4.6.

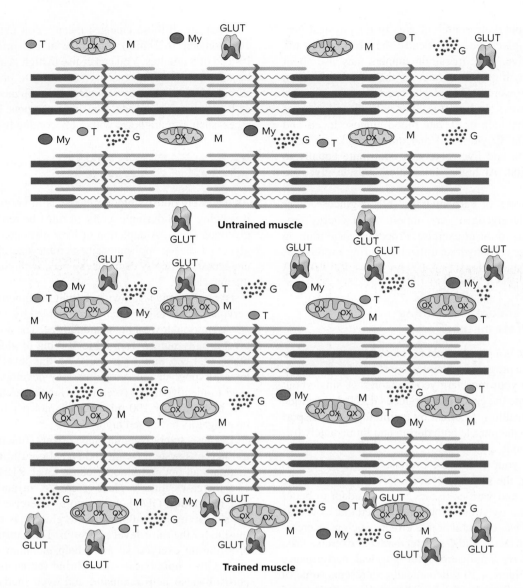

FIGURE 4.10 Some of the effects of aerobic or endurance training upon skeletal muscle. Increases in glycogen (G) and triglyceride (T) provide a greater energy store, increased levels of GLUT-4 receptors (GLUT) provide the potential to increase glucose delivery to the muscle as needed, while the increase in mitochondria size and number (M), myoglobin content (My), oxidative enzymes (ox), and slow-twitch muscle fiber size facilitates the use of oxygen for production of energy.

TABLE 4.6 Major hormones involved in regulation of blood glucose levels

Hormone	Gland	Stimulus	Action
Insulin	Pancreas	Increase in blood glucose	Helps transport glucose into cells; decreases blood glucose levels
Glucagon	Pancreas	Decrease in blood glucose; exercise stress	Promotes gluconeogenesis in liver; helps increase blood glucose levels
Epinephrine	Adrenal	Exercise stress; decrease in blood glucose	Promotes glycogen breakdown and glucose release from the liver; helps increase blood glucose levels
Cortisol	Adrenal	Exercise stress; decrease in blood glucose	Promotes breakdown of protein and resultant gluconeogenesis; helps increase blood glucose levels

Hypoglycemia may be a concern of athletes in several situations. One possibility is a reactive hypoglycemia following the consumption of a high-carbohydrate meal 30–60 minutes or more prior to an athletic event. If hypoglycemia develops just prior to or during the early stages of the event, the effect could impair performance. At one time, hypoglycemia as a consequence of pre-exercise carbohydrate ingestion was believed to be a large concern. However, as described by Jeukendrup and Killer, and as discussed in depth later in the chapter, there appears to be no good reason to avoid pre-exercise carbohydrate consumption.

Hypoglycemia may also develop during prolonged exercise tasks, but it may be dependent upon the intensity level of the exercise. In low-intensity exercise, such as 30–50 percent of VO_2 max, the primary fuel is fat, and hence the use of carbohydrate is minimized. Moreover, at this low intensity level, gluconeogenesis can help maintain blood glucose above hypoglycemic levels.

During the early part of prolonged moderate- to high-intensity aerobic exercise, muscle glycogen is the major source of energy derived from carbohydrate, although some blood glucose is utilized. However, Weltan and others found that as muscle glycogen levels get low in the latter stages of an endurance task, the muscle increases its fat oxidation and blood glucose, derived from liver glycogen, now accounts for most of the muscular energy from carbohydrate. Gluconeogenesis is increased, but Hargreaves indicates that it cannot completely compensate for decreased liver glycogen availability. Thus, the blood glucose levels fall toward hypoglycemia.

Whether hypoglycemia impairs physical performance may depend upon the individual. In their study, Utter and others reported that a lower rating of perceived exertion (RPE) during prolonged running was associated with higher blood glucose, suggesting that maintenance of optimal blood glucose levels could help prevent psychological distress. Some earlier research reported that exercise-induced hypoglycemia led to the expected symptoms, including dizziness and partial blackout. However, more contemporary research from three different laboratories has revealed that a number of subjects may become hypoglycemic during the latter stages of a prolonged exercise task to exhaustion at 60–75 percent of their VO_2 max and yet are able to continue exercising while hypoglycemic, even at levels as low as 25 mg per 100 ml. It appears that the role hypoglycemia plays in the etiology of fatigue in prolonged exercise has not been totally elucidated, although there appears to be individual susceptibility.

Nevertheless, it is well documented that with increased exercise duration, there is a progressive decrease in muscle glycogen and a progressive increase in blood glucose uptake by the muscle. However, liver supplies of glycogen are limited, and thus blood glucose levels eventually fall. Prevention of hypoglycemia is one of the major objectives of carbohydrate consumption during prolonged exercise, because all individuals will eventually suffer ill-effects when they reach their minimum blood glucose threshold.

How is lactic acid production related to fatigue?

In review, as noted in chapter 3, lactic acid is an end product of anaerobic glycolysis. Anaerobic glycolysis represents the lactic acid energy system, found primarily in the type IIb white muscle fibers, but also the type IIa red fibers. Anaerobic glycolysis is increased at the onset of high-intensity exercise, such as 200- to 400-meter track events, as a means to rapidly replenish ATP for muscle contraction or for the rapid resynthesis of PCr. The process of aerobic glycolysis can also generate ATP, but it is too slow during high-intensity exercise. Thus, lactic acid, or lactate, is produced when the production of pyruvate from glycolysis exceeds the oxidative capacity of the mitochondria.

Blood lactic acid (lactate) levels increase during high-intensity exercise and for years have been thought to be the cause of fatigue. However, Coyle notes that the lactate molecule *per se* does not cause fatigue, but rather that its accumulation in blood reflects a disturbance of muscle cell homeostasis. One factor that may disturb muscle cell homeostasis is an increased concentration of hydrogen ions, reflecting an increased acidity. Debold notes that even after 100 years of research on muscle fatigue, the molecular basis is still poorly understood. Using in vitro studies, Debold has demonstrated that high levels of hydrogen ions and phosphate inhibit the molecular motions of muscle proteins such as myosin, troponin, and tropomyosin, which leads to decreased force production and potentially fatigue. Fitts noted that it is now generally thought that the component of fatigue correlated with lactate results from the effects of an increased free hydrogen ion rather than lactate or the undissociated lactic acid. The hydrogen ion and associated increased acidity could elicit fatigue by inhibiting a number of physiological processes in the muscle cell associated with contraction. As noted in chapter 13, sodium bicarbonate, a buffer of acidity in the muscle cell, may be an effective means to enhance performance in high-intensity exercise tasks.

The lactate produced during exercise is not a waste product. Lactate is a carbohydrate; one molecule of lactate contains about half the energy of one molecule of glucose. Years ago, George Brooks, from the University of California at Berkeley, proposed the lactate shuttle, whereby the lactate produced during exercise in white muscle fibers would be shuttled to other tissues, such as the heart and red oxidative muscle fibers, where it could be oxidized for energy. Hashimoto and Brooks also hypothesize the lactate produced in the cell cytoplasm may be oxidized by mitochondria in the same cell. Research supports the lactate shuttle hypothesis and, as discussed later in this chapter, some sports scientists have actually tested lactate salt supplementation as a means to provide energy to enhance exercise performance.

How is low muscle glycogen related to the development of fatigue?

Low muscle glycogen may impair both aerobic and anaerobic exercise performance.

Low Muscle Glycogen and Aerobic Exercise Muscle glycogen is the major energy source for prolonged, moderately high- to high-intensity aerobic exercise. Elite marathon runners can maintain a fast race pace primarily through oxidation of carbohydrate, primarily muscle glycogen, and to a lesser extent fatty acids stored in the muscle. Coyle indicates that exercise at 70–85 percent of VO_2 max cannot be maintained without sufficient carbohydrate oxidation, and thus the severe lowering of muscle glycogen, often coupled with hypoglycemia, results in the need to reduce exercise intensity to 40–60 percent of VO_2 max.

A number of studies have shown that physical exhaustion was correlated with very low muscle glycogen levels, but others have shown some glycogen remaining even though subjects were exhausted. Several mechanisms have been postulated to explain the development of fatigue even with some muscle glycogen remaining.

- Location of glycogen. Costill has indicated that performance would be adversely affected only when muscle glycogen levels went below 40 mmol/kg of muscle tissue. It may be that complete depletion of muscle glycogen is not necessary for performance to suffer, for glycolysis may be impaired with lower glycogen levels or the glycogen in the muscle fiber may be located where it is not readily available for glycolysis. Ørtenblad and colleagues have described that glycogen is not homogeneously distributed in muscle fibers; it is localized in separate pools. Additionally, glycogen granules have their own glycolytic enzymes and regulating proteins and it may be the depletion of these complexes localized in the myofibrils that is related to fatigue.
- Rate of energy production. Shulman and Rothman propose a model in which energy is supplied in milliseconds via glycogenolysis, and indicate that one possible mechanism for muscle fatigue is that at low but nonzero glycogen concentrations, there is not enough glycogen to supply millisecond energy needs. In a related vein, Fitts notes that low levels of muscle glycogen may interfere with maintenance of optimal levels of Krebs cycle intermediates, which can reduce the rate of aerobic ATP production, and further notes that the metabolism of blood-borne substrates (blood glucose and free fatty acids(FFA)) is simply too slow to maintain heavy exercise intensities.
- Muscle fiber type. The fatigue that develops may be related to the depletion of muscle glycogen from specific muscle fiber types. In prolonged exercise at 60–75 percent of VO_2 max, type I fibers (red, oxidative slow twitch) and type IIa fibers (red, oxidative-glycolytic fast twitch) are recruited during the early stages of the task, but as muscle glycogen is depleted, the athlete must recruit type IIb fibers (white, glycolytic fast twitch) to maintain the same pace. However, it takes more mental effort to recruit the type IIb fibers, which will be more stressful to the athlete. Type IIb fibers also are more likely to produce lactic acid, increasing the acidity, which may increase the perceived stress of the exercise. In a study, Krustrup and others reported that glycogen depletion of the slow-twitch muscle fibers, necessitating recruitment of fast-twitch muscle fibers and increased energy demands, is a factor that may predispose to fatigue.
- Use of fat for energy. As muscle glycogen becomes depleted in the slow-twitch muscle fibers, the muscle cell will rely more on fat as the primary energy source. Because fat is a less-efficient fuel than carbohydrate, the pace will slow down.
- Role of the brain. Signals sent from peripheral tissues to the brain may regulate energy metabolism. A low glycogen level in exercising muscle may be such a signal and may invoke neural responses causing fatigue. Matsui and colleagues recently

showed decreased liver and muscle glycogen after 30 and 60 minutes of running, and a decrease in glycogen in five areas of the brain after 120 minutes of running. The interactions between decreased muscle and brain glycogen and fatigue need to be further studied.

Low Muscle Glycogen and Anaerobic Exercise Fatigue in very high-intensity, anaerobic-type exercise generally is attributed to the detrimental effects of the acidity in the muscle cell associated with lactic acid production. Research has now shown that maximal high-intensity exercise, lasting only about 60 seconds, is not impaired by a very low muscle glycogen concentration, approximately 30 mmol/kg muscle. However, it is possible that performance in such very high-intensity, short-term exercise tasks may be impaired with extremely low muscle glycogen in the fast-twitch muscle fibers. Moreover, with somewhat longer anaerobic tasks, approximating 3 minutes, one laboratory study reported a reduced performance in the time to exhaustion test after 4 days of a low-carbohydrate, high-fat diet when compared to a normal, mixed diet and a high-carbohydrate diet. Although muscle glycogen levels were not measured, a logical assumption is that they were lower on the low-carbohydrate diet.

In addition, field research has suggested that slower overall sprint speed, such as in the latter parts of prolonged athletic contests like soccer and ice hockey, may be due to muscle glycogen depletion. Muscle biopsies of these athletes revealed very low glycogen levels, which were attributed not only to the strenuous exercise in the contest but also to the fact that these athletes were consuming diets low in carbohydrates. In support of these field studies, Balsom and others reported that low muscle glycogen levels impaired laboratory exercise performance in repeated bouts of very high-intensity intermittent exercise, 6-second cycle ergometer performance followed by 30 seconds of rest. Krustrup and others reported that almost 50 percent of muscle fibers were completely or almost empty of glycogen following a soccer game, and suggested that slower sprint performance in the latter part of a game may be explained by low glycogen levels in individual muscle fibers. Also, low muscle glycogen stores may lead to a decrease in exercise intensity during training.

In summary, low levels of glycogen in the white, fast-twitch IIb muscle fibers may limit performance in intermittent, anaerobic-type exercise tasks. Both hypoglycemia and low glycogen in the red muscle fiber types, most likely a combination of the two, may be contributing factors to fatigue in prolonged endurance exercise.

Train low compete high Although the importance of dietary carbohydrate to support exercise performance is clear, alternating between periods of high and low carbohydrate availability may offer advantages as well. John Hawley, an expert in promoting training adaptation by manipulating carbohydrate availability, a concept that has been referred to as "train low," has recently reviewed the research in this area. The concept is based on the theory that making carbohydrate less available at critical times will improve adaptations to training better than if carbohydrate was available at all times.

One way to reduce carbohydrate availability is to train twice-a-day with the second session conducted under "low glycogen availability." Essentially, an athlete would train intensely, not replace carbohydrate post-exercise, and then conduct a second bout of exercise while muscle glycogen was decreased. Research supports that this method will result in positive training adaptations as measured by an increase in several enzymes involved in mitochondrial biogenesis. However, although this has been proven effective in improving training adaptations (e.g., increased muscle enzyme activity), it can result in decreased power output during subsequent training sessions, an outcome that is undesirable for athletes. Another approach is to extend the duration of low carbohydrate availability during the overnight period (train high and sleep low). Essentially, an athlete would train intensely in the evening (high glycogen availability), go to bed fasted and complete a submaximal morning exercise session before re-feeding (low glycogen availability). This method is being actively studied, but data are unavailable at this time. A final method is to reduce exogenous carbohydrate availability before or during exercise. In this scenario, exercise occurs fasted or without carbohydrate available during exercise. Studies that have investigated this concept have shown similar improvements in enzymatic activities, suggesting that training adaptations are not impaired by decreased exogenous carbohydrate availability. However, the effects on performance outcomes are unclear.

According to Hawley, there are can be discrepancies between training adaptation (assessed with cellular variables) and performance (assessed with whole body exercise) outcomes. There are several reasons to support this perspective. As Hawley notes, there may not be a direct relationship between athletic performance and training-induced cellular adaptations. Through training, well-trained athletes may have already maximized the muscle adaptations that support athletic performance, and remaining adaptations may not play an important role. Small gains in performance (<1%) are difficult if not impossible to measure in a laboratory. Finally some "train low" approaches might impede performance during training causing unfavorable muscular adaptations. For instance, reduced training intensity, due to low glycogen availability, may alter muscle fiber recruitment and substrate utilization. Thus, athletes and sports dietitians must consider both physiological and performance outcomes when evaluating a dietary intervention.

Hawley reported that during short-term training programs (3 to 10 weeks) in which half of the workouts occurred when muscle glycogen or exogenous carbohydrate availability was low, training adaptations were improved or similar to training with normal muscle glycogen. Despite the supportive research on muscular adaptations, Hawley states that there is no clear evidence that "training low" improves athletic performance, and that it is probably unlikely that an athlete would choose a diet plan that compromised training intensity. At this time, many studies are under way to further investigate the effects of manipulating carbohydrate availability on exercise performance.

How are low endogenous carbohydrate levels related to the central fatigue hypothesis?

As noted previously, hypoglycemia and low muscle glycogen levels may impair exercise performance, and one mechanism for each involves adverse effects on brain function. Collectively, they may contribute to central fatigue in a different way.

In the latter stages of prolonged exercise bouts, low muscle glycogen, in combination with decreased blood glucose levels, will stimulate gluconeogenesis from muscle protein. In particular, branched-chain amino acids (BCAAs) in the muscle will be catabolized to provide energy. Because BCAA release from the liver may be decreased, or uptake by the muscle may increase, blood levels of BCAA decline. The *central fatigue hypothesis* during prolonged exercise suggests that this decline in blood BCAA may contribute to fatigue. In general, fatigue is hypothesized to occur when BCAA levels drop and the concentration of another amino acid—tryptophan—increases in its free form, or free tryptophan (fTRP). BCAAs compete with fTRP for similar receptors that facilitate their entry into the brain, so high BCAA levels prevent brain uptake of fTRP. With an increased fTRP:BCAA ratio, entry of fTRP into the brain cells will be facilitated. Increased brain levels of tryptophan may stimulate the formation of serotonin, a neurotransmitter in the brain that may be related to fatigue sensations (see figure 4.11). Preventing the increase in the fTRP:BCAA ratio is theorized to prevent the premature development of fatigue, and the use of BCAA supplements in this regard will be covered in chapter 6. Meeusen has noted that

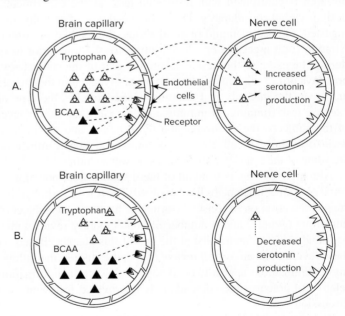

FIGURE 4.11 BCAA and the central fatigue hypothesis. (A) An increased level of serum free-tryptophan (fTRP ▲) resulting in a high fTRP:BCAA ratio will bind to receptors in the capillary for transport to nerve cells and increased serotonin formation, which may be associated with central fatigue. (B) An increased level of BCAAs (▲) will compete with the fTRP for receptors, blocking them from entering the nerve cell and decreasing production of serotonin, helping to prevent central fatigue.

postponing central fatigue with nutritional interventions, including amino acids, water, carbohydrate, and caffeine, has been studied. Although carbohydrate (discussed later in this chapter) and caffeine show promise in reducing central fatigue, other nutrients do not appear as promising. However, carbohydrate intake during exercise may also be helpful, as discussed later in this section.

Will eating carbohydrate immediately before or during an event improve physical performance?

Because hypoglycemia or muscle glycogen depletion may be a cause of fatigue during endurance exercise, supplementation with glucose or other forms of carbohydrate before or during exercise may be theorized to delay the onset of fatigue and improve performance. Thousands of studies have been conducted on this topic ever since carbohydrates were identified as the most efficient energy source for exercise (more than 80 years ago), and researchers' interest in this topic remains unabated today. In recent years, the research designs have usually been highly sophisticated as investigators have attempted to provide specific answers relative to the type, amount, and timing of carbohydrate ingestion before and during performance. Although some problems remain in providing quantitative data, the use of stable isotopes of ingested carbohydrates (referred to as *exogenous* carbohydrates in comparison to *endogenous* stores in the body), as detailed by Wolfe and George, has enhanced our understanding of their metabolic fate when ingested prior to or during exercise.

However, the reviewer attempting to synthesize the available research is confronted with a difficult task, as the experimental designs varied considerably. The amount and type of carbohydrate ingested, the use of liquid or solid forms, the method of administration (oral ingestion or venous infusion), the time prior to or during the exercise that it was taken, the diet of the subject several days prior to the study, the amount of glycogen in the muscle and liver, the intensity and duration of the exercise, the type of exercise task (running, swimming, cycling, etc.), the fitness level of the subjects, the environmental temperature, and the method used to evaluate blood glucose and muscle glycogen utilization are some of the important differences between studies.

Although the results from all of these studies were not similar, some general consistencies have evolved. The role of carbohydrate supplementation on exercise performance has been the subject of numerous reviews, and a number of contemporary reviews may be found in the reference list at the end of this chapter. Based on these reviews and an overall review of specific studies, the following generalizations appear to be logical. More specific information relative to practical recommendations is provided following this discussion.

Use of the Ingested Carbohydrate   Using labeled carbohydrate sources and analyzing the expired carbon dioxide for radioactivity, investigators have shown that some of the ingested, or exogenous, carbohydrate may be used as an energy source within 5–10 minutes, indicating that it may empty rapidly from the stomach, be absorbed from the small intestine into the blood, and enter into metabolic pathways. Peak use of exogenous carbohydrate appears to occur 75 to 90 minutes after ingestion. A number of studies have shown that the ingested carbohydrate may contribute a significant percentage of the carbohydrate energy source during exercise, ranging from 20 to 40 percent in some studies, but as much as 60 to 70 percent during the latter stages of exercise, when endogenous liver and muscle glycogen stores become depleted.

Possible Fatigue-Delaying Mechanisms   The precise mechanism whereby glucose ingestion helps delay the onset of fatigue during moderate- to high-intensity exercise (i.e., >65 percent VO_2 max) has not been totally elucidated, but several theories have been studied.

Maintenance of blood glucose levels   The available data suggest that the ability of carbohydrate intake to delay fatigue may be related to the maintenance of higher blood glucose levels, possibly by sparing liver glycogen until late in the exercise and the prevention of hypoglycemia in susceptible individuals; blood glucose would be available to enter the muscle and provide a source of energy for aerobic glycolysis and may provide glucose to the brain to prevent premature central fatigue. As noted, exogenous glucose is used increasingly as the exercise task becomes prolonged.

Reduction of psychological effort   Some research has shown that glucose ingestion could make an endurance task psychologically easier and suggested that the physiological effects of the glucose, either in the brain or in the muscles, reduced the stressful effects of exercise. Several studies by Utter and others found that carbohydrate ingestion reduced the ratings of perceived exertion during prolonged running and cycling. For example, they reported that marathoners ingesting carbohydrate compared to placebo beverages were able to run at a higher intensity during a competitive marathon, and yet the ratings of perceived exertion (RPE) were similar in both groups of runners, suggesting that the carbohydrate may have permitted them to run at a faster rate with similar psychological effort. However, it has not been determined whether these ergogenic effects may be attributed to the effect of glucose as a source of energy in the muscle or to its effect on the central nervous system, either as a direct energy source for brain metabolism or through its effect on BCAA levels. In an effort to improve endurance performance, Jeukendrup pioneered a method of rinsing, but not ingesting, carbohydrate in the mouth. It has been shown that the presence of carbohydrate in the mouth activates several areas of the brain. In a recent review, he highlighted 12 studies that examined the effects of carbohydrate mouth rinse on endurance exercise performance (30 to 70 minutes) and reported that 9 studies showed significant improvements. These improvements were of a similar magnitude as would be expected with carbohydrate ingestion. The carbohydrate mouth rinse methods might be particularly useful for athletes who experience gastrointestinal upset with carbohydrate ingestion or in those attempting to reduce energy intake to manage their body mass.

In several studies, carbohydrate supplementation during exercise has been reported to prevent the decrease in serum BCAA during the later stages of prolonged exercise, possibly by mitigating secretion of cortisol. According to the central fatigue hypothesis, preventing an increase in the fTRP:BCAA ratio would deter the onset of mental fatigue.

Sparing of muscle glycogen Although sparing of muscle glycogen could be another benefit of carbohydrate ingestion before or during moderate- to high-intensity exercise, research findings are equivocal.

In a unique experiment from the University of Texas, subjects received venous glucose infusions to maintain a hyperglycemic state during 2 hours of exercise at 73 percent of VO_2 max, but the net rate of muscle glycogen utilization was not affected compared to control conditions. Arkinstall and Chryssanthopoulos and their colleagues also noted no muscle glycogen sparing effect with carbohydrate supplementation during the exercise task.

In contrast, Yaspelkis and others, also from the University of Texas, noted that during low-intensity exercise (i.e., <50 percent VO_2 max) or during low- to moderate-intensity exercise tasks, carbohydrate supplementation during exercise could spare use of muscle glycogen in slow-twitch muscle fibers and enhance performance. They noted that during low-intensity exercise the serum levels of both glucose and insulin were elevated, which could promote muscle use of serum glucose and sparing of muscle glycogen. Bosch and others, as well as Tsintzas and others, reported that carbohydrate intake during prolonged exercise at about 70 percent VO_2 max did spare muscle glycogen use, and the Tsintzas group reported that the sparing effect occurred in the type I, slow-twitch muscle fibers, but not in the type II, fast-twitch fibers. Williams noted that although other reviewers concluded that consuming carbohydrate during exercise did not spare use of muscle glycogen in cyclists, research findings from his laboratory did find glycogen sparing in runners who consumed carbohydrate drinks throughout prolonged exercise, and the glycogen sparing occurred early in the exercise task. Hargreaves noted also that the breakdown of muscle glycogen may be slowed because the supply of blood glucose is improved when carbohydrate is consumed.

Limitations to Prevent Fatigue Although glucose ingestion may help delay fatigue during moderately high-intensity exercise, it cannot totally prevent the onset of fatigue. It appears that a maximum of about 1.5 to 1.7 grams of the ingested carbohydrate may be available each minute, which is much lower than the required energy needs at 65–85 percent of VO_2 max. Jeukendrup and Jentjens indicate that the intestines and liver may be limiting factors, the intestines being unable to absorb the ingested carbohydrate at a faster rate, while the liver may limit the amount of glucose released into the blood. When blood glucose, BCAA, and/or muscle glycogen levels are eventually reduced to a critical level, fatigue occurs.

Initial Endogenous Stores If the individual has normal liver and muscle glycogen stores, glucose feedings are unnecessary for continuous, moderately high-intensity exercise bouts lasting 60–90 minutes or less but may be beneficial for high-intensity exercise tasks of similar duration, as noted below. Because the body can store carbohydrate in the muscles and liver, the usefulness of glucose or other carbohydrate intake before or during exercise depends on the adequacy of those supplies already in the muscle and liver to meet energy needs. For competition, the muscle and liver glycogen stores should be adequate to meet carbohydrate energy needs. The critical point is to consume substantial amounts of carbohydrates a day or two prior to the event and to decrease the duration and intensity of training to assure ample endogenous glycogen supplies.

The available research has shown that the consumption of glucose, fructose, sucrose, maltodextrin (a glucose polymer), or other carbohydrate combinations immediately prior to events of short or moderate duration has a negligible effect upon performance. Adding a gallon of gas to a full tank will not make a car go faster during a short ride. The same is true of sugar to a muscle already filled with glycogen. If, however, muscle glycogen levels are low and the exercise task is somewhat prolonged, then ingestion of carbohydrate just prior to the exercise bout may improve performance. It is important to note, however, that to enhance performance, the exogenous carbohydrate source must be able to delay the onset of fatigue that might otherwise occur as a result of premature depletion of endogenous carbohydrate sources, a viewpoint also proposed by Tsintzas and Williams.

Exercise Intensity and Duration The potential beneficial effects of carbohydrate supplementation depend on the interaction of exercise intensity and duration, which, of course, are interrelated. The shorter the duration, the greater the exercise intensity can be. Stellingwerff and Cox have written the most comprehensive review of the effects of carbohydrate ingestion on exercise performance that takes into account the influence of exercise intensity and duration. They reported that of 61 total studies, 50 (82 percent) showed a performance-enhancing effect of carbohydrate ingestion. Of 10 studies that assessed the effects of carbohydrate ingestion on exercise tasks lasting less than 1 hour, 6 showed a performance enhancement. Of 13 studies of the effects of carbohydrate mouth rinse on exercise performance lasting less than 1 hour, 10 showed a beneficial effect. During exercise tasks lasting from 60 to 120 minutes, 15 of 18 studies showed a performance-enhancing effect of carbohydrate ingestion. Finally, in studies with exercise tests lasting more than 120 minutes in duration, 16 of 17 studies showed a performance-enhancing effect of carbohydrate supplementation. Overall, there was a positive relationship between total exercise time and percent increase in performance, indicating that carbohydrate ingestion was more effective in longer tasks. The authors noted that the primary mechanisms through which carbohydrate improves performance probably differ based on exercise intensity and duration. For instance, during brief, intense exercise carbohydrate acts on the receptors in the mouth and works through the central nervous system to enhance performance; thus, the type of carbohydrate may not be important. In longer exercise tasks, rapidly absorbed carbohydrates, possibly greater than 90 grams/hour, are needed to replenish depleting muscle glycogen stores. The authors stressed that recommendations should be tailored to individual tolerance.

The following sections provide more details about some of the individual studies that have evaluated the effects of carbohydrate ingestion on exercise performance. The time frames are representative of those that have been well studied, and science-based recommendations for carbohydrate intake pre-, during, and postexercise are presented in table 4.7.

TABLE 4.7 Some recommended guidelines for carbohydrate intake as a means to help optimize exercise/sports performance. Carbohydrate intake before and during exercise may help optimize performance, whereas carbohydrate intake after exercise may facilitate recovery for subsequent training or competition. In general, the lower the intensity and the shorter the duration of exercise, the less the need for additional carbohydrate. Recommendations are based on scientific studies. Physically active individuals should consume various types and amounts of carbohydrate before and during exercise and sport training to determine personal optimal dietary strategies. See the text for additional information and guidelines.

Exercise intensity/sport	Duration	Before exercise*	During exercise**	After exercise***
Very high-intensity aerobic (5K run)	<30 minutes	None needed	None needed	None needed
High-intensity aerobic (10K run)	30–90 minutes	20–25 grams	30–60 grams carbohydrate. Mouth rinse 1.5 grams/ml for 5 to 10 sec every 8 to 10 min of exercise	60–80 grams/hour for 3–4 hours
Intermittent high-intensity (team sports, such as soccer)	60–90 minutes	20–25 grams	30–60 grams carbohydrate. Mouth rinse 1.5 grams/ml for 5 to 10 sec every 8 to 10 min of exercise	60–80 grams/hour for 3–4 hours
Moderate- to high-intensity aerobic (half-marathon; marathon)	>90 minutes	20–50 grams Carbohydrate loading	60–80 grams/hour	60 grams/hour for 3–4 hours
Moderate-intensity aerobic (ironman-distance triathlon; 140 miles; 226 kilometers)	>6 hour	20–50 grams Carbohydrate loading	60–80 grams/hour	60–80 grams/hour for 3–4 hours
High-intensity resistance training (lifting weights)	1–2 hours	None needed	None needed	60–80 grams/hour for 3–4 hours

*Within 10–15 minutes of the start of exercise. All individuals should consume a pregame meal sometime between 1–4 hours prior to exercise in order to ensure normal muscle glycogen and blood glucose levels. Carbohydrate intake 3–4 hours before should average about 3–4 grams per kilogram body weight, but only 1–2 grams per kilogram body weight if consumed within 1–2 hours of exercise.

**Fluids such as sports drinks are recommended. Drinking about 8 ounces (240 milliliters) of a typical sports drink every 15 minutes will provide about 60 grams of carbohydrate per hour.

***For most athletes, consuming a diet with substantial amounts of healthful carbohydrates over the course of 24 hours will replace muscle glycogen levels to normal. For those who want a speedy recovery of muscle glycogen for subsequent intense training or competition the same or following day, using this rapid muscle glycogen replacement protocol may be recommended. Athletes may also benefit by consuming some protein with the carbohydrate, about 1 gram of protein for every 4 grams of carbohydrate.

Very high-intensity exercise for less than 30 minutes Research suggests that carbohydrate supplementation will not enhance performance in high-intensity exercise bouts less than 30 minutes in length. For example, Palmer and others noted that consuming carbohydrate 10 minutes before competing in a 20-kilometer cycle time trial did not enhance performance in well-trained cyclists. Nevertheless, if carbohydrate supplements could ameliorate a muscle or liver glycogen deficiency, performance could improve. For example, Walberg-Rankin reported that carbohydrate supplementation improved high-intensity anaerobic exercise performance in wrestlers following a drastic weight-reduction program with very limited carbohydrate intake. Presumably, the carbohydrate supplement, consumed in a 5-hour period before testing, increased muscle glycogen levels, particularly in fast-twitch fibers, enhancing carbohydrate utilization and subsequent performance.

Very high-intensity resistance exercise training While the performance-enhancing benefits of carbohydrate ingestion on endurance exercise performance are well accepted, less is known about the effects of carbohydrate on resistance exercise performance. As strength and conditioning training programs are an integral part of success in most sports, properly fueling resistance training workouts is essential. A bout of resistance exercise can reduce muscle glycogen by up to 40 percent, indicating the importance of glycogen as a fuel for resistance training and raising the possibility that carbohydrate ingestion or mouth rinsing may improve resistance exercise performance. A few studies, mostly conducted by Haff and colleagues, have shown that carbohydrate supplementation prior to (1.0 g/kg body mass) and during (0.5 g/kg body mass) resistance exercise enhanced resistance exercise performance. However, this has not been shown in every study. Recently, Jensen and colleagues were able to show an improvement in maximal strength following carbohydrate mouth rinse in athletes who were fatigued by prior exercise. At this point in time, there are no specific recommendations for athletes to consume carbohydrate before or during resistance exercise (see table 4.7).

High-intensity exercise for 30 to 90 minutes Within this time frame, the potential benefit of carbohydrate consumption may depend on the duration of the exercise, intensity of exercise, and training level of the athlete. For example, two studies found that neither consumption of a 6 percent carbohydrate solution nor infusing glucose at the rate of 1 gram per minute improved performance in a 1-hour maximal cycling protocol. Additionally, Burke and others reported no effect of a commercial gel supplying about 1.1 grams of carbohydrate per kilogram body weight on half-marathon performance compared to the placebo. However, in a review, Karelis and colleagues examined studies with exercise times ranging between 30 and 60 minutes. They noted a beneficial effect of carbohydrate ingestion with exercise lasting at least 40–50 minutes. Moreover, supplementation may benefit well-trained athletes who may be able to exercise at high intensity for about an hour. For example, Jeukendrup and el-Sayed, with their associates, reported that cyclists exercising for about an hour at high intensity significantly improved their performance following ingestion of a carbohydrate supplement, as compared to a placebo. Also, Ball and others reported that carbohydrate intake during a simulated time trial improved performance in a sprint at the end of 50 minutes of high-intensity cycling. In such cases, it is possible that the ingested carbohydrates may help provide glucose to the fast-twitch muscle fibers or prevent premature depletion in the slow-twitch fibers.

As indicated earlier, the presence of carbohydrate in the oral cavity has been shown to improve the performance by stimulating the central nervous system. Exercises lasting about an hour have been the most well studied, and it appears that the type or sweetness of carbohydrate is not relevant. Currently, the most practical advice points toward swishing 1.5 grams of carbohydrate per milliliter of water for 5 to 10 seconds during every 8 to 10 minutes of exercise. At this time, a great deal more work needs to be done to learn how carbohydrate mouth rinsing improves exercise performance and what conditions (e.g., fasting, fed, inclusion of other nutrients) may enhance or reduce these effects. Importantly, as noted by Stellingwerff and Cox, several practical concerns need to be considered. For instance, can an athlete find time to swish with carbohydrate for 10 seconds every 8 to 10 minutes, and how will this affect breathing? The authors suggested a "sports confectionary" (concentrated carbohydrate, like a jelly bean) in the cheek cavity, but depending on the sport, this might be against the rules or present a choking hazard.

Intermittent, high-intensity exercise for 60 to 90 minutes Research has shown that individuals engaged in endurance-type contests with intermittent bouts of sprinting, such as soccer, ice hockey, or tennis, may benefit from carbohydrate supplements taken before and during the game. In a controlled laboratory protocol representative of a 60-minute intermittent, high-intensity competitive sport such as soccer or field hockey, Welsh and colleagues, from Mark Davis's laboratory, reported that carbohydrate intake before and during the exercise task resulted in significant improvements in various tests of physical and mental functions performed throughout the experimental trial. Toward the end of the 60-minute period, the carbohydrate trial resulted in faster 20-meter sprint time, longer time to fatigue in a shuttle run, enhanced whole body motor skills, and decreased self-reported perceptions of fatigue. The results suggested a beneficial role of carbohydrate-electrolyte ingestion on physical and mental functions during intermittent exercise similar to that of many competitive team sports. Similar findings

were reported by Winnick and others. Other field research studies, although not universally supportive, have shown similar benefits of carbohydrate intake under game conditions. Several reviewers, such as Kirkendall and Kovacs, indicate that carbohydrate intake before and during prolonged, intermittent, high-intensity exercise sports may enhance performance.

High- to moderate-intensity exercise greater than 90 minutes Research generally supports a beneficial effect of carbohydrate intake on exercise performance tasks greater than 90 minutes (if the exercise intensity is high enough), particularly so when the task is more prolonged, such as 2 hours or more. For example, Kimber and others reported a significant inverse correlation between the amount of carbohydrate consumed and the finishing time of male triathletes in an Ironman triathlon, suggesting that increasing carbohydrate consumption during such a prolonged event may enhance performance. Jeukendrup indicates that the performance benefits of carbohydrate ingestion are likely achieved by maintaining or raising plasma glucose concentrations to help sustain high rates of carbohydrate oxidation.

When, how much, and in what form should carbohydrates be consumed before or during exercise?

The most common athletic events or physical performance activities that may benefit from carbohydrate feedings are those associated with long duration (90–120 minutes or more) at moderate- to high-intensity levels. Marathon running, cross-country skiing, and endurance cycling are common sports of this kind. Other sports that require intermittent bouts of intensive activity over a prolonged period, such as soccer, may also benefit. However, the individual participating in these activities, particularly under warm or hot environmental conditions, also needs to replenish fluid losses incurred through sweating. In such cases, fluid replenishment is more critical than carbohydrate. The topic of fluid replacement during exercise is covered in more detail in chapter 9, but because carbohydrate is one of the contents in the majority of the sports drinks developed as fluid replacements for athletes, its role is discussed briefly here.

Many studies have been conducted to determine the best carbohydrate feeding regimen to prevent fatigue during prolonged exercise. A number of different variables have been studied, such as the timing of the feeding and the type, amount, and concentration of carbohydrate.

Again, based on current reviews by the primary investigators regarding carbohydrate supplementation for exercise performance and a careful analysis of individual studies, the following points represent the general conclusions and recommendations for individuals who may be exercising at 60–80 percent of their VO_2 max or greater for 1–2 hours or longer. These points may also be applicable to athletes engaged in intermittent, high-intensity exercise sports that last an hour or more. But remember, individuals may have varied reactions to carbohydrate intake, so athletes should experiment in training before using these recommendations in actual competition.

Pre-exercise: When and How Much?

Four hours or less before exercise Carbohydrate intake 60–240 minutes prior to prolonged exercise tasks (longer than 90 minutes) may enhance performance. Research has demonstrated improved performance when adequate carbohydrate was consumed either 1, 3, or 4 hours prior to a prolonged exercise task involving simulated racing conditions during the latter stage. Other research revealed no significant differences in 30-kilometer run performance when equal amounts of carbohydrate were supplemented either 4 hours before or during the run, suggesting the ingested carbohydrate was available for energy production using either strategy.

The amount of carbohydrate ingested 4 hours prior to performance should be based upon body weight. Several studies have used 4–5 grams/kg (1.8–2.3 grams/pound) with good results. For an athlete who weighs 60 kg (132 pounds), the recommended amount would be 240–300 grams. The carbohydrates could be consumed in any of several forms, including fluids such as juices or glucose polymer solutions, or solid carbohydrates such as fruits or starches. The fiber content should be minimized to prevent possible intestinal problems during exercise. Keep in mind that 300 grams of carbohydrate is about 1,200 Calories, a somewhat substantial meal. You may consult appendix E for an expanded list of foods high in carbohydrate. Table 4.8 presents a quick estimate of carbohydrates in the various Food Exchanges and sports products.

The guidelines presented on pages xxxxx relative to precompetition meals provide appropriate guidelines.

Less than 1 hour before exercise Jeukendrup and Killer reviewed the myths surrounding pre-exercise carbohydrate feedings. They found that the ingestion of carbohydrates in the hour before exercise either improved performance or had no impact on performance. Based on these findings, there is little evidence to abstain from carbohydrate ingestion in the hour prior to exercise, for those who do not experience symptoms of hypoglycemia. Prudence suggests that individuals who may be prone to reactive hypoglycemia should avoid carbohydrate intake, particularly high-glycemic-index foods, 15–60 minutes prior to performance. Simple sugars ingested within this time frame may actually impair physical performance in such individuals because of the adverse effects of reactive hypoglycemia, such as muscular weakness. Moreover, this same insulin response may speed up muscle glycogen utilization. This may be a disadvantage to the marathoner, whose glycogen levels may be depleted too early in the race. Several earlier studies showed that run time to exhaustion was shorter by about 20–25 percent after athletes consumed 2–3 ounces of glucose within an hour before the endurance test.

However, not all individuals experience reactive hypoglycemia. Kuipers and others noted that about one-third of well-trained subjects experienced hypoglycemia following the ingestion of 50 grams of glucose after a 4-hour fast. However, the hypoglycemia was transient, as blood glucose levels returned to normal after 20 minutes of exercise at 60 percent VO_2 max. No performance data were measured. In a study by Seifert and others, subjects were given various carbohydrate solutions to raise their insulin levels; when their insulin levels peaked, they undertook an exercise task at 60 percent of VO_2 max for 50 minutes. No hypoglycemia developed, nor were there any adverse sensory or psychological responses.

If carbohydrate is consumed approximately 1 hour prior to performance, about 1–2 grams/kg (60–120 grams for a 60-kg athlete) may be recommended, for these levels have been shown to enhance performance in several studies. One study using only

TABLE 4.8	Grams of carbohydrate in selected Food Exchanges and sports products

1 fruit exchange = 15 grams carbohydrate
  1 apple
  1 orange
  1/2 banana
  4 ounces orange juice
1 starch exchange = 15 grams carbohydrate
  1 slice bread
  1/2 cup cereal
  1/4 large bagel
  1/2 cup cooked pasta
  1 small baked potato
Sports drinks: 7–8 ounces = 15 grams carbohydrate
  Gatorade
  PowerAde
  SportAde
Sports bars = 20–50 grams carbohydrate
  1 PR Bar
  1 Power Bar
Sports gels = 20–30 grams carbohydrate
  1 Power Gel packet
  1 ReLode packet
Energy drinks: 8 ounces = 25–50 grams carbohydrate
  Gatorade Energy Drink
  SoBe Energy

12 grams 1 hour prior to performance showed no beneficial effect. Both glucose polymers and foods with a low glycemic index have been used successfully.

Immediately before exercise As noted previously, consuming carbohydrate immediately before exercise of short duration, and even exercise tasks of less than 90 minutes or so, normally will not enhance performance. For example, Marjerrison and others found that the ingestion of a carbohydrate solution 30 minutes before undertaking four 30-second anaerobic Wingate tests had no effect on power output; Smith and others reported no significant effect on swim time performance of ingesting a 10 percent glucose solution 5 minutes before a 4-kilometer swim of approximately 70 minutes. However, carbohydrate intake immediately prior to (within 5–10 minutes) prolonged endurance exercise tasks of 2 hours or more may help delay the development of fatigue and improve performance if the athlete is exercising at a level greater than 50 percent VO_2 max, such as 60–75 percent. The majority of the studies, including controlled laboratory investigations and field research involving different types of endurance athletes, support this point of view. At this level of exercise intensity, the insulin response to glucose ingestion is suppressed; in addition, the secretion of epinephrine is increased. These two hormonal responses interact to help maintain or elevate the blood glucose level and prevent the hypoglycemic response that typically may occur in reactive individuals if more time elapses between the ingestion of the carbohydrate and the initiation of exercise.

If carbohydrates are consumed immediately before exercise, that is, within 10 minutes of the start, about 50–60 grams of a glucose polymer in a 40–50 percent solution has been used effectively in some studies. Dry glucose polymers are available commercially. One tablespoon is about 15 grams. To make a 50 percent solution containing 50 grams of the polymer, put about 3 level tablespoons of the polymer into 100 milliliters (about 3–4 ounces) of water. To make a 7.5 percent solution containing 15 grams, put 1 tablespoon of the polymer into 200 milliliters (about 7 ounces) of water. Several commercial "energy" drinks contain 25–50 grams of carbohydrate per 8 fluid ounces, which are about 10–20 percent solutions.

During exercise Carbohydrate ingested during prolonged exercise can help maintain blood glucose levels and reduce the psychological perception of effort, as measured by the ratings of perceived exertion, during the latter stages of an endurance task. As the exercise task continues and the muscle glycogen level falls, the amount of energy derived from the ingested carbohydrates increases. Most research supports the benefits of consuming carbohydrates early in and throughout the exercise task, but even a single carbohydrate feeding late in a prolonged exercise bout may help replenish blood glucose levels, increase carbohydrate oxidation, and delay fatigue.

All major investigators, including Asker Jeukendrup, Trent Stellingwerff, Louise Burke, and Naomi Cermak, conclude that carbohydrate intake during prolonged exercise enhances performance. Studies have been undertaken in both laboratory and field settings, using different types of exercise modalities, and on both men and women.

During Exercise: When and How Much? During exercise, feedings every 15–20 minutes appear to be a reasonable schedule, but possibly more frequently when attempting to maximize carbohydrate intake or to obtain fluids when exercising under warm or hot environmental conditions. Although you may consume considerable quantities of carbohydrate during exercise, your ability to use this exogenous source for energy is limited. The reason is not known, but as noted previously, may be related to insufficient intestinal absorption or impaired delivery from the liver.

Sports drinks averaging 6–10 percent carbohydrate have been found to enhance prolonged endurance performance. A typical serving of a sports drink (8 ounces) would contain about 14–24 grams of carbohydrate, so depending on the concentration, an athlete who wanted to maximize utilizable carbohydrate intake would need to drink about 32–56 ounces to obtain about 100 grams of carbohydrate per hour. Drinking 8 ounces every 15 minutes would provide 32 ounces (1 quart) over the course of an hour, but consumption would have to be more frequent to obtain 56 ounces. Consuming 56 ounces of fluid over the course of an hour might be difficult and may pose a potential health risk for some individuals. Although the fluids could provide the desired amount of carbohydrate, excessive fluid consumption could lead to overhydration and a serious medical condition known as hyponatremia, as shall be discussed in chapter 9.

Several other protocols have been effective. One involved consumption of a high concentration (about 1 gram carbohydrate/kg body weight) immediately before or during the first 20 minutes of the exercise, and then use of lower concentrations such as found in commercial sports drinks at regular intervals. Other investigators have noted that taking a single, more concentrated dose of carbohydrate, such as 100–200 grams total, in the latter stages of prolonged exercise may be beneficial. Additionally, because of the nature of their sport, soccer players and other such athletes may need to consume a high concentration before the game and during halftime, or breaks in the game as they occur.

It should be noted that consumption of carbohydrate solutions above 10 percent during exercise may cause gastrointestinal distress, as may other high concentrations of simple carbohydrates. However, some athletes may learn to tolerate larger concentrations, such as 15–20 percent. Ultradistance athletes, who exercise at a lower intensity, may tolerate even higher concentrations ranging from 20 to 50 percent.

Asker Jeukendrup, Naomi Cermak, and Luc van Loon recommend the following guidelines for carbohydrate intakes during exercise to maximize performance and minimize gastrointestinal distress. For athletes engaged in very short, high-intensity exercise lasting less than 0.5 hour: no carbohydrate is necessary during exercise. For short, high-intensity exercise or intermittent team sports lasting 0.5 to 1.25 hours: very little carbohydrate is required, possibly just a mouth rinse. For intermittent team sports of moderate duration from 1 to 1.5 hours: up to 60 grams per hour is recommended. For intermittent team sports of long duration beyond 2 hours: up to 90 grams per hour of multiple transportable carbohydrates (mixed sugars) are recommended. For endurance/continuous exercise lasting 1 to 3 hours, up to 60 grams per hour of carbohydrate are recommended. Finally, for prolonged endurance exercise beyond 2.5 hours in duration: up to 90 grams per hour of multiple transportable carbohydrates are recommended. Additionally, it is recommended that if an athlete is going to exercise for more than 2 hours, but is starting exercise with suboptimal carbohydrate levels, they consume up to 90 grams of multiple transportable carbohydrates per hour.

Athletes may learn to tolerate higher amounts of carbohydrate (i.e., train the gut), so these recommendations, although based in research, allow for some adjustment. Athletes should experiment with different doses of carbohydrate during training or practice, but not competition.

Optimal Supplementation Protocol Several studies have indicated that although the intake of carbohydrate either before or during exercise may separately enhance performance, the best effect was observed when carbohydrate was consumed both before and during exercise. For example, Chryssanthopoulos and others had subjects run to exhaustion at 70 percent VO_2 max and found that although a high-carbohydrate meal 3 hours prior to performance improved endurance time, the combination of the meal and a carbohydrate-electrolyte solution during exercise further improved endurance running capacity.

Type of Carbohydrate A number of different types of carbohydrates have been studied, including glucose, fructose, galactose, sucrose, maltose, glucose polymers such as maltodextrins, both individually and in various combinations, as well as soluble starch (a very long polymer), high-glycemic-index foods such as potatoes, and low-glycemic-index foods such as legumes. In general, there appears to be no difference between these different types of carbohydrates as a means to enhance endurance performance when used appropriately. However, there may be some important considerations relative to the use of various carbohydrate combinations, fructose, solid carbohydrates, and low-glycemic-index foods.

Carbohydrate combinations Jeukendrup noted studies showing that a single carbohydrate ingested during exercise will be oxidized at rates up to about 1 gram/minute, even when large amounts of carbohydrate are ingested. However, combinations of carbohydrate (coined multiple transportable carbohydrates), particularly glucose and fructose, that use different intestinal transporters for absorption have been shown to result in higher oxidation rates (see figure 4.12). This seems to be the way to increase exogenous carbohydrate oxidation rates, up to 1.7 grams/minute. Combinations of carbohydrates are recommended to increase glucose oxidation at a rate of more than 60 grams per hour. Currell and Jeukendrup reported that ingestion of a drink containing multiple carbohydrates (glucose and fructose), as compared to either a glucose drink or water, improved performance by 8 and 19 percent, respectively, in time-trial performance following a 2-hour bout of cycling. Power output was greater throughout the approximate 1-hour time trial with the glucose/fructose drink. Single sources of carbohydrate, such as glucose, appear to be adequate when less is needed. Thus, check food labels for ingredients to ensure that the chosen sports drink contains such combinations.

Fructose Most people can tolerate small amounts of fructose. It is found naturally in fruits and is an ingredient in some sports drinks. However, consuming larger amounts may pose problems. Because fructose is absorbed slowly from the intestinal tract, it can create a significant osmotic effect in the intestines, leading to diarrhea and gastrointestinal distress in some individuals. Research has indicated that a 6 percent solution of fructose, when compared to similar solutions of glucose and sucrose, caused significant gastrointestinal distress and an impairment in exercise performance. The athlete should be cautious in using fructose as the sole source of carbohydrate before or during exercise. Sports drinks containing fructose include it in small concentrations.

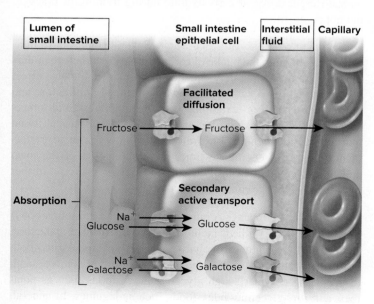

FIGURE 4.12 The villi in the intestines contain different receptors for the monosaccharides, which may increase carbohydrate absorption when multiple sources of carbohydrate are ingested.

Fructose is generally not the preferred carbohydrate for postexercise muscle glycogen resynthesis. However, relative to muscle glycogen repletion, little is known about liver glycogen repletion. One classic human study from Eric Hultman showed that, when compared to glucose, a fructose infusion caused greater liver glycogen repletion rates and no increase in hepatic glucose output. More recently, Décombaz and others showed that, following glycogen-depleting exercise, fructose or galactose plus maltodextrin ingestion caused twice the liver glycogen repletion rate as glucose plus maltodextrin ingestion. So although there are few data available on liver glycogen repletion, it is possible that postexercise carbohydrate consumption that includes some fructose and galactose may enhance liver glycogen accumulation. Additionally, high-fructose corn syrup, although rich in fructose, is treated as an added sugar. The health risks of added sugars are covered later in this chapter.

Carbohydrate Form In a review, Cermak and van Loon concluded that there is no influence of the form in which carbohydrates are ingested (i.e., liquid, solid, semisolid [slurry]) on exercise performance. A small number of studies have been conducted that support this viewpoint. For instance, Pfeiffer and colleagues found no differences in oxidation rates between liquid, solid, and semisolid carbohydrates. Campbell and others studied the effect of different forms of carbohydrate (liquid, gel, and jellybeans) on endurance exercise performance and found no differences in blood glucose maintenance during exercise or exercise performance.

Importantly, an athlete's preference of carbohydrate form could have a greater effect on performance than carbohydrate form, so the important factors to consider in carbohydrate choice have little to do with form and a great deal to do with preference, dose, gastric emptying, and fluid and electrolyte needs

Low-glycemic-index foods Although research on glycemic index (GI) and performance has been conducted for 20 years, the data are far from conclusive. Several reviews from experts in the topic are available. Donaldson and colleagues concluded in a review that there is still a lack of agreement on the benefits of consuming low vs. high GI carbohydrates on exercise performance. In their review, they noted that only 5 of 13 relevant investigations of pre-exercise carbohydrate consumption measured performance and that of the 5 that did, performance only improved in the low GI condition in 2 studies. In a similar analysis, O'Reilly and others evaluated 13 studies on pre-exercise high vs. low GI carbohydrate intake. Only 2 demonstrated a beneficial effect of consuming a low GI carbohydrate prior to exercise; however, this effect is attenuated if carbohydrate is consumed during exercise, which is common in most sports.

Ormsbee and others reported that consuming a low GI carbohydrate before exercise does cause a reduced blood glucose/insulin response (7 studies). Metabolically, this may cause an increase in fat oxidation or help to maintain normal blood glucose levels during exercise (7 studies); however, this was not shown in 2 other studies. So a measurable metabolic benefit is commonly found, although researchers have found it difficult to translate this into a clear performance benefit. For instance, Ormsbee notes that time to exhaustion and time trial performance has been enhanced by ingestion of low GI carbohydrate (5 studies), but this has not been shown in other studies (6 studies). There are considerable methodological differences between these studies, which makes interpretation of a small body of literature (<20 studies) difficult. Of note is that there are no reports of performance decrements due to pre-exercise consumption of low GI carbohydrates, so athletes may experiment in practice to determine if there is a benefit. Additional research is needed to evaluate the effect of pre-exercise low GI carbohydrate consumption on endurance exercise performance.

Carbohydrate with protein Studies have been conducted to determine the impact on performance of consuming protein with carbohydrate during exercise. McCleave and others found time to exhaustion to be 15.2 percent longer for female competitive cyclists and triathletes when a 3 percent carbohydrate/1.2 percent protein supplement was consumed every 20 minutes, compared to a 6 percent carbohydrate supplement. Using similar supplementation, Ferguson-Stegall found that total time to exhaustion was greater for cyclists and triathletes for intensities at or below the ventilatory threshold. Subjects cycling to exhaustion above the ventilatory threshold demonstrated no difference in performance with the supplements. In a review, van Loon noted that of 13 studies that investigated the effects of protein ingestion during exercise, only three showed a significant improvement in endurance performance. Still, some of the improvements were quite large (up to 30 percent) so at least in some individuals, during exercise protein ingestion may be ergogenic. However, the mechanism for improved performance is unknown. More importantly, protein ingestion during exercise does increase protein synthesis, before the exercise session is finished. So small amounts of protein consumed before or during exercise might aid in recovery.

Several studies have compared the effects of carbohydrate supplementation alone to carbohydrate/protein supplementation on performance following recovery from previous exercise. Betts and others had subjects complete a 90-minute run at 70 percent of VO_2 max, followed by a 4-hour recovery period, during which they consumed either a carbohydrate or a carbohydrate/protein mixture. The subjects then ran to exhaustion at 85 percent of VO_2 max, but there was no difference between treatments. Romano-Ely and others investigated the effect of a carbohydrate-protein-antioxidant drink, as compared to an isocaloric carbohydrate drink, on cycling time to exhaustion at 70 percent VO_2 max and, 24 hours later, at 80 percent VO_2 max. The drinks were consumed every 15 minutes during exercise and immediately afterward. There were no significant differences between the treatments on performance time during either of the cycling tests. Conversely, Bernardi and others had subjects complete a 60-minute time trial followed by a 6-hour recovery period, during which the subjects consumed either carbohydrate or carbohydrate/protein. The subjects then repeated the 60-minute time-trial ride. Ingestion of carbohydrate/protein increased fat oxidation, increased recovery, and improved performance relative to isoenergetic carbohydrate ingestion. In a meta-analysis, Stearns and colleagues demonstrated an average 9 percent improvement in subsequent endurance performance with co-ingestion of protein and carbohydrate compared

to carbohydrate alone. They also found an ergogenic effect when supplements were matched for carbohydrate content.

The use of chocolate milk has been reviewed by Roy and others as a more economical alternative to sports drinks during recovery from exercise. Benefits to this beverage include a ratio of carbohydrates to protein in the range recommended by the International Society of Sports Nutrition and its naturally high concentrations of electrolytes; it also affords a greater feeling of fullness compared to water or carbohydrate beverages. Karp and colleagues had highly trained cyclists perform an interval workout followed by 4 hours of recovery and then an endurance trial to exhaustion at 70 percent VO_2 max. During recovery, subjects consumed the same volume of chocolate milk, fluid replacement drink, or carbohydrate replacement drink. The carbohydrate content was equivalent for the chocolate milk and the carbohydrate replacement drink. Total time to exhaustion and total work were significantly greater for chocolate milk and fluid replacement subject compared to the carbohydrate replacement drink group. These results are supported by research done by Pritchett, Thomas, and Gilson, who also found at least as effective muscle recovery responses with chocolate milk and carbohydrate recovery drinks.

Individuality Probably the most important recommendation is for the athlete to experiment with different types and amounts of carbohydrate during training before using them in competition. Just as it is important for you to know your optimal race pace for an endurance event, so, too, must you know how well you can tolerate different amounts and concentrations and types of carbohydrates. Williams noted that the type of event may influence the amount of carbohydrate ingested, as runners may be more prone to gastrointestinal distress than cyclists. "Runner's trots" is a form of diarrhea that may be associated with excess consumption of highly concentrated sugar solutions, such as "energy" drinks.

Just as you train your muscles to learn their capacity, you may also be able to train your digestive system to know its limits. During training, experiment with various types and concentrations of carbohydrate, both before and during exercise. Ron Maughan, an internationally respected authority in sports nutrition, indicated that the optimal strategy relative to carbohydrate utilization is to use your own subjective experience, which you can gain during training.

What is the importance of carbohydrate replenishment after prolonged exercise?

There are several possible applications of this question. One is the athlete who may be involved in a prolonged exercise bout, have a rest period of 1–4 hours, and then must exercise again, such as athletes who train two or three times daily. Benefits may accrue to anaerobic endurance-, aerobic endurance-, and resistance-trained individuals. A second application is the athlete who trains intensely every day and must have an adequate recovery in the one-day rest interval. A third application, covered in the next section, is the technique of carbohydrate loading.

After prolonged exercise, increased levels of GLUT-4 receptors in the muscle cell membrane help move available blood glucose into the muscle for resynthesis to muscle glycogen. Several studies have shown that ingesting carbohydrate during the rest interval between two prolonged exercise bouts improves performance in the second bout. This finding is comparable to the beneficial effects of carbohydrate intake during prolonged exercise bouts. The carbohydrate can help restore blood glucose levels but may also be used to resynthesize muscle glycogen. In cases such as this, where the rate of muscle glycogen resynthesis is important, high-glycemic-index foods, such as potatoes, bread, glucose, or glucose polymers, would be the preferred source of carbohydrate, for they apparently lead to a faster restoration of muscle glycogen than does a meal rich in low-glycemic-index foods. For repeat prolonged exercise tasks with about a 4-hour interval, a general recommendation is to consume 1 gram of carbohydrate per kilogram body weight immediately after the first event and again 2 hours prior to the second event. Additional carbohydrate may also be consumed immediately before and during the second event.

Carbohydrate with protein Carbohydrate has been combined with other nutrients, particularly protein, in attempts to enhance muscle glycogen resynthesis. Protein and some amino acids, such as arginine, may stimulate the release of insulin, which, if added to the effects of carbohydrate-mediated insulin release, could increase the rate at which glucose is transported into the muscle cell. In a review, Beelen and colleagues concluded that the inclusion of protein or amino acids with carbohydrates does not further enhance postexercise muscle glycogen synthesis when an adequate amount of carbohydrate (1.2 g/kg/hr) is ingested at frequent intervals (every 15–30 minutes). They added that this combination may accelerate postexercise muscle glycogen synthesis rates when less carbohydrate is provided (<1.0 g/kg/hr). Kerksick and others recently published the International Society of Sports Nutrition position stand on nutrient timing. It states that adding protein to carbohydrate (ratio of 1:3–4) may increase endurance performance and maximally promotes glycogen synthesis during acute and subsequent endurance exercise. Several studies, such as those by Baty and Romano-Ely and their colleagues, have shown that carbohydrate/protein supplementation may also reduce the incidence of muscle soreness following exercise, including lower levels of serum enzymes used as markers of muscle tissue damage. Moreover, as shall be noted in chapter 6, consuming some additional protein following strenuous exercise may have some beneficial effects, such as improved muscle protein balance.

If rapid resynthesis of muscle glycogen is not important, it is good to note that studies have shown that consumption of adequate amounts of carbohydrate over a 24-hour period will restore muscle glycogen levels to normal. For athletes who train intensely on a daily basis with either resistive or aerobic exercise that leads to muscle glycogen depletion, sports nutritionists normally recommend that approximately 8–10 grams of carbohydrate per kilogram body weight should be consumed daily to restore muscle glycogen levels to normal. For an individual who weighs 70 kilograms, this approximates 560–700 grams of carbohydrate, or 2,240–2,800 carbohydrate Calories. This amount of carbohydrate would represent about 65–80 percent of the daily caloric intake of an athlete consuming 3,500 Calories. Over the 24-hour period, the rate of muscle glycogen recovery is approximately 5–7 percent per hour. Sports drinks

may be a convenient means to consume carbohydrate immediately after exercise. The remaining carbohydrate should be derived from other natural sources in the diet, including both simple carbohydrates in fruits and complex carbohydrates in grains, potatoes, and other foods with adequate dietary fiber and other nutrients. The inclusion of high-glycemic-index foods in the daily diet will help speed resynthesis of muscle glycogen over the 24-hour period and may be very compatible with the Prudent Healthy Diet. Regular meals consumed during the 24-hour recovery period should include healthful low-glycemic-index foods with adequate amounts of protein.

Following prolonged, high-intensity competitive exercise performance, such as running a marathon, the resulting muscle damage will limit muscle glycogen replenishment for several days. Rest is important during this time, and muscle glycogen levels may return to normal following seven or more days of high-carbohydrate meals.

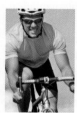

Will a high-carbohydrate diet enhance my daily exercise training?

Most scientists and sports nutritionists who study carbohydrate metabolism in athletes recommend a high-carbohydrate diet for most athletes, particularly endurance athletes, because success in athletic competition is contingent upon optimal training, and for the endurance athlete, optimal training may be contingent upon adequate nutrition, primarily the ingestion of sufficient carbohydrate every day. Louise Burke, a prominent sports nutritionist, and her associates recommended that athletes in general training consume daily approximately 5–7 grams of carbohydrate per kilogram body weight, but endurance athletes should consume about 7–10 grams per kilogram. These recommendations are comparable to those of Melinda Manore, another sports nutrition expert. Burke and others noted that most male athletes may be meeting these needs, but many female endurance athletes, particularly those attempting to lose weight for competition, may not. Older athletes may need to ensure adequate carbohydrate intake during training. According to Mittendorfer and Klein, aging causes a shift in energy substrate use during exercise with an increased oxidation of glucose and less fat, presumably caused by age-related changes in skeletal muscle.

There are some limited data supporting the concept of enhanced training following a high-carbohydrate diet. A number of field and laboratory studies with athletes have attempted to mimic actual sport conditions. For example, one group of soccer players improved performance on an intermittent exercise task designed to mimic physical activity in a game, while another group improved performance in a standardized intermittent running task and a run to exhaustion. In other studies, runners were able to endure longer on a treadmill run to exhaustion; swimmers were better able to maintain 400-meter swim velocity; and triathletes experienced a significant improvement in treadmill endurance following 30 minutes of swimming, cycling, and running. Based on the available data, Edward Coyle, an international authority in carbohydrate metabolism during exercise, indicated that physical performance seems better maintained with a high- versus moderate-carbohydrate diet.

In general, the normal carbohydrate intake of athletes in training studies was increased from approximately 40–45 percent to 55–70 percent of the daily Calories for varying periods, but usually a week or more. This level of carbohydrate approximates the upper levels of the AMDR for carbohydrate.

Not all athletes, including endurance athletes, need high-carbohydrate diets all the time. In a meta-analysis, Erlenbusch and others indicated that subjects following a high-carbohydrate diet could exercise longer until exhaustion, but this finding applied more to untrained individuals than trained individuals. As you may recall, aerobic exercise training improves the ability of the muscles to use fat as an energy source, so they may be somewhat less dependent on carbohydrate for a given training protocol. Thus, a moderate-carbohydrate diet may be adequate for trained athletes. For example, obtaining 45 percent of daily energy needs from carbohydrate might be considered moderate, as it is at the lower end of the AMDR. On such a diet, an endurance athlete who consumes 3,000 Calories per day during training would derive 1,350 Calories from carbohydrate ($0.45 \times 3,000$), which is about 340 grams of carbohydrate. For a 60-kilogram athlete, this is about 5.6 grams of carbohydrate per kilogram body weight. Although this is slightly less than that recommended for endurance athletes, research has shown that such amounts may be sufficient to maintain training on a daily basis.

However, training may appear more stressful psychologically. In several studies, the psychological status of athletes, as measured by the vigor and fatigue components of the Profile of Mood States (POMS) questionnaire and their rating of perceived exertion (RPE) during exercise, was improved when they switched from moderate- to higher-carbohydrate diets. In his review, Coyle concluded that mood state seems better maintained with a high-rather than moderate-carbohydrate diet. Utter and others reported reduced ratings of perceived exertion in subjects involved in prolonged (2.6 hours), intermittent cycling following ingestion of carbohydrate before and during the exercise bout.

Coyle also indicates that a high-carbohydrate diet may help reduce symptoms of overreaching and, possibly, overtraining. Gleeson and others note that heavy, prolonged exertion is associated with numerous hormonal and biochemical changes in the body, many of which may have detrimental effects on immune function. A well-balanced diet helps promote optimal immune function, and reviews by Gleeson and Nieman indicate that consuming carbohydrate during exercise attenuates rises in stress hormones such as cortisol and appears to limit the degree of exercise-induced immunosuppression. An impaired immune response is one possible factor associated with the overtraining syndrome. Carbohydrate intake following exercise also promotes protein synthesis via the insulin effect, which may enhance muscle and overall recovery.

Some nutritionists indicate that many athletes do not eat high-carbohydrate diets because it may be impractical for them to do so. Selecting foods high in carbohydrate content, highlighted earlier in this chapter, provides a sound guide to increase the carbohydrate content of the diet, as do some of the recommendations in the following section regarding carbohydrate loading. Chapter 11 will provide additional information specific to daily caloric intake for planning a diet.

In summary, as Coyle notes, athletes do not train hard every day, so they do not require a high intake of carbohydrate every day of training. Nevertheless, a diet rich in healthful carbohydrates not only may have several major health benefits but may also help guarantee optimal energy sources for daily exercise training. Moreover, as Louise Burke points out, experts in the field of energy metabolism indicate that there is no evidence that diets which are restricted in carbohydrate, such as the "zone" diet discussed in chapters 5 and 6, enhance training. Carbohydrate is the major fuel for most athletes in training. The slogan *Train high and compete high* refers to the concept of training and competing with high carbohydrate intake.

Key Concepts

▶ Carbohydrate is the most important energy source for moderately high- to high-intensity exercise.

▶ Regular training increases the ability of the muscles to store and use carbohydrate for energy production.

▶ Low levels of blood glucose or muscle glycogen may be contributing factors in the premature onset of fatigue in prolonged exercise.

▶ Low levels of muscle glycogen may contribute to impaired performance in prolonged, moderate- to high-intensity endurance exercise and in sports involving intermittent, high-intensity exercise for 60–90 minutes.

▶ Consuming carbohydrate before and during prolonged, intermittent, high-intensity or continuous exercise may help delay the onset of fatigue, but unless carbohydrate intake corrects a muscle glycogen deficiency, such practices will not improve performance in most athletic events of shorter duration.

▶ Combinations of carbohydrates, such as glucose and fructose, consumed during exercise appear to optimize the amount of exogenous carbohydrate that can be oxidized.

▶ Athletes should experiment with different carbohydrate supplementation strategies during training to help determine the amount, type, and timing of intake that may be suitable for them in competition.

▶ Glucose, sucrose, glucose polymers, and solid carbohydrates appear to be equally effective as a means of enhancing performance, but fructose may be more likely to cause gastrointestinal distress if used alone.

▶ Carbohydrates with a high glycemic index may facilitate muscle glycogen replenishment when consumed immediately after exercise and every 2 hours thereafter.

▶ To maintain the quality of training, athletes who train at moderate to high intensity on a daily basis should eat a healthful diet rich in complex carbohydrates, complemented with some high-glycemic-index foods, to replenish muscle glycogen.

Check for Yourself

▶ Given the recommendation to consume about 1.0 to 1.5 grams of carbohydrate per kilogram body weight per hour for 4–5 hours after exercise in order to rapidly replenish muscle glycogen, calculate how much carbohydrate you would need per hour and list specific foods, and amounts, that you might need to consume each hour.

Carbohydrate Loading

What is carbohydrate, or glycogen, loading?

Because carbohydrate becomes increasingly important as a fuel for muscular exercise as the intensity of the exercise increases, and because the amount of carbohydrate stored in the body is limited, muscle and liver glycogen depletion could be factors that limit performance capacity in distance events characterized by high levels of energy expenditure for prolonged periods. **Carbohydrate loading**, also called *glycogen loading* and *glycogen supercompensation,* is a dietary technique designed to promote a significant increase in the glycogen content in both the liver and the muscles in an attempt to delay the onset of fatigue. It is generally used for 3–7 days in preparation for major athletic competitions.

What type of athlete would benefit from carbohydrate loading?

In general, carbohydrate loading is primarily suited for individuals who will sustain high levels of continuous energy expenditure for prolonged periods, such as long-distance runners, swimmers, bicyclists, triathletes, cross-country skiers, and similar athletes. In addition, athletes who are involved in prolonged stop-and-go activities, such as soccer, lacrosse, and tournament-play sports like tennis and handball, may benefit. For example, Rico-Sanz and others concluded that exhaustion during soccer-specific performance is related to the capacity to use muscle glycogen, underlying the importance of glycogen loading. In essence, carbohydrate loading may be effective for athletes engaged in events that use muscle glycogen as the major energy source and that may lead to a depletion of glycogen in the muscle fibers. Athletes who compete in sports involving high-intensity, short-duration energy expenditure will not benefit from carbohydrate loading. For example, Hatfield and others reported no effects of carbohydrate loading on performance in resistance training involving multiple sets of maximal jump squats. However, bodybuilders have been reported to carbohydrate load in attempts to appear more muscular owing to increased muscle glycogen levels and associated water retention.

Recall from chapter 3 that humans have several different types of skeletal muscle fibers. In general, the slow-twitch red and fast-twitch red fibers are used mainly during long, continuous activities and are aerobic in nature, whereas the fast-twitch white fibers are used for short, fast activities and are anaerobic in nature. Consider the differences between a distance runner and a soccer player. The former may run at a steady pace for hours, whereas the latter will constantly be changing speeds, with many bouts of full speed interspersed with recovery periods of slower running. Research has shown that glycogen depletion patterns of the two different muscle fiber types are related to the type of exercise. Long, continuous exercise depletes glycogen principally in the slow-twitch red and fast-twitch red fibers, whereas fast, intermittent bouts of exercise with periods of rest—actually a form of interval training—primarily deplete glycogen in the fast-twitch white fibers. However, it should be noted that glycogen depletion may occur in all types of fibers in either prolonged, continuous or intermittent exercise and may be quite appreciable, depending upon intensity and duration of the exercise bouts. If carbohydrate loading works for the specific muscle fiber involved, then both types of athletes may benefit. Both should have greater glycogen stores in the latter stages of their respective athletic contests.

How do you carbohydrate load?

As you might suspect, the key to carbohydrate loading is to switch from the normal, balanced diet to one very high in carbohydrate content. The original, classic carbohydrate loading technique, emanating from earlier Scandinavian research, involved a glycogen depletion stage induced by prolonged exercise and a restricted diet. For example, a runner might go for an 18- to 20-mile run to use as much stored glycogen as possible, and then ingest very little carbohydrate in the following 2- to 3-day period. Exercise is continued during this 2- to 3-day period to keep glycogen stores low. Following the depletion stage, the loading stage began. During this phase, carbohydrate may contribute 70 or more percent of the caloric intake. The intensity and duration of exercise during this phase were reduced considerably. The usual case was to rest fully for 2 to 3 days. Thus, the classic carbohydrate loading pattern involved three stages: depletion, carbohydrate deprivation (high-fat/protein diet), and carbohydrate loading. However, this original method may be particularly difficult to tolerate, especially if one tries to exercise at high levels during the depletion phase. The lack of carbohydrate in the diet combined with the exercise bouts may elicit symptoms of hypoglycemia (weakness, lethargy, irritability). Moreover, prolonged exhaustive exercise may lead to muscle trauma, which may actually impair the storage of extra glycogen. This classic, original method is presented in table 4.9.

Although some early research supported this technique, more recent data suggest that this strict routine may be unnecessary, particularly the total program of depletion. For example, in trained runners, research has shown that simply changing to a very high-carbohydrate diet, combined with 1 or 2 days of rest or reduced activity levels (tapering), will effectively increase muscle and liver glycogen. Well-controlled research has revealed that exhaustive running is not necessary to achieve muscle glycogen supercompensation. It appears to be important to continue endurance training, or other high-intensity training specific to the sport, during the 7–14 days prior to competition. Such training will maintain adequate levels of GLUT-4 receptors to transfer blood glucose into the muscle cell and of glycogen synthase, the enzyme in the muscle that synthesizes glycogen from glucose. Evidence also suggests that if the total carbohydrate content is consumed over the entire week, in contrast to concentrating it in 2–3 days, there will be little difference in the muscle glycogen content between the two techniques.

Although there may be a number of variations in the carbohydrate loading protocol, a generally recommended format is also presented in table 4.9. The interested athlete may want to experiment with both techniques and make adjustments through experience.

Sports scientists have generally recommended that carbohydrate intake during carbohydrate loading be about 8–10 grams

TABLE 4.9 Different methods for carbohydrate loading

A recommended method		Original, classic method	
1st day:	tapering exercise	1st day:	depletion exercise
2nd day:	mixed diet, moderate carbohydrate; tapering exercise	2nd day:	high-protein/fat diet; low carbohydrate; tapering exercise
3rd day:	mixed diet, moderate carbohydrate; tapering exercise	3rd day:	high-protein/fat diet; low carbohydrate; tapering exercise
4th day:	mixed diet, moderate carbohydrate; tapering exercise	4th day:	high-protein/fat diet; low carbohydrate; tapering exercise
5th day:	high-carbohydrate diet; tapering exercise	5th day:	high-carbohydrate diet; tapering exercise
6th day:	high-carbohydrate diet; tapering exercise or rest	6th day:	high-carbohydrate diet; tapering exercise or rest
7th day:	high-carbohydrate diet; tapering exercise or rest	7th day:	high-carbohydrate diet; tapering exercise or rest
8th day:	competition	8th day:	competition

High-carbohydrate diet: 400–800 g per day depending on body weight; about 70–80 percent of dietary Calories should be carbohydrate.

per kilogram body weight, and Louise Burke, from the Australian Institute of Sport, recommended that marathon runners consume about 10–12 grams per kilogram body weight over the 36–48 hours prior to the race. These recommendations could total about 400–800 grams per day, depending on the size of the individual, which is not too different from the generally recommended dietary content of carbohydrate for the endurance athlete in regular training; Burke recommends that marathoners consume 7–12 grams of carbohydrate per kilogram body mass during training. It is important to note that the athlete should not change his or her diet drastically prior to competition. Consuming a high-carbohydrate diet during training will condition the body to metabolize carbohydrate properly during this loading phase. Table 4.10 represents a general dietary plan for carbohydrate loading. The total caloric value and grams of carbohydrate should be adjusted to individual needs. They are dependent upon the size of the individual and daily energy expenditure in exercise. It is important not to consume excess Calories, for they may be converted into body fat if in excess of the maximal storage capacity of the muscle and liver for glycogen.

Some guidelines for replenishment of glycogen were presented earlier. Because glycogen loading for long-distance events occurs over two to three days, it would be wise to stress complex carbohydrates in the diet because of their higher nutrient content. However, simple carbohydrates may also be used effectively to increase muscle glycogen stores, as can high-carbohydrate sports drinks such as Gatorade energy drink. Moreover, the diet should also include the daily requirements for protein and fat.

If, for some reason, the athlete cannot carbohydrate load over the 3- to 7-day period, a rapid protocol may be effective. Fairchild and others found that one day of a high-carbohydrate intake, approximately 10 grams of high-glycemic-index carbohydrate per kilogram body mass, nearly doubled the muscle glycogen concentration, from 109 to 198 mmol/kg wet weight muscle. The carbohydrate feeding was preceded by a short bout of near maximal-intensity exercise for 3 minutes. They reported that these muscle glycogen levels were comparable to those achieved over a 2- to 6-day regimen.

Most prolonged endurance events begin in the morning. The last large meal should be about 15 hours prior to race time, possibly topped off with a simple carbohydrate snack before retiring for the night. Some athletes drink a glucose polymer for the last major meal to avoid the presence of intestinal residue the morning of competition. A carbohydrate breakfast such as orange juice, toast, jelly, or other carbohydrates along with some protein may be eaten 3 to 4 hours prior to competition. Review the discussion of precompetition meals in chapter 2. This overall dietary regimen should help maximize muscle and liver glycogen stores. The athlete should then follow the guidelines presented previously relative to carbohydrate intake before and during performance.

Will carbohydrate loading increase muscle glycogen concentration?

Most, but not all, studies show that an appropriate carbohydrate loading protocol, compared to normal or low dietary carbohydrate intake, will substantially increase muscle glycogen levels. Although some previous research found that muscle glycogen levels in the early phases of loading did not increase as much in females as in males, more recent, better-controlled research by James, Paul, and Tarnopolsky, with their associates, revealed that carbohydrate loading increased muscle glycogen concentration in both men and women, provided that total energy intake was adequate. No gender differences were noted. McLay and others noted that women generally have lower resting muscle glycogen levels during the midfollicular phase of the menstrual cycle, as compared to the midluteal phase, but the lower glycogen storage in the midfollicular phase could be overcome by carbohydrate loading. In general, carbohydrate intakes of 8 grams or more per kilogram body weight will provide optimal muscle glycogen concentrations for both males and females.

TABLE 4.10 Daily food plan for carbohydrate loading

Dietary sources of fats, proteins, and carbohydrates	Amount and calories	Grams of carbohydrate, protein, and fat
Meat, fish, poultry, eggs, cheese, select low-fat items	6–8 oz Calories: 330–440	0 grams carbohydrate* 42–56 grams protein 18–24 grams fat
Breads, cereals, and grain products	10–20 servings Calories: 800–1,600	150–300 grams carbohydrate 24–60 grams protein
Vegetables, high Calorie (such as corn)	4 servings Calories: 280	60 grams carbohydrate 8 grams protein
Fruits	4 servings Calories: 240	60 grams carbohydrate
Fats and oils	2–4 teaspoons Calories: 90–180	10–20 grams fat
Milk, skim	2 servings Calories: 180	24 grams carbohydrate 16 grams protein
Desserts, such as pie	2 servings Calories: 700	102 grams carbohydrate 6 grams protein 30 grams fat
Beverages, naturally sweetened	8–24 ounces Calories: 80–240	20–60 grams carbohydrate
Water	8 or more servings Calories: 0	
TOTAL KCAL	2,700–3,860	

TOTAL GRAMS AND APPROXIMATE % OF DIETARY CALORIES

Carbohydrate	416–606	65%
Protein	96–146	15%
Fat	58–74	20%

Consult table 4.2 for specific high-carbohydrate foods in each of the food sources.

*Beans are listed in the meat group because of their high protein content; however, they are also low in fat and high in carbohydrates, so they are an excellent selection from this food group. Substitution of beans for meat will increase the total grams of carbohydrate and the percentage of dietary Calories from carbohydrate.
Including high-carbohydrate drinks, such as glucose polymers, can add significant amounts of carbohydrate to the diet and may substitute for other foods.
Source: Adapted from M. Forgac, "Carbohydrate Loading: A Review" in *Journal of the American Dietetic Association* 75:42–5, 1979.

Glycogen content in the muscle has been reported to increase about two to three times beyond normal and liver glycogen content nearly doubled following a carbohydrate loading regimen, and this increase may last at least 3 days in a rested athlete. However, it may be important to taper and rest about 2 days prior to the event. Fogelholm and others reported no increase in muscle glycogen following the classic loading protocol if athletes continued to train 45–60 minutes per day, even though the training was easy. This finding merits confirmation, as other studies have shown muscle glycogen supercompensation when individuals tapered, although most studies use at least 1 day of rest before the competitive exercise test.

Carbohydrate loading has been shown to increase muscle glycogen stores after exhaustive exercise, but apparently the process does not work repeatedly within a short time frame. McInerney and others reported that muscle glycogen supercompensation did not occur when subjects attempted to increase muscle glycogen levels repeatedly during a 5-day period while performing exhaustive exercise every other day.

In general, the full carbohydrate loading procedure should be used sparingly, mainly in preparation for a peak event. However, athletes should experiment with the procedure, or at least experiment with various forms of carbohydrate to be used, sometime during training before using it in competition.

How do I know if my muscles have increased their glycogen stores?

The most accurate way would be to have a muscle biopsy taken (a needle is inserted into the muscle and a small portion is extracted and analyzed), but this is not very practical. A practical method that has been recommended is to monitor changes in body weight. Kreitzman and others noted that glycogen is stored in the liver, muscles, and fat cells in hydrated form (three to four parts water), and weight gain may occur with carbohydrate loading. Thus, keeping an accurate record of your body weight, which should be recorded every morning as you arise and after you urinate, may help you determine the answer to this question. Approximately 3 grams of water are bound to each gram of stored glycogen. If your body stores an additional 300–400 grams of glycogen, along with 900–1,200 grams of water, your body weight will increase about 1,200–1,600 grams, or 2.5–3.5 pounds, above your normal training weight during the loading phase. The weight gain would be greater with additional glycogen storage. This is indicative that the carbohydrate loading has been effective, because rapid weight gains from one day to another are usually due to changes in body water content.

Will carbohydrate loading improve exercise performance?

Although athletes in most sports may benefit from an increased carbohydrate content in the diet, the full procedure of carbohydrate loading is not necessary for the vast majority of athletes.

In general, carbohydrate loading has not been found to enhance performance in single, high-intensity exercise tasks ranging up to 60 minutes or so. For example, Vandenberghe and others found no effect of muscle glycogen levels (manipulated by carbohydrate loading) on muscle glycolytic rate during very high-intensity exercise (125 percent VO_2 max) or on all-out performance at this exercise intensity, a time approximating 3 minutes. Various other studies have reported that carbohydrate loading does not increase the speed of runners in events ranging from 10 kilometers to the half-marathon or in cycling time trials up to 60 minutes. However, Pizza and others, using an exercise task consisting of a 15-minute submaximal run followed by a run to exhaustion at 100 percent VO_2 max, reported an increase in performance associated with carbohydrate loading. The run to exhaustion approximated 5 minutes. In general, this finding is an exception to the rule, so additional research is warranted.

Carbohydrate loading may benefit athletes involved in prolonged, intermittent, high-intensity exercise tasks. Akermark and others, using elite Swedish ice hockey players on two competitive teams as subjects, reported that the team that carbohydrate loaded between two games had higher muscle glycogen levels, which were associated with improvement in distance skated, number of shifts skated, and skating speed in the second game.

Carbohydrate loading has been studied most extensively as a means to improve performance in more prolonged aerobic endurance exercise tasks. In general, the results are supportive of an ergogenic effect. Laboratory studies have shown that exercise time to exhaustion is closely associated with the amount of muscle glycogen available or the amount of carbohydrate in the diet. When endurance performance is compared after subjects have been on either a high-fat/high-protein diet, a mixed, balanced diet, or a high-carbohydrate diet for 4–7 days, performance on the high-fat/high-protein diet is worse than on the other two. However, research findings comparing a mixed, balanced diet with a high-carbohydrate diet have been equivocal, with some results favoring the high-carbohydrate diet and others revealing no difference between the two.

A number of studies have shown that carbohydrate loading, as compared to a normal carbohydrate intake, does not enhance endurance performance. However, in many of these studies the performance tests may not have been long enough for the individual to derive the full benefit from carbohydrate loading, as the duration was less than 2 hours. However, one of the best-designed placebo-controlled studies also found no beneficial effect of carbohydrate loading. Using a cycling exercise protocol designed to be similar to a competitive 100-km road race (about 2.5 hours), Burke and others found that a 3-day carbohydrate loading regimen (9 grams carbohydrate/kg), as compared to a moderate-carbohydrate diet (6 grams carbohydrate/kg), did not enhance performance even though muscle glycogen content increased significantly. They also provided carbohydrate (1 gram per kilogram body mass) during the exercise test and suggested that the availability of blood glucose during exercise may offset any detrimental effects on performance of lower pre-exercise muscle and liver glycogen concentrations. Additionally, the authors noted that carbohydrate loading may be effective in prolonged endurance events in which the exercise intensity is relatively more constant. In this study, the exercise task included repeated high-intensity sprints, which are common in cycling races but not in other events, such as marathon running. Additionally, the cyclists consumed more than 60 grams of carbohydrate per hour, which though recommended for runners as well, is often more difficult to do in running than cycling. Finally, the investigators also indicated that although the time to finish the 100-km ride (about 1.6 minutes faster with carbohydrate loading) was not statistically significant, such an effect, if real, could make a difference in the finishing order of top cyclists.

In contrast, a number of studies suggest that carbohydrate loading may be an effective technique to enhance endurance exercise performance. However, it should be noted that most of these studies have not used a true placebo, as was done in the aforementioned study by Burke and others.

Hargreaves and others note that the increased muscle glycogen associated with carbohydrate loading may be used more readily in exercise tasks approximating 65–70 percent VO_2 max, which might be a reasonable pace for an average runner competing in a marathon. If muscle glycogen were used more rapidly during the early stages of a marathon, theoretically carbohydrate loading would provide no advantage during the latter stages of the race. However, Bosch and others note that although carbohydrate loading may reduce the relative contribution of blood glucose to overall carbohydrate oxidation, the improved performance may be attributed to the initially greater amount of muscle glycogen as a means to spare the premature use of blood glucose and liver glycogen.

A supportive study was conducted by Clyde Williams in England. Male and female runners performed a 30-kilometer (18.6-mile) run on a treadmill and then were divided into two groups. One used a carbohydrate loading technique for a week, while the other group maintained their normal carbohydrate intake. Although there were no significant differences between the groups for overall performance time in the 30 kilometers, the carbohydrate loading group ran the last 5 kilometers significantly faster compared to their initial trial.

In another cycling study, Walker and others studied the effect of a carbohydrate loading and exercise tapering regimen in well-trained women on performance of a cycling test to exhaustion at 80 percent VO_2 max. The high-carbohydrate diet (approximately 78 percent carbohydrate), as compared to the moderate diet (approximately 48 percent carbohydrate), induced a 13 percent greater muscle glycogen content and an 8 percent improvement in cycling time.

Moreover, several field studies with runners and cross-country skiers have shown improved performances with carbohydrate loading. In general, carbohydrate loading, in contrast to a mixed diet, did not enable these athletes to go faster during the early stages of their events, but the high glycogen levels enabled them to perform longer at a given speed. The end result was an overall faster time. Failure to carbohydrate load has also been identified as one of the factors contributing to collapse of runners in an ultramarathon. Indeed, in a review, Peters noted that current evidence continues to support high carbohydrate intakes for ultraendurance athletes to increase muscle glycogen stores before the event.

Based on studies published prior to that of Burke and others, several major reviews support the performance-enhancing effectiveness of carbohydrate loading. Clyde Williams reported that an International Consensus Conference on sports nutrition concluded that the most significant influence on performance was the amount of carbohydrate stores in the athlete's body prior to heavy endurance exercise, which is the purpose of carbohydrate loading. Hawley and others concluded that carbohydrate loading would postpone fatigue in endurance events lasting more than 90 minutes and may improve performance in events where a set distance is covered as fast as possible, such as cycling and running, by about 2–3 percent according to some scientists. In their review, Williams and Lamb generally support these viewpoints relative to male athletes. However, they note that although carbohydrate loading can increase muscle glycogen stores in women, it appears to offer no benefit to their endurance performance; Tarnopolsky indicates that women oxidize more lipid and less carbohydrate compared to men during endurance exercise, a finding that may underlie this viewpoint.

Although carbohydrate loading may be an effective technique to enhance performance in prolonged aerobic endurance events, research suggests the most effective protocol is to carbohydrate load and use carbohydrate supplements during the event. Kang and others noted that this method can exert an additional ergogenic effect by preventing a decline in blood glucose levels and maintaining carbohydrate metabolism during the later stages of prolonged aerobic exercise. Given the findings of Burke and others, this method appears to be the most appropriate, as it will help provide increases in muscle glycogen before exercise as well as replenishment of blood glucose during exercise, two factors that may be associated with enhancement of endurance performance.

Are there any possible detrimental effects relative to carbohydrate loading?

From a performance standpoint, the extra body weight associated with the increased water content may be a disadvantage. In activities where moving the body weight is important, extra energy will be required to lift the extra 2–3 pounds of body water. However, in most performance events for which carbohydrate loading is advocated, the benefits from the energy aspects of the increased glycogen should more than offset the additional water weight. Moreover, if the individual is performing in a hot environment, the extra water, even small amounts, could be available as a source of sweat and may be helpful in controlling body temperature during exercise in the heat. Although one study suggested that the water stored with glycogen did not confer any advantage in regulation of body temperature while exercising in heat, the duration of the exercise, only 45 minutes, would not be sufficient to benefit from the increased water levels. Another study conducted in South

Africa revealed no beneficial or detrimental effects of carbohydrate loading on body temperature during 2.5 hours of exercise in a moderate environment (70° Fahrenheit; 21° Celsius). However, performance in longer exercise tasks with greater levels of water losses might be enhanced. Additional research is needed to study the potential effects of increased muscle glycogen levels on body water availability and temperature regulation during prolonged exercise under warm environmental conditions.

From a health standpoint, there may be some hazards to individuals with certain conditions. Although diabetics have been known to carbohydrate load, they should consult their physicians prior to using the technique. Individuals with high blood lipid or cholesterol levels might avoid the high-fat/high-protein diet phase of the depletion stage if, for some reason, they prefer the original, classic method of carbohydrate loading. Blood serum lipids and cholesterol have been reported to rise significantly during this phase. In addition, these individuals should eat mostly low-glycemic-index carbohydrates during the loading phase, because an increased intake of high-glycemic-index carbohydrates may raise blood lipid levels. Furthermore, hypoglycemia may occur during the high-fat/high-protein phase.

Several laboratory studies and one case study have reported electrocardiographic (ECG) abnormalities in individuals who used the classic carbohydrate loading technique. Although no cause-and-effect relationship was determined, these investigators speculated that hypoglycemia or glucose intolerance may be involved. In contrast, other well-controlled research with marathoners and typical joggers revealed no ECG changes following the classic method of carbohydrate loading.

Several investigators theorized that carbohydrate loading could lead to destruction of muscle fibers by excessive glycogen storage, but no data were presented to support their contentions. It appears that the muscle has a maximal capacity to store glycogen, approximately 4 grams/100 grams of muscle, and beyond that level excess carbohydrate would apparently be converted to fat and stored in adipose tissues.

Other potential problems with the high-carbohydrate phase are diarrhea, nausea, and cramping, particularly when the diet is changed drastically or large amounts of simple carbohydrates are consumed. Individuals who wish to carbohydrate load should experiment with such diets during their training and not just before competition.

In general, however, the recommended carbohydrate loading technique presented in table 4.9, which at the most is only a 7-day dietary regimen, poses no significant health hazards to the normally healthy individual.

Key Concepts

▶ Carbohydrate loading is not a technique for all types of athletes, but it may benefit athletes involved in long-distance competition such as marathoning.
▶ Various carbohydrate loading techniques may effectively increase muscle glycogen stores, but tapering exercise or rest and a high-carbohydrate diet are the essential points.

Carbohydrates: Ergogenic Aspects

Throughout this chapter you have learned that carbohydrate intake, in a variety of ways, may be used to enhance physical performance. Truly, carbohydrates represent one of our most important ergogenic nutrients. In this brief section we shall look at several forms of carbohydrate that might possess ergogenic properties. Additionally, numerous carbohydrate-based products, such as the sports "energy" drinks, have been marketed to athletes and many contain purported ergogenic substances, such as caffeine, ephedrine, and amino acids. These specific nutritional ergogenics will be discussed in later chapters where appropriate.

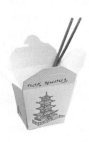

Do the metabolic by-products of carbohydrate exert an ergogenic effect?

Recall that the primary mechanism in the transformation of muscle glycogen into energy is glycolysis. The end product during aerobic metabolism is normally pyruvate. However, glycolysis leading to the formation of pyruvate involves production of a number of metabolic by-products in a chain of about a dozen sequential steps, each step being controlled by an enzyme (see appendix G, figure G.1). One theory of fatigue is that if one of these steps is blocked by inactivation of an enzyme, glycolysis may not continue at an optimal rate, since a necessary metabolic by-product may be in short supply. This blocked step could represent a weak link in the chain, possibly reducing the formation of pyruvate and subsequent ATP production. Pyruvate has been studied as a potential ergogenic aid, as have other metabolic by-products of carbohydrate metabolism.

Pyruvate Pyruvate is a three-carbon metabolic by-product of glycolysis. Although the mechanism of its underlying potential as an ergogenic aid is unknown, pyruvate is theorized to accelerate the Krebs cycle or use glucose more efficiently, both of which could enhance exercise performance. DHAP is a combination of pyruvate and dihydroxyacetone, another three-carbon metabolic by-product of glycolysis.

Pyruvate administered alone has been used in attempts to decrease body fat and increase muscle mass, possibly by speeding up Krebs cycle activity. Kalman and others also reported a significant decrease in body weight and fat mass in healthy, overweight men and women following 6 weeks of pyruvate supplementation (6 grams per day). Ostojic and Ahmetovic had healthy male soccer players supplement their diets with 4 grams of pyruvate for 4 weeks and found no impact on body mass, fat mass, or muscle mass. No exercise performance data were reported from these studies. Although these findings may be important to the obese, they may not be applicable to the healthy, nonobese, well-trained individual as a means of shedding additional body fat for sports competition.

Research investigating the ergogenic effect of pyruvate supplementation is very limited and generally has not shown any beneficial effects on exercise performance in either untrained or trained subjects. Koh-Banerjee and others studied the effects of supplementation with calcium pyruvate (5 grams daily for 30 days) on body composition and metabolic responses to submaximal and maximal exercise in untrained females undertaking exercise training. No beneficial effects were noted. In a double-blind, crossover study, Morrison and others found that pyruvate supplementation (7 grams/day for one week) did not enhance cycle time to exhaustion in well-trained male cyclists in an aerobic endurance test. According to Kreider and others, the International Society of Sports Nutrition has included calcium pyruvate in the category of apparently not effective and/or dangerous. This is attributed to the lack of evidence that ingesting the amount typically found in pyruvate supplements has any positive effect on body composition and on some blood lipids. In a recent review, Onakpoya and colleagues concluded that the evidence to show that pyruvate supplementation can help reduce body weight is not convincing. Additionally, they noted limited available evidence on the safety of pyruvate supplementation but that there are reports of adverse effects such as gas, bloating, diarrhea, and increased low-density lipoprotein (LDL) cholesterol. At this time, pyruvate supplementation would not be recommended.

Previous studies with animals have shown that DHAP increases muscle glycogen content, so Ronald Stanko and his associates at the University of Pittsburgh investigated the potential ergogenic effect of DHAP in humans. Two studies were conducted, both using untrained males as subjects. The dosage of DHAP in both studies was 100 grams per day for 7 days; DHAP was prepared in a 3:1 ratio of dihydroxyacetone (75 g) to sodium pyruvate (25 g) and administered either in Jello or artificially sweetened fluids. The placebo in both studies was 100 grams of Polycose, a carbohydrate. The DHAP or Polycose was substituted for a portion of the carbohydrate in the diet. Both studies were well designed, using a double-blind, placebo, repeated-measures crossover approach. In the first study, the diet was standardized at 55 percent carbohydrate of the daily caloric intake. The criterion test was an arm ergometer exercise task to exhaustion at 60 percent VO_2 peak following a week of supplementation. DHAP significantly increased endurance time, attributed primarily to an increased muscle glycogen concentration and increased extraction of blood glucose, both factors providing more glucose to the exercising muscle. In the second experiment, subjects consumed a high-carbohydrate diet (70 percent of the daily caloric intake). The criterion test was a cycle ergometer exercise task to exhaustion at 70 percent VO_2 peak. DHAP improved performance in an identical fashion to the first study, the effect being attributed to increased blood glucose extraction by the exercising muscle. The results of these two well-controlled studies indicate an ergogenic effect of DHAP with untrained subjects, but confirming data are needed with well-trained athletes.

Lactate Salts As noted previously, lactic acid is a metabolic by-product of anaerobic glycolysis. We also indicated that although lactic acid is often associated with fatigue, most sport scientists theorize it is the hydrogen ion release that increases the acidity and impairs performance, not the lactate itself. Lactate is actually a small metabolite of glucose; its formula is $C_3H_5O_3$, about half of that of glucose, $C_6H_{12}O_6$. Thus, lactate still possesses considerable energy and, as Van Hall noted, may be converted back to pyruvate to enter the energy pathway in the skeletal muscles. Lactate may also be converted back to glucose by the liver.

Various lactate supplements have been studied as a means to enhance endurance performance. For example, Cytomax™ is a sports drink that contains lactate in a patented form, alpha-L-Polylactate. Cytomax™ also contains fructose, glucose, and a glucose polymer.

In an early study, Fahey and others investigated the effect of polylactate (80 percent polylactate, 20 percent sodium lactate, in 7 percent solution with water), a glucose polymer, and an artificially sweetened placebo on various psychological, physiological, and metabolic parameters during cycling at 50 percent of VO_2 max for 3 hours. The fluids were consumed 5 minutes before exercise and at 20-minute intervals during exercise. There were no differences between treatments in perceived exertion, lactate, heart rate, oxygen consumption, rectal temperature, or selected skin temperatures.

Moreover, Fred Brouns and his colleagues at Maastricht in the Netherlands reported that 3 weeks of supplementation with oral lactate salts did not influence the removal of lactate during and following exercise, suggesting no value to lactate supplementation in this regard. Bryner and others compared the effects of four sports drinks (2 percent lactate; 8 percent carbohydrate; 2 percent lactate/8 percent carbohydrate combination; placebo) on performance in a cycle ergometer exercise test to exhaustion that also incorporated a 30-second Wingate cycle power test. Subjects consumed 100 grams of carbohydrate several hours before the test, and then consumed the sport drinks during the test. There were no significant differences among the sports drinks for endurance time, peak power, glucose, insulin, or blood pH, indicating that lactate supplementation, either alone or in combination with carbohydrate, provided no advantage over carbohydrate alone.

More recently, Azevedo and others compared the effects of Cytomax™ with a leading sports drink (containing glucose and fructose) on performance of experienced cyclists. In a crossover study, the subjects consumed either drink both before and during the cycling task, which consisted of cycling at 62 percent VO_2 peak for 90 minutes, followed by high-intensity cycling to exhaustion at 86 percent VO_2 peak. The investigators reported that lactate was used more rapidly and to a greater extent than fructose or glucose, and endurance time with Cytomax™ more so than other sports drinks was 25 percent longer in the high-intensity cycling test.

Based on the current data, it would appear that lactate preparations may provide additional energy, somewhat comparable to carbohydrate sources. The preliminary research findings showing a more ergogenic effect of Cytomax™ over other sports drinks need confirmation from other research laboratories.

Ribose Ribose is a 5-carbon monosaccharide found throughout body cells as part of various compounds, such as RNA (ribonucleic acid) in the cell nucleus. Ribose also comprises the sugar portion of adenosine, the nucleotide found in ATP (adenosine triphosphate). ATP, as you recall, is the immediate source of energy for muscle contraction, both in the heart and in skeletal muscles.

Although found in nature, very little ribose is consumed in a natural diet. Instead, a specific metabolic pathway (pentose phosphate pathway) produces ribose from glucose to meet our body needs. Recently, ribose supplements (made from corn sugar) have been marketed to physically active individuals as a means to promote faster recovery in heart and skeletal muscles, presumably by facilitating the formation of adenosine, one of the major components of ATP.

Research indicates that strenuous exercise may necessitate rapid recovery of adenosine within muscle cells, which might benefit from adequate ribose. Pliml and others found that ribose ingestion (60 grams daily for 3 days) improved exercise performance time in patients with severe coronary artery disease, while other studies have suggested that ribose, when supplemented, could serve as an energy source and promote adenosine synthesis in various patient groups.

The effect of ribose supplementation has been evaluated using healthy, physically active individuals and athletes. Several studies used an acute supplementation protocol. Kerksick and others reported that 3 grams of ribose, provided to moderately trained male cyclists about 25 minutes prior to exercise, had no effect on five maximal 30-second anaerobic capacity cycling tests with a 3-minute recovery. In a crossover study, Peveler and others also found no effect of an acute 625-milligram dose of ribose on peak power, mean power, or rate of fatigue in three intermittent 30-second Wingate tests of anaerobic capacity in healthy males.

Research using chronic supplementation of ribose also does not support an ergogenic effect. Berardi and Ziegenfuss studied the effect of oral ribose supplementation (32 grams over a 36-hour period) on high-intensity, intermittent, anaerobic cycle ergometer performance; the exercise task consisted of six 10-second sprints with a 60-second recovery. They concluded that ribose supplementation does not have a consistent or substantial effect on anaerobic cycle sprinting as evaluated by peak and mean power output. Hellsten and others reported that 3 days of ribose supplementation (based on body weight, approximately 45 grams daily) elicited a greater resynthesis of ATP compared to the placebo. However, the slight increase in ATP availability did not enhance performance, as there were no differences between the placebo and ribose supplement for mean and peak power outputs. The authors note that a small reduction in muscle ATP does not appear to limit high-intensity exercise performance. In a well-designed study, Op 'T Eijnde and others evaluated the effect of oral ribose supplementation (16 grams/day for days) on two maximal knee-extension exercise protocols and ATP recovery. The exercise bouts were separated by a 60-minute rest period. They concluded that oral ribose supplementation had no effect on maximal intermittent exercise performance or ATP recovery. In the longest supplementation protocol, Dunne and others compared the effects of ribose or dextrose (10 grams each before and after practice) supplementation for weeks on 2,000-meter rowing performance in female collegiate rowers. Over the course of the 8 weeks, performance in both groups improved, but the dextrose group (about 10 seconds faster) showed significantly more improvement at 8 weeks than the ribose group. The investigators thought that the ribose did not impair performance, but the dextrose simply may have elicited a greater improvement. In their review, Dhanoa and Housner note that although ribose manufacturers claim it provides an ergogenic benefit, scientific research does not support this claim.

Current data do not support an ergogenic effect of ribose supplementation.

Multiple Carbohydrate By-Products Sports supplements manufacturers often combine multiple nutrients in a single supplement on the theory that each may exhibit an ergogenic effect, but the effect will be amplified with multiple components. Limited research is available with multiple by-products of carbohydrate metabolism, but Brown and others investigated the ergogenic potential of a multinutrient supplement composed primarily of intermediates of the Krebs cycle, which may be derived from carbohydrate, fat, or protein. Three weeks of supplementation did not improve cycling time to exhaustion at approximately 70–75 percent VO_2 max, nor did it improve the rate of recovery.

Key Concept

▶ Metabolic by-products of carbohydrate metabolism have been tested as ergogenics. Most have been found to be ineffective, although research with physically trained individuals is limited with several purported ergogenic products.

Check for Yourself

▶ Go to a health food store that sells sports supplements and ask the clerk for carbohydrate products, including metabolites, that may help you train or compete more effectively. Evaluate the supplement fact labels for content and performance claims. What is your judgment?

Dietary Carbohydrates: Health Implications

Although improving somewhat, the diet of the typical American and Canadian still appears to be unbalanced. In general, we consume too many Calories for the level of physical activity we do, and we eat too much of the unhealthy fats and carbohydrates. Such a diet may pose several health problems. As we shall see in chapter 5,

excessive consumption of total and saturated fat appears to be of major concern relative to the development of several chronic diseases. In this section, we discuss the health aspects of dietary carbohydrates. In general, the health effects associated with various sugars and starches is not in the substances themselves, but rather in the nutrients that accompany them in the foods we eat. For example, sugar in orange juice is little different from sugar in a soda, but the orange juice contains substantial amounts of vitamin C, potassium, and other nutrients, whereas the soda has none unless fortified. Whole grains contain more fiber and more of some micronutrients than refined grains.

In the recent past, low-carbohydrate diets have been all the rage. As shall be noted in chapter 10, research has indicated that such diets may have some health benefits, but these health benefits appear to be attributed more to decreased caloric intake than to diet composition. The pendulum, rightfully so, has shifted toward a diet rich in carbohydrate, specifically healthier carbohydrate choices.

Nutritional objectives in *Healthy People 2020* and in the *2010 Dietary Guidelines for Americans* recommend that we consume more grains, making whole grains half of all grains consumed. We should also reduce the consumption of refined carbohydrates and added sugars, often referred to as *bad carbs*. Although no foods, or carbohydrates, are inherently good or bad, following these two general guidelines may produce some significant health benefits. Additionally, an appropriate exercise program may have a healthful influence on carbohydrate metabolism.

How do refined sugars and starches affect my health?

As noted previously, sugars may be found naturally in foods, or they may be manufactured from starches, such as high-fructose corn syrup, and added to foods. Refined starches are predominant in many foods, such as white bread, pasta, and rice. Consumption of refined sugars and starches in excess may be associated with various health risks, attributed mainly to their high glycemic index.

Dental Caries One of the most common health problems that has been associated with dietary sugar is tooth decay, or dental caries. However, the National Institutes of Health, in its consensus statement on management of dental caries throughout life, noted that effective preventive practice involves a number of factors, including proper oral hygiene (brushing, flossing, use of fluoride) and dietary modifications (use of sugarless products). Tooth decay is not necessarily a matter of how much sugar one eats, but in what form and how often. Dental erosion is increasing and is associated with dietary acids, a major source of which is soft drinks. Sticky, chewy, sugary foods eaten often between meals increase the risk of developing dental caries. Starchy foods that adhere to teeth, such as bread, are also cariogenic. Such foods may increase the presence of dental plaque, which may lead to periodontal infection. Seymour and others cite epidemiological research supporting a relationship between periodontal infection and various systemic diseases, such as coronary heart disease, stroke, and diabetes. The infection may lead to systemic inflammation, which may induce adverse effects, such as atherosclerosis. Seymour and others indicate that the control of oral disease is essential in the prevention and management of these systemic conditions.

Of particular interest to athletes, von Fraunhofer and Rogers reported far greater enamel dissolution in flavored and energy (sports) drinks than previously noted for water. They noted that sipping sports drinks over long periods of time may erode tooth enamel; therefore, drink quickly. In contrast, Mathew and others reported no relationship between consumption of sports drinks and dental erosion in university athletes. Nevertheless, scientists have developed a prototype sports drink, containing substantial amounts of calcium and maltodextrins, which is alleged to cause less dental enamel erosion than the typical commercial sports drink.

Chronic Diseases Over the years, dietary intake of refined sugar has been alleged to contribute to a wide variety of health problems, including obesity, diabetes, heart disease, and cancer, as well as various psychological afflictions such as hyperactivity in children, premenstrual syndrome (PMS), and seasonal affective disorder (SAD). Such allegations have been based mainly on theoretical considerations, but with support from some recent epidemiological studies. A habitual diet rich in high-glycemic-index foods theoretically may lead to insulin resistance and high serum triglyceride levels, risk factors for diabetes and heart disease, respectively. This may be especially so in individuals who are obese, and will be discussed in detail in chapter 10. Bantle also indicated that fructose, which is a low-glycemic-index sugar, may increase serum triglycerides and may be a contributing factor to obesity. Individuals should avoid high-fructose corn syrup, but eating fruits with naturally occurring fructose is not a cause for concern. Added sugars can increase caloric intake and predispose to obesity.

As a part of the National Health and Nutrition Examination Survey (NHANES 2003–2006) of 4,258 healthy adults, fructose intake was calculated and blood pressure was directly measured. Jalal and colleagues determined a median fructose intake of 74 g/d (equivalent to 2.5 sugary soft drinks per day). They also found this fructose intake to be associated with a 26, 30, and 77 percent higher risk for blood pressure values of $\geq 135/85$, $\geq 140/90$, and $>160/100$ mmHg, respectively. Fung and others conducted a 24-year follow-up with the Nurses' Health Study cohort and identified a significant positive association between sugar-sweetened beverage intake and coronary heart disease risk.

High sugar intake has been associated with development of cancer. Two large epidemiological studies by Larsson and Stattin and their associates found that increased consumption of sugar and high-sugar foods, particularly sugar-sweetened sodas, increases the risk of pancreatic cancer. The increased sugar intake may cause the pancreas to produce more insulin, which may cause hyperinsulinemia and increased insulin-like growth factor, factors that may stimulate cell division in the pancreas and lead to cancer.

Additionally, as discussed previously, a high-carbohydrate diet can affect the fTRP:BCAA ratio and formation of the neurotransmitter serotonin. Serotonin may influence mood and behavior associated with PMS and SAD or other psychological states.

The National Academy of Sciences, in its DRI recommendations for carbohydrate, noted that, given the currently available scientific evidence relative to the effect of dietary sugar on dental caries, psychological behavior, cancer, risk of obesity, and risk of hyperlipidemia, there is insufficient evidence to set a UL for total or added sugar in the diet. Nevertheless, the Academy noted that the theory linking a high glycemic index to certain health problems, such as diabetes and CHD, appears to be valid and supported by some studies, but the evidence at this time appears to be insufficient to substantiate the theory. Furthermore, the Academy noted that individuals who consume excess amounts of added sugars may not obtain sufficient amounts of various micronutrients, and that this may lead to adverse health effects. Johnson and others, in the American Heart Association scientific statement on dietary sugars intake and cardiovascular health, recommend an upper limit of half the discretionary Calorie allowance from added sugars. For most American women, this is no more than 100 Calories per day, and for most American men it is no more than 150 Calories per day from added sugars.

Given these considerations, and the fact that many health organizations recommend a reduced intake of refined sugars to about 10 percent or less of the daily caloric intake, it appears to be prudent to moderate your consumption of refined sugars and starches.

Suggestions to decrease intake of refined starches and sugars were presented in chapter 2.

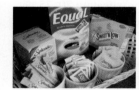 **Are artificial sweeteners safe?**

Artificial sweeteners are products designed to provide sweetness but little or no Calories. Theoretically, these sweeteners could be used to reduce intake of refined sugars, but as Liebman noted, the consumption of both artificial sweeteners and refined sugars has increased over the past ten years. A number of artificial sweeteners have been produced and approved, and they have been incorporated into foods, dietary supplements, sports nutrition products, energy drinks, and diet products. Table 4.11 provides a list of artificial sweeteners currently approved for use in the United States. Acesulfame-K is a naturally occurring potassium salt; Advantame is derived from aspartame and vanillin; Aspartame is made from the two amino acids aspartic acid and phenylalanine; Neotame is derived from the same amino acids; Saccharin is a non-caloric derivative of coal tar; *Siraitia grosvenorii* is an extract of Swingle fruit (also known as Luo Han Guo or monk fruit); Stevia is a derivative of the plant *Stevia rebaudiana;* and Sucralose is produced by altering the sugar molecule with chlorine.

Some artificial sweeteners have Calories (for instance, Aspartame has 4 Calories per gram); however, the amount typically consumed to provide the desired sweetness usually reduces the Calories to near zero per serving. Artificial sweeteners are ubiquitous and are often combined with natural sugars to provide sweetness with fewer Calories. For example, Coca-Cola markets Coca-Cola Life, a reduced-sugar soda that is partially sweetened with Stevia; Chobani markets several flavors of reduced-Calorie yogurts in its Simply 100 series that are flavored with Stevia; and Arnold Whole Wheat Sandwich thins also contain Stevia.

Each of these sweeteners has undergone the necessary safety testing to be approved by the US government; however, some still question the safety. As new artificial sweeteners are developed and incorporated into foods, sports nutrition, low-calorie, and low-carbohydrate products, and because the use and approval of artificial sweeteners differ between countries, it is wise for consumers to consult with a regulatory body for the most up-to-date information. The interested reader should consult the website of the United States Food and Drug Administration www.fda.gov) and search under the food additives section. Here one can easily find currently approved artificial sweeteners, a summary of available safety data, acceptable daily intake (ADI) levels, and whom to contact to report adverse effects.

Sugar alcohols, which are mentioned early in the text, are another class of sweeteners. Common examples include sorbitol, xylitol, mannitol, and maltitol, but there are several others. The sweetness of sugar alcohols varies from one-quarter to one-half as sweet as sugar up to about the same sweetness as sugar. Sugar alcohols do contain energy, about 1.5 to 2.5 Calories per gram, but cause a smaller increase on blood glucose, which is why they are often found in diabetic candies, gums, and sugarfree chocolate.

Sugar alcohols are only partially digested and metabolized and can lead to flatulence, diarrhea, and other gastrointestinal symptoms or discomfort. While these issues are typically associated with high intakes of sugar alcohols, some athletes may inadvertently consume large amounts of sugar alcohols because they are unaware that they are used in a wide variety of sports nutrition and diet products. For instance, on a given day, an athlete may consume chewable vitamin C with breakfast and have a low-carbohydrate protein bar as a snack, a low-sugar energy drink before a workout, and a protein shake postworkout. Chewable vitamins, low-carbohydrate sports bars, low-sugar energy drinks, and protein powders often contain several artificial sweeteners and sugar alcohols to make them more palatable. Athletes are encouraged to read labels closely to identify sugar alcohols and to avoid intake prior to or during competition. One helpful tip is to search labels for the term "net carbohydrates." For example, the EAS Advantage Carb Control Bar contains 26 grams of carbohydrate with 2 to 4 grams of "net carbs." This product contains 26 grams of carbohydrate as 5 grams of fiber, 2 grams of sugar, and 19 grams of sugar alcohols. Although this product is marketed as a snack or meal replacement, an athlete who ingests 10 to 20 grams of sugar alcohols per day may experience gastrointestinal distress. In terms of sweeteners, the product contains maltitol syrup, fructo-oligosaccharides, maltitol, xylitol, and sucralose.

The Academy of Nutrition and Dietetics has published a position stand on non-nutritive sweeteners. Perhaps the most hotly debated question about artificial sweeteners at this point in time is do they increase appetite or body weight? In the position stand, Fitch and Keim did not find evidence to suggest that non-nutritive/artificial sweeteners cause weight gain or increased appetite, but many questions remain to be answered.

TABLE 4.11   Artificial sweeteners approved for use in the United States

Name	Brand name	Times sweeter than sugar	Acceptable daily intake in packets per day
Acesulfame-K	Sunett® Sweet One®	200	165
Advantame	*	20,000	4,000
Aspartame	Equal® NutraSweet®	200	165
Neotame	Newtame®	7,000–13,000	200
Saccharin	Sweet and Low® Sweet Twin® Sweet'N Low® Necta Sweet®	200–700	250
Siraitia grosvenorii Swingle (Luo Han Guo) fruit extracts (SGFE)	Nectresse® Monk Fruit in the Raw® PureLo®	100–250	Not determined
Stevia Certain high purity steviol glycosides purified from *Stevia rebaudiana* leaves	Truvia	200–400	29
Sucralose	Splenda®	600	165

*No brand name yet.

Source:Table adapted from summary table of high-intensity sweeteners at: http://www.fda.gov/Food/IngredientsPackagingLabeling/FoodAdditivesIngredients/ucm397725.htm.

Why are complex carbohydrates thought to be beneficial to my health?

To increase consumption of total carbohydrate in the diet while reducing the consumption of refined sugars, one must increase the consumption of complex carbohydrates. Some diet plans developed for health, such as the Pritikin program, recommend that 80 percent of the dietary Calories be supplied by carbohydrates, mostly complex and unrefined. More recently, the OmniHeart diet focused on healthy carbohydrates, fats, and proteins. The OmniHeart diet plan includes the following tips for increasing consumption of healthier carbohydrates:

- Eat 1–2 servings of fruit at every meal and have an extra fruit at breakfast.
- Have 2–3 servings of vegetables at lunch and dinner.
- Create a fruit and nut trail mix for snacks: ¼ cup dried fruit with 1 oz. unsalted nuts.
- Use whole grains rather than refined grains as often as possible.
- Select legumes for a carbohydrate and protein source several times a week.

A diet rich in complex carbohydrates may reduce the percentage contribution from fats if excessive, which may confer significant health benefits, as noted in chapter 5. Complex carbohydrates are found primarily in starchy vegetables, whole grains, and legumes, but small amounts are also found in fruits.

Whole-grain products are one of the best sources of healthy carbohydrates. As defined by the FDA, whole grains contain all three ingredients of a cereal grain, namely the outer bran and the inner germ and endosperm, and in the same proportion as found in nature (see figure 4.13). Seal noted that an increasing body of evidence from both epidemiological and prospective studies supports an inverse relationship between consumption of whole-grain foods and risk of coronary heart disease. For example, Djoussé and Gaziano found that those who ate the most whole-grain cereals over the course of the week had the greatest reduction in risk of heart failure. Over the course of approximately 20 years, those who consumed no whole-grain cereals weekly had a relative risk (RR) of heart failure of 1.0; those who consumed 2–6 servings weekly had an RR of 0.79, and those who consumed 7 or more servings had an RR of 0.71, which represents about a 22–28 percent lower risk of heart failure.

When shopping, look for products labeled 100% Whole Wheat or 100% Whole Grains. Products labeled 100% wheat, multigrain, or stone ground may be made primarily from refined grains. The first ingredient listed should be whole oats, whole rye, whole wheat, or other whole grains such as brown rice, bulgur, or oatmeal. Many vitamins, minerals, phytonutrients, antioxidants, and fiber may be lost in processing of whole grain to refined grain. Some, but not all, may be replaced during processing, so you may not get the synergistic health effects of the multiple nutrients. In your efforts to increase fiber intake, look at the 10 Tips to Help You Eat Whole Grains on the www.ChooseMyPlate.gov site.

Current thinking supports the concept that the beneficial health effects of a diet rich in complex carbohydrates, which may be considered to be a low-glycemic-index diet, may be linked to several

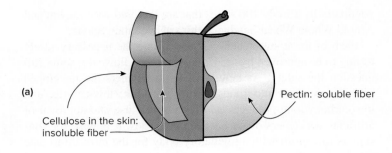

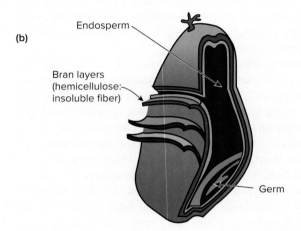

FIGURE 4.13 Various forms of fiber. (a) The skin of an apple consists of the insoluble fiber cellulose, which provides structure for the fruit. The soluble fiber pectin "glues" the fruit cells together. (b) The outside layer of a wheat kernel is made of layers of bran—insoluble fiber—making this grain a good source of fiber. Fruits, vegetables, whole grains, and legumes such as beans are rich in fiber.

important attributes of such a diet, including the collective presence of various phytochemicals, vitamins, minerals, and dietary fiber. The health benefits of phytochemicals were discussed in chapter 2, while the benefits of vitamins and minerals will be covered in chapters 7 and 8. Most research relative to the healthful benefits of complex carbohydrates has focused on dietary fiber.

Why should I eat foods rich in fiber?

The current AI recommendation by the National Academy of Sciences for total fiber has been set at 14 grams per 1,000 Calories, or 38 grams for men and 25 grams for women up to age 50 and slightly lower amounts thereafter. Recall that total fiber consists of both dietary fiber and functional fiber, and various specific forms of fiber are found in each category; some specific forms of fiber may be classified as both dietary and functional fiber. Although the Academy indicates that specific forms of fiber have properties that result in different physiological effects that may impact health, it did not feel that the evidence was sufficient to establish separate recommendations for each type of fiber. Nevertheless, some feel that the use of the water-solubility classifications system, as discussed previously, might be useful conceptually to illustrate the potential health benefits of certain forms of fiber. As noted earlier, dietary fiber is found naturally in various plant foods.

Exactly how dietary fiber may be protective is not known, but several mechanisms have been proposed that may help in the prevention of certain forms of cancer, coronary heart disease, obesity, diabetes, hypertension, and various disorders of the gastrointestinal tract. Here are some of the theories relative to the potential health benefits of total fiber:

1. Water-insoluble fibers are considered to be those with the greatest effect on fecal bulk. Adding bulk to the contents of the large intestine stimulates peristalsis and speeds up the transit time of food through the intestines. The increased bulk has been shown to dilute any possible cancer-causing (carcinogens) that might attack cell walls, while faster transit diminishes the time carcinogens may have to act. Increased bulk—and peristalsis—also decreases the incidence rate of diverticulitis, an inflammatory disorder in the large intestine that may cause rupture, leading to serious complications.

2. Fiber-rich foods are low-glycemic-index foods, and they may increase insulin sensitivity and prevention of weight gain. Fiber slows down gastric (stomach) emptying and thereby slows glucose absorption in the small intestine. The high viscosity of soluble fiber also decreases intestinal absorption. These effects may lead to better control of blood sugar and may lengthen the sensation of fullness, or satiety, which may be important to individuals on weight-loss diets. Fiber-rich diets are frequently lower in fat and added sugars, and thus contain fewer Calories. So high-fiber diets may be useful in the prevention or treatment of obesity and obesity-related chronic diseases such as diabetes and hypertension.

3. Fiber, particularly gummy forms of water-soluble fiber such as beta-glucans in oats, may bind with various substances in the gastrointestinal tract. Soluble fiber may bind with carcinogens so that they are excreted by the bowel. Soluble fibers may also bind with and lead to the excretion of bile salts, which contain cholesterol; normally bile salts are reabsorbed into the body, but excretion of bile salts, along with their cholesterol content, may help reduce serum cholesterol levels. This effect may decrease the risk of coronary heart disease. (Lower serum cholesterol levels decrease the risk of atherosclerosis, a major cause of heart disease.)

4. Some water-soluble fibers may be fermented in the large intestine to form short-chain fatty acids (SCFAs). Zeng and others noted that several of these SCFAs are theorized to help prevent gastrointestinal disorders, cancer, and cardiovascular disease. Some act in the colon; others are absorbed into the blood, are delivered to the liver, and may help decrease synthesis of cholesterol.

Although it may be illustrative to view the health benefits of fiber based on its water solubility, Joanne Slavin, a scholar on the health effects of dietary fiber, notes that it is difficult to generalize as to the physiological effects of fiber based on this classification system. For example, she notes that rice bran, which is devoid of soluble fiber, has been shown to reduce serum cholesterol, while recent research has also supported the effect of insoluble fiber to reduce the risk of heart disease. Thus, health benefits may be attributable to total fiber.

Numerous studies, including major epidemiological studies and clinical trials, have investigated the effect of total fiber on reducing the risk or incidence of chronic diseases. Based on these studies, the National Academy of Sciences established the AI for total fiber because it may reduce the risk of coronary heart disease, and more recent research supports this concept.

The Academy cited studies showing a beneficial effect of total fiber and a low-glycemic-index diet on other health problems, particularly in individuals with diabetes or hyperlipidemia, but the evidence was not as convincing as that for prevention of heart disease.

Although there is not complete consistency in the research, a large number of studies demonstrate beneficial effects of a diet that is high in fiber. In terms of the effects of dietary fiber on mortality, in the most important meta-analysis to date, Yang and colleagues analyzed 17 prospective studies that included 982,411 individuals. When comparing persons with dietary fiber intakes in the top third with persons whose intakes were in the bottom third, there was a 16 percent decrease in risk of mortality. Further, for every 10 grams/day increase in dietary fiber intake, there was a 10 percent reduction in mortality risk. There are many other meta-analytical reviews that demonstrate the benefits of dietary fiber. For instance, as recently reported in a meta-analysis by Kim and Je, cereal and vegetable, but not fruit, fiber intake was associated with reduced risk of mortality. In their meta-analysis, Threapleton and colleagues reported that dietary fiber intake from cereal and vegetable sources was associated with lower risk of cardiovascular and coronary heart disease, while fruit fiber intake was associated with decreased risk of cardiovascular disease. In a meta-analysis of randomized controlled trials of patients with type 2 diabetes, Silva and others reported that high-fiber diets (from food or supplement sources) reduced glycated hemoglobin and fasting blood glucose. The authors acknowledged that increased fiber intake improved glycemic control and should be considered in the treatment of type diabetes. In their systematic review and meta-analysis, Aune and co-authors reported that at least 2 servings of whole grains per day should be consumed to reduce the risk of type 2 diabetes. In this analysis, a decreased risk was associated with whole-grain intake, while an increased risk was found for refined grains such as white rice. In a systematic review and meta-analysis, Aune and colleagues reported that a high intake of dietary fiber was associated with decreased risk of colon cancer but that future research should include information on fiber subtypes. As Clark and Slavin have indicated, dietary fiber intake is associated with a lower body weight in many epidemiological studies. However, the majority of studies that investigate the effects of fiber intake on satiety or food intake do not support an effect.

Even though there may be debate over the usefulness of the glycemic index as a means to design a healthful diet for chronic diseases other than heart disease, consuming a fiber-rich diet is certainly prudent dietary behavior, given that coronary heart disease is the number one cause of death in Western societies. And although the National Academy of Sciences indicates that the relationship of fiber intake to other health problems is the subject of ongoing investigation and currently unresolved, there appear to be no adverse health effects associated with a fiber-rich or low-glycemic-index diet. Indeed, a fiber-rich diet may be useful for other possible health benefits.

Prevention of colon cancer has been one of the main theories underlying the promotion of a high-fiber diet. Rock has indicated that the relationship between dietary fiber intake and colorectal cancer has been inconsistent. However, she noted that no significant relationship between fiber intake (or major food sources of fiber) and risk for colorectal cancer was observed in a recently reported, large, pooled analysis of several studies. Nevertheless, she notes limitations in epidemiological studies and indicates that the effect of increased dietary fiber intake on risk for colorectal cancer has not been adequately addressed in studies conducted to date. More research, including longer-term trials and higher levels of fiber intake, is needed to increase knowledge in this area.

As the different types of fiber appear to convey health benefits in different ways, a balanced intake of total fiber appears to be the best approach. The Academy notes that although the AI are based on total fiber, the greatest health benefits may come from the ingestion of cereal fibers and various viscous fibers, including gums and pectins, which are found in fruits and vegetables. Obtaining 25–38 grams of fiber daily is not difficult, but you have to eat more whole grains, fruits, vegetables, and legumes. Total fiber is listed on food labels. In particular, check food labels on breads and cereals, staples of the daily diet. According to the *2010 Dietary Guidelines for Americans,* although Americans eat adequate amounts of total grains, most of these come from refined sources rather than whole grains. Additionally, on average Americans eat less than 1 ounce-equivalent of whole grains per day, and less than 5 percent consume the minimum amount of whole grains. Refined grains contain little or no fiber, whereas whole grains are usually rich in fiber. Some brands of bread contain 3 grams of fiber per slice, and only 50 Calories. Breakfast cereals may also be very high in fiber, some containing 10 or more grams per serving.

Here are some suggestions from *Consumer Reports on Health* for ten easy ways to eat more fiber:

- Look for "good sources" of fiber (~3 grams per serving).
- Choose whole grains (100 percent whole wheat or 100 percent whole grain).
- Start the day right (oatmeal or a high-fiber cereal).
- Choose fiber-filled snacks (raw carrots or celery, popcorn, or fiber-rich crackers).
- Drink it up (blend chunks of fruit or vegetables with yogurt, juice, or soy milk).
- Look for fiber-fortified pastas.
- Don't forget legumes (add beans or lentils).
- Keep the skin on (wash but don't peel skins of fruits and vegetables).
- Bake it in (add crushed bran cereal or flax or sesame seeds to baked items).
- Consider a supplement (if foods are not enough).

According to one physician, a good way to see if you are eating enough fiber is to observe the buoyancy of your stool in the toilet.

It should float, or at least appear flaky and break apart. If it sinks or does not break apart, you are not eating enough fiber.

There appear to be few or no health disadvantages to a high-fiber diet. As we shall see in chapter 8, there has been some concern that high-fiber diets could lead to increased losses of certain minerals, such as iron and zinc, but research has shown that such concerns are generally unwarranted if one follows the recommendations just given.

Schneeman, discussing development of a scientific consensus on the importance of dietary fiber, notes that fiber serves as a marker for diets rich in plant foods, which provide additional benefits for maintaining health. Liebman notes that it is important to recognize that the health benefits attributed to dietary fiber may be associated with the form in which the fiber is consumed—as part of a whole, natural food containing other potential health-promoting nutrients such as vitamins and phytochemicals, rather than by consumption of a purified supplement form. This is in accord with the position stand of the American Dietetic Association, written by Marlett and others, on dietary fiber. Get more plant foods in your diet!

Do some carbohydrate foods cause food intolerance?

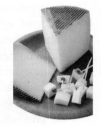

About one in nine Americans may develop gastrointestinal distress when they consume dairy products containing substantial amounts of lactose, particularly milk. African-Americans are more likely to suffer lactose intolerance. Such individuals lack the enzyme lactase and hence cannot metabolize lactose in the digestive tract. The most common symptoms of **lactose intolerance** are gas, bloating, abdominal pain, and diarrhea, although headache and fatigue may also occur.

Individuals may be diagnosed as being lactose intolerant through a lactose tolerance test administered by a physician. A self-detection technique may be an effective approach. If you experience problems such as gas and diarrhea after consuming milk, abstain from all dairy products for 2 weeks and then evaluate the results. If the symptoms resolve, and then reoccur when you resume dairy food consumption, you may need to reduce the amount of lactose in your diet. Unfortunately, usually this means a reduced intake of dairy foods, which are considered to be the main dietary source of not only lactose but calcium as well. Di Stefano and others indicated that lactose intolerance may prevent the achievement of adequate peak bone mass in young adults and may, therefore, predispose them to severe osteoporosis.

Calcium will be discussed in detail in chapter 8, but here are several strategies lactose-intolerant individuals may use to obtain adequate calcium intake. In an extensive review of 33 studies, including nearly 3,000 children, MacGillivray and others concluded that lactose-free foods can help reduce the duration of diarrhea when compared to lactose-containing foods. Thus, changing to lactose-free milk and milk products may be a viable alternative that allows calcium intake to remain adequate. In a meta-analysis of well-designed studies, Savaiano and others indicated that symptoms of lactose intolerance may be minimal with small amounts of dairy foods, such as 1 cup or less. Consuming small amounts of milk over the course of the day may provide significant amounts of calcium. Dairy products that have been fermented, such as yogurt, may be tolerated and provide a good calcium source. Cheese may also be a good source of calcium, although it is high in fat. Dark green, leafy vegetables, tofu, sardines, salmon, and calcium-fortified fruit juices are all nondairy sources of calcium. Additionally, calcium supplements may be useful either in tablet form or as added to various foods, such as soy milk, rice milk, or orange juice.

Wheat products may produce gastrointestinal symptoms comparable to lactose intolerance. The problem is not the wheat itself but rather a protein called gluten. Gluten is found in wheat, rye, and barley, which are the main constituents in most of the grain-based products we eat, such as cereals, breads, and pasta. **Gluten intolerance** represents a sensitivity to gluten; the immune system recognizes gluten as a foreign substance, but does not induce an allergic response. Some sports nutritionists note that simple gluten intolerance can be uncomfortable, but the symptoms are fleeting. Symptoms may vary from none to severe. Simple gluten intolerance could be problematic for endurance athletes. Alternate sources of carbohydrate, such as corn, potatoes, rice, soybeans, and similar foods, will be needed to replace grain-based foods. Gluten-free products are currently available in the marketplace.

Gluten intolerance is also known as celiac disease, which, as described by Guandalini and Assiri, is the most common genetically based food intolerance in the world, with a prevalence of about 70 million people. In severe cases, the gluten damages the lining of the small intestine, which can lead to impaired nutrient absorption and a variety of nutrient-deficiency diseases, including weight loss, anemia, and osteoporosis. Celiac disease necessitates medical treatment and a lifelong gluten-free diet.

Does exercise exert any beneficial health effects related to carbohydrate metabolism?

As noted in chapter 1, an appropriate exercise program may provide a variety of health benefits. In subsequent chapters, we shall detail the preventive health effects of exercise as related to several major health problems, such as obesity, diabetes, hypertension, and coronary heart disease. Some of these beneficial effects may be attributed to the effect of exercise on carbohydrate metabolism.

Aging is normally associated with impaired glucose tolerance, which is associated with decreased insulin sensitivity. As shall be noted in chapter 10, such effects may contribute to metabolic aberrations associated with the development of coronary heart disease. However, Holloszy and Greiwe noted that these deleterious changes are not inevitable but are most likely related to a sedentary lifestyle and increased body weight. They found

that athletic individuals 60 years and older had glucose tolerance and insulin action as good as young athletes nearly half their age.

Exercise may enhance glucose tolerance and insulin sensitivity in several ways. In their review, Asano and colleagues reported that a single bout of exercise increases bioavailability of nitric oxide, a potent vasodilator, which decreases postexercise blood pressure. Additionally, increased carbohydrate oxidation during exercise can lead to increased fat oxidation postexercise and at rest. Finally, a single bout of exercise improves glucose tolerance and insulin sensitivity and reduces glycemia for up to 72 hours. Chronic exercise training potentiates the effect of exercise on insulin sensitivity through multiple adaptations in glucose transport and metabolism. Frøsig and others suggested that improved insulin-stimulated glucose uptake associated with endurance training may result from hemodynamic adaptations, such as greater blood flow to the muscle, as well as increased cellular protein content of individual insulin signaling components and molecules involved in glucose transport and metabolism. Exercise plays an important, if not essential, role in the prevention and treatment of impaired insulin sensitivity.

Given the epidemic of obesity and type 2 diabetes in the United States and other industrialized nations, these beneficial effects of exercise on carbohydrate metabolism underscore its importance as preventive medicine. More details are presented in chapter 10.

Key Concepts

▶ Added sugars should be limited in the diet. The maximal recommended amount is 25 percent of daily energy intake, but some health professionals recommend lower amounts of about 10 percent. Intake of refined starches should also be limited.

▶ An increase in the amount of total fiber to about 25–38 grams per day may be helpful as a protective measure against the development of heart disease, and possibly other chronic diseases. Consuming more whole grains, more fresh fruits, more nonstarchy vegetables, and more legumes, which are low GI foods, will help ensure adequate fiber intake.

Check for Yourself

▶ Check the food labels of various breads for fiber content. Do some brands have significantly more than others? What impact could switching breads have on meeting the recommended daily fiber intake of 25 grams for females and 38 grams for males?

If you are not currently eating enough fiber, try this experiment. Keep a record of your appetite and your bowel movements for a week or so, and then switch to a high-fiber diet, consuming fruits and vegetables, whole wheat and whole-grain breads, and other high-fiber foods as documented by food labels. Record approximate grams of total fiber consumed daily. Also record an increase (↑), a decrease (↓), or no change (NC) for appetite, and record the number of daily bowel movements. Compare your appetite and bowel movements to the previous week. Did the high-fiber diet influence either?

Week 1 (normal diet)

	Sunday	Monday	Tuesday	Wednesday	Thursday	Friday	Saturday
Breakfast							
Lunch							
Dinner							
Snacks							
Appetite							
Bowel Movement(s)							

Week 2 (high-fiber diet)

	Sunday	Monday	Tuesday	Wednesday	Thursday	Friday	Saturday
Breakfast							
Lunch							
Dinner							
Snacks							
Appetite							
Bowel Movement(s)							

Review Questions—Multiple Choice

1. Which of the following statements relative to carbohydrate loading is false?
   a. It is beneficial primarily for athletes involved in prolonged endurance events, such as the typical marathon (26.2 miles).
   b. It involves the intake of about 500–600 grams of carbohydrate each day for several days prior to competition.
   c. Research generally supports its effectiveness as a means of improving performance by helping to delay the onset of fatigue in the latter stages of prolonged exercise tasks.
   d. The major advantage of carbohydrate loading is the increased storage of glycogen in the adipose cells for use during exercise.
   e. The increase in carbohydrate stores in the body may be detected by the increased body weight attributed to the water-binding effect of stored glycogen.

2. If you were to recommend to a runner a fluid replacement protocol, including carbohydrate content, for use during a marathon, which of the following would you *not* recommend?
   a. Use a 50–60 percent solution of galactose.
   b. Provide approximately 10–15 grams of carbohydrate per feeding.
   c. Provide feedings about every 15–20 minutes.
   d. Limit the amount of fructose in the solution.
   e. Choose a combination of carbohydrates.

3. Which of the following statements relative to the intake of carbohydrates and physical performance is false?
   a. If an individual has normal glycogen levels in the muscle and liver, carbohydrate feedings are usually not necessary if the exercise task is only about 60–90 minutes.
   b. The intake of concentrated sugar solutions may actually impair performance if they lead to osmosis of fluids into the stomach and precipitate the feeling of gastric distress.
   c. Carbohydrate intake may help delay the onset of fatigue in prolonged exercise by either preventing the early onset of hypoglycemia or delaying the depletion of muscle glycogen levels.
   d. Carbohydrate intake prior to and during endurance exercise tasks lasting more than 2 hours may be helpful as a means of enhancing performance.
   e. If consumed during exercise, it takes approximately 60–90 minutes for the carbohydrate to find its way into the muscle and be used as an energy source.

4. Following a meal high in simple carbohydrate, which of the following is most likely to occur in the next 1–2 hours?
   a. suppression of insulin with a resultant hyperglycemia
   b. hyperglycemia, which stimulates insulin secretion followed by possible hypoglycemia
   c. hypoglycemia, which stimulates insulin secretion and a return to normal blood glucose levels
   d. hyperglycemia with a suppression of insulin and movement of blood glucose into the liver and muscle tissues
   e. no change in blood glucose level

5. Which of the following is *not* one of the potential health benefits of dietary fiber?
   a. It may increase the bulk in the large intestine and dilute possible carcinogens.
   b. It may increase the bulk in the large intestine and help speed up intestinal transit.
   c. It may bind with carcinogens and help to excrete them.
   d. It may help excrete bile salts and reduce serum cholesterol levels.
   e. It may bind with certain minerals such as zinc and help to excrete them.

6. Which of the following Food Exchanges is least likely to be high in dietary fiber?
   a. vegetable
   b. starch/bread
   c. milk
   d. fruit
   e. legumes (meat exchange)

7. What two tissues in the body store the most carbohydrate?
   a. adipose and kidney
   b. kidney and liver
   c. liver and muscles
   d. muscles and kidney
   e. adipose and muscles

8. Common table sugar is
   a. glucose.
   b. dextrose.
   c. fructose.
   d. sucrose.
   e. maltose.

9. The total amount of carbohydrate, as a percentage of the daily calories, that represents the Acceptable Macronutrient Distribution Range (AMDR) for Americans and Canadians is
   a. 12–15.
   b. 20–30.
   c. 30–45.
   d. 45–65.
   e. 85–90.

10. The glycemic index represents
   a. the degree to which an athlete suffers from hypoglycemia.
   b. the amount of glucose released into the blood in response to exercise.
   c. the effect a particular food has on the rate and amount of increase in the blood glucose level.
   d. the amount of stored glycogen in the muscle and liver.
   e. the total amount of insulin released in response to food intake.

Answers to multiple choice questions:
1. d; 2. a; 3. e; 4. b; 5. e; 6. c; 7. c; 8. d; 9. d; 10. c

Review Questions—Essay

1. Differentiate between dietary fiber and functional fiber, and contrast the new AI for total fiber with the current Daily Value (DV) used on food labels.
2. You have eaten a high-carbohydrate meal for lunch. Explain the digestion and metabolic fate of this carbohydrate over the next 5 hours, including an hour of running at the end of this time frame.
3. Explain three possible mechanisms of fatigue due to inadequate carbohydrate intake prior to and during the running of a 26.2-mile marathon.
4. Identify athletes who might benefit from carbohydrate loading, and present details of the dietary and exercise training protocol.
5. Discuss the possible health benefits associated with a diet rich in complex carbohydrates and low to moderate in refined carbohydrates.

Books

American Institute of Cancer Research. 2007. *Food, Nutrition, Physical Activity and the Prevention of Cancer: A Global Perspective.* Washington, DC: American Institute of Cancer Research.

Houston, M. 2006. *Biochemistry Primer for Exercise Science.* Champaign, IL: Human Kinetics.

Maughan, R., and Murray, R. 2001. *Sports Drinks.* Boca Raton, FL: CRC Press.

National Academy of Sciences. 2005. *Dietary Reference Intakes for Energy, Carbohydrates, Fiber, Fat, Fatty Acids, Cholesterol, Protein and Amino Acids.* Washington, DC: National Academies Press.

U.S. Department of Health and Human Services Public Health Service. 2010. *Healthy People 2020.* Washington, DC: U.S. Government Printing Office.

Reviews and Specific Studies

Achten, J., et al. 2004. Higher dietary carbohydrate content during intensified running training results in better maintenance of performance and mood state. *Journal of Applied Physiology* 96:1331–40.

Akermark, C., et al. 1996. Diet and muscle glycogen concentration in relation to physical performance in Swedish elite ice hockey players. *International Journal of Sport Nutrition* 6:272–84.

Appel, L., et al. 2005. Effects of protein, monounsaturated fat, and carbohydrate intake on blood pressure and serum lipids: Results of the OmniHeart randomized trial. *Journal of the American Medical Association* 294:2455–64.

Arkinstall, M., et al. 2001. Effect of carbohydrate ingestion on metabolism during running and cycling. *Journal of Applied Physiology* 91:2125–34.

Asano, R., et al. 2014. Acute effects of physical exercise in type 2 diabetes: A review. *World Journal of Diabetes* 5:659–65.

Aune, D., et al. 2013. Whole grain and refined grain consumption and the risk of type 2 diabetes: A systematic review and dose-response meta-analysis of cohort studies. *European Journal of Epidemiology* 28:845–58.

Azevedo, J., et al. 2007. Lactate, fructose and glucose oxidation profiles in sports drinks and the effect on exercise performance. *PLoS ONE* 26; 2 (9):e927.

Ball, T., et al. 1995. Periodic carbohydrate replacement during 50 min of high intensity cycling improves subsequent sprint performance. *International Journal of Sport Nutrition* 5:151–58.

Balsom, P., et al. 1999. High-intensity exercise and muscle glycogen availability in humans. *Acta Physiologica Scandinavica* 165:337–45.

Bangsbo, J., et al. 2006. Physical and metabolic demands of training and match-play in the elite football player. *Journal of Sports Sciences* 24:665–74.

Bantle, J. 2006. Is fructose the optimal glycemic index sweetener? *Nestle Nutrition Workshop Series: Clinical & Performance Programme* 11:83–91.

Baty, J. 2007. The effect of a carbohydrate and protein supplement on resistance exercise performance, hormonal response, and muscle damage. *Journal of Strength & Conditioning Research* 21 (2): 321–29.

Beelen, M., et al. 2010. Nutritional strategies to promote postexercise recovery. *International Journal of Sport Nutrition & Exercise Metabolism* 20:515–32.

Berardi, J., and Ziegenfuss, T. 2003. Effects of ribose supplementation on repeated sprint performance in men. *Journal of Strength Conditioning Research* 17:47–52.

Berardi, J., et al. 2008. Recovery from a cycling time trial is enhanced with carbohydrate-protein supplementation vs. isoenergetic carbohydrate supplementation. *Journal of the International Society of Sports Nutrition* 5:24.

Betts, J., et al. 2005. Recovery of endurance running capacity: Effect of carbohydrate-protein mixture. *International Journal of Sport Nutrition* 15:590–609.

Blair, S., et al. 1980. Blood lipid and ECG response to carbohydrate loading. *Physician & Sports Medicine* 8:69–75.

Bosch, A., et al. 1994. Influence of carbohydrate ingestion on fuel substrate turnover and oxidation during prolonged exercise. *Journal of Applied Physiology* 76:2364–72.

Braun, B. 2008. Effects of high altitude on substrate use and metabolic economy: Cause and effect? *Medicine & Science in Sports & Exercise* 40:1495–500.

Brooks, G. 2007. Lactate: Link between glycolytic and oxidative metabolism. *Sports Medicine* 37:341–43.

Brouns, F., et al. 1995. Chronic oral lactate supplementation does not affect lactate disappearance from blood after exercise. *International Journal of Sport Nutrition* 5:117–24.

Brown, A., et al. 2004. Tricarboxylic-acid-cycle intermediates and cycle endurance capacity. *International Journal of Sport Nutrition & Exercise Metabolism* 14:720–29.

Brown, L., et al. 1999. Cholesterol-lowering effects of dietary fiber: A meta-analysis. *American Journal of Clinical Nutrition* 69:30–42.

Bryner, R., et al. 1998. Effect of lactate consumption on exercise performance. *Journal of Sports Medicine & Physical Fitness* 38:116–23.

Burke, L., et al. 2000. Carbohydrate loading failed to improve 100-km cycling performance in a placebo-controlled trial. *Journal of Applied Physiology* 88:1284–90.

Burke, L., et al. 2001. Guidelines for daily carbohydrate intake: Do athletes achieve them? *Sports Medicine* 31:267–99.

Burke, L. 2001. Nutritional practices of male and female endurance cyclists. *Sports Medicine* 31:521–32.

Burke, L., et al. 2004. Carbohydrates and fat for training and recovery. *Journal of Sports Sciences* 22:15–30.

Burke, L., et al. 2005. Effect of carbohydrate intake on half-marathon performance of well-trained runners. *International Journal of Sport Nutrition & Exercise Metabolism* 5:573–89.

Burke, L., et al. 2006. Energy and carbohydrate for training and recovery. *Journal of Sports Sciences* 24:675–85.

Burke, L. 2007. Nutrition strategies for the marathon. *Sports Medicine* 37:344–47.

Burke, L. M., 2014. Carbohydrate needs of athletes in training. In *Sports Nutrition. The Encyclopedia of Sports Medicine,* ed. R. J. Maughan. Oxford, UK: Wiley Blackwell.

Campbell, C., et al. 2008. Carbohydrate-supplement form and exercise performance. *International Journal of Sport Nutrition & Exercise Metabolism* 18:179–90.

Carter, J., et al. 2004. The effect of carbohydrate mouth rinse on 1-h cycle time trial performance. *Medicine & Science in Sports & Exercise* 36:2107–11.

Carter, J., et al. 2004. The effect of glucose infusion on glucose kinetics during a 1-h time trial. *Medicine & Science in Sports & Exercise* 36:1543–50.

Chryssanthopoulos, C., et al. 2002. Influence of a carbohydrate-electrolyte solution ingested during running on muscle glycogen utilization in fed humans. *International Journal of Sports Medicine* 23:279–84.

Chryssanthopoulos, C., et al. 2002. The effect of a high carbohydrate meal on endurance running capacity. *International Journal of Sport Nutrition & Exercise Metabolism* 12:157–71.

Clark, M. J., and Slavin, J. L. 2013. The effect of fiber on satiety and food intake: A systematic review. *Journal of the American College of Nutrition* 32:200–11.

Consumers Union. 2005. Sweeteners can sour your health. *Consumer Reports on Health* 17 (1):8–9.

Consumers Union. 2009. 10 easy ways to eat more fiber. *Consumer Reports on Health* 21 (12):7.

Costill, D. 1988. Carbohydrates for exercise: Dietary demands for optimal performance. *International Journal of Sports Medicine* 9:1–18.

Coyle, E. 1995. Substrate utilization during exercise in active people. *American Journal of Clinical Nutrition* 61 (Supplement): 968S–79S.

Coyle, E. 2000. Physical activity as a metabolic stressor. *American Journal of Clinical Nutrition* 72:512S–20S.

Coyle, E. 2004. Highs and lows of carbohydrate diets. *Sports Science Exchange* 17 (2):1–6.

Coyle, E. 2007. Physiological regulation of marathon performance. *Sports Medicine* 37:306–11.

Currell, K., and Jeukendrup, A. 2008. Superior endurance performance with ingestion of multiple transportable carbohydrates. *Medicine & Science in Sports & Exercise* 40:275–81.

Davis, J. 1996. Carbohydrates, branched-chain amino acids and endurance: The central fatigue hypothesis. *Sports Science Exchange* 9(2):1–6.

Debold, E. 2012. Recent insights into the molecular basis of muscular fatigue. *Medicine and Science in Sports and Exercise* 44:1440–52.

Desbrow, B., et al. 2004. Carbohydrate-electrolyte feedings and 1-h time trial cycling performance. *International Journal of Sport Nutrition & Exercise Metabolism* 14:541–49.

Dhanoa, T., and Housner, J. 2007. Ribose: More than a simple sugar? *Current Sports Medicine Reports* 6:254–57.

Di Stefano, M., et al. 2002. Lactose malabsorption and intolerance and peak bone mass. *Gastroenterology* 122:1793–99.

Djoussé, L., and Gaziano, J. 2007. Breakfast cereals and risk of heart failure in the physicians' health study I. *Archives of Internal Medicine* 167:2080–85.

Donaldson, C., et al. 2010. Glycemic index and exercise endurance. *International Journal of Sport Nutrition & Exercise Metabolism* 20:154–65.

Dunne, L., et al. 2006. Ribose versus dextrose supplementation, association with rowing performance: A double-blind study. *Clinical Journal of Sport Medicine* 16:68–71.

Décombaz, J., et al. 2011. Fructose and galactose enhance post-exercise human liver glycogen synthesis. *Medicine and Science in Sports and Exercise* 43:1964–71.

Edgerton, V., and Roy, R. 2006. The nervous system and movement. In *ACSM's Advanced Exercise Physiology,* ed. C. M. Tipton. Philadelphia: Lippincott Williams & Wilkins.

el-Sayed, M., et al. 1997. Carbohydrate ingestion improves performance during a 1-h simulated cycling trial. *Journal of Sports Sciences* 15:223–30.

Erlenbusch, M., et al. 2005. Effect of high-fat or high-carbohydrate diets on endurance exercise: A meta-analysis. *International Journal of Sport Nutrition and Exercise Metabolism* 15:1–14.

Fahey, T., et al. 1991. The effects of ingesting polylactate or glucose polymer drinks during prolonged exercise. *International Journal of Sport Nutrition* 1:249–56.

Fairchild, T., et al. 2002. Rapid carbohydrate loading after a short bout of near maximal-intensity exercise. *Medicine & Science in Sports & Exercise* 34:980–86.

Febbraio, M. 2001. Alterations in energy metabolism during exercise and heat stress. *Sports Medicine* 31:47–59.

Fehm, H., et al. 2006. The selfish brain: Competition for energy resources. *Progress in Brain Research* 153:129–40.

Ferguson-Stegall, L., et al. 2010. The effect of a low carbohydrate beverage with added protein on cycling endurance performance in trained athletes. *Journal of Strength & Conditioning Research* 24 (10): 2577–86.

Fitch, C., et al. 2012. Use of nutritive and nonnutritive sweeteners. *Journal of the Academy of Nutrition and Dietetics* 112:739–58.

Fogelholm, M., et al. 1991. Carbohydrate loading in practice: High muscle glycogen concentration is not certain. *British Journal of Sports Medicine* 25:41–44.

Food and Drug Administration. 2006. Artificial sweeteners: No calories . . . Sweet! *FDA Consumer* 40 (4):27–28.

Frøsig, C., et al. 2007. Effects of endurance exercise training on insulin signaling in human skeletal muscle: Interactions at the level of phosphatidylinositol 3-kinase, Akt, and AS160. *Diabetes* 56:2093–102.

Fung, T., et al. 2009. Sweetened beverage consumption and risk of coronary heart disease in women. *American Journal of Clinical Nutrition* 89:1037–42.

Gallus, S., et al. 2007. Artificial sweeteners and cancer risk in a network of case-control studies. *Annals of Oncology* 18:40–44.

Gilson, S., et al. 2010. Effects of chocolate milk consumption on markers of muscle recovery following soccer training: A randomized cross-over study. *Journal of the International Society of Sports Nutrition* 7:19.

Gleeson, M. 2006. Can nutrition limit exercise-induced immunodepression? *Nutrition Reviews* 64:119–31.

Gleeson, M., et al. 2004. Exercise, nutrition and immune function. *Journal of Sports Sciences* 22:115–25.

Greenwood, D., et al. 2013. Glycemic index, glycemic load, carbohydrates, and type 2 diabetes: Systematic review and dose-response meta-analysis of prospective studies. *Diabetes Care* 36:4166–71.

Grotz, V., and Munro, I. 2009. An overview of the safety of sucralose. *Regulatory Toxicology & Pharmacology* 55:1–5.

Guandalini, S., and Assiri, A. 2014. Celiac disease: A review. *Journal of the American Medical Association Pediatrics* 168:272–78.

Haff, G., et al. 1999. The effect of carbohydrate supplementation on multiple sessions and bouts of resistance exercise. *Journal of Strength and Conditioning Research* 13:111–17.

Haff, G., et al. 2001. The effects of supplemental carbohydrate ingestion on intermittent isokinetic leg exercise. *Journal of Sports Medicine and Physical Fitness* 41:216–22.

Haff, G., et al. 2003. Carbohydrate supplementation and resistance training. *Journal of Strength and Conditioning Research* 17:187–96.

Hargreaves, M., et al. 1995. Influence of muscle glycogen on glycogenolysis and glucose uptake during exercise in humans. *Journal of Applied Physiology* 78:288–92.

Hashimoto, T., and Brooks, G. 2008. Mitochondrial lactate oxidation complex and an adaptive role for lactate production. *Medicine & Science in Sports & Exercise* 40:486–94.

Hatfield, D., et al. 2006. The effects of carbohydrate loading on repetitive jump squat power performance. *Journal of Strength Conditioning & Research* 20:167–71.

Hawley, J. A. 2014. Manipulating carbohydrate availability to promote training adaptation. *Gatorade Sports Science Exchange* 27:1–7.

Hawley, J., et al. 1997. Carbohydrate-loading and exercise performance: An update. *Sports Medicine* 24:73–81.

Hellsten, Y., et al. 2004. Effect of ribose supplementation on resynthesis of adenine nucleotides after intense intermittent training in humans. *American Journal of Physiology. Regulatory, Integrative, & Comparative Physiology* 286:R182–88.

Holloszy, J. 2005. Exercise-induced increase in muscle insulin sensitivity. *Journal of Applied Physiology* 99:338–43.

Holloszy, J., and Greiwe, J. 2001. Overview of glucose metabolism and aging. *International Journal of Sport Nutrition & Exercise Metabolism* 11:S58–63.

Holloszy, J., et al. 1998. The regulation of carbohydrate and fat metabolism during and after exercise. *Frontiers in Science* 3:D1011–27.

Jalal, D., et al. Increased fructose associates with elevated blood pressure. *Journal of the American Society of Nephrology* 21:1543–49.

James, A., et al. 2001. Muscle glycogen supercompensation: Absence of a gender-related difference. *European Journal of Applied Physiology* 85:533–58.

Jensen, M., et al. in press. Carbohydrate mouth rinse counters fatigue related strength reduction. *International Journal of Sport Nutrition and Exercise Metabolism.*

Jentjens, R., et al. 2006. Exogenous carbohydrate oxidation rates are elevated after combined ingestion of glucose and fructose during exercise in the heat. *Journal of Applied Physiology* 100:807–16.

Jeukendrup, A. 2004. Carbohydrate intake during exercise and performance. *Nutrition* 20:669–77.

Jeukendrup, A. 2007. Carbohydrate supplementation during exercise: Does it help? How much is too much? *Sports Science Exchange* 20 (3):1–6.

Jeukendrup, A. 2014. Carbohydrate ingestion during exercise. In *Sports Nutrition. The Encyclopedia of Sports Medicine,* ed. R. J. Maughan. Oxford, UK: Wiley Blackwell.

Jeukendrup, A., and Jentjens, R. 2000. Oxidation of carbohydrate feedings during prolonged exercise: Current thoughts, guidelines and directions for future research. *Sports Medicine* 29:407–24.

Jeukendrup, A., and Killer, S. 2010. The myths surrounding pre-exercise carbohydrate feeding. *Annals of Nutrition & Metabolism* 57 (suppl. 2):18–25.

Jeukendrup, A., et al. 1997. Carbohydrate-electrolyte feedings improve 1-h time trial cycling performance. *International Journal of Sports Medicine* 18:125–29.

Jeukendrup, A., et al. 2006. Exogenous carbohydrate oxidation during ultraendurance exercise. *Journal of Applied Physiology* 100:1134–41.

Jeukendrup, A., et al. 2013. Multiple Transportable Carbohydrates and Their Benefits. *Gatorade Sports Science Exchange.* 26:1–8.

Johnson, R., et al. 2009. Dietary sugars intake and cardiovascular health: A scientific statement from the American Heart Association. *Circulation* 120:1011–20.

Kalman, D., et al. 1999. The effects of pyruvate supplementation on body composition in overweight individuals. *Nutrition* 15:337–40.

Kang, J., et al. 1995. Effect of carbohydrate ingestion subsequent to carbohydrate supercompensation on endurance performance. *International Journal of Sport Nutrition* 5:329–43.

Karelis, A., et al. 2010. Carbohydrate administration and exercise performance: What are the mechanisms involved? *Sports Medicine* 40 (9):747–63.

Karp, J., et al. 2006. Chocolate milk as a post-exercise recovery aid. *International Journal of Sport Nutrition & Exercise Metabolism* 16:78–91.

Kavouras, S., et al. 2004. The influence of low versus high carbohydrate diet on a 45-min strenuous cycling exercise. *International Journal of Sport Nutrition & Exercise Metabolism* 14:62–72.

Keim, N., et al. 2006. Carbohydrates. In *Modern Nutrition in Health and Disease,* eds. M. Shils, et al. Philadelphia: Lippincott Williams & Wilkins.

Kerksick, C., et al. 2005. Effects of ribose supplementation prior to and during intense exercise on anaerobic capacity and metabolic markers. *International Journal of Sport Nutrition & Exercise Metabolism* 15:653–64.

Kerksick, C., et al. 2008. International Society of Sports Nutrition position stand: Nutrient timing. *Journal of the International Society of Sports Nutrition* 5:17.

Kim, Y., and Je, Y. 2014. Dietary fiber intake and total mortality: A meta-analysis of prospective cohort studies. *American Journal of Epidemiology* 180:565–73.

Kimber, N., et al. 2002. Energy balance during an Ironman triathlon in male and female triathletes. *International Journal of Sport Nutrition & Exercise Metabolism* 12:47–62.

Kirkendall, D. 2004. Creatine, carbs, and fluids: How important in soccer nutrition? *Sports Science Exchange* 17 (3):1–6.

Kjaer, M. 1998. Hepatic glucose production during exercise. *Advances in Experimental Medicine & Biology* 441:117–27.

Koh-Banerjee, P., et al. 2005. Effects of calcium pyruvate supplementation during training on body composition, exercise capacity, and metabolic responses to exercise. *Nutrition* 21:312–19.

Kovacs, M. 2006. Carbohydrate intake and tennis: Are there benefits? *British Journal of Sports Medicine* 40 (5):e13.

Kreider, R., et al. 2010. International Society of Sports Nutrition exercise and sport nutrition review: Research and recommendations. *Journal of the International Society of Sports Nutrition* 7:7.

Kreitzman, S., et al. 1992. Glycogen storage: Illusions of easy weight loss, excessive weight regain, and distortions in estimates of body composition. *American Journal of Clinical Nutrition* 56:292S–93S.

Krustrup, P., et al. 2004. Slow-twitch fiber glycogen depletion elevates moderate-exercise fast-twitch fiber activity and O_2 uptake. *Medicine & Science in Sports & Exercise* 36:973–82.

Krustrup, P., et al. 2006. Muscle and blood metabolites during a soccer game: Implications for sprint performance. *Medicine & Science in Sports & Exercise* 38:1165–74.

Kuipers, H., et al. 1999. Pre-exercise ingestion of carbohydrate and transient hypoglycemia during exercise. *International Journal of Sports Medicine* 20:227–31.

Larsson, S., et al. 2006. Consumption of sugar and sugar-sweetened foods and the risk of pancreatic cancer in a prospective study. *American Journal of Clinical Nutrition* I84:1171–76.

Liebman, B. 1998. Sugar: The sweetening of the American diet. *Nutrition Action Health Letter* 25 (9):1–8.

Liebman, B. 2008. Fiber free-for-all: Not all fibers are equal. *Nutrition Action Health Letter* 35 (6):1–7.

Lim, U., et al. 2006. Consumption of aspartame-containing beverages and incidence of hematopoietic and brain malignancies. *Cancer Epidemiology, Biomarkers & Prevention* 15:1654–59.

Lupton, J., and Trumbo, P. 2006. Dietary fiber. In *Modern Nutrition in Health and Disease,* eds. M. Shils, et al. Philadelphia: Lippincott Williams & Wilkins.

Ma, Y., et al. 2005. Association between dietary carbohydrates and body weight.

American Journal of Epidemiology 161:359–67.

MacGillivray, S., et al. 2013. Lactose avoidance for young children with acute diarrhoea. *Cochrane Database of Systematic Reviews.* Oct 31;10:CD005433.

Magnuson, B., et al. 2007. Aspartame: A safety evaluation based on current use levels, regulations, and toxicological and epidemiological studies. *Critical Reviews in Toxicology* 37:629–727.

Marjerrison, A., et al. 2007. Preexercise carbohydrate consumption and repeated anaerobic performance in pre- and early-pubertal boys. *International Journal of Sport Nutrition & Exercise Metabolism* 17:140–51.

Marlett, J., et al. 2002. Position of the American Dietetic Association: Health implications of dietary fiber. *Journal of the American Dietetic Association* 102:993–1010.

Mathew, T., et al. 2002. Relationship between sports drinks and dental erosion in 304 university athletes. *Caries Research* 36:281–87.

Matsui, T., et al. 2011. Brain glycogen decreases during prolonged exercise. *Journal of Physiology* 589:3383–93.

Maughan, R., and Burke, L. 2015. Carbohydrates. In *Nutritional Supplements in Sport, Exercise, and Health. An A–Z Guide,* ed. L. M. Castell, S. J. Stear, and L. M. Burke. New York: Routledge.

Maughan, R., et al. 1997. Diet composition and the performance of high-intensity exercise. *Journal of Sports Sciences* 15:265–75.

Mazzeo, R., and Fulco, C. 2006. Physiological systems and their responses to conditions of hypoxia. In *ACSM's Advanced Exercise Physiology,* ed. C. M. Tipton. Philadelphia: Lippincott Williams & Wilkins.

McCleave, E., et al. 2011. A low carbohydrate-protein supplement improves endurance performance in female athletes. *Journal of Strength & Conditioning Research* 25 (4):879–88.

McInerney, P., et al. 2005. Failure to repeatedly supercompensate muscle glycogen stores in highly trained men. *Medicine & Science in Sports & Exercise* 37:404–11.

McLay, R., et al. 2007. Carbohydrate loading and female endurance athletes: Effect of menstrual-cycle phase. *International Journal of Sport Nutrition & Exercise Metabolism* 17:189–205.

Meeusen, R. 2014. Exercise, nutrition and the brain. *Sports Medicine* 44:S47–S56.

Mirrahimi, A., et al. 2014. The role of glycemic index and glycemic load in cardiovascular disease and its risk factors:
A review of the recent literature. *Current Atherosclerosis Reports* 16 (381):1–10.

Mittendorfer, B., and Klein, S. 2001. Effect of aging on glucose and lipid metabolism during endurance exercise. *International Journal of Sport Nutrition & Exercise Metabolism* 11:S86–91.

Morrison, M., et al. 2000. Pyruvate ingestion for 7 days does not improve aerobic performance in well-trained individuals. *Journal of Applied Physiology* 89:549–56.

Murray, R., et al. 1989. The effects of glucose, fructose, and sucrose ingestion during exercise. *Medicine & Science in Sports & Exercise* 21:275–82.

National Institutes of Health. 2001. Diagnosis and management of dental caries throughout life. *NIH Consensus Statement* 18(1):1–23.

Nieman, D. 2007. Marathon training and immune function. *Sports Medicine* 37:412–15.

Nieman, D., and Bishop, N. 2006. Nutritional strategies to counter stress to the immune system in athletes, with special reference to football. *Journal of Sports Sciences* 24:763–72.

Nilsson L., and Hultman, E. 1974. Liver and muscle glycogen in man after glucose and fructose infusion. *Scandinavian Journal of Laboratory and Clinical Investigation* 33:5–10.

O'Reilly, J., et al. 2010. Glycaemic index, glycaemic load and exercise performance. *Sports Medicine* 40:27–39.

Onkapaya, I. 2014. Pyruvate supplementation for weight loss: A systematic review and meta analysis of randomized clinical trials. *Critical Reviews in Food Science and Nutrition* 54:17–23.

Op 'T Eijnde, B., et al. 2001. No effects of oral ribose supplementation on repeated maximal exercise and de novo ATP resynthesis. *Journal of Applied Physiology* 91:2275–81.

Ormsbee, M., et al. 2014. Pre-exercise nutrition: The role of macronutrients, modified starches and supplements on metabolism and endurance performance. *Nutrients* 6:1782–808.

Ørtenblad, N., et al. 2013. Muscle glycogen stores and fatigue. *Journal of Physiology* 15:4405–13.

Ostojic, S., and Ahmetovic, Z. 2009. The effect of 4 weeks treatment with a 2-gram daily dose of pyruvate on body composition in healthy trained men. *International Journal for Vitamin & Nutrition Research* 79 (3):173–79.

Palmer, G., et al. 1998. Carbohydrate ingestion immediately before exercise does not improve 20 km time trial performance in
well-trained cyclists. *International Journal of Sports Medicine* 19:415–18.

Paul, D., et al. 2001. Carbohydrate during the follicular phase of the menstrual cycle: Effects on muscle glycogen and exercise performance. *International Journal of Sport Nutrition & Exercise Metabolism* 11:430–31.

Peters, H., et al. 1995. Exercise performance as a function of semi-solid and liquid carbohydrate feedings during prolonged exercise. *International Journal of Sports Medicine* 16:105–13.

Peveler, W., et al. 2006. Effects of ribose as an ergogenic aid. *Journal of Strength & Conditioning Research* 20:519–22.

Pfeiffer, B., et al. 2010. CHO oxidation from a CHO gel compared with a drink during exercise. *Medicine & Science in Sports & Exercise* 42 (11):2038–45.

Pi-Sunyer, F. 2002. Glycemic index and disease. *American Journal of Clinical Nutrition* 76:290S–98S.

Pizza, F., et al. 1995. A carbohydrate loading regimen improves high intensity, short duration exercise performance. *International Journal of Sport Nutrition* 5:110–16.

Pliml, W., et al. 1992. Effects of ribose on exercise-induced ischaemia in stable coronary artery disease. *Lancet* 340:507–10.

Pritchett, K., et al. 2009. Acute effects of chocolate milk and a commercial recovery beverage on postexercise recovery indices and endurance cycling performance. *Applied Physiology, Nutrition, & Metabolism* 34:1017–22.

Rauch, H., et al. 2005. A signalling role for muscle glycogen in the regulation of pace during prolonged exercise. *British Journal of Sports Medicine* 39:34–38.

Richter, E., et al. 2001. Regulation of muscle glucose transport during exercise. *International Journal of Sport Nutrition & Exercise Metabolism* 11:S71–77.

Rico-Sanz, J., et al. 1999. Muscle glycogen degradation during simulation of a fatiguing soccer match in elite soccer players examined noninvasively by 13C-MRS. *Medicine & Science in Sports & Exercise* 31:1587–93.

Rock, C. 2007. Primary dietary prevention: Is the fiber story over? *Recent Results in Cancer Research* 173:171–77.

Romano-Ely, B., et al. 2006. Effect of an isocaloric carbohydrate-protein-antioxidant drink on cycling performance. *Medicine & Science in Sports & Exercise* 38:1608–16.

Roy, B. 2008. Milk: The new sports drink? A review. *Journal of the International Society of Sports Nutrition* 5:15.

Sacks, F., et al. 2014. Effects of high vs. low glycemic index of dietary carbohydrate on cardiovascular disease risk factors and insulin sensitivity. 2014. The OmniCarb randomized clinical trial. *Journal of the American Medical Association* 312:2531–41.

Saris, W. 1989. Study of food intake and energy expenditure during extreme sustained exercise: The Tour de France. *International Journal of Sports Medicine* 10:S26–S31.

Savaiano, D., et al. 2006. Lactose intolerance symptoms assessed by meta-analysis: A grain of truth that leads to exaggeration. *Journal of Nutrition* 136:1107–13.

Sawka, M., and Young, A. 2006. Physiological systems and their responses to conditions of heat and cold. In *ACSM's Advanced Exercise Physiology,* ed. C. M. Tipton. Philadelphia: Lippincott Williams & Wilkins.

Schneeman, B. 1999. Building scientific consensus: The importance of dietary fiber. *American Journal of Clinical Nutrition* 69:30–42.

Seal, C. 2006. Whole grains and CVD risk. *Proceedings of the Nutrition Society* 65:24–34.

Seifert, J., et al. 1994. Glycemic and insulinemic response to preexercise carbohydrate feedings. *International Journal of Sport Nutrition* 4:46–53.

Seymour, G., et al. 2007. Relationship between periodontal infections and systemic disease. *Clinical Microbiology & Infection* 13 (Supplement 4):3–10.

Short, S. 1993. Surveys of dietary intake and nutrition knowledge of athletes and their coaches. In *Nutrition in Exercise and Sport,* ed. I. Wolinsky and J. Hickson. Boca Raton, FL: CRC Press.

Shulman, R., and Rothman, D. 2001. The "glycogen shunt" in exercising muscle: A role of glycogen in muscle energetics and fatigue. *Proceedings of the National Academy of Sciences* 98:457–61.

Silva, F. M., et al. 2013. Fiber intake and glycemic control in patients with type 2 diabetes mellitus: A systematic review with meta-analysis of randomized controlled trials. *Nutrition Reviews* 71:790–801.

Smith, G., et al. 2002. The effect of preexercise glucose ingestion on performance during prolonged swimming. *International Journal of Sport Nutrition & Exercise Metabolism* 12:136–44.

Spriet, L. 2007. Regulation of substrate use during the marathon. *Sports Medicine* 37:332–36.

Stanko, R., et al. 1990. Enhanced leg exercise endurance with a high-carbohydrate diet and dihydroxyacetone and pyruvate. *Journal of Applied Physiology* 69:1651–56.

Stanko, R., et al. 1990. Enhancement of arm exercise endurance capacity with dihydroxyacetone and pyruvate. *Journal of Applied Physiology* 68:119–24.

Stattin, P., et al. 2007. Prospective study of hyperglycemia and cancer risk. *Diabetes Care* 30:561–67.

Stearns, R., et al. 2010. Effects of ingesting protein in combination with carbohydrate during exercise on endurance performance: A systematic review with meta-analysis. *Journal of Strength & Conditioning Research* 24 (8):2192–202.

Stellingwerff, T., and Cox, G. 2014. Systematic review: Carbohydrate supplementation on exercise performance or capacity of varying durations. *Applied Physiology Nutrition and Metabolism* 39:998–1011.

Tarnopolsky, M. 2000. Gender differences in substrate metabolism during endurance exercise. *Canadian Journal of Applied Physiology* 25:312–27.

Tarnopolsky, M. 2008. Sex differences in exercise metabolism and the role of 17-beta estradiol. *Medicine & Science in Sports & Exercise* 40:648–54.

Tarnopolsky, M., et al. 2001. Gender differences in carbohydrate loading are related to energy intake. *Journal of Applied Physiology* 91:225–30.

Thomas, K., et al. 2009. Improved endurance capacity following chocolate milk consumption compared with 2 commercially available sport drinks. *Applied Physiology, Nutrition, & Metabolism* 34:78–82.

Threapleton, D., et al. 2013. Dietary fibre intake and risk of cardiovascular disease: Systematic review and meta-analysis. *British Medical Journal* 347:f6879.

Tsintzas, K., and Williams, C. 1998. Human muscle glycogen metabolism during exercise: Effect of carbohydrate supplementation. *Sports Medicine* 25:7–23.

Tsintzas, K., et al. 2001. Phosphocreatine degradation in type I and type II muscle fibers during submaximal exercise in man: Effect of carbohydrate ingestion. *Journal of Physiology* 537:305–11.

Tufts University. 2007. Five new reasons to get whole grains. *Health & Nutrition Letter* 25 (6):1–2.

Van Hall, G. 2000. Lactate as fuel for mitochondrial regeneration. *Acta Physiologica Scandinavica* 168:643–56.

van Loon, L. C. 2013. Is there a need for protein ingestion during exercise? *Gatorade Sports Science Exchange* 109:1–6.

van Loon, L., et al. 2001. The effects of increasing exercise intensity on muscle fuel utilisation in humans. *Journal of Physiology* 536:295–304.

Vandenberghe, K., et al. 1995. No effect of glycogen level on glycogen metabolism during high intensity exercise. *Medicine & Science in Sports & Exercise* 27:1278–83.

Venables, M., et al. 2005. Erosive effect of a new sports drink on dental enamel during exercise. *Medicine & Science in Sports & Exercise* 37:39–44.

von Fraunhofer, J., and Rogers, M. 2005. Effects of sports drinks and other beverages on dental enamel. *General Dentistry* 53:28–31.

Walberg-Rankin, J. 2000. Dietary carbohydrate and performance of brief, intense exercise. *Sports Science Exchange* 13 (4):1–4.

Walker, J., et al. 2000. Dietary carbohydrate, muscle glycogen content, and endurance performance in well-trained women. *Journal of Applied Physiology* 88:2151–58.

Wallis, G., et al. 2007. Dose-response effects of ingested carbohydrate on exercise metabolism in women. *Medicine & Science in Sports & Exercise* 39:131–38.

Welsh, R., et al. 2002. Carbohydrates and physical/mental performance during intermittent exercise to fatigue. *Medicine & Science in Sports & Exercise* 34:723–31.

Weltan, S., et al. 1998. Influence of muscle glycogen content on metabolic regulation. *American Journal of Physiology* 274:E72–E82.

Weltan, S., et al. 1998. Preexercise muscle glycogen content affects metabolism during exercise despite maintenance of hyperglycemia. *American Journal of Physiology* 274:E83–E88.

Williams, C. 2006. Nutrition to promote recovery from exercise. *Medicine & Science in Sports & Exercise* 19:1–6.

Winnick, J., et al. 2005. Carbohydrate feedings during team sport exercise preserve physical and CNS function. *Medicine & Science in Sports & Exercise* 37:306–15.

Wolfe, R., and George, S. 1993. Stable isotopic tracers as metabolic probes in exercise. *Exercise & Sports Science Reviews* 21:1–31.

Wong, J., et al. 2006. Colonic health: Fermentation and short chain fatty acids. *Journal of Clinical Gastroenterology* 40:235–43.

Yang, Y., et al. 2015. Association between dietary fiber and lower risk of all-cause mortality: A meta-analysis of cohort studies. *American Journal of Epidemiology* 181:83–91.

Yaspelkis, B., et al. 1993. Carbohydrate supplementation spares muscle glycogen during variable-intensity exercise. *Journal of Applied Physiology* 75:1477–85.

Zeng, H. 2014. Mechanisms linking dietary fiber, gut microbiota and colon cancer prevention. *World Journal of Gastrointestinal Oncology* 6:41–51.

Zierler, K. 1999. Whole body glucose metabolism. *American Journal of Physiology* 276:E409–26.

Fat: An Important Energy Source during Exercise

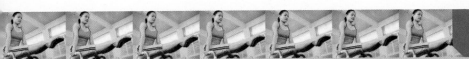

CHAPTER FIVE

LEARNING OBJECTIVES

After studying this chapter, you should be able to:

1. List the different types of dietary fatty acids and identify general types of foods in which they are found.

2. Calculate the approximate amount, in grams or milligrams, of total fat, saturated fat, and cholesterol that should be included in your daily diet.

3. Describe how dietary fat is absorbed, how it is distributed in the body, and what its major functions are in human metabolism.

4. Explain the role of fat in human energy systems during exercise and how endurance exercise training affects exercise fat metabolism.

5. Explain the theory underlying the role of increased fat oxidation to enhance prolonged aerobic endurance performance.

6. List the various dietary fat strategies and dietary supplements that have been investigated as a means of enhancing exercise performance, and highlight the major findings.

7. Describe the proposed process underlying the development of atherosclerosis and cardiovascular disease, including the role that dietary fat and cholesterol may play in its etiology.

8. List and describe at least eight of the ten dietary strategies that are proposed to help treat or prevent the development of atherosclerosis and cardiovascular disease.

9. Explain the role of exercise as a means of helping prevent the development of atherosclerosis and cardiovascular disease.

Introduction

From a health standpoint, dietary fat is the nutrient of greatest concern to the American Heart Association because excessive consumption of certain types of fat has been associated with the development of coronary heart disease. Excessive consumption of dietary fat may also contribute to the development of obesity, a risk factor for several other chronic diseases, such as diabetes. Thus, one of the major recommendations advocated in Healthy People 2020 *for a healthier diet is to reduce the amount of dietary fat intake to a reasonable level. Part of the rationale for this recommendation and some general guidelines for implementing it are presented in this chapter, but additional information may also be found in chapters 2 and 11.*

We need some fat in our diet. Despite its potential health hazards when consumed in excess, dietary fat contains several essential nutrients that serve a variety of important functions in human nutrition. The National Academy of Sciences has set an Acceptable Macronutrient Distribution Range (AMDR) for total fat of 20–35 percent of daily energy intake. Because some types of fat may confer various health benefits, the Academy also set Adequate Intakes (AI) for several fatty acids. Moreover, in its position statement regarding nutrition and athletic performance, the American Dietetic Association, Dietitians of Canada, and the American College of Sports Medicine noted that, overall, diets should provide moderate amounts of energy from fat (20 to 35 percent of energy) and that there is no health or performance benefit to consuming a diet containing less than 20 percent energy from fat. For the endurance athlete, one of the most important functions of fat is to provide energy during exercise, and researchers have explored a variety of techniques in attempts to improve endurance performance by increasing the ability of the muscle to use fat as a fuel.

To clarify the role of dietary fat in health and its possible relevance to sports, this chapter presents information on the basic nature of dietary fats and associated lipids, the metabolic fate and physiological functions of fats and cholesterol in the body, the role of fat as an energy source during exercise, the use of various dietary practices or ergogenic aids in attempts to improve fat metabolism and endurance performance, and possible health problems associated with excessive dietary fat.

Dietary Fats

What are the different types of dietary fats?

What we commonly call fat in our diet actually consists of several substances classified as lipids. **Lipids** represent a class of organic substances that are insoluble in water but soluble in certain solvents such as alcohol or ether. The three major dietary lipids of importance to humans are triglycerides, cholesterol, and phospholipids. All three have major functions in the body.

What are triglycerides?

The **triglycerides**, also known as the true fats or the neutral fats, are the principal form in which fats are eaten and stored in the human body. Triglycerides are composed of two different compounds—fatty acids and glycerol. When an acid (fatty acid) and an alcohol (glycerol) combine, an **ester** is formed, the process being known as *esterification*. (Three fatty acids are attached to each glycerol molecule.) Figure 5.1 is a diagram of a triglyceride. Another term

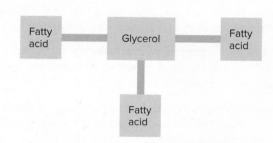

FIGURE 5.1 Structure of a triglyceride. Three fatty acids combine with glycerol to form a triglyceride.

used for triglyceride is *triacylglycerol*. Some triglycerides may be modified commercially to contain only two fatty acids, known as diglycerides, or diacylglycerols.

Fatty acids, one of the components of fat, are chains of carbon, oxygen, and hydrogen atoms that vary in length and in the degree of saturation of carbon with hydrogen. Short-chain fatty acids (SCFAs) contain fewer than 6 carbons, medium-chain fatty acids (MCFAs) have 6 to 12 carbons, and long-chain fatty acids (LCFAs) have 14 or more carbons.

Fatty acids may be saturated or unsaturated. A **saturated fatty acid** contains a full quota of hydrogenated ions so that all of its carbon bonds are full; saturated fats such as butter are solid at room temperature. Carbon molecules in unsaturated fatty acids may incorporate more hydrogen because they have some unfilled bonds, or double bonds. These unsaturated fatty acids may be classified as **monounsaturated**, having a single double bond and capable of incorporating two hydrogen ions, and **polyunsaturated**, having two or more double bonds and capable of incorporating four or more hydrogen ions; monounsaturated and polyunsaturated fats as oils are liquid at room temperature.

Polyunsaturated fatty acids are further identified according to the location of the first carbon double bond from the last, or omega, carbon. **Omega-3** and **omega-6 fatty acids** are the two major types, and the numeric represents the location of the first double bond. Other terminology to identify these two fatty acids are ω-3 and n-3 and ω-6 and n-6. Adequate amounts of omega-3 and omega-6 fatty acids may confer health benefits, as noted later in the chapter. At room temperature, saturated fats are usually solid, while unsaturated fats are usually liquid. **Partially hydrogenated fats** or oils have been treated by a process that adds hydrogen to some of the unfilled bonds, thereby hardening the fat or oil. In essence, the fat becomes more saturated. During the hydrogenation process, the normal position of hydrogen ions at the double bond is on the "same side" (*cis*). This is known as a *cis* **fatty acid**, but if partially hydrogenated so that hydrogen ions are on opposite sides of the double bond, it results in a *trans* **fatty acid**. Figure 5.2 represents the structural difference among a saturated, a monounsaturated, a polyunsaturated (*cis* and *trans*), and an omega-3 polyunsaturated fatty acid. The health implications of these different types of fats are discussed later in this chapter. In general, though, excess intake of saturated and *trans* fatty acids is associated with increased health risks, whereas adequate intake of monounsaturated, polyunsaturated, and omega-3 fatty acids may be associated with neutral or some beneficial health effects.

Glycerol is an alcohol, a clear, colorless, syrupy liquid. It is obtained in the diet as part of triglycerides, but it also may be produced in the body as a by-product of carbohydrate metabolism. On the other hand, glycerol can be converted back to carbohydrate in the process of gluconeogenesis in the liver.

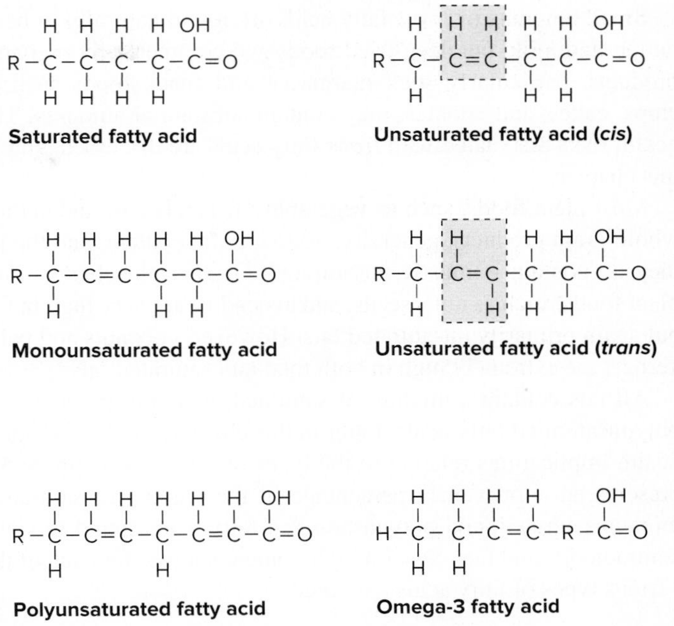

What are some common foods high in fat content?

The fat content in foods can vary from 100 percent, as found in most cooking oils, to minor trace amounts, less than 5–10 percent, as found in most fruits and vegetables. Some foods obviously have a high-fat content: butter, oils, shortening, mayonnaise, margarine, and the visible fat on meat. However, in other foods, the fat content may be high but not as obvious. This is known as **hidden fat**. Whole milk, cheese, nuts, desserts, crackers, potato chips, and a wide variety of commercially prepared foods may contain considerable amounts of hidden fat. For example, a 5-ounce baked potato contains 145 Calories with about 3 percent fat, while a 5-ounce

FIGURE 5.2 Structural differences between saturated, monounsaturated, and polyunsaturated fatty acids (including the *cis* and *trans* forms) and the omega-3 fatty acid. Note there is a single double bond between carbon atoms in the monounsaturated fatty acid and two or more in the polyunsaturated fatty acid. In the omega-3 fatty acid, the double bond is located three carbons from the last, or omega, carbon. The R represents the radical, or the presence of many more C—H bonds. In the *trans* configuration, one of the hydrogen ions is moved to the opposite side.

serving of potato chips contains 795 Calories, more than 60 percent of them from fat.

In general, animal foods found in the meat and milk groups are high in fat, particularly saturated fat. Hamburger meat contributes the most saturated fat to the typical American diet. However, careful selection and preparation of foods in these groups will considerably reduce fat content. The percentage of fat in meat and milk products may vary considerably; beef, pork, and cheese products usually contain considerable amounts of fat, up to 70 percent or more fat Calories. The meat and dairy industries are responding to dietary modifications by many Americans and are making low-fat red meats and low-fat cheeses available to consumers. For example, 3 ounces of beef eye of round or pork tenderloin contain about 140 Calories, 4 grams of total fat, and 1.5 grams of saturated fat; both cuts of meat contain fewer than 30 percent of their Calories as fat. Lean cuts of poultry and fish have much lower levels of fat. Trimming the fat from meats or removing the skin from poultry drastically reduces the fat content. Some fish, such as flounder and tuna, are remarkably low in fat, whereas others, such as salmon and mackerel, are higher in total fat content but contain greater amounts of omega-3 fatty acids. Look for foods in the very lean meat exchange list in appendix D. In the milk group, whole milk contains about 8 grams of fat per cup; skim milk contains about 0.5–1.0 gram, which is much less than whole milk. Low-fat cheese alternatives containing soy or rice are available.

Small amounts of *trans* fatty acids are found naturally in beef, butter, and milk, but deep-fried foods and commercially prepared products, particularly stick margarine and snack foods such as chips, cakes, and cookies, may contain substantial amounts. The health risks associated with *trans* fatty acids are discussed later in this chapter.

Most plant foods, such as vegetables, fruits, beans, and natural whole-grain products, generally are low in fat content, and the fat they do contain is mostly unsaturated. On the other hand, some plant foods, such as nuts, seeds, and avocados, are very high in fat, but again primarily unsaturated fats. However, coconuts and palm kernels are extremely high in both total and saturated fats.

All fats contain a mixture of saturated, monounsaturated, and polyunsaturated fatty acids. Later in this chapter, we discuss some health implications relating to the types of fats we eat; figure 5.3 presents an approximate percentage of the amount of saturated, monounsaturated, and polyunsaturated fatty acids found in some common oils and fats. Several high-content sources for each of the various types of fatty acids are noted.

How do I calculate the percentage of fat Calories in a food?

It is important to realize that a product advertised as 95 percent fat free (or only 5 percent fat) may contain a considerably higher percentage of its Calories as fat: The advertised percentage refers to the *weight of the product, not its caloric content*. The product may contain a considerable amount of water, which contains no Calories. Thus, luncheon meat advertised as 95 percent fat free may actually contain more than 40 percent of its Calories from fat depending on the water weight. Foods with a high water content contain even higher percentages of fat Calories. A striking example is whole milk, which is only 3.5 percent fat by weight; however, one glass of milk contains about 150 Calories and 8 grams of fat, which accounts for 48 percent of the caloric content ($8 \times 9 = 72$; $72/150 = 48$). Even low-fat milk (2 percent fat) contains about 37 percent fat Calories.

If you want to calculate the percentage of fat calories in most foods you eat, you can get the information you need from the food

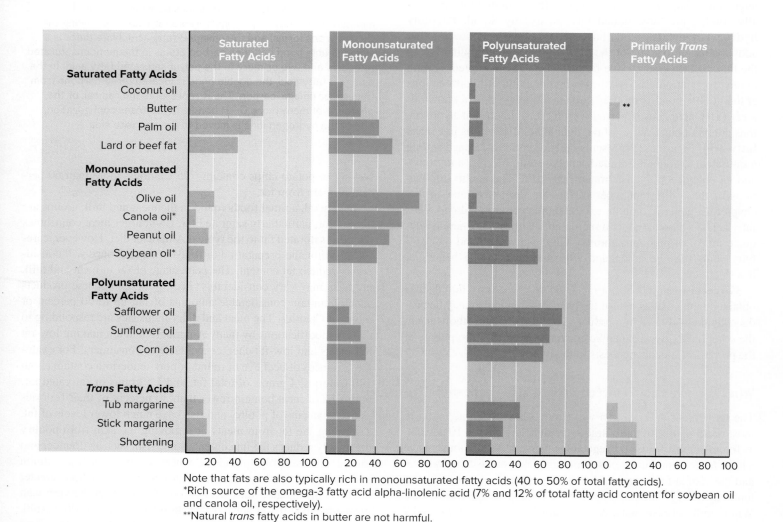

Note that fats are also typically rich in monounsaturated fatty acids (40 to 50% of total fatty acids).
*Rich source of the omega-3 fatty acid alpha-linolenic acid (7% and 12% of total fatty acid content for soybean oil and canola oil, respectively).
**Natural *trans* fatty acids in butter are not harmful.

FIGURE 5.3 Saturated, monounsaturated, polyunsaturated, and *trans* fatty acid composition of common fats and oils (expressed as % of all fatty acids in the product.

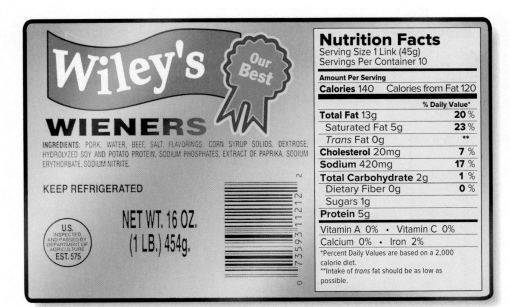

FIGURE 5.4 Reading labels helps locate hidden fat. Who would think that wieners (hot dogs) can contain about 85 percent of energy content as fat? Looking at the hot dog itself does not suggest that almost all its energy content comes from fat, but the label shows otherwise. Do the math: 120/140 Calories = 0.85, or 85 percent.

label, which will include the total Calories and the Calories from fat; additional mandatory information is the total fat, saturated fat, and *trans* fatty acid content. The label optionally may list the Calories from saturated fat and the amounts of polyunsaturated and monounsaturated fat. Figure 5.4 presents a food label to help illustrate the hidden fat in a hot dog (wiener). If you do not have a food label, then you will need to know the Calories and grams of fat for the food. Both of these values can be obtained from a food composition table found in most basic nutrition texts or online. Table 5.1 presents the methods for calculating the percent of fat Calories and percent of saturated fat Calories from either a food label or food composition table. Table 5.2 represents the percentage of food energy that is derived from fat in some common foods; the percentages are indicated for both total fat and saturated fat. Additional information is presented in chapter 11, where the focus is on reducing high-fat foods in the diet as a means to Calorie control.

What are fat substitutes?

Fat substitutes, or fat replacers, are supposedly designed to provide the taste and texture of fats, but without the Calories (9 Calories per gram), saturated fat, or cholesterol. They are found in many normally high-fat products, such as ice cream, that are marketed as fat free. Fat substitutes may be manufactured from carbohydrate, protein, or fats. Although a number of fat substitutes are under development, the following are commonly used.

Some carbohydrates, such as starches and gums, provide thickness and structure and are useful as fat substitutes. Guar gum, gum arabic, and cellulose gel are examples. Oatrim, made from oats, is being used to replace fat in milk. Depending on the form used, the caloric content may range from 0 to 4 Calories per gram. Simplesse is manufactured from milk or egg protein by a microparticulation process so that it has the taste and texture of fat. The caloric value of Simplesse is only 1.3 Calories per gram. The use of Simplesse has been approved by the FDA. Salatrim, which

TABLE 5.1	Calculation of the percentage of Calories in foods that are derived from fat

Method A. Data from food label

Amount per serving

Calories = 90
Calories from fat = 30
To calculate percentage of food Calories that consist of fat, simply divide the Calories from fat by the Calories per serving and multiply by 100 to express as a percent.
30/90 = 0.33   0.33 × 100 = 33 percent fat Calories

Method B. Data from food composition table

Amount per serving

Calories = 90
Total fat, grams = 8
Saturated fat, grams = 3
To calculate percentage of food Calories that consist of total fat or saturated fat, use the caloric value for fat of 1 gram = 9 Calories.
Total fat = 8 grams
Total fat Calories = 8 grams × 9 Calories/gram = 72 Calories
Use the same procedure as in Method A.
72/90 = 0.80   0.80 × 100 = 80 percent fat Calories
Saturated fat = 3 grams
Saturated fat Calories = 3 grams × 9 Calories/gram = 27 Calories
27/90 = 0.30   0.30 × 100 = 30 percent saturated fat Calories

is an acronym for *short- and long-chain fatty acid triglyceride molecule,* is a modified fat containing only 5 Calories per gram. Olestra is an ester of sucrose with long-chain fatty acids, a structure that cannot be hydrolyzed by digestive enzymes or absorbed by the gastrointestinal tract and therefore supplies no Calories to the body.

TABLE 5.2 Percentage of total fat Calories and saturated fat Calories in some common foods*

Food	% Calories total fat	% Calories saturated fat	Food	% Calories total fat	% Calories saturated fat
Meat group			*Vegetables*		
Bacon	80	30	Asparagus	8	2
Beef, lean and fat (untrimmed)	70	32	Beans, green	7	1.5
			Broccoli	12	1.5
Beef, lean only (trimmed)	35	15	Carrots	4	<1
			Potatoes	1	<1
Hamburger, regular	62	29	*Fruits*		
Chicken, breast (with skin)	35	11			
			Apples	5	<1
Chicken, breast (without skin)	19	5	Bananas	5	2
			Oranges	4	<1
Luncheon meat (bologna)	82	35	*Starches/breads/cereals*		
Salmon	37	7	Bread		
Flounder, tuna	8	2	White	12	2
Egg, white and yolk	67	22	Whole wheat	12	2
Egg, white	0	0	Crackers	30	12
Milk group			Doughnuts	43	7
			Macaroni	5	<1
Milk, whole	45	28	Macaroni and cheese	46	20
Milk, skim	5	2.5	Oatmeal	13	2
Cheese, cheddar	74	47	Pancakes, wheat	30	7
Cheese, mozzarella, part skim	56	35	Spaghetti	5	<1
Ice cream	49	28	*Fats and oils*		
Ice milk	31	18	Butter	99	62
Yogurt, partially skim milk	29	14	Lard	99	40
Dried beans and nuts			Margarine	99	21
			Oil, corn	100	13
Beans, dry, navy	4	<1	Oil, coconut	100	87
Beans, navy, canned with pork	28	12	Salad dressings		
			French	95	15
Peanuts	77	17	French, special dietary low fat	14	<1
Peanut butter	76	19			

<1 = less than 1 percent
*Percentages may vary. See food labels for specific information when available.

What is cholesterol?

Cholesterol is one of the lipids known as *sterols*. It is not a fat, but it is a fat-like, pearly substance found in animal tissues. Cholesterol is not an essential nutrient for humans because it is manufactured naturally in the liver from fatty acids and from the breakdown products of carbohydrate and protein—glucose and amino acids.

What foods contain cholesterol?

Cholesterol is found only in animal products and is not found in fruits, vegetables, nuts, grains, or other nonanimal foods. Table 5.3 presents some foods from the meat and milk groups

with the cholesterol content in milligrams. Several foods from the bread/cereal group are also included, indicating that the preparation of some bread/cereal products may add cholesterol by including some animal product containing cholesterol, mainly eggs.

Some plants contain various products that resemble cholesterol. Plant sterols and stanols may possess some health benefits, as noted later in this chapter.

What are phospholipids?

Chemically, **phospholipids** are somewhat comparable to triglycerides. They have a glycerol base, one or two attached fatty acids, and an additional structure that contains a phosphate group. One

TABLE 5.3	Cholesterol content, in milligrams, for some common foods	
	Amount	**Cholesterol**
Meat group		
Beef, pork, ham	1 oz	25
Poultry	1 oz	23
Fish	1 oz	21
Shrimp	1 oz	45
Lobster	1 oz	25
Eggs	1	220
Liver	1 oz	120
Milk group		
Milk, whole	1 cup	27
Milk, 2%	1 cup	15
Milk, skim	1 cup	7
Butter	1 tsp	12
Margarine	1 tsp	0
Cream cheese	1 tbsp	18
Ice milk	1 cup	10
Ice cream	1 cup	85
Bread/cereal group		
Bread	1 slice	0
Biscuit	1	17
Pancake	1	40
Sweet roll	1	25
French toast	1 slice	130
Doughnut	1	28
Cereal, cooked	1 cup	0

Fruits, vegetables, grains, and nuts have no cholesterol.

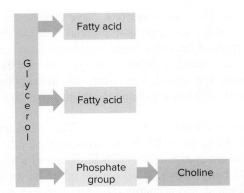

FIGURE 5.5 Simplified diagram of the phospholipid lecithin.

of the most common phospholipids is **lecithin**, whose structure is depicted as a simple diagram in figure 5.5. Phospholipids are not essential nutrients, as the body can make them from triglycerides. As discussed later in this chapter, some phospholipids have been studied as potential ergogenic aids.

What foods contain phospholipids?

Egg yolks provide substantial amounts of lecithin, and other good sources include liver, wheat germ, and peanuts. However, lecithin may be degraded in the digestive tract to smaller constituents. Your body can make all of the phospholipids it needs. Because dietary phospholipids are not associated with any health risks, there is little concern with dietary intake.

How much fat and cholesterol do we need in the diet?

In a review, Jequier indicated that we need dietary fat for three reasons: to meet energy needs, to provide essential fatty acids, and to provide essential fat-soluble vitamins.

Dietary fats are a concentrated source of energy, and adequate dietary intake is very important during the growth and development years. Dietary fats also provide several essential fatty acids, without which various health problems would develop. Dietary fats also provide the fat-soluble vitamins A, D, E, and K.

These factors, along with possible implications for health, were taken into consideration in the development of Dietary Reference Intakes for dietary fats, which may be found in the DRI table for macronutrients in the front inside cover. For the purpose of developing its DRI, the National Academy of Sciences classified fat into the following categories:

Total fat
Saturated fatty acids (SFAs)
Cis monounsaturated fatty acids (MUFAs)
Cis polyunsaturated fatty acids (PUFAs)
   n-6 fatty acids (omega-6)
   n-3 fatty acids (omega-3)
Trans fatty acids

The abbreviations for the various fatty acids, as well as the omega classification, will be used interchangeably with the respective fat or fatty acids.

Total Fat The Academy developed an AMDR of 20–35 percent of daily energy intake from total fat, which is an estimate based on adverse effects that may occur from consuming either a low-fat or high-fat diet. Individuals should obtain sufficient but not excessive amounts of dietary fat within this range of energy intake. No RDA, AI, or UL have been developed for total fat because of insufficient evidence, but diets higher than 35 percent dietary fat are not recommended because saturated fat intake may be increased beyond this level. Other health professional groups have recommended 30 percent of daily energy intake as the maximal from fat.

Saturated Fatty Acids and *Trans* Fatty Acids The Academy did not develop an RDA, AI, or UL for saturated fat or *trans* fat. However, increased intake of both of these fats is associated with increased risk of coronary heart disease. Although the Academy notes that because most diets contain fats and because most fats contain a mixture of fatty acids, it is not possible to consume a diet devoid of saturated and *trans* fats. Nevertheless, the prevailing undertone in this DRI report is to minimize the dietary intake of these two types of fat. Other health organizations suggest a maximum of 7–10 percent of the daily energy intake be derived from the combination of saturated and *trans* fats. In the popular media, saturated and *trans* fats are often referred to as *bad* fats.

Cis Monounsaturated Fatty Acids The Academy did not develop an RDA, AI, or UL for monounsaturated fats, indicating that they are not essential fatty acids because they may be synthesized by the body. About 20–40 percent of the fat we consume is monounsaturated, and primarily olive oil. Although no DRI have been set for monounsaturated fat, the Academy notes that they may have some benefit in the prevention of chronic disease. Olive oil is a staple in the Mediterranean diet and its alleged health benefits will be discussed later in this chapter. In the popular media, monounsaturated fats are often referred to as *good* fats.

Cis Polyunsaturated Fatty Acids The Academy developed an AI for polyunsaturated fatty acids because there may be some health benefits associated with such dietary intakes. AI were set for both omega-6 and omega-3 fatty acids. In the popular media, some polyunsaturated fats, particularly omega-3 fatty acids, are often referred to as *good* fats.

Omega-6 fatty acids Linoleic acid, an essential omega-6 polyunsaturated fatty acid, must be supplied in the diet because the body cannot produce it from other fatty acids. The AI for adult males age 19–50 is 17 grams of linoleic acid daily, 12 grams/day for females. For males and females age 51 and over, the AI are 14 and 11 grams daily, respectively. Somewhat smaller AI have been developed for children and adolescents age 9–18. Linoleic acid is found in vegetable and nut oils—such as corn, sunflower, peanut, and soy oils—that constitute food products such as margarine, salad dressings, and cooking oils. **Conjugated linoleic acid (CLA)**, an isomer of linoleic acid, has been suggested to be ergogenic and possess health benefits, which will be discussed in later sections of this chapter.

Omega-3 fatty acids Alpha-linolenic acid, an omega-3 polyunsaturated fatty acid, is also considered to be an essential fatty acid. The AI for adult males age 19 and older is 1.6 grams of alpha-linolenic acid daily, 1.1 grams/day for females. Somewhat smaller AI have been developed for children and adolescents age 9–18. Alpha-linoleic acid is found in green leafy vegetables, canola oil, flaxseed oil, soy products, some nuts, and fish. The potential health benefits of omega-3 fatty acids, including several derived from fish oils (eicosapentaenoic acid, EPA; docosahexaenoic acid, DHA), are discussed later in this chapter.

Cholesterol Cholesterol is vital to human physiology in a variety of ways, so the body needs an adequate supply. Because cholesterol may be manufactured in the body from either fats, carbohydrate, or protein, however, there is apparently little need for us to obtain large amounts, if any, in the foods we eat. Also, because a positive relationship has been established between high

blood cholesterol levels and coronary heart disease, reduction of dietary cholesterol has been advocated by a number of health-related associations. The American Heart Association, in its set of dietary guidelines, recommends that cholesterol intake be less than 300 milligrams/day, or about 100 milligrams of cholesterol for every 1,000 Calories you eat.

The 2015 Dietary Guidelines for Americans are currently being developed. In a surprising decision, the 2015 Dietary Guidelines Advisory Committee decided not to forward the previous recommendation about limiting cholesterol intake to 300 milligrams/day. The committee identified dietary cholesterol as a nutrient "not of concern for overconsumption" and noted that there is no relationship between dietary and serum cholesterol. This controversial recommendation has been criticized but demonstrates the complex relationship between dietary fat and cholesterol and health. Practically speaking, foods that are high in cholesterol are often high in Calories and saturated fat. Therefore, a diet that is low cholesterol may still be beneficial for health.

Table 5.4 indicates the grams of fat and saturated fat and milligrams of cholesterol that may be consumed daily on a diet containing 30 percent of the Calories as fat and less than 300 milligrams of cholesterol. For the 30 percent recommendation, a very simple method to determine the grams of total fat you may consume on a given caloric diet is to simply drop the zero from the daily caloric total and divide by 3—for example,

$$2,100\text{-Calorie diet}$$
$$2,100 = 210$$
$$210/ = 70 \text{ grams total fat}$$

For lower percentages of fat Calories, say 20 percent, simply multiply the daily caloric intake by the percentage desired and divide by 9 to get the grams of fat allowed per day. For example, 20 percent of 2,500 Calories would permit 500 Calories from fat, or about 55 grams/day.

As we shall see later in this chapter and in chapter 10, excessive consumption of dietary fat and cholesterol may be linked to a variety of chronic diseases, including heart disease and obesity. In certain individuals with blood lipid abnormalities, the recommended reduction in dietary fats and cholesterol is even greater than the Prudent Healthy Diet, with the total dietary Calories from fat being 20 percent or lower in some diet plans, as in the Ornish diet plan.

TABLE 5.4	Daily allowance for grams of fat and saturated fat, and milligrams of cholesterol*			
Total Calories	Fat Calories	Grams of fat	Grams of saturated fat	mg of cholesterol
1,000	300	33	11	100
1,500	450	50	16	150
2,000	600	66	22	200
2,500	750	83	27	250
3,000	900	100	33	300

*Based on a diet containing 30 percent of Calories as fat with 100 milligrams of cholesterol per 1,000 Calories.

Theoretically, high-fat diets may be deleterious to physical performance in several ways. The fat may displace carbohydrate in the diet, may lead to excessive caloric intake and body weight, and may cause gastrointestinal distress if consumed as part of a pregame meal. All of these factors could impair physical performance. On the other hand, some investigators have contended that high-fat diets may enhance exercise performance. These issues will be discussed later in this chapter.

Key Concepts

▶ The three major lipids in human nutrition are triglycerides, cholesterol, and phospholipids.

▶ Triglycerides, which consist of fatty acids and glycerol, account for about 98 percent of the lipids we eat. Fatty acids may be saturated or unsaturated. Unsaturated fatty acids may be monounsaturated or polyunsaturated. Polyunsaturated fatty acids exist in two forms, *cis* and *trans*. Omega-3 fatty acids are also polyunsaturated.

▶ The fat content of foods varies considerably, but generally the fruit, vegetable, and starch food exchanges are good sources of unsaturated fats and are low in total fat, whereas the meat and milk food exchanges contain foods that may have a high total fat and saturated fat content.

▶ Cholesterol is a nonfat substance vital to human metabolism, and although it may be obtained in the diet only from animal foods, the body can produce its own supply from other dietary nutrients such as saturated fats.

▶ The AMDR for dietary fat is 20–35 percent of daily caloric intake. Although some fat is essential in the diet as a source of essential fatty acids (linoleic and alpha-linolenic) and the fat-soluble vitamins (A, D, E, K), these nutrients may be obtained from polyunsaturated fats. The total amount of saturated and *trans* fats in the diet should be less than 10 percent, preferably 7 percent of daily caloric intake, while monounsaturated and polyunsaturated fats should constitute the majority of the AMDR.

Check for Yourself

▶ Peruse food labels of some of your favorite foods and check the fat content. Pay particular attention to percent Daily Value for total fat, saturated fat, and cholesterol. Check also for *trans* fat content.

Metabolism and Function

In this section we briefly cover the digestion of dietary lipids, their metabolic disposal in the body, interactions with carbohydrate and protein, the major functions of fats in the body, and energy stores of fat.

How does dietary fat get into the body?

The major dietary sources of lipids are the triglycerides, comprising about 98 percent, while the other 2 percent consists mainly of sterols and phospholipids. Most of the dietary triglycerides contain long-chain fatty acids (14 or more carbons). Lipids are insoluble in water, and therefore their digestion and absorption is somewhat more complicated than that of carbohydrates; a broad overview is presented in figure 5.6. As lipids enter the small intestine, they stimulate hormonal secretion by the intestine that culminates in the secretion of bile from the gallbladder and lipases from the pancreas into the intestinal lumen. The bile salts serve as emulsifiers, breaking up the lipid droplets into smaller segments that may be hydrolyzed by the lipid enzymes, pancreatic lipases, and cholesterases. In essence, lipids are hydrolyzed into free fatty acids (FFAs), glycerol, cholesterol, and phospholipids, which through an intricate process are then absorbed into the cells of the intestinal mucosa. Here they are combined into a fat droplet called a **chylomicron**, which contains a large amount of triglyceride and smaller amounts of cholesterol, phospholipids, and protein. The chylomicron is one form of a **lipoprotein**, which, by its name, you can see is composed of lipids and protein. A diagram of a lipoprotein is presented in figure 5.7. The chylomicron then leaves the intestinal cell and is absorbed by the lacteal in the villi, where it is eventually transported in the lymphatic system to the blood. A schematic of the absorption process is presented in figure 5.8.

Medium-chain triglycerides (MCTs) release medium-chain fatty acids (MCFAs) with shorter carbon chain lengths (6–12 carbons), enabling them to be absorbed directly into the blood without being converted into chylomicrons. They are transported directly to the liver. Because of this rapid processing, MCTs have been theorized to possess ergogenic potential, and their efficacy in this regard will be discussed in a later section. Short-chain fatty acids (SCFAs) derived from triglycerides are also absorbed like MCFAs.

What happens to the lipid once it gets in the body?

The digestion of lipids into chylomicrons is slow, and the absorption after a high-fat meal can last several hours. As the chylomicron circulates in the blood, it reacts with various cells in the body, particularly cells in the muscle and adipose tissues. Specific proteins in the outer coat of lipoproteins are known as apolipoproteins. **Apolipoproteins**, or *apoproteins,* increase lipid solubility and enable the various lipoproteins to react with specific receptors in cells throughout the body. The apolipoproteins in the chylomicron interact with an enzyme, lipoprotein lipase, which is produced in the muscle and adipose cells and released to the capillary blood vessels surrounding the cells. The lipoprotein lipase releases fatty acids and glycerol from the chylomicron. The fatty acids are absorbed into the cells by simple diffusion and receptors for some LCFAs, while the glycerol is transported primarily to the liver for conversion to glucose. The remains of the chylomicron, the chylomicron remnant, are transported to the liver for disposal.

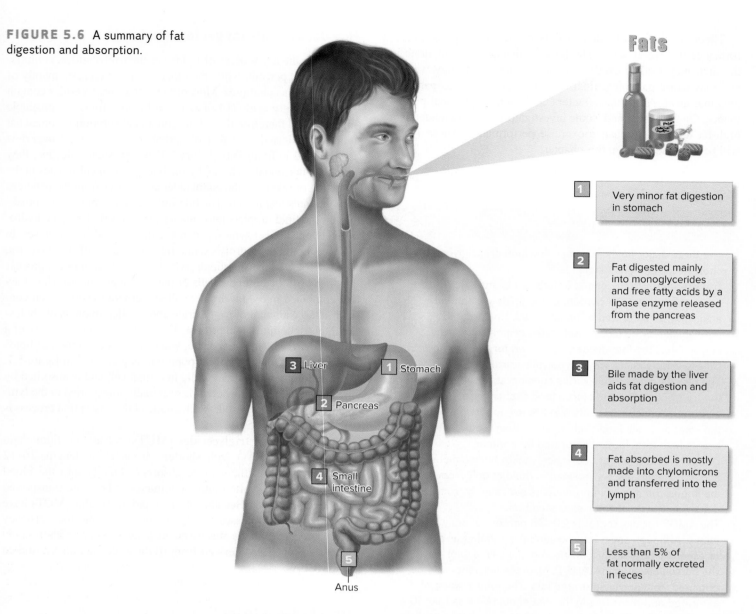

FIGURE 5.6 A summary of fat digestion and absorption.

Fats

| 1 | Very minor fat digestion in stomach |

| 2 | Fat digested mainly into monoglycerides and free fatty acids by a lipase enzyme released from the pancreas |

| 3 | Bile made by the liver aids fat digestion and absorption |

| 4 | Fat absorbed is mostly made into chylomicrons and transferred into the lymph |

| 5 | Less than 5% of fat normally excreted in feces |

3 Liver   1 Stomach

2 Pancreas

4 Small intestine

5

Anus

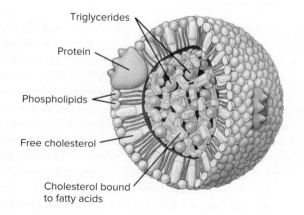

Triglycerides

Protein

Phospholipids

Free cholesterol

Cholesterol bound to fatty acids

FIGURE 5.7 Schematic of a lipoprotein. Lipoproteins contain a core of triglycerides and cholesterol esters surrounded by a coat of apoproteins, cholesterol, and phospholipids. The proportion of protein, cholesterol, triglycerides, and phospholipids varies among the different types of lipoproteins.

In the muscle, the fatty acids may either be used as a source of energy or combine with newly generated glycerol, which is derived as a metabolic by-product of glycolysis, leading to the formation and storage of muscle triglycerides. In exercise science literature, intramuscular triglycerides are often referred to as *intramyocellular triacylglycerol (IMTG)*. In the adipose cell, most of the fatty acids combine with glycerol and are stored as adipose cell triglycerides.

The key organ in the body for the metabolism of most nutrients is the liver. It is a clearinghouse in human metabolism. As blood passes through the liver, its cells take the basic nutrients and convert them into other forms. As mentioned in chapter 4, the liver is able to manufacture glucose from a variety of other nutrients, including glycerol. Pertinent to our discussion here is its role in lipid metabolism. As noted previously, glycerol and chylomicron remnants, including phospholipids, are transported to the liver, as are the MCFAs and SCFAs directly from the intestinal tract. Adipose cells are metabolically active in the sense that they are constantly releasing fatty acids for use by the body, including

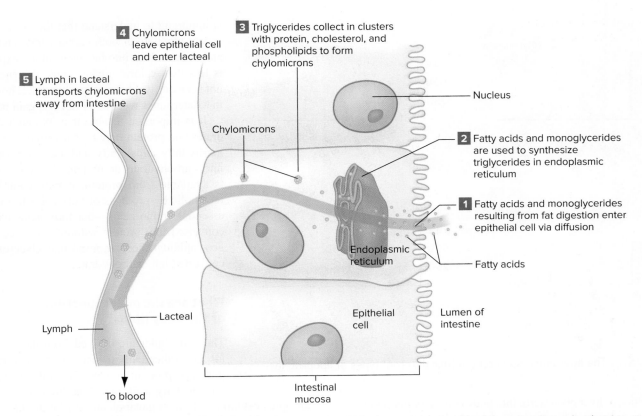

4 Chylomicrons leave epithelial cell and enter lacteal

3 Triglycerides collect in clusters with protein, cholesterol, and phospholipids to form chylomicrons

5 Lymph in lacteal transports chylomicrons away from intestine

Chylomicrons

Nucleus

2 Fatty acids and monoglycerides are used to synthesize triglycerides in endoplasmic reticulum

1 Fatty acids and monoglycerides resulting from fat digestion enter epithelial cell via diffusion

Endoplasmic reticulum

Fatty acids

Lacteal

Epithelial cell

Lumen of intestine

Lymph

To blood

Intestinal mucosa

FIGURE 5.8 The absorption of lipids. In the lumen of the intestine, several lipases, assisted by bile salts, digest lipids to various forms of fatty acids, phospholipids, cholesterol, and glycerol, which are absorbed by an intricate process into the epithelial cells of the intestinal mucosa. Here they are combined with protein to form chylomicrons, a form of lipoprotein, which are transported out of the cell and into the lacteal, where the lymph eventually carries them to the blood. Medium-chain triglycerides (MCTs) may be absorbed directly into the blood (not depicted).

the liver. The major role of the liver is to combine these various components (fatty acids, glycerol, cholesterol, and phospholipids), along with protein, into various forms of lipoproteins.

What are the different types of lipoproteins?

After the chylomicrons have been cleared from the blood, which may take several hours, other lipoproteins constitute approximately 95 percent of the serum lipids. The metabolism of lipoproteins is complex, for they are constantly being synthesized and catabolized by the liver and other body tissues. As a result, there is an exchange of protein and lipid components among the different classes of lipoproteins, which can lead to the conversion of one form into another.

The classification of lipoproteins may be determined by several methods. One of the methods is by the type of apolipoprotein present and its functions. Lipoproteins have a number of different apoproteins, which enable them to react with different tissues. The letters *A, B, C, D,* and *E,* including subdivisions such as *A-I* and *A-II,* are common designations. The second method, most popularly known, is based on the density of the lipoprotein particle. Designations range from high to very low density.

The chylomicron is one form of lipoprotein, but it is relatively short-lived because it is derived from dietary fat intake. For our

purposes in this book, the major classifications of lipoproteins along with their suggested composition and function are listed next; a graphical depiction is presented in figure 5.9. However, it should be noted that a wide variety of lipoproteins exists, based on their specific lipid and protein content. Additionally, their metabolism and complete functions have not been totally elucidated.

VLDL (very low-density lipoproteins). **VLDL** consist primarily of triglycerides formed in the liver from endogenous sources, whereas chylomicrons contain triglycerides from exogenous sources, that is, the diet. Like chylomicrons, VLDL are transported to the tissues to provide fatty acids and glycerol. The loss of some triglycerides to the liver or tissues produces VLDL remnants, referred to as IDL (intermediate-density lipoprotein) or TRL (triglyceride-rich lipoprotein). These remnants are either taken up by the liver or converted into LDL. Apoprotein B is the major apoprotein associated with both VLDL and IDL.

LDL (low-density lipoproteins). **LDL** contain a high proportion of cholesterol and phospholipids, but little triglycerides. LDL are formed after the VLDL and IDL release most of their stores of triglycerides. LDL size may be important. One form of LDL, a small, dense LDL, with important health implications has been identified. LDL, interacting with cell membrane

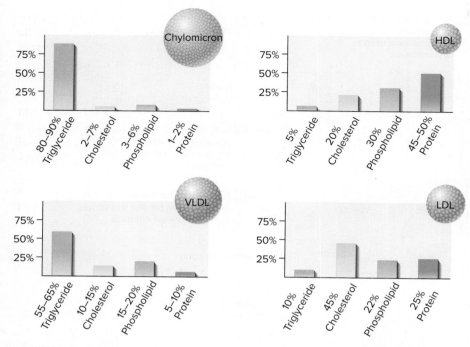

FIGURE 5.9 The approximate content of four different types of lipoproteins.

receptors, deliver cholesterol into body cells. Apolipoprotein B is the major apolipoprotein associated with LDL.

HDL (high-density lipoproteins). **HDL** contain a high proportion of protein (about 45–50 percent), moderate amounts of cholesterol and phospholipids, and very little triglycerides. Various HDL are produced in the liver and intestinal tract. Several subclasses of HDL have been identified, most notably HDL$_2$ and HDL$_3$. HDL transport cholesterol from peripheral cells to the liver, known as *reverse cholesterol transport.* Apolipoprotein A is the major apolipoprotein associated with HDL.

Lipoprotein (a). **Lipoprotein (a)** is very similar to the LDL, being in the upper LDL density range. The principal apolipoprotein associated with lipoprotein (a) is apolipoprotein (a).

Other apolipoproteins constitute the structure of lipoproteins. For example, apolipoprotein E is formed in the liver and present in all lipoproteins. These lipoproteins are needed to bind with cell membrane receptors.

A simplified schematic of fat metabolism is presented in figure 5.10. A more detailed diagram of lipoprotein interactions is presented in appendix G, figure G.4B.

Can the body make fat from protein and carbohydrate?

You may recall that glycogen is made up of many individual glucose molecules and is a glucose polymer. In essence, fatty acids are polymers of acetyl CoA, the primary substrate for the Krebs cycle.

As noted in figure 4.9, the amino acids of protein may be converted into acetyl CoA, which can then be converted into fat. Carbohydrates also may be converted into fat via acetyl CoA. It is important to understand that the body will take excess amounts of both carbohydrate and protein and convert them into fat when caloric expenditure is less than caloric intake. Thus, in general, it is not necessarily what you eat, but rather how much, that determines whether or not you gain body fat.

It is important to note that although carbohydrates and protein may be converted into fat (primarily fatty acids), fatty acids cannot be converted into carbohydrate or protein. If excess nitrogen is available from protein, it may combine with metabolic by-products of fatty acids to form nonessential amino acids—but fatty acids cannot be converted into protein without this excess nitrogen, although keep in mind that glycerol can be converted into carbohydrate.

What are the major functions of the body lipids?

The body lipids are derived from the dietary lipids and other carbon sources, namely carbohydrate and protein; however, with the exception of linoleic fatty acid and alpha-linolenic fatty acid, all lipids essential to human metabolism may be produced by the liver. The body lipids serve a variety of functions, including all three purposes of food: They form body structures, help regulate metabolism, and provide a source of energy.

Structure The structure of virtually all cell membranes, including the nerve membranes, consists partly of lipids, notably cholesterol and phospholipids. Lipids form myelin, an important component in the sheath covering nerve fibers. The structural fat deposits in the adipose tissues are used as insulators to conserve body heat and shock absorbers to protect various organs.

Metabolic Regulation Various fatty acids interact with proteins, the major metabolic regulators in the body. Essential fatty acids are found in cell membranes and are involved in various intracellular metabolic pathways, including regulation of gene expression. Cholesterol is a component of several hormones, such as testosterone and estrogen, which have diverse effects in the regulation of human metabolism. The majority of cholesterol in the body is used by the liver to produce bile salts, essential for the digestion of fats. Phospholipids are also instrumental for blood clotting.

Adipose cells produce various substances called **adipokines** (adipocytokines) and release them into the bloodstream. These adipokines may function as hormones, affecting tissues in other parts of the body. Leptin is one such adipokine that we will discuss in chapter 10.

Some derivatives of the omega-6 and omega-3 fatty acids formed by oxidation have some potent biological functions in the body. These derivatives—prostaglandins, prostacyclins, thromboxanes, and leukotrienes—are collectively known as **eicosanoids**. These eicosanoids possess local hormone-like properties that influence a number of physiological functions, including

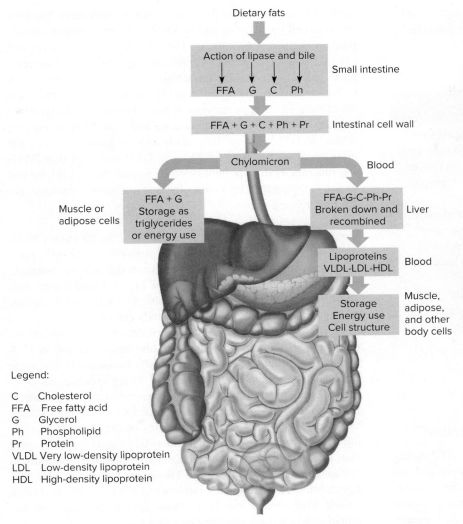

Dietary fats

Action of lipase and bile — Small intestine

FFA   G   C   Ph

FFA + G + C + Ph + Pr — Intestinal cell wall

Chylomicron — Blood

Muscle or adipose cells — FFA + G Storage as triglycerides or energy use

FFA-G-C-Ph-Pr Broken down and recombined — Liver

Lipoproteins VLDL-LDL-HDL — Blood

Storage Energy use Cell structure — Muscle, adipose, and other body cells

Legend:

C   Cholesterol
FFA   Free fatty acid
G   Glycerol
Ph   Phospholipid
Pr   Protein
VLDL Very low-density lipoprotein
LDL   Low-density lipoprotein
HDL   High-density lipoprotein

FIGURE 5.10 Simplified diagram of fat metabolism. After digestion, most of the fats are carried in the blood as chylomicrons. Through the metabolic processes in the body, fat may be utilized as a major source of energy, used to help develop cell structure, or stored as a future energy source.

several that may have implications for health or physical performance. Several important eicosanoids are derived from omega-3 fatty acids, and the theorized health and performance implications will be discussed in later sections of this chapter.

Energy Source   In general, the function of the majority of the body lipids, the triglycerides, is to provide energy to drive metabolic processes. The majority of the triglycerides in the body are stored in the adipose tissue. They break down to free fatty acids (FFA) and glycerol, which are released into the blood, with the FFA being transported to the tissues and the glycerol going to the liver. In the tissues, the FFA are reduced to acetyl CoA and enter the Krebs cycle to produce energy via the oxygen system. The glycerol is used by the liver to form other lipids or glucose. This energy-yielding process is illustrated in appendix G, figure G.4A.

During rest, nearly 60 percent of the energy supply is provided by the metabolism of fats when the individual consumes a

mixed diet, but it may be higher when blood glucose is low, as after an overnight fast. Most of the energy provided is presented to cells as fatty acids, either FFA delivered via the blood or fatty acids from stored intracellular triglycerides. Inside the cell, the metabolism of fatty acids into acetyl CoA (a 2-carbon molecule) is known as **beta-oxidation**, for the beta carbon is the second carbon on the fatty acid chain. The acetyl CoA is then processed through the citric acid (Krebs) cycle and associated electron transport system for production of energy as ATP. At rest, a high-fat meal will increase the proportion of energy derived from fat. In general, the greater the amount of fatty acids available in the plasma, the greater their use as a source of energy. For example, the heart muscle may derive 100 percent of its energy needs from fatty acids after a lipid-rich meal.

Ketones, ketoacids that are metabolic by-products of excess fatty acid metabolism, may also serve as an energy source for body cells. Ketones diffuse from the liver into the blood and are transported to the body tissues, where they can eventually be used as a source of energy. The major ketones are acetoacetic acid, beta-hydroxybutyric acid, and acetone. These ketones usually are produced in small amounts, but when the use of fatty acids as an energy source is high (such as with fasting, high-fat diets, and diabetes) ketone levels in the blood will increase. Ketones are an important energy source during fasting or starvation. However, excessive accumulation may lead to acidosis (ketosis) in the blood, a condition which may cause coma and death, such as in uncontrolled diabetes.

How much total energy is stored in the body as fat?

The greatest amount of energy stored in the body is fat in the form of triglycerides. Fat is a very efficient, compact means to store energy, for several reasons. First, fat has 9 Calories per gram, more than twice the value of carbohydrate and protein. Also, there is very little water in body fat compared to the 3–4 grams of water stored with each gram of carbohydrate or protein. In essence, based on weight, body fat may be about five to six times as efficient an energy store as carbohydrate and protein. If the average 154-pound man had to carry all the potential energy of his fat stores as carbohydrate, he would weigh nearly 300 pounds.

Most of the triglycerides are stored in the adipose tissues, approximately 80,000–100,000 Calories of energy in the average adult male with normal body fat. The triglycerides within and between the muscle cells may provide approximately 2,500–2,800 Calories, while those in the blood provide only about 70–80 Calories. The free fatty acids (FFA) in the blood total about 7–8 Calories. The liver also contains an appreciable store of triglycerides.

Thus, you can see that the human body contains a huge reservoir of energy Calories in the form of fat. A summary is presented in chapter 3, table 3.3.

Key Concepts

▶ Fats are transported in the blood primarily as lipoproteins. Lipoproteins may be classified by their density and have various functions. In general, VLDL transport fats to the tissues, LDL transport cholesterol to the tissues, and HDL transport cholesterol from the tissues.

▶ Dietary lipids may serve the three major functions of nutrients. They may be utilized as an energy source: they may be used as part of body-cell structure; and by-products of fat metabolism, known as eicosanoids, may act as local hormones and affect a variety of metabolic functions.

▶ The vast majority of dietary fats are stored as triglycerides in the adipose cells, but significant amounts may also be stored in the muscles as intramuscular triglycerides, also known as intramyocellular triacylglycerols.

Fats and Exercise

Are fats used as an energy source during exercise?

The two major energy sources for the production of ATP during exercise are carbohydrates in the form of muscle glycogen and fats in the form of fatty acids, mainly LCFA. In steady-state exercise, both can be converted into acetyl CoA for subsequent oxidation in the citric acid cycle. In general, a mixture of both fuel sources is used during exercise, although the quantitative values may vary depending on a variety of factors, including the intensity and duration of the exercise bout, the diet, and the training status of the individual. The use of fat as an energy source during endurance exercise, including the marathon, has been the subject of several recent symposia and reviews, including those by Hawley, Jeukendrup, Roepstorff, Spriet, and Spriet and Hargreaves, and several key studies, such as those by Romijn and associates. The following discussion represents some of the key findings from these reviews and studies.

Fat Energy Sources The fatty acids used by the muscle cells during exercise may be derived from a variety of sources, including the plasma triglycerides in the chylomicrons and VLDL, but these sources are considered to be minor, providing less than 10 percent of fat energy.

The two major energy sources are the plasma FFA and the fatty acids derived from intramuscular triglycerides (IMTG). The plasma FFA are in very short supply, so they must be replenished by the vast stores of triglycerides in the adipose tissue. An enzyme in the adipose cells, known as hormone-sensitive lipase (HSL), catabolizes the intracellular triglycerides to FFA and glycerol. The FFA are released into the blood, bound to the protein albumin as a carrier and transported to the muscle cells or other cells. The FFA enter the cell by diffusion and by specific protein receptors (transporters) in the cell membrane. The FFA are activated in the cell cytoplasm, transported into the mitochondria by an enzyme complex containing the amine **carnitine**, metabolized to acetyl CoA by beta-oxidation, and produce energy via the citric acid cycle and the associated electron transport system. The muscle triglycerides may also be metabolized to fatty acids and glycerol by an enzyme similar to HSL, and the fatty acids may be transported into the mitochondria. (See figure 5.11.) van Loon indicated that IMTG can function as an important substrate source during exercise and its use is determined by various factors, including exercise intensity and training status.

Use during Exercise During rest, most of the fat energy needs of the body are met by the supply of plasma FFA to the cells. Fatty acids are constantly being mobilized from the adipose tissues to replenish the plasma FFA. Most of the FFA released during rest, about 70 percent, are actually re-esterified back into triglycerides, the remainder being delivered to the body cells for energy.

During exercise, only about 25 percent of these FFA are re-esterified, so this alone provides a substantial increase in FFA delivery to the muscle cells. Additionally, hormones that activate HSL, such as epinephrine, are secreted during exercise, stimulating the breakdown of adipose cell triglycerides and the release of FFA into the blood for transport and entrance to the muscle cell. Spriet noted that fatty acid proteins may be important in regulating the FFA transport into cells, and as Glatz and others reported, muscle contraction activates the fatty transporters in the muscle cell membrane, thus increasing FFA uptake into the muscle cell. Epinephrine also stimulates intramuscular lipases to catabolize muscle triglycerides into FFA. These fatty acids then enter the mitochondria and are degraded to acetyl CoA.

During mild exercise at about 25 percent of VO_2 max, 20 percent or less of the total energy cost is derived from carbohydrate, while

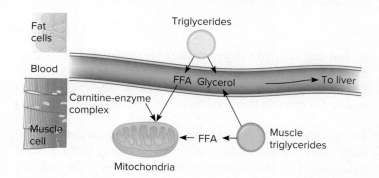

FIGURE 5.11 Fat as an energy source during exercise. Free fatty acids (FFA) are an important energy source during endurance exercise. They may be released by the adipose tissue triglycerides and travel by the blood to the muscle cells, and also may be derived from the muscle cell triglycerides. A carnitine-enzyme complex is needed to transport the FFA into the mitochondria. The glycerol that is released from the triglycerides may be transported to the liver for gluconeogenesis. (See appendix G, figure G.4A, for more details.)

the other 80 percent or more comes from fat. Wolfe indicates that exercise-induced lipolysis normally provides FFA at a rate in excess of that needed during exercise. Thus, the plasma FFA provided by the adipose tissue appear to be the major source of fat energy during mild exercise, but their percentage use decreases and that of muscle triglycerides increases as the exercise intensity increases up to about 65 percent VO_2 max. At this point, fats and carbohydrates appear to contribute equally to the energy expenditure, and the plasma FFA and muscle triglycerides contribute equally to the energy derived from fats. Carbohydrate increasingly becomes the predominant fuel as exercise exceeds 65 percent of VO_2 max. At high-intensity exercise levels, about 85 percent VO_2 max, the percentage contribution from fats (mostly muscle triglycerides) diminishes to 25 percent or less as muscle glycogen becomes the preferential energy source. These percentages are relevant to trained athletes and will be somewhat lower in untrained individuals. A summary of fat utilization during exercise is presented in table 5.5.

Limiting Factors   In a review, Lange stated that the human being is far from optimally designed for fat oxidation during exercise, noting that fat oxidation alone can sustain a metabolic rate corresponding to only 50–60 percent of VO_2 max. Although researchers contend that factors limiting fatty acid utilization during high-intensity exercise are largely unknown, several have been suggested. First, inadequate FFA mobilization from adipose tissue may limit FFA delivery to the muscle. Wolfe indicates that fat oxidation is increased significantly at exercise intensities of 85 percent VO_2 max when lipid is infused, but carbohydrate still remains the most significant source of energy. Second, suboptimal intramuscular processes may also limit fat oxidation. For example, Wolfe indicated that the high rate of carbohydrate oxidation during high-intensity exercise may inhibit fatty acid oxidation by limiting transport into the mitochondria, possibly by inhibition of the carnitine-enzyme complex.

In his review, Spriet noted that these two factors may limit fat utilization during high-intensity exercise, but other regulatory factors may be involved as well, such as limited transport of fatty acids into the muscle cell and the optimal muscle triglyceride

lipase activity. Frayn, in a review, concluded that there is a problem with delivery of sufficient fatty acids to muscle from adipose tissue only during high-intensity exercise. This limitation may be due to feedback inhibition of lipolysis, possibly due to lactate or catecholamine concentrations. As noted by Spriet, research is needed to determine what down-regulates fat use during exercise intensity above 85 percent of VO_2 max.

Dietary Effects   As noted in previous chapters, the amount of energy that may be obtained from muscle and liver glycogen is rather limited. Feeding carbohydrate before and during exercise may reduce fat utilization. Spriet and Hargreaves indicated that the reduction in fat metabolism following glucose ingestion appears to be the result of increased plasma insulin levels. Insulin may decrease adipose tissue lipolysis, thus decreasing FFA availability in the plasma. Also, insulin may reduce fatty acid oxidation in the muscle, possibly by inhibiting fatty acid transport into the mitochondria. Although fat oxidation may be reduced, the available carbohydrate would provide a more efficient energy source. In one study, Larson-Meyer and others found that reducing intramuscular lipid levels with a low-fat diet over the course of 3 days had no effect on endurance running performance, as measured by a 2-hour run at 62 percent of VO_2 max followed by a 10-kilometer time trial.

Carbohydrate intake before and during prolonged exercise helps, but within 90–120 minutes or more of high-intensity aerobic exercise, glycogen stores approach very low levels and the body shifts to an increasing usage of FFA, leading to a decrease in the intensity of the exercise. In cases such as prolonged endurance tasks like ultramarathons, FFA may provide nearly 90 percent of the energy in the latter stages of the event when muscle glycogen and blood glucose levels are inadequate to sustain higher-intensity exercise.

Use of Ketones   Although ketones may be utilized by the muscle, they do not appear to contribute significantly to energy production during exercise.

However, Jeff Volek, a leading expert on high-fat diets and nutritional ketosis, notes that there is a need for longer-term studies on performance. Volek contends that allowing an athlete to keto adapt, or allowing the atlete to spend long enough on a low-carbohydrate/high-fat diet to achieve very high fat oxidation rates, could have many health and performance benefits. However, this is controversial and a great deal more research needs to be conducted.

TABLE 5.5	Fat energy sources during exercise
Plasma chylomicrons	Not a major source
Plasma VLDL	Not a major source
Plasma FFA	Major source; replenished by adipose cell release of FFA; used in exercise at low to moderate intensity, i.e., 25–65 percent VO_2 max; use decreases as exercise intensity increases toward 65 percent VO_2 max
Muscle FFA	Major source; released from intramuscular triglycerides; low use during mild exercise; used increasingly as exercise intensity increases toward 65 percent VO_2 max

Note: With high-intensity exercise, 65 percent VO_2 max or higher, total fat oxidation falls.

Does gender or age influence the use of fats as an energy source during exercise?

Gender   Women possess a greater percentage of body fat than men, and several writers for popular runners' magazines have suggested that women could process this fat more efficiently and thus be more effective in ultramarathon events. Tarnopolsky indicated some theoretical rationale supports this viewpoint, as both the muscle lipid content and the maximal activity of a key enzyme in fat metabolism are higher in females.

The greater fat oxidation for women during submaximal endurance exercise compared with men seems to occur partly through a sex hormone–mediated enhancement of lipid-oxidation pathways. In several studies Tarnopolsky and his associates, using the respiratory exchange ratio to evaluate energy substrate utilization following carbohydrate loading, reported that women oxidized significantly more fat and less carbohydrate than men when exercising at 65 or 75 percent VO_2 max. Similar findings were presented in studies headed by Knechtle and Venables. Roepstorff noted that some sport scientists think women may use more IMTG during exercise than men, possibly attributed to gender differences in skeletal muscle HSL regulation.

However, other studies have shown similar utilization of fat as an energy source by men and women during exercise, particularly when matched for their aerobic capacity. Replicating their previous study with males, Romijn and others studied substrate metabolism in well-trained females at 25, 65, and 85 percent of VO_2 max. As with the men, carbohydrate oxidation in women increased progressively with exercise intensity, whereas the highest rate of fat oxidation was during exercise at 65 percent of VO_2 max. They concluded that the patterns of use of carbohydrate and fat during moderate- and high-intensity exercise are similar in trained men and women.

Whether or not women oxidize fat more efficiently than men appears to be debatable, and whether or not it improves ultraendurance performance is also questionable. For example, in one of their studies, cited previously, Tarnopolsky and others found that although the women oxidized more fat and less carbohydrate than the men, the men improved their performance in the exercise task following carbohydrate loading but the women did not.

Age   Young children may use more fat for energy during exercise compared to older, postpubertal children and adults. Aucouturier and others suggested that a low activity of glycolytic enzymes in children may lead to greater use of lipid for energy during submaximal exercise. In a 60-minute cycling task at 70 percent VO_2 max, Timmons and others reported a higher utilization of fat in 12-year-old preadolescent girls as compared to adolescent 14-year-old girls. In another comparably designed study, they reported similar findings between 12-year-old boys in various stages of puberty and 14-year-old pubertal boys. Stephens and others also found that young males in the early and middle stages of puberty, as compared to males in late puberty and early adulthood, used more fat and less carbohydrate during exercise at intensities ranging from 30 to 70 percent of VO_2 peak. However, they indicated that the conversion to an adult-like metabolic profile of fuel utilization during exercise appears to be complete by the end of puberty in males.

What effect does exercise training have on fat metabolism during exercise?

A single bout of exercise influences fat utilization during exercise. Tunstall and others found that a single endurance exercise session led to an increased expression of genes in the skeletal muscle that increase the capacity for fat oxidation, and 9 days of training augmented this effect.

TABLE 5.6	Possible mechanisms associated with the increased use of fat as an energy source during aerobic endurance exercise following exercise training

- Increased blood flow and capillarization to the muscle, delivering more plasma FFA
- Increased muscle triglyceride content, possibly associated with increased insulin sensitivity. Insulin regulates movement of FFA into muscle cells; exercise training may also increase the activity of lipoprotein lipase or fatty acid transporters at the muscle cell membrane
- Increased sensitivity of both adipose and muscle cells to epinephrine, resulting in increased FFA release to the plasma and within the muscle from triglycerides
- Increased number of fatty acid transporters in the muscle cell membrane to move fatty acids from the plasma into the muscle cell
- Improved ability to use ketones as an energy source
- Increased number and size of mitochondria, and associated oxidative enzymes for processing of activated FFA
- Increased activation of FFA and transport across the mitochondrial membrane
- Increased activity of oxidative enzymes

In general, research indicates that trained athletes use more fat than untrained athletes during a standardized exercise task. For example, if you ran an 8-minute mile both before and after a 2-month endurance training program, you would use the same amount of caloric energy each time. However, after training, more of that energy would be derived from fat. Hence, training helps you become a better fat burner, so to speak, which may help spare some of the glycogen in your muscles. Although the exact mechanisms have not been identified, the reviews by Horowitz and Klein and Jeukendrup and his colleagues document multiple factors, as presented in table 5.6.

Overall, according to Martin, the increased content and use of muscle triglycerides may be the primary mechanism underlying the greater capacity of trained muscle to oxidize fatty acids during exercise. Increased utilization of fat during exercise is one of the major effects of training experienced by the endurance athlete.

Although carbohydrate becomes more important as an energy source during high-intensity exercise, Coggan and others found highly trained endurance athletes may be able to use fats more efficiently at exercise intensity levels of 75–80 percent VO_2 max, and in a review Spriet noted that IMTG is an important energy source during prolonged, moderate dynamic exercise up to about 85 percent of VO_2 max in well-trained athletes. The ability to derive a substantial proportion of the energy demands of intensive exercise from fatty acids is extremely important for athletes such as marathoners who may be able to save some of their muscle glycogen for utilization in the latter stages of the race. An optimal mixture of fatty acids and glycogen for energy will enable them to sustain their pace, whereas the total depletion of muscle glycogen and subsequent reliance on fatty acids as the sole energy supply would force them to slow down. Thus, it is important for the endurance athlete to become a better "fat burner," and a variety of ergogenic aids have been proposed to enhance this effect.

Key Concepts

▶ One of the major functions of fat is to provide energy. Although fat may be an important energy source for low- to moderate-intensity exercise, it is not the optimal energy source during high-intensity aerobic or anaerobic exercise. Nevertheless, well-trained athletes may use IMTG as an energy source up to 85 percent of VO_2 max.

▶ Some research suggests that when compared to adult males, adult females may use more fat as a source of energy during endurance exercise; however, research with similarly well-trained male and female athletes reveals no differences in fuel utilization endurance exercise.

▶ Endurance exercise training, by enacting multiple mechanisms, enhances the use of fat for energy during aerobic exercise. Endurance athletes are better *fat burners*.

Fats: Ergogenic Aspects

Because exercise training leads to an increased utilization of fatty acids as an energy source and improved performance in prolonged endurance events (theoretically by sparing muscle glycogen), a variety of dietary practices, dietary supplements, and pharmacological agents have been employed in attempts to facilitate this metabolic process during exercise. In a review of the proposed mechanism, Jeukendrup noted that the increased availability and oxidation of fatty acids would generate more acetyl CoA, which in turn would inhibit a cascade of events that would essentially decrease the activity of enzymes involved in carbohydrate breakdown. Such an effect could spare the use of muscle glycogen and enhance endurance performance. As noted in chapter 4, preliminary studies from Clyde Williams's laboratory at Loughborough suggest that an increased fat metabolism may be the mechanism underlying enhanced endurance performance following a low-glycemic-index diet.

Both acute and chronic dietary strategies have been used to increase the concentration of muscle triglycerides or serum level of FFA. Such strategies include high-fat diets, fasting, and even infusion of lipids into the bloodstream. Dietary supplements and drugs have been used to either increase the supply of oxidizable fats or the rate of fat metabolism. Dietary supplements include medium-chain triglycerides, lecithin, glycerol, omega-3 fatty acids, carnitine, hydroxycitrate, conjugated linoleic acid, and phosphatidylserine. Caffeine also has been theorized to enhance fat oxidation, and its role as an ergogenic aid is covered in chapter 13.

High-fat diets

High-fat diets are among the most popular and controversial diets in nutrition. First, a great deal of research points to diets high in fat as disease promoting; this will be discussed later in the chapter.

Second, if one macronutrient is increased, and Calories are held constant, the amount of another macronutrient in the diet must decrease. The beneficial effect of high-carbohydrate diets on exercise performance, as described in the previous chapter, has been well documented, so if an increase in dietary fat results in a decrease in dietary carbohydrate, performance could be compromised. High-fat diets may be used on an acute or chronic basis. Some people refer to acute high-fat diets as **fat loading**.

Acute fat loading involves dietary strategies immediately before exercise. Hargreaves notes that elevated plasma FFA levels are associated with reduced muscle glycogenolysis, which could help spare muscle glycogen. Because the rate at which FFA are oxidized in the muscle is dependent in part upon their concentration in the blood plasma, several different acute dietary techniques have been tried in attempts to increase plasma FFA levels.

Chronic fat loading involves dietary strategies about a week or so prior to endurance exercise. These strategies are designed to increase lipid metabolism and gene expression in skeletal muscle, resulting in an increased ability of the skeletal muscle to use fat as an energy source during exercise. In a review, Roepstorff and others indicated that ingestion of a fat-rich diet induces an increase in intramuscular triglyceride (IMTG) content, primarily in the type I muscle fibers used for oxidative energy production. Spriet and Hargreaves reported that IMTG levels can be increased by 50 to 80 percent following the consumption of a high-fat diet. Thus, chronic high-fat diets are designed primarily to increase IMTG. Some investigators have also evaluated the effect of chronic fat loading prior to 1–2 days of carbohydrate loading to see if there were any additional benefits associated with this dietary protocol. This latter dietary protocol is similar to the classic carbohydrate-loading protocol discussed in chapter 4.

Acute High-Fat Diets Lipid digestion and absorption are slow, so one strategy is to infuse a lipid solution (such as Intralipid) directly into the blood along with heparin, a substance that stimulates lipoprotein lipase activity and increases plasma FFA levels. Such a strategy increases fat oxidation and reduces carbohydrate oxidation, which may enhance endurance exercise performance. However, after a lipid solution was used by a national team in the Tour de France, the entire team withdrew from the race allegedly due to adverse reactions. No research has been uncovered that supports this ergogenic technique.

A second strategy is to ingest a high-fat meal prior to exercise performance. For example, in two studies, Okano and others reported no significant differences between a high-fat meal (61 percent fat content) and a control or low-fat meal on performance in a cycling test to exhaustion at 78–80 percent VO_2 max following 2 hours of riding at 60–67 percent VO_2 max. Additionally, Rowlands and Hopkins investigated the effect of a high-fat (85 percent fat energy) meal, as compared to a high-carbohydrate (85 percent carbohydrate energy) meal and high-protein (30 percent protein energy) meal consumed 90 minutes before an endurance cycling test, which involved a 1-hour preload at 55 percent VO_2 max, five 10-minute incremental loads from 55–82 percent of peak power, and a 50-kilometer time trial that included several 1-km and 4-km sprints. Subjects consumed a carbohydrate supplement during the cycling protocol. The meal composition had no clear effect on sprint or 50-kilometer cycle performance.

An acute high-fat dietary strategy does not appear to enhance performance and, in fact, may actually impair performance if it contributes to gastrointestinal distress because of the delayed gastric emptying associated with fats. Research has shown that consuming a high-fat diet for 1 or 2 days, another acute approach, may actually impair performance in high-intensity exercise tasks.

One of the principles behind keto-adaptation is that athletes must be consuming high-fat diets for long enough to gain an effect. Thus, the lack of a benefit seen on exercise performance in studies of acute high-fat diets is not surprising.

Chronic High-Fat Diets Several investigators have challenged the dogma that endurance athletes need high-carbohydrate diets and suggest that endurance performance may benefit from diets containing about 50 percent or more energy from fat. Brown and Cox note that athletes can adapt to such a diet and maintain physical endurance capacity, will increase their muscle triglyceride levels, and may increase the use of fat and decrease use of carbohydrate during exercise. Stellingwerff and others recently reported that 5 days of a high-fat diet while training increases rates of whole body fat oxidation and decreases carbohydrate oxidation during aerobic cycling. In general, research has shown that when an individual is placed on a chronic low-carbohydrate and high-fat diet for about a week or more, the body adjusts its metabolism to use fats more efficiently. However, metabolic improvements do not necessarily correlate with or guarantee performance improvements. According to Yeo and others, it appears that there are responders and nonresponders to this practice. Thus, preliminary screening may be helpful to determine which athletes may benefit from this dietary intervention. But do such changes lead to enhanced endurance exercise performance?

Studies showing ergogenic effect Several studies support an ergogenic effect of chronic fat loading. Pendergast and Horvath, along with their associates, conducted several of the first contemporary studies. Although two studies from their laboratory have shown that adapting to a high-fat diet (38–41 percent fat content) over a 1- to 4-week period improved treadmill running time to exhaustion, both studies had problems with the experimental design, such as no random assignment of the diet conditions and no counterbalancing of diet order. Moreover, the diets were not exceptionally high in fat content. Muoio and others acknowledged the limitations to experimental design in their prototype study, and the interested reader is referred to the other study by Venkatraman and Pendergast.

More recently, Horvath and others had male and female runners consume diets of 16 and 31 percent fat for 4 weeks and then about half the subjects increased their dietary fat intake to 44 percent. All diets were designed to be isocaloric, but the runners actually consumed about 19 percent fewer Calories on the low-fat (16 percent) diet. There were no differences among the diets for VO_2 max, anaerobic power, or body mass, but the endurance run after the low-fat diet was reduced compared to the medium- and high-fat diets. However, it is possible that decreased energy intake contributed to this decrease in performance.

Lambert and her colleagues also found some ergogenic effects in several studies. In one study, they placed athletes on a high-fat (70 percent fat Calories) diet or low-fat (12 percent fat Calories) diet for 2 weeks, testing the effects on three performance tests done in consecutive order with 30 minutes rest between each. The three exercise tests included a Wingate high-power test, a high-intensity test to exhaustion at 90 percent VO_2 max, and a moderate-intensity test to exhaustion at 60 percent VO_2 max. Although there were no significant effects between the two diets for performance in the first two exercise tests, the cyclists rode significantly longer on the moderate-intensity test following adaptation to the high-fat diet. The investigators noted that adaptation to the high-fat diet decreased the reliance on carbohydrate as an energy source during exercise and thus suggested the improved performance was due to muscle-glycogen sparing.

In a subsequent study, Lambert and others evaluated the effect of a 10-day high-fat diet, prior to 3 days of a carbohydrate-loading regimen, on cycling performance in a trial consisting of 150 minutes at 70 percent VO_2 max followed by a 20-kilometer time trial. Compared to their habitual diet with carbohydrate loading, the high-fat diet enabled the endurance cyclists to increase total fat oxidation and reduce carbohydrate oxidation, as well as significantly improve time trial performance by 1.4 minutes.

Studies showing no ergogenic effect Conversely, other well-controlled research suggests that chronic high-fat diets do not benefit endurance performance. The most often cited study used to argue the beneficial effects of a low-carbohydrate, high-fat diet on endurance performance was published in 1983 by Phinney and colleagues. After 4 weeks of keto-adaptation, there were dramatic increases in fat oxidation (on average 90 g/hour) and decreases in exercise RQ (from 0.83 to 0.72) in five cyclists. Interestingly, pre-exercise muscle glycogen levels at the end of the study were half of what they were at baseline (143 vs. 76 mmol/kg). However, there were no changes in VO_2 max and no improvements in endurance performance as a result of the diet. Using well-trained cyclists as subjects, Havemann and others reported no significant differences in 100-kilometer time-trial performance when consuming either a high-fat (68 percent fat) or high-carbohydrate (68 percent carbohydrate) diet for 6 days, followed by 1 day of carbohydrate loading, but the high-fat diet impaired 1-kilometer sprint power. The authors noted that although the high-fat diet increased fat oxidation, it compromised high-intensity sprint performance.

Several studies have shown no effect of chronic fat loading on endurance performance in trained individuals. Brown and Cox, in a randomized study using 32 endurance-trained cyclists, reported no difference in 20-km road time performance over a period of 12 weeks when subjects consumed either a high-fat (47 percent of energy) or a high-carbohydrate (69 percent of energy) diet. Burke and her associates found no beneficial effects in two studies. In the first study they investigated the effects of a high-fat diet for 5 days, followed by a 1-day high-carbohydrate diet, on an endurance cycling protocol involving cycling at 70 percent VO_2 max for 2 hours followed by an intense time trial. Compared to a high-carbohydrate diet, the high-fat diet induced greater utilization of fat with an associated muscle glycogen sparing, but there was no significant improvement in the cycling time trial, even though performance following the high-fat phase was about 3.4 minutes faster. In a subsequent study using a similar protocol, Burke and her associates reported no significant effect on endurance performance.

In a similar vein, Rowlands and Hopkins compared the effects of three different 14-day dietary regimens on 100-kilometer cycling performance. One of the diets was high-carbohydrate, one was high-fat, and one was high-fat before 2.5 days of carbohydrate loading. Both high-fat diets increased fat oxidation during the cycling trial, and although there were no significant differences between the three trials, the 100-kilometer performance was approximately 3–4 percent faster with the high-fat diets. Interestingly, power output in the last 5 kilometers of the time trial was significantly greater for the high-fat with carbohydrate-loading trial as compared to the high-carbohydrate trial. The authors noted that although the main effects of the study were not significant, there was some evidence for enhanced ultraendurance cycling with a high-fat diet compared to a high-carbohydrate diet. Carey and others compared the effects of two 6-day diets, either high-carbohydrate or high-fat, on a prolonged cycling task involving 4 hours at 65 percent VO_2 peak followed by a 1-hour time trial. In both diets, a high-carbohydrate diet was consumed on the day prior to testing. Similar to other studies, the high-fat diet increased total fat oxidation and reduced carbohydrate oxidation, but there was no effect on cycling performance. However, the power output was 11 percent higher during the time trial after the high-fat diet as compared to the high-carbohydrate condition, but this difference was not statistically significant.

It is interesting to note that in three of these contemporary studies, although the chronic fat-loading protocol was not shown statistically to improve performance, the investigators did note that performance was generally improved compared to the other diets.

In a crossover design study, Holloway and others recently placed healthy men on 5-day diets of high fat (70 percent fat, 4 percent carbohydrates, and 26 percent protein) and a control (24 percent fat, 50 percent carbohydrates, and 26 percent protein). Men in the study ingested one diet and following a 2-week washout period consumed the other diet. The high-fat diet impaired cognitive function in the areas of attention, speed, and mood. A decrement in any one of these areas could affect an individual's ability to train and compete, particularly in activities that require an athlete to react to an opponent or conditions.

Reviews concluding no ergogenic effect Conversely, other reviewers concluded that chronic high-fat diets are not ergogenic. In her review, Bente Kiens noted that varying periods of fat adaptation followed by a carbohydrate-rich diet, despite an increased fat oxidation and a concomitant decrease in carbohydrate oxidation during submaximal exercise, exerts no beneficial effects on subsequent time trial endurance cycling performance.

In their review, Burke and Hawley indicated that endurance athletes who consume chronic high-fat diets, as compared to iso-caloric high-carbohydrate diets, may increase fat oxidation and spare use of muscle glycogen during submaximal exercise. They noted that these effects persist even under conditions in which carbohydrate availability is increased, either by consuming a high-carbohydrate meal before exercise and/or ingesting glucose solutions during exercise. Yet despite marked changes in the patterns of fuel utilization that favor fat oxidation, they conclude that this strategy does not provide clear benefits to the performance of prolonged endurance exercise.

Trent Stellingwerff, an expert in nutrition and athletic performance, reviewed the data on the effects of ketogenic diets on exercise performance. He noted that out of 21 published studies, 12 showed a performance decrease and 7 showed no benefit of a ketogenic diet. Only two studies are available that show improved performance. Stellingwerff estimates, via the rates of energy expenditure, ATP production, and available fuel stores, that an elite endurance athlete can "complete" a marathon while on a ketogenic diet but that the athlete's time to complete the race will be dramatically slower.

One of the questions that must be addressed when considering a low-carbohydrate, high-fat diet is not if you can finish the race but how fast you can finish the race. Volek and others correctly point out that a keto-adapted endurance athlete is able to oxidize up to 1.5 g of fat/min during an Ironman triathlon, and so would not need to ingest exogenous fuels such as carbohydrate to complete the race. However, Stellingwerff points out that under keto-adapted circumstances and based on the caloric requirements to complete a marathon, an athlete would only be able to complete the race in 3 to 4 hours. Thus, low-carbohydrate, high-fat diets may allow athletes to perform, but possibly not at their best and far from an elite level. In a *New York Times* article, Louise Burke, an expert on low-carbohydrate, high-fat/ketogenic diets, noted that "sports performance requires metabolic flexibility," which means that athletes need to be able to use one system well, not just fat oxidation.

Several things are not known and must be clearly defined for research on low-carbohydrate, high-fat/ketogenic diets to progress:

1. How much dietary fat and dietary carbohydrate constitute a low-carbohydrate, high-fat/ketogenic diet in terms of exercise performance?
2. How long does one have to stay on a low-carbohydrate, high-fat/ketogenic diet for beneficial effects to occur?
3. Is there a biological marker (e.g., blood ketones) that can be used to indicate when one is keto-adapted?
4. Are the effects of a low-carbohydrate, high-fat/ketogenic diet different based on training status, athletic event, body size, or any other variables?
5. Are low-carbohydrate, high-fat/ketogenic diets healthy for extended periods of time?

High-fat diets and weight loss

Despite the popularity of low-carbohydrate, high-fat/ketogenic diets in the media, the role of this style of diet in the long-term management of body mass is unclear. In a meta-analysis of 13 studies containing almost 1,600 individuals, Bueno and colleagues concluded that low-carbohydrate, high-fat diets result in greater reductions in body mass, triglycerides, and diastolic blood pressure. However, as has been described elsewhere in this text, care must be taken when interpreting the results of a meta-analysis. For instance, only 4 of the studies included lasted longer than 12 months, and weight loss relapse typically happens after this point in time. Importantly, although some cardiovascular risk factors improved, the authors point out that pathological markers such as hepatic lipids, endothelial function, cardiovascular events, and renal function, which are important when describing the safety of a diet, were not assessed. Also, compliance to these diets is an important factor, some studies had participant dropout rates as high as 50 percent, and by the end of the study, dietary carbohydrate intake from participants was higher than allowed in many studies. Finally, average BMI in the sample indicates that subjects were obese, so it is unclear what the effects of a low-carbohydrate, high-fat diet in normal-weight people might be.

The popularity of low-carbohydrate, high-fat diets continues to be very high, but a great deal more research needs to be conducted regarding the safety and efficacy of this style of eating. For instance, if people lose more weight when restricting carbohydrates, is it because they are eating less due to their displeasure with the diet plan? If so, it would seem that this style of eating may not be effective in the long run. Also, if this style of eating is sustainable, what are the long-term effects on health outcomes such as cancer or other diseases?

Often, when describing the effects of diet on health, we use proxy markers such as serum cholesterol, LDL, or blood pressure to estimate health. However, these markers do not perfectly predict or correlate with health. Ultimately, to answer a question about health, one must consider mortality as an outcome. Noto and colleagues reported analyzed 17 low-carbohydrate diet studies and found that low-carbohydrate diets were associated with increased risk of mortality but that they did not increase risk of cardiovascular disease mortality.

Does exercising on an empty stomach or fasting improve performance?

A controversial area related to dietary fat intake is the issue of fasting for a limited period of time prior to exercise. Some people contend that this will improve training adaptations and subsequently performance. Indeed, fasting, even an overnight fast, can increase FFA availability and, theoretically, increase fat oxidation, spare glycogen, and improve performance. On the other hand, if fasting reduces muscle glycogen or causes hypoglycemia, it could impair performance. Another popular theory is that training while fasted will encourage greater weight loss either through metabolic adaptations or reductions in appetite. Despite the large amount of available research on the benefits of carbohydrate ingestion before exercise, several research groups have examined exercising after various durations of fasting. The following is a summary.

Gutierrez and others reported decreased aerobic endurance physical working capacity in young men following a 3-day fast. Data from Peter Hespel's lab showed that following a 6-week endurance training program, training in a fasted state increased oxidative enzymes, such as citrate synthase and β-hydroxyacyl coenzyme A dehydrogenase, and intramyocellular lipid breakdown more than training in a fed state. Other work from this group showed that Glut-4 and proteins involved with fatty acid transport increased when training in the fasted state. However, following the endurance training program, there were no differences in VO_2 max between those who trained under fasted or fed conditions. Stannard and colleagues compared 4 weeks of fasted or fed endurance training and showed greater increases in VO_2 max in fasted subjects and greater increases in muscle glycogen in fed subjects. There were no differences in citrate synthase and β-hydroxyacyl coenzyme A dehydrogenase between groups. The reader is cautioned that beneficial metabolic changes may not lead to beneficial performance changes.

Some believe that training while fasted improves weight loss more than training in a fed state. Schonfeld and others examined the effects of 4 weeks of training in a fed or fasted state while on a hypocaloric diet. Both groups decreased body mass and fat mass, but there were no differences between groups. The authors acknowledge that a longer period of time may be needed for any differences between protocols to take effect. In acute studies, both Gonzalez and Deighton showed that there was no advantage of exercising after an overnight fast or after a meal on subsequent appetite or daily energy intake. Thus, there are no convincing data that athletes should train while in the fasted state. However, many Muslim athletes may be training or competing while fasting for religious reasons during Ramadan. Trabelsi and others showed that resistance training was unaffected by fasting during Ramadan but that fasted athletes were more likely to be dehydrated. In a similar study, endurance training while fasting during Ramadan resulted in changes to various metabolic parameters related to hydration and kidney function. Although it is not currently known if sports performance *per se* is negatively impacted by fasting during Ramadan, athletes should be aware that proper hydration might be compromised.

Can the use of medium-chain triglycerides improve endurance performance or body composition?

It has been suggested that medium-chain triglycerides (MCTs) are ergogenic, possibly because they are water soluble, which may confer two advantages: They can be absorbed by the portal circulation and delivered directly to the liver instead of via the chylomicron route in the lymph, and they more readily enter the mitochondria in the muscle cells, as they do not need carnitine. MCTs have been marketed commercially. Research has shown that MCTs do not inhibit gastric emptying, as common fat does, and may be absorbed rapidly in the small intestine. Also, Massicotte and his associates reported that exogenous MCTs are oxidized at a rate comparable to exogenous glucose, being oxidized within the first 30 minutes of exercise. MCT supplements are available as a liquid, which can be added to food, or soft gel capsules. MCTs are also added to meal-replacement powders, energy, and protein bars. Recently, possibly due to an interest in low-carbohydrate, high-fat diets or in foodstuffs such as coconut oil, there has been a resurgence in MCT use.

Bueno and colleagues recently completed a meta-analysis of the effects of replacing at least 5 grams of dietary long-chain fatty acids with medium-chain fatty acids in 16 studies that included 399 participants. Reportedly, replacement with MCTs resulted in greater reductions in body mass, body fat, and waist circumference. But the authors stated that their results should be taken with caution until longer-duration and better-quality research trials are completed. Mumme and others also conducted a meta-analysis of the effects of MCTs on weight loss and body composition, studying 13 trials with 749 individuals. MCT ingestion resulted in greater decreases in body mass, body fat, and subcutaneous and visceral fat, but these changes were small. Consuming MCTs resulted in about a 0.51-kg extra decrease in body mass over a 10 week period. More importantly, the authors systematically identified several areas of concern with the studies they included in their analysis. They expressed concerns over how well the MCT products were blinded, if data were selectively reported, and if there was a commercial bias. Bueno and colleagues also note that the blinding of the source of the fat in their analysis was rated "low" or "unclear" for every study.

Some early research found that MCT supplementation alone may actually impair endurance exercise performance, whereas an MCT-carbohydrate supplement might be ergogenic. Van Zyl and others, using endurance-trained cyclists, compared the effects of three supplements on an endurance performance task consisting of a 2-hour ride at 60 percent VO_2 max followed by a 40-kilometer performance ride. The three supplements, consumed throughout the performance task, were carbohydrate only, MCTs only, and carbohydrate with MCTs; the MCT dose was about 86 grams. Compared to the carbohydrate supplement, the MCT supplement actually impaired 40-kilometer performance, whereas the combination carbohydrate-MCT supplement improved performance. These investigators suggested that the carbohydrate-MCT supplement improved performance in the 40-kilometer performance ride by decreasing oxidation of muscle glycogen during the preliminary submaximal 2-hour ride, thus sparing the glycogen for the more intense exercise task.

However, most studies have not shown any beneficial effects of MCT supplementation, either alone or combined with carbohydrate, on endurance exercise performance. One such study was conducted by Goedecke and others, from Tim Noakes's laboratory in South Africa. Nine endurance-trained cyclists cycled for 2 hours at 63 percent of VO_2 peak, then completed a 40-kilometer time trial under three conditions: glucose, glucose and low-dose MCTs, and glucose and high-dose MCTs, all in solution. The solutions were ingested immediately before and every 10 minutes during exercise. Although MCT ingestion increased serum FFA concentration, there were no beneficial effects on performance as compared to the glucose trial. In a well-designed crossover study, Angus and others compared the effects of carbohydrate to carbohydrate plus MCT on 100-kilometer cycling time trial in eight endurance-trained males. The beverages were provided during the trial at about every 15 minutes and consisted of a 6 percent carbohydrate solution with and without a 4.2 percent MCT solution. They found that compared to the placebo trial, the carbohydrate enhanced 100-kilometer cycling performance, but the addition of MCT did not provide any further performance enhancement. In a similar study with ultraendurance athletes, but with carbohydrate or MCTs provided before an ultradistance ride, Goedecke and others reported that MCT supplementation actually impaired periodic sprint performance within the event. Using muscle biopsies, Horowitz and others have also shown that a carbohydrate-MCT solution does not spare muscle glycogen during high-intensity aerobic exercise.

Using a chronic MCT feeding protocol, Misell and others had 12 trained male endurance runners consume either corn oil (LCT) or MCT (60 grams) daily for 2 weeks. The runners then performed an endurance treadmill test consisting of a 30-minute run at 85 percent VO_2 max followed by a run to exhaustion at 75 percent VO_2 max. The investigators reported that chronic MCT consumption neither enhances endurance performance nor significantly alters exercise metabolism in trained male runners. Louise Burke states that there is no evidence of benefits of chronic MCT ingestion for athletes. Also, the effectiveness of MCT is limited by the inability of athletes to tolerate the amount necessary to have an effect. So if there were any possible beneficial effects on endurance performance, they would likely be outweighed by gastrointestinal distress.

Is the glycerol portion of triglycerides an effective ergogenic aid?

As you may recall, glycerol is one of the by-products of triglyceride breakdown. Burelle and others have noted that exogenous glycerol can be oxidized during prolonged exercise, presumably following conversion into glucose in the liver. Thus, researchers theorized that it could be an efficient energy source during exercise. However, in well-controlled research, glycerol feedings did not prevent either hypoglycemia or muscle glycogen depletion patterns in several prolonged exercise tasks. Apparently the rate at which the human liver converts glycerol to glucose is not rapid enough to be an effective energy source during strenuous prolonged exercise. However, as noted in chapter 9, glycerol may be used to increase body water stores, including plasma volume, prior to exercise, and has been theorized to be ergogenic for endurance athletes performing under warm environmental conditions.

Are phospholipid dietary supplements effective ergogenic aids?

Lecithin Lecithin, also known as *phosphatidylcholine,* is a phospholipid that occurs naturally in a variety of foods, such as beans, eggs, and wheat germ. Because it is an important component of many types of human body tissues, contains choline needed for the synthesis of acetylcholine (an important neurotransmitter), and contains phosphorus, it has been theorized to be ergogenic. Several German studies conducted more than 50 years ago reported increases in power and strength following several days of supplementation with 22–83 milligrams of lecithin. However, these early studies have been discredited because of poor experimental design. In a study with better experimental design, Staton reported that 30 grams of lecithin supplementation daily for 2 weeks had no effect upon grip strength.

Although lecithin does not appear to be an effective ergogenic aid, several of its constituents have been theorized to enhance exercise performance. Choline, an amine associated with vitamin-like activity, has been studied independently or as part of lecithin for potential ergogenic effects on endurance performance and is discussed in chapter 7. Phosphate salts are covered in chapter 8.

Phosphatidylserine **Phosphatidylserine**, like phosphatidylcholine, is a naturally occurring phospholipid found in cell membranes. Food products that are good sources of phosphatidylserine include green leafy vegetables, rice, fish, and soybeans. Dietary supplements, some marketed as Phosphatidyl Serine, are derived primarily from soybeans and are marketed to improve brain health, claiming to be essential for normal functioning of neuronal cell membranes.

Several studies have evaluated the effect of phosphatidylserine supplementation on various responses to exercise and exercise performance. Kingsley notes that phosphatidylserine may serve as an antioxidant, which may help reduce muscle tissue damage. It also may help promote optimal balance of calcium and other minerals in the cell during exercise, which might influence exercise performance, because of its role in promoting transport of substances across cell membranes. Kingsley also notes early research indicating that oral supplementation with phosphatidylserine moderated exercise-induced changes in the hypothalamic-pituitary-adrenal axis, which could affect hormonal responses to exercise that may influence performance.

In one of the first studies, Kingsley and others provided male soccer players with 750 milligrams of soy phosphatidylserine daily for 10 days. The players engaged in intermittent exercise designed to simulate soccer match play, immediately followed by an exhaustive run. The supplement had no effect on muscle soreness or markers of muscle damage and lipid peroxidation following exhaustive running; however, supplementation tended to increase running time to exhaustion, but the difference between the treatment and placebo groups was not statistically significant. In another study with a similar supplementation protocol, Kingsley and others reported no significant effect of phosphatidylserine supplementation on markers of muscle tissue damage, inflammation, and oxidative stress, or on delayed onset of muscle soreness following downhill running for nearly an hour.

Although phosphatidylserine supplementation appears to have little effect on reducing markers of muscle damage or soreness after severe exercise, Kingsley and others did find improved exercise performance in one study. Using a similar supplementation protocol (750 milligrams for 10 days), phosphatidylserine supplementation significantly increased cycling time to exhaustion at 85 percent VO_2 max, and the authors suggested that phosphatidylserine supplementation might possess ergogenic potential.

These findings are interesting, but research with phosphatidylserine supplementation and exercise performance is in its preliminary stages and additional research is merited.

Omega-3 fatty acid and fish oil supplements

There is a great deal of interest in the health-promoting, or ergogenic, effects of omega-3 polyunsaturated fatty acids. It is well known that populations who consume diets high in these fatty acids have decreased risk of cardiovascular disease. In particular, eicosapentaenoic (EPA) and docosahexaenoic (DHA) acid have been studied because of their potential anti-inflammatory effect. People who do not regularly consume oily fish probably consume less than 200 milligrams/day, and fish oil supplements are an easy way to increase omega-3 fatty acid intake.

Omega-3 fatty acids are theorized to be ergogenic not because of their energy content but because they may elicit favorable physiological effects relative to several types of physical performance. One theory is based on the finding that omega-3 fatty acids may be incorporated into the membrane of the red blood cell (RBC), making the RBC less viscous and less resistant to flow. Another theory is based on the role of certain by-products—the eicosanoids mentioned previously—whose production in the body cells is related to omega-3 fatty acid metabolism. In particular, two specific forms of the eicosanoids, prostaglandin E_1 (PGE_1) and prostaglandin I_2 (PGI_2), may elicit a vasodilation effect on the blood vessels. Walser and others noted that 6 weeks of EPA and DHA (total 5 grams/day) supplementation enhances blood flow during exercise in healthy individuals. Theoretically, the less viscous RBC and the vasodilative effect should enhance blood flow, facilitating the delivery of blood and oxygen to the muscles during exercise, benefiting the endurance athlete.

Unfortunately, although the ergogenic potential of omega-3 fatty acids is an interesting hypothesis, there are few supportive scientific data. Results from well-controlled, peer-reviewed scientific research indicate that omega-3 fatty acids do not affect energy metabolism during exercise. For example, Bortolotti and others recently reported that supplementation with 7.2 grams of fish oil daily, containing 1.1 grams/day eicosapentaenoic acid and 0.7 grams/day docosahexaenoic acid, for 14 days exerted no effect on glucose or lipid energy metabolism during 30 minutes of cycling at 50 percent VO_2 max.

Research also indicates that omega-3 fatty acid supplementation has no effect on aerobic endurance performance. Buckley and others supplemented the diets of 25 professional Australian Football League players for 5 weeks in a randomized, double-blind study. The players were matched for performance of a 2,200-meter running time trial and provided either 6×1 gram capsules of either sunflower oil (placebo) or DHA-rich fish oil (1.56 grams DHA and 0.36 gram eicosapentaenoic acid). At the end of the 5 weeks of supplementation, the fish oil group had lower serum triglycerides and lower heart rate during submaximal exercise. Buckley and others did not find improvements in endurance exercise performance, as determined by time to exhaustion, or recovery. In a slightly longer study, Peoples and colleagues supplemented the diets of 16 well-trained male cyclists for 8 weeks with either 8×1 grams of olive oil (control) or fish oil in a double-blind, parallel design. The fish oil supplementation lowered heart rate during VO_2 peak testing and steady-state submaximal exercise, as well as whole-body oxygen consumption and rate pressure product. Time to voluntary fatigue was not influenced by fish oil supplementation.

Suggested doses of fish oil supplements would be about 1 to 2 grams/day, with the goal being reduced exercise-induced inflammation and general health. Mickleborough recently reviewed the effects of omega-3 supplements on performance and stated that in terms of performance, the human data are inconclusive. This viewpoint is supported by Calder and Lindley in their review. Thus, the ingestion of omega-3 fats/fish oil supplements to enhance athletic performance is not supported at this point. Importantly, Mickleborough noted the following potential safety issues related to fish oil supplementation:

- Supplements could be made from fish that are contaminated with heavy metals. This is theoretical and has not been reported in the literature, but as discussed throughout this textbook, dietary supplement quality control can be a concerning issue.
- Fish oil supplements can cause increased bleeding due to decreased platelet stickiness. This could be an issue, especially at higher doses.
- Digestive problems, such as flatulence and diarrhea, are possible. Ingesting fish oil supplements before or during exercise performance could be ergolytic due to gastrointestinal distress.
- High doses of fish oil may increase LDL-cholesterol.
- Fish oil supplements can decrease blood pressure, which could be a problem for an athlete who is already hypotensive.
- Fish oil supplements can result in a fishy taste in the month.

Can carnitine improve performance or weight loss?

Carnitine is a water-soluble, vitamin-like compound that facilitates the transport of long-chain fatty acids into the mitochondria. There are basically two forms of carnitine, L-carnitine and D-carnitine, but other forms are available, such as L-propionylcarnitine. L-carnitine is the physiologically active form in the body, so in the following discussion, carnitine will refer mostly to L-carnitine, but in some studies L-propionylcarnitine has been used.

Dietary Sources   Carnitine is not an essential dietary nutrient because it may be formed in the liver from other nutrients—principally two amino acids, lysine and methionine. Also, carnitine is found in substantial amounts in animal foods. Meat products, particularly beef and pork, are good sources of carnitine; much less is found in fish and poultry, and even lower amounts in dairy products. Only minimal amounts of carnitine are found in fruits, vegetables, and grains. For example, for similar weights, beef has about 300 times as much carnitine as bread; 3 ounces of beef contains about 60 mg of carnitine. There is no RDA for carnitine. Most individuals consume enough carnitine in the daily diet, and the body has an effective conservation system. The typical non-vegetarian diet provides about 100–300 milligrams/day. Carnitine deficiencies are very rare.

Theory as an Ergogenic Aid   Carnitine supplementation has been theorized to enhance physical performance and weight loss because of several of its metabolic functions in the muscle cell. Approximately 90 percent of the body supply of carnitine is located in the muscle tissues, where it is part of an enzyme (carnitine palmitoyl transferase) important for transport of long-chain fatty acids into the mitochondria for oxidation. Theoretically, supplemental carnitine might facilitate the transport of LCFAs into the mitochondria for oxidation, which would be an important consideration if the oxidation of fatty acids were limited by their transport into the mitochondria.

Effects on Performance   Although these are logical theories and interesting medical applications, the available scientific evidence is somewhat equivocal and in general does not appear to support an ergogenic effect of carnitine supplementation. Major reviews regarding the effect of carnitine supplementation on physical performance have been published, and the following are the key points regarding the ergogenic effects of carnitine supplementation emanating from these reviews and studies:

1. Supplementation will increase plasma levels of carnitine, but much of this will be excreted by the kidneys. Stephens and Greenhaff state that the bioavailability of carnitine is <15 percent of a 2- to 6-gram dose. They estimate that it would take about 100 days of supplementation to increase muscle carnitine 10 percent. Several earlier studies showed that oral carnitine supplementation cannot increase muscle carnitine levels. However, Wall and others were able to increase muscle carnitine 21 percent in 168 days when combined with 80 grams of carbohydrate twice daily. These data must be reproduced, and athletes should consider the effects of an extra 640 Calories of sugar per day, particularly if they are attempting to lose weight.
2. The primary theory underlying carnitine supplementation is enhanced fat utilization. If muscle carnitine does not increase with supplementation, no increase in fat oxidation should be expected, and this has been reported. However, in the study by Wall and others in which muscle carnitine did increase, muscle glycogen use decreased 55 percent, muscle lactate was 44 percent lower, and work output improved. Numerous studies have reported no ergogenic effect under a variety of exercise tests conditions, likely because muscle carnitine did not increase in those trials. As the number of studies showing no metabolic or ergogenic effect of carnitine far outweigh the number that have shown an effect, carnitine cannot be recommended until more research is conducted.
3. Preliminary data, from William Kraemer's research group, suggest that combining carnitine with tartrate may have some beneficial effects for individuals engaged in resistance training. Tartrate, a salt, possesses antioxidant properties. Spiering and others reported that carnitine supplementation, either 1- or 2-gram doses for 3 weeks, reduced markers of metabolic stress and perceived muscle soreness following a resistance training workout. Kraemer and others noted that carnitine/tartrate supplementation may increase responses of androgenic receptors that help muscle formation, which they suggest may help promote recovery from resistance exercise. These preliminary findings are interesting and merit additional research, possibly evaluating the effects of carnitine and tartrate separately.

4. Both Asker Jeukendrup and Melinda Manore, two experts on dietary supplements and sports nutrition, have reviewed the purported effects of carnitine on weight loss. Neither finds any evidence that carnitine is effective for weight loss.

5. D-carnitine may be toxic, as it can deplete L-carnitine, leading to a carnitine deficiency. L-carnitine appears to be a safe supplement, but some reviewers recommend no more than 2–5 grams per day, possibly for only 1 month at a time.

Carnitine is generally thought of as an ineffective ergogenic aid, but this is probably because it is difficult to increase muscle carnitine. Until a way to increase muscle carnitine becomes available and more practical, supplementation cannot be recommended, although more research needs to be done.

Can hydroxycitrate (HCA) enhance endurance performance?

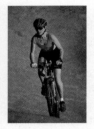

Hydroxycitric acid is derived from a tropical fruit and marketed as a dietary supplement, hydroxy-citrate (HCA). Kriketos and others noted that as a competitive inhibitor of citrate lysase, HCA has been hypothesized to modify citric acid cycle metabolism to promote fatty acid oxidation. Although some studies with mice suggest that HCA supplementation may enhance endurance performance, human studies do not support such an ergogenic effect.

Kriketos and others, in an excellent crossover study, reported no significant effect of HCA supplementation (3.0 grams/day for 3 days) on blood serum energy substrates, fat metabolism, or energy expenditure either during rest or during moderately intense exercise. However, the subjects were sedentary males. Using endurance-trained cyclists as subjects, van Loon and others evaluated the effect of HCA supplementation (3.1 ml/kilogram body mass of a 19 percent HCA solution) given twice to the cyclists before and during 2 hours of cycling at 50 percent VO_2 max. They concluded that HCA supplementation, even in large quantities, does not increase total fat oxidation in endurance-trained cyclists.

Melinda Manore, an expert in sports nutrition, recently reviewed several common weight-loss supplements. Regarding HCA, she stated that there is no benefit of HCA on weight loss, fat oxidation, or appetite. Additionally, there have been several safety issues raised with HCA, including liver injuries, although it is unknown if this is related to poor quality control or the plant extract itself. Saito, using an animal model, reported that HCA was toxic to and caused atrophy of the testes. In their review, Márquez and others state that most HCA supplementation studies in humans have been small and short in duration (e.g., not longer than 12 weeks). They concluded that there is little evidence to support the effectiveness HCA.

Can conjugated linoleic acid (CLA) enhance exercise performance or weight loss?

Conjugated linoleic acid (CLA) has been marketed as a sports dietary supplement to resistance-trained individuals, mainly as a means to promote weight loss and gain muscle mass. For similar and other reasons, CLA also has been marketed as a means to improve health.

Research regarding its ergogenic effect on exercise-trained individuals is very limited. Using resistance-trained athletes as subjects, Kreider and others investigated the effect of CLA supplementation (6 grams prescribed daily dose; 28 days) on body composition and muscular strength, and reported no significant effects on total body mass, fat mass, fat-free mass, or strength as measured by a single maximal repetition in the bench press and leg press. Pinkoski and others, in a crossover design, also found that CLA supplementation (5 grams daily for 7 weeks) resulted in minimal changes in body composition and no changes in the strength tests in males and females involved in resistance training. However, in the first phase of the study, which did not involve a crossover design, male subjects receiving CLA experienced significant increases in bench press strength compared to the placebo group. The crossover phase of the study, as the authors note, is a stronger experimental design.

Macaluso and others recently reviewed seven studies on CLA supplementation and exercise performance and noted that more than half showed no beneficial effect. Onkapoya and colleagues, in their meta-analysis, concluded that CLA supplementation results in a statistically significant, albeit small and possibly clinically irrelevant, decrease in body mass relative to placebo ingestion. Presently, adverse reactions to CLA supplementation are mild, with gastrointestinal distress being most commonly reported. Based on limited research, CLA supplementation does not currently appear to be an effective ergogenic aid for trained individuals, but confirming research is needed. Its role in health is discussed later in this chapter.

What's the bottom line regarding the ergogenic effects of fat burning diets or strategies?

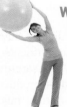

As noted in this section, numerous fat burning strategies have been employed in attempts to enhance prolonged endurance exercise performance. Theoretically, such strategies would increase the oxidation of fat, decrease the utilization of carbohydrate, and thus spare some muscle glycogen for use in the later stages of exercise. As muscle glycogen is a more efficient fuel compared to fats, performance should be enhanced.

However, John Hawley, an international sports science scholar, reviewed all such fat burning strategies and concluded that endurance exercise capacity is not systematically improved with increases in serum FFA availability, even in some studies with substantial muscle glycogen sparing. He noted that for some reason, exercise capacity is remarkably resistant to change. Other studies suggest that high-fat diets may impair performance in some events, such as high-intensity surges during a race or sprints to the finish. Moreover, individuals may find it difficult to adhere to a high-fat diet.

Dietary Fats and Cholesterol: Health Implications

As noted in previous chapters, the etiology of chronic diseases such as cancer and coronary heart disease is complex and involves multiple risk factors. Eliminating or reducing as many risk factors as possible is the best approach to optimize your health. Your diet is one of the most important risk factors that can be modified to promote good health, particularly the amount and composition of fat you eat. Every few years the American Dietetic Association provides a review of the evidence regarding various dietary practices and effects on cardiovascular disease, the most recent being the review by Van Horn and others. In this section, we shall focus on the role of dietary fat in the etiology of coronary heart disease (CHD), and in chapter 10, we shall discuss the possible role of dietary fat in obesity and related health problems, such as diabetes, high blood pressure, and various forms of cancer.

CHD is still the number one cause of death in industrialized nations. In its recommendations regarding dietary fat, the National Academy of Sciences indicated that although very high-fat diets may predispose to CHD, so, too, may very low-fat diets. For example, Siri and Krauss reported that increased dietary carbohydrates, particularly simple sugars and starches with high glycemic index, can modify the serum lipid profile in ways that may also be conducive to CHD. Lipid expert Penny Kris-Etherton and her associates recently noted that the main message regarding dietary fat is very simple: Avoid diets that are *very low* and *very high* in fat. The guiding principle is that moderation in total fat is the defining benchmark for a contemporary diet that reduces risk of chronic disease. Moreover, within the range of a moderate-fat diet, it is still important to individualize the total fat prescription. Fats are not all equal. Some are better for your health than others, and, as noted, the terms *good* and *bad* fats have been popularized. Remember, however, that even some *bad* fats can fit into a healthy diet. The key is moderation.

Because the available evidence relating dietary lipids to cardiovascular disease is so compelling, we shall treat this subject in some detail. However, note that the dietary and exercise recommendations advanced later in this chapter for the prevention of cardiovascular disease may also help prevent other chronic diseases, such as obesity and certain forms of cancer.

How does cardiovascular disease develop?

Nearly one out of every two deaths in the United States is due to diseases of the heart and blood vessels. Each year, approximately 1 million Americans die from some form of cardiovascular disease, including coronary heart disease, stroke, hypertensive disease, rheumatic heart disease, and congenital heart disease.

Coronary heart disease is the major disease of the cardiovascular system; of the million deaths noted previously, it is responsible for more than half. Although the total percentage of deaths due to coronary heart disease has been declining in recent years, it is still an epidemic and the number one cause of death among both males and females.

Coronary heart disease (CHD) is also known as **coronary artery disease (CAD)** because obstruction of the blood flow in the coronary arteries is responsible for the pathological effects of the disease. The coronary arteries, which nourish the heart muscle, are illustrated in figure 5.12. The major manifestation of CHD is a heart attack, which results from a stoppage of blood flow to parts of the heart muscle. A decreased blood supply, known as **ischemia**, will deprive the heart of needed oxygen. In some individuals, ischemia results in **angina**, a sharp pain in the chest, jaw, or along the inside of the arm indicative of a mild heart attack. Other terms often associated with a heart attack include **coronary thrombosis**, a blockage of a blood vessel by a clot (thrombus); **coronary occlusion**, which simply means blockage; and **myocardial infarct**, death of heart cells that do not get enough oxygen due to the blocked coronary artery. The major cause of blocked arteries is atherosclerosis.

Arteriosclerosis is a term applied to a number of different pathological conditions wherein the arterial walls thicken and lose their elasticity. It is often defined as hardening of the arteries. **Atherosclerosis**, one form of arteriosclerosis, is characterized by the formation of **plaque**, an accumulation of fatty acids, oxidized LDL-cholesterol, macrophages (white blood cells that oxidize LDL), foam cells (macrophages that consume cholesterol),

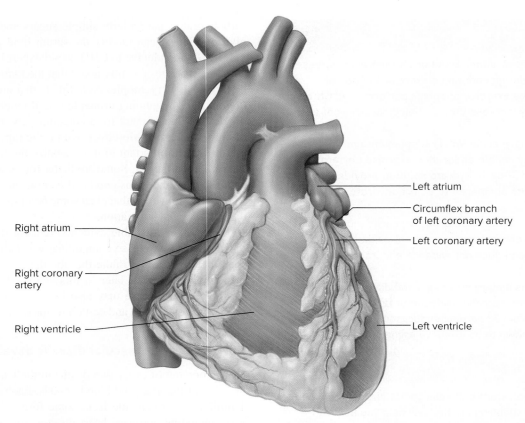

Right atrium

Right coronary artery

Right ventricle

Left atrium

Circumflex branch of left coronary artery

Left coronary artery

Left ventricle

FIGURE 5.12 The heart and the coronary arteries. The heart muscle itself receives its blood supply from the coronary arteries. The main coronary arteries are the left coronary artery, one of its branches named the circumflex, and the right coronary artery. Atherosclerosis of these arteries leads to coronary heart disease.

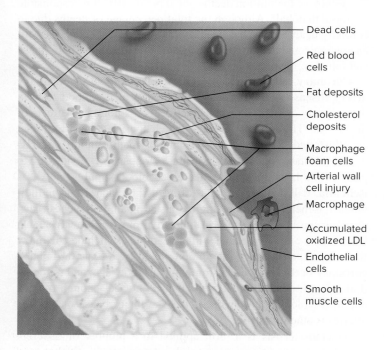

Dead cells

Red blood cells

Fat deposits

Cholesterol deposits

Macrophage foam cells

Arterial wall cell injury

Macrophage

Accumulated oxidized LDL

Endothelial cells

Smooth muscle cells

FIGURE 5.13 An enlargement of atherosclerotic plaque. Oxidized LDL-cholesterol, macrophages, foam cells, fibrous material, and other debris collect beneath the endothelial cells lining the coronary artery. The site of the plaque may be initiated by some form of injury to the cell lining, possibly an ulceration as shown.

cytokines (immune system mediators of inflammation), cellular debris, fibrin, and calcium on the inner lining of the coronary artery wall. A cap of smooth muscle cells forms around the plaque to prevent contact with the arterial wall. Figure 5.13 presents a schematic of the content of arterial plaque.

Inflammatory processes precipitated by cytokines are now recognized to play a central role in the pathogenesis of atherosclerosis by interacting with serum cholesterol and serving as an initiating factor in plaque buildup. As the plaque accumulates, the diameter of the artery is diminished, decreasing blood flow to the heart muscle. Foam cells continue to accumulate, becoming a major component of plaque. The foam cells secrete a substance that can weaken the muscle cap. If the muscle cap ruptures, plaque will leak into the bloodstream and trigger the formation of a clot, which partially or completely blocks blood flow to a section of heart muscle, leading to death of cardiac cells due to inadequate oxygen and nutrients. The process is depicted in figure 5.14.

Atherosclerosis is a slow, progressive disease that begins in childhood and usually manifests itself later in life. Because of its prevalence in industrialized society, scientists throughout the world have been conducting intensive research to identify the cause or causes of atherosclerosis and coronary heart disease. The actual cause has not yet been completely identified, but considerable evidence has identified factors that may predispose an individual.

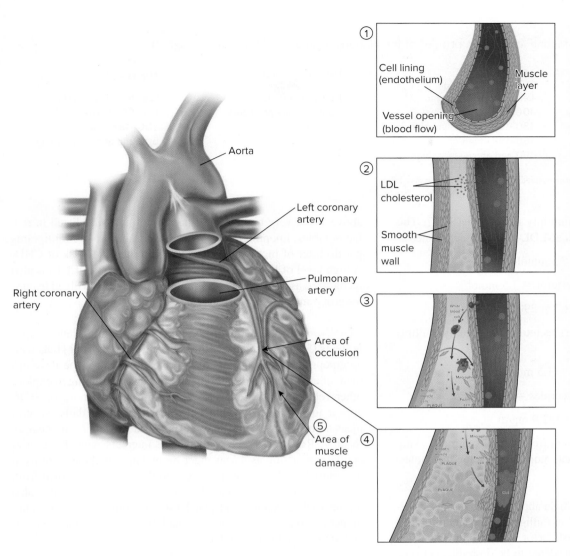

FIGURE 5.14 The developmental process of atherosclerosis and thrombosis. (1) Normal coronary artery. (2) LDL-cholesterol seeps through the endothelium into the smooth muscle wall. (3) Immune system responds, sending macrophages (white blood cells) to ingest the LDL-cholesterol; macrophages become foam cells, a major component of plaque; a smooth muscle cap forms to protect the endothelium. (4) Foam cells accumulate, secreting a substance that weakens the cap; the cap ruptures; plaque leaks into the bloodstream, triggering clot formation. (5) Blocked artery leads to a decrease or cessation of blood flow to a section of heart tissue, leading to heart attack, which may be mild or fatal depending on the severity of the blockage.

As noted previously, a risk factor represents a statistical relationship between two items such as high serum cholesterol and heart attack. This does not mean that a cause-and-effect relationship exists, although such a relationship is often strongly supported by the available evidence. The three principal risk factors associated with CHD are high blood pressure, high serum cholesterol levels, and cigarette smoking. Several major professional and governmental health organizations also believe that physical inactivity is a fourth principal risk factor. Other interacting risk factors are heredity, diabetes, diet, obesity, age, gender, and stress. Elevated blood levels of homocysteine and C-reactive protein (CRP) have been associated with CHD, and their role as risk factors continues to be studied. Homocysteine is discussed in chapter 7. CRP is a marker for inflammation.

www.americanheart.org/riskassessment Use this questionnaire to assess your risk of developing coronary heart disease. Knowing your cholesterol levels and blood pressure is helpful but not required. Some information about risk factors is also presented.

How do the different forms of serum lipids affect the development of atherosclerosis?

In atherosclerosis, the plaque that develops in the arterial walls is composed partly of fats and cholesterol. Hence, high levels of blood lipids (triglycerides and cholesterol) are associated with increased plaque formation. However, as you recall, triglycerides and cholesterol may be transported in the blood in a variety of ways, but primarily as constituents of lipoproteins. Considerable research has been devoted to identifying those specific lipoproteins and other lipid components that may predispose to CHD, and although there is some debate about the meaningfulness of specific serum lipid profiles, some theories prevail.

The four main serum lipid factors associated with increased risk of atherosclerosis are total cholesterol, LDL-cholesterol, HDL-cholesterol, and triglycerides. The guidelines for the fasting blood serum level profile recommended by the National Cholesterol Education Program are presented in table 5.7.

Serum lipid levels are normally given in milligrams per deciliter (mg/dl), as shown in table 5.7. A deciliter is 100 milliliters. However, you may see cholesterol and triglyceride levels expressed as millimole per liter (mmol/L). To convert mmol/L

TABLE 5.7   Recommended fasting lipoprotein profile* of the National Cholesterol Education Program

Total cholesterol	LDL-cholesterol	HDL-cholesterol	Triglycerides
Less than 200—desirable 200–239—borderline high 240 or above—high	Less than 100—optimal 100–129—near optimal 130–159—borderline high 160–189—high 190 and above—very high	Less than 40—low 60 or above—protective	Less than 150—normal 151–199—borderline high 200–499—high 500 and above—very high

*Fasting levels expressed in mg/dl; testing recommended every 5 years for those over 20.

of cholesterol to mg/dl, simply multiply mmol/L by 38.67. This applies to total cholesterol as well as LDL- and HDL-cholesterol.

Example: Total cholesterol = 7.5 mmol/L

Example: Total cholesterol = 7.5 mmol/l

7.5 mmol/L × 38.67 = 290 mg/dL

To convert mmol/L of triglycerides into mg/dl, simply multiply by 88.57.

Example: Serum triglycerides = 1.5 mmol/L

Example: Serum triglycerides = 1.5 mmol/l

1.5 × 88.57 = 132.9 mg/dl

To convert in the opposite direction, from mg/dl to mmol/L, simply divide mg/dl by the appropriate numerical factor for cholesterol or triglycerides.

Total Cholesterol   The major villain appears to be serum cholesterol. Total cholesterol, expressed in milligrams per 100 milliliters of blood (mg/dl), is a significant risk factor. As noted in table 5.7, a cholesterol level below 200 is considered to be desirable, between 200 and 239 is borderline-high, and above 240 is high. However, you should be aware that there is a rather large standard error of measurement involved in some tests of cholesterol, being on the order of 30 milligrams. What this means is that if your blood cholesterol is reported as 220 (borderline high), you may actually have a cholesterol level of 190 (desirable) or 250 (high) if you vary, respectively, one standard error below or above your actual measurement of 220. For this reason, it may be a good idea to have a second test completed if you are concerned about your total cholesterol level.

LDL-Cholesterol   The form by which cholesterol is transported in your blood may also be related to the development of atherosclerosis. In general, a high level of low-density lipoproteins (LDL) is the major risk factor associated with atherosclerosis. A current theory suggests various forms of LDL, such as small, dense LDL and the variant lipoprotein (a), may be more prone to oxidation by macrophages at an injured site in the arterial epithelium, leading to an influx into the cell wall and the formation of plaque. The presence of oxygen free radicals has been suggested to accelerate this process. Other mechanisms, such as increased clotting ability, may be operative. As noted in table 5.7, LDL levels less than 100 are optimal, while those above 160 pose a high risk and those

above 190 a very high risk. Although not normally listed in risk factor tables, lipoprotein (a) values greater than 25–30 milligrams per deciliter of blood are associated with increased risk of CHD. A high level of IDL (which some consider a form of LDL) is also recognized as a risk factor, as is apolipoprotein B, involved in cholesterol transport to the tissues.

HDL-Cholesterol   Conversely, high levels of high-density lipoproteins (HDL), particularly the subfraction HDL_2 and HDL with apolipoprotein A-I, appear to be protective against the development of atherosclerosis, although research is continuing to explore other relationships. Levels of 60 milligrams or more of HDL appear to be protective, but because HDL varies daily, several measurements over time may be required to obtain an accurate reading. Research suggests that HDL interacts with the arterial epithelium, acting as a scavenger by picking up cholesterol from the arterial wall and transporting it to the liver for removal from the body, known as *reverse cholesterol transport*. HDL may also inhibit LDL oxidation and platelet aggregation. HDL_2 levels are higher in women until menopause and then decrease, with an associated increased risk for CHD.

Triglycerides   Jacobson and others noted that elevated triglyceride levels may be a significant independent risk factor for coronary heart disease. Also, it is often associated with increased levels of LDL, particularly the small, dense LDL, and decreased levels of HDL. Current guidelines from the National Cholesterol Education Program (NCEP) indicate that triglyceride levels below 150 milligrams per deciliter are normal, whereas the risk associated with progressively increasing levels goes from borderline high to very high (see table 5.7). Jacobson and others indicate increasing concern over the increasing rate of hypertriglyceridemia, which is associated with overweight and obesity.

A summary of serum lipid factors associated with increased risk of atherosclerosis is presented in table 5.8.

Cholesterol Ratios and Other Tests   If your total blood cholesterol is borderline or high, a determination of the LDL and HDL levels may be desirable, for they provide additional information relative to your risk. Based on epidemiological data, several ratios have been developed to assess risk of CHD, with the lower the ratio, the lower the risk.

One common comparison is the ratio of total cholesterol (TC) to the HDL level, or TC/HDL. A ratio of about 4.5 is associated

TABLE 5.8 Serum lipid factors associated with increased risk of atherosclerosis

High levels of total cholesterol
High levels of LDL-cholesterol
High levels of dense form of LDL-cholesterol
High levels of IDL-cholesterol
High levels of abnormal lipoprotein, lipoprotein (a)
High levels of apolipoprotein B
High levels of triglycerides
Low levels of HDL-cholesterol
Low levels of HDL_2-cholesterol
Low levels of apolipoprotein A-I

with an average risk for CHD. For example, an individual with a total cholesterol of 200 and an HDL of 60 would have a ratio of 3.33 (200/60), or a lower risk, while someone with the same total cholesterol but an HDL of 20 would have a much higher risk with a ratio of 10 (200/20).

Another comparison is the ratio of LDL to HDL or LDL/HDL. An LDL to HDL ratio of about 3.5 is considered to be an average risk for CHD. Thus, a ratio of 140/60, or 2.3, would be a much lower risk than 140/20, or 7.0.

Additional tests are merited for those at high risk for CHD. Special lipoprotein tests may measure density levels of the various lipoproteins. Tests for other markers of atherosclerosis, such as homocysteine and CRP, will add to the diagnosis. For example, Ridker and others noted that high CRP levels may be more effective predictors of heart attacks than high LDL-cholesterol levels, but the greatest risk is when both are high.

http://cvdrisk.nhlbi.nih.gov   If you know your total and HDL-cholesterol levels, as well as your systolic blood pressure, you may check your risk of having a heart attack in the next 10 years.

Can I reduce my serum lipid levels and possibly reverse atherosclerosis?

Lowering your serum cholesterol, particularly your LDL-cholesterol, is a very effective means to help prevent CHD. LaRosa indicated that for each 1 percent reduction in LDL-cholesterol, there is a corresponding 1 percent reduction in coronary heart disease risk. Several approaches may help you improve your serum lipid levels and reduce the risk of atherosclerosis. A healthy lifestyle is one, and appropriate drug therapy is another. However, even with a healthy lifestyle some individuals may have poor serum lipid profiles. Certain forms of hypercholesteremia are genetic. In the future, gene therapy may be the treatment of choice for such individuals, possibly manipulating genes to decrease LDL and increase HDL.

Currently, drug therapy may be required to reduce serum lipid levels in genetically predisposed individuals, as well as in those with poor diets. Some drugs stimulate liver degradation and excretion of cholesterol, others increase lipoprotein lipase activity or LDL receptor function to decrease serum triglyceride levels, while still others bind with bile salts in the intestines so that they are not reabsorbed; because bile salts are derived from cholesterol, it is effectively excreted from the body. Statins, drugs that inhibit an enzyme (HMG-CoA reductase) that regulates cholesterol, have been particularly effective to reduce serum LDL-cholesterol. For more detail on current and proposed medicinal means to help lower serum lipids, the interested reader is referred to the review by Jain.

The National Cholesterol Education Program indicated that individuals at high risk for cardiovascular disease might consider getting their LDL levels as low as possible and could explore with their doctor the possibility of taking lipid-lowering drugs; table 5.9 provides some guidelines. However, even if on drug therapy, individuals should not abandon a healthy lifestyle.

Adopting a healthier lifestyle is the first step in attempts to improve one's serum lipid profile. A healthy lifestyle may not only help to prevent the development of atherosclerosis but also lead to regression of coronary artery blockage. In their review, Greg Brown and others noted that the available data support the hypothesis that lowering of serum lipids may lead to the regression of atherosclerotic lesions and elicit improved clinical effects. For those who are interested in preventing the development of atherosclerosis or reversing its progress, an appropriate diet and exercise program, as discussed below, are two key elements of a healthy lifestyle that are recommended by health professionals. Both factors may have favorable effects not only on serum lipid levels but on other risk factors for CHD as well, such as obesity and hypertension.

TABLE 5.9 National serum cholesterol guidelines

Risk category	Heart disease risk factors	Target LDL in milligrams/deciliter	Take drugs if LDL is
Low	Those with zero or one heart disease risk factor	Less than 160	190 or higher
Moderate	Those with two or more risk factors and less than a 10% to 20% risk of heart attack within 10 years	Less than 130	160 or higher
Moderately high	Those with two or more risk factors and a 10% to 20% risk of heart attack within 10 years	Less than 130 (optional goal 100)	130 or higher
High	Those who have heart disease or diabetes, or have two or more risk factors that give them greater than a 20% chance of a heart attack within 10 years	Less than 100 (optional goal 70)	100 or higher

Source: National Cholesterol Education Program Guidelines.

What should I eat to modify my serum lipid profile favorably?

The National Cholesterol Education Program was developed with the general goal of reducing the prevalence of high serum cholesterol in the United States. One of the first steps is to identify those individuals with high serum cholesterol by various simplified screening techniques, such as the measurement of total cholesterol by small samples of blood obtained through fingertip capillary blood. If this measure is borderline high (200–239 mg/dl) or high (>240 mg/dl), venous blood samples may be taken to determine LDL and HDL levels. If high serum cholesterol levels are detected, dietary modifications and other appropriate lifestyle changes may be recommended.

Figure 5.15 illustrates the composition of the average American diet and the Step 1 diet of the NCEP. Although the differences between the two diets appear to be small, such changes may reduce serum lipids. A sensible plan to reduce serum lipid levels is presented in figure 5.16, and representative results are shown in figure 5.17. If the original dietary plan is not effective after several months, the Step 2 NCEP diet may be recommended, which is essentially the same as the Step 1 diet but with less than 7 percent of the dietary Calories from saturated fat and less than 200 milligrams of cholesterol per day. Two meta-analyses revealed that the NCEP diet plan significantly decreased total blood cholesterol and may have multiple beneficial effects on major cardiovascular risk factors.

Several health organizations, including the American Heart Association, the National Institutes of Health, and the National Heart, Lung, and Blood Institute, have recommended a number of dietary guidelines that have been shown to lower serum cholesterol or serum triglycerides. Moreover, recent studies using the DASH (Dietary Approaches to Stop Hypertension) and OmniHeart (Optimal MacroNutrient Intake for Heart Health) diet plans have also helped refine dietary recommendations for healthy eating.

Based on the available scientific evidence, the following guidelines appear to be prudent and are consistent with the National Academy of Sciences recommendations for dietary fat. Although these guidelines have been developed to help individuals reduce high serum lipid profiles, they will also help to maintain normal levels and thus may be regarded as preventive medicine. As you may note, these recommendations are extensions of some guidelines for the Prudent Healthy Diet. Each guideline may be used to select foods that appeal to personal tastes. King and Gibney noted that individuals are more likely to eat a healthful diet if it includes foods they enjoy. It should be noted that in the near future the application of nutrigenomics may permit individualized dietary recommendations. Menus may be tailored to the genetic profile of each individual to maximize dietary effects favorable to the lipid profile and prevention of CHD, as well as prevention of other chronic diseases.

1. *Adjust caloric intake to achieve and maintain ideal body weight.* One of the most common causes of high triglyceride levels is too much body fat, particularly in the abdominal region. The health risks of obesity are detailed in chapter 10.

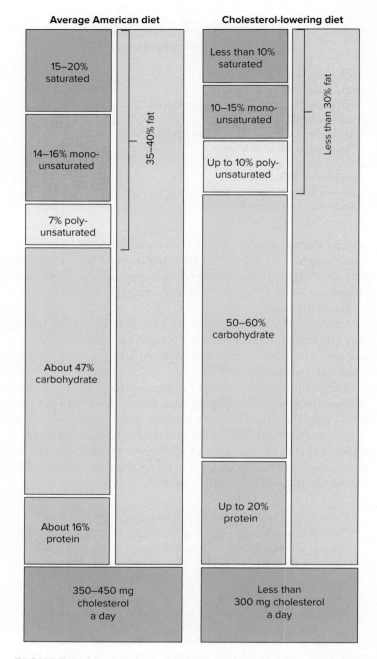

FIGURE 5.15 Comparison of the composition of the average American diet to the National Cholesterol Education Program Step 1 cholesterol-lowering diet.

Source: U.S. Department of Health and Human Services.

In many cases, simply losing body weight or reducing caloric intake will reduce these levels.

2. *Reduce the total amount of fats in the diet.* The American Heart Association recently increased the upper limit of dietary fat intake from 30 percent to 35 percent. Keep in mind that is the upper limit. Reducing the total amount of fat will usually reduce the amount of Calories, but nutrient content will actually improve. Reducing total fat intake to 20 percent or lower of total daily Calories, as recommended in some healthy

Measuring your progress: A sensible plan

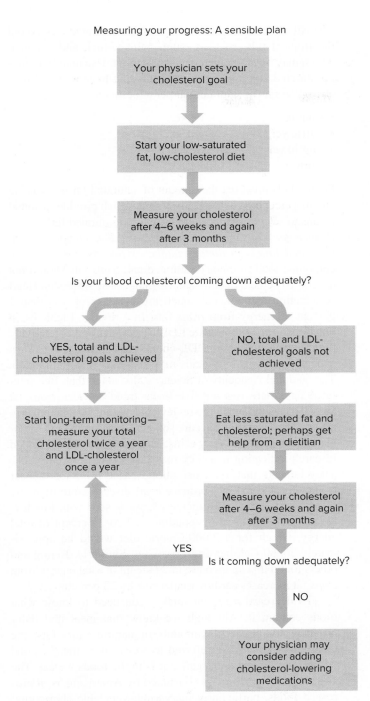

FIGURE 5.16 A sensible plan to monitor the effects of a cholesterol-lowering diet. The initial diet plan may involve the National Cholesterol Education Program Step 1 diet, but if unsuccessful, the Step 2 diet may be implemented. In individuals highly resistant to dietary modifications, drug therapy may be prescribed.

Source: U.S. Department of Health and Human Services.

diet plans, will reduce total and LDL-cholesterol even more. However, a very low-fat diet (10 percent fat Calories) may actually cause a negative lipid profile in some individuals. To help prevent this, the carbohydrate Calories that replace the fat Calories should *not* be derived from refined carbo-

Expected changes in blood cholesterol level

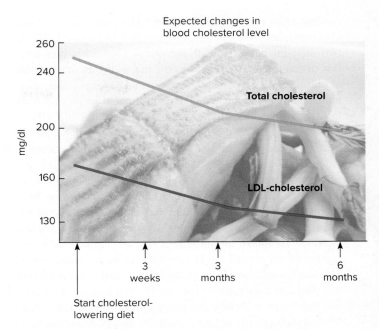

FIGURE 5.17 Representative expected changes in total serum cholesterol and LDL-cholesterol associated with appropriate dietary modifications, such as switching from the typical American diet to the Step 1 diet of the National Cholesterol Education Program (NCEP).

Source: U.S. Department of Health and Human Services.

hydrates but rather from complex carbohydrates containing dietary fiber.

However, for a style of eating to be effective at improving health, it must be sustainable. Gibson and others, in their meta-analysis, demonstrated that individuals on low-carbohydrate, high-fat/ketogenic diets were less hungry, had a decreased desire to eat, and had a greater feeling of satiety/fullness. Over the long term, decreased appetite could lead to weight loss, which would improve cardiovascular health. Johnston and others recently analyzed 48 randomized weight-loss trials with dietary fat intakes ranging from low fat (<20 percent of daily Calories) up to high fat (55 percent of total Calories). They determined that the differences between the diets were too small to be important to affect weight loss; thus, low fat or high fat was not an important factor for determining weight loss. However, long-term diet-induced weight-loss studies are among the most difficult type of research studies to complete, and participants often have poor compliance to the dietary intervention. Because weight loss will only occur if the diet is maintained, the authors recommended that the diet that promotes the best adherence is the ideal diet.

3. *Reduce the amount of saturated fat to less than 7 percent of dietary Calories.* The American Heart Association decreased the upper limit of saturated fat intake from 10 percent to 7 percent. As a matter of fact, scientists recommend reducing intake of saturated fats as low as possible while consuming a nutritionally adequate diet. The National Academy of Sciences indicated that there is a positive linear trend between total saturated fatty acid intake and total and LDL-cholesterol

concentration and increased risk of CHD. Saturated fats may also increase blood clotting, another risk factor for CHD. In two meta-analyses, Howell and others found that consumption of saturated fatty acids was the major dietary determinant of plasma cholesterol response to diet, while Clarke and others indicated that reducing the intake of saturated fat produced the most significant benefits regarding the prevention of CHD.

The effects of dietary fat intake on human health are extremely complex, and not as straight forward as saturated fats are bad and must be avoided. As an example, Volk and colleagues from Jeff Volek's lab placed obese volunteers on 3-week diets, with dietary carbohydrate increasing from 47 grams/day to 346 grams/day and saturated fat decreasing from 84 grams/day to 32 grams/day over the study. Dietary saturated fat intake had no effect on the saturated fatty acid content of any plasma lipids. However, as dietary carbohydrate increased, palmitoleic acid, which is associated with poor health outcomes, also increased. This study, which showed no relationship between dietary and plasma saturated fat, but instead showed a potentially negative aspect of dietary carbohydrate in obese patients with metabolic syndrome, highlights the complex relationship between diet and health. The same team studied the effects of 12 weeks of consuming three whole eggs per day vs. a yolk-free substitute while on a low- (25 to 30 percent of Calories) carbohydrate diet in patients with metabolic syndrome. Although both groups lost weight and improved certain aspects of metabolic health, the group consuming whole eggs improved more in some inflammatory markers, plasma insulin, VLDL, and HDL-cholesterol. This research demonstrates that fat intake interacts with carbohydrate intake, body mass, weight loss, and existing metabolic disease.

On the other hand, a recent article in the *Nutrition Action Health Letter* that featured some of the world's leading experts on diet and health reported that red meat intake is associated with decreased longevity, increased risk of heart disease, colon and rectal cancer, stroke, and diabetes. Whether or not this results from the saturated fat content of the meat, reducing red meat intake in the American diet seems sensible. The biggest contributor of saturated fat to the American diet is hamburger meat, even if it is labeled lean. However, extra lean hamburger may be low in total fat and saturated fat. Note the following comparison for 1 serving (4 ounces) of hamburger (ground beef) containing various percentages of fat:

> Regular hamburger (25%) = 331 Calories, 28 grams of fat (10.7 grams saturated fat)
> Lean hamburger (15%) = 243 Calories, 17 grams of fat (6.6 grams saturated fat)
> Extra lean hamburger (5%) = 155 Calories, 5.6 grams of fat (2.5 grams saturated fat)
> Extra lean hamburger (3%) = 136 Calories, 4.5 grams of fat (1.5 grams saturated fat)

Processed meats, such as most luncheon meats, are relatively high in fat. In contrast, fish, chicken, turkey, and very lean cuts of beef (eye of round) and pork (tenderloin) contain much less fat and saturated fat.

All oils contain saturated fats and unsaturated fats. Avoid the tropical oils, such as palm, palm kernel, and coconut, which may be 50–90 percent saturated fat. Use mainly monounsaturated and polyunsaturated oils that have no more than about 2 grams of saturated fat per tablespoon:

- Canola
- Safflower
- Sunflower
- Corn
- Olive
- Sesame
- Soybean
- Peanut

Food labels must list the amount of saturated fat per serving and its percentage of the Daily Value, which provides a sound means to select products with little to no saturated fat.

4. *Reduce the consumption of* trans *fats and, comparable to saturated fat, keep dietary intake as low as possible.* The combined total of dietary saturated and *trans* fats should not exceed 10 percent of daily caloric intake. The American Heart Association recommends much lower intake of less than 1 percent of energy from *trans* fats. In a review, Lichtenstein noted that *trans* fats elevate LDL-cholesterol and at relatively high intakes decrease HDL-cholesterol levels. Some data suggest that *trans* fatty acids may also trigger inflammation. The National Academy of Sciences also noted that, like saturated fats, there is a positive linear trend between *trans* fat and CHD. Although some reviewers contend that the adverse effects of *trans* fatty acids are somewhat less than those associated with saturated fatty acids, Mozaffarian and others cited research indicating that they may be as bad, or even worse. They indicate that, on a per-calorie basis, *trans* fats appear to increase the risk of coronary heart disease more than any other macronutrient. An increased risk is seen with low levels of consumption corresponding to 1 to 3 percent of total energy, which for a 2,000-Calorie diet would be approximately 20–60 Calories from *trans* fat. Similarly, Remig and others found that an increase in 2 percent of total energy from *trans* fat increases cardiovascular risk by 23 percent.

To decrease *trans* fat intake, you need to know what foods contain it. Although we know that meat and dairy products contain small amounts of natural *trans* fats, the Consumers Union has referred to *trans* fat as the "stealth" fat because we may not realize it is in the foods we eat. The vast majority of *trans* fat consumed by Americans is in processed foods, particularly margarine; vegetable shortening; white bread; packaged goods such as cookies, crackers, potato chips, and cakes; and fried fast foods such as french fries. The major component of each of these foods that adds *trans* fatty acids is usually partially hydrogenated vegetable oil. *Trans* fatty acid content per serving is now listed in the Nutrition Facts food label. However, the food label may list 0 grams of *trans* fat if there is less than 0.5 gram per serving. Thus, consuming multiple servings of such products daily may accumulate, totaling several grams or more of *trans* fat. In late 2015, the FDA decided that *trans* fat is not "generally recognized as safe" for use in human food and that manufacturers must remove partially hydrogenated oils from their products within 3 years.

5. *Substitute monounsaturated fats for saturated fats and simple or refined carbohydrates.* Consume about 10–15 percent of Calories from monounsaturated fats. Although no DRI have been set for monounsaturated fats, the National Academy of Sciences notes that they may have some benefit in the prevention of chronic disease.

Epidemiological research has indicated that the Mediterranean diet is associated with reduced risk of CHD. Olive oil, the primary source of dietary fat, is a staple of the Mediterranean diet. It is rich in monounsaturated fatty acids, is a good source of various phytochemicals, and contains the antioxidant vitamin E. In separate reviews, Covas and Perez-Jimenez and others highlighted various mechanisms, such as improved serum lipoprotein profile and reduced inflammation, whereby olive oil may reduce the risk of heart disease. However, they noted that the specific mechanisms underlying the beneficial effects of olive oil need further research. Nevertheless, the FDA has approved a *qualified* health claim for olive oil, indicating that eating 2 tablespoons of olive oil daily may, due to its monounsaturated fat content, reduce the risk of CHD. Keep in mind that *qualified* health claims are based on limited, not conclusive, evidence.

Walter Willett, the renowned nutrition research scientist from Harvard University, reported that both epidemiological and metabolic studies suggest that individuals can benefit greatly by adopting elements of the Mediterranean diet. Although olive oil is one of those elements, others include a diet rich in vegetables, whole grains, and seafood, all of which may confer health benefits in the prevention of CHD.

Dietary fats can have powerful effects on metabolic health. One recent example is the study from Wang and colleagues in which obese individuals were placed on a low-fat diet (24 percent of energy from fat), a moderate-fat diet (34 percent of energy from fat), and a moderate-fat diet with one Hass avocado per day (also 34 percent of energy from fat). After 5 weeks, the decrease in LDL was greater in the avocado group than in the other moderate-fat or the low-fat group. Additionally, LDL particle number, small-density LDL-cholesterol, and LDL/HDL ratio were all decreased in the avocado group. Avocados, olive oil, and nuts are rich sources of MUFAs.

The American Heart Association provided its stamp of approval to diets rich in MUFAs, provided saturated fatty acid intake is limited to a minimum and caloric intake is in balance. These two points may be the key to the role of MUFAs, such as olive oil, in helping prevent CHD.

Additionally, the OmniHeart study by Appel and others found that substituting monounsaturated fats, mainly olive oil, canola oil, and nuts, for simple carbohydrates, primarily desserts, may help promote heart health. For example, in a pooled analysis of 25 intervention trials, Sabaté and others found that 67 grams (2.4 oz.) of nuts consumed daily lowered triglyceride and LDL-cholesterol levels. These effects were dose related and more marked in those with higher LDL-cholesterol levels. Thus, consumption of nuts may lower the risk of CHD. The OmniHeart plan provides the following tips to enrich the diet with monounsaturated fats.

- Have a teaspoon per day of olive or canola oil–based margarine on bread at lunch.
- Have 1 or 2 tablespoons of salad dressing made with olive or canola oil and vinegar in salads each day.
- Add a teaspoon of olive or canola oil or margarine in vegetables at dinner.
- Use olive or canola oil to sauté or stir-fry vegetables and add to recipes.
- Have 1 ounce of unsalted nuts rich in monounsaturated fat, such as almonds, peanuts, and pecans, as a snack or add to cereals.

6. *Consume adequate amounts of polyunsaturated fatty acids.* As indicated previously, the National Academy of Sciences developed an AI for both the omega-6 and omega-3 polyunsaturated fatty acids because there may be some health benefits associated with such dietary intakes. Both types of fatty acids help promote healthy skin and are a source of various eicosanoids that may influence health processes. When substituted for saturated fat, polyunsaturated fat may reduce total serum cholesterol, including LDL-cholesterol. In their study of pooled data from 11 American and European studies, Jakobsen and others examined associations between type of fat consumed and risk of CHD. They found that when polyunsaturated fats were substituted for saturated fats, there was a reduced risk of both coronary events and coronary deaths.

One of the most controversial papers published on dietary fat intake and health was the meta-analysis by Chowdhury and colleagues mentioned in chapter 1. The limitations of the meta-analysis procedure are described earlier in the text. Essentially, in their analysis of more than 70 studies with over 500,000 people, Chowdhury and others concluded that encouraging high consumption of polyunsaturated fats and low consumption of saturated fats was not supported by evidence, so should not be recommended for cardiovascular health. However, this analysis had some errors that were corrected in a subsequent article. Also, the authors did not include some studies that would not have supported their conclusions. In fact, several leading nutrition researchers called for the article to be retracted, but it was not.

A great deal can be learned from such controversial papers. One important point is if dietary saturated fat is reduced, what is it replaced with? Replacing dietary saturated fat with polyunsaturated fats or carbohydrate could yield different effects on health. One thing that can be learned from this controversial article is to focus not on nutrients (e.g., eat less saturated fat and more polyunsaturated fat) but on whole foods (e.g., eat more avocados and less butter). If this whole-foods approach is used over an entire diet plan, it is likely there will be an overall consumption of health-promoting nutrients and a decrease in anti-health-promoting nutrients.

Essential fatty acids Polyunsaturated fatty acids should constitute about 10 percent of the daily caloric intake, and if foods are selected wisely this should provide adequate amounts of both omega-6 and omega-3 fatty acids. The essential omega-6 linoleic fatty acid is found in various vegetable oils that constitute food products such as margarine, salad dressings, and cooking oils. Several sources are listed in table 5.10. The essential omega-3 alpha-linolenic fatty acid is found in green leafy vegetables, canola oil, flaxseed oil, soy products, some nuts, and fish. Some nuts are especially rich in both the omega-3 and omega-6 fatty acids. Although both essential fatty acids may confer separate health benefits, the omega-3 fatty acids are thought to be more important for the prevention of CHD.

Omega-3 fatty acids The three principal omega-3 fatty acids—alpha-linolenic, EPA (eicosapentaenoic acid), and DHA (docosahexaenoic acid)—are believed to reduce the risk of CHD, but EPA and DHA are believed to be more potent. EPA and DHA may be formed in the body from alpha-linolenic acid, but this process appears to be limited. However, both EPA and DHA are found in substantial quantities in various fish oils, as highlighted in table 5.11. Eggs from chickens fed a special diet may contain DHA in amounts ranging from 0.05 to 0.15 gram, but the eggs are still high in cholesterol. Fish oil supplements may contain 0.3–0.5 gram.

As mentioned earlier, omega-3 fatty acids have been theorized to be ergogenic because of the production of specific eicosanoids. Omega-3 fatty acids are also being studied for their potential health benefits, which also may be related to specific eicosanoids that are produced. Although the health-related role of omega-3 fatty acids and eicosanoids is complex and has not been totally determined, here is a simple summarization. The cell membrane contains a variety of molecular compounds, including phospholipids and their associated fatty acids. When the diet is high in linoleic acid, one of the main fatty acids in the phospholipids is arachidonic acid, which produces one form of eicosanoids when it is metabolized. When the diet is high in fish oils, EPA and DHA become the major source of eicosanoids, which are different in nature compared to those derived from arachidonic acid. In essence, the different forms of eicosanoids function as local hormones in body cells affecting metabolism and gene expression, and the effects associated with omega-3 fatty acid–derived eicosanoids appear to provide some health benefits. Metcalf and others found that dietary omega-3

TABLE 5.11	Grams of EPA and DHA in fish per 3-ounce edible fish portion and in fish oils per gram of oil	
>1 gram/ 3 ounces	0.5–1.0 gram/ 3 ounces	<0.5 gram/ 3 ounces
Herring	Halibut	Catfish
Oysters, Pacific	Omega-3	Cod
Salmon, Atlantic, farmed	concentrate*	Cod liver oil*
Salmon, Atlantic, wild	Salmon, sockeye	Crab
Salmon, chinook	Trout	Flounder/sole
Sardines	Tuna, fresh	Haddock
	Tuna, white, canned in water	Lobster
		Oysters, Eastern
		Scallops
		Shrimp
		Tuna, light, canned in water

*Note: Omega-3 content in fish oils or supplements is per gram of oil. Check supplement labels for content.

Source: Adapted from USDA Nutrient Data Laboratory. Ranges listed are rough estimates because oil content can vary markedly with species, season, diet, and packaging and cooking methods.

fatty acids are rapidly incorporated into the phospholipids of human heart muscle cells, displacing arachidonic acid.

The effects of fish intake on cardiovascular health is less controversial than research on the effects of saturated fat intake on health. Chowdhury found that fish consumption is associated with decreased risk of cerebrovascular disease, such as strokes. This points to the beneficial effects of omega-3 fats on health. Epidemiological research has suggested that populations consuming diets rich in fish products have a lower incidence rate of CHD, and experimental research has suggested a number of possible mechanisms underlying this relationship:

- Reduce serum triglycerides
- Increase HDL-cholesterol
- Prevent clot formation
- Decrease platelet aggregation and stickiness
- Improve vascular tone
- Decrease blood viscosity
- Optimize blood pressure
- Promote anti-inflammatory activity
- Decrease abnormal heart rhythms

Most research has focused on the effects of fish oil or omega-3 fatty acid supplementation on CHD, and the reviews of published studies are contradictory. Robinson and Stone noted that epidemiological studies show more consistent reductions in the incidence of nonfatal myocardial infarction and ischemic stroke than do the clinical trials of increased omega-3 fatty acid intake, which suggests important confounding factors in the observational studies. In this regard, Cundiff and others found that individuals who consumed more EPA and DHA also consumed fewer Calories, fewer Calories from total

TABLE 5.10	Alpha-linolenic content of selected oils, nuts, and seeds

Oils, nuts, and seeds	Alpha-linolenic content, grams/tablespoon
Olive oil	0.1
Walnuts, English	0.7
Soybean oil	0.9
Canola oil	1.3
Walnut oil	1.4
Flaxseed	2.2
Flaxseed (linseed) oil	8.5

Source: USDA Nutrient Data Laboratory.

fat and saturated fat, and more dietary fiber. They suggested that the benefit of fish or omega-3 fatty acids may be due to the association of greater fish intakes with an overall healthier dietary pattern. In a recent systematic review of 48 randomized controlled trials and 41 cohort studies, which provide stronger evidence than epidemiological studies, Hooper and others concluded that there is no clear effect of omega-3 fatty acid intake on total mortality or cardiovascular events.

Wallin and others reported geographic differences in the effect of fish consumption on Type 2 Diabetes risk, such that there were small increases (United States), no effect (Europe), or decreases in risk (Asia). This is another example of how a meta-analysis of different types of studies can add to the confusion around dietary fat and health. Szostak-Wegierek and others point out that an increase in omega-6 polyunsaturated fats without regard to omega-3 fats might be problematic in terms of cardiovascular disease. They claim a healthy Mediterranean diet has an omega 6 to omega 3 ratio of 2:1 and that this is not being adhered to in countries that increased omega-6 fat intake. Nevertheless, other contemporary reviews and meta-analyses indicate that increased consumption of fish oils and omega-3 fatty acids is cardioprotective. For example, Konig and others, in a meta-analysis, concluded that consuming small quantities of fish is associated with a risk reduction for both nonfatal myocardial infarction (27 percent reduction) and CHD mortality risk (17 percent reduction). In another meta-analysis, Studer and others concluded that consumption of omega-3 fatty acids was effective as a means of preventing mortality from cardiovascular disease. Mori and Woodman also concluded that prospective studies demonstrate an inverse association between fish intake and CHD mortality. Harris even proposed an omega-3 fatty acid index as a new marker or risk factor for CHD. The National Institutes of Health (NIH) indicates that there is significant scientific evidence supporting the claim that increased dietary omega-3 intake improves outcomes in hypertriglyceridemia, hypertension, and secondary cardiovascular disease prevention. The NIH also concluded that there is supportive, but not conclusive, evidence in the primary prevention of cardiovascular disease, which is the basis for the *qualified* health claim on food labels that consumption of conventional foods containing omega-3 fatty acids may reduce the risk of CHD.

Tufts University, one of the leading international nutrition research universities, noted that the predominance of the medical literature continues to support eating fish for cardiovascular health. Based on the available evidence, Kris-Etherton and others provided some dietary guidelines in the American Heart Association Scientific Statement: Fish Consumption, Fish Oil, Omega-3 Fatty Acids, and Cardiovascular Disease. The key points are

- Eat fish, particularly fatty fish, at least two times a week. Fatty fish such as mackerel, lake trout, herring, sardines, albacore tuna, and salmon are high in EPA and DHA.
- Eat plant foods rich in the alpha-linolenic acid, an omega-3 fatty acid that may be converted into EPA and DHA in the body.

- Individuals who have high serum triglycerides may benefit from a fish oil supplement of 2–4 grams of EPA and DHA per day. Patients with CHD may benefit but should consult with their physicians.

Although eating more fish and fish oils is a healthful recommendation, a report by the Institute of Medicine, *Seafood Choices: Balancing Benefits and Risks,* raises some caveats. Some types of fish may contain significant amounts of mercury, as methylmercury, which if consumed in excess may harm the nervous system and impair neurodevelopment in the fetus or young children. Sushi is generally made from large blue fin, or *ahi,* tuna, which may contain mercury. Some types of fish, particularly older, larger predatory fish such as shark and farmed fish such as Atlantic salmon, may contain environmental contaminants such as dioxins and polychlorinated biphenyls.

In a major review, Mozaffarian and Rimm concluded that the benefits of fish intake exceed the potential risks. However, along with the AHA, FDA, and Consumers Union, caution is recommended depending on a person's stage in life:

- For women of childbearing age, benefits of modest fish intake, excepting a few selected species, outweigh risks. The FDA indicates that pregnant women should limit the intake of shark, swordfish, king mackerel, and tilefish and limit consumption of other fish to no more than 12 ounces per week. The FDA indicates that shrimp, salmon, pollock, and catfish are generally low in mercury. Based on new FDA data showing that some canned light tuna may contain as much mercury as white (albacore) tuna, the Consumers Union recommends that women who are pregnant avoid canned tuna entirely. Women of childbearing age should also limit weekly consumption of canned tuna: no more than three 6-ounce cans of light tuna or no more than one can of white tuna.
- Young children should also limit consumption of fish that may be high in mercury, including tuna. The Consumers Union recommends that young children who weigh up to 45 pounds should eat less than one can of tuna a week. Young children may also eat salmon, tilapia, shrimp, and clams daily but should limit intake of other fish to several times a week or less.
- The health effects of low-level methylmercury in adults are not clearly established. Adults should consume a variety of seafood. Select fresh, local seafood where available. The Consumers Union recommends the following safe fish consumption for adult men and women:

Daily	Several times a week
Salmon	Flounder
Tilapia	Sole
Pollock	Herring
Sardine	Mackerel
Oyster	Croaker
Shrimp	Scallop
Clam	Crab
Crawfish	

Environmentalists recommend choosing safe, sustainable fish, such as wild Alaska salmon, canned pink or sockeye salmon, sardines, Atlantic mackerel, and farmed oysters.

http://seafood.edf.org/ The Environmental Defense Fund provides information on fish that are safe to eat and offers substitutes for overfished choices.

Although consuming fish is the recommended means to obtain EPA and DHA, fish oil supplements are also available. Weber and others noted that the possible higher mercury content of some fish may make the intake of omega-3 fatty acids as capsules the better choice. Mercury accumulates in the muscle of the fish, not the fat tissues that is the source of fish oils. Although some health professionals recommend higher amounts for individuals with high levels of serum triglycerides or heart disease, one recommendation for healthy individuals is 500 to 1,300 milligrams a day of EPA and DHA combined. This is more liberal than the recommendation from Lee and colleagues in their review. They propose at least 1 gram of long-chain omega-3 fatty acids daily for patients with known CHD, and 250–500 mg daily for those without disease. The amount of EPA and DHA in a typical fish oil capsule varies, but generally a 1,000-milligram fish oil softgel will contain about 180 mg of EPA and 120 mg of DHA or a total of 300 mg of omega-3 fatty acids. Consuming two to four capsules a day would provide the recommended amount. Some capsules may contain more than 500 mg of omega-3 fatty acids. However, Brunton and Collins note that many types of omega-3 fatty acid dietary supplements are available, but the efficacy, quality, and safety of these products are open to question because they are not regulated by the same standards as pharmaceutical agents. Health professionals recommend that you discuss the benefits and risks of taking fish oil supplements with your doctor. If you do take supplements, do so with food to help absorption.

You may also see omega-3 fatty acids prominently displayed on many food labels, such as cereals, pasta, yogurt, and soy milk. However, check the ingredient list for the source. If it is soybean, canola, or flaxseed oil, the omega-3 fatty acid is alpha-linolenic, which is a good choice but not considered to be as healthful as EPA and DHA.

Conjugated linoleic acid (CLA) Conjugated linoleic acid (CLA), a polyunsaturated omega-6 fatty acid found naturally in small amounts in dairy foods and beef, has been studied for its potential to reduce body fat. Whigham and others conducted a meta-analysis of 18 human studies and concluded that CLA supplementation in a dose of about 3.2 grams daily produces a modest loss of body fat in humans, about 0.1 pound per week. Although this may be meaningful over time, the Consumers Union reports some research suggesting that CLA supplementation may induce some effects, such as impaired blood glucose regulation and inflammation, that might contribute to chronic health problems. The role of CLA in weight control will be discussed further in chapter 10, but currently those at risk for CHD might be advised not to use it.

7. *Limit the amount of dietary cholesterol.* In recent years, some have contended that dietary cholesterol does not influence serum cholesterol and the development of CHD. For example, Hasler noted that it is now known that there is little if any connection between dietary cholesterol and blood cholesterol levels, and consuming up to one or more eggs per day does not adversely affect blood cholesterol levels. In contrast, in a meta-analysis covering 17 studies that evaluated cholesterol intake for at least 14 days, Weggemans and others noted that the addition of 100 milligrams of dietary cholesterol per day would increase slightly the ratio of total cholesterol to HDL-cholesterol, an adverse effect on the serum cholesterol profile. They concluded that the advice to limit cholesterol intake by reducing consumption of eggs and other cholesterol-rich foods may still be valid.

Limiting cholesterol intake is particularly important for cholesterol responders, those individuals with a genetic predisposition whose body production of cholesterol does not automatically decrease when the dietary intake increases. The average U.S. daily intake is approximately 400–500 milligrams or more.

Although some countries, such as Canada and the United Kingdom, do not provide specific recommendations regarding dietary cholesterol, the United States government does, as do some health professional organizations. The amount specified in the Daily Value for food labels is 300 milligrams. The American Heart Association recommends a cholesterol intake of 300 milligrams/day or less or 100 milligrams per 1,000 Calories consumed.

8. *If you consume foods with artificial fats, do so in moderation.* The fat substitutes discussed earlier in this chapter are generally recognized as safe and have been approved by the Food and Drug Administration (FDA). Although olestra has been approved by the FDA, some contend that its use may interfere with the absorption of several fat-soluble vitamins and beta-carotene. However, the FDA requires that products containing olestra-type fat substitutes be enriched with fat-soluble vitamins to offset potential losses.

Snack foods containing olestra, particularly when consumed in large amounts, may cause intestinal cramps and loose stools. McRorie and others reported that although olestra-containing potato chips induced a gradual stool softening effect after several days of consumption, when consumed in smaller amounts, such as 20–40 grams, there were no objective measures of diarrhea or increased gastrointestinal symptoms. Nevertheless, the Center for Science in the Public Interest noted that the FDA received more than 18,000 adverse-reaction reports from people who had eaten olestra-containing foods. Sales of such foods have dropped dramatically.

In its position statement, the American Dietetic Association (ADA) concludes that the majority of fat replacers, when used in moderation by adults, can be safe and useful adjuncts to lowering the fat content of foods and may play a role in decreasing total dietary energy and fat intake. However, the ADA notes that they are effective only if they lower the total caloric content of the food and if the consumer uses these foods as part of a balanced meal plan, such as that promoted in the 2010 *Dietary Guidelines for Americans.*

Some fat is needed in the diet to provide the essential fatty acids and fat-soluble vitamins, and this fat should be obtained easily through natural, wholesome foods such as whole grains, fruits, and vegetables. Following such appropriate guidelines, the American Diabetes Association indicated that foods with fat replacers have the potential to help people with diabetes reduce total and saturated fat intake and may help improve the serum lipid profile. Another possible health benefit of fat substitutes may be their application in weight-loss programs. This topic will be covered in chapter 11.

9. *Reduce intake of refined carbohydrates and increase consumption of plant foods high in complex carbohydrates and dietary fiber, particularly water-soluble fiber.* Refined sugar and starches provoke higher triglyceride concentrations more than complex carbohydrates with fiber do. Again, the value of complex carbohydrates in the diet is stressed, particularly high-fiber foods, as a means to help reduce serum cholesterol. Research has suggested that without adequate amounts of fiber, a diet low in saturated fats and cholesterol has only modest effects on lowering CHD risk. Thus, replace high-fat foods with high-fiber foods. Legumes, such as beans, are an excellent source of carbohydrate and water-soluble fiber. Beans also contain protein, and soy protein, as found in products such as tofu, has been shown to reduce cholesterol in men with both normal and high serum cholesterol. Oat products, such as found in oatmeal, may effectively lower serum cholesterol. Increased consumption of fruits and vegetables is recommended as well, for they may provide substantial amounts of the antioxidant vitamins (C, E, and beta-carotene) that may help to prevent undesired oxidations in the body. Guidelines presented in the preceding chapter are helpful to increase carbohydrate intake, and the role of antioxidant vitamins will be discussed in chapter 7.

Some plant foods, such as almonds and oats, may also contain various sterols and stanols, which are known to reduce serum cholesterol. Devaraj and Jialal indicated that about 2 grams of stanols or sterols per day may lower total and LDL-cholesterol, possibly by interfering with the uptake of both dietary and biliary cholesterol from the intestinal tract. Commercial margarines such as Benecol and Take Control contain such plant stanols and sterols. In a meta-analysis of six well-designed studies, Moruisi and others concluded that fat spreads (margarines) providing about 2.5 grams of phytosterols/stanols daily over the course of 1 to 3 months reduced both total cholesterol and LDL-cholesterol. As noted in chapter 2, a diet rich in plant sterols and stanols may reduce the risk of heart disease. Plant foods also contain several phytochemicals that may reduce serum cholesterol. Many food manufacturers, such as those who produce breakfast cereals and orange juice, are fortifying their products with sterols, stanols, phytochemicals, and other nutrients, creating functional foods designed to reduce serum cholesterol and provide other health benefits as well.

10. *Nibble food throughout the day.* Interestingly, David Jenkins showed a significant reduction in serum LDL-cholesterol if subjects consumed their daily Calories, actually the same food, throughout the day rather than in three concentrated meals at breakfast, lunch, and dinner. In particular, it may be wise to avoid eating a high-fat meal. Nicholls and others reported that a single meal rich in saturated fats may impair blood vessel function and reduce the anti-inflammatory potential of HDL-cholesterol. The Consumers Union noted that a single high-fat meal significantly increased serum triglycerides and decreased blood flow through the heart. Jakulj and others found that a single high-fat meal could increase the blood pressure response to a stressful situation, such as public speaking. All of these factors may increase the short-term risk of a heart attack in susceptible individuals.

In simple, practical terms, what do all of these recommendations mean? Some, such as Lawrence and Harcombe and others, claim that the adverse health effects associated with saturated fat intake are incorrect and that advice on dietary fat consumption and health should never have been introduced to the public. This is likely an oversimplification and can be misleading. It is best to focus on an overall healthy lifestyle that includes adequate amounts of physical activity, acceptable levels of physical fitness, proper weight management, and a diet that is not extreme in terms of the intake of specific nutrients. You should not eliminate all fat from your diet but simply reduce the amount of fat that you eat. In essence, eat less butter, fatty meats, organ foods such as liver and kidney, egg yolks, whole milk, cheeses, ice cream, gravies, creamed foods, high-fat desserts, and refined sugar. Eat more very lean meats, fish, poultry, egg whites, skim and low-fat milk products, fruits and vegetables, beans, and whole-grain products, or the Prudent Healthy Diet. Table 5.12 provides some specifics.

You may have noted that alcohol intake was not one of these recommendations. As detailed in chapter 13, low-risk alcohol intake may provide some protection against CHD for those who do drink. However, most health professionals do not recommend that nondrinkers begin to consume alcohol for its potential health benefits because of other health risks associated with drinking in excess.

Can exercise training also elicit favorable changes in the serum lipid profile?

Physical inactivity, or lack of exercise, has been identified as one of the primary risk factors associated with an increased incidence of atherosclerosis and cardiovascular disease. Hence, exercise programs stressing aerobic endurance-type activities have been advocated as a means of reducing the incidence levels of these conditions, possibly via direct beneficial effects on the heart or blood vessels. However, the precise mechanism whereby exercise may help reduce the morbidity and mortality of CHD has not been identified. Therefore, many authorities believe that the beneficial effect may not be due to exercise itself but rather the possible associated effects, such as reductions in body fat and blood pressure. Although some investigators believe that endurance exercise may

TABLE 5.12   General food selections to decrease total dietary fat, saturated fat, and cholesterol

	Choose	Go easy on	Decrease
Meat, poultry, fish and shellfish (up to 6 ounces a day)	Lean cuts of meat with fat trimmed, such as beef—round, sirloin, chuck, loin lamb—leg, arm, loin, rib pork—tenderloin, leg (fresh), shoulder (arm or picnic) veal—all trimmed cuts except ground poultry without skin fish, shellfish		"Prime" grade fatty cuts of meat such as beef—corned beef brisket, regular ground short ribs pork—spareribs, blade roll Goose, domestic duck Organ meats such as liver, kidney, sweetbreads, brain Highly processed meats such as sausage, bacon, frankfurters, regular luncheon meats Caviar, roe
Dairy products (2 servings a day; 3 servings for women who are pregnant or breast-feeding)	Skim milk, 1% milk, low-fat buttermilk, low-fat evaporated or nonfat milk Low-fat yogurt and low-fat frozen yogurt Low-fat soft cheeses such as: cottage, farmer, pot Cheese labeled no more than 2 to 6 grams of fat an ounce	2% milk Part-skim ricotta Part-skim or imitation hard cheeses, such as part-skim mozzarella "Light" cream cheese "Light" sour cream	Whole milk, such as regular, evaporated, condensed Cream, half-and-half, most nondairy creamers and products, real or nondairy whipped cream Cream cheese, sour cream, ice cream, custard-style yogurt Whole-milk ricotta High-fat cheeses, such as Neufchatel, Brie, Swiss, American, mozzarella, feta, cheddar, Muenster
Eggs (no more than 3 egg yolks a week)	Eggs whites Cholesterol-free egg substitutes		Egg yolks
Fats and oils (up to 6 to 8 teaspoons a day)	Unsaturated vegetable oils, such as corn, olive, peanut, rapeseed (canola oil), safflower, sesame, soybean Margarine or shortening made with unsaturated fats listed above: liquid, tub, stick Diet mayonnaise, salad dressings made with unsaturated fats listed above Low-fat dressings	Nuts and seeds Avocados and olives	Butter, coconut oil, palm kernel oil, palm oil, lard, bacon fat Margarine or shortening made with saturated fats listed above Dressings made with egg yolk
Breads, cereals, pasta, rice, dried peas and beans (6 to 11 servings a day)	Breads, such as whole wheat, pumpernickel, and rye breads; sandwich buns; dinner rolls; bagels; English muffins; rice cakes; focus on whole wheat products Low-fat crackers, such as matzo, pita, bread sticks, rye krisp, saltines, zwieback Hot cereals, most cold dry cereals Pasta such as plain noodles, spaghetti, macaroni; all with low-fat sauces Wild rice Dried peas and beans, such as split peas, black-eyed peas, chickpeas, kidney beans, navy beans, black beans, lentils, soybeans, soybean curd (tofu)	Store-bought pancakes, waffles, biscuits, muffins, cornbread; refined grains	Croissants, butter rolls, sweet rolls, Danish pastry, doughnuts Most snack crackers, such as cheese crackers, butter crackers, those made with saturated fats Granola-type cereals made with saturated fats Pasta and rice prepared with cream, butter, or cheese sauces, egg noodles

(Continued)

TABLE 5.12 Continued

	Choose	Go easy on	Decrease
Fruits and vegetables (2 to 4 servings of fruit and 3 to 5 servings of vegetables)	Fresh, frozen, canned, or dried fruits and vegetables		Vegetables prepared in butter, cream, or sauce Fruits in high-sugar syrup
Sweets and snacks (avoid too many sweets)	Low-fat frozen desserts, such as sherbet, sorbet, Italian ice, frozen yogurt, popsicles Low-fat cakes, such as angel food cake Low-fat cookies, such as fig bars, gingersnaps Low-fat candy, such as jelly beans, hard candy Low-fat snacks, such as plain popcorn, pretzels Nonfat beverages, such as carbonated drinks, juices, tea, coffee	Frozen desserts, such as ice milk Homemade cakes, cookies, and pies using unsaturated oils sparingly Fruit crisps and cobblers Potato and corn chips prepared with unsaturated vegetable oil	High-fat frozen desserts, such as ice cream, frozen tofu High-fat cakes, such as: most store-bought, pound, and frosted cake Store-bought pies, most store-bought cookies Most candy, such as chocolate bars Potato and corn chips prepared with saturated fat Buttered popcorn High-fat beverages, such as frappes, milkshakes, floats, eggnogs
Label ingredients (To avoid too much fat, saturated fat, or cholesterol, go easy on products that list first any fat, oil, or ingredients higher in saturated fat or cholesterol. Choose more often those products that contain ingredients lower in fat, saturated fat, and cholesterol.)	Ingredients lower in saturated fat or cholesterol: Carob, cocoa Oils, like: corn, cottonseed, olive, safflower, sesame, soybean, sunflower Nonfat dry milk, nonfat dry milk solids, skim milk		Ingredients higher in saturated fat or cholesterol: chocolate Animal fat, such as bacon, beef, ham, lamb, meat, pork, chicken or turkey fats, butter, lard Coconut, coconut oil, palm-kernel or palm oil Cream Egg and egg-yolk solids Hardened fat or oil Hydrogenated vegetable oil Shortening or vegetable shortening, unspecified vegetable oil (could be coconut, palm-kernel, palm)

Source: Adapted from "Report of the Expert Panel of Detection, Evaluation, and Treatment of High Blood Cholesterol in Adults." National Heart, Lung, and Blood Institutes of Health.

have a preventive function independent of these associated effects, it also exerts a significant beneficial influence on the serum lipid profile, which, like blood pressure, is one of the major risk factors.

An acute bout of exercise may reduce risk factors for CHD. For example, Thompson and others recently noted that acute exercise may reduce blood pressure and serum triglycerides, increase HDL-cholesterol, and improve insulin sensitivity and glucose homeostasis. Thus, some of the beneficial effects of exercise on risk factors for CHD, including the serum lipid profile, may be attributed to recent exercise bouts. However, some of these benefits may become long-lasting with a chronic exercise training program.

Chronic exercise training has been shown to affect favorably the serum lipid profile. Hundreds of epidemiological and experimental studies have been conducted over the past several decades to investigate the effects of exercise on serum lipids. Space does not permit a detailed analysis of each, but major reviews of the worldwide literature have been reported by prominent authorities such as Stefanik and Wood, Leon and Sanchez, Durstine, and Williams. Although most of these reviews involved males, similar reviews have evaluated the effects of exercise training on women, such as those by Dowling and the meta-analysis by Kelley and others. These reviews have noted a rather consistent pattern relating exercise and blood lipids, and some of the benefits have been associated with concomitant body weight control. In general, increased levels of exercise are associated with lower plasma levels of triglycerides and higher levels of HDL, as documented in several recent meta-analyses by Kelley and Kelley. However, Durstine and others note that exercise training seldom alters total and LDL-cholesterol, although some studies have shown small decreases in the latter. Moreover, research has shown that exercise may not improve the lipid profile of some individuals, primarily in those with genetic defects. These individuals may receive other health benefits of exercise but may need drug therapy to control elevated serum lipid levels.

In an attempt to quantify the serum lipid changes with the amount of exercise, Durstine and his associates conducted a meta-analysis of well-controlled studies. One of the dose-response findings from their analysis indicated that an exercise training volume of 1,200–2,200 Calories per week is often effective at elevating HDL-C levels from 2–8 mg/dl and lowering triglyceride levels by 5–38 mg/dl. Their analysis also suggests that greater increases in HDL-cholesterol can be expected with additional increases in exercise training volume. This amount of physical activity is reasonable and attainable for most individuals and is within the ACSM recommended range for healthy adults. Lifetime aerobic exercise appears to be the key, and moderately intense leisure-time activity, such as brisk walking, may elicit beneficial effects in men, women, children, and adolescents. As noted by Kelley and others, walking favorably affects the adult serum lipid profile independent of changes in body composition.

However, in women, extreme amounts of exercise combined with insufficient energy intake and leading to amenorrhea may reverse these benefits. The effects of exercise-induced amenorrhea will be discussed further in chapters 8 and 10, but it appears that the lower levels of estrogen associated with this condition may lead to lower levels of HDL-cholesterol.

As noted previously, a single high-fat meal may increase the risk of heart attack. However, Katsanos indicates that expending about 500 Calories or more through moderate-intensity exercise within 16 hours before the meal will minimize adverse changes in the lipid profile. As discussed below, this supports the finding that endurance athletes who consume diets rich in fat maintain normal serum lipid profiles.

Although the precise biochemical mechanisms underlying the beneficial effects of exercise on serum lipids have not been identified, researchers have found that in physically trained males and females, activity levels of several enzymes, such as hepatic lipase and lipoprotein lipase, are modified in such a way as to promote a more rapid catabolism of triglycerides and a greater production of HDL. The muscle cell membrane may be modified favorably to become more insulin sensitive, helping clear lipids from the blood into the muscle. Exercise may also favorably modify the serum lipid levels by helping the individual lose body fat or influencing changes in other aspects of his or her lifestyle, such as diet.

Research has revealed that the beneficial effects of exercise training are additive to a diet modified in fat content, such as one reduced in total and saturated fat. A low-fat diet will reduce total cholesterol and LDL-cholesterol but may also undesirably decrease HDL-cholesterol. Exercise may prevent or attenuate the decrease in HDL-cholesterol on such diets, but when combined with omega-3 fatty acid supplementation may actually increase serum HDL-cholesterol, as reported in a study by Thomas and others. Thus, the combination of both dietary modifications and exercise is the recommended approach to modify favorably serum lipid levels.

Research also reveals that highly trained endurance runners who increase their dietary fat to about 40 percent or more of daily caloric intake for 4 weeks do not experience any adverse effects in their blood lipid profiles. Although this type of diet is not recommended on a long-term basis, the review by Brown and Cox illustrates some of the protective effects of exercise training on serum lipid changes associated with short-term increases in dietary fat. They suggest that the strenuous physical training seems to metabolize the increased fat intake for energy and prevents adverse changes in the lipid profile.

www.americanheart.org Use this site to obtain information to help reduce the risk of heart disease and stroke. There are sections on diet and nutrition, healthy cooking, and exercise.

Key Concepts

▶ Low-density forms of lipoproteins (LDL) may predispose certain individuals to coronary heart disease, whereas high-density forms (HDL) may be protective.

▶ In general, a low- to moderate-fat diet is recommended for both health and physical performance. One should consume less high-fat meat and dairy products and more fruits, vegetables, whole-grain products, dietary fiber, lean meats, and skim milk. Fish, including fatty fish such as salmon, is part of a heart-healthy diet.

- Diets rich in saturated fats, *trans* fats, and cholesterol may increase the risk of coronary heart disease. In the United States, in general, the recommended dietary intake of total fat is 35 percent or less of the total caloric intake, with saturated and *trans* fats at less than 7 percent of the total. The recommended cholesterol intake is less than 300 milligrams/day or 100 milligrams per 1,000 Calories.
- Aerobic exercise training increases the ability of the muscles to use fat as an energy source and can be an important adjunct to diet in beneficially modifying the serum lipid profile and reducing body fat, two factors that may reduce the risk of coronary heart disease (CHD). Relative to the serum lipid profile, aerobic exercise training is most effective in reducing serum triglycerides and increasing serum HDL-cholesterol.

Check for Yourself

- Major professional health organizations, such as the American Heart Association, the National Cancer Society, and the American Diabetes Association, all have pamphlets or Internet sites providing dietary recommendations to help prevent related diseases. Obtain pamphlets or visit Websites for several such organizations and evaluate the findings relative to dietary fat. Compare your findings.

APPLICATION EXERCISE

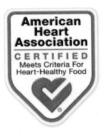

American Heart Association, Inc.

The American Heart Association established its Food Certification Program in 1995 to provide consumers an easy and reliable way to identify heart-healthy foods. Foods that display the distinctive red heart with the white check mark are evaluated to meet the program's standards.

Go to your local supermarket and look for foods with labels that display the American Heart Association *heart-check mark,* as displayed here. Try to find foods in the different food groups, such as grains, fruits, vegetables, meats, and dairy. Make a list of foods you find in each of the food categories, and visit www. heartcheckmark.org to review the nutritional criteria these products must meet to be certified. You may notice that desserts do not have the AHA symbol. In an effort to reduce sugar intake, desserts have been taken off the list of packaged foods, according to Tufts University.

Review Questions—Multiple Choice

1. If a 2,000-Calorie diet contains 100 grams of fat, the percentage of fat Calories in the diet is which of the following?
   a. 20 percent
   b. 25 percent
   c. 35 percent
   d. 45 percent
   e. 60 percent

2. Which of the following dietary supplements has been proven to increase fat utilization during exercise, store muscle glycogen, and enhance endurance exercise performance?
   a. carnitine
   b. conjugated linoleic acid
   c. omega-3 fatty acids
   d. hydroxycitrate
   e. medium-chain triglycerides
   f. a and b
   g. none of the above

3. Which of the following is most conducive to the development of atherosclerosis?
   a. a total cholesterol of 190 milligrams
   b. a low level of very low-density lipoprotein cholesterol
   c. a high-density lipoprotein cholesterol of 70 milligrams
   d. a low-density lipoprotein cholesterol of 170 milligrams
   e. a total cholesterol/high-density lipoprotein cholesterol ratio of less than 3.5

4. Which lipid dietary component appears to be most likely to cause an increase in serum cholesterol and the development of atherosclerosis?
   a. saturated fats
   b. polyunsaturated fats
   c. monounsaturated fats
   d. omega-3 fatty acids
   e. phospholipids

5. What compound in the diet cannot be used to form fat if it is consumed in excess?
   a. fat
   b. complex carbohydrate
   c. simple carbohydrate
   d. protein
   e. alcohol
   f. All are capable of forming fat.

6. Which essential fatty acids are needed in the diet?
   a. linoleic and alpha-linolenic
   b. oleic and linoleic
   c. stearic and alpha-linolenic
   d. palmitic and stearic
   e. palmitoleic and stearic

7. Which of the following statements relative to fats is false?
   a. Hydrogenation of fats makes them more saturated.
   b. Saturated fats are found primarily in animal foods.

c. Vegetable fats are primarily unsaturated fats.

d. Polyunsaturated fats are theorized to be more healthful than saturated fats.

e. Saturated fats appear to help lower blood cholesterol levels.

8. Which of the following is not good advice in attempts to reduce *serum* cholesterol?

a. Limit whole egg consumption to about two to four per week.

b. Eat fish and white poultry meat in place of saturated fat meat.

c. Drink skim milk instead of whole milk.

d. Use butter instead of soft tub, non-*trans* fatty acid margarine.

e. Eat more fruits, vegetables, and whole-grain products.

9. Fats may be a significant source of energy during exercise of low intensity and long duration. What is the main form of fats used for energy production during low-intensity exercise?

a. phospholipids derived from the cell membrane

b. chylomicrons from the liver

c. free fatty acids from the adipose cells and muscle cells

d. VLDL from the liver

e. cholesterol from the kidney

10. Aerobic endurance exercise may have some beneficial effects on the serum lipid profile and help to prevent coronary heart disease (CHD). In particular, what aspects of the serum lipid profile are improved from exercise to help reduce risk of CHD?

a. lower both total cholesterol and LDL-cholesterol

b. lower total cholesterol and increase LDL-cholesterol

c. lower both triglycerides and LDL-cholesterol

d. lower both triglycerides and HDL-cholesterol

e. lower triglycerides and increase HDL-cholesterol

Answers to multiple choice questions: 1. d; 2. g; 3. d; 4. a; 5. f; 6. a; 7. e; 8. d; 9. c; 10. e

Review Questions—Essay

1. List the major classes of dietary fatty acids and discuss their relative importance to cardiovascular health. Include in your discussion specific fatty acids as deemed relevant.

2. Describe the role that the blood lipoproteins play in the etiology of atherosclerosis and cardiovascular disease.

3. What is carnitine and how is it theorized to enhance endurance exercise performance? Does research support the theory?

4. Describe the process of chronic fat loading as a strategy to enhance endurance exercise performance, and provide a synthesis of research findings relative to its efficacy.

5. List at least five dietary strategies that may help reduce the risk of atherosclerosis and cardiovascular disease, including specific foods in the diet.

References

Books

American Institute of Cancer Research. 2007. *Food, Nutrition, Physical Activity, and the Prevention of Cancer: A Global Perspective,* Washington, DC: AICR.

Houston, M. 2006. *Biochemistry Primer for Exercise Science.* Champaign, IL: Human Kinetics.

Institute of Medicine. 2006. *Seafood Choices: Balancing Benefits and Risks.* Washington, DC: National Academies Press.

Jeukendrup, A. 1997. *Aspects of Carbohydrate and Fat Metabolism during Exercise.* Haarlem the Netherlands: De Vriesborch.

Moffatt, R., and Stamford, B. 2006. *Lipid Metabolism and Health.* Boca Raton, FL: CRC Press.

National Academy of Sciences. 2005. *Dietary Reference Intakes for Energy, Carbohydrates, Fiber, Fat, Protein and Amino Acids* (Macronutrients). Washington, DC: National Academies Press.

U.S. Department of Health and Human Services Public Health Service. 2001. *Third Report of the National Cholesterol Education Program of the Expert Panel on Population Strategies for Blood Cholesterol Reduction.* Bethesda, MD: National Institutes of Health.

U.S. Department of Health and Human Services Public Health Service. 2010. *Healthy People 2020: National Health Promotion and Disease Prevention Objectives.* Washington, DC: U.S. Government Printing Office.

Wardlaw, G., and Hampl, J. 2007. *Perspectives in Nutrition.* New York: McGraw-Hill.

Reviews and Specific Studies

Achten, J., and Jeukendrup, A. 2004. Optimizing fat oxidation through exercise and diet. *Nutrition* 20:716–27.

American College of Sports Medicine, et al. 2009. Position of the American Dietetic Association, Dietitians of Canada, and the American College of Sports Medicine: Nutrition and athletic performance. *Medicine & Science in Sports & Exercise* 41:709–31.

American Diabetes Association. 2000. Role of fat replacers in diabetes medical nutrition therapy. *Diabetes Care* 23:S96–97.

American Dietetic Association, et al. 2000. Position of the American Dietetic Association, Dietitians of Canada, and the American College of Sports Medicine: Nutrition and athletic performance. *Journal of the American Dietetic Association* 100:1543–56.

American Dietetic Association. 2005. Position of the American Dietetic Association: Fat replacers. *Journal of the American Dietetic Association* 105:266–75.

American Heart Association. 1999. Monounsaturated fatty acids and risk of cardiovascular disease. *Circulation* 100:1253–8.

American Heart Association. 2006. Diet and lifestyle recommendations revision 2006: A scientific statement from the American Heart Association Nutrition Committee. *Circulation* 114:82–96.

Angus, D., et al. 2000. Effect of carbohydrate or carbohydrate plus medium-chain triglyceride ingestion on cycling time trial performance. *Journal of Applied Physiology* 88:113–19.

Appel, L., et al. 2005. Effects of protein, monounsaturated fat, and carbohydrate intake on blood pressure and serum lipids: Results of the OmniHeart randomized trial. *Journal of the American Medical Association* 294:2455–64.

Aucouturier, J., et al. 2008. Fat and carbohydrate metabolism during submaximal exercise in children. *Sports Medicine* 38:213–38.

Blesso, C., et al. 2013. Effects of carbohydrate restriction and dietary cholesterol provided by eggs on clinical risk factors in metabolic syndrome. *Journal of Clinical Lipidology* 7:463–71.

Blesso, C., et al. 2013. Whole egg consumption improves lipoprotein profiles and insulin sensitivity to a greater extent than yolk-free egg substitute in individuals with metabolic syndrome. *Metabolism* 62:400–10.

Bortolotti, M., et al. 2007. Fish oil supplementation does not alter energy efficiency in healthy males. *Clinical Nutrition* 26:225–30.

Brilla, L., and Landerholm, T. 1990. Effect of fish oil supplementation and exercise on serum lipids and aerobic fitness. *Journal of Sports Medicine & Physical Fitness* 30:173–80.

Brown, G., et al. 1993. Lipid lowering and plaque regression: New insights into prevention of plaque disruption and clinical events in coronary disease. *Circulation* 87:1781–89.

Brown, R., and Cox, C. 2000. High-fat versus high-carbohydrate diets: Effect on exercise capacity and performance of endurance trained cyclists. *New Zealand Journal of Sports Medicine* 28:55–59.

Brown, R., and Cox, C. 2001. Challenging the dogma of dietary carbohydrate requirements for endurance athletes. *American Journal of Medicine & Sports* 3:75–86.

Brunton, S., and Collins, N. 2007. Differentiating prescription omega-3-acid ethyl esters (P-OM3) from dietary-supplement omega-3 fatty acids. *Current Medical Research & Opinion* 23:1139–45.

Buckley, J., et al. 2009. DHA-rich fish oil lowers heart rate during submaximal exercise in elite Australian Rules footballers. *Journal of Science & Medicine in Sport* 12:503–7.

Bueno, N. B., et al. 2015. Dietary medium-chain triacylglycerols versus long-chain triacylglycerols for body composition in adults: Systematic review and meta-analysis of randomized controlled trials. *Journal of the American College of Nutrition* 34:175–83.

Bueno, N., et al. 2013. Very-low-carbohydrate ketogenic diet v. low-fat diet for long-term weight loss: A meta-analysis of randomised controlled trials. *British Journal of Nutrition* 110:1178–87.

Burelle, Y., et al. 2001. Oxidation of [(13) C]-glycerol ingested along with glucose during prolonged exercise. *Journal of Applied Physiology* 90:1685–90.

Burke, L. M. 2015. Medium-chain triglycerides. In *Nutritional Supplements in Sport, Exercise, and Health. An A–Z Guide*, ed. L. M. Castell, S. J. Stear, and L. M. Burke. New York: Routledge.

Burke, L., and Hawley, J. 2002. Effects of short-term fat adaptation on metabolism and performance of prolonged exercise. *Medicine & Science in Sports & Exercise* 34:1492–98.

Burke, L., et al. 2000. Effect of fat adaptation and carbohydrate restoration on metabolism and performance during prolonged cycling. *Journal of Applied Physiology* 89:2413–21.

Burke, L., et al. 2002. Adaptations to short-term high-fat diet persist during exercise despite high carbohydrate availability. *Medicine & Science in Sports & Exercise* 34:83–91.

Carey, A., et al. 2001. Effects of fat adaptation and carbohydrate restoration on prolonged endurance exercise. *Journal of Applied Physiology* 91:115–22.

Center for Science in the Public Interest. 1999. Olean times at P & G. *Nutrition Action Health Letter* 26 (8):2.

Center for Science in the Public Interest. 2013. Six reasons to eat less meat. *Nutrition Action Health Letter* (June):1–7

Cheuvront, S. 1999. The zone diet and athletic performance. *Sports Medicine* 27:213–28.

Chowdhury, R., et al. 2012. Association between fish consumption, long chain omega 3 fatty acids, and risk of cerebrovascular disease: Systematic review and meta-analysis. *BMJ* 345:e6698.

Chowdhury, R., et al. 2014. Association of dietary, circulating, and supplement fatty acids with coronary risk: A systematic review and meta-analysis. *Annals of Internal Medicine* 160:398–406.

Clarke, R., et al. 1997. Dietary lipids and blood cholesterol: Quantitative meta-analysis of metabolic ward studies. *British Medical Journal* 314:112–17.

Coggan, A., et al. 2000. Fat metabolism during high-intensity exercise in endurance-trained and untrained men. *Metabolism* 49:122–28.

Consumers Union. 2002. Chest pain after eating? *Consumer Reports on Health* 14 (7):3.

Consumers Union. 2006. Mercury in tuna. *Consumer Reports* 71 (7):20–21.

Costill, D., et al. 1979. Lipid metabolism in skeletal muscle of endurance trained males and females. *Journal of Applied Physiology* 47:787–91.

Covas, M. 2007. Olive oil and the cardiovascular system. *Pharmacological Research* 55:175–86.

Cundiff, D., et al. 2007. Relation of omega-3 fatty acid intake to other dietary factors known to reduce coronary heart disease risk. *American Journal of Cardiology* 99:1230–33.

De Bock, K., et al. 2008. Effect of training in the fasted state on metabolic responses during exercise with carbohydrate intake. *Journal of Applied Physiology* 104:1045–55.

Decombaz, J., et al. 1993. Effect of L-carnitine on submaximal exercise metabolism after depletion of muscle glycogen. *Medicine & Science in Sports & Exercise* 25:733–40.

Deighton, K., et al. 2012. Appetite, energy intake and resting metabolic responses to 60 min treadmill running performed in a fasted versus a postprandial state. *Appetite* 58:946–54.

Devaraj, S., and Jialal, I. 2006. The role of dietary supplementation with plant sterols and stanols in the prevention of cardiovascular disease. *Nutrition Reviews* 64:348–54.

Dowling, E. 2001. How exercise affects lipid profiles in women. *Physician and Sportsmedicine* 29 (9):45–52.

Durstine, J., et al. 2001. Blood lipid and lipoprotein adaptations to exercise: A quantitative analysis. *Sports Medicine* 31:1033–62.

Erlenbusch, M., et al. 2004. Effect of high-fat or high-carbohydrate diets on endurance exercise: A meta-analysis. *International Journal of Sport Nutrition & Exercise Metabolism* 15:1–14.

Franco, O., et al. 2005. Effects of physical activity on life expectancy with cardiovascular disease. *Archives of Internal Medicine* 165:2355–60.

Frayn, K. 2010. Fat as fuel: Emerging understanding of the adipose tissue-skeletal muscle axis. *Acta Physiologica* 199:509–18.

Gibson, A., et al. 2015. Do ketogenic diets really suppress appetite? A systematic review and meta-analysis. *Obesity Reviews* 16:64–76.

Glatz, J., et al. 2002. Exercise and insulin increase muscle fatty acid uptake by recruiting putative fatty acid transporters to the sarcolemma. *Current Opinion in Clinical Nutrition & Metabolic Care* 5:365–70.

Goedecke, J., et al. 1999. Effect of medium-chain triacylglycerol ingested with carbohydrate on metabolism and exercise performance. *International Journal of Sports Medicine* 9:35–47.

Goedecke, J., et al. 2005. The effects of medium-chain triacylglycerol and carbohydrate ingestion on ultra-endurance exercise performance. *International Journal of Sport Nutrition & Exercise Metabolism* 15:15–27.

Gonzalez, J., et al. 2013. Breakfast and exercise contingently affect postprandial metabolism and energy balance in physically active males. *British Journal of Nutrition* 110:721–32.

Grundy, S. 2006. Nutrition in the management of disorders of serum lipids and lipoproteins. In *Modern Nutrition in Health and Disease,* ed. M. Shils, et al. Philadelphia: Lippincott Williams & Wilkins.

Gutierrez, A., et al. 2001. Three days fast in sportsmen decreases physical work capacity but not strength or perception-reaction time. *International Journal of Sport Nutrition & Exercise Metabolism* 11:420–29.

Harcombe, Z., et al. 2015. Evidence from randomised controlled trials did not support the introduction of dietary fat guidelines in 1977 and 1983: A systematic review and meta-analysis. *Open Heart* 2015;2: doi:10.1136/openhrt-2014-000196

Hargreaves, M. 2006. The metabolic systems: Carbohydrate metabolism. In *ACSM's Advanced Exercise Physiology,* ed. C. M. Tipton. Philadelphia: Lippincott Williams & Wilkins.

Harris, W. 2004. Are omega-3 fatty acids the most important nutritional modulators of coronary heart disease risk? *Current Atherosclerosis Reports* 6:447–52.

Harris, W. 2007. Omega-3 fatty acids and cardiovascular disease: A case for omega-3 index as a new risk factor. *Pharmacological Research* 55:217–23.

Hasler, C. 2000. The changing face of functional foods. *Journal of the American College of Nutrition* 19:499S–506S.

Havemann, L., et al. 2006. Fat adaptation followed by carbohydrate loading compromises high-intensity sprint performance. *Journal of Applied Physiology* 100:194–202.

Hawley, J. 2002. Effect of increased fat availability on metabolism and exercise capacity. *Medicine & Science in Sports & Exercise* 34:1485–91.

Hawley, J., et al. 2000. Fat metabolism during exercise. In *Nutrition in Sport,* ed. R. Maughan. Oxford: Blackwell Scientific.

Heinonen, O. 1996. Carnitine and physical exercise. *Sports Medicine* 22:109–32.

Holloway, C., et al. 2011. A high-fat diet impairs cardiac high-energy phosphate metabolism and cognitive function in healthy human subjects. *American Journal of Clinical Nutrition* 93:748–55.

Hooper, L., et al. 2006. Risks and benefits of omega-3 fats for mortality, cardiovascular disease, and cancer: Systematic review. *British Medical Journal* 332:752–60.

Horowitz, J., and Klein, S. 2000. Lipid metabolism during endurance exercise. *American Journal of Clinical Nutrition* 72:558S–63S.

Horowitz, J., et al. 2000. Preexercise medium-chain triglyceride ingestion does not alter muscle glycogen use during exercise. *Journal of Applied Physiology* 88:219–25.

Horvath, P., et al. 2000. The effect of varying dietary fat on performance and metabolism in trained male and female runners. *Journal of the American College of Nutrition* 19:52–60.

Howell, W., et al. 1997. Plasma lipid and lipoprotein responses to dietary fat and cholesterol: A meta-analysis. *American Journal of Clinical Nutrition* 65:1747–64.

Huffman, D., et al. 2004. Effect of *n*-3 fatty acids on free tryptophan and exercise fatigue. *European Journal of Applied Physiology* 92:584–91.

Hulbert, A. 2005. Dietary fats and membrane function: Implications for metabolism and disease. *Biological Reviews of the Cambridge Philosophical Society* 80:155–69.

Jacobson, T., et al. 2007. Hypertriglyceridemia and cardiovascular risk reduction. *Clinical Therapy* 29:763–77.

Jain, K., et al. 2007. The biology and chemistry of hyperlipidemia. *Bioorganic & Medical Chemistry* 15:4674–99.

Jakobsen, M., et al. 2009. Major types of dietary fat and risk of coronary heart disease: A pooled analysis of 11 cohort studies. *American Journal of Clinical Nutrition* 89:1425–32.

Jakulj, F., et al. 2007. A high-fat meal increases cardiovascular reactivity to psychological stress in healthy young adults. *Journal of Nutrition* 137:935–39.

Jenkins, D., et al. 1989. Nibbling versus gorging: Metabolic advantages of increased meal frequency. *New England Journal of Medicine* 321:929–34.

Jequier, E. 1999. Response to and range of acceptable fat intake in adults. *European Journal of Clinical Nutrition* 53:S84–S88.

Jeukendrup, A. 2002. Regulation of fat metabolism in skeletal muscle. *Annals of the New York Academy of Sciences* 967:217–35.

Jeukendrup, A. E., et al. 1998. Fat metabolism during exercise: A review. Part II: Regulation of metabolism and the effects of training. *International Journal of Sports Medicine* 19:293–302.

Jeukendrup, A., and Aldred, S. 2004. Fat supplementation, health, and endurance performance. *Nutrition* 20:678–88.

Jeukendrup, A., and Randell, R. 2011. Fat burners: Nutrition supplements that increase fat metabolism. *Obesity Reviews* 12:841–51.

Jeukendrup, A., et al. 1996. Effect of endogenous carbohydrate availability on oral medium-chain triglyceride oxidation during prolonged exercise. *Journal of Applied Physiology* 80:949–54.

Jeukendrup, A., et al. 1998. Effect of medium-chain triacylglycerol and carbohydrate ingestion during exercise on substrate utilization and subsequent cycling performance. *American Journal of Clinical Nutrition* 67:397–404.

Johnson, E., and Schaefer, E. 2006. Potential role of dietary *n*-3 fatty acids in the prevention of dementia and macular degeneration. *American Journal of Clinical Nutrition* 84:1494S–98S.

Johnston, B., et al. 2014. Comparison of weight loss among named diet programs in overweight and obese adults: A meta-analysis. *Journal of the American Medical Association* 312:923–33.

Jones, P., and Kubow, S. 2006. Lipids, sterols, and their metabolites. In *Modern Nutrition in Health & Disease,* eds. M. Shils, et al. Philadelphia: Lippincott Williams & Wilkins.

Katsanos, C. 2006. Prescribing aerobic exercise for the regulation of postprandial lipid metabolism: Current research and recommendations. *Sports Medicine* 36:547–60.

Kelley, G., and Kelley, K. 2006. Aerobic exercise and HDL$_2$-C: A meta-analysis of randomized controlled trials. *Atherosclerosis* 184:207–15.

Kelley, G., and Kelley, K. 2007. Aerobic exercise and lipids and lipoproteins in children and adolescents: A meta-analysis of randomized controlled trials. *Atherosclerosis* 191:447–53.

Kelley, G., et al. 2004. Aerobic exercise and lipids and lipoproteins in women: A meta-analysis of randomized controlled trials. *Journal of Women's Health* 13:1148–64.

Kelley, G., et al. 2004. Walking, lipids, and lipoproteins: A meta-analysis of randomized controlled trials. *Preventive Medicine* 38:651–61.

Kiens, B., and Helge, J. 2000. Adaptations to a high fat diet. In *Nutrition in Sport,* ed. R. Maughan. Oxford: Blackwell Scientific.

King, S., and Gibney, M. 1999. Dietary advice to reduce fat intake is more successful when it does not restrict habitual eating patterns. *Journal of the American Dietetic Association* 99:685–89.

Kingsley, M. 2006. Effects of phosphatidylserine supplementation on exercising humans. *Sports Medicine* 36:657–69.

Kingsley, M., et al. 2005. Effects of phosphatidylserine on oxidative stress following intermittent running. *Medicine & Science in Sports & Exercise* 37:1300–06.

Kingsley, M., et al. 2006. Effects of phosphatidylserine on exercise capacity during cycling in active males. *Medicine & Science in Sports & Exercise* 38:64–71.

Kingsley, M., et al. 2006. Phosphatidylserine supplementation and recovery following downhill running. *Medicine & Science in Sports & Exercise* 38:1617–25.

Knechtle, B., et al. 2004. Fat oxidation in men and women endurance athletes in running

and cycling. *International Journal of Sports Medicine* 25:38–44.

Kodama, S., et al. 2007. Effect of aerobic exercise training on serum levels of high-density lipoprotein cholesterol: A meta-analysis. *Archives of Internal Medicine* 167:999–1008.

Konig, A., et al. 2005. A quantitative analysis of fish consumption and coronary heart disease mortality. *American Journal of Preventive Medicine* 29:335–46.

Kraemer, W., et al. 2006. Androgenic responses to resistance exercise: Effects of feeding and L-carnitine. *Medicine & Science in Sports & Exercise* 38:1288–96.

Kreider, R., et al. 2002. Effects of conjugated linoleic acid supplementation during resistance training on body composition, bone density, strength and selected hematological markers. *Journal of Strength Conditioning Research* 16:325–34.

Kriketos, A., et al. 1999. ($-$)-Hydroxycitric acid does not affect energy expenditure and substrate oxidation in adult males in a post-absorptive state. *International Journal of Obesity & Related Metabolic Disorders* 23:867–73.

Kris-Etherton, P., et al. 2002. AHA scientific statement: Fish, fish oils and omega-3 fatty acids. *Circulation* 106:2747–57.

Kris-Etherton, P., et al. 2002. Dietary fat: Assessing the evidence in support of a moderate-fat diet: The benchmark based on lipoprotein metabolism. *Proceedings of the Nutrition Society* 61:287–98.

Lambert, E., et al. 1994. Enhanced endurance in trained cyclists during moderate intensity exercise following 2 weeks adaptation to a high fat diet. *European Journal of Applied Physiology* 69:287–93.

Lambert, E., et al. 2001. High-fat diet versus habitual diet prior to carbohydrate loading: Effects of exercise metabolism and cycling performance. *International Journal of Sport Nutrition & Exercise Metabolism* 11:209–25.

Lange, K. 2004. Fat metabolism in exercise—With special reference to training and growth hormone administration. *Scandinavian Journal of Medicine & Science in Sports* 14:74–99.

LaRosa, J. 2007. Low-density lipoprotein cholesterol reduction: The end is more important than the means. *American Journal of Cardiology* 100:240–42.

Larsen, T., et al. 2006. Conjugated linoleic acid supplementation for 1 y does not prevent weight or body fat regain. *American Journal of Clinical Nutrition* 83:606–12.

Larson-Meyer, D., et al. 2008. Effect of dietary fat on serum and intramyocellular lipids and running performance. *Medicine & Science in Sports & Exercise* 40:892–902.

Lawrence, G. 2013. Dietary fats and health: Dietary recommendations in the context of scientific evidence. *Advances in Nutrition* 4:294–302.

Lee, J., et al. 2009. Omega-3 fatty acids: Cardiovascular benefits, sources, and sustainability. *Nature Reviews: Cardiology* 6:753–8.

Leon, A., and Sanchez, O. 2001. Response of blood lipids to exercise training alone or combined with dietary interventions. *Medicine & Science in Sports & Exercise* 33:S502–15.

Lichtenstein, A. 2000. Trans fatty acids and cardiovascular disease risk. *Current Opinion in Lipidology* 11:37–42.

Macaluso, F., et al. 2013. Do fat supplements increase physical performance? *Nutrients* 5:509–24.

Manore, M. 2012. Dietary supplements for improving body composition and reducing body weight: Where is the evidence? *International Journal of Sports Nutrition and Exercise Metabolism* 22:139–54.

Márquez, F., et al. 2012. Evaluation of the safety and efficacy of hydroxycitric acid or *Garcinia cambogia* extracts in humans. *Critical Reviews in Food Science and Nutrition* 52:585–94.

Martin, W. 1997. Effect of endurance training on fatty acid metabolism during whole body exercise. *Medicine & Science in Sports & Exercise* 29:635–39.

Massicotte, D., et al. 1992. Oxidation of exogenous medium-chain free fatty acids during prolonged exercise: Comparison with glucose. *Journal of Applied Physiology* 73:1334–39.

McRorie, J., et al. 2000. Effects of olestra and sorbitol consumption on objective measures of diarrhea: Impact of stool viscosity on common gastrointestinal symptoms. *Regulatory Toxicology & Pharmacology* 31:59–67.

Metcalf, R., et al. 2007. Effects of fish-oil supplementation on myocardial fatty acids in humans. *American Journal of Clinical Nutrition* 85:1222–28.

Mickleborough, T. 2008. A nutritional approach to managing exercise-induced asthma. *Exercise & Sport Science Reviews* 36:135–44.

Misell, L., et al. 2001. Chronic medium-chain triacylglycerol consumption and endurance performance in trained runners. *Journal of Sports Medicine & Physical Fitness* 41:210–15.

Mora-Rodriguez, R., and Coyle, E. 2000. Effects of plasma epinephrine on fat metabolism during exercise: Interactions with exercise intensity. *American Journal of Physiology Endocrinology & Metabolism* 278:E669–76.

Mori, T., and Woodman, R. 2006. The independent effects of eicosapentaenoic acid and docosahexaenoic acid on cardiovascular risk factors in humans. *Current Opinion in Clinical Nutrition & Metabolic Care* 9:95–104.

Moruisi, K., et al. 2006. Phytosterols/stanols lower cholesterol concentrations in familial hypercholesterolemic subjects: A systematic review with meta-analysis. *Journal of the American College of Nutrition* 25:41–48.

Mozaffarian, D., and Rimm, E. 2006. Fish intake, contaminants, and human health: Evaluating the risks and the benefits. *Journal of the American Medical Association* 296:1885–99.

Mozaffarian, D., et al. 2006. *Trans* fatty acids and cardiovascular disease. *New England Journal of Medicine* 354:1601–16.

Mumme, K., and Stonehouse, W. 2015. Effects of medium-chain triglycerides on weight loss and body composition: A meta-analysis of randomized controlled trials. *Journal of the Academy of Nutrition and Dietetics* 115:249–63.

Muoio, D., et al. 1994. Effect of dietary fat on metabolic adjustments to maximal VO$_2$ and endurance in runners. *Medicine & Science in Sports & Exercise* 26:81–88.

Nicholls, S., et al. 2006. Consumption of saturated fat impairs the anti-inflammatory properties of high-density lipoproteins and endothelial function. *Journal of the American College of Cardiology* 48:715–20.

Noakes T., et al. 2014. Low-carbohydrate diets for athletes: What evidence? *British Journal of Sports Medicine* 48:1077–78.

Noto, H., et al. 2013. Low-carbohydrate diets and all-cause mortality: A systematic review and meta-analysis of observational studies. *PLoS One* 8:e55030.

Okano, G., et al. 1996. Effect of 4 h preexercise high carbohydrate and high fat meal ingestion on endurance performance and metabolism. *International Journal of Sports Medicine* 17:530–34.

Okano, G., et al. 1998. Effect of elevated blood FFA levels on endurance performance after a single fat meal ingestion.

Medicine & Science in Sports & Exercise 30:763–68.

Onakpoya, I., et al. 2012. The efficacy of long-term conjugated linoleic acid (CLA) supplementation on body composition in overweight and obese individuals: A systematic review and meta-analysis of randomized clinical trials. *European Journal of Nutrition* 51:127–34.

Oostenbrug, G., et al. 1997. Exercise performance, red blood cell deformability, and lipid peroxidation: Effects of fish oil and vitamin E. *Journal of Applied Physiology* 83:746–52.

Peoples, G., et al. 2008. Fish oil reduces heart rate and oxygen consumption during exercise. *Journal of Cardiovascular Pharmacology* 52:540–47.

Perez-Jimenez, F., et al. 2005. International conference on the healthy effect of virgin olive oil. *European Journal of Clinical Investigation* 35:421–24.

Phinney, S. D., et al. 1983. The human metabolic response to chronic ketosis without caloric restriction: Preservation of submaximal exercise capability with reduced carbohydrate oxidation. *Metabolism* 32:769–76.

Pinkoski, C., et al. 2006. The effects of conjugated linoleic acid supplementation during resistance training. *Medicine & Science in Sports & Exercise* 38:339–48.

Raastad, T., et al. 1997. Omega-3 fatty acid supplementation does not improve maximal aerobic power, anaerobic threshold and running performance in well-trained soccer players. *Scandinavian Journal of Medicine & Science in Sports* 7:25–31.

Remig, V., et al. 2010. *Trans* fats in America: A review of their use, consumption, health implications, and regulation. *Journal of the American Dietetic Association* 110: 585–92.

Reynolds, G. 2015. Should athletes eat fat or carbs? *New York Times,* February 25, http://well.blogs.nytimes.com/2015/02/25/should-athletes-eat-fat-or-carbs/?_r=0

Ridker, P., et al. 2002. Comparison of C-reactive protein and low-density-lipoprotein cholesterol levels in the prediction of first cardiovascular events. *New England Journal of Medicine* 347:1557–65.

Robinson, J., and Stone, N. 2006. Antiatherosclerotic and antithrombotic effects of omega-3 fatty acids. *American Journal of Cardiology* 98:39i–49i.

Roepstorff, C., et al. 2005. Intramuscular triacylglycerol in energy metabolism during exercise in humans. *Exercise & Sport Sciences Reviews* 33:182–88.

Romijn, J., et al. 1993. Regulation of endogenous fat and carbohydrate metabolism in relation to exercise intensity and duration. *American Journal of Physiology* 265:E380–E391.

Romijn, J., et al. 2000. Substrate metabolism during different exercise intensities in endurance-trained women. *Journal of Applied Physiology* 88:1707–14.

Rowlands, D., and Hopkins, W. 2002. Effect of high-fat, high-carbohydrate, and high-protein meals on metabolism and performance during endurance cycling. *International Journal of Sport Nutrition & Exercise Metabolism* 12:318–35.

Rowlands, D., and Hopkins, W. 2002. Effects of high-fat and high-carbohydrate diets on metabolism and performance in cycling. *Metabolism* 51:678–90.

Sabaté, J., et al. 2010. Nut consumption and blood lipid levels. *Archives of Internal Medicine* 170:821–27.

Saito, M., et al. 2005. High dose of *Garcinia cambogia* is effective in suppressing fat accumulation in developing male Zucker obese rats, but highly toxic to the testis. *Food Chemistry Toxicology* 43:411–9.

Schoenfeld, B. J., et al. 2014. Body composition changes associated with fasted versus nonfasted aerobic exercise. *Journal of the International Society of Sports Nutrition* 11:54.

Shrier, I. 2005. Mediterranean diet for reducing mortality and easing the metabolic syndrome. *Physician and Sportsmedicine* 33 (5):8–9.

Shulman, D. 2002. Fuel on fat for the long run. *Marathon & Beyond* 6 (5):128–36.

Siri, P., and Krauss, R. 2005. Influence of dietary carbohydrate and fat on LDL and HDL particle distributions. *Current Atherosclerosis Reports* 7:455–59.

Spiering, B., et al. 2007. Responses of criterion variables to different supplemental doses of L-carnitine L-tartrate. *Journal of Strength & Conditioning Research* 21:259–64.

Spriet, L. 2002. Regulation of skeletal muscle fat oxidation during exercise in humans. *Medicine & Science in Sports & Exercise* 34:1477–84.

Spriet, L. 2006. The metabolic systems: Lipid metabolism. In *ACSM's Advanced Exercise Physiology,* ed. C. Tipton. Philadelphia: Lippincott Williams & Wilkins.

Spriet, L. 2007. Regulation of substrate use during the marathon. *Sports Medicine* 37:332–36.

Spriet, L., and Gibala, M. 2004. Nutritional strategies to influence adaptations to training. *Journal of Sports Sciences* 22:127–41.

Spriet, L., and Hargreaves, M. 2006. The metabolic systems: Interaction of lipid and carbohydrate metabolism. In *ACSM's Advanced Exercise Physiology,* ed. C. Tipton. Philadelphia: Lippincott Williams & Wilkins.

Stannard, S. R., et al. 2010. Adaptations to skeletal muscle with endurance exercise training in the acutely fed versus overnight-fasted state. *Journal of Science and Medicine in Sport* 13:645–9.

Staton, W. 1951. The influence of soya lecithin on muscular strength. *Research Quarterly* 22:201–7.

Stefanik, M., and Wood, P. 1994. Physical activity, lipid and lipoprotein metabolism, and lipid transport. In *Physical Activity, Fitness, and Health,* ed. C. Bouchard, et al. Champaign, IL: Human Kinetics.

Stellingwerff, T., et al. 2006. Decreased PDH activation and glycogenolysis during exercise following fat adaptation with carbohydrate restoration. *American Journal of Physiology. Endocrinology & Metabolism* 290:E380–88.

Stephens, B., et al. 2006. The influence of biological maturation on fat and carbohydrate metabolism during exercise in males. *International Journal of Sport Nutrition & Exercise Metabolism* 16:166–79.

Stephens, F., and Greenhaff, P. 2015. L-carnitine. In *Nutritional Supplements in Sport, Exercise, and Health. An A–Z Guide,* ed. L. M. Castell, S. J. Stear, and L. M. Burke. New York: Routledge.

Studer, M., et al. 2005. Effect of different antilipidemic agents and diets on mortality: A systematic review. *Archives of Internal Medicine* 165:725–30.

Szostak-Wegierek, D., et al. 2013. The role of dietary fats for preventing cardiovascular disease. A review. *Roczniki Panstwowego Zakladu Higieny* 64:263–9.

Tarnopolsky, M. 2000. Gender differences in metabolism: Nutrition and supplements. *Journal of Science & Medicine in Sport* 3:287–98.

Tarnopolsky, M. 2000. Gender differences in substrate metabolism during endurance exercise. *Canadian Journal of Applied Physiology* 25:312–27.

Tarnopolsky, M. 2008. Sex differences in exercise metabolism and the role of 17-beta estradiol. *Medicine & Science in Sports & Exercise* 40:648–54.

Tarnopolsky, M., et al. 1995. Carbohydrate loading and metabolism during exercise in men and women. *Journal of Applied Physiology* 68:302–8.

Tartibian, B., et al. 2010. The effects of omega-3 supplementation on pulmonary function of young wrestlers during intensive training. *Journal of Sciences & Medicine in Sport* 13:281–86.

Taylor, J., et al. 2006. Conjugated linoleic acid impairs endothelial function. *Arteriosclerosis, Thrombosis & Vascular Biology* 26:307–12.

Thomas, T., et al. 2004. Effects of omega-3 fatty acid supplementation and exercise on low-density lipoprotein and high-density lipoprotein subfractions. *Metabolism* 53:749–54.

Thompson, P., et al. 2001. The acute versus the chronic response to exercise. *Medicine & Science in Sports & Exercise* 33:S438–45.

Timmons, B., et al. 2007. Energy substrate utilization during prolonged exercise with and without carbohydrate intake in pre-adolescent and adolescent girls. *Journal of Applied Physiology* 103:995–1000.

Timmons, B., et al. 2007. Influence of age and pubertal status on substrate utilization during exercise with and without carbohydrate intake in healthy boys. *Applied Physiology, Nutrition & Metabolism* 32:416–25.

Trabelsi, K., et al. 2012. Effect of resistance training during Ramadan on body composition and markers of renal function, metabolism, inflammation, and immunity in recreational bodybuilders. *International Journal of Sport Nutrition and Exercise Metabolism* 22:267–75.

Trabelsi, K., et al. 2012. Effects of fed- versus fasted-state aerobic training during Ramadan on body composition and some metabolic parameters in physically active men. *International Journal of Sport Nutrition and Exercise Metabolism* 22:11–18.

Tufts University. 2007. Studies find new omega-3 benefits. *Tufts University Health & Nutrition Letter* 25 (5):4–5.

Tufts University. 2010. No dessert for heart checkmark program. *Tufts University Health & Nutrition Letter* 28 (2):3.

Tunstall, R., et al. 2002. Exercise training increases lipid metabolism gene expression in human skeletal muscle. *American Journal of Physiology. Endocrinology & Metabolism* 283:E66–72.

Van Horn, L., et al. 2008. The evidence for dietary prevention and treatment of cardiovascular disease. *Journal of the American Dietetic Association* 108:287–331.

van Loon, L. 2004. Use of intramuscular triacylglycerol as a substrate source during exercise in humans. *Journal of Applied Physiology* 97:1170–87.

van Loon, L., et al. 2000. Effects of acute (-)-hydroxycitrate supplementation on substrate metabolism at rest and during exercise in humans. *American Journal of Clinical Nutrition* 72:1445–50.

Van Proeyen, K., et al. 2010. Training in the fasted state improves glucose tolerance during fatrich diet. *Journal of Physiology* 588:4289–302.

Van Proeyen, K., et al. 2011. Beneficial metabolic adaptations due to endurance exercise training in the fasted state. *Journal of Applied Physiology* 110:236–45.

Venables, M., et al. 2005. Determinants of fat oxidation during exercise in healthy men and women: A cross-sectional study. *Journal of Applied Physiology* 98:160–67.

Venkatraman, J., and Pendergast, D. 1998. Effect of the level of dietary fat intake and endurance exercise on plasma cytokines in runners. *Medicine & Science in Sports & Exercise* 30:1198–204.

Volek, J. S., et al. 2015. Rethinking fat as a fuel for endurance exercise. *European Journal of Sport Science* 15:13–20.

Volk, B., et al. 2014. Effects of step-wise increases in dietary carbohydrate on circulating saturated fatty acids and palmitoleic acid in adults with metabolic syndrome. *PLoS One* 9:e113605.4.

Vukovich, M., et al. 1994. Carnitine supplementation: Effect on muscle carnitine and glycogen content during exercise. *Medicine & Science in Sports & Exercise* 26:1122–29.

Wall, B., et al. 2011. Chronic oral ingestion of L-carnitine and carbohydrate increases muscle carnitine content and alters muscle fuel metabolism during exercise in humans. *Journal of Physiology* 589:963–73.

Wallin, A., et al. 2012. Fish consumption, dietary long-chain n-3 fatty acids, and risk of type 2 diabetes: Systematic review and meta-analysis of prospective studies. *Diabetes Care* 35:918–29.

Walser, P., et al. 2006. Supplementation with omega-3 polyunsaturated fatty acids augments brachial artery dilation and blood flow during forearm contraction. *European Journal of Applied Physiology* 97:347–54.

Wang, L., et al. 2015. Effect of a moderate fat diet with and without avocados on lipoprotein particle number, size and subclasses in overweight and obese adults: A randomized, controlled trial. *Journal of the American Heart Association* 4:e001355.

Warber, J., et al. 2000. The effects of choline supplementation on physical performance. *International Journal of Sport Nutrition & Exercise Metabolism* 10:170–81.

Weber, H., et al. 2006. Prevention of cardiovascular diseases and highly concentrated *n*-3 polyunsaturated fatty acids (PUFAs). *Herz* 31 (Supplement 3):24–30.

Weggemans, R., et al. 2002. Dietary cholesterol from eggs increases the ratio of total cholesterol to high-density lipoprotein cholesterol in humans: A meta-analysis. *American Journal of Clinical Nutrition* 73:885–91.

Whigham, L., et al. 2007. Efficacy of conjugated linoleic acid for reducing fat mass: A meta-analysis in humans. *American Journal of Clinical Nutrition* 85:1203–11.

Whitten, P. 1993. Stanford's secret weapon: New nutrition program lifts Cardinal swimmers to record-breaking year. *Swimming World & Junior Swimmer* 34 (March/April): 28–33.

Willett, W. 2006. The Mediterranean diet: Science and practice. *Public Health & Nutrition* 9:105–10.

Williams, P. 2001. Health effects resulting from exercise versus those from body fat loss. *Medicine & Science in Sports & Exercise* 33:S611–21.

Wolfe, R. 1998. Fat metabolism in exercise. *Advances in Experimental Medicine & Biology* 441:147–56.

Yeo, W., et al. 2011. Fat adaptation in well-trained athletes: Effects on cell metabolism. *Applied Physiology, Nutrition, & Metabolism* 36:12–22.

Zderic, T., et al. 2004. High-fat diet elevates resting intramuscular triglyceride concentration and whole body lipolysis during exercise. *American Journal of Physiology. Endocrinology & Metabolism* 286:E217–25.

Protein:
The Tissue Builder

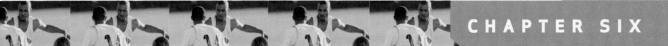

CHAPTER SIX

LEARNING OBJECTIVES

After studying this chapter, you should be able to:

1. Distinguish between complete and incomplete protein and identify foods that may be one or the other.

2. Calculate the approximate grams of protein that should be included in your daily diet.

3. Name the nine essential amino acids.

4. Describe the digestion of protein, its metabolic fate and distribution in the body, and its major functions in human metabolism.

5. Explain the role of protein in human energy systems during exercise.

6. Understand the rationale underlying the judgment of some investigators that both strength and endurance athletes need more dietary protein than the amount provided by the RDA. State general recommendations to various athletes based on grams of protein per kilogram body weight.

7. Based on current research findings, describe the dietary strategies involving protein intake (amount, type, and timing) before and/or after exercise that may help provide the substrate and hormonal milieu conducive to muscle tissue anabolism during recovery.

8. Explain the theory underlying the use of protein supplements, specific amino acids, and other dietary supplements, such as creatine and HMB, as ergogenic aids, and highlight the major research findings relative to their efficacy.

9. Identify the potential health risks associated with either inadequate or excess dietary intake of protein or individual amino acids.

Protein is one of our most essential nutrients for optimal health. Additionally, it has a wide variety of physiological functions that are essential to optimal physical performance. For example, protein forms the structural basis of muscle tissue, is the major component of most enzymes in the muscle, and can serve as a source of energy during exercise. Because protein is so important to the development and function of muscle tissue, and because most feats of human physical performance involve strenuous muscular activity in one form or another, it is no wonder that protein has persisted throughout the years as the food of the athlete. Indeed, surveys have revealed that many high school and college athletes believe that athletic performance is improved by a high-protein diet. Protein is one of the best-selling sports supplements. A best-selling diet book suggests that protein is the key macronutrient for the athlete, and for health as well.

Companies that market nutritional supplements for athletes have capitalized on this belief. Probably the athletic groups most susceptible to the lure of protein supplements are bodybuilders and strength-type athletes, such as weight lifters and football players. Numerous high-protein products have been developed for these athletes in attempts to exploit the protein-muscle strength relationship. In recent years, specific amino acids have been theorized to maximize muscle mass and strength gains and have been advertised extensively on the Internet and in magazines for bodybuilders. Some advertisements even suggest that certain amino acid mixtures have an effect similar to drugs such as anabolic steroids, which have been used to stimulate muscle development.

Protein supplements are marketed for other types of athletes as well. Although protein is not regarded as a major energy source during exercise, research has suggested that endurance athletes may use some specific amino acids for energy production under certain conditions. Protein supplements, often combined with carbohydrate, are marketed in sport drinks to endurance athletes. Additionally, specific amino acids have been theorized to delay the onset of fatigue during prolonged exercise through their effect on neurotransmitters in the brain.

There is no doubt that an adequate amount of dietary protein and related essential amino acids is required by all individuals. However, the advertisements directed toward athletes imply that additional protein, usually in the form of protein or amino acid supplements, is necessary for optimal performance. Although the National Academy of Sciences has indicated that the Recommended Daily Allowance (RDA) provides sufficient protein to athletes, some investigators recommend that athletes in training increase their protein intake. However, these investigators usually recommend that the protein be derived from natural food sources and the amount of protein recommended is well within the Acceptable Macronutrient Dietary Range (AMDR).

Other dietary supplements related to protein or amino acids, such as amines or various metabolic by-products, have become increasingly popular in recent years. One of the current hot sellers is creatine, but other supplements such as inosine and HMB are also available. In most cases these dietary supplements have been marketed to strength-trained athletes as a means to foster muscle growth and strength development, but some are intended for use by athletes involved in other sports, such as aerobic endurance events.

Does the physically active individual need more protein or related dietary supplements in the diet? The information presented in this chapter should provide a general answer to this question. Topics to be covered include dietary needs and sources of protein; metabolic fates and functions in the body; the effects of exercise on protein metabolism and dietary requirements; the ergogenic potential of protein, amino acids, or other related supplements; and health aspects of dietary protein.

Dietary Protein

What is protein?

Protein is a complex chemical structure containing carbon, hydrogen, and oxygen—just as carbohydrates and fats do. Protein has one other essential element—nitrogen, which constitutes about 16 percent of most dietary protein. These four elements are combined into a number of different structures called **amino acids**, each one possessing an amino group (NH_2) and an acid group (COOH), with the remainder being different combinations of carbon, hydrogen, oxygen, and in some cases sulfur. There are 20 amino acids, all of which can be combined in a variety of ways to form the proteins necessary for the structure and functions of the human body. The body may also modify the structure of dietary amino acids, such as converting proline to hydroxyproline, to meet its needs. Figure 6.1 depicts the formula of **alanine**, an amino acid discussed later.

Proteins are created when two amino acids link and form a peptide bond; hence, a dipeptide is formed. As more amino acids are added, a polypeptide is formed. Most proteins are polypeptides, combining up to 300 amino acids. Figure 6.2 depicts the building of a protein.

Protein is contained in both animal and plant foods. Humans obtain their supply of amino acids from these two general sources.

Is there a difference between animal and plant protein?

To answer this question, let us first look at a basic difference between two groups of amino acids. Humans can synthesize some amino acids in their bodies but cannot synthesize others. The nine amino acids that cannot be manufactured in the body are called **essential**, or **indispensable, amino acids** and must be supplied in the diet. Those that may be formed in the body are called **nonessential**, or **dispensable, amino acids**. Six of the dispensable amino acids are conditionally indispensable, which means that they must be obtained through the diet when endogenous synthesis cannot meet metabolic demands, such as in severe catabolic states. Although nutrition scientists prefer the terms *indispensable* and *dispensable*, this text uses the terms *essential* and *nonessential* because they are most commonly used.

It should be noted that all 20 amino acids are necessary for protein synthesis in the body and must be present simultaneously for optimal maintenance of body growth and function. The use of the terms *essential* and *indispensable* in relation to amino acids is to distinguish those that must be obtained in the diet. Table 6.1 presents the dietary essential, nonessential, and conditionally essential amino acids.

TABLE 6.1   The dietary amino acids

Essential amino acids	Nonessential amino acids
Histidine	Alanine
Isoleucine*	Arginine**
Leucine*	Asparagine
Lysine	Aspartic acid
Methionine	Cysteine**
Phenylalanine	Glutamic acid
Threonine	Glutamine**
Tryptophan	Glycine**
Valine*	Proline**
	Serine
	Tyrosine**

*Branched-chain amino acids.
**Conditionally essential.

The National Academy of Sciences indicates that different dietary sources of protein vary widely in their composition and nutritional value. The quality of a source of protein is an expression of its ability to provide the nitrogen and amino acid requirements for growth, maintenance, and repair. The key factors are digestibility and the ability to provide the indispensable amino acids. All natural, unprocessed animal and plant foods contain all 20 amino acids. However, the amount of each amino acid in specific foods varies. Over the years a number of different techniques have been used, usually with animals, to assess the quality of protein in selected foods. One of the most widely used is the Protein Digestibility-Corrected Amino Acid Score (PDCAAS), which incorporates real-life variables, including the amino acid content and digestibility of the protein. Scores can range from 1.0 to 0.0, with 1.0 being the highest quality. We need not go into a detailed discussion of all techniques to evaluate protein quality, but essentially they focus on the concept of **nitrogen balance**, the ability of the body to retain nitrogen. In essence, nitrogen balance is protein balance. In positive nitrogen balance the body is retaining protein to adequately support growth and development, whereas in negative nitrogen balance the body is losing protein, with possible

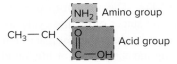

FIGURE 6.1 The chemical structure of alanine, an amino acid. The amino group (NH_2) contains nitrogen, while the acid group is represented by COOH.

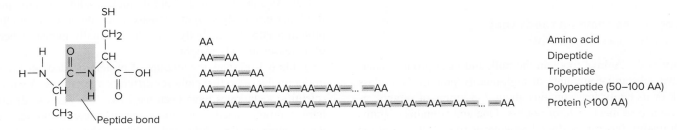

FIGURE 6.2 Formation of peptides and polypeptides from amino acids, with eventual formation of proteins.

impairment in growth and development. The quality of the protein in foods we eat may affect nitrogen balance.

In general, those foods that contain an adequate content of all nine essential amino acids to support both life and growth are known as **complete proteins**, or high-quality proteins, and will have a high PDCAAS score, while those that have a deficiency of one or more essential amino acids and are unable to support life or growth are called **incomplete proteins**, or low-quality proteins, and have a lower score. Relative to human requirements, an essential amino acid that is in limited supply in a particular food is labeled a **limiting amino acid**.

The proteins ingested as animal products are generally regarded to be of a higher quality than those found in plants. This is not to say that an amino acid found in a plant is inferior to the same amino acid found in an animal. They are the same. When we look at the distribution of all the amino acids in the two food sources, however, we can then see two major reasons animal protein is called a high-quality protein, whereas plant protein is of lower quality. The PDCAAS for egg white and meat is, respectively, 1.0 and 0.92, while the score for kidney beans and whole wheat is, respectively, 0.68 and 0.40.

Animal protein is a complete protein because it contains each essential amino acid in the proper proportion to human requirements. As noted, all 20 amino acids must be present simultaneously for the body to synthesize them into necessary body proteins. If 1 amino acid is in short supply, protein construction may be blocked. Having the proper amount of animal protein in the diet is a good way to ensure receipt of a balanced supply of amino acids. Some protein supplements marketed to athletes are made from animal protein, including milk, egg, and whey protein.

Plant proteins can provide you with all the protein and amino acids you need for optimal growth and development. However, proteins usually exist in smaller concentrations in plant foods. For example, 2 ounces of fish contain about 14 grams of protein, while 2 ounces of cooked macaroni have only 2 grams; 2 ounces of beans, which are generally regarded to be good sources of protein, have only 5 grams. In addition, most plant proteins have insufficient amounts of 1 or more of the essential amino acids (i.e., limiting amino acids). Grain products are usually deficient in lysine, whereas legumes are low in methionine. An exception to this generality is the protein isolated from soybeans, which when processed properly is comparable to animal protein. As noted in chapter 2, vegetarians who eat plant foods in proper combinations over the course of the day will receive a balanced supply of amino acids. Some populations receive most of their protein from plant sources.

What are some common foods that are good sources of protein?

Animal Foods Animal foods in the milk and meat groups generally have substantial amounts of high-quality protein. One glass of milk or its equivalent contains about 7–8 grams of protein, as does 1 ounce of meat, fish, or poultry. One egg contains 6 grams of high-quality protein, as does 1 serving of Egg Beaters, but the latter has half the Calories and no fat or cholesterol.

Plant Foods and Supplements **Legumes**, such as dry beans (black, garbanzo, great northern, kidney, lima, navy, pinto, soybeans), lentils, and peas (black-eyed, split), are relatively good sources of protein. Legumes also are high in carbohydrate and for this reason are currently classified as a starch Food Exchange. However, because of their relatively high protein content, legumes may be included within the meat and meat substitutes Exchange List. One-half cup contains about 7–9 grams of protein. Nuts contain fair amounts of protein but are high in fat. Fruits, vegetables, and grain products all have some protein, but the content varies; generally speaking, the protein content is low, ranging from less than 1 gram to about 3 grams of protein per serving, although some products may contain more, such as protein-enriched pasta. Some sports drinks and sports bars contain significant amounts of protein. Protein supplements targeted to strength-trained individuals may contain substantial amounts of protein, but may also be expensive.

Table 6.2 and figure 6.3 present some common foods in each of several food groups, with the number of grams of protein in each. Notice the effect combination-type foods have on protein content: for example, macaroni and cheese versus plain macaroni. Most food labels today list the grams of protein per serving. For plant foods commonly eaten in a vegan diet, review table 2.10 in chapter 2.

How much dietary protein do I need?

Humans actually do not need protein *per se* but rather an adequate amount of nitrogen and essential amino acids. However, because all nine essential amino acids and almost all dietary nitrogen are derived from dietary protein, it serves as the basis for our daily requirements. Bilsborough and Mann note that three ways of defining protein intake are absolute intake in grams per day, relative intake based on grams per unit body weight (the basis of the RDA), and as percentage of daily energy intake (the basis of the AMDR).

In the United States, the recommended dietary intake of protein is based upon the RDA. The amount of protein necessary in the diet varies in different stages of the life cycle, as may be noted in the Dietary Reference Intakes table for macronutrients in the front inside cover. During the early years of life, children manufacture protein tissue during rapid growth stages, with the rate of growth (and thus the protein needs) varying from infancy through late adolescence. In young adulthood, the protein requirement stabilizes. Throughout the life cycle, however, the protein requirement established in the RDA is based upon the body weight of the individual. As a person passes from infancy to adulthood, the protein RDA per unit body weight decreases, but the absolute amount of protein needed by the body as a whole actually increases because of increases in body weight.

Table 6.3 presents the amount of protein needed per kilogram or per pound of body weight for different age groups. A variety of scientific techniques have been used over the years to determine human protein needs, and more recent research has reaffirmed these estimates for adults and children. The values for the first year of life are AI, while the remainder are RDA. The values in

TABLE 6.2 Protein content in some common foods

Food	Amount	Protein (grams)	Food	Amount	Protein (grams)
Milk list			*Fruit list*		
Milk, whole	1 c	8	Banana	1	1
Milk, skim	1 c	8	Orange	1	1
Cheese, cheddar	1 oz.	7	Pear	1	1
Yogurt	1 c	8			
Meat list			*Starch list*		
			Bread, wheat	1 slice	3
Beef, lean	1 oz.	8	Bran flakes	1 c	4
Chicken breast	1 oz.	8	Doughnuts	1	1
Luncheon meat	1 oz.	5	Macaroni	1/2 c	3
Fish	1 oz.	7	Macaroni and cheese	1/2 c	9
Eggs	1	6	Peas, green	1/2 c	4
Navy beans, cooked*	1/2 c	7	Potato, baked	1	3
Peanuts, roasted	1/4 c	9	Quinoa	1 c	8
Peanut butter	1 tbsp	4			
			Sports drinks and bars		
Vegetable list			Gatorade Nutrition Shake	11 oz.	20
			Power Bar Protein Plus	1	30
Broccoli	1/2 c	2	Endurox R4 Recovery Drink	12 oz.	11
Carrots	1	1			
			Protein sports supplements		
			GNC Pro Performance 100% Whey Protein	31 g	20

Protein (grams) may vary slightly from the Food Exchange Lists because these data were derived from food analyses reported by the United States Department of Agriculture. Some data were obtained from company Websites.

*Found in both the meat and meat substitutes and starch lists in appendix E.

this table are dependent upon adequate daily energy intake (i.e., Calories), because a low-energy diet will increase protein needs. To calculate your requirement, simply determine your body weight in kilograms or pounds and multiply by the appropriate figure for your age group. Recall that 1 kilogram is equal to 2.2 pounds. As an example, compute the protein requirement for a 154-pound, or 70-kg, average 23-year-old male:

$$0.36 \text{ g protein/pound} \times \text{pounds} = 55.4 \text{ or } 56 \text{ g protein/day}$$
$$0.8 \text{ g protein/kg} \times 70 \text{ kg} = 56 \text{ g protein/day}$$

On a protein-free diet, the average individual loses approximately 0.34 g protein/kg body weight per day, which could be replaced by a similar amount of high-quality egg protein. However, allowances are made in the RDA for the fact that individual protein needs vary, that the biological quality of all dietary protein is not as good as egg protein, and that the efficiency of utilization decreases at higher dietary protein-intake levels. Hence, the RDA is adjusted upward to account for these factors.

The RDA for protein, as noted, is based upon body weight of the individual at different ages. If you took the recommended energy intake in Calories for each age group, say 2,500 C for the average adult male, and calculated the percentage of this value that the RDA for protein supplies, the values approximate 10 percent for each age group. The National Academy of

Sciences indicated that the AMDR should not be set below levels for the RDA for protein, which is about 10 percent of energy. Mathematically, 56 grams of protein, at 4 Calories per gram, total 224 Calories, which is about 9 percent of 2,500, or near the lower limit of the AMDR.

As noted in previous chapters, the Acceptable Macronutrient Distribution Ranges (AMDR) for individuals have been set based on evidence from interventional trials, with support of epidemiological evidence, to suggest a role in the prevention of increased risk of chronic disease and based on ensuring sufficient intakes of essential nutrients. The AMDR for protein is 10–35 percent of energy for adults and 5–20 and 10–30 percent for young and older children, respectively. The health implications of the AMDR will be discussed later in this chapter.

It is important to note, as Millward indicated in a review, that protein needs are determined by overall food energy intake. If energy intake is inadequate, as may be the case in those on weight-loss diets or the elderly, dietary protein may be used for energy instead of its core purpose of building tissue. Thus, some individuals may need more or higher-quality protein because their energy intake may be low. In particular, some exercise scientists recommend adequate protein for the elderly as a means to prevent sarcopenia (loss of muscle mass) and osteoporosis (loss of bone mass).

How much of the essential amino acids do I need?

The Academy also established RDA for the nine essential amino acids. The amounts for adults age 19 and over are found in table 6.4. Slightly larger amounts are recommended for children and adolescents. For the average adult, about 25 percent of the total protein requirement should consist of the essential amino acids; this amounts to about 14–15 grams. Phenylalanine is an essential amino acid, whereas tyrosine is normally listed as a nonessential amino acid. The two are of similar chemical structure so that when substantial quantities of tyrosine are contained in the diet, the need for phenylalanine will decrease somewhat. The same holds true for the essential sulfur-containing amino acid methionine and its chemically related counterpart, cysteine. Individuals who obtain the RDA for protein should have no problem obtaining these recommended values.

Fortunately, we do not need to memorize these amino acids and check our food products to see if they are present. A few general rules can help ensure that we receive a balanced supply in our diet.

What are some dietary guidelines to ensure adequate protein intake?

To answer in one sentence: Eat a wide variety of animal and plant foods. The high-quality, complete proteins are obtained primarily from animal foods. Meat, fish, eggs, poultry, milk, and cheese contain the type and amount of the essential amino acids necessary for maintaining life and promoting growth and development. They are high-nutrient-density foods, particularly if fat content is low to moderate. Because animal protein is of high quality, you do not need as much of it to satisfy your RDA. For example, for a male who needs about 56 grams of protein per day, only 45 grams are needed if it is animal protein. One glass of milk, with 8 grams of protein, will provide almost 20 percent of his protein RDA. Two glasses of milk, one egg, and 3 ounces of lean meat, fish, or poultry will provide 100 percent of his RDA. In addition, a substantial proportion of daily vitamin and mineral needs will also be supplied in these foods. As noted in chapter 5, selection of low-fat foods will enhance the nutrient density by reducing Calories.

Currently, adults in the United States consume only 3.5 ounces of fish per week. There is moderate evidence that consumption of seafood is associated with reduced risk of heart disease.

TABLE 6.3	Grams of protein needed per kilogram or per pound body weight during the life cycle	
Age in years	Grams/kg body weight	Grams/pound body weight
0.0–0.5	1.52	0.69
0.5–1.0	1.10	0.50
1–3	1.10	0.50
4–8	0.95	0.43
9–13	0.95	0.43
14–18	0.85	0.39
19 and up	0.8	0.36

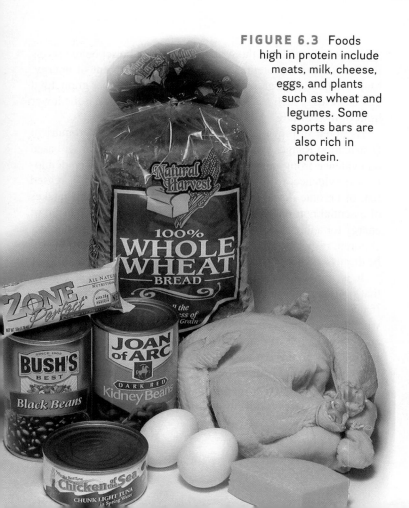

FIGURE 6.3 Foods high in protein include meats, milk, cheese, eggs, and plants such as wheat and legumes. Some sports bars are also rich in protein.

TABLE 6.4	RDA for the essential amino acids in an adult male (70 kg)	
	RDA (mg/kg)	Total mg
Histidine	14	980
Isoleucine	19	1,260
Leucine	42	2,940
Lysine	38	2,660
Methionine plus cysteine	19	1,260
Phenylalanine plus tyrosine	33	2,310
Threonine	20	1,400
Tryptophan	5	350
Valine	24	1,680
Total		14,840

Therefore, in the 2010 *Dietary Guidelines for Americans*, there is a quantitative recommendation for seafood intake of 8 or more ounces per week from a variety of seafood. You can also go to www.ChooseMyPlate.gov. Click on Food Groups, then Protein Foods Group, to learn more about what foods are healthy choices for each of the food groups. The Food Gallery links may also help in determining serving sizes. From the www.ChooseMyPlate.gov main page, select *10 Tips*. Here you will find easy-to-follow tips for consumers and professionals in a convenient format, including "With Protein Foods, Variety Is Key."

Plant foods also may provide good sources of protein. Grain products such as wheat, rice, and corn, as well as soybeans, peas, beans, and nuts, have a substantial protein content. However, most plant foods contain incomplete proteins because they lack a sufficient quantity of some essential amino acids. For this reason, the protein RDA for the adult male is 65 grams per day when plant proteins are the primary source. However, Craig and Mangels, in the position stand on vegetarian diets by the American Dietetic Association, state that if certain plant foods are eaten over the course of a day, such as grains and legumes, they may supply all the essential amino acids necessary for human nutrition and be as complete a protein as animal protein.

Some research has suggested that if the daily dietary protein is obtained through a mixture of animal and plant foods in a ratio of 30:70, that is, 30 percent of the protein from animal foods and 70 from plant foods, the protein quality would be similar to the use of animal foods alone. Mixing animal and plant foods in the same meal is common and is healthful and nutritious. Animal foods provide excellent sources of essential minerals, such as iron, zinc, and calcium, while plant foods provide carbohydrate, dietary fiber, and various phytochemicals.

Key Concepts

- Protein contains nitrogen, an element essential to the formation of 20 different amino acids, the building blocks of all body cells. All 20 amino acids are necessary for protein formation in the body.
- Essential, or indispensable, amino acids cannot be adequately synthesized in the body and thus must be obtained through dietary protein, whereas nonessential, or dispensable, amino acids may be synthesized in the body. Conditionally indispensable amino acids may be synthesized from other amino acids under normal conditions, but their synthesis may be limited under certain conditions when insufficient amounts of their precursors are available.
- The RDA for protein is based upon the body weight of the individual, and the amount needed per unit body weight is greater during childhood and adolescence than during adulthood. The adult RDA is 0.8 gram of protein per kilogram body weight, or 0.36 gram per pound body weight.
- The Acceptable Macronutrient Distribution Range (AMDR) for protein indicates that dietary intake should be no less

than 10 percent and no greater than 35 percent of daily energy needs.
- The human body needs a balanced mixture of essential amino acids, and although animal protein provides all of the essential amino acids in the proper blend, a combination of certain plant proteins, such as grains and legumes, will satisfy this dietary requirement.
- Although animal foods in the meat and milk groups have high protein content, they may also be high in fat. Increasing the proportion of dietary protein intake from plant sources is recommended. Combining animal and plant proteins in one meal, such as milk and cereal or stir-fry vegetables and meat, will increase the protein quality of the meal.

Check for Yourself

- Peruse food labels of some of your favorite foods and check the protein content. Check both animal and plant foods and compare the grams of protein provided by a serving. The percent of the Daily Value (DV) is not required, but it may be found on some labels.

Metabolism and Function

What happens to protein in the human body?

Dietary protein consists of long, complex chains of amino acids. In the digestive process, enzymes (proteases) in the stomach and small intestine break the complex protein down into polypeptides and then into individual amino acids. The amino acids are absorbed through the wall of the small intestine, pass into the blood, and then pass to the liver via the portal vein (see figure 6.4). The digestion of protein takes several hours, but once the amino acids enter the blood they are cleared within 5 to 10 minutes. There is a constant interchange of amino acids among the blood, the liver, and the body tissues. The liver is a critical center in amino acid metabolism. It is continually synthesizing a balanced amino acid mixture for the diverse protein requirements of the body. These amino acids are secreted into the blood and carried as free amino acids or as plasma proteins such as albumin. All these functions consume energy, and the thermic effect (TEF) is greater for protein than for carbohydrate and fat. Whether or not this plays an important role in weight control is discussed in chapter 10.

The most important metabolic fate of the amino acids is the formation of specific proteins, including the structural proteins such as muscle tissue and the functional proteins such as enzymes. Body cells obtain amino acids from the blood, and the genetic apparatus in the cell nucleus directs the synthesis of proteins specific to the cell needs. The body cells may also use some of the nitrogen from the amino acids to form nonprotein nitrogen compounds, such as creatine. For example, the muscle cells will form

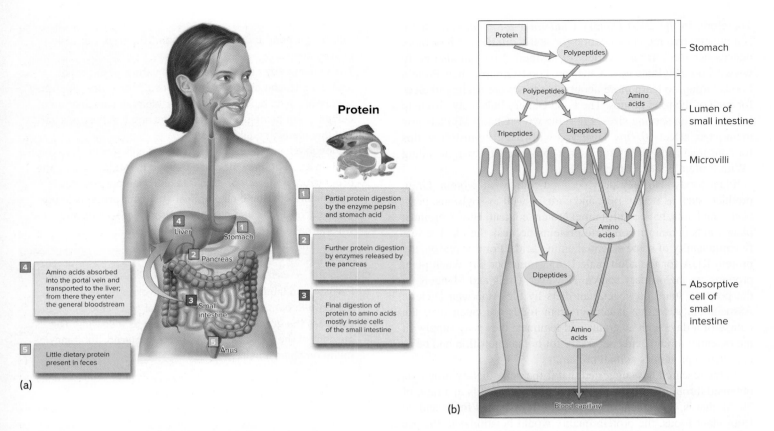

Protein

1. Partial protein digestion by the enzyme pepsin and stomach acid

2. Further protein digestion by enzymes released by the pancreas

3. Final digestion of protein to amino acids mostly inside cells of the small intestine

4. Amino acids absorbed into the portal vein and transported to the liver; from there they enter the general bloodstream

5. Little dietary protein present in feces

(a)

Stomach —
Lumen of small intestine —
Microvilli —
Absorptive cell of small intestine —

Protein → Polypeptides
Polypeptides → Amino acids
Polypeptides → Tripeptides, Dipeptides
Amino acids
Dipeptides
Amino acids
Blood capillary

(b)

FIGURE 6.4 (*a*) A summary of protein digestion and absorption. (*b*) Stomach acid and enzymes contribute to protein digestion. Enzymatic protein digestion begins in the stomach and ends in the absorptive cells of the small intestine, where the last peptides are broken down into single amino acids.

contractile proteins as well as the enzymes and creatine phosphate necessary for energy production. The body cells will use only the amount of amino acids necessary to meet their protein needs. They cannot store excess amino acids to any significant amount, although the protein formed may be catabolized to release amino acids back to the blood.

Because the human body does not have a mechanism to store excess nitrogen, it cannot store amino acids *per se*. Through the process of **deamination**, the amino group (NH_2) containing the nitrogen is removed from the amino acid, leaving a carbon substrate known as an **alpha-ketoacid**. The excess nitrogen must be excreted from the body. In essence, the liver forms **ammonia** (NH_3) from the excess nitrogen; the ammonia is converted into **urea**, which passes into the blood and is eventually eliminated by the kidneys into the urine.

The alpha-ketoacid that is released may have several fates. For one, this carbon substrate may be oxidized for the release of energy. For another, it may accept another amino group and be reconstituted to an amino acid. It also may be channeled into the metabolic pathways of carbohydrate and fat. The liver is the main organ where this conversion occurs. In essence, some of the amino acids are said to be **glucogenic amino acids**, that is, glucose forming. At various stages of the energy transformations within the liver, the glucogenic amino acids may be converted to glucose. As noted in chapter 4, this process is called *gluconeogenesis*. The

ketogenic amino acids are metabolized in the liver to acetyl CoA, which may be used for energy production via the Krebs cycle or converted to fat. The glucose and fat produced may be transported to other parts of the body to be used. Thus, although excess protein cannot be stored as amino acids in the body, the energy content is not wasted, for it is converted to either carbohydrate or fat.

Protein turnover represents the process by which all body proteins are being continuously broken down and resynthesized, and it is an ongoing process. The National Academy of Sciences indicates that about 250 grams of body protein turns over daily in an adult, or about 0.5 pound of body mass. Figure 6.5 presents a summary of the fates of protein in human metabolism. See also appendix G, figure G.5.

Can protein be formed from carbohydrates and fats?

Yes, but with some major limitations. Protein has one essential element, nitrogen, which is not possessed by either carbohydrate or fat. However, if the body has an excess of amino acids, the liver may be able to use the nitrogen-containing amino groups from these excess amino acids and combine them with alpha-ketoacids derived from either carbohydrate or fat metabolism. A key alpha-ketoacid from carbohydrate is pyruvic acid, while fat yields acetoacetic acid. The net result is the formation in the body of some of the nonessential amino acids using carbohydrates and fats as part

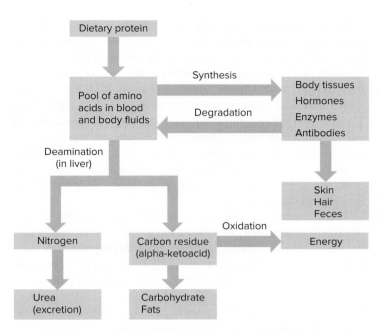

FIGURE 6.5 Simplified diagram of protein metabolism. Following the digestion of dietary proteins, one of the major functions of the amino acids is the synthesis of body tissues, enzymes, hormones, and antibodies. However, protein also is constantly being degraded by the liver. The excess nitrogen is excreted as urea, while the carbon residue may be converted into carbohydrate or fat or used to produce energy.

of the building materials. Keep in mind that nitrogen must be present for this to occur, and its source is dietary protein.

What are the major functions of protein in human nutrition?

Dietary protein may be utilized to serve all three major functions of food. Through the action of the individual amino acids, protein serves as the structural basis for the vast majority of body tissues,

is essential for regulating metabolism, and can be used as an energy source. In one way or another protein is involved in almost all body functions. Its individual roles are beyond the scope of this text, so the following discussion represents just some of its major functions of importance to health and fitness. Table 6.5 highlights the major functions of protein in the body.

Protein is the main nutrient used in the formation of all body tissues. This role is extremely important in periods of rapid growth, such as childhood and adolescence. Athletes who attempt to gain muscle tissue also need an adequate dietary supply of protein to create a positive protein balance. Certain amino acids, such as the branched-chain amino acids (BCAA) leucine, isoleucine, and valine, constitute a significant amount of muscle tissue.

Protein is critical in the regulation of human metabolism. It is used in the formation of almost all enzymes, many hormones, and other compounds that control body functions. Insulin, hemoglobin, and the oxidative enzymes in the mitochondria are all proteins that have important roles in regulating metabolism during exercise. Other metabolic roles of protein include the maintenance of water balance and acid-base balance, regulation of the blood clotting process, prevention of infection, and development of immunity to disease. Proteins also serve as carriers for nutrients in the blood, such as the free fatty acids (FFA) and the lipoproteins, and help transport nutrients into the body cells.

Although protein is not a major energy source for humans at rest, it can serve such a function under several conditions. In nutritional energy balance, the priority use of dietary protein is to promote synthesis of body proteins essential for optimal structure and function. However, as noted previously, excess dietary protein may be deaminated and used for energy, or it may be converted to carbohydrate or fat and then enter metabolic pathways for energy production or storage. During periods of starvation or semistarvation, adequate amounts of dietary or endogenous carbohydrates and dietary fats may not be available. Both dietary protein and the body protein stores are used for energy purposes in such a situation, because energy production takes precedence over tissue

TABLE 6.5	Summary of the functions of proteins and amino acids in human metabolism
1. Structural function	Form vital constituents of all cells in the body, such as contractile muscle proteins
2. Transport function	Transport various substances in the blood, such as the lipoproteins for conveying triglycerides
3. Enzyme function	Form almost all enzymes in the body to regulate numerous, diverse physiological processes
4. Hormone and neurotransmitter function	Form various hormones, such as insulin; form various neurotransmitters, or neuropeptides, that function in the central nervous system, such as serotonin
5. Immune function	Form key components of the immune system, such as antibodies
6. Acid-base balance function	Buffer acid and alkaline substances in the blood to maintain optimal pH
7. Fluid balance function	Exert osmotic pressure to maintain optimal fluid balance in body tissues, particularly the blood
8. Energy function	Provide source of energy to the Krebs cycle when deaminated; excess protein may be converted to glucose or fat for subsequent energy production
9. Movement function	Provide movement when structural muscle proteins use energy to contract

building in metabolism. Hence, if the active individual desires to maintain lean body mass, it is essential to have not only adequate protein intake but also sufficient carbohydrate Calories in the diet to provide a **protein-sparing effect**. In other words, carbohydrate Calories will be used for energy production, thus sparing utilization of protein as an energy source and allowing it to be used for its more important structural and metabolic functions.

Although body proteins are composed of all 20 amino acids, individual amino acids may have important specific effects in the body. For example, the amino acid glycine is a neurotransmitter substance; tryptophan and tyrosine are important for the formation of several chemical transmitters in the brain; and the branched-chain amino acids (leucine, isoleucine, and valine) are major components of muscle tissue that may provide a source of energy.

Because of the diverse roles of protein and amino acids in the body, athletes have used protein supplements for years in attempts to improve performance. Amino acid supplements have also been used for this purpose. The effectiveness of such supplements is evaluated in later sections.

Key Concept

▶ The major function of dietary protein is to build and repair tissues and to synthesize hormones, enzymes, and other body compounds essential in human metabolism, but it also may be used as a significant source of energy under certain conditions.

Proteins and Exercise

Protein has always been considered one of the main staples of an athlete's diet. In this section we discuss several topics regarding protein and exercise, including its use as an energy source, possible avenues for protein loss, protein metabolism during recovery, and dietary requirements and recommendations for strength and endurance athletes.

Are proteins used for energy during exercise?

The average individual consumes about 10 percent or more of daily energy intake from protein. For individuals in protein and energy balance, this protein intake must be balanced through energy expenditure and other body losses. In general, scientists suggest that about 5 percent of daily protein intake may be used directly for energy. Protein in excess of tissue needs may be converted to carbohydrate or fat, which may also be used for energy. Protein may also be lost from the body in various ways, such as creatinine and urea excreted in the urine and sloughed body cells. In one review, Gibala noted that protein is regarded as a minor source of fuel during rest, usually accounting for less than 5 percent of total daily energy expenditure. However, given its nutritional importance, researchers have attempted to determine the effect of exercise on protein balance and needs.

Scientists have used a variety of techniques to study protein metabolism during exercise. Because urea is a by-product of protein metabolism, its concentration in the urine, blood, and sweat has been analyzed. Also, the presence in the urine of a marker for muscle protein breakdown, known as 3-methylhistidine, a modified amino acid, has been studied to evaluate protein catabolism. The nitrogen balance technique consists of precisely measuring nitrogen intake and excretion to determine whether the individual is in positive or negative protein balance. Finally, labeled isotopes of amino acids have been ingested or injected to study their metabolic fate during exercise, not only in the whole body but also in isolated muscle groups.

Using these techniques, investigators have evaluated the use of protein during both resistance exercise and aerobic endurance exercise. Although both types of exercise affect protein metabolism, the use of protein as an energy source appears to be more prevalent in aerobic exercise, particularly when prolonged.

Resistance Training   In a review, Rennie and Tipton noted that resistance exercise causes little change in amino acid oxidation, but probably depresses protein synthesis and elevates breakdown acutely. In this regard, Evans suggested that the eccentric muscle contraction associated with resistance training may produce ultrastructural damage that may stimulate this protein turnover. However, Wolfe noted that factors regulating muscle protein breakdown in human subjects are complex and interactive, and proposed that muscle protein breakdown is paradoxically elevated in the anabolic state following resistance exercise. Thus, while it appears that resistance exercise does not increase protein or amino acid oxidation, it may provoke muscle tissue breakdown.

Aerobic Endurance Exercise   Poortmans has noted that although protein may be used to produce significant amounts of ATP in the muscle, during aerobic endurance exercise the rate of production is much slower than with carbohydrate and fat, the preferred fuels. On the other hand, Rennie and Tipton noted that sustained dynamic exercise stimulates amino acid oxidation, mainly by activating an enzyme (BCAA dehydrogenase, or BCAAD) that oxidizes BCAA and increases ammonia production in proportion to exercise intensity. If the exercise is intense enough, there is a net loss of muscle protein as a result of decreased protein synthesis, increased catabolism, or both. Some of the amino acids are oxidized as fuel, and the rest provide substrates for gluconeogenesis. In this regard, prolonged exercise may be comparable to a state of starvation. As the endurance athlete depletes the endogenous carbohydrate stores, the body catabolizes some of its protein for energy or eventual conversion to glucose. Protein catabolism has been shown to increase significantly even when muscle glycogen is depleted by only about 33–55 percent.

Mechanisms and By-products   In general, a brief session of exercise lowers the rate of protein synthesis and speeds protein breakdown. The exact mechanisms of protein metabolism during exercise have not been determined, though several mechanisms have been proposed. Parkhouse has reported that exercise, particularly exercise to exhaustion, activates specific proteolytic enzymes in the muscle that degrade the myofibrillar protein. Fitts and Metzger found elevated levels of proteolytic enzymes in fatigued muscle. In a review, Wagenmakers indicated that six amino acids (BCAA; asparagine, aspartate, glutamate) may be metabolized in the muscle, providing the nitrogen needed for the synthesis of ammonia, alanine, and glutamine. During exercise, particularly prolonged aerobic exercise, Graham and MacLean noted significant muscle efflux of ammonia, glutamine, and alanine. These three products carry excess nitrogen from the muscle to other parts of the body, most notably the liver, for recycling or conversion to urea.

Ammonia, a nitrogen by-product of protein catabolism, is an indicator of increased muscle amino acid breakdown. Although no underlying mechanism has been identified, increasing levels of ammonia in the body have been associated with fatigue, somewhat comparable to the accumulation of lactic acid. One theory is that increased ammonia levels in the muscle may impair oxidative processes, thus decreasing energy production, while another theory suggests that increased plasma ammonia may impair brain functions and induce central fatigue. Because ammonia is formed in the muscle from the amino group, removal of the amino group by alanine or glutamine may help decrease the production of ammonia and delay the onset of fatigue.

Glutamine release from the muscle also increases during exercise, and it is an important fuel for various cells in the body, particularly those in the immune system. As we shall see later, glutamine supplementation has been studied as a means to enhance immune function in athletes.

Leucine and the Glucose-Alanine Cycle

Although a number of amino acids may be used as energy substrate during exercise, the major research effort has focused on the fate of leucine. Wagenmakers noted that the increase in BCAA oxidation during prolonged exercise seems to be specific for leucine only. In essence, the amino group of leucine catabolism eventually combines with pyruvate in the muscle cell to form alanine and leaves the residual alpha-ketoacid. The alpha-ketoacid may enter the Krebs cycle and be used for energy production. The alanine is released into the bloodstream and transported to the liver, where it is converted into glucose. The glucose may then be released into the blood to be used by the central nervous system and may eventually find its way to the contracting muscle to be used as an energy source. Alanine appears to be the most important means of transporting the amino group to the liver for excretion as urea. This overall process involving gluconeogenesis, known as the glucose-alanine cycle, is depicted graphically in figure 6.6. Some investigators have noted that during the latter part of endurance exercise, the blood levels of alanine increase, presumably because more is released from the muscle. However, the estimated glucose production approximates only 4 grams per hour, which might make a limited contribution in mild-intensity exercise but is possibly insignificant during high-intensity exercise when carbohydrate use may approximate 3 grams or more per minute. Additionally, several investigators have reported an increased release of branched-chain amino acids (BCAAs) from the liver during endurance exercise, with subsequent uptake by the muscle cells.

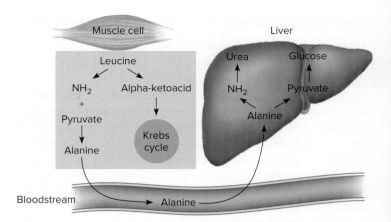

FIGURE 6.6 Glucose-alanine cycle. Alanine may be produced in the muscle tissue from the breakdown of other amino acids, most notably leucine. The alanine is then released into the blood and travels to the liver for eventual conversion to glucose through the process of gluconeogenesis. (See appendix G, figure G.5, for other amino acids that may enter energy pathways.)

Protein Use and Importance of Carbohydrate

Protein (amino acids) can be utilized during exercise to provide energy directly in the muscle and via glucose produced in the liver, particularly when the body stores of glycogen and glucose are low. In earlier research, Lemon reported that in the latter stages of prolonged endurance exercise, protein could contribute up to 15 percent of the total energy cost. However, less protein would be used for energy during the early stages of prolonged exercise when carbohydrate is adequate. Thus, Gibala suggested that the contribution of amino acid oxidation to total energy expenditure is negligible during short-term, intense exercise and accounts for 3–5 percent of the total energy production during prolonged exercise. In his review, Tarnopolsky cited similar figures, indicating that protein oxidation could account for 1 to 6 percent of the energy cost of aerobic exercise. Tarnopolsky also noted that women oxidize less protein compared with men and show lower leucine oxidation during aerobic exercise.

It is important to note how dietary carbohydrate influences protein as an energy source during exercise. A low-carbohydrate diet leading to decreased muscle glycogen levels will lead to increased dependence on protein as an energy source. However, adequate carbohydrate intake before and during prolonged exercise will help reduce the use of body protein for this purpose, because the presence of adequate muscle glycogen appears to inhibit enzymes that catabolize muscle protein. Scientists from the University of Maastricht in the Netherlands noted that high-carbohydrate diets may have a protein-sparing effect for endurance athletes.

Although the available evidence suggests that metabolism of protein and its use as an energy source are increased during exercise, the magnitude of its contribution may depend on a variety of factors, such as the intensity and duration of exercise and the availability of other fuels, such as carbohydrate, either as stored muscle glycogen or consumed during exercise.

Does exercise increase protein losses in other ways?

Other than loss of protein from oxidation, exercise has been shown to increase protein losses from the body in several other ways.

Urinary Losses   Exercise may cause an elevated level of protein in the urine, a condition known as **proteinuria**. This condition has been observed following competition in a wide variety of sports, including running, football, basketball, and handball. Research suggests that the greater the intensity of the exercise, such as a high-intensity 400-meter sprint versus a lower-intensity 3,000-meter run, the greater the loss of protein in the urine. Prolonged aerobic exercise, such as the triathlon, has also increased urinary protein loss. Yaguchi and others suggested that heavy, prolonged exercise, such as a triathlon, may induce some transient kidney damage in some individuals. Such damage may explain the findings of Poortmans, who reported a decreased reabsorption of protein in the kidney tubules following intense exercise. However, the total amount of protein lost in this manner appears to be rather negligible, amounting to less than 3 grams per day.

Sweat Losses   Protein also may be lost in the sweat. Several investigators have reported the presence of both amino acids and proteins in exercise-induced sweat, with both sweat rate and sweat nitrogen losses increasing with greater exercise intensities. Again, the losses are relatively minor, on the order of 1 gram per liter of sweat in adult males. This avenue could account for 2–4 grams of protein in an endurance athlete training in a warm environment.

Gastrointestinal Losses   As shall be noted in chapter 8, prolonged, intense exercise may also increase gastrointestinal losses of iron, which may be bound to blood proteins. Again, however, these protein losses would be relatively minor.

What happens to protein metabolism during recovery after exercise?

Although net protein breakdown occurs during exercise, in general protein synthesis is believed to predominate during the recovery period. In a review, Tipton and Wolfe noted that whole body protein breakdown is generally reduced following aerobic endurance exercise, while whole body protein synthesis is either increased or unchanged. However, they note that whole body protein synthesis may not represent changes in specific muscle groups. Muscle groups that have been exercised may experience protein synthesis, as they may be especially insulin sensitive after exercise. In another review, Walberg-Rankin notes that although leucine may be oxidized during moderate aerobic exercise, leucine balance returns to normal in 24 hours, indicating a reduced leucine catabolism over this time frame.

Tipton and Wolfe report that resistance exercise induces protein breakdown in the exercised muscles, which may persist in the immediate recovery period. However, over the next 24–48 hours, protein anabolism appears to predominate and the net effect is increased protein synthesis. Wolfe notes that anabolic states appear to be due more to stimulation of synthesis rather than a decrease in breakdown. This is especially so if adequate amino acids are available.

Eccentric exercise, such as lowering weights during resistance exercise or running downhill rapidly, puts tremendous stress on muscle tissue, and often induces muscle soreness in the following days. Tipton and Wolfe note that following eccentric exercise, whole body protein breakdown is increased. Microtears in muscle fibers may impair protein synthesis and delay recovery from such exercise. The muscle fiber microtears are believed to be the causative factor underlying the muscle soreness that, because its onset is usually delayed for 1–2 days, is referred to as **delayed onset of muscle soreness (DOMS)**.

What effect does exercise training have upon protein metabolism?

Rennie noted that protein metabolism may also become more efficient as a result of training, noting that the response of muscle protein turnover to habitual exercise is comparable to other metabolic changes in the muscle associated with exercise training. Although an initial bout of exercise may markedly elevate protein breakdown and synthesis in an untrained individual, the effect would be much less in one who has trained habitually. Tarnopolsky indicated that training induces a decreased *activity* in BCAAD, the enzyme that oxidizes BCAAs, when exercising at a standardized workload of the same absolute intensity.

As mentioned, protein synthesis appears to predominate in the muscles during recovery. With training, or repeated bouts of exercise on a regular basis, changes in the muscle structure and function are additive. Numerous studies have found that after resistance or endurance exercise, protein balance becomes positive. Trained individuals, during rest, have been shown to experience a preferential oxidation of fat and a sparing of protein, as measured by leucine metabolism and the respiratory quotient. The specific exercise task apparently stimulates the DNA in the muscle cell nucleus to increase the synthesis of protein, and the type of protein that is synthesized is specific to the type of exercise. Aerobic exercise stimulates syntheses of mitochondria and oxidative enzymes, which are composed of protein and are necessary for energy production in the oxygen system. Resistance training promotes synthesis of the contractile muscle proteins. These adaptations are the key factors underlying improved performance (see figure 6.7).

Other than its beneficial effects in increasing structural and functional protein important to resistance or aerobic endurance exercise, training may influence protein metabolism in other ways to help prevent premature fatigue. You may recall from previous chapters that there is substantial research to support the conclusion that aerobic endurance training improves the ability of the muscle cell to use both carbohydrate and fat as energy sources during exercise. Although extensive evidence is not available, in a review, Graham and others noted that following endurance training, enzymes in the muscles appear to develop the potential for increased capacity for oxidation of leucine and the other

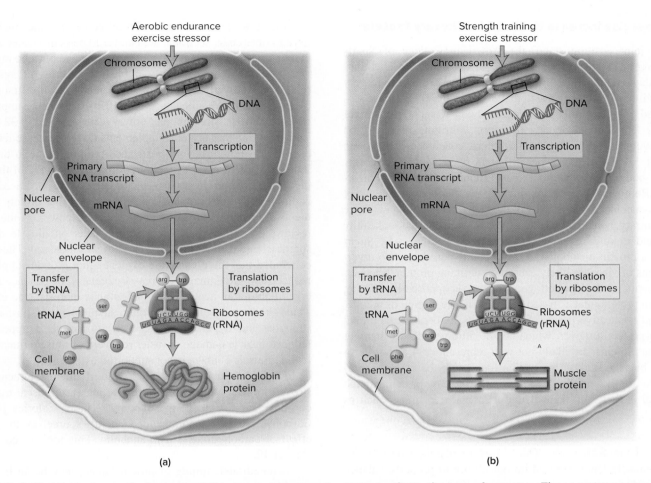

FIGURE 6.7 Adaptations in body tissues following exercise training are specific to the type of exercise. The exercise stressor influences the genes to initiate the formation of protein synthesis through the transcription, transfer, and translation processes. The transcription process provides the template (messenger RNA:mRNA) for the specific protein; the transfer (transfer RNA) process moves specific amino acids to the ribosome; the translation process by the ribosomes (ribosomal RNA) forms the protein. (*a*) Aerobic exercise training will lead to an increase in serum hemoglobin levels, which transport oxygen to the muscle cells. (*b*) Resistance training will lead to an increase in skeletal muscle protein.

BCAAs, which are an abundant source of energy in the muscles. Thus, endurance training may increase the capacity of the muscle to derive energy from protein in a fashion similar to the increased utilization of fat, another possible means to spare the use of carbohydrates such as blood glucose, to help protect the main energy source for the brain, and muscle glycogen. Although these changes do not appear to spare the use of muscle protein, they would appear to spare the use of carbohydrate, and thus may help prevent fatigue when carbohydrate levels are decreased during exercise.

Additionally, when exercising at a standardized workload before and after training, training may also decrease the production or accumulation of ammonia. Extrapolating from animal research, some investigators theorize that instead of forming ammonia, the nitrogen is incorporated into other amino acids, such as alanine, for transportation from the muscle to the liver. Theoretically, reduced plasma ammonia levels may be associated with less fatigue.

Training properly may also help prevent muscle injury associated with eccentric exercise. Research shows that physically trained individuals, when compared to untrained individuals, do not experience as much muscle tissue damage during prolonged, eccentric exercise tasks. However, specificity of training is also important, and individuals preparing for a race with a significant downhill component, such as the Boston Marathon, should gradually incorporate increasing intensities of eccentric exercise into their training.

In general, these changes associated with appropriate training appear to represent another means whereby the body adapts to endurance training in an attempt to prevent fatigue. However, some research indicates that excessive training leading to the overtraining syndrome is associated with a persistent decrease in plasma amino acids, particularly glutamine.

The effect of training in producing a positive nitrogen balance or a positive protein balance, and possibly the effect of preventing the overtraining syndrome, depends on an adequate dietary supply of protein and Calories.

Does exercise Increase the Need for Dietary Protein?

In their joint position stand, the American College of Sports Medicine, the Academy of Nutrition and Dietetics, and Dietitians of Canada concluded that protein requirements are higher in very active individuals and suggested that endurance and resistance athletes need 1.2–1.7 grams per kilogram body weight. In a similar vein, the International Society of Sports Nutrition, in a position stand developed by Campbell and others, concluded that protein intake of 1.4 to 2.0 grams per kilogram body weight daily may improve body adaptations to exercise training. Conversely, in its Dietary Reference Intakes for protein, the National Academy of Sciences concluded that in view of the lack of compelling evidence to the contrary, no additional dietary protein is suggested for healthy adults undertaking resistance or endurance exercise. As Stuart Phillips, a protein metabolism expert, points out, these two divergent points of view are likely caused by defining protein "needs or requirements" with body nitrogen balance, as opposed to defining "optimum protein intake" based on maintenance or gain of muscle, bone, and connective tissues. Skeletal muscle, bone, tendon, and ligament protein turnover, which can be 50 times slower than gut or plasma proteins, are likely not well represented in a short-term nitrogen balance study. This section focuses on the optimum protein intake for those individuals seeking to increase or maintain the functional capacity of skeletal muscle/connective tissue, such as athletes.

Strength-Type Activities   Our ability to maintain or increase skeletal muscle mass is based on our ability to properly balance two processes, muscle protein synthesis (MPS) and muscle protein breakdown (MPB). Following the ingestion of a high-protein meal (from either food or protein supplement), there is a period of time when blood levels of amino acids increase dramatically. This aminoacidemia stimulates MPS, while the resulting increase in blood insulin (hyperinsulinemia) inhibits MPB. In this scenario, which fluctuates throughout a normal day, a positive protein balance occurs when MPS is greater than MPB, which can stimulate muscle hypertrophy and increase strength. As described by Devries and Phillips, two factors that greatly influence MPS and MPB are resistance training and energy intake. Following a resistance exercise workout, both MPS and MPB are increased, with positive protein balance achieved when protein is consumed following the exercise. When energy intake is restricted, which occurs in athletes as well as the general population, MPS decreases, which can cause a negative protein balance and subsequently a decrease in muscle mass. As discussed later in the chapter, the addition of protein to the diet may help to prevent negative protein balance and muscle loss during times of energy restriction.

A common question by those attempting to increase muscle mass and strength with resistance training is whether or not additional dietary protein will cause a further increase in muscle hypertrophy and strength. The answer to this is unequivocally yes. A recent meta-analysis by Cermak and colleagues supports the need for additional protein to promote the best adaptations to resistance training. In young adults, the ingestion of additional protein (>1.2 g of protein/kg of body weight/d) during resistance training (6 to 24 weeks) caused a 50 percent greater increase in muscle fiber cross-sectional area and a 20 percent greater increase in maximal strength than resistance training and placebo ingestion.

Harris Lieberman recently published a series of systematic reviews specifically on protein supplements. In the first review, by Lieberman and colleagues, the effects of protein supplements on muscle mass, strength, and power were assessed in 32 studies. They reported that protein supplements do not increase lean mass or muscle strength beyond resistance training alone in untrained individuals. However, as the duration and frequency of the training was increased, lean mass and strength were increased by the addition of protein supplements. It appeared that protein supplements did not improve aerobic or anaerobic power. In the second review, the effects of protein supplements on muscle damage, soreness, and recovery from 27 studies was assessed. The authors concluded that there was little evidence that protein supplements reduced muscle damage, decreased soreness, or enhanced recovery following an acute bout of endurance or resistance exercise. Thus, although the effects of protein supplements on post-exercise strength, and hypertrophy are well supported, it appears that reduced muscle damage or faster recovery of muscle function following muscle damage is not supported by research.

In addition to protein, Gail Butterfield recommends that strength-trained athletes attempting to increase muscle mass also consume additional energy, about 200 more Calories per day. Carbohydrate is a recommended energy source, as the insulin effect of carbohydrate is also anabolic. This topic is covered in chapter 12.

As noted later, timing of protein intake may be an important consideration for strength-trained individuals. Additionally, some dietary protein suggestions for strength-trained individuals are presented in chapter 12.

Endurance-Type Activities   It is important to reinforce the viewpoint that carbohydrate is the main energy source for endurance-type athletes. Besides its efficiency as a metabolic fuel during exercise, carbohydrate also provides a potent protein-sparing effect. Consuming sufficient carbohydrate will decrease reliance on protein during aerobic endurance exercise, reduce the formation of ammonia, and better maintain normal protein status in the body.

Nevertheless, additional dietary protein has been recommended for endurance athletes because they may utilize protein as an energy source during exercise and may need protein to synthesize oxidative enzymes and mitochondria. Athletes involved in prolonged, intermittent, high-intensity sports, such as soccer, field or ice hockey, lacrosse, and basketball, may also fall into this category. Additionally, extra protein has been recommended to prevent development of anemia during the early stages of training. In brief, **sports anemia** is thought to occur because the body uses dietary protein for these aforementioned purposes at the expense of hemoglobin formation, leading to anemia. Sports anemia also has been associated with iron nutriture and will be discussed in more detail in chapter 8.

Moore and colleagues recently reviewed the dietary protein needs of endurance athletes and noted that muscle remodeling is needed to break down old and damaged proteins and synthesize new proteins. Acute endurance exercise and chronic endurance exercise training cause an increase in MPS, and this adaptive response to endurance training can be enhanced by providing additional dietary protein.

As with strength-trained individuals, various investigators have also estimated the protein requirement of endurance-trained individuals. In a review based on protein balance studies, Lemon recommends that individuals involved in vigorous aerobic endurance exercise consume 1.1 to 1.4 g/kg/day; slightly higher amounts, about 1.4–1.7 grams per kilogram body weight, have been recommended for individuals involved in intermittent, high-intensity sports because these include a balance of endurance and power activities.

Given these divergent opinions, what are some prudent recommendations regarding dietary protein intake for physically active individuals?

What are some general recommendations relative to dietary protein intake for athletes?

Tipton and Witard, in a review of protein requirements for athletes, concluded that athletes are frequently put into general categories of strength and endurance athletes within research studies. A difficulty with these categories is they may not be specific enough to examine the protein requirements of many athletes. In fact, there are gaps in our knowledge that do not allow for meaningful recommendations for athletes in sports such as football, rugby, or decathlon. Additionally, Tipton and Witard state that few data exist on protein intakes and performance measures with respect to gender. Nevertheless, recent reviews by some of the most prominent investigators in protein metabolism during exercise provide the basis for some reasonable guidelines. All of the recommendations are consistent with the AMDR for protein.

The following mathematical presentations are possible scenarios for various athletes who wish to maintain or increase protein balance. The protein needs are based upon the RDA, a rough estimate of the amount of protein used during strenuous exercise, and additional protein needs for the individual who wants to gain weight.

Let us look first at the young resistance-trained athlete who wants to gain body weight, preferably in the form of muscle tissue, through a weight-training program. The protein RDA for an adult male is 0.80 gram per kilogram. At moderate activity levels, the average 70-kg male would be in protein balance with about 56 grams daily. However, according to the suggested upper recommendation of about 1.7 grams per kilogram, he would need about 119 g daily if involved in a strenuous training program. Is this a reasonable amount?

One pound of muscle tissue is equal to 454 grams, and its composition is approximately 70 percent water, 7 percent lipids, and 22 percent muscle tissue. Hence, 1 pound of muscle contains about 100 grams of protein (454 × 0.22). If the desired weight gain is 1 pound of lean body mass per week, a reasonable goal, then this

young male would need to assimilate an additional 14 grams of protein per day (100 grams/7 days) to supply the amount in 1 pound of muscle tissue. A gain of 2 pounds per week, although probably more difficult to accomplish, would require the assimilation of 28 additional grams of protein per day. Let us be liberal and estimate an additional 22 grams of protein per day to cover losses due to exercise. In summary, assuming that a portion of these protein needs are not covered by the safety margin incorporated in the RDA, this young athlete would need approximately 106 grams of protein per day (56 + 28 + 22) to gain 2 pounds of lean body tissue per week, or about 1.5 grams of protein per kilogram body weight. This value falls within the recommended range for resistance-trained athletes.

Endurance athletes are not necessarily interested in gaining weight, but they may need to replenish the protein that may serve as an energy source during training. Running 10 miles per day would expend approximately 1,000 Calories or more. Again, let us be liberal and assume that if 6 percent of this energy cost, or 60 Calories, was derived from protein, then approximately 15 grams of protein (60 Calories/4 Calories per gram of protein) would have to be replaced. With a liberal estimated additional loss of 10 grams of protein in the urine and sweat, the total daily protein requirement for a 70-kg young male, again assuming that these additional needs are not accounted for by the safety margin in the RDA, would be 81 grams (56 + 15 + 10), or 1.2 g/kg. Again, this value falls within the recommended range.

1. *Obtain about 15 percent or more of daily energy intake from protein.* As do most investigators, Peter Lemon indicates that it is possible to get these recommended amounts from natural food sources in the daily diet. For example, the average caloric intake for a moderately active young male averages 2,500–3,000 C. This caloric intake may be increased through physical training as more Calories are expended. Thus, caloric intake would be increased to approximately 3,500–4,000 C. It is important to note that adequate energy intake, primarily in the form of carbohydrates, will improve protein balance. In essence, an increased energy intake appears to decrease protein requirements somewhat.

   If the protein portion of the dietary Calories averaged 12 percent, a general recommended level of protein intake, then the intake of protein would approximate 1.5–1.7 grams per kilogram body weight, which parallels the amounts estimated in the examples cited previously. Currently, the protein content of the average American diet is 12 to 16 percent, and Walberg-Rankin noted that most athletes consume this much or more in their daily diets. Consuming a diet with a protein content of 15 percent could provide a value of 2.0 grams or more per kilogram body weight, and other surveys among strength-type athletes indicate that they obtain this amount. These values approach or exceed the higher amounts recommended by some investigators for individuals in training. The calculations are presented in table 6.6.

   Some athletes may need to increase the percentage of protein in their daily caloric intake. Athletes in weight-control sports, such as wrestlers and gymnasts, may be in greater

TABLE 6.6	Calculation of grams protein/kilogram body weight	
Body weight: 70 kg One gram protein = 4 Calories		
Daily caloric intake:	3,500–4,000	3,500–4,000
Percent protein:	15	12
Calories in protein:	525–600	420–480
Grams of protein:	131–150	105–120
Grams protein/kg:	1.9–2.1	1.5–1.7

need of protein because of low caloric intake. Endurance athletes, particularly ultraendurance athletes, are susceptible to overtraining and chronic fatigue. Such athletes have been found to have depressed plasma levels of amino acids, which Kingsbury and others indicated appeared to be associated with inadequate protein intake.

Maintaining muscle mass during weight loss is critical for athletes and nonathletes alike, as muscle mass is a major determinant of basal metabolic rate, is the primary site of glucose disposal, and is necessary to perform sporting activities. In his review, Phillips noted that a high-protein diet (25 to 35 percent of energy intake) is more effective at attenuating the loss of lean body mass that occurs on low-Calorie diets than a normal-protein diet (12 to 15 percent of energy intake).

Helms and others reached a similar conclusion, noting that 2.3 to 3.1 g of protein/kg of body mass/day was needed to offset losses in lean body mass. Churchward-Venne and colleagues reports that overfeeding energy in the form of protein (about 1.8 to 3.0 g/kg/d, 15 to 25 percent of Calories) results in gains in lean body mass even without resistance training. As a note of caution, increasing the protein content of the diet, without increasing the Calorie content, could displace another important macronutrient (e.g., carbohydrate). One way that higher-protein diets can encourage weight loss is by promoting satiety (i.e., feeling of fullness). In a review, Leidy and others reported that 1.2 to 1.6 g of protein/kg body mass/day improves appetite and body weight management. Thus, although the exact dose is not known, dietary protein intake above recommended levels, and at least at what has been reported to maximize MPS in hard-training athletes, may be important in athletes in weight-control sports or those actively trying to lose weight.

Young athletes have high protein needs to support growth and development. Volek indicates that female strength athletes may require more protein than their endurance-training counterparts to attain positive nitrogen balance and promote protein synthesis. Also, some female endurance athletes may need more protein because of inadequate energy intake, and low dietary protein intake has been associated with amenorrhea, a topic discussed further in chapters 8 and 10.

Increasing the protein percentage of daily energy intake may help such athletes obtain adequate protein. For example, a young wrestler attempting to lose weight to compete in a lower weight category might be on a diet of 1,600 Calories per day. With an RDA of 0.85 gram of protein per kilogram body weight, a 60-kilogram (132- pound) wrestler would need 51 grams of protein to meet the RDA and up to 102 grams to meet the highest recommendation for strength-type athletes. To consume 51 grams of protein, the wrestler would need to obtain about 13 percent of daily energy intake from protein, but to obtain 102 grams of protein he would need to obtain about 25 percent of daily energy intake from protein. These amounts are well within the AMDR for protein.

Wise selection of high-quality protein foods will provide adequate amounts through a balanced diet to meet bodily needs during the early and continued stages of training. It is not difficult to increase the protein content of the diet. For example, 8 ounces of roasted, skinless chicken breast and two glasses of skim milk, a total of less than 600 Calories, will provide more than 70 grams of high-quality protein, the RDA for our typical 70-kg adolescent and more than half of the 125 grams that may be recommended for such an athlete attempting to gain muscle mass. Perusal of table 6.2 and appendix E will help you select high-protein foods. Additional points on this subject are covered in chapter 12 under the topic of gaining weight as muscle.

2. *Consume protein, preferably with carbohydrate, before and after workouts.* Eating strategies may also be an important consideration, particularly timing of protein intake. Most research has focused on amino acid or protein ingestion following exercise, but some studies have also studied the effect of pre-exercise protein intake. The feedings usually occurred immediately before or within an hour of exercise. Many studies have used **protein hydrolysate**, a high-protein dietary supplement containing a solution of amino acids and peptides prepared from protein by hydrolysis. Wolfe noted that the protein supplement should contain all the essential amino acids, and many studies also added carbohydrate.

Protein intake before exercise In separate reviews, Tipton and Wolfe both noted research studies suggesting that ingestion of free amino acids plus carbohydrates before exercise results in a superior anabolic response to exercise than if ingested after exercise. Lemon indicates that the practice of consuming nutrients prior to exercise may be beneficial by providing fuel and/or minimizing catabolic processes. However, in his review Tipton noted that the difference in anabolic response between pre-exercise and postexercise ingestion of protein is not apparent. In 2008, the International Society of Sports Nutrition published its position stand on nutrient timing. As a part of this position stand, Kerksick and others stated that the optimal pre-exercise meal is dependent on several factors, including exercise duration and fitness level. General guidelines they suggest are ingestion of 1–2 grams of carbohydrate per kilogram body weight and 0.15–0.25 gram of protein per kilogram body weight in the 3–4 hours prior to competition.

Protein intake after exercise Perhaps the two most frequently asked questions by those interested in adding protein to their diet are "what is the best time to eat protein?" and "is one protein better than another?" These questions are often in reference to which time and what type of protein will cause the greatest increase in MPS, muscle hypertrophy, and strength. As reviewed by van Loon, many proteins, including whey, casein, soy, casein hydrolysate, egg, whole milk, and fat-free milk have been shown to improve postexercise protein balance or MPS. However, the goal of an athlete is maximal or optimal MPS. There are a wide variety of protein supplements available for athletes and other consumers to choose from, including whey, casein, egg, soy, and collagen. During the past few years, experts in protein metabolism from the laboratories of Stuart Phillips, Kevin Tipton, and Luc van Loon have published research studies that have helped to answer these two important questions about protein.

The two most commonly consumed protein supplements are the two proteins in milk: casein and whey. Data from the Phillips group have demonstrated that whey protein stimulates MPS more than casein or soy protein, both at rest and postexercise. It makes sense that whey protein causes the largest increase in MPS because (1) whey is rapidly digested, exits the stomach quickly, and results in a large increase in blood amino acids; (2) whey is a complete protein, containing all the essential amino acids; and (3) whey is high in the amino acid leucine with about 3 grams of leucine per 25 grams of whey protein. Conversely, soy protein has lower levels of essential amino acids, branched-chain amino acids, and leucine. Also, soy protein is less bioavailable than whey or casein and when consumed, is more likely to be oxidized or involved with organ protein catabolism and urea synthesis. Casein, although it is digested and absorbed more slowly than soy, has higher levels of essential amino acids, branched-chain amino acids, and leucine than soy. Collagen is an incomplete protein; is low in essential amino acids, branched-chain amino acids, and leucine; and is a poor choice for a protein supplement.

It appears that the branched-chain amino acid leucine is an important factor in the MPS response to a particular type of protein. The powerful effect of leucine on MPS is referred to as the leucine trigger or leucine threshold. Essentially, muscle leucine levels must reach a critical level for protein ingestion to cause the greatest increase in MPS. The exact amount of leucine needed to maximally stimulate MPS is not known, because it varies based on age and physical activity level. However, a range of leucine doses can be suggested based on recent studies. Moore and Witard achieved the highest rates of MPS following ingestion of 20 grams of whey protein containing 1.7 to 2.4 grams of leucine. In a follow-up study, by Churchward-Venne, MPS was equal following ingestion of 25 grams of whey protein or 6.25 grams of whey protein plus 5 grams of leucine.

Several groups are conducting research in an attempt to determine the optimal dosing pattern of postexercise protein consumption. Atherton has described the "muscle full effect," where MPS returns to baseline values after 2 hours, even if amino acids are still provided. Should protein be ingested as a single bolus, for example, 20 grams, or as several small servings, for example, 5 grams every 15 minutes? Also, how long should postexercise protein ingestion last to get the maximal MPS response? Areta showed that the timing and distribution of whey protein can modify MPS over 12 hours of recovery. Four servings of 20 grams of whey protein, ingested every 3 hours, caused the largest increase in MPS compared to 8 servings of 10 grams ingested every 1.5 hours, and 2 servings of 40 grams ingested every 6 hours.

The existence of a postexercise anabolic window and importance of postexercise protein ingestion in general has recently been called into question by Schoenfeld, an expert in muscle hypertrophy. In a meta-analysis, Schoenfeld showed a beneficial effect of postexercise protein consumption on muscle hypertrophy, but this effect was not evident when total protein intake was considered. He contends that the benefit of postexercise protein ingestion was not necessarily due to timing but simply to greater protein consumption. Also, Aragon and Schoenfeld have pointed out that much of the postexercise protein consumption research is conducted with volunteers in a fasted state. This is unlikely to be the case with real athletes. They suggest pre- or postexercise protein ingestion of about 0.4 to 0.5 g of protein/kg of lean body mass as a general guideline to create the optimal anabolic effect.

Practically speaking, an inexpensive, nutrient-dense food such as fat-free milk or cottage cheese would be an excellent choice for a high-quality/high essential amino acid, high-leucine food. However, athletes often seek the optimal adaptive training response and may choose to consume a protein supplement at certain times during the day. Additionally, if an athlete is attempting to optimize muscular adaptations to training as well as decrease body fat, a postexercise leucine-enriched, low-dose whey protein supplement might be the logical choice. Finally, the constraints of sport can influence dietary protein intake behaviors. Some athletes compete multiple times per day, which would necessitate a fast-digesting protein, while others travel a great distance to a training facility or competition and may not have access to a refrigerator.

Are protein supplements necessary?

Few researchers would argue that protein supplements are necessary; rather, it is optimal to consume a high-quality protein several times per day to support positive protein balance. This can be achieved with high-protein foods, protein supplements, or a combination of the two. However, in any discussion of protein supplements vs. high-protein foods, it is worth noting that humans shouldn't focus on eating individual nutrients, but rather whole foods that supply a variety of essential nutrients. For example, a protein supplement may contain high amounts of essential amino acids. A food such as milk may also contain high amounts of essential amino acids, as well as important vitamins such as vitamin D, important minerals such as calcium, important macronutrients that support human performance such as carbohydrate, and much more. Similarly, a food such as lean beef contains high concentrations of essential amino acids, but also high amounts of the minerals iron and zinc. Also, as demonstrated in table 6.8, protein supplements generally cost much more than high-protein foods. Although there is nothing inherently wrong with protein supplements, they should be treated as just that, supplements to a healthy diet.

Protein and carbohydrate intake after exercise Carbohydrate alone may have some effect on protein synthesis following exercise, as it may help to decrease secretion of cortisol, a hormone that promotes protein catabolism. Moreover, Lemon has noted that the insulin response to dietary carbohydrate has been shown to enhance the already elevated protein synthetic rate in muscle following a strength-training session. However, van Loon, Drummond, and others indicate that if adequate protein is available, there is no need for carbohydrates to promote muscle protein synthesis, but also noted that because resistance exercise uses muscle glycogen, the carbohydrate could help replenish muscle glycogen.

Several studies and reviews have suggested that such protein intake soon *after* exercise, possibly combined with carbohydrate, was beneficial. Anton Wagenmakers, an international authority on protein metabolism during exercise, noted that protein provides the amino acids and carbohydrate increases insulin secretion. Wagenmakers noted that the effect of amino acids and insulin on protein synthesis is substantially larger after exercise, suggesting that exercise potentiates the anabolic effect of insulin and amino acids. Levenhagen and others reported that consuming protein immediately after exercise enhanced accretion of whole body and leg protein as compared to protein consumption several hours later. These findings were supported in more recent studies by Koopman and others, who used a protein/carbohydrate solution during exercise and added leucine to a protein/carbohydrate feeding after exercise. Esmarck also found that consumption of protein with carbohydrate soon after exercise also benefits muscle protein synthesis in the elderly as well.

Nutrient timing and performance Based on available research findings, the ratio of carbohydrates to protein requires additional investigation, as concluded by the International Society of Sports Nutrition in its position stand on nutrient timing. In this position stand, Kersick et al. conclude that the approach often used is to consume a supplement containing a ratio of 3–4 grams of carbohydrate per gram of protein within 30 minutes following exercise. Although commercial protein/carbohydrate sport drinks and supplements are available, Phillips and others recommend high-quality protein food sources, such as dairy protein, eggs, and lean meat, which provide an abundance of essential amino acids. In their review, Rennie and others note that a solution of mixed amino acids will increase human muscle protein synthesis to about the same extent as complete meals. A turkey breast sandwich on whole-wheat bread consumed with a glass of chocolate skim milk provides a good balance of protein and carbohydrate. Karp and Elliot, along with their associates, indicated that milk, including chocolate milk, may be an effective recovery drink for athletes and provides an alternative to supplements.

It should be noted that although these dietary practices may provide the nutrients necessary for an anabolic response in the muscle, Gibala indicates it remains to be determined if the acute effects of such supplementation eventually lead to greater gains in muscle mass following habitual training. In a study involving a 10-week resistance training program, Cribb and Hayes found that consuming a supplement containing protein, creatine, and glucose (1 gram/kg body weight) immediately before and after training, as compared to consuming the same supplement in the morning and evening, resulted in greater increases in lean body mass, muscle cross-section area, and muscular strength. Although this study would appear to support anabolic effects of protein and carbohydrate intake immediately before and after exercise training, the supplement also contained creatine, which as noted later in this chapter may by itself increase muscle mass and strength. Most investigators in this area indicate that more research is needed to determine the optimal combination of protein and timing for the various types of exercise training adaptations.

Before Sleep Protein Intake

van Loon and colleagues have pioneered research in the area of protein consumption prior to sleep, with the goal of optimizing protein synthesis during the overnight period. Historically, strength and power athletes have instinctively ingested protein during the middle of the night to aid in recovery and encourage muscle hypertrophy. This has not been studied until very recently. van Loon's team showed a 22 percent higher rate of muscle protein synthesis during the overnight period when 40 grams of casein protein was consumed 30 minutes before sleep. In a 12 week resistance training study, the same group showed increased strength and muscle cross sectional area in participants ingesting 27.5 grams of protein each night before sleep compared to those ingesting a placebo. Although there are few studies, it appears that protein ingestion before sleep is an effective dietary strategy to optimize protein synthesis, and increase strength and muscle mass in young men.

3. *Be prudent regarding protein intake.* Whether or not athletes in training need additional protein is not clear at this time. Two experts in protein metabolism, Kevin Tipton and Robert Wolfe, noted that given sufficient energy intake, lean body mass can be maintained within a wide range of protein intakes. They note that since a high protein intake is not likely harmful, and since there is a metabolic rationale for the efficacy of an increase in dietary protein if muscle hypertrophy is the goal, a higher protein intake within the context of an athlete's overall dietary requirements may be beneficial. However, they also note that there are few convincing data to indicate that the ingestion of a high amount of protein (2–3 grams per kilogram body weight) is necessary. Based on current literature, they conclude that it may be too simplistic to rely on recommendations of a particular amount of protein per day, because the amount depends on energy intake, type of protein, and timing of intake.

    Consuming additional protein within the AMDR is both safe and prudent. Table 6.7 presents a summary of some prudent daily protein intakes for sedentary and physically active individuals. These recommendations are in accord with those of the U.S. Anti-Doping Agency in its nutrition guide to athletes, *Optimal Dietary Intake.*

TABLE 6.7	Prudent protein intakes in grams per kilogram body weight for sedentary and physically active individuals
	Grams of protein/kg body weight
Sedentary	0.8
Strength-trained, maintenance	1.2–1.4
Strength-trained, gain muscle mass	1.6–1.7
Endurance-trained	1.2–1.4
Intermittent, high-intensity training	1.4–1.7
Weight-restricted	1.4–1.8

The values presented represent a synthesis of those recommended by leading researchers involved in protein metabolism and exercise. Teenagers should add 10 percent to the calculated values.

To calculate body weight in kilograms, simply multiply your weight in pounds by 0.454. Then, multiply your weight in kilograms by the appropriate value in the grams per kilogram body weight column to determine the range of grams of protein intake per day. Teenagers should increase this amount by 10 percent.

Protein: Ergogenic Aspects

Given the potential importance of protein to optimal physical performance, a wide variety of ergogenic aids associated with protein nutrition have been used in attempts to enhance performance. Such supplements remain popular. As Lawrence and Kirby noted, protein, amino acids, and creatine were among the top five most popular sports supplements.

What types of special protein supplements are marketed to physically active individuals?

As already discussed, some investigators suggest that athletes involved in weight training to gain weight or in strenuous endurance exercise may need somewhat more than the RDA for protein to maintain or increase protein balance, particularly if energy intake (Calories) is not adequate to meet daily energy expenditure.

To provide additional protein to the diet, investigators have used high-protein diets, powdered protein sources, canned liquid meals high in protein and energy, sports drinks and bars, or special foods and concoctions high in protein content. However, the protein content is actually derived from natural protein, such as milk, egg, or soy protein. As Bucci has indicated, supplements of intact proteins, such as the proteins found in these products, offer no advantages over protein found in other food sources, since these supplements are in fact derived from natural foods. In addition, many of these protein supplements are expensive when compared to natural protein that may be obtained easily in high-protein foods such as powdered milk, skim milk, eggs, and chicken. Blending powdered milk into a glass of skim milk, with some vanilla or other flavoring, will provide substantial amounts of high-quality protein—your own personal protein supplement. Some comparative costs for different sources of protein are presented in table 6.8.

Nevertheless, commercial supplements may be a convenient means for some busy athletes to secure additional protein in the diet. Many of these products contain high-quality protein, such as milk, whey, or egg protein; provide a balanced mixture of protein, carbohydrate, and fat for additional Calories; and may also contain supplemental vitamins and minerals. Although these products do not contain all of the nutrients of natural foods, they may be useful adjuncts to a balanced diet. Certain brands have been available for years, such as Nutrament, but several companies have marketed products specifically for physically active individuals, such as Mega Whey by GNC and Nutrition Shake by Gatorade. It is important to reemphasize the point that these supplements should be used as an adjunct to an otherwise balanced nutritional plan, not as a substitute.

Whey and colostrum are two forms of protein that are sold as dietary supplements and marketed as a means to enhance sport performance. Whey proteins are extracted from the liquid whey that is produced during the manufacture of cheese or casein. Whey protein isolates are more than 90 percent protein. Hayes and Cribb note that whey proteins are a rich source of essential amino acids, thus providing the foundations for preservation of muscle mass. Walzem and others note that bovine whey may contain other substances, including growth factors. Colostrum, or

TABLE 6.8 Costs of protein found in various food sources

Source	Serving size	Grams of protein/serving	Cost per serving	Cost per 8 grams of protein
Powdered milk	23 grams	8	$0.13	$0.13
Egg	1	6	$0.10	$0.13
Turkey breast	4 ounces	28	$0.75	$0.21
Skim milk	8 fluid ounces	8	$0.20	$0.20
Protein capsules	8 capsules	8	$1.20	$1.20
MetRx Bar	3.5-ounce bar	27	$2.50	$0.74
Boost	8 fluid ounces	10	$1.10	$0.88
Avalanche Power Drink	16 fluid ounces	40	$3.00	$0.60
Whey Pro	1 scoop	23	$1.01	$0.34

bovine colostrum, is the first milk secreted by cows. Standardized preparations of colostrum are available as dietary supplements. Brinkworth and others indicate that colostrum is a rich source of protein, carbohydrates, vitamins, minerals, and various biologically active components, also including growth factors. Although no mechanism has been identified, one theory involves increased levels of serum insulin-like growth factor (IGF-1), which could be anabolic. However, Kuipers and others provided 60 grams of colostrum daily for 4 weeks to endurance-trained males and found no effect on blood IGF-1 or IGF binding protein levels.

Other protein substances, such as spirulina (algae), brewer's yeast, specific enzymes, and even DNA and RNA, have been advocated as means to improve physical performance. Spirulina and brewer's yeast are good sources of protein and a variety of vitamins and minerals but convey no magical ergogenic qualities. The enzymes DNA and RNA would be degraded in the digestive process and thus could not be utilized for the purpose for which they were ingested.

Protein/carbohydrate solutions, some marketed as sports drinks, have been theorized to enhance endurance performance above and beyond that provided by carbohydrate alone. As noted in chapter 4, carbohydrate-containing sports drinks may enhance performance in prolonged endurance exercise, but does adding protein provide any additional benefits?

Do high-protein diets or protein supplements increase muscle mass and strength in resistance-trained individuals?

Some athletes in training may need more protein, and as noted below, some may increase muscle mass and strength with resistance training and protein supplementation. Moreover, some studies suggest that protein/carbohydrate beverages consumed during resistance exercise may help reduce muscle tissue damage and soreness.

High-Protein Diets Several earlier laboratory studies have compared the effect of normal protein intake, about 0.8–1.4 grams per kilogram, to higher levels, such as 1.6–2.8 grams per kilogram, on body composition changes during a weight-training program. In general, these studies revealed that although protein balance could be maintained or even be positive with the consumption of a normal amount of protein, the body protein balance was even more positive with the larger amounts. The additional body weight also appears to be in the form of lean body mass.

Other well-designed studies have not shown any ergogenic effects on strength-type performance. Weideman and others, using nuclear magnetic resonance to measure leg volume, reported no significant increase in leg muscle hypertrophy following 13 weeks of weight training with 2.94 grams of protein per kilogram per day, nor did Lemon and others find increased muscle mass when subjects consumed 2.62 grams of protein per kilogram per day, as compared to 1.35 grams per kilogram. Additionally, neither of these two studies reported a significant effect of the high-protein intake on measures of strength. In a review, Garlick and others noted an absence of strong evidence that high-protein diets confer any advantage in terms of strength.

More recent research also indicates that protein supplementation does not appear to increase muscular strength. Andersen and others provided either protein or carbohydrate before and after resistance training over the course of 14 weeks. The protein group showed significant hypertrophy in both type I and II muscle fibers, while the carbohydrate group experienced little change from baseline. However, there were no differences between the groups regarding increases in muscle strength. Hoffman and others studied collegiate strength/power athletes stratified into three groups depending on their daily intake of protein as either below (1.0–1.4 g/kg), at (1.6–1.8 g/kg), or above (>2.0 g/kg) recommended levels. No differences in body composition or strength were noted after 12 weeks of resistance training. In a study with older men (59–76 years), Candow and others reported that although 12 weeks of resistance training increased muscle size and strength, protein supplementation (0.3 g/kg) provided either before or after each training bout had no additional effects.

As noted previously, some investigators recommend protein intake immediately following exercise. Several studies have evaluated the effect of protein supplementation on possible muscle damage during resistance training. Kraemer and others reported that amino acid supplementation may be effective as a means to attenuate muscle strength loss during a period of increased intensity of resistance training designed to produce overreaching, possibly by providing substrate for muscle anabolism and reducing muscle damage. One study reported that 15 grams of protein consumed immediately after exercise enhanced muscle repair, as measured by changes in enzyme status associated with muscle damage.

More recent research suggests that combining carbohydrate with protein may be more effective. Several studies by Bird and others have found that providing a supplement containing both carbohydrate and essential amino acids (6 grams), as compared to a placebo or carbohydrate and essential amino acids alone, reduced markers of muscle protein catabolism 48 hours after resistance training. They suggested that such a supplement may induce an anticatabolic effect and better favor conservation of muscle protein following intense resistance exercise.

Given the possibility of enhanced muscle repair, consuming some of the recommended daily amount of protein immediately following exercise may be a prudent behavior.

Whey and Colostrum   Research findings reveal mixed, but generally positive, effects relative to the ergogenic potential of whey supplementation to resistance-trained individuals. However, other protein sources were often combined with the whey protein. Cribb and others found that whey isolate (1.5 g/kg/d), as compared to the same amount of casein, over the course of 10 weeks of resistance training significantly increased lean body mass and strength improvements in recreational bodybuilders. In another study, Cribb and others compared the effects of supplementation with creatine, whey protein, creatine with whey protein, or carbohydrate placebo during 11 weeks of resistance training using four groups of trained subjects; the whey protein content was approximately 100 grams. Compared to the carbohydrate group, the whey protein group and the other two groups increased muscle strength. Kerksick and others studied the effects of whey protein supplementation in resistance-trained males engaged in 10 weeks of resistance training. Three groups consumed either a carbohydrate placebo, 40 grams/day of whey protein plus casein, or 40 grams of whey protein and several other amino acids. All groups experienced similar significant increases in muscle strength, but the combination whey/casein group experienced the greatest increases in fat-free mass. Candow and others compared the effects of whey protein (1.2 g/kg) and soy protein (1.2 g/kg) versus a placebo on changes in body composition and strength over 6 weeks of resistance training in untrained individuals. They found that both the whey and soy protein supplements, compared to the placebo, induced small but significant increases in lean tissue mass and strength, but there was no difference between the two sources of protein. Finally, Coburn and others reported that supplementation with a leucine/whey combination over the course of 8 weeks of resistance training of the knee extensors significantly increased muscle strength, but had no effect on muscle hypertrophy.

Several studies have evaluated the ergogenic effect of colostrum supplementation, using whey protein as a placebo to reveal whether colostrum supplementation produced any benefits beyond those attributed to whey protein alone. Hofman and others evaluated the effect of bovine colostrum on body composition and four tests of exercise performance in elite male and female field hockey players. The tests included two shuttle sprints (50 and 300 meters total for time), a shuttle sprint test to exhaustion, and a vertical jump. The subjects consumed 60 grams of colostrum daily for 8 weeks and whey protein served as the placebo. The colostrum had no effect on body composition or three of the four exercise tests, but did appear to improve performance in the 50-meter shuttle sprint test. Antonio and others investigated the effect of 20 grams of bovine colostrum, given daily during 8 weeks of aerobic and heavy-resistance exercise training, on body composition, strength, and aerobic endurance. Whey protein was the placebo. There were no effects of the colostrum on exercise performance. The whey group significantly increased total body mass, whereas the colostrum group, although not increasing total body mass, did increase lean body mass, which was attributed to a slight decrease in body fat. Brinkworth and others, studying the effect of either bovine colostrum or whey protein supplementation (60 grams daily) during 8 weeks of resistance training, found that subjects in the colostrum group increased arm circumference and cross-sectional area, but the increase was due principally to a greater increase in skin and subcutaneous fat.

Do high-protein diets or protein supplements improve aerobic endurance performance in endurance-trained individuals?

Protein supplementation may also help reduce muscle tissue damage and soreness during aerobic endurance training, but there is little evidence to support a performance-enhancing, or ergogenic, effect on aerobic endurance following acute or prolonged protein supplementation.

High-Protein Diets or Meals   The 40:30:30 "zone diet" alluded to in chapter 5 may be considered to be a high-protein diet because 30 percent of the daily Calories are derived from protein (high end of the AMDR), 40 percent are derived from carbohydrate, and 30 percent are derived from fat. The premise underlying the "zone diet" is a change in hormonal activity, resulting in vasoactive eicosanoids that permit greater oxygen delivery to the muscle, a condition referred to as the "zone." In a review, Cheuvront criticized the "zone diet" book, noting that the claims of improved sport performance are based on anecdotal reports and selectively quoted research, not on sound scientific evidence. Cheuvront states that, in actuality, reliable and abundant peer-reviewed literature is in opposition to the suggestion that such a diet can support competitive athletic endeavors, much less improve them, and even suggests that the "zone diet" may actually be ergolytic in nature. Some evidence does indicate that high-protein diets, at the expense of carbohydrate, may impair endurance performance. Jarvis and others evaluated the effects of a 7-day zone diet, compared with a normal diet, on body composition and run time to exhaustion in recreational endurance athletes. Daily energy intake was significantly reduced by about 300 Calories on the zone diet, as was body mass and run time to exhaustion at 80 percent of VO_2 max. These investigators do not recommend the zone diet for athletes unless future research validates its proposed ability to enhance athletic performance. It should be noted that subjects consumed fewer Calories while on the zone diet, a factor that may have impeded performance. However, Macdermid and Stannard conducted a study in which the caloric energy was the same in both the high-carbohydrate and high-protein diets: In a crossover design, for 7 days subjects received either a high-carbohydrate diet or a high-protein–moderate-carbohydrate diet and then completed an individually based cycling time trial that lasted more than 2 hours. Although there were no differences in various physiological measures, the high-protein diet significantly impaired cycling endurance performance by 20 percent, indicating an ergolytic effect. The subjects also indicated that it was difficult to train on the high-protein diet.

Nevertheless, for weight-restricted athletes attempting to lose body fat or maintain a low body weight for sports competition, some investigators recommend increased protein intake. With a 1,500-Calorie diet, a 30 percent protein allotment would be 450 Calories, or approximately 112 grams of protein. For a lean athlete, this amount of protein may help ensure protein adequacy and may fall in the range of recommended protein intake.

In summary, Lemon notes that although endurance athletes may need a higher protein intake (1.2–1.4 grams per kilogram body weight) than sedentary individuals, these recommendations are based on protein balance studies. Lemon further states that there are no data to indicate that such a protein intake, as compared to the RDA of 0.8 grams per kilogram, will enhance sport performance. Such studies are needed.

Protein/Carbohydrate Preparations Various sports drinks containing both protein and carbohydrate have been marketed as a means to enhance performance when consumed during exercise and to facilitate recovery and improve subsequent exercise performance when consumed after exercise. In one of the first studies, Ivy and others compared the effects of adding protein to a carbohydrate solution on aerobic endurance performance. Trained cyclists, consuming 200 milliliters of solution every 20 minutes, exercised for 3 hours at intensities varying from 45 to 75 percent of VO_2 max and then exercised to exhaustion at 85 percent of VO_2 max. The carbohydrate solution (7.75 percent) significantly improved endurance performance compared to the placebo, but the carbohydrate/protein combination (7.75/1.94 percent) enhanced performance even more than the carbohydrate solution. Saunders, in a review, indicated that other studies report similar findings. However, Saunders did note limitations to these studies; the main factor was that in the studies showing improved performance, the protein supplied in the beverage was in addition to the carbohydrate, thus providing more energy.

Other studies do not support an ergogenic effect of protein/carbohydrate supplementation when compared to carbohydrate supplements containing equal energy. For example, van Essen and others reported that when trained athletes ingested a sports drink during exercise at a rate considered optimal for carbohydrate delivery, protein provided no additional performance benefit during an 80-kilometer cycling trial, an event that simulated "real life" competition. Romano-Ely and others also compared the effects of a protein/carbohydrate drink, which also included antioxidants, to an isocaloric carbohydrate drink on cycling time to exhaustion at 70 percent VO_2 max; the drinks were consumed every 15 minutes during exercise. There was no significant difference between the treatments on performance time. In his review, Gibala indicated that there is no established mechanism by which protein intake during exercise should improve acute endurance performance, and these latter studies support this viewpoint.

As noted previously, consuming protein and carbohydrate following exercise provides a milieu conducive to enhanced anabolism and muscle recovery. Some have contended that ingesting carbohydrate plus protein following prolonged exercise may restore exercise capacity more effectively than ingestion of carbohydrate alone. For example, compared to a standard commercial carbohydrate/electrolyte sports drink, Karp and others found that both low-fat chocolate milk and a commercial protein/carbohydrate sports drink, each of which contain about 34 grams of carbohydrate and 9 grams of protein per 8 fluid ounces, enhanced performance in a cycling test to exhaustion 4 hours after a hard interval workout. However, although the subjects consumed the same amount of fluid in each trial, the two protein/carbohydrate drinks contained more than twice as much carbohydrate and more than three times as much caloric energy as the carbohydrate/electrolyte sports drink.

When the energy content is similar, consuming protein/carbohydrate meals or supplements during recovery, as compared to carbohydrate alone, has no effect on subsequent exercise performance. In two separate studies, Betts and others had physically active males complete a 90-minute run at 70 percent of VO_2 max followed by a 4-hour recovery, during which they consumed either a carbohydrate or carbohydrate/protein solution with similar energy content. The recovery was followed by a run to exhaustion at either 70 or 85 percent of VO_2 max, but there was no difference between the two recovery diets. Studies by Rowlands and Millard-Stafford, along with their colleagues, have shown that consuming high-protein/carbohydrate meals or fluid supplements following intense exercise training, as compared to comparable carbohydrate feedings, does not enhance performance in intermittent, high-intensity (10 maximal 2.5-minute cycling sprints) or aerobic endurance (5-kilometer track run) the following day. In a systematic review, Lieberman and colleagues assessed the effects of protein plus carbohydrate ingestion on acute and repeated endurance exercise performance in 26 studies. This review included studies of protein and carbohydrate ingestion during an acute exercise bout, and protein and carbohydrate ingestion during and after exercise and the effects on a subsequent bout of exercise. The authors concluded that the addition of protein to a carbohydrate supplement had no effect on endurance exercise performance.

In his review, Saunders also noted that consumption of protein/carbohydrate solutions has been associated with reduced markers of muscle damage and less muscle soreness. Several studies support this viewpoint. In their study cited earlier, which involved a 21-kilometer outdoor run at a set pace followed by a treadmill run to exhaustion at 90 percent of VO_2 max, Millard-Stafford and others reported that the carbohydrate/protein mixture resulted in less muscle soreness. Romano-Ely and others also reported that subjects experienced less muscle soreness on the carbohydrate/protein drink, and blood enzyme tests indicated less muscle tissue damage. Conversely, Green and others found that a carbohydrate-protein drink consumed following an exercise task (downhill running) designed to induce muscle injury and soreness had no effect on quadriceps strength recovery or muscle soreness.

Overall these preliminary findings are promising. Nancy Rodriguez, a sports-nutrition scientist at the University of Connecticut, indicates that long-term, well-controlled diet and exercise intervention studies are essential for clarification of the relation between protein intake, endurance exercise, and skeletal-muscle protein turnover.

Colostrum   Several studies evaluated the effect of colostrum on endurance exercise performance. Brinkworth and others supplemented the daily diet of elite rowers during 9 weeks of training for the world championships with 60 grams of bovine colostrum. Whey protein was used as the placebo. Subjects completed several bouts of a rowing protocol involving both submaximal and a 4-minute maximal test. They found that although the colostrum supplement increased the estimated buffer capacity, it had no effect on rowing performance. Coombes and others evaluated the effect of different colostrum dosages on two tests of aerobic capacity in competitive cyclists. The dosages included 60 grams of colostrum, 20 grams of colostrum plus 40 grams of whey protein, and 60 grams of whey protein, which was the placebo group. The exercise tests included two VO_2 max tests with a 20-minute interval between each, and a cycle time-trial test following 2 hours of cycling at 65 percent of VO_2 max. Although performance in the VO_2 max tests was not improved by colostrum, it did provide a small but significant improvement in the time-trial performance. Shing and others also reported some ergogenic effects of colostrum supplementation. Over the course of 10 weeks of training, including a final 5 days of high-intensity cycling, highly trained male road cyclists consumed either a placebo or a daily supplement containing 10 grams of bovine colostrum protein concentrate (CPC). A 40-kilometer time trial was done periodically to evaluate performance. The effects of the colostrum supplement on cycling time-trial performance during the first 9 weeks of regular training was unclear, but performance of the colostrum group was enhanced significantly following the 5 days of high-intensity training. They reported that the CPC helped to maintain the ventilatory threshold. As with the effects of colostrum on strength-type activities, these too should be considered preliminary data; confirmation with additional research is needed. Shing has stated that there is limited evidence supporting an ergogenic effect of colostrum, an that because it may contain prohibited substances, it could affect the outcome of doping tests.

Are amino acid, amine, and related nitrogen-containing supplements effective ergogenic aids?

As noted previously, providing all essential amino acids during recovery from exercise may be associated with enhanced muscle protein synthesis, but whether or not this translates into enhanced exercise performance has not been determined. In recent years, however, specific amino acids have become increasingly available and popular in certain athletic circles.

Weight lifters are consuming various amino acids in attempts to stimulate the release of growth hormone from the pituitary gland, hoping that the growth hormone will then stimulate muscle development. Amino acids have also been used to stimulate the release of insulin from the pancreas; insulin is also considered to be an anabolic hormone because it facilitates the uptake of amino acids by the muscle cells. Indeed, certain amino acid mixtures have been advertised to be more potent than anabolic steroids, one of the most popular drugs used by strength and power athletes. Anabolic steroids and related substances are discussed in chapter 13. Other amino acids have been advertised in magazines for endurance athletes, suggesting that they may be utilized as a fuel during training or help prevent fatigue by altering the formation of neurotransmitters in the brain. Still other amino acid mixtures and related compounds such as creatine and inosine have been used in attempts to increase ATP or PCr levels in the muscle or to help athletes lose body weight for competition.

Scientific research has shown that individual amino acid supplements may induce specific physiological responses in the body, particularly the formation of certain chemicals in the brain needed for nerve impulse transmission as well as secretion of hormones. However, amino acid metabolism is very complex. It depends on a variety of factors, such as the concentration in the blood, competition with other amino acids, feedback control mechanisms, and the presence in the diet of other nutrients. Consumption of specific amino acid mixtures or even high-protein diets may actually lead to nutritional imbalances, as an overload of one amino acid may inhibit the absorption of others into the body.

Because purified amino acids, known as free-form amino acids, amines such as creatine, and other nitrogen-containing substances have become commercially available for athletes, they have been the focus of increased research activity by sports medicine scientists. However, although the number of studies is increasing relative to the effect of amino acid supplementation upon physical performance, with the exception of creatine the data are still somewhat limited. Moreover, some investigators combine several amino acids or use commercial supplements that may contain not only several amino acids but other nutrients as well, which may cloud the possible ergogenic effect of any one specific amino acid. The following discussion highlights some of the current key findings regarding specific amino acids, various combinations of amino acids, amines, and nitrogen-containing compounds that have been studied for their potential ergogenic effect.

Arginine and Citrulline   Arginine, a conditionally essential amino acid, has several functions in human metabolism. One of its most important is to serve as a precursor for nitric oxide

(NO) synthesis. NO acts as a vasodilator to increase blood flow. Citrulline also is an amino acid, but is not one of the 20 essential or nonessential amino acids because it is not involved in protein synthesis. However, dietary citrulline is eventually taken up by the kidney and metabolized to generate large amounts of arginine. Hickner and others noted that citrulline supplementation increases plasma arginine levels to a higher level than arginine supplementation.

Arginine infusion and oral supplementation are being studied for possible health benefits, particularly in individuals with circulatory problems, because arginine may function to promote vasodilation. In their earlier review, Cheng and others reported that oral arginine supplementation has been shown to improve exercise ability in CHD patients. More recent research supports this viewpoint. For example, Doutreleau and others reported that 6 weeks of arginine supplementation to patients with chronic stable heart failure enhanced endurance exercise performance, reducing heart rate and blood lactate responses. Conversely, Wilson and others noted no beneficial effects of arginine supplementation, compared to a placebo, on treadmill walking distance to the onset of pain in patients with peripheral arterial disease. They also noted no increase in NO synthesis with arginine supplementation, which may underlie this negative finding.

There is limited research regarding the effect of arginine and citrulline supplementation on exercise performance in healthy individuals. Hickner and others used two supplementation protocols with citrulline, one using two different protocols, either 9 grams in three 3-gram doses over 24 hours or 3 grams once every 3 hours before exercise testing, which consisted of a variable speed and grade treadmill run time to exhaustion. There were no differences in treadmill run times between placebo and L-citrulline supplementation when the data were analyzed separately by dose protocol. However, the authors reported a higher rating of perceived exertion associated with citrulline supplementation and when the data from the two protocols were combined, the run time to exhaustion was actually impaired with citrulline supplementation. Jeacoke and others pointed out that there are a dearth of investigations into the effects of citrulline on exercise performance. They note that there are a small number of randomized controlled trials of the effects of citrulline supplementation on exercise performance available, but that data are mixed or show no effect. Certainly, more research needs to be conducted, but if drinking beetroot juice or eating green leafy vegetables is more effective at increasing nitric oxide levels, than the ingestion of citrulline supplements may be unnecessary. In a related vein, Buchman and others provided arginine or a placebo to marathon runners and speculated that arginine may be ergolytic, as the predicted times of the runners receiving arginine were slower than those receiving the placebo.

Other studies show no ergogenic or ergolytic effects of arginine supplementation. McConell and others infused arginine to endurance-trained cyclists during exercise (30 grams in 1 hour). Although the cyclists experienced a decrease in blood glucose, there was no effect on performance in a 15-minute maximal cycling time trial following 2 hours of cycling at 72 percent VO_2 max. Using a chronic supplementation protocol, Abel and others reported that 4 weeks of supplementation with arginine aspartate (5.7 g arginine; 8.7 g aspartate) had no effect on endocrine or metabolic responses, peak oxygen uptake, or cycling endurance to exhaustion. As noted later, aspartate salts have also been theorized to be ergogenic.

Arginine, Lysine, and Ornithine Research has shown that infusing any of a number of amino acids into the blood potentiates the release of **human growth hormone (HGH)**, a polypeptide. HGH is released from the pituitary gland into the bloodstream, affecting all tissues. One of its effects is to stimulate the production of another hormone, insulin-like growth factor-1, that spurs growth of tissue, including muscle tissue. Some amino acids may also stimulate the release of insulin, an anabolic hormone, from the pancreas. McConell reported that arginine infusion increased HGH and insulin. Such effects could be ergogenic for strength-trained individuals, and Cynober indicates that arginine and its related amino acids such as ornithine are found in dietary supplements for bodybuilders.

Although more than a half-dozen amino acids may stimulate HGH release when infused, the effect of oral supplementation is less clear. However, Jacobson has reported that the oral administration of selected amino acids may lead to HGH release similar to that promoted by infusion. Bucci, in his book on nutritional ergogenics, also notes that oral intake of amino acids, particularly arginine and ornithine, may increase HGH release, while others have suggested that lysine may elicit similar effects.

Arginine supplementation may increase HGH secretion at rest, but impair it during exercise. In one study, Collier and others found that oral arginine supplementation (7 grams) increases secretion of HGH, but not as much as a bout of resistance exercise. In a review, Kanaley concluded that arginine alone increases HGH levels by about 100 percent, while exercise can increase HGH levels by 300–500 percent. However, when arginine and exercise are combined, the increase is less than seen with exercise alone, suggesting that arginine supplementation does not augment and may actually decrease the HGH response to exercise.

Research by Bucci and his colleagues has supported the effect of ornithine to increase serum HGH levels. Using dosages of 40, 100, and 170 milligrams per kilogram body weight, only the highest dose of ornithine increased HGH levels, but it caused intestinal distress (osmotic diarrhea) in many of the subjects, and thus its use at this effective dose may be impractical. Moreover, in a related study, Bucci and others noted that ornithine did not increase the secretion of insulin.

Arginine, lysine, and ornithine, separately or in various combinations, have received the most research attention regarding an ergogenic effect for strength/power-type athletes. They have been advertised in bodybuilding magazines as being more powerful than anabolic steroids, potent drugs used by some athletes to increase muscle mass. The advertisers apparently are capitalizing on the potential of these amino acids to enhance HGH release.

Two of the earliest published studies by Elam collectively reported that arginine and ornithine supplementation in conjunction with a weight-training program reduced body fat, increased lean body mass, and increased strength over a 5-week period.

The dosage was 2 grams per day (1 gram each of arginine and ornithine), 5 days per week. Unfortunately, both studies have been criticized in the literature on the grounds of the statistical procedure by which the experimental and control groups were compared. A different analysis of the same data revealed no significant difference between the experimental and control groups in the first study. The studies have also been criticized for questionable measurement techniques and for making assumptions without adequate supporting data.

Several studies with better experimental designs have not shown any significant ergogenic effect of arginine and lysine, or other similar amino acid combinations. Lambert and others, using combinations of arginine/lysine and ornithine/tyrosine, reported no significant increases in HGH, while Fogelholm and his associates noted no significant increases in HGH or insulin secretion following supplementation with arginine, ornithine, and lysine in competitive weight lifters. Hawkins and associates, using experienced male weight lifters as subjects, reported no beneficial effects of oral arginine supplementation on various measures of muscle function, including peak torque and endurance. Suminski and others reported that although a bout of weight training would increase HGH levels in noncompetitive weight lifters, supplementation with arginine and lysine provided no additional benefit. Mitchell and others, also using experienced weight lifters, reported that 8 weeks of supplementation with arginine and lysine elicited no significant effect on HGH secretion, body composition, or various strength measures. As discussed in chapter 13, increased HGH may not induce an ergogenic effect in young, resistance-trained males.

One study by Campbell and others did find some ergogenic effects of arginine supplementation when combined with alpha-ketoglutarate. Resistance-trained men consumed either a placebo or 12 grams daily (3 equal doses) of arginine alpha-ketoglutarate during 8 weeks of periodized resistance training. Compared to the placebo, the supplement group improved performance in bench press strength and anaerobic peak power in a Wingate test. However, there were no effects between groups in body composition and isokinetic quadriceps muscle endurance.

In their review, Chromiak and Antonio indicated that oral doses of arginine, lysine, and ornithine that are great enough to induce significant growth hormone release are likely to cause gastrointestinal discomfort. Moreover, they reported no studies finding that such supplementation augments HGH release, nor do any studies support an ergogenic effect to increase muscle mass and strength to a greater extent than strength training alone.

Cynober notes that, to date, there have been no studies on the safety of long-term administration of these amino acids in healthy subjects. However, Böger notes that doses of 3–8 grams per day of arginine appear to be safe and do not appear to cause acute pharmacologic effects in humans.

Tryptophan   Although tryptophan is one of the amino acids that may increase the release of HGH, its theoretical ergogenic effect is based upon another function. A neurotransmitter in the brain, serotonin (5-hydroxytryptamine), is derived from tryptophan. This neurotransmitter may induce sleepiness and elicit a mellow mood,

and Segura and Ventura hypothesize that it may help to decrease the perception of pain. They postulate that individuals who show the best tolerance of or resistance to pain may be able to delay the onset of fatigue, and that tryptophan supplementation therefore might improve exercise performance. In their study, 12 healthy athletes exercised to exhaustion on a treadmill at 80 percent of their VO_2 max under two conditions: A placebo was compared with a dosage of 1,200 milligrams of L-tryptophan consumed in 300-mg doses over the 24 hours prior to testing. They reported no significant improvement in peak oxygen uptake or heart rate response, but did note a significant improvement in time to exhaustion (49 percent) and a decreased rating of perceived exertion (RPE) following the L-tryptophan trial. The times to exhaustion were extremely variable among the individual subjects, ranging from 2.5–18 minutes, suggesting that some of the individuals may not have been well trained. In another study with untrained individuals, Cunliffe and others reported that tryptophan supplementation (30 mg per kilogram body weight) increased both subjective and objective measures of fatigue. Although tryptophan supplementation had no effect on grip strength, work output on a wrist ergometer increased significantly.

Stensrund and his associates challenged the results of the Segura and Ventura study, noting that a 49 percent increase in performance would be rather phenomenal in trained athletes. Thus, they decided to replicate this study using 49 well-trained male runners and better control conditions, although they had their subjects run to exhaustion at 100 percent VO_2 max, not 80 percent. In contrast to the study by Segura and Ventura, they reported no significant effect of tryptophan supplementation on performance. Other research from the University of Maastricht revealed no effect of tryptophan supplementation on endurance performance at 70–75 percent of VO_2 max, and research with horses reported a decrease in endurance performance at 50 percent of VO_2 max.

Based on these limited data, tryptophan does not appear to be an effective ergogenic in either short-term or prolonged exercise tasks in exercise-trained individuals, a finding also supported in the review by Anton Wagenmakers. Some adverse health effects have been associated with tryptophan supplementation and are discussed in the next section.

Branched-Chain Amino Acids (BCAAs)   The three BCAAs are leucine, isoleucine, and valine. BCAA supplementation has been theorized to enhance exercise performance in a variety of ways. BCAAs, particularly leucine, could be used as a fuel during exercise to prevent adverse changes in neurotransmitter function, to spare the use of muscle glycogen, and to prevent or decrease the net rate of protein degradation. These effects could influence mental and physical performance, and may also favorably affect body composition, but most research has focused on the central fatigue hypothesis.

Central fatigue hypothesis   Eric Newsholme, a biochemist at Oxford University, proposed the central fatigue hypothesis, postulating that high levels of serum free-tryptophan (fTRP) in conjunction with low levels of BCAA, or a high fTRP:BCAA ratio, may be a major factor in the etiology of fatigue during prolonged endurance exercise. Research with animals has shown that a high fTRP:BCAA ratio may lead to an increased production of serotonin. Newsholme suggested that serum BCAA levels eventually decrease in endurance exercise, such as marathon running, because they may be used for energy production. Such an effect would possibly increase the fTRP:BCAA ratio, facilitating the transport of tryptophan into the brain and increasing serotonin production, which could lead to fatigue because increased serotonin levels may depress central nervous system functions. Some, but not all, research with humans supports this finding. Blomstrand and others have shown in several studies that prolonged endurance exercise, such as the 26.2-mile (42.2-kilometer) marathon, increases the fTRP:BCAA ratio, but Conlay and others noted no change in this ratio in experienced runners immediately following completion of the Boston Marathon. Tanaka and others also noted no change in the fTRP:BCAA ratio in a 6-week study designed to induce overtraining.

The central fatigue hypothesis and BCAA supplementation have received considerable research attention since Newsholme proposed his hypothesis in the late 1980s, and these studies have served as the basis for several reviews. Based on these reviews, and research studies published subsequent to these reviews, the following appear to be the key points regarding the central fatigue hypothesis and the effects of nutritional interventions, particularly BCAA and carbohydrate supplementation.

Support for the hypothesis Animal studies support the concept of central fatigue during prolonged exercise tasks. Fatigue appears to be associated with increases in brain serotonin, but fatigue is also correlated with changes in other brain neurotransmitters as well, such as dopamine. Some human data also suggest that serotonin may be involved in the development of fatigue. Several drugs, approved for use with humans, may block the removal of serotonin from its active sites, thus magnifying its effects. In several studies involving running or cycling at 70 percent VO_2 max, these drugs either impaired performance or increased the psychological perception of effort, both negative findings.

However, J. Mark Davis of the University of South Carolina points out that although the central fatigue hypothesis has some support from experimental data, the underlying mechanism has not been determined. Investigators are studying this issue, looking not only at mechanisms associated with serotonin, but other brain neurotransmitters as well, such as dopamine.

BCAA supplementation and the fTRP:BCAA ratio If serum BCAAs fall during prolonged exercise, then BCAA supplementation might be a preventive measure. It is known that BCAAs are metabolized primarily in the muscle, not the liver, and thus may provide an energy source during exercise. Some research has shown that oral supplementation with BCAAs or leucine will increase the serum levels of BCAA, the BCAAs may possibly be used as an energy source during exercise, the BCAAs may prevent or decrease the rate of endogenous protein degradation during exercise, and the BCAAs may help to maintain a normal fTRP:BCAA ratio during prolonged exercise. However, Rennie and others indicated that the total contribution of BCAAs to fuel provision during exercise is minor and insufficient to increase dietary protein requirements.

BCAA supplementation and mental performance Several sports, such as tennis and soccer, involve prolonged, high-intensity intermittent bouts of exercise in which mental alertness must be maintained. In such events, the fTRP:BCAA ratio may increase, as documented by Struder and associates in a study involving nationally ranked tennis players involved in 4 hours of continuous tournament tennis.

As evaluated by various tests of cognitive performance, reviews by Blomstrand and Meeusen and others reported that BCAA supplementation improved mental performance in national-class soccer players after a game and in runners after a 30-kilometer race. However, other investigators reported no effect of BCAA supplementation on mental acuity following a 40-kilometer cycle performance test. These are interesting field studies, and additional similar research is merited, complemented by well-controlled laboratory studies.

BCAA supplementation and perceived exertion Somewhat related to mental performance is the psychological perception of effort, or how mentally stressful the subject perceives a given exercise task to be. This psychological effort is usually evaluated by Borg's Rating of Perceived Exertion Scale, or RPE (see page 482). In their research, Blomstrand and others reported that BCAA supplementation, compared to a placebo trial, reduced the RPE and mental fatigue of endurance-trained cyclists during a 60-minute ride at 70 percent VO_2 max followed by another 20 minutes of maximal exercise. The fTRP:BCAA ratio increased in the placebo trial, but remained unchanged or even decreased in the BCAA trial. Conversely, other well-controlled studies have reported no significant effect of BCAA supplementation on RPE during intense exercise, such as during a 40-kilometer cycling performance test and 90 minutes of exercise at a 2-millimole lactate threshold.

BCAA supplementation and physical performance Investigators have studied BCAA supplementation with acute dosages administered to subjects just before and during the exercise task, and chronic dosages provided to the subject for several weeks prior to and during the exercise task. Dosages have varied, ranging from 5–20 grams per day. When provided with liquids, the dosages ranged up to 7 grams per liter.

Acute supplementation In one of the first reports of acute supplementation, Blomstrand and her colleagues studied the performance of 193 marathoners, separated into placebo and BCAA supplement groups. Overall, there was no significant difference in marathon performance between the placebo group and the BCAA group. However, using some debatable statistical tactics, they reported that BCAA supplementation significantly improved performance in the "slower" runners in the race (3:05–3:30 hours) but had no effect on the performance of the "faster" runners (<3:05 hours). They suggested that the slower runners may have depleted their muscle glycogen earlier, therefore decreasing their serum BCAA levels earlier in the race and benefiting more from the supplementation. Although this was an interesting field study, it has been criticized by Davis for several problems with experimental methodology.

Most well-controlled laboratory studies and field studies involving acute BCAA supplementation have reported no significant ergogenic effects on exercise performance. In many of these studies, the BCAA supplement was compared to a carbohydrate supplement, usually involving three trials: carbohydrate alone, BCAA alone, and BCAA with carbohydrate. An analysis of about ten studies revealed that acute BCAA supplementation, particularly when compared to carbohydrate solutions, had no effect on time to exhaustion in running or cycling tests ranging in intensities from 70–85 percent VO_2 max; performance cycling tests of 40 kilometers and 100 kilometers; intermittent, prolonged high-intensity 20-second anaerobic running performance; and prolonged shuttle-run performance tasks comparable to energy expenditure in soccer, basketball, and hockey. Even the study by Blomstrand and others that reported decreased RPE and mental fatigue in endurance-trained cyclists did not find any significant improvement in performance as measured by the total work done in the 20-minute maximal test.

An earlier well-controlled study conducted under heat stress conditions did report an ergogenic effect of BCAA supplementation. Mittleman and others, providing BCAAs (9.4–15.8 grams) as part of a carbohydrate-free drink before and during exercise, reported an increase of 12 percent in cycle time to exhaustion at 40 percent VO_2 peak. Plasma BCAA levels were elevated, but cardiovascular, thermoregulatory, and psychological data were unchanged compared to the placebo condition. They noted that comparison of this study with others must be made with caution because the environmental stress ($95°F$), low exercise intensity, and form of BCAA supplement (without glucose) were unique. Moreover, no specific mechanism underlying the improved performance was proposed. A lack of effect on the RPE does not support the central fatigue hypothesis. Two subsequent studies reported no beneficial effect of BCAA supplementation on exercise in the heat. Watson and others had subjects consume BCAAs in solution before (12 grams) and during (1.8 grams every 15 minutes) a cycling trial to exhaustion at 50 percent VO_2 max in the heat. They reported no effect in performance time, or on heart rate, core or skin temperature. Cheuvront and others induced muscle glycogen depletion and hypohydration in subjects prior to 60 minutes of cycling at 50 percent of VO_2 peak followed by a 30-minute time trial in the heat. A BCAA/carbohydrate solution was consumed during the trial, and although the plasma BCAAs increased 2.5 fold, compared to the carbohydrate solution there was no effect on time-trial performance, nor were cognitive performance, mood, perceived exertion, or perceived thermal comfort affected. These studies indicate that BCAA supplementation does not enhance prolonged exercise performance under warm environmental conditions.

Several earlier reviews provide conflicting opinions regarding the ergogenic effects of acute BCAA supplementation. Davis indicates that most studies show no effects of BCAA supplementation on performance, and Hargreaves and Snow note that BCAA supplementation does not appear to affect fatigue during prolonged exercise. In a review, Meeusen and Wilson conclude that although there is good evidence that brain neurotransmitters can play a role in the development of fatigue during prolonged exercise, nutritional manipulation of these systems through the provision of amino acids has proven largely unsuccessful. Conversely, Blomstrand indicates that ingestion of BCAAs reduces the perceived exertion and mental fatigue during prolonged exercise and improves cognitive performance after the exercise. She suggests also that in some situations BCAA ingestion may improve physical performance, such as during actual competitive races where central fatigue may be more pronounced than in laboratory experiments. Nevertheless, she also notes that more research is needed.

Chronic supplementation   Research regarding the effects of chronic BCAA supplementation on exercise performance is more limited, but in one study conducted at the University of Virginia, researchers reported an improvement in 40-kilometer cycling performance following 14 days of BCAA supplementation. Several other studies used a commercial supplement containing BCAAs along with glutamine and carnitine. In general, these laboratory studies reported no significant effects on total time to complete a simulated half-Ironman triathlon (2-km swim; 90-km bike; 21-km run), prolonged aerobic endurance exercise at 65 percent VO_2 max, or cycle ergometer time to exhaustion at 120 percent VO_2 peak. Although these last three studies have shown no beneficial effect, subjects in the triathlon study ran the last segment 12.8 minutes faster while on the supplement, but this time was not significant due to highly variable performances.

In a more recent study, Crowe and others studied the effect of chronic leucine supplementation, one of the BCAAs, on performance in competitive outrigger canoeists. In a placebo-controlled study, the canoeists who consumed leucine (45 mg/kg/day) over the course of 6 weeks significantly increased upper body power and rowing time to exhaustion at 70–75 percent maximal aerobic power. The average RPE also decreased. These research findings should be considered to be preliminary, and additional research is merited.

Importance of carbohydrate   Although research with BCAA supplementation is merited to help understand the underlying causes of fatigue in prolonged aerobic endurance exercise, endurance athletes apparently do not need to take BCAA supplements in attempts to enhance performance if carbohydrate is available. In most studies that compared carbohydrate solutions, carbohydrate/BCAA solutions, and placebo solutions, both solutions with carbohydrate improved endurance performance compared to the placebo solution, but there were no differences between the carbohydrate solution and the carbohydrate/BCAA solution. In general, the carbohydrate solution attenuates the increase in the fTRP:BCAA ratio, which reduces tryptophan uptake by the brain. However, Davis points out that the mechanism whereby carbohydrate supplementation prevents fatigue during prolonged exercise is not clear; it may prevent fatigue centrally by ameliorating brain functions, or it may prevent fatigue peripherally by providing energy substrate for the contracting muscle.

Most recent reviews evaluating exercise and the central fatigue hypothesis have concluded that although the data are equivocal, in general they suggest that BCAA supplementation is neither ergogenic nor ergolytic. Carbohydrate still appears to be the preferential fuel for athletes to consume before and during prolonged intermittent and continuous endurance exercise tasks.

BCAA supplementation and body composition BCAA supplementation has been theorized to decrease muscle protein breakdown during exercise. In an earlier review, Williams cited some evidence that chronic BCAA supplementation, as part of a low-Calorie diet, was more effective than three other diets as a means for elite wrestlers to lose body fat over a 19-day period. No changes in muscular strength or aerobic and anaerobic capacities were noted, suggesting that exercise performance was maintained even with the greater body fat losses. More recently, Gleeson indicated that no valid scientific evidence supports the commercial claims that orally ingested BCAAs have an anticatabolic effect during and after exercise in humans or that BCAA supplements may accelerate the repair of muscle damage after exercise. Conversely, Blomstrand reported that BCAAs have been found to have anabolic effects in human muscle during recovery from endurance exercise, suggesting that BCAAs activate signaling pathways controlling protein synthesis. In support of this viewpoint, Greer and others reported that consuming 50 grams of BCAAs in a drink, both before and during 90 minutes of cycling at 55 percent VO_2 max, reduced markers of muscle damage and ratings of perceived soreness for 1–2 days in untrained college males. These findings do not appear to be applicable to trained individuals or athletes. Additional research may be desirable.

Glutamine Glutamine, a nonessential amino acid, is the most abundant amino acid in the plasma. Houston indicates that it represents about 60 percent of the body's amino acid pool. Glutamine, like alanine, is synthesized in the muscle tissue, where it is found in high concentrations, and is a major means for removing excess amino groups from the muscle, delivering the amino groups to the liver and kidneys for excretion or reuse of excess nitrogen. It is also an important fuel for the immune system.

Glutamine supplementation, muscle mass, and strength Glutamine appears to be involved in the regulation of a number of metabolic processes important to exercise. Oral glutamine supplementation has been shown to increase HGH levels, and glutamine may also stimulate protein synthesis by increasing muscle cell volume. Abcouwer and Souba noted that patients may be provided nutritional support including glutamine or glutamine precursors to help spare muscle mass. However, several studies indicate that neither short-term nor long-term glutamine supplementation has an ergogenic effect on muscle mass or strength performance. In a double-blind, placebo, short-term crossover study, Antonio and others studied the effects of high-glutamine supplementation (0.3 grams per kilogram) of glycine on exercise performance in resistance-trained men. One hour after ingestion, subjects performed four total sets of exercise to fatigue, but the glutamine supplementation had no significant effect on performance. In another well-designed study, Candow

and others provided glutamine (0.9 grams/kilogram lean tissue mass) or placebo to two groups undertaking 6 weeks of total body resistance training. Although the training increased lean muscle mass and strength, the glutamine supplementation provided no additional benefits. Additionally, alpha-ketoglutarate, a precursor of glutamine, has been theorized to be anabolic, but no data are available to support this theory.

Glutamine supplementation and muscle glycogen Glutamine is also gluconeogenic, and is also involved in glycogen synthesis, two factors that could influence energy production from carbohydrate during prolonged aerobic endurance exercise. However, the limited available data are conflicting. In one study, adding glutamine to a glucose drink did not provide any additional benefits on muscle glycogen resynthesis following muscle glycogen depletion. In another study, adding glutamine to a glucose polymer solution appeared to provide an additive effect on total body carbohydrate storage during recovery from prolonged exercise, possibly increasing liver glycogen levels. However, as noted previously, adding protein to carbohydrate may increase glycogen levels during recovery, and although glutamine may stimulate muscle glycogen synthesis, Hargreaves and Snow noted that it provides no advantage over ingestion of adequate carbohydrate alone.

Glutamine supplementation and immune function Glutamine also is a major fuel for key cells, notably lymphocytes and macrophages, of the immune system. Melis and others indicated that glutamine has a major impact on the functionality of the immune system. In sports, a healthy immune system is theorized to prevent overtraining. In their review, Abcouwer and Souba indicated that glutamine may be considered a conditionally essential amino acid because it may be needed in individuals, such as burn patients, suffering a catabolic insult. This might also include athletes undertaking strenuous exercise and inducing microtrauma to the muscles, a possible contributing factor to the overtraining syndrome.

Overtraining, or staleness, in athletes is characterized by a number of signs and symptoms, referred to as the *overtraining syndrome*. Subjective symptoms such as fatigue, irritability, sleep disturbance, heaviness, and depression are associated with decreases in physical performance. Overtrained athletes are also thought to be more susceptible to various infections, particularly upper respiratory tract infections, possibly because of an impaired immune system.

Several studies have reported a positive association between decreased plasma glutamine levels and overtraining. Parry-Billings and others studied 40 overtrained, international-class athletes at the British Olympic Medical Centre; most of the overtrained athletes were involved in endurance-type events. The investigators noted a decreased plasma glutamine level compared to control athletes not regarded as being overtrained. Kingsbury and others reported similar findings for overtrained elite track and field athletes, as compared to other elite athletes without symptoms of overtraining. In a review, Williams cited research indicating that plasma glutamine levels are decreased in athletes who participate in sport activities predisposing to overtraining, including marathon running and repeated bouts of intensive training. One research group indicated that plasma glutamine may be useful as an indicator of the overtrained state.

Most research with glutamine supplementation in athletes has focused on its role to affect favorably markers of immune function or to prevent signs and symptoms of overtraining, particularly upper respiratory tract infections. Williams notes that both animal and human studies provide conflicting data regarding beneficial effects of glutamine supplementation before, during, or after exercise. For example, some research revealed a lower incidence of infections during the 7 days following intense exercise bouts in various athletic groups who consumed a glutamine-supplemented drink (81 percent with no infections) compared to those taking a placebo drink (49 percent with no infections) immediately after and 2 hours after the exercise bout. The investigators suggested these effects are possibly associated with an apparent increase in specific lymphocyte cells. However, this same investigative group reported no beneficial effects of glutamine supplementation on lymphocyte distribution following the Brussels Marathon. Additionally, other investigators reported that although glutamine supplementation helped to maintain plasma glutamine levels following prolonged aerobic exercise, no beneficial effects on lymphocyte function were noted.

Although some investigators have suggested that carbohydrate intake may counter glutamine depletion, a well-controlled study by van Hall and others indicated that carbohydrate intake during prolonged exercise (cycling to exhaustion) did not prevent the normal decrease in plasma glutamine concentration during recovery. In contrast, Gleeson and others indicated that a low-carbohydrate diet over 3 days is associated with a greater fall in plasma glutamine levels during recovery from exercise. Thus, as documented previously, adequate daily carbohydrate intake appears to be a sound dietary strategy for most athletes.

Castell cited some preliminary data indicating that glutamine supplementation may reduce the self-reported incidence of illness in endurance athletes following prolonged exercise. Based on such findings, Antonio and Street speculated that glutamine has potential utility as a dietary supplement for athletes engaged in heavy exercise training. Although such a recommendation may be prudent, confirming data are needed to provide more solid scientific support. In reviews, Hargreaves and Snow, Nieman, along with Akerström and Pedersen, indicated that there is little support from controlled studies to recommend glutamine supplementation for enhanced immune function and prevention of upper respiratory tract infections.

In summary, Phillips notes that although glutamine is a popular dietary supplement consumed for purported ergogenic benefits of increased strength, quicker recovery, decreased frequency of respiratory infections, and prevention of overtraining, the available studies regarding glutamine supplementation and exercise performance show a lack of evidence for such benefits.

Aspartates Potassium and magnesium aspartate are salts of aspartic acid, a nonessential amino acid. Although the mechanism has not been clearly documented, these substances have been postulated to improve aerobic and anaerobic exercise performance, possibly by enhancing fatty acid metabolism and thereby sparing glycogen, by reducing accumulation of ammonia (metabolic by-product of protein), or simply by improving psychological motivation. The ammonia hypothesis has been tested in several studies since increases in serum ammonia have been associated with muscular fatigue, although, as noted previously, the mechanism is not clear.

Research findings relative to the ergogenic effect of acute short-term supplementation of aspartates are equivocal. A number of both early and contemporary studies have reported no beneficial effects of aspartate supplementation. For example, Maughan and Sadler had eight males ride to exhaustion on a bicycle ergometer at 75–80 percent of their VO_2 max following either a placebo or 3,000 milligrams each of potassium and magnesium aspartate consumed in the 24 hours prior to testing. No beneficial effects upon blood concentrations of energy substrates or ammonia were found, nor were any significant effects on physiological or psychological variables important to aerobic exercise performance reported. In an anaerobic exercise task, Tuttle and others reported no significant effect of aspartate supplementation (approximately 10 grams) on plasma ammonia concentrations, ratings of perceived exertion during a resistance training workout, or performance in a bench press repetition test to failure at 65 percent of maximal bench press strength. As noted earlier, chronic supplementation with aspartate (8.7 grams/day for 4 months) had no effect on peak oxygen uptake or cycling endurance to exhaustion.

However, an equal number of early and contemporary studies have found some beneficial applications of aspartates. Although several of these studies possessed flaws in experimental design, increases in aerobic endurance of 21–50 percent have been reported. Wesson and others, using a double-blind, placebo protocol, revealed that the ingestion of 10 grams of aspartates over a 24-hour period increased endurance capacity by more than 15 percent when subjects exercised at 75 percent of their VO_2 max. These researchers also reported increased blood levels of free fatty acids and decreased levels of blood ammonia.

In a review, Trudeau noted that the effect of aspartate supplementation on endurance seems generally favorable in humans, but the underlying mechanism for performance enhancement has not been confirmed. It appears that additional quality research is needed to evaluate the ability of aspartates to exert an ergogenic effect. Dosage may be a key factor, as dosages of about 10 grams have usually been associated with improved performance.

Glycine Glycine is a nonessential amino acid. Because it is involved in the formation of creatine, and hence phosphocreatine (PCr), it could theoretically be an ergogenic aid. Gelatin, an incomplete protein, is composed of approximately 25 percent glycine, and thus also has been ascribed ergogenic qualities. Several studies conducted more than a half-century ago suggested a beneficial effect of glycine or gelatin supplementation on various measures of strength, but the experiments were poorly designed. More contemporary research with proper experimental design and relatively large doses of glycine revealed no beneficial effects on physical performance. However, although glycine supplementation has not been shown to be ergogenic, direct supplementation with creatine may induce favorable effects, as noted below.

Glycine is the first-listed ingredient in glycine-arginine-alpha-ketoisocaproic acid (GAKIC), which has been theorized to enhance muscle performance by favorably modifying protein metabolism by use of amino acids (glycine, arginine) combined with ketoacids (alpha-ketoisocaproic acid). Previous research has supported its use to increase muscle strength, and a well-designed study by Buford and Koch also provides some support for its potential to enhance anaerobic performance. Subjects consumed 11.2 grams of GAKIC prior to five supramaximal 10-second cycle ergometer sprints, separated by 1-minute rest intervals. The GAKIC treatment produced a greater retention of mean power between sprints 1 and 2, but no significant differences were noted among the other trials. The investigators suggested that the data supported an ergogenic effect of GAKIC. However, these data should be considered preliminary, and additional research is merited to support these findings.

Chondroitin and Glucosamine Chondroitin and glucosamine are derived from connective tissue, and each has been marketed as a dietary supplement, either separately or in combination, to help promote healthy joints in individuals who exercise. Gelatin, also derived from connective tissue, has also been advertised to promote joint health. Although weight-bearing or resistance exercise training has not been shown to cause excessive wear-and-tear on healthy joints, and may actually improve joint health, some dietary supplement entrepreneurs may suggest otherwise. In a sense, if a dietary supplement could prevent joint pain, and thus promote optimal exercise training, it could be considered ergogenic.

Both chondroitin and glucosamine may be synthesized in the human body from amino acids and other nutrients, and both are found in human cartilage, one of the main components involved in joint health. Glucosamine is believed to help form compounds, such as proteoglycans, that form the structural basis for cartilage, while chondroitin is part of a protein that helps cartilage hold water to give it elasticity and resiliency. Cartilage serves as a kind of shock absorber, and prevents bone-to-bone contact. Excessive wear of cartilage leads to osteoarthritis, a painful joint condition. Dietary supplements of chondroitin are made from cattle cartilage, while those of glucosamine are made from shellfish. Different salt forms of supplements are available, such as sulfate and hydrochloride. Theoretically, such supplements will help maintain normal cartilage levels and prevent development of osteoarthritis. Schardt notes that by 2030, one out of every four American adults will have doctor-diagnosed arthritis.

Numerous studies have investigated the role of chondroitin and/or glucosamine supplementation on symptoms of arthritic pain. However, the results are equivocal. For example, Hughes and Carr found that glucosamine sulfate (1,500 milligrams daily for 6 months) was no more effective than a placebo in modifying pain symptoms in patients with osteoarthritis of the knee. In contrast, in a well-controlled, 3-year study using American College of Rheumatology criteria, Pavelka and others evaluated the progression of knee osteoarthritis following either ingestion of glucosamine sulfate (1,500 mg daily) or a placebo. Given some

beneficial effects on joint space narrowing and symptoms including pain, function, and stiffness, they concluded that long-term treatment with glucosamine sulfate retarded the progression of knee osteoarthritis.

The National Institutes of Health funded a large multicenter clinical study called GAIT (Glucosamine/Chondroitin Arthritis Intervention Trial) designed to provide a clearer picture of the role that these dietary supplements, both separately and in combination, may play in the treatment of osteoarthritis. Nearly 1,600 subjects, with an average age of 59 and experiencing arthritic knee pain, were assigned to receive daily either 1,500 mg of glucosamine hydrochloride, 1,200 mg of chondroitin sulfate, both glucosamine hydrochloride and chondroitin sulfate, 200 mg of an anti-inflammatory drug, or placebo for 24 weeks. Although the glucosamine/chondroitin combination did provide relief to a subset of patients with moderate-to-severe knee pain, the investigators considered these findings to be preliminary and recommended additional research. However, overall the findings indicated that glucosamine, chondroitin, or the glucosamine/chondroitin combination did not reduce knee pain in patients with osteoarthritis more than a placebo.

The NIH study was designed to provide a definitive answer regarding the efficacy of such dietary supplements to reduce arthritic pain, but it did not. In a review designed to determine why studies with glucosamine came up with such divergent findings, Vlad and others found that trials using glucosamine sulfate produced more positive results than studies using glucosamine hydrochloride. They concluded that glucosamine hydrochloride was not effective. In a meta-analysis with a similar purpose, Reginster and others noted that one of the major differences between studies with different results was the form of glucosamine, and they noted that glucosamine sulfate supplementation provided the most compelling evidence as a potential for providing symptomatic relief and inhibiting the progression of osteoarthritis. Herrero-Beaumont and others note that although the mechanism of action of glucosamine sulfate still remains to be clearly defined, it may help by reducing the effects of pro-inflammatory agents present in osteoarthritis cartilage.

In a meta-analysis of studies regarding the effects of chondroitin supplementation for osteoarthritis of the knee or hip, Reichenbach and others concluded that the benefit of chondroitin supplementation is minimal or nonexistent, and recommended that its use in clinical practice be discouraged. If these findings are valid, the supplements used in the NIH study, particularly glucosamine hydrochloride, may not have been the best choices. Current research suggests that glucosamine sulfate may possess the greatest therapeutic potential.

Most of these supplement studies have been conducted with older people; for example, the average age in the NIH study was almost 60. Few studies have been conducted with younger, athletic subjects. In a well-controlled study, Ostojic and others evaluated the effect of glucosamine sulfate administration on the functional ability and the degree of pain intensity in competitive male athletes after suffering an acute knee injury. More than 100 athletes, with an average age of 25.1 years, received either glucosamine (1,500 mg per day) or a placebo for 28 days. Testing was done weekly. The investigators found no significant differences between the glucosamine and placebo group in mean pain intensity scores for resting and walking and degree of knee swelling at any time. Knee flexibility was unaffected during the first 3 weeks, but in the final test the glucosamine group demonstrated significant improvement in knee flexion and extension as compared with the placebo group. In general, these results suggest that glucosamine supplementation is not effective as a means to treat an acute knee injury, which is not the same as arthritis. In a study of Navy Seals in training, who could certainly be considered fit athletes, a commercial supplement containing both glucosamine and chondroitin did relieve knee pain symptoms in a small group of men with arthritic pain.

Other related dietary supplements have been studied as a means to treat osteoarthritis. SAM-e, short for S-adenosylmethionine, is derived from the essential amino acid methionine, and plays some important metabolic functions in the body, including serving as a possible anti-inflammatory agent. In a recent meta-analysis of 11 studies, Soeken and others concluded that SAM-e appears to be comparable to NSAIDs for treatment of pain and functional limitations, and less likely to report adverse effects. Schardt reiterated these points, but also noted that the doses used were high and could cost as much as $20 daily. Schardt also indicated that the quality of SAM-e dietary supplements available in the United States is variable, with some brands containing less than listed on the label.

Currently, chondroitin, glucosamine, and related supplements are being marketed to those with existing arthritic pain. To our knowledge, there are no data that these supplements will prevent the development of joint pain or osteoarthritis in young, healthy athletes. However, they may be of some benefit to older athletes experiencing joint pain that limits training or competition.

For anyone, particularly those with osteoarthritis, who may want to experiment with chondroitin and glucosamine, Tufts University offers several caveats. First, although these supplements are believed to be safe, they may cause mild side effects, such as bloating or a touch of diarrhea. Second, check with your doctor because there may be some complications. For example, diabetics may react adversely to glucosamine because it may increase insulin resistance. Third, a reasonable dose would be 1,500 milligrams of glucosamine sulfate and 1,200 milligrams of chondroitin daily for about 2–4 months. If pain symptoms have not improved, they probably are not going to. Finally, remember as with most dietary supplements, purity, safety, and effectiveness are not guaranteed.

http://dietarysupplements.nlm.nih.gov/ Type in glucosamine or chondroitin in the search box. Then select the specific brand or active ingredient. Provides details on product ingredients and other information. You may use this Website to research any dietary supplement mentioned in this and other chapters.

Creatine **Creatine** is not an amino acid, but a nitrogen-containing compound known as an *amine*. Creatine is found in some foods, particularly meat products, and it may be formed in the kidney and liver from glycine and arginine. Creatine may be delivered to the muscle, where it may combine readily with phosphate to form phosphocreatine, a high-energy phosphagen in the ATP-PCr energy system that is stored in the muscle. As you may recall, the ATP-PCr energy system is important for rapid energy production, such as in speed and power events. Sahlin and others noted that during very high-intensity exercise, within 10 seconds maximal power output decreases considerably and coincides with depletion of PCr.

Creatine supplements have been marketed to athletes at all levels. They come in various forms (powder, pills, candy, chews, gum, gels, serum, micronized) for both strength and endurance athletes, including products specifically for men, women, and adolescent athletes age 11–19. Relative to the latter, Metzl and others, in a survey of middle and high school athletes ages 10–18 in a New York City suburb, found that creatine is being used by middle and high school athletes at all grades. Use increases with grade level and the prevalence of use by athletes in grades 11 and 12 approaches levels reported among college athletes. The most cited reasons for taking creatine were enhanced performance and appearance. Indeed, creatine continues to be one of the most popular sports supplements of all time.

Although creatine has been known for years to play an important role in energy metabolism, it is only within the past 15 years or so that considerable research has been devoted to evaluate the potential ergogenic effect of creatine supplementation. Numerous studies, several major reviews, and a book focusing on creatine supplementation have been published, and the following represent some of the key points.

Supplementation protocol, effects on total muscle creatine and phosphocreatine (PCr), and theory The average individual needs to replace about 2 grams of creatine per day to maintain normal total creatine and creatine phosphate (PCr). The normal daily intake of creatine approximates 1 gram for those who consume meat, but may be virtually zero for pure vegetarians. Endogenous formation of creatine helps complement dietary sources to achieve 2 grams, but because of inadequate dietary intake, vegetarians may have lower amounts of total creatine in the body. For example, Lukaszuk and others found that switching from a meat-eating diet to a lactoovovegetarian diet for 3 weeks significantly reduced muscle total creatine.

Several supplementation strategies have been used in attempts to increase total body creatine stores. One very effective strategy is to consume a total of 20–30 grams of creatine, usually pure creatine monohydrate, in four equal doses (5–7 grams per dose) over the course of the day (morning, noon, afternoon, evening). Significant effects have been observed even after only 2 days of creatine loading. Paul Greenhaff, one of the pioneering researchers with creatine, noted that this supplementation protocol will enhance muscle creatine storage. Excessive amounts will not be stored but, as noted by Burke and others, excesses will be excreted unchanged in the urine. Longer-term supplementation with lower doses, such as 4 weeks at a dose of 3 grams per day, has been shown to be as equally effective. However, one study providing 2 grams per day for 6 weeks showed no beneficial effects on either muscle creatine stores or PCr levels.

Subjects may be responders or nonresponders. Research by Burke and others, in a study with vegetarians, found that individuals with initially low levels of intramuscular creatine are more responsive to supplementation, while Syrotuik and Bell identified several characteristics of nonresponders, such as higher initial levels of creatine and phosphocreatine before loading and fewer type II muscle fibers. However, Green and others have shown that combining creatine with a simple carbohydrate, such as glucose, will increase creatine transport into the muscle even in subjects with near-normal levels of muscle creatine, possibly via an insulin-mediated effect. The solution used in Green's study consisted of 5 grams of creatine and about 90 grams of simple carbohydrate, consumed 4 times per day. However, Preen and others found that a smaller amount of glucose (1 gram per kilogram body weight), taken with only two of four daily 5-gram creatine doses, increased muscle creatine stores significantly more than creatine supplementation alone. This loading protocol may be useful for those who may want to cut the carbohydrate intake by 50 percent or more. Once creatine is in the muscle, it is locked there and gradually disappears over several weeks.

In general, although not all studies are in agreement, well-controlled research by Greenhaff, Harris, Casey, and their associates has shown that an appropriate creatine-loading protocol will increase total muscle creatine, including free creatine and PCr. In their book, Williams, Kreider, and Branch reviewed more than 20 studies, and reported an average 18.5 percent increase in total muscle creatine, and an average 20.7 percent increase in PCr. Preen and others found that, once loaded, total muscle creatine levels could be maintained with creatine doses of 2–5 grams per day.

Most of the creatine in the body is found in the muscles, and Casey and others suggest that any performance benefits may be related to increased creatine within type II muscle fibers. About 60 percent of the total muscle creatine is PCr, and the remainder is free creatine. Theoretically, according to Casey and Greenhaff, increasing the amount of PCr will provide more substrate for generating ATP during high-intensity exercise, and higher levels of free creatine will help resynthesize PCr. Additionally, Yquel and others, using magnetic resonance to evaluate PCr levels during repeated bouts of maximal plantar flexion exercise, found that creatine supplementation increased muscle power by about 5 percent. They noted that this effect could be attributed to a higher rate of phosphocreatine resynthesis, which would provide more PCr for ATP resynthesis.

In essence, increased muscle phosphocreatine and free creatine may enhance the potential of the ATP-PCr energy system and provide the athlete with an edge in competitive events involving very high-intensity exercise performance. Moreover, the enhanced ATP-PCr energy system may permit more intensive training. Volek and others found that creatine supplementation appears to be effective for maintaining muscular performance during the initial phase of high-volume resistance training, possibly deterring overreaching and the associated small decrements in performance. Enhanced training should translate into enhanced competitive performance.

Effect on exercise performance Research regarding the effects of creatine supplementation on exercise performance continues at a solid pace. Most research has investigated the effect of creatine supplementation on short-term, maximal exercise tasks of less than 30 seconds, those highly dependent on the ATP-PCr energy system, which may be referred to as *anaerobic power*. Many studies also incorporated repetitive exercise tasks with short recovery intervals, which could evaluate the possible effect of enhanced PCr resynthesis during recovery. However, some research has also investigated the effect of creatine supplementation on exercise performance tasks of somewhat longer duration, including anaerobic endurance, that would be dependent on the lactic acid energy system (anaerobic glycolysis) and aerobic endurance that would be dependent on the oxygen energy system (aerobic glycolysis).

ATP-PCr energy system Research involving the effects of creatine supplementation on strength and power continues at a steady pace. As with most research evaluating the effectiveness of ergogenic aids, all studies are not in agreement. However, many studies with creatine, conducted at some leading universities throughout the world, have provided some strong evidence supportive of a positive ergogenic effect of creatine supplementation in certain exercise endeavors, primarily those characterized by repetitive high-intensity exercise bouts with brief recovery periods. Using appropriate research methodology, recent studies have shown significant improvement in the following exercise tasks following creatine supplementation.

- Improvement in total and maximal force in repetitive isometric muscle contractions
- Improvement in muscular strength and endurance in isotonic strength tests, including 1-RM tests
- Improvement in muscular force/torque and endurance in isokinetic strength testing
- Improvement in cycle ergometer performance in maximal tests ranging from 6 to 30 seconds

In their book, Williams, Kreider, and Branch note that approximately 75 percent of the studies reported beneficial effects of creatine supplementation on isotonic strength and endurance and cycle ergometer power and endurance, while about 50 percent of the studies revealed ergogenic effects on isometric and isokinetic tests of muscular strength, power, and endurance. All of these test protocols involved laboratory procedures, although some of the isotonic strength tests, such as the bench press, could be analogous to the sport of competitive weightlifting. Most studies involved males, but studies with females also reported improved performance. Studies continue to provide supportive evidence of the ergogenicity of creatine supplementation.

The effects of creatine supplementation on field performance tests, such as jumping, running, swimming, skating, and other miscellaneous events, are less consistent, but overall still generally favorable. For example, of 15 studies evaluating the effect of creatine supplementation on single or repetitive sprint-run, sprint-swim, or sprint-cycle performance ranging from 5 to 100 meters or up to 30 seconds duration, creatine supplementation improved performance in 8 of the trials, but had no effect in the other 7. For example, Skare and others, using a standard creatine-loading protocol with well-trained male sprinters as subjects, reported significant improvements in 100-meter sprint velocity and time to complete 6 intermittent 60-meter sprints. Additionally, Preen and others studied the effect of a 5-day creatine-loading protocol on long-term repetitive sprints, doing 10 sets of multiple 6-second bike sprints with varying periods of recovery in an 80-minute time frame. Muscle biopsies revealed increased total creatine and PCr following supplementation, and both peak power and total work production were increased significantly. Conversely, Op 'T Eijnde and others reported no significant improvement in a 70-meter shuttle run sprint power test by well-trained tennis players following a standard 5-day creatine-loading protocol.

Some of these findings have a direct application to sports competition, such as an increased 1-RM performance in weight lifting, faster 50-yard swim times, and faster 100-meter sprint run times. The laboratory findings for other types of exercise performance are also rather strong, and do support a possible application to actual field competitions. For example, Preen and others noted that the findings from their study could suggest improved performance in intermittent high-intensity sports, such as soccer.

In this regard, several investigators have designed laboratory-controlled exercise protocols designed to mimic an actual sport event. Romer and others, in a well-controlled placebo, crossover study with competitive squash players, found that creatine loading for 5 days enhanced performance in an exercise protocol involving high-intensity, intermittent exercise involving 10 sets of simulated positional play to mimic squash. Creatine supplementation improved mean set sprint time by 3.2 percent compared to the placebo condition. The authors concluded that this study provides evidence that oral creatine supplementation improves exercise performance in competitive squash players. In one of the few studies with creatine supplementation conducted with young athletes, Ostojic reported enhanced performance in various soccer-related performance tests, such as sprint-power times and dribble test times, in 16-year-old soccer players. In a related study, Cox and others studied the effects of creatine supplementation on an exercise test protocol designed to simulate match play in soccer. The test involved 5 blocks of 11-minute exercise involving sprint running, agility runs, and a precision ball-kicking drill interspersed with recovery walks, jogs, and runs. Creatine supplementation improved performance in some repeated sprint and agility tasks even though the subjects increased body mass, but the creatine had no effect on ball-kicking accuracy.

Thus, creatine supplementation might improve speed in repetitive sprints, important for many sports, but may not necessarily enhance sports skills. In support of this viewpoint, Op 'T Eijnde and others, in the study cited previously with well-trained tennis players, reported no significant effects of creatine loading on tennis stroke performance as measured by power and precision of their serves.

Kirkendall suggests the available research is not applicable to the actual style of running in soccer and indicates that because so much of the running in soccer is at less than maximal sprinting speed, creatine supplementation likely provides no benefit for match performance. It certainly is difficult to study the effect of nutritional interventions on actual game performance. However, one might rationalize that if additional phosphocreatine could provide a slight advantage in speed at a critical point during a match, it might make the difference in the outcome of the contest. In their review, Hespel and others indicated that creatine may be useful for soccer.

Available research suggests that prolonged supplementation with maintenance doses of creatine may not provide any additional performance-enhancing advantage compared to a 5-day creatine-loading protocol. Peyrebrune and others reported that 5 days of creatine loading (20 grams/day) improved performance time of elite swimmers in eight 50-yard repeat swims. Swimmers were then assigned to either a creatine-maintenance dose (3 grams/day) or placebo for 22–27 weeks of additional swim training. Following the training period, all subjects again followed the creatine-loading protocol and repeated the 50-yard swim protocol. There was no statistically significant difference in performance times between the two groups, suggesting that the maintenance protocol was not necessary if the athlete undergoes a creatine-loading protocol prior to performance.

Lactic acid energy system Theoretically, increasing muscle PCr concentration could possibly buffer acidity and mitigate the effect of lactic acid production on muscle contraction, thus improving anaerobic endurance performance in events of maximal exercise ranging from about 30 to 150 seconds. Fewer studies are available, but creatine supplementation has been reported to benefit performance in some anaerobic endurance tests, including maximal isometric and isotonic muscular work output, cycle ergometer work output, running performance in 300 meters, and treadmill run to exhaustion at intensities greater than 100 percent VO_2 max. However, the vast majority of the studies reported no beneficial effect of creatine supplementation on 100-meter swim performance.

Overall, approximately 50 percent of the studies evaluating anaerobic endurance have shown some improvement in performance following creatine supplementation. The results are not as consistent as those shown for anaerobic power, but do provide some evidence that creatine supplementation may be helpful in more prolonged anaerobic endurance events, such as a 400- or 800-meter track race. More research is needed to document this effect.

Oxygen system There appears to be little theoretical support for a beneficial effect of creatine supplementation on more prolonged exercise endeavors, those lasting more than several minutes and depending primarily upon aerobic endurance capacity. However, some investigators have suggested that creatine supplementation could modify substrate availability to improve performance, or could benefit athletes who perform repeated sprints during their overall aerobic endurance events, such as cycling sprints during a triathlon.

Several studies have reported ergogenic effects on exercise performance tasks greater than 3 minutes in duration, such as repeat 1,000-meter runs and a 1,000-meter rowing event. However, these tasks may still depend somewhat on anaerobic metabolism, particularly in sprints near the end, and thus performance may be improved as noted previously. Some evidence also indicates that creatine supplementation may benefit anaerobic sprint performance within an overall aerobic endurance event, but confirming data are needed.

There is little scientific support for the idea that creatine supplementation benefits VO$_2$ max, energy metabolism when running or cycling at 50–90 percent of VO$_2$ max, or performance in exercise tasks of longer duration—those that depend primarily on aerobic glycolysis or lipolysis, such as endurance cycling. However, endurance sports such as cycling, often have periods of sprinting either during or at the end of a race. For example, Vandebuerie and colleagues showed improved sprint capacity after a 2.5 hour endurance ride following creatine ingestion. Similarly, Engelhardt and others reported increased sprint power during and endurance ride in creatine supplemented subjects. More recently, Hickner and colleagues reported that creatine supplementation caused a 10 percent decrease in oxygen consumption near the end of a 2 hour cycling ride, but no increase in performance in the sprint that followed. Although there are few studies, it appears that there may be a benefit of creatine supplementation for some endurance athletes, such as cyclists, who must also sprint as part of their sport.

As noted previously, creatine supplementation has been shown to improve performance in interval run repeats of 300 and 1,000 meters. If creatine supplementation could help an athlete train more effectively at shorter distances, conceivably performance in longer distances might eventually be improved. However, the available research does not support this hypothesis. In a placebo-controlled study, Syrotuik and others trained competitive rowers for 6 weeks with both rowing and resistance training. The creatine group consumed a standard 5-day loading protocol followed by a 5-week standard maintenance dose. Although the training significantly improved body composition, VO$_2$ max, repeated power interval performance, and 2,000-meter rowing times in both groups, the creatine provided no additional advantage.

One possible application of creatine loading for the endurance athlete, as reported by Santos and others, is prevention of muscle soreness. Following a typical creatine-loading protocol with experienced marathon runners, they found reduced markers of muscle cell damage and inflammation after a 30-kilometer race. No performance difference between the creatine and control group was noted. Confirmation of these findings is recommended.

Effect on body mass The effect of creatine supplementation on body mass has been studied on both a short-term and long-term basis. More than 50 studies have shown an increase in body mass during the first week of creatine supplementation, and most of these studies suggest that the gains in body mass may be associated with water retention in the muscles. Increased creatine content in the muscle draws water.

Evaluation of the effects of long-term creatine supplementation on body mass has been conducted primarily with strength-trained individuals, or athletes training specific to their sport. Of approximately 20 studies, 80 percent provided evidence of significant gains in either total body mass or lean body mass. Many of these studies used carbohydrate as the placebo, but Tarnopolsky and others were one of the first to use protein, which may be a more appropriate placebo. They compared a creatine-dextrose supplement (10 grams creatine; 75 grams dextrose) with a protein-dextrose supplement (10 grams casein; 75 grams dextrose) on body mass, body composition, and strength over 8 weeks of resistance training in untrained young men. Both groups increased lean body mass and strength in a similar fashion, but the creatine-dextrose group experienced a significantly greater gain in body mass (4.3 kilograms) compared to the protein-dextrose group (1.9 kilograms). The authors note that the greater body mass gains may have implications for certain sports.

The increase in muscle mass may be associated with a creatine supplementation-induced ability to do more repetitions during training, which may induce favorable genetic adaptations. Willoughby and Rosene studied the effect of 12 weeks of creatine supplementation and resistance training on muscular strength and myosin heavy chain (MHC) mRNA and protein expression. Compared to both a control and placebo group, the creatine group significantly increased fat-free mass and strength. Additionally, they found that in general the MHC mRNA and protein expression were significantly higher in the creatine group compared to the other groups, and suggested that the increased strength and muscle size associated with creatine supplementation may be attributed to increased MHC synthesis. Olsen and others found that strength training increased the proportion of satellite cell number and myonuclei concentration in human skeletal muscle fibers, thereby allowing enhanced muscle fiber growth, but significantly greater enhancements were observed with creatine supplementation during the early phases of training. Other research, such as the study by Deldicque and others, indicated that creatine supplementation may favorably affect signaling pathways, such as those involving insulin-like growth factor (IGF), in the muscle. These cellular mechanisms may underline the research finding, as determined by muscle biopsy techniques, that creatine supplementation augments the increases in muscle cell diameter normally found after weeks of resistance training.

Rockwell and others found that during voluntary weight loss, creatine supplementation maintained anaerobic performance better than a placebo. However, in another study, creatine supplementation made it more difficult for weight-control athletes to lose weight for competition. This could produce adverse health effects if athletes would resort to more drastic weight-cutting methods, a topic covered in chapter 10.

Caffeine and creatine In research from Peter Hespel's laboratory in Belgium, Vandenberghe and others have shown that when caffeine, about 2.5 milligrams per kilogram body weight, is consumed with creatine, the caffeine negates the potential ergogenic effect of creatine. In their studies, both creatine and creatine with caffeine increased muscle creatine and PCr stores, but muscular performance improved only with the creatine supplement. In subsequent research, Hespel and others found that caffeine intake prolongs muscle relaxation time following muscle contraction and thus overrides the shortening of the relaxation time due to creatine supplementation. However, some of the early studies that revealed an ergogenic effect of creatine supplementation reportedly used coffee, with naturally occurring caffeine, as the mixing solution to deliver the creatine. Moreover, Doherty and others found that caffeine still provided an ergogenic effect in subjects who had followed a standard creatine-loading protocol and abstained from daily caffeine during the conduct of the study. Subjects performed three treadmill runs to exhaustion at 125 percent of VO_2 max, including a baseline test before creatine supplementation and a placebo and caffeine trial after supplementation. Compared to the baseline and placebo trials, caffeine significantly increased run time to exhaustion, and the rating of perceived exertion was also lower at 90 seconds during the treadmill run, suggesting the ergogenic effects were attributed partly to psychological effects. However, one might note that this exercise protocol primarily involves anaerobic glycolysis, not the ATP-PCr energy system, which might be more dependent on rapid rates of muscle relaxation during very high intensity, repetitive exercise tasks.

Because some athletes may take both creatine and caffeine in attempts to enhance performance, these preliminary findings merit additional research to substantiate this possible detrimental effect of caffeine.

Formulation A number of different formulations and types of creatine supplements are available for sale (e.g. liquid, complexed with other compounds, etc.). Typically, these products are marketed as having better absorption than creatine monohydrate, of which >99 percent is absorbed. Many of these products are also marketed as being safer than creatine monohydrate, which has an excellent and well documented safety profile. Typically, these products are also advertised as being more effective than creatine monohydrate. These claims are largely unsubstantiated. The most comprehensive review of different creatine supplement formulations was published by Jäger and others. They note that although products are marketed with claims of better bioavailability, safety, or efficacy, compared to creatine monohydrate there is little to no evidence to support these claims. Additionally, while creatine monohydrate is well absorbed and tolerated, some of these creatine supplements are pro-creatinine or contain very little creatine at all. At this point in time, given the enormous amount of data on the safety and efficacy of creatine monohydrate, it is unadvisable to recommend a different creatine formulation.

Safety The safety of creatine monohydrate supplementation has been thoroughly reviewed by several experts including Persky and Rawson, Gualano and others, and Casa, Armstrong, Maresh and colleagues. Gualano and colleagues note that there are several hundred published studies and millions of exposures to creatine monohydrate supplements, and creatine supplementation maintains an excellent record of safety. Although creatine monohydrate supplements are viewed as safe when taken in recommended doses, misinformation persists about the safety of creatine supplements. The interested reader can refer to these comprehensive reviews, which cover the safety of creatine supplementation on renal, muscular, and thermoregulatory systems. Below are summaries of some of the individual studies that have investigated the effects of creatine monohydrate supplementation.

Kidney and liver function The breakdown product of creatine is creatinine, which is excreted by the kidneys. Individuals with impaired kidney function may be at risk, but there appears to be little danger to those with healthy kidneys who follow recommended supplementation protocols. None of the studies using creatine

supplements for up to 12 weeks have reported any acute adverse side effects, nor did several long-term studies. Schilling and others evaluated the health effects of creatine supplementation on 3 groups of athletes from various sports. Groups included those who did not use creatine, those who used it about a year, and those who used it more than a year. The mean loading dose was 13.7 grams and the mean maintenance dose was 9.7 grams. All group means for standard clinical examination of complete blood count, 27 blood chemistries, and hormone levels fell within normal clinical range. Mayhew and others recruited 10 American football players who consumed, on an average, about 14 grams of creatine per day for approximately 3 years. They reported no differences in tests of kidney or liver function as compared to a control group of football players, and concluded that long-term creatine supplementation has no detrimental effects on kidney or liver functions in highly trained college athletes. Poortmans and Francaux, in a study that evaluated kidney function in several individuals who consumed creatine over a period of 10 months to 5 years, also reported no adverse effects. Although some individual case studies have associated kidney problems with creatine supplementation, Poortmans noted that these studies did not show definitively that creatine supplementation was the cause. For example, in one case study the individual had a preexisting kidney problem.

In a review, Kim and colleagues concluded that liver and kidney function are not affected in healthy subjects supplemented with creatine, even after several months. However, those with pre-existing renal disease or those with potential risk of renal malfunction are cautioned not to consume creatine supplements at a dosage of more than 3–5 grams/day.

Gastrointestinal distress Creatine supplementation has also been associated with gastrointestinal (GI) distress, including nausea, vomiting, and diarrhea. However, most studies do not report such effects with recommended creatine-loading protocols. Ostojic and Ahmetovic examined the GI effects on top-level soccer players after providing them with either creatine (2×5 grams or 1×10 grams) or a placebo for 28 days. There was a significantly higher incidence of diarrhea with the 10-gram creatine dose (55.6 percent) compared to the 2×5 gram dose (28.6 percent) and the placebo (35 percent). Thus, GI stress of creatine may depend on the dose consumed. Creatine is often consumed along with glucose, and high glucose loads can cause GI distress. Consuming a large dose of creatine just before an event may also cause problems. It should be noted that there is no need to use such a practice, as it has not been shown to enhance performance.

Dehydration, muscle cramps and tears Bailes and others suggested that creatine supplementation could contribute to subclinical dehydration and heatstroke in selected individuals. Theoretically, an increase in intramuscular water content could dilute electrolytes, possibly leading to cramps, and a tightened musculature associated with intracellular swelling could predispose to muscle tears. Although some anecdotal reports indicate that creatine supplementation may lead to these health problems, most controlled studies do not. For example, Jeff Volek, an expert on creatine metabolism, studied the effect of a 7-day creatine-loading protocol on physiological responses to exercise in the heat and reported no adverse effects on thermoregulatory processes or other heat-related health problems, such as muscle cramping. Mendel and others also reported that a standard 5-day loading protocol did not have a negative effect on thermoregulatory responses during exercise in the heat at 39°C (102°F). In their study cited previously, Schilling and others also reported no differences in the reported incidence of muscle injury, cramps, or other adverse side effects. In their review, Lopez and others found no substantial evidence of detrimental effects on heat dissipation or body fluid balance with creatine supplementation (20–25 g/day) taken over 5–28 days. Moreover, Kilduff and others found that creatine supplementation, by inducing greater water retention, reduced the heart rate and rectal temperature during prolonged exercise in the heat, resulting in a more efficient thermoregulatory response. Dalbo and others examined creatine supplementation leading to muscle cramps and dehydration. In their review, they found no evidence that creatine supplementation increases the risk or dehydration or muscle cramps. Instead, they found that creatine supplementation may decrease the risk of dehydration during exercise by enhancing total body water, decreasing exercise core temperature, and lowering exercise heart rate and sweat rate.

However, Schroeder and others found that creatine supplementation (6 days of loading and 28 days of maintenance) with typical dosages significantly increased anterior compartment pressure in the lower leg after the 6-day loading protocol, both at rest and following 20 minutes of running, and these pressures remained elevated during the maintenance period. The authors noted that these pressures were abnormal. Hile and colleagues supplemented the diet of subjects with 21.6 grams of creatine per day for 7 days. On day 7, the subjects performed 2 hours of submaximal cycling followed by an 80-minute heat tolerance test. This loading dose of creatine increased anterior compartment pressures, but these pressure changes were temporary. Additionally, the 7-day loading dose did not produce symptoms associated with anterior compartment syndrome, such as aching, cramping, burning pain, or tightness in the lower leg or anterior compartment.

Medical applications Gualano and others report that creatine monohydrate supplementation can benefit individuals suffering from a variety of diseases, including myopathies, neurodegenerative disorders, cancer, rheumatic diseases, and type 2 diabetes. Although the progression of some diseases is not slowed by creatine supplements, for instance Parkinson's disease, the safety profile remains good, even in vulnerable patient populations. Certainly, more research needs to be conducted on the effects of creatine supplements on patient populations who can benefit from increased strength, resistance to fatigue, or increase is body mass. The world's leading creatine researchers meet about every 5 years to discuss advancements in the field. Typically, a summary article or review articles are published highlighting new findings. The interested reader can visit "http://www.creatineconference2015.com/" www.creatineconference2015.com to examine the latest research topics on medical applications of creatine supplements, and then watch for publications from the conference to be published in a peer reviewed journal in the future.

Creatine supplementation may be useful in rehabilitation from musculoskeletal injury, including athletic injuries. Peter Hespel, a renowned creatine researcher, and his associates evaluated the potential of creatine supplementation during the rehabilitation process for disuse atrophy. In a remarkable double-blind, placebo-controlled study, they casted the right leg of subjects for 2 weeks to induce disuse atrophy. The subjects then participated in a 10-week rehabilitation program for knee extension, with some subjects taking creatine and others the placebo. As expected, the casting decreased both the cross-sectional area of the quadriceps muscle and knee extension strength. During the rehabilitation period, the creatine subjects recovered muscle size and strength at a faster rate than the placebo group, suggesting that creatine supplementation may be an effective adjunct in various forms of rehabilitative therapy. However, creatine supplementation may not facilitate the rehabilitative process for all injuries; Tyler and others reported no effect on recovery from anterior cruciate ligament (ACL) reconstruction.

Creatine supplementation may also be important to help prevent the loss of muscle mass, or sarcopenia, associated with aging. Bemben and Lamont indicate that creatine supplementation affects muscle strength development regardless of sex or age, and Candow and Chilibeck suggest that creatine supplementation may be an important consideration in resistance training programs for older individuals as a means to preserve muscle mass, muscular strength, and muscular endurance to help prevent falls and fractures and to enhance performance in activities of daily living.

Given these overall findings, the role of creatine supplementation as medical therapy appears to hold promise, but additional controlled research is needed to substantiate some of these preliminary findings.

Summary Several major reviews have appeared in recent years, and most suggest that creatine supplementation may enhance performance in events where the amount of PCr may be a limiting factor. The ergogenic effect of creatine appears to be due to the greater stores of PCr, but may also involve a greater resynthesis of PCr during recovery between exercise bouts. The International Society of Sports Nutrition, in a position stand developed by Buford and others, stated that creatine monohydrate is the most effective ergogenic nutritional supplement currently available to athletes in terms of increasing high-intensity exercise capacity, such as those primarily dependent on PCr, and increasing lean body mass during training. For additional details on the effects of creatine supplementation on strength, resistance to fatigue, muscle mass, and exercise performance, the interest reader is referred to meta-analyses by Branch and by Lanhers, narrative reviews by Kreider, Rawson and Clark on, Rawson and Volek, and Volek and Rawson, and the book by Williams, Kreider, and Branch.

HMB (Beta-Hydroxy-Beta-Methylbutyrate) Beta-hydroxy-beta-methylbutyrate (**HMB**) is not a nutrient per se, but a by-product of leucine metabolism in the human body. The body produces about 0.2–0.4 gram of HMB per day depending on dietary leucine intake. HMB is marketed as a dietary supplement in the form of calcium-HMB or HMB free acid (HMB-FA), mostly to strength power athletes. HMB supplementation is theorized to increase lean muscle mass, decrease body fat, increase muscle strength, and reduce muscle damage. Although the underlying mechanism is not known, investigators who developed HMB speculate that it may inhibit the breakdown of muscle tissue during strenuous exercise. Initially, in attempts to increase the nutritional quality of animal meat, research with various farm animals indicated that HMB supplementation may increase lean muscle mass and decrease body fat.

About 40 human HMB supplementation studies have been published, and several extensive reviews are available. Compared to creatine monohydrate and beta alanine (discussed later in this chapter), which have consistently been shown to be ergogenic, the literature on HMB is much more difficult to interpret. One reason for this is that there are large differences in the methods and populations used to study HMB supplementation. Another reason is that some of the studies focus n muscle damage, while others focus on outcomes like gains in lean body mass or strength.

Several years ago, in a small meta-analysis of 9 studies, Nissen and Sharp concluded that HMB supplementation reduced muscle damage and increased strength and lean body mass. However, subsequent studies failed to support these initial conclusions. More recently, Molfino and colleagues reviewed the effects of HMB supplementation in young adults from 22 studies and reported that HMB supplementation increased lean body mass and strength in only about half of the studies. Similar findings from the review by Zanchi and colleagues make it difficult to recommend HMB supplementation for young adults seeking to increase lean body mass or strength. The recommended daily dosage of HMB is about 3 grams per day appears safe, but there are few safety data available.

Recently, in a controversial study, Wilson and colleagues reported significant, but very large gains in lean body mass (7.4 kg) and strength (1RM bench press + squat + deadlift: 77 kg), in trained males ingesting HMB-FA during resistance training. As these gains rival those of high–dose anabolic steroids combined with resistance training, they should be interpreted cautiously. Wilkinson and colleagues described that HMB-FA supplementation stimulated muscle protein synthesis, increased anabolic signaling, and attenuated muscle protein breakdown, which could explain how HMB supplementation might benefit resistance training athletes. Although HMB- FA is absorbed better than calcium HMB, there are very few data available on HMB-FA supplementation, and the findings need to be replicated. Slater concluded that the beneficial of HMB supplementation on adaptations to resistance training are small in untrained individuals and negligible in athletes. Much more research needs to be conducted on HMB before it can be recommended.

Beta-Alanine and Carnosine   Beta-alanine has recently been marketed as a dietary supplement for athletes. Some contend that it may be more effective than creatine at delaying fatigue in high-intensity exercise.

Beta-alanine (β-alanine) is a naturally occurring amino acid, but unlike the normal form of alanine (L-alpha alanine) it is not used in the formation of any major proteins or enzymes. However,

beta-alanine can be taken up by muscle cells and combined with histidine to form a peptide, **carnosine**. Carnosine is highly concentrated in muscle tissue and is a robust intracellular buffer. Although carnosine only accounts for about 7 percent of the buffering capacity of skeletal muscle, this can be doubled through beta-alanine supplementation. The seminal research on beta-alanine, as was the case with creatine supplementation, was conducted by Roger Harris and colleagues. Since that time, many studies of the effects of beta-alanine supplementation on muscle carnosine content and on exercise performance have been conducted. Although these studies used different methods to tests the efficacy of beta-alanine ingestion, enough studies have been conducted for the data to be synthesized and published in several extensive reviews. Craig Sale, of Nottingham Trent University, is a leading authority on muscle carnosine and beta alanine supplementation.

In a meta-analysis from his lab, a 2.85 percent improvement in exercise performance from beta-alanine supplementation was noted, which, although small, would be very valuable to an athlete. Of note was that when studies were categorized into three distinct time periods, exercise performance lasting >240 seconds and from 60 to 240 seconds was improved with supplementation, but not during tasks lasting less than 60 seconds. As the cause of fatigue in exercise lasting less than 60 seconds is unlikely to be acidosis, it appears that very brief, intense tasks may not improve subsequent to beta alanine supplementation. Sale and Harris rate beta- alanine as a supplement that has "Level IV" or the highest level of evidence available to show efficacy of a supplement. Jones agrees that beta-alanine supplements can increase muscle carnosine levels and improve exercise performance during high-intensity exercise.

In a systematic review of 19 studies, Quesnele and colleagues also concluded that beta alanine is ergogenic, but noted a concern with the available data. As the range of supplement doses was 2.0 to 6.4 grams per day and duration was 4 to 13 weeks, it is clear that more work needs to be conducted on optimal dosing. Based on the available data, a sensible supplementation protocol suggested by Jones and supported by research is 3 to 6 grams of beta alanine per day for 4 to 8 weeks. This could increase muscle carnosine content by about 40 to 50 percent, with muscle carnosine levels remaining elevated for about 3 months after supplementation is stopped. The only known side effect of beta-alanine is paresthesia (flushing), but this appears to have been fixed with timed-release supplements, or by ingesting smaller doses more frequently throughout the day. One intriguing possibility is the potential combination of dietary supplements such as creatine monohydrate, beta alanine, and sodium bicarbonate (discussed in Chapter 13), that are effective in improving performance of brief, intense exercise, but that work through different mechanisms.

Some data are available, but much more research needs to be conducted.

Tyrosine   Tyrosine is a precursor for the catecholamine hormones and neurotransmitters, specifically epinephrine, norepinephrine, and dopamine. Some have suggested that inadequate production of these hormones or transmitters could compromise optimal physical performance. Thus, as a precursor for the formation of these hormones and neurotransmitters, tyrosine has been suggested to be ergogenic.

However, research is very limited. Sutton and others, in a well-designed, placebo-controlled, crossover study, had subjects consume tyrosine (150 milligrams/kilogram body weight) 30 minutes prior to taking a series of physical performance tests. Although the tyrosine supplementation significantly increased plasma tyrosine levels, there were no significant ergogenic effects on aerobic endurance, anaerobic power, or muscle strength.

Taurine   Taurine is synthesized from amino acids, mainly methionine and cysteine, and is found only in animal foods. Taurine is a vitamin-like compound that has multiple functions in the body, including effects on heart contraction, insulin actions, and antioxidant activity that could be of interest to the athlete. Taurine is an ingredient in several energy drinks, such as Red Bull.

Relative to sports performance, Cuisinier and others reported increased concentrations of urinary taurine following a marathon. Based on these observations, they theorized that the increased taurine secretion could be a marker for muscle damage and speculated as to whether taurine supplementation would minimize such changes. da Silva and colleagues demonstrated decreased levels of some post-eccentric exercise muscle damage markers (e.g. strength, soreness, muscle serum proteins), but not antioxidant enzymes or inflammatory markers in young men who ingested taurine for 2 weeks. Ra and colleagues showed decreased muscle soreness in young men ingesting 2 g of taurine per day for 2 weeks prior to a high-intensity eccentric exercise protocol. However, no other measures of muscle damage (e.g. swelling, muscle serum proteins, range of motion) were affected.

Lawrence Spriet, an expert in taurine supplementation, noted that human skeletal muscle are resistant to large, prolonged increases in plasma taurine, which can prevent muscle Taurine uptake. This is the opposite of rodent skeletal muscle, so animal research must be interpreted cautiously. If there are benefits of taurine supplementation on human skeletal muscle, this likely occurs outside the muscle cell. Much more research is needed before taurine transport into the muscle is well understood and also before taurine can be recommended as a supplement. Spriet states that supplemental taurine is not ergogenic in humans. Rutherford and others examined the effects of 1.66 grams of taurine compared to a placebo in a randomized, crossover blinded study. One hour after consumption of the beverage, the endurance-trained men cycled at 66 percent VO_2 max for 90 minutes, followed by a cycling time trial. Taurine supplementation resulted in increased fat oxidation during only the 90-minute ride. Taurine supplementation had no effect on carbohydrate oxidation, fat oxidation, or performance in the time trial, however.

Inosine   **Inosine** is not an amino acid but is classified as a nucleoside. It is included for discussion here because it is associated with the development of **purines**, nonprotein nitrogen compounds that have important roles in energy metabolism. On the basis of animal research and studies of blood storage techniques, writers in popular magazines have theorized that inosine may be an effective ergogenic aid for a variety of athletes. Advertisements have

suggested that inosine may improve ATP production in the muscle and thus be of value to strength-type athletes. Additionally, inosine is thought to enhance oxygen delivery to the muscles, thus being beneficial to aerobic endurance athletes.

There are no data to support these claims. No studies investigating the effect of inosine upon strength or power have been uncovered. Research from our laboratory at Old Dominion University has revealed no ergogenic effect of inosine on aerobic endurance, but on the contrary, a possible decrement in performance. Nine highly trained runners consumed either a placebo or 6 grams of inosine prior to several tests of performance, including a peak oxygen uptake test and a 3-mile run on the treadmill conducted to simulate an all-out race. Although there were no differences in 3-mile run performance, peak oxygen uptake, or a variety of hematological and psychological variables, time to exhaustion during the peak oxygen uptake test was longer in the placebo condition. We speculated that inosine may impair the ability of fast-twitch muscle to function optimally in very high intensity exercise, which occurs in the latter stages of tests of maximal or peak oxygen uptake. Research from Ball State University revealed similar findings. Starling and his colleagues investigated the effect of 5,000 milligrams of inosine daily for 5 days on the performance of competitive male cyclists on three tests: a Wingate bike test, a 30-minute self-paced cycling performance test, and a supramaximal cycling sprint to fatigue. Compared to the placebo trial, they reported no significant effect of inosine supplementation on any performance measures in the three tests, and actually reported an impaired performance in the supramaximal test following inosine supplementation. In the most recent double-blind, placebo, crossover study, McNaughton and others studied the effect of inosine supplementation on cycling performance in highly trained cyclists. The subjects consumed 10 grams of inosine daily for 10 days, with a 6-week washout period between trials. Subjects were tested at baseline, after 5 days, and after 10 days on three cycle-performance tests designed to measure different energy systems. The first test included five repetitions of a 6-second sprint; the second test was a 30-second sprint; and the last test was a 20-minute time trial. Inosine supplementation had no effect on any of the tests. Thus, on the basis of the available data, inosine does not appear to be an effective ergogenic aid.

One of the by-products of inosine is uric acid, a compound that may accumulate in the joints and cause gout. In both the Starling and McNaughton studies, inosine supplementation increased serum uric acid levels. Individuals predisposed to gout should be aware of this possible complication.

Dietary Nitrate   It is generally accepted that a diet rich in vegetables is associated with a healthy, long life. Nitrate is found in all vegetables, particularly in leafy greens and beetroot. It has been examined lately for its potential benefits to the cardiovascular system.

In an effort to examine the effects of dietary nitrate supplementation on performance, Lansley and others supplemented the diets of club-level competitive cyclists with 0.5 liters of beetroot juice or nitrate-depleted beetroot juice. Following a 2.5-hour rest period, the cyclists performed a 4-km and a 16.1-km time trial. Power output by those who had consumed the beetroot juice was significantly higher during the time trials, although there was no difference in the VO_2 response to exercise between the treatments. Moreover, the researchers found beetroot juice to result in improved performances in both the 4-km (2.8 percent) and 16.1-km (2.7 percent) time trials.

Bailey and others provided 0.5 liters of beetroot juice or blackcurrant cordial as placebo to men daily for 6 days. Along with an elevation of plasma nitrate on days 4–6, they documented a 6 mmHg lower systolic blood pressure with beetroot supplementation compared with the placebo. The oxygen cost of cycling at a fixed submaximal level was significantly reduced (23 percent) and increased the time to task failure (16 percent) during severe exercise. The supplement produced no ill side effects, although subjects experienced beeturia (red urine) and red stools. These side effects are consistent with those reported in other studies.

In a balanced, randomized crossover study, Vanhatalo and colleagues supplemented the diets of subjects with either 0.5 liters of organic beetroot juice per day or blackcurrant juice as a placebo for 15 days. The supplementation was well tolerated, with beeturia being a reported side effect. A significant reduction of systolic (4 mmHg) and diastolic (4 mmHg) blood pressures was demonstrated at 2.5 hours after supplementation, and this was maintained for the 15-day period. The oxygen cost of moderate-intensity exercise was reduced 2.5 hours after supplementation and was maintained for the 15-day protocol.

The world authority on dietary nitrate and beetroot juice supplementation is Andrew Jones at the University of Exeter. As he notes in two recent reviews, dietary nitrate supplementation at a dose of about 5 to 7 mmol nitrate (about 0.1 mmol/kg body mass) increases plasma nitrite, reduces the oxygen cost of exercise, enhances exercise performance, and decreases blood pressure. The benefits are obtained quickly, approximately 3 hours after ingestion, and can be maintained for up to about 2 weeks if nitrate ingestion is continued. Longer term studies are not available. The amount of dietary nitrate needed for an effect is easily achieved by consuming 0.5 L of beetroot juice, but other high nitrate foods, such as leafy vegetables, can be used as well. Currently, data showing the benefits of nitrate ingestion on exercise performance have focused on continuous exercise lasting 5 to 25 minutes in duration. Clements et al., in their review of 31 studies with over 300 volunteers, agreed that nitrate supplementation is an effective ergogenic aid, but more research is needed. The effects of nitrate supplementation on very brief and intense exercise, team sports and other intermittent activities, and long term continuous exercise have not been well studied to date.

A meta-analysis on 16 studies of dietary nitrate and blood pressure by Siervo and colleagues revealed that beetroot juice and inorganic nitrate supplementation significantly reduce blood pressure. While this is great news from a public health perspective, people taking prescribed medication for hypertension should consult with their doctor about nitrate, to avoid a potentially dangerous hypotensive episode. Similarly, athletes may be ingesting dietary supplements that already contain nutrients that may alter blood pressure (e.g. pre-workout supplements), and the addition of nitrate or more nitrate could cause a dangerous hypotensive response. More research needs to be conducted on the efficacy and safety of dietary nitrate, but current data supports a performance and anti-hypertensive effect.

Summary A balanced diet containing 12–15 percent of the Calories as protein will provide amounts of the individual amino acids more than adequate to obtain the estimated RDA, even for those who exercise extensively. For example, some reports suggest that endurance athletes need more leucine because they may use about 850 mg, or 29 percent of the estimated leucine RDA, in a 2-hour workout. However, one glass of milk contains 950 mg of leucine, and more than 5,000 mg are consumed in a normal daily diet. Similar comparisons could be made with other amino acids.

In one study, Tipton and others indicated that net muscle protein synthesis following exercise was similar whether amino acids were infused or taken orally. However, we are unaware of any research indicating that amino acid preparations taken orally are, over the course of a day, more effective than amino acids consumed as natural components of protein-rich foods. Nevertheless, companies that market amino acid supplements for athletes indicate that amino acids found in food are liberated slowly in the digestive processes, somewhat like a time-release tablet, and may not elicit similar effects compared to consumption of free-form amino acids. Whether or not such individual amino acids confer any ergogenic effect is still questionable at best. Although several amino acids have received some research attention, the available reputable scientific data are still somewhat limited. Additional research is merited with several purported ergogenic amino acids, particularly aspartic acid salts and the BCAAs. Creatine supplementation appears to be an effective ergogenic aid for repetitive, high-intensity, short-duration exercise tasks, but additional research is needed to evaluate the effectiveness of acute or chronic creatine supplementation as applied to specific sport events. Moreover, more research is needed to explore the effect of creatine supplementation on performance in events characterized by anaerobic and aerobic glycolysis. Research findings regarding the ergogenic effect of HMB are ambiguous. Additional research is needed to study the effect of HMB supplementation on body composition, strength, power, and related sports events. Inosine supplementation appears to be an ineffective ergogenic aid.

Key Concepts

▶ Although consumption of adequate protein or protein/carbohydrate preparations during exercise training may provide a milieu conducive to muscle protein anabolism, current research is preliminary and insufficient to support an ergogenic effect of such preparations, including whey protein and colostrum, on resistance or aerobic endurance exercise performance.

- Central fatigue during prolonged aerobic exercise is hypothesized to occur when BCAA levels are decreased. BCAAs normally compete with free-tryptophan (fTRP) for entry into the brain. fTRP increases serotonin production, which is believed to induce fatigue. Thus, an increased fTRP:BCAA ratio may induce central fatigue.
- Although several interesting hypotheses have been proposed, individual amino acid supplements are not currently considered to be effective as a means of improving physical performance.
- Creatine loading may be an effective means to increase muscle levels of both phosphocreatine (PCr) and free creatine. Consuming about 20 grams daily, in four equal doses of 5 grams each, for 4–5 days has been shown to be an effective loading protocol. Increased muscle creatine levels may be maintained with a dose of 2–5 grams daily.
- Research with laboratory-controlled, repetitive, short-duration, high-intensity exercise tasks designed to mimic sports competition suggests that creatine may be an effective ergogenic aid. Research findings are somewhat equivocal regarding the ergogenic effect of other protein-related supplements, such as HMB and beta-alanine. Additional research is needed to document an ergogenic effect of creatine in actual sport competition and to help resolve the ambiguity with other related supplements.

Check for Yourself

- Using table 6.8 as a guide, go to a health food store that sells sports supplements and check the cost of various protein supplements. Calculate the cost per serving and the average cost per 8 grams of protein. Compare to the table.

Dietary Protein: Health Implications

The Acceptable Macronutrient Distribution Range for individuals has been set for protein based on evidence from interventional trials, with support of epidemiological evidence, to suggest a role in the prevention of increased risk of chronic diseases and based on ensuring sufficient intakes of essential nutrients. As noted previously, the AMDR for protein is 10–35 percent of energy, and slightly lower percentages were set for children (5–20 percent for young and 10–30 percent for older children). There may be several possible adverse health effects from consuming a diet which is consistently outside the AMDR for protein, either too low or too high. Excess intake of individual amino acids may also pose health risks. You can also go to www.ChooseMyPlate.gov. Click on Tips and Resources, then Go Lean With Protein and the Nutrients and Health Implications for more information on protein food choices and your health.

Does a deficiency of dietary protein pose any health risks?

A short-term protein deficiency (several days) is not likely to cause any serious health problems, mainly because body metabolism adjusts to conserve its protein stores. However, because protein is the source of the essential amino acids, and because protein-rich foods also contain an abundance of essential vitamins and minerals, a prolonged deficiency could be expected to cause serious health problems. Such is the case in certain parts of the world where protein intake is inadequate for political, economic, or other reasons. Protein–Calorie malnutrition is one of the major nutritional problems in the world today, particularly for young children. Infections develop because the immune system, which depends on adequate protein, is weakened. Death is common. For children who survive, physical and mental growth may be permanently retarded. Protein deficiency may also occur in individuals who abuse sound nutritional practices, such as drug addicts, chronic alcoholics, and extreme food faddists, but adults are more likely to recover fully with adequate nutrition.

Elderly individuals, those over 65 years, may be more prone to protein undernutrition because they may eat less protein-rich food and may use protein less efficiently. Houston and others reported that in elderly men, protein intakes greater than the RDA seemed to help conserve lean body mass, particularly skeletal muscle tissue. Lesourd indicated that protein undernutrition in the elderly may impair immune function, making them more susceptible to infections. Adequate protein also plays an important role in bone development, thereby influencing peak bone mass. Bonjour and others note that low protein intake can be detrimental for both the acquisition of bone mass during growth and its conservation during adulthood. Low protein intake impairs both the production and action of IGF-I, an essential factor for bone longitudinal growth. Protein intake is especially important during childhood, but is very important during adulthood as well. According to a review by Gaffney-Stomberg and colleagues, between 32 percent and 41 percent of women 50 years of age and older consume less than the current RDA of 0.8 g of good-quality protein per kilogram body weight per day. This is higher than the 22–38 percent of men in the same age group who do not meet the protein RDA. This is of particular concern given the loss of muscle mass, or *sarcopenia*, seen with aging. Genaro and Martini found that sarcopenia in the elderly is associated with decreased metabolic rate, increased risk of falls and fractures, and thus an increased morbidity and loss of independence.

Individuals who are on a low-protein diet plan, or young athletes who are on modified starvation diets to lose weight for such sports as gymnastics, ballet, or wrestling, may experience periods of protein insufficiency. During this time, the individual may be in negative nitrogen balance; that is, more nitrogen is being excreted from the body than is being ingested. Body tissues such as muscles and hemoglobin may be lost, with a possible reduction in strength and endurance capacity. Adequate protein intake is essential for proper physiological functioning and health, both in the inactive and active individual.

Several major health problems associated with excessive weight loss, both in nonathletes and athletes, are related to both energy and protein balance. The role of protein in weight control, both weight loss and gain, will be discussed in chapters 10 through 12. In brief, diets rich in protein could help promote weight loss by increasing satiety and curbing the appetite while also increasing thermogenesis and energy expenditure; protein may also help promote weight gain by maintaining muscle mass.

Does excessive protein intake pose any health risks?

As noted in previous chapters, the intake of even small amounts of food protein may be hazardous to individuals susceptible to food allergies or food intolerance. Certain proteins found in common foods such as milk, fish, eggs, shellfish, peanuts, and wheat may cause symptoms such as abdominal pain, gas, bloating, and diarrhea and even an anaphylactic reaction, which may be fatal. However, dietary protein intake normally does not cause any health problems with most individuals.

Bilsborough and Mann noted some dangers of excessive protein intake, such as elevated blood levels of ammonia and insulin, but note that healthy individuals appear to adapt well to highly variable dietary protein intakes; frank signs of symptoms of amino acid excess are observed rarely, if at all, under usual dietary conditions.

Although the National Academy of Sciences did not establish a UL for protein, the upper level of the AMDR is 35 percent of daily energy intake from protein. Recent American and Canadian survey data reveal that adult males consume about 71–100 grams of protein per day, while women consume about 55–62 grams. Protein constitutes approximately 12–16 percent of the daily energy intake, which is within the AMDR for protein. However, some individuals may consume much greater percentages of their caloric intake as protein, particularly athletes and individuals on weight-loss diets. Even though the Academy did not set a UL for protein, it did note that high protein intakes have been implicated in various chronic diseases. The health effects of dietary protein may depend on its source. As noted previously in several chapters, a plant-based diet may confer some health benefits.

Cardiovascular Disease and Cancer The National Academy of Sciences reported that high-protein diets *per se* do not appear to increase the risk for CHD, and even suggested that such diets may be more healthful because of possible beneficial effects on blood pressure and lowering of LDL-cholesterol and triglycerides. The Academy also noted that no clear role has emerged for total dietary protein in the development of cancer. However, the Academy did note that the dietary source of protein may be involved. For example, excessive consumption of animal foods such as meat may be a contributing factor to the development of disease, possibly because of a relationship to the potential high total and saturated fat content or the method of preparation.

A reduction in animal-derived dietary protein has been recommended for various reasons. One point to consider is that protein in many animal foods is often accompanied by substantial quantities of saturated fat and cholesterol, which have been associated with an increased risk of atherosclerosis and coronary heart disease. Interestingly, an epidemiological study by Hu and others reported

that after controlling for specific types of fat in the diet, women consuming high-protein diets did not experience an increase in heart disease risk. Moreover, Hu indicated that high-protein diets are thought to increase satiety and facilitate weight loss, which could improve cardiovascular risk factors. Nevertheless, the researchers recommended caution in consuming high-protein diets given the saturated fat/cholesterol connection.

The worldwide report of the American Institute of Cancer Research (AICR), as discussed in chapter 2, indicated that the evidence that red meats and processed meats are a cause of colorectal cancer is convincing. The AICR also indicated that there is limited evidence suggesting that red meat and processed meat may cause other cancers, and that methods of preparation (grilled and barbecued) that may char meats are a cause of stomach cancer.

In the United States, approximately 70 percent of dietary protein is obtained from animal products, with most coming from meat, fish, and poultry, and smaller amounts from dairy products and eggs. Although such a diet assures adequate protein, it is not in accord with general healthful guidelines to consume less meat and derive more protein from plant foods. This ratio of animal:plant protein of 70:30 might be more healthful if reversed to 30:70.

The OmniHeart diet plan, as discussed in previous chapters, focuses on *good* carbohydrates and *good* fats, but it also stresses the importance of *good* proteins, such as those derived from plants and low-fat animal products. Table 6.9 provides some of the OmniHeart diet plan tips to increase your intake of *good* protein-rich foods. For example, a glass of whole milk and a glass of skim milk both have 8 grams of protein, but whole milk also has 8 grams of fat compared to less than 1 gram in the skim milk. Nutritionally, skim milk is 40 percent protein Calories while whole milk is 22.5 percent.

Soy protein has been recommended as a meat substitute and, as noted in chapter 2, foods rich in soy protein may carry a health claim suggesting benefits in preventing heart disease. Modern processing techniques, fortifying soybeans with methionine, have helped to make soy a complete protein. Soy products derived from soybeans include tofu, tempeh, miso, soy nuts, soy nut butter, and soy milk. Many of these products have been added to school lunches—as soy-based burgers and hot dogs—to decrease

---

TABLE 6.9 Omniheart diet plan tips to increase healthier protein-rich foods

- Have a serving of legumes, nuts, seeds, or whole and high-protein grains (such as bulgur wheat, or millet), or lean meats, fish, and poultry with skin removed in at least 2 meals.
- Have a serving of fat-free or low-fat milk products at 3 meals or at 2 meals and a snack.
- Use egg whites or egg substitutes at breakfast and other meals and in recipes.
- Top whole-grain cereals with 1 oz unsalted nuts.
- Spread unsalted peanut butter on whole-grain toast.
- Add different kinds of beans in salads, recipes, and main dishes.
- Try vegetarian meat substitutes in sandwiches, salads, and mixed dishes such as chili, and as main-course entrees.

fat intake. For health benefits, the FDA-approved health claim is based on an intake of about 25 grams of soy protein a day.

Other than containing high-quality protein and being virtually free of saturated fat and sodium, soy contains a number of substances that might confer health benefits, including isoflavones, phytosterols, and omega-3 fatty acids. Some have suggested that most health benefits are believed to be due to the isoflavones (genistein and daidzien), as they may function as phytoestrogens, or weak estrogen-like substances, and possibly have protective effects against heart disease. However, as we will see, research indicates that the soy protein and soy isoflavones provide greater benefits when combined than when either occurs alone. Whole soy foods are recommended, as they naturally contain about 2 milligrams of isoflavones for every gram of soy protein. Isoflavones may be lost in highly processed foods, and isoflavone supplements may not contain protein. Check the food label; soy should be one of the first three ingredients.

Clarkson noted that dietary soy protein has been shown to have several beneficial effects on cardiovascular health. This viewpoint is supported by Reynolds and others, who conducted a meta-analysis of 41 randomized, controlled trials and concluded that dietary soy protein was associated with a significant reduction in mean serum total cholesterol, low-density lipoprotein cholesterol, and triglycerides, and a significant increase in high-density lipoprotein cholesterol. Several recent studies have shown that whole soy protein, not the isolated isoflavones, induces the beneficial effects on serum lipids. In a randomized, crossover study, Jenkins and others studied the cholesterol-lowering effect of a soy protein-based diet (about 50 grams daily) that contained either low or high amounts of isoflavones. Although both soy diets reduced total and LDL-cholesterol, the isoflavone content had no effect. Lichtenstein and others found that relatively high levels of soy protein (>50 grams per day) induced a small but significant drop in total and LDL-cholesterol in mildly hypercholesterolemic individuals, but soy-derived isoflavones had little effect. In a review of 22 studies, Sacks and others reported a relatively small decrease (3 percent) in LDL-cholesterol relative to the large amount of soy protein consumed, and also noted no effect of isolated isoflavones on serum cholesterol.

In his review, Schardt noted that soy products have been marketed as a means of preventing several forms of cancer, most notably breast and prostate cancer. Natural estrogen is believed to contribute to the development of breast cancer. It is thought that isoflavones functioning as phytoestrogens may block this cancer-causing effect. However, Skibola and Smith noted that at high levels, flavonoids may act as mutagens, or pro-oxidants that generate free radicals. In this regard, Schardt reported that some investigators suggest that adding an estrogen-like compound in excess may act like estrogen and actually cause cancer. He further notes that some researchers believe that the isoflavones in soy may be protective prior to menopause when serum estrogens are high, but may become harmful after menopause when serum estrogens are lower. Based on these considerations, some recommend that women who have a family history of estrogen-dependent breast cancer should limit soy food intake to only several servings per week.

In an FDA review, Henkel indicated that adverse health concerns focus on specific components of soy, such as the isoflavones,

not the whole food or intact soy proteins. This recommendation is supported in an American Heart Association Scientific Advisory by Sacks and others, recommending against isoflavone supplements because their efficacy or safety are not established and cautioning against possible adverse effects. For any potential health benefits, scientists agree with the general recommendation to incorporate soy foods into the diet in moderation rather than consuming soy or isoflavone supplements. Moreover, investigators note that although those with hypercholesterolemia may benefit slightly from a diet rich in soy protein, they might be better advised to use other therapy to reduce serum cholesterol and the risk of heart disease.

Liver and Kidney Function As you may recall, the liver is the major organ involved in protein metabolism. Excess dietary protein may be converted to carbohydrate or fat, with the excess nitrogen being converted to urea for excretion from the body via the kidneys. High-protein diets may also lead to excessive production of ketones, which also must be excreted by the kidneys to prevent an increase in blood acidity, known as *ketosis.* Thus, excess dietary protein would appear to stress the liver and kidney.

Diets containing moderate amounts of protein do not appear to adversely affect liver or kidney function. Although kidney function progressively declines with aging, according to the National Academy of Sciences the protein content of the diet is not responsible for this decline. Some research has also shown that athletes on somewhat high-protein diets might not be adversely affected. For example, in their study Poortmans and Dellalieux reported no evidence of kidney damage, as evaluated by renal clearance tests, in male bodybuilders who had protein intakes of less than 2.8 g protein/kg body weight daily.

However, certain individuals should be concerned with the protein content in their diet. Eisenstein and others noted that caution with high-protein diets is recommended in those individuals who may be predisposed to kidney disease, particularly in those with diabetes mellitus. The American Diabetes Association recommends that diabetics consume no more than the daily RDA for protein. Individuals with chronic kidney disease need to monitor protein intake under guidance from health professionals.

Individuals prone to kidney stones should also moderate protein intake. High-protein diets may lead to more acidic urine—and the more acidic the urine, the greater the excretion of calcium. The Academy notes that the most common form of kidney stones is composed of calcium oxalate, and its formation is promoted by an acidic urine with high concentrations of calcium and oxalate.

Bone and Joint Health As noted, excess dietary protein may increase urine acidity, which may be attributed to the increased acids in the blood associated with the oxidation of the sulfur amino acids. The National Academy of Sciences indicates that calcium might be absorbed from the bones to help buffer this acidity. If so, excess calcium losses could lead to decreased bone density. However, the Academy indicates that whether this bone resorption leads to bone loss and osteoporosis is controversial, but does cite recent studies showing no association between protein intake and bone mineral density. The Academy suggests that the diet may be the key.

Studies present conflicting data as to whether animal protein, as contrasted to plant protein, decreases bone density with an increased risk of osteoporosis and bone fractures. Protein is needed for bone development at all stages of life, but excessive intake may lead to increased calcium losses. Krall and Dawson-Hughes indicate that over a wide range of protein intake, an average increase in dietary protein of 1 gram leads to the loss of 1 milligram of calcium in the urine. Although this does not seem too substantial a loss given the RDA for calcium, it could be significant for those on a high-protein and low-calcium diet. Cao and colleagues fed a group of postmenopausal women low protein + low potential renal acid load and high protein + high potential renal acid load diets. Their analysis revealed no adverse effects on bone health with the high-protein diet. The Academy notes that inadequate protein intake itself leads to bone loss, but increased protein intake may lead to increased calcium intake and bone loss does not occur if calcium intake is adequate. Dawson-Hughes and Harris reiterate these points, noting that there is currently no consensus on the effect of dietary protein intake on the skeleton. However, they also note that there is some indication that low calcium intakes adversely influence the effect of dietary protein on fracture risk. In a review, Heaney and Layman add another perspective. They note that loss of bone mass and loss of muscle mass that occur with age are closely related, so helping to maintain muscle mass with increased dietary protein may also help promote bone health. They also concur that dietary intake of both calcium and protein must be adequate to fully realize the benefit of each nutrient on bone.

Bonjour notes that experimental and clinical published data concur to indicate that low protein intake negatively affects bone health, and indicates that dietary proteins are as essential as calcium and vitamin D for bone health and osteoporosis prevention. The key appears to be getting enough of both protein and calcium. The topic of calcium balance is presented in chapter 8.

Gout, a painful inflammation of the joints, may be aggravated by high-protein diets containing substantial quantities of purines, which are metabolized to uric acid (not the same as urea). The uric acid may accumulate in the joints and cause inflammation.

Heat Illnesses Because both urea and ketone bodies must be eliminated by the kidneys, dehydration could occur from excessive fluid losses. Such an effect could compromise the ability to deal with exercise in the heat. Additionally, Johnson and others found that increasing the protein content of the diet from 17 to 31 percent of energy would significantly increase the resting energy expenditure, an effect they suggested could contribute to the development of heat illnesses when exercising under warm environmental conditions. Both of these are possibilities, and the implications are discussed in chapter 9 when we discuss fluid balance and temperature regulation during exercise.

Does the consumption of individual amino acids pose any health risks?

Amino acids do not exist free in foods we eat, but are complexed with other amino acids to form protein. The National Academy of Sciences noted no evidence that amino acids derived from usual or even high intakes of protein from foodstuffs present any health risk. Although no UL has been established for amino acids, the Academy indicated that the absence of a UL means that caution is warranted in using any single amino acid at levels significantly above that normally found in food. Extreme consumption of individual amino acid supplements may pose a health risk.

Free amino acids have been manufactured to serve as a drug, to be given to patients intravenously for adequate protein nutrition. They may also be used as food additives to enhance the protein quality of foods deficient in specific amino acids. They are also marketed as dietary supplements and sold separately, or in combination with other amino acids. As dietary supplements, purity and safety are not guaranteed. In 1989 a serious epidemic of eosinophilia-myalgia syndrome (EMS), a neuromuscular disorder characterized by weakness, fever, edema, rashes, bone pain, and other symptoms, was attributed to an L-tryptophan supplement contaminated during manufacturing.

Slavin and her colleagues have noted that amino acids taken in large doses are essentially drugs with unknown effects. The long-term effects of even moderate doses are also unknown, as noted previously in regard to arginine and its effect on HGH secretion. One problem is that excessive reliance on free-form amino acids, in comparison to dietary protein, may lead to a diet deficient in key vitamins and minerals that are normally found in protein foods, such as iron and zinc in meat, fish, and poultry. Some evidence from human and animal research indicates individual amino acids may interfere with the absorption of other essential amino acids; suppress appetite and food intake; precipitate tissue damage; contribute to kidney failure; lead to osteoporosis; cause gastrointestinal distress such as nausea, vomiting, and diarrhea; or create unfavorable psychological changes.

In a review, Barrett and Herbert indicated that the Federation of American Societies for Experimental Biology (FASEB) criticized the widespread use of amino acids in supplements, noting that they were being used as drugs for pharmacologic purposes, not for nutritive purposes. In this regard, FASEB notes that there is little scientific support for the use of amino acid supplements for their stated purposes and that safety levels for amino acid use have not been established.

So what's the bottom line? At present, there are inadequate scientific data to support either an ergogenic or a health benefit of supplementation with individual amino acids in the healthy individual. Adequate amounts of each amino acid may be obtained in a diet containing protein in amounts consistent with the Prudent Healthy Diet, and because such a diet may confer some benefits relative to physical performance and health, it should be the source of amino acid nutrition. Additional research is needed to evaluate both the ergogenic effectiveness and the health implications of supplementation with individual amino acids.

Key Concept

▸ Dietary deficiencies, as well as dietary excesses, of protein and amino acids may interfere with optimal physiological efficiency, which may lead to impairment of health status.

Obtain a supply of creatine monohydrate—about 100 grams, enough to provide 20 grams a day for 5 days. Measure your weight accurately in the morning after arising and your normal bathing routine, but before eating breakfast. Consume 20 grams of creatine per day for the 5 days, taking it in 4 equal doses of 5 grams at breakfast, at lunchtime, late afternoon, and before bed. Weigh yourself again the morning after taking the last dose. Did your body weight change? Record your weight again next week, and the following three weeks. Did your body weight change again? Compare your findings to the text discussion.

Creatine Monohydrate Trial

	Day 1	Day 6	1 Week Later	2 Weeks Later	3 Weeks Later
Morning Weight					

Review Questions—Multiple Choice

1. A high-quality protein is best described as one that:
   a. contains 10 grams of protein per 100 grams of food.
   b. contains all of the essential amino acids in the proper amounts and ratio.
   c. contains all of the nonessential amino acids.
   d. contains adequate amounts of glucose for protein sparing.
   e. contains the amino acids leucine, isoleucine, and valine.

2. Which of the following statements involving the interaction of protein and exercise training is false?
   a. Small amounts of protein may be used as an energy source during endurance exercise but usually account for less than 5 percent of the energy cost of the exercise.
   b. Small amounts of protein may be lost in the urine and sweat during exercise.
   c. Resistance weight-training programs usually result in the development of a positive nitrogen balance in most athletes who are attempting to gain body weight in the form of muscle mass.
   d. Although weight lifters and endurance athletes may need slightly more protein than accounted for by the RDA, such increased protein may be obtained readily and more economically through a planned diet.
   e. Research has shown conclusively that all amino acid supplements and other protein supplements will enhance performance in sports.

3. Which of the following has the least amount of dietary protein?
   a. one ounce of chicken breast
   b. one-half cup of baked beans
   c. one slice of whole wheat bread
   d. one orange
   e. one-half glass of skim milk

4. Which of the following statements relative to protein and exercise is false?
   a. Protein may be catabolized during exercise and used as an energy source, but the contribution is less than 10 percent.
   b. Carbohydrate intake may exert a protein-sparing effect during exercise.
   c. Very low levels of protein intake during training may lead to the development of a condition known as sports anemia.
   d. Research has shown that individuals who are training to gain weight need about 6 to 8 grams of protein per kilogram body weight.
   e. In general, research has shown that protein supplementation above the RDA will not improve physiological performance capacity during aerobic endurance exercise.

5. In the recommendations for a healthy diet from the National Academy of Sciences, what is the Acceptable Macronutrient Distribution Range for protein as a percent of daily energy intake in Calories?
   a. 15–20
   b. 10–35
   c. 4–6
   d. 12–14
   e. 40–65

6. Which of the following statements relative to protein metabolism is false?
   a. Excess protein may be converted to glucose in the body.
   b. The liver is a critical center for the control of amino acid metabolism.
   c. Essential amino acids can be formed in the liver from carbohydrate and nitrogen from nonessential amino acids.
   d. Excess protein may be converted to fat in the body.
   e. Urea is a waste product of protein metabolism.

7. Which is most likely to be a complete, high-quality protein food?
   a. cheddar cheese
   b. peanut butter
   c. green peas
   d. corn
   e. macaroni

8. Supplementation with some amino acids has been theorized to decrease the formation of serotonin in the brain and possibly help delay the onset of central nervous system fatigue in prolonged aerobic endurance exercise. Which amino acids are theorized to do this?
   a. leucine, isoleucine, and valine
   b. arginine, ornithine, and inosine
   c. tryptophan, arginine, and creatine
   d. inosine, creatine, and alanine
   e. asparagine, aspartic acid, and glutamine

9. If an adult weighed 176 pounds, the RDA for protein would be what, in grams?
   a. 176
   b. 140.8
   c. 80
   d. 64
   e. 309.7

10. Research has suggested that creatine supplementation may enhance performance in which of the following types of physical performance tasks?
    a. an all-out power lift in 1 second
    b. high-intensity exercise lasting 6–30 seconds
    c. 10-kilometer race lasting about 30 minutes
    d. marathon running (26.2 miles)
    e. ultramarathons, such as Ironman-type triathlons

Answers to multiple choice questions:
1. b; 2. e; 3. d; 4. d; 5. b; 6. c; 7. a; 8. a; 9. d; 10. b.

Review Questions—Essay

1. Differentiate between complete and incomplete proteins as related to essential and nonessential amino acids and indicate several specific foods that are considered to contain either complete or incomplete protein.

2. Describe the process of gluconeogenesis from protein.

3. Explain why some scientists recommend that both strength and endurance athletes may need more dietary protein than the RDA. Provide some recommended values and calculate the recommended grams of protein for a 70-kilogram athlete.

4. Explain the central fatigue hypothesis as related to BCAA supplementation for endurance athletes and summarize the research findings as to the related ergogenic efficacy of BCAA supplementation.

5. Discuss the concept of the *good* proteins in the OmniHeart diet plan and the underlying rationale as to how they may be more beneficial in helping protect against cardiovascular disease. Discuss also how the form of food protein and its preparation may influence risk for certain cancers.

References

Books

American Institute of Cancer Research. 2007. *Food, Nutrition, Physical Activity, and the Prevention of Cancer: A Global Perspective.* Washington, DC: AICR.

Bucci, L. 1993. *Nutrients as Ergogenic Aids for Sports and Exercise.* Boca Raton, FL: CRC Press.

Houston, M. 2006. *Biochemistry Primer for Exercise Science.* Champaign, IL: Human Kinetics.

National Academy of Sciences. 2005. *Dietary Reference Intakes for Energy, Carbohydrates, Fiber, Fat, Fatty Acids, Cholesterol, Protein and Amino Acids (Macronutrients).* Washington, DC: National Academies Press.

United States Anti-Doping Agency. 2005. *Optimal Dietary Intake.* Colorado Springs, CO.

Williams, M., Kreider, R., and Branch, J. 1999. *Creatine: The Power Supplement.* Champaign, IL: Human Kinetics.

Reviews and Specific Studies

Abcouwer, S., and Souba, W. 1999. Glutamine and arginine. In *Modern Nutrition in Health and Disease,* eds. M. Shils, et al. Baltimore: Williams & Wilkins.

Abel, T., et al. 2005. Influence of chronic supplementation of arginine aspartate in endurance athletes on performance and substrate metabolism: A randomized, double-blind, placebo-controlled study. *International Journal of Sports Medicine* 26:344–49.

Akerström, T., and Pedersen, B. 2007. Strategies to enhance immune function for marathon runners: What can be done? *Sports Medicine* 37:416–19.

American College of Sports Medicine, American Dietetic Association, Dietitians of Canada. 2009. Joint position statement: Nutrition and athletic performance. *Medicine & Science in Sports & Exercise* 41:709–31.

Andersen, L., et al. 2005. The effect of resistance training combined with timed ingestion of protein on muscle fiber size and muscle strength. *Metabolism* 54:151–56.

Antonio, J., and Street, C. 1999. Glutamine: A potentially useful supplement for athletes. *Canadian Journal of Applied Physiology* 24:1–14.

Antonio, J., et al. 2001. The effects of bovine colostrum supplementation on body composition and exercise performance in active men and women. *Nutrition* 17:243–47.

Antonio, J., et al. 2002. The effects of high-dose glutamine ingestion on weightlifting performance. *Journal of Strength & Conditioning Research* 16:157–60.

Appel, L., et al. 2005. Effects of protein, monounsaturated fat, and carbohydrate intake on blood pressure and serum lipids: Results of the OmniHeart randomized trial. *JAMA* 294:2455–64.

Aragon, A., and Schoenfeld, B. 2013. Nutrient timing revisited: Is there a post-exercise anabolic window? *Journal of the International Society of Sport Nutrition.* 10:5.

Areta, J., et al. 2013. Timing and distribution of protein ingestion during prolonged recovery from resistance exercise alters myofibrillar protein synthesis. *Journal of Physiology* 591:2319–31.

Artioli, G., et al. 2010. Role of β-alanine supplementation on muscle carnosine and exercise performance. *Medicine & Science in Sports & Exercise* 42(6):1162–73.

Bailes, J., et al. 2002. The neurosurgeon in sport: Awareness of the risks of heatstroke and dietary supplements. *Neurosurgery* 51:283–86.

Barrett, S. and Herbert, V. 1999. Fads, frauds, and quackery. In *Modern Nutrition in Health and Disease,* eds. M. Shils et al. Baltimore: Williams & Wilkins.

Begum, G., et al. 2005. Physiological role of carnosine in contracting muscle. *International Journal of Sport Nutrition & Exercise Metabolism* 15:493–514.

Betts, J., et al. 2005. Recovery of endurance running capacity: Effect of carbohydrate-protein mixture. *International Journal of Sport Nutrition & Exercise Metabolism* 15:590–609.

Betts, J., et al. 2007. The influence of carbohydrate and protein ingestion during recovery from prolonged exercise on subsequent endurance performance. *Journal of Sports Sciences* 13:1–12.

Bilsborough, S., and Mann, N. 2006. A review of issues of dietary protein intake in humans. *International Journal of Sport Nutrition & Exercise Metabolism* 16:129–52.

Bird, S., et al. 2006. Independent and combined effects of liquid carbohydrate/essential amino acid ingestion on hormonal and muscular adaptations following resistance training in untrained men. *European Journal of Applied Physiology* 97:225–38.

Bird, S., et al. 2006. Liquid carbohydrate/protein amino acid ingestion during a short-term bout of resistance exercise suppresses myofibrillar protein degradation. *Metabolism* 55:570–77.

Blomstrand, E. 2001. Amino acids and central fatigue. *Amino Acids* 20:25–34.

Blomstrand, E. 2006. A role for branched-chain amino acids in reducing central fatigue. *Journal of Nutrition* 136: 544S–47S.

Blomstrand, E., et al. 1991. Administration of branched-chain amino acids during sustained exercise—Effects on performance and on plasma concentration of some amino acids. *European Journal of Applied Physiology* 65:83–88.

Blomstrand, E., et al. 1997. Influence of ingesting a solution of branched-chain amino acids on perceived exertion during exercise. *Acta Physiologica Scandinavica* 159:41–49.

Blomstrand, E., et al. 2006. Branched-chain amino acids activate key enzymes in protein synthesis after physical exercise. *Journal of Nutrition* 136:269S–73S.

Böger, R. 2007. The pharmacodynamics of L-arginine. *Journal of Nutrition* 137:1650S–55S.

Bonjour, J. 2005. Dietary protein: An essential nutrient for bone health. *Journal of the American College of Nutrition* 24: 526S–36S.

Bonjour, J., et al. 2000. Protein intake and bone growth. *Canadian Journal of Applied Physiology* 26:S153–66.

Branch, J. 2003. Effect of creatine supplementation on body composition and performance: A meta-analysis. *International Journal of Sport Nutrition & Exercise Metabolism* 13:198–226.

Brinkworth, G., et al. 2002. Oral bovine colostrum supplementation enhances buffer capacity, but not rowing performance in elite female rowers. *International Journal of Sport Nutrition & Exercise Metabolism* 12:349–63.

Brinkworth, G., et al. 2004. Effect of bovine colostrum supplementation on the composition of resistance trained and untrained limbs in healthy young men. *European Journal of Applied Physiology* 91:53–60.

Bucci, L., et al. 1990. Ornithine ingestion and growth hormone release in bodybuilders. *Nutrition Research* 10:239–45.

Bucci, L., et al. 1992. Ornithine supplementation and insulin release in bodybuilders. *International Journal of Sport Nutrition* 2:287–91.

Buchman, A. L., et al. 1999. The effect of arginine or glycine supplementation on gastrointestinal function, muscle injury, serum amino acid concentrations and performance during a marathon run. *International Journal of Sports Medicine* 20:315–21.

Budgett, R., et al. 1998. The overtraining syndrome. In *Oxford Textbook of Sports Medicine,* eds. M. Harries, et al. Oxford: Oxford University Press.

Buford, B., and Koch, A. 2004. Glycine-arginine-alpha-ketoisocaproic acid improves performance of repeated cycling sprints. *Medicine & Science in Sports & Exercise* 36:583–87.

Buford, T., et al. 2007. International Society of Sports Nutrition position stand: Creatine supplementation and exercise. *Journal of the International Society of Sports Nutrition* 4:6.

Burke, D., et al. 2001. The effect of 7 days of creatine supplementation on 24-hour urinary creatine excretion. *Journal of Strength & Conditioning Research* 15:59–62.

Burke, D., et al. 2001. The effect of whey protein supplementation with and without creatine monohydrate combined with resistance training on lean tissue mass and muscle strength. *International Journal of Sport Nutrition & Exercise Metabolism* 11:349–64.

Burke, D., et al. 2003. Effect of creatine and weight training on muscle creatine and performance in vegetarians. *Medicine & Science in Sports & Exercise* 36:1946–55.

Butterfield, G. 1991. Amino acids and high protein diets. In *Perspectives in Exercise Science and Sports Medicine. Ergogenics: Enhancement of Sports Performance,* eds. D. Lamb and M. Williams. Indianapolis, IN: Benchmark Press.

Campbell, B., et al. 2006. Pharmacokinetics, safety, and effects on exercise performance of l-arginine alpha-ketoglutarate in trained adult men. *Nutrition* 22:872–81.

Campbell, B., et al. 2007. International Society of Sports Nutrition position stand: Protein and exercise. *Journal of the International Society of Sports Nutrition* 4:8.

Candow, D., and Chilibeck, P. 2007. Effect of creatine supplementation during resistance training on muscle accretion in the elderly. *Journal of Nutrition, Health & Aging* 11(2):185–8.

Candow, D., et al. 2001. Effect of glutamine supplementation combined with resistance training in young adults. *European Journal of Applied Physiology* 86:142–49.

Candow, D., et al. 2006. Effect of whey and soy protein supplementation combined with resistance training in young adults. *International Journal of Sport Nutrition & Exercise Metabolism* 16:233–44.

Candow, D., et al. 2006. Protein supplementation before and after resistance training in older men. *European Journal of Applied Physiology* 97:548–56.

Cao, J., et al. 2011. A diet high in meat protein and potential renal acid load increases fractional calcium absorption and urinary calcium excretion without affecting markers of bone resorption or formation in postmenopausal women. *Journal of Nutrition* 141:391–7.

Casey, A., and Greenhaff, P. 2000. Does dietary creatine supplementation play a role in skeletal muscle metabolism and performance? *American Journal of Clinical Nutrition* 72:607S–17S.

Casey, A., et al. 1996. Creatine ingestion favorably affects performance and muscle metabolism during maximal exercise in humans. *American Journal of Physiology* 271:E31–E37.

Castell, L. 2003. Glutamine supplementation in vitro and in vivo, in exercise and in immunodepression. *Sports Medicine* 33:323–45.

Cermak, N., et al. Protein supplementation augments the adaptive response of skeletal muscle to resistance-type exercise training: A meta-analysis. *American Journal of Clinical Nutrition* 96:1454–64.

Cheng, J., et al. 2001. L-arginine in the management of cardiovascular disease. *Annals of Pharmacotherapy* 35:755–64.

Cheuvront, S. 1999. The zone diet and athletic performance. *Sports Medicine* 27:213–28.

Cheuvront, S., et al. 2004. Branched-chain amino acid supplementation and human performance when hypohydrated in the heat. *Journal of Applied Physiology* 97:1275–82.

Chromiak, J., and Antonio, J. 2002. Use of amino acids as growth-hormone releasing agents by athletes. *Nutrition* 18:657–61.

Churchward-Venne, T., et al. 2013. Role of protein and amino acids in promoting lean mass accretion with resistance exercise and attenuating lean mass loss during energy deficit in humans. *Amino Acids* 45:231–40.

Clarkson, T. 2002. Soy, soy phytoestrogens and cardiovascular disease. *Journal of Nutrition* 132:566S–69S.

Clegg, D., et al. 2006. Glucosamine, chondroitin sulfate, and the two in combination for painful knee arthritis. *New England Journal of Medicine* 354:795–808.

Clegg, D., et al. 2006. Glucosamine, chondroitin sulfate, and the two in combination for painful knee osteoarthritis. *New England Journal of Medicine* 354:795–808.

Clements, W., et al. 2014. Nitrate ingestion: A review of the health and physical performance effects. *Nutrients* 6:5224–64.

Coburn, J., et al. 2006. Effects of leucine and whey protein supplementation during eight weeks of unilateral resistance training. *Journal of Strength & Conditioning Research* 20:284–91.

Collier, S., et al. 2006. Oral arginine attenuates the growth hormone response to resistance exercise. *Journal of Applied Physiology* 101:848–52.

Conlay, L., et al. 1989. Effects of running the Boston marathon on plasma concentrations of large neutral amino acids. *Journal of Neural Transmission* 76:65–71.

Coombes, J., et al. 2002. Dose effects of oral bovine colostrum on physical work capacity in cyclists. *Medicine & Science in Sports & Exercise* 34:1184–88.

Cox, G., et al. 2002. Acute creatine supplementation and performance during a field test simulating match play in elite soccer players. *International Journal of Sport Nutrition & Exercise Metabolism* 12:33–46.

Craig, W., and A. Mangels. 2009. Position of the American Dietetic Association: Vegetarian diets. *Journal of the American Dietetic Association* 109:1266–82.

Cribb, P., and Hayes, A. 2006. Effects of supplement timing and resistance exercise on skeletal muscle hypertrophy. *Medicine & Science in Sports & Exercise* 38:1918–25.

Cribb, P., et al. 2006. The effect of whey isolate and resistance training on strength, body composition, and plasma glutamine. *International Journal of Sport Nutrition & Exercise Metabolism* 16:494–509.

Cribb, P., et al. 2007. Effects of whey isolate, creatine, and resistance training on muscle hypertrophy. *Medicine & Science in Sports & Exercise* 39:298–307.

Crowe, M., et al. 2006. Effects of leucine supplementation on exercise performance. *European Journal of Applied Physiology* 97:664–72.

Cuisinier, C., et al. 2001. Changes in plasma and urinary taurine and amino acids in runners immediately and 24h after a marathon. *Amino Acids* 20:13–23.

Cunliffe, A., et al. 1998. A placebo controlled investigation of the effects of tryptophan or placebo on subjective and objective measures of fatigue. *European Journal of Clinical Nutrition* 52:425–30.

Cynober, L. 2007. Pharmacokinetics of arginine and related amino acids. *Journal of Nutrition* 137:1646S–49S.

da Silva, L. 2014. Effects of taurine supplementation following eccentric exercise in young adults. *Applied Physiology Nutrition and Metabolism* 39:101–4.

Dalbo, V., et al. 2008. Putting to rest the myth of creatine supplementation leading to muscle cramps and dehydration. *British Journal of Sports Medicine* 42:567–73.

Davis, J. 1996. Carbohydrates, branched-chain amino acids and endurance: The central fatigue hypothesis. *Sports Science Exchange* 9(2):1–5.

Davis, J. 2000. Nutrition, neurotransmitters and central nervous system fatigue. In *Nutrition in Sport,* ed. R. J. Maughan. Oxford: Blackwell Science.

Davis, J., et al. 1999. Effects of branched-chain amino acids and carbohydrate on fatigue during intermittent, high-intensity running. *International Journal of Sports Medicine* 20:309–14.

Davis, J., et al. 2000. Serotonin and central nervous system fatigue: Nutritional considerations. *American Journal of Clinical Nutrition* 72:573S–78S.

Dawson-Hughes, B., and Harris, S. 2002. Calcium intake influences the association of protein intake with rates of bone loss in elderly men and women. *American Journal of Clinical Nutrition* 75:773–79.

Deldicque, L., et al. 2005. Increased IGF mRNA in human skeletal muscle after creatine supplementation. *Medicine & Science in Sports & Exercise* 37:731–36.

Devries, M., and Phillips, S. 2015. Supplemental protein in support of muscle mass and health: Advantage whey. *Journal of Food Science* 80:A8–A15.

Doherty, M., et al. 2002. Caffeine is ergogenic after supplementation of oral creatine monohydrate. *Medicine & Science in Sports & Exercise* 34:1785–92.

Doutreleau, S., et al. 2006. Chronic L-arginine supplementation enhances endurance tolerance in heart failure patients. *International Journal of Sport Medicine* 27:567–72.

Drummond, M., et al. 2009. Nutritional and contractile regulation of human skeletal muscle protein synthesis and mTORC1 signaling. *Journal of Applied Physiology* 106:1374–84.

Eisenstein, J., et al. 2002. High-protein weight-loss diets: Are they safe and do they work? A review of the experimental and epidemiologic data. *Nutrition Reviews* 60:189–200.

Elam, R. 1988. Morphological changes in adult males from resistance exercise and amino acid supplementation. *Journal of Sports Medicine & Physical Fitness* 28:35–39.

Elam, R., et al. 1989. Effects of arginine and ornithine on strength, lean body mass and urinary hydroxyproline in adult males. *Journal of Sports Medicine & Physical Fitness* 29:52–56.

Elliot, T., et al. 2006. Milk ingestion stimulates net muscle protein synthesis following resistance exercise. *Medicine & Science in Sports & Exercise* 38:667–74.

Engelhardt, M., et al. 1998. Creatine supplementation in endurance sports. *Medicine and Science in Sports and Exercise* 30:1123–9.

Esmarck, B. 2001. Timing of postexercise protein intake is important for muscle hypertrophy with resistance training in elderly humans. *Journal of Physiology* 535:301–11.

Evans, W. 2001. Protein nutrition and resistance exercise. *Canadian Journal of Applied Physiology* 26:S141–52.

Fielding, R., and Parkington, J. 2002. What are the dietary protein requirements of physically active individuals? New evidence on the effects of exercise on protein utilization during post-exercise recovery. *Nutrition in Clinical Care* 5:191–96.

Fitts, R., and Metzger, J. 1993. Mechanisms of muscular fatigue. In *Principles of Exercise Biochemistry,* ed. J. Poortmans. Basel, Switzerland: Karger.

Fogelholm, G., et al. 1993. Low-dose amino acid supplementation: No effects on serum human growth hormone and insulin in male weightlifters. *International Journal of Sport Nutrition* 3:290–97.

Gaffney-Stomberg, E., et al. 2009. Increasing dietary protein requirements in elderly people for optimal muscle and bone health. *Journal of the American Geriatrics Society* 57:1073–79.

Garlick, P., et al. 1999. Adaptation of protein metabolism in relation to limits to high dietary protein intake. *European Journal of Clinical Nutrition* 53:S34–S43.

Genaro, Pde, S., and Martini, L. 2010. Effect of protein intake on bone and muscle mass in the elderly. *Nutrition Reviews* 68:616–30.

Gibala, M. 2001. Regulation of skeletal muscle amino acid metabolism during exercise. *International Journal of Sport Nutrition & Exercise Metabolism* 11:87–108.

Gibala, M. 2002. Dietary protein, amino acid supplements, and recovery from exercise. *Sports Science Exchange* 15(4):1–4.

Gibala, M. 2007. Protein metabolism and endurance exercise. *Sports Medicine* 37:337–40.

Gleeson, M. 2005. Interrelationship between physical activity and branched-chain amino acids. *Journal of Nutrition* 135:1591S–95S.

Gleeson, M., et al. 1998. Effect of low- and high-carbohydrate diets on the plasma glutamine and circulating leukocyte responses to exercise. *International Journal of Sport Nutrition* 8:45–59.

Graham, T., and MacLean, D. 1998. Ammonia and amino acid metabolism in skeletal muscle: Human, rodent and canine models. *Medicine & Science in Sports & Exercise* 30:34–46.

Graham, T., et al. 1997. Effect of endurance training on ammonia and amino acid metabolism in humans. *Medicine & Science in Sports & Exercise* 29:646–53.

Green, A., et al. 1996. Carbohydrate ingestion augments creatine retention during creatine feeding in humans. *Acta Physiologica Scandinavica* 158:195–202.

Green, M., et al. 2008. Carbohydrate-protein drinks do not enhance recovery from exercise-induced muscle injury. *International Journal of Sport Nutrition & Exercise Metabolism* 18:1–18.

Greenhaff, P. 1997. Creatine supplementation and implications for exercise performance. In *Advances in Training and Nutrition for Endurance Sports,* eds. A. Jeukendrup, M. Brouns, and F. Brouns. Maastricht, the Netherlands: Novartis Nutrition Research Unit.

Greenhaff, P., et al. 1994. Effect of oral creatine supplementation on skeletal muscle phosphocreatine resynthesis. *American Journal of Physiology* 266:E725–E730.

Greer, B., et al. 2007. Branched-chain amino acid supplementation and indicators of muscle damage after endurance exercise. *International Journal of Sport Nutrition & Exercise Metabolism* 17:595–607.

Gualano, B., et al. 2012. In sickness and in health: The widespread application of creatine supplementation. *Amino Acids* 43 (2):519–29.

Hargreaves, M., and Snow, R. 2001. Amino acids and endurance exercise. *International Journal of Sport Nutrition & Exercise Metabolism* 11:133–45.

Harris, R., et al. 2006. The absorption of orally supplied beta-alanine and its effect on muscle carnosine synthesis in human vastus lateralis. *Amino Acids* 30:279–89.

Harris, R., et al. 1992. Elevation of creatine in resting and exercised muscle on normal subjects by creatine supplementation. *Clinical Science* 83:367–74.

Harris, R., et al. 1993. The effect of oral creatine supplementation on running performance during maximal short term exercise in man. *Journal of Physiology* 467:74P.

Hartman, J., et al. 2007. Consumption of fat-free fluid milk after resistance exercise promotes greater lean mass accretion than does consumption of soy or carbohydrate in young, novice, male weightlifters. *American Journal of Clinical Nutrition* 86:373–81.

Hawkins, C., et al. 1991. Oral arginine does not affect body composition or muscle function in male weight lifters. *Medicine & Science in Sports & Exercise* 23:S15.

Hayes, A., and Cribb, P. 2008. Effect of whey protein isolate on strength, body composition and muscle hypertrophy during resistance training. *Current Opinion in Clinical Nutrition & Metabolic Care* 11:40–44.

Heaney, R., and Layman, D. 2008. Amount and type of protein influences bone health. *American Journal of Clinical Nutrition* 87:1567S–70S.

Hefler, S., et al. 1995. Branched-chain amino acid (BCAA) supplementation improves endurance performance in competitive cyclists. *Medicine & Science in Sports & Exercise* 27:S149.

Helms, E., et al. 2014. A systematic review of dietary protein during caloric restriction in resistance trained lean athletes: A case for higher intakes. *International Journal of Sport Nutrition and Exercise Metabolism* 24:127–38.

Henkel, J. 2000. Soy: Health claims for soy protein, questions about other components. *FDA Consumer* 34(3):13–20.

Hernandez, M., et al. 1996. The protein efficiency ratios of 30:70 mixtures of animal: Vegetable protein are similar or higher than those of the animal foods alone. *Journal of Nutrition* 126:574–81.

Herrero-Beaumont, G., et al. 2007. The reverse glucosamine sulfate pathway: Application in knee osteoarthritis. *Expert Opinion on Pharmacotherapy* 8:215–25.

Hespel, P., et al. 2001. Oral creatine supplementation facilitates the rehabilitation of disuse atrophy and alters the expression of muscle myogenic factors in humans. *Journal of Physiology* 536:625–33.

Hespel, P., et al. 2002. Opposite actions of caffeine and creatine on muscle relaxation time in humans. *Journal of Applied Physiology* 92:513–18.

Hespel, P., et al. 2006. Dietary supplements for football. *Journal of Sports Sciences* 24:749–61.

Hickner, R., et al. 2006. L-citrulline reduces time to exhaustion and insulin response to a graded exercise test. *Medicine & Science in Sports & Exercise* 38:660–66.

Hickner, R., et al. 2010. Effect of 28 days of creatine ingestion on muscle metabolism and performance of a simulated cycling road race. *Journal of the International Society of Sport Nutrition* 7:26.

Hile, A., et al. 2006. Creatine supplementation and anterior compartment pressure during exercise in the heat in dehydrated men. *Journal of Athletic Training* 41:30–5.

Hobson, R., et al. 2012. Effects of beta-alanine supplementation on exercise performance: A meta-analysis. *Amino Acids* 43:25–37.

Hoffman , J., et al. 2006. Effect of protein intake on strength, body composition and endocrine changes in strength/power athletes. *Journal of the International Society of Sport Nutrition* 3(2): 12–18.

Hofman, Z., et al. 2002. The effect of bovine colostrum supplementation on exercise performance in elite field hockey players. *International Journal of Sport Nutrition & Exercise Metabolism* 12:461–69.

Houston, D., et al. 2008. Dietary protein intake is associated with lean mass change in older, community-dwelling adults: The Health, Aging, and Body Composition (Health ABC) Study. *American Journal of Clinical Nutrition* 87:150–55.

Hu, F. 2005. Protein, body weight, and cardiovascular health. *American Journal of Clinical Nutrition* 82:242S–47S.

Hu, F. B., et al. 1999. Dietary protein and risk of ischemic heart disease in women. *American Journal of Clinical Nutrition* 70:221–27.

Hughes, R., and Carr, A. 2002. A randomized, double-blind, placebo-controlled trial of glucosamine sulfate as an analgesic in osteoarthritis of the knee. *Rheumatology* 41:279–84.

Hultman, E., et al. 1996. Muscle creatine loading in men. *Journal of Applied Physiology* 81:232–37.

Ivy, J., et al. 2003. Effect of a carbohydrate-protein supplement on endurance performance during exercise of varying intensity. *International Journal of Sport Nutrition & Exercise Metabolism* 13:382–95.

Jacobson, B. 1990. Effect of amino acids on growth hormone release. *Physician & Sportsmedicine* 18 (January):63–70.

Jacobson, B., et al. 2001. Nutrition practices and knowledge of college varsity athletes: A follow-up. *Journal of Strength & Conditioning Research* 15:63–68.

Jarvis, M., et al. 2002. The acute 1-week effects of the Zone diet on body composition, blood lipid levels, and performance in recreational endurance athletes. *Journal of Strength & Conditioning Research* 16:50–57.

Jeacocke, N., et al. 2015. L-citrulline. In *Nutritional Supplements in Sport, Exercise, and Health. An A–Z Guide,* ed. L. M. Castell, S. J. Stear, and L. M. Burke. New York: Routledge.

Jenkins, D., et al. 2002. Effects of high- and low-isoflavone soy foods on blood lipids, oxidized LDL, homocysteine, and blood pressure in hyperlipidemic men and women. *American Journal of Clinical Nutrition* 76:365–72.

Johnson, C., et al. 2002. Postprandial thermogenesis is increased 100% on high-protein, low-fat diet versus a high-carbohydrate, low-fat diet in healthy, young women. *Journal of the American College of Nutrition* 21:55–61.

Jones, A. 2013. Dietary nitrate: The next magic bullet? *Gatorade Sports Science Exchange* 110:1–5.

Jones, A. 2014. Buffers and their role in the nutritional preparation of athletes. *Gatorade Sports Science Exchange* 124:1–5.

Jones, A. 2014. Dietary nitrate supplementation and exercise performance. *Sports Medicine* 44:S35–45.

Jäger, R., et al. 2011. Analysis of the efficacy, safety, and regulatory status of novel forms of creatine. *Amino Acids* 40:1369–83.

Kanaley, J. 2008. Growth hormone, arginine and exercise. *Current Opinion in Clinical Nutrition & Metabolic Care* 11:50–54.

Karp, J., et al. 2006. Chocolate milk as a post-exercise recovery aid. *International Journal of Sport Nutrition & Exercise Metabolism* 16:78–91.

Kerksick, C., et al. 2006. The effects of protein and amino acid supplementation on performance and training adaptations during ten weeks of resistance training. *Journal of Strength & Conditioning Research* 20:643–53.

Kerksick, C., et al. 2008. International Society of Sports Nutrition position stand: Nutrient timing. *Journal of the International Society of Sports Nutrition* 5:17.

Kilduff, L., et al. 2004. The effects of creatine supplementation on cardiovascular, metabolic, and thermoregulatory responses during exercise in the heat in endurance-trained humans. *International Journal of Sport Nutrition & Exercise Metabolism* 14:443–60.

Kim, H., et al. 2011. Studies on the safety of creatine supplementation. *Amino Acids* 40:1409–1418.

Kingsbury, K., et al. 1998. Contrasting plasma free amino acid patterns in elite athletes. *British Journal of Sports Medicine* 32:25–32.

Kirkendall, D. 2004. Creatine, carbs, and fluids: How important in soccer nutrition? *Sports Science Exchange* 17(3):1–6.

Koopman, E., et al. 2004. Combined ingestion of protein and carbohydrate improves protein balance during ultra-endurance exercise. *American Journal of Physiology-Endocrinology & Metabolism* 287: E712–20.

Koopman, R. 2007. Role of amino acids and peptides in the molecular signaling in skeletal muscle after resistance exercise. *International Journal of Sport Nutrition & Exercise Metabolism* 17:S47–S57.

Koopman, R., et al. 2005. Combined ingestion of protein and free leucine with carbohydrate increases postexercise muscle protein synthesis in vivo in male subjects. *American Journal of Physiology. Endocrinology & Metabolism* 288:E645–53.

Kraemer, W., et al. 2006. The effects of amino acid supplementation on hormonal responses to resistance training overreaching. *Metabolism* 55:282–91.

Krall, E., and Dawson-Hughes, B. 1999. Osteoporosis. In *Modern Nutrition in Health and Disease,* eds. M. Shils et al. Baltimore: Williams and Wilkins.

Kreider, R. 2003. Effects of creatine supplementation on performance and training adaptations. *Molecular & Cellular Biochemistry* 244:89–94.

Kreider, R., et al., 2010. ISSN exercise & sport nutrition review: Research and recommendations. *Journal of the International Society of Sports Nutrition* 7:7.

Kuipers, H., et al. 2002. Effects of oral bovine colostrum supplementation on serum insulin-like growth factor-I levels. *Nutrition* 18:566–67.

Lambert, M., et al. 1993. Failure of commercial oral amino acid supplements to increase serum growth hormone concentrations in male bodybuilders. *International Journal of Sport Nutrition* 3:298–305.

Lanhers, C. ,et al. 2015. in press. Creatine supplementation and lower limb strength performance: A systematic review and meta-analyses. *Sports Medicine.*

Lansley, K., et al. 2011. Acute dietary nitrate supplementation improves cycling time trial performance. *Medicine & Science in Sports & Exercise* 43:1125–31.

Lawrence, M., and Kirby, D. 2002. Nutrition and sports supplements: Fact or fiction? *Journal of Clinical Gastroenterology* 35:299–306.

Layman, D., et al. 2008. Protein in optimal health: Heart disease and type 2 diabetes.

American Journal of Clinical Nutrition 87:1571S–75S.

Leidy, H., et al. 2015. The role of protein in weight loss and maintenance. *American Journal of Clinical Nutrition* 101:1320S–29S.

Lemon, P. 1998. Effects of exercise on dietary protein requirements. *International Journal of Sport Nutrition,* 8:426–47.

Lemon, P. 2000. Effects of exercise on protein metabolism. In *Nutrition in Sport,* ed. R. J. Maughan. Oxford: Blackwell Science.

Lemon, P. 2000. Protein metabolism during exercise. In *Exercise and Sport Science,* eds. W. E. Garrett and D. T. Kirkendall. Philadelphia: Lippincott Williams & Wilkins.

Lemon, P., et al. 1992. Protein requirements and muscle mass/strength changes during intensive training in novice bodybuilders. *Journal of Applied Physiology* 73:767–75.

Lesourd, B. 1995. Protein undernutrition as the major cause of decreased immune function in the elderly: Clinical and functional implications. *Nutrition Reviews* 53:S86–S94.

Levenhagen, D., et al. 2001. Postexercise nutrient intake timing in humans is critical to recovery of leg glucose and protein homeostasis. *American Journal of Physiology. Endocrinology & Metabolism* 280:E982–93.

Levenhagen, D., et al. 2002. Postexercise protein intake enhances whole-body and leg protein accretion in humans. *Medicine & Science in Sports & Exercise* 34:828–37.

Liappis, N., et al. 1979. Quantitative study of free amino acids in human eccrine sweat excreted from the forearms of healthy trained and untrained men during exercise. *European Journal of Applied Physiology* 42:227–34.

Lichtenstein, A., et al. 2002. Lipoprotein response to diets high in soy or animal protein with and without isoflavones in moderately hypercholesterolemic subjects. *Arteriosclerosis, Thrombosis, & Vascular Biology* 22:1852–58.

Lopez, R., et al. 2009. Does creatine supplementation hinder exercise heat tolerance or hydration status? A systematic review with meta-analyses. *Journal of Athletic Training* 44:215–23.

Lopez, R., et al. 2009. Does creatine supplementation hinder exercise heat tolerance or hydration status? A systematic review with meta-analyses. *Journal of Athletic Training* 44:215–23.

Lukaszuk, J., et al. 2002. Effect of creatine supplementation and a lactoovovegetarian diet on muscle creatine concentration. *International Journal of Sport Nutrition & Exercise Metabolism* 12:336–48.

Macdermid, P., and Stannard, S. 2006. A whey-supplemented, high-protein diet versus a high-carbohydrate diet: Effects on endurance cycling performance. *International Journal of Sport Nutrition & Exercise Metabolism* 16:65–77.

Madsen, K., et al. 1996. Effects of glucose, glucose plus branched-chain amino acids, or placebo on bike performance over 100 km. *Journal of Applied Physiology* 81:2644–50.

Matthews, D. 2006. Proteins and amino acids. In *Modern Nutrition in Health and Disease,* eds. M. Shils, et al. Philadelphia: Lippincott Williams & Wilkins.

Maughan, R., and Sadler, D. 1983. The effects of oral administration of salts of aspartic acid on the metabolic response to prolonged exhausting exercise in man. *International Journal of Sports Medicine* 4:119–23.

Mayhew, D., et al. 2002. Effects of long-term creatine supplementation on liver and kidney functions in American college football players. *International Journal of Sport Nutrition and Exercise Metabolism* 12:453–60.

McConell, G. 2007. Effects of L-arginine supplementation on exercise metabolism. *Current Opinion in Clinical Nutrition & Metabolic Care* 10:46–51.

McConell, G., et al. 2006. L-arginine infusion increases glucose clearance during prolonged exercise in humans. *American Journal of Physiology. Endocrinology & Metabolism* 290:E60–E66.

McLellan, T., et al. 2014. Effects of protein in combination with carbohydrate supplements on acute or repeat endurance exercise performance: A systematic review. *Sports Medicine* 44:535–50.

McNaughton, L., et al. 1999. Inosine supplementation has no effect on aerobic or anaerobic cycling performance. *International Journal of Sport Nutrition* 9:333–44.

Meeusen, R., and Wilson, P. 2007. Amino acids and the brain: Do they play a role in "central fatigue"? *International Journal of Sport Nutrition & Exercise Metabolism* 17:S37–S46.

Meeusen, R., et al. 2006. The brain and fatigue: New opportunities for nutritional interventions? *Journal of Sports Sciences* 24:773–82.

Melis, G., et al. 2004. Glutamine: Recent developments in research on the clinical significance of glutamine. *Current Opinion in Clinical Nutrition & Metabolic Care* 7:59–79.

Mendel, R., et al. 2005. Effects of creatine on thermoregulatory responses while exercising in the heat. *Nutrition* 21:301–307.

Metzl, J., et al. 2001. Creatine use among young athletes. *Pediatrics* 108:421–25.

Millard-Stafford, M., et al. 2005. Recovery from run training: Efficacy of a carbohydrate-protein beverage. *International Journal of Sport Nutrition & Exercise Metabolism* 15:610–24.

Miller, B. 2007. Human muscle protein synthesis after physical activity and feeding. *Exercise & Sport Sciences Reviews* 35:50–55.

Millward, D. 2004. Macronutrient intakes as determinants of dietary protein and amino acid adequacy. *Journal of Nutrition* 134:1588S–96S.

Mitchell, M., et al. 1993. Effects of supplementation with arginine and lysine on body composition, strength and growth hormone levels in weightlifters. *Medicine & Science in Sports & Exercise* 25:S25.

Mitchell, W., et al. 2015. A dose- rather than delivery profile-dependent mechanism regulates the "muscle-full" effect in response to oral essential amino acid intake in young men. *Journal of Nutrition* 145:207–14.

Mittleman, K., et al. 1998. Branched-chain amino acids prolong exercise during heat stress in men and women. *Medicine & Science in Sports & Exercise* 30:83–91.

Moore, D., et al. 2009. Ingested protein dose response of muscle and albumin protein synthesis after resistance exercise in young men. *American Journal of Clinical Nutrition* 89:161–68.

Moore, D., et al. 2014. Beyond muscle hypertrophy: Why dietary protein is important for endurance athletes. *Applied Physiology Nutrition and Metabolism* 39:987–97.

Mujika, I., et al. 2000. Creatine supplementation and sprint performance in soccer players. *Medicine & Science in Sports & Exercise* 32:518–25.

Newsholme, E., and Blomstrand, E. 1996. The plasma level of some amino acids and physical and mental fatigue. *Experientia* 52:413–15.

Newsholme, E., and Castell, L. 2000. Amino acids, fatigue and immunodepression in exercise. In *Nutrition in Sport,* ed. R. J. Maughan. Oxford: Blackwell Science.

Newsholme, E., et al. 1992. Physical and mental fatigue: Metabolic mechanisms and importance of plasma amino acids. *British Medical Bulletin* 48:477–95.

Nieman, D. 2001. Exercise immunology: Nutrition countermeasures. *Canadian Journal of Applied Physiology* 26:S45–55.

Olsen, S., et al. 2006. Creatine supplementation augments the increase in satellite cell and myonuclei number in human skeletal muscle induced by strength training. *Journal of Physiology* 573:525–34.

Op 'T Eijnde, B., et al. 2001. Creatine loading does not impact on stroke performance in tennis. *International Journal of Sports Medicine* 22:76–80.

Ostojic, S. 2004. Creatine supplementation in young soccer players. *International Journal of Sport Nutrition & Exercise Metabolism* 14:95–103.

Ostojic, S., and Ahmetovic, Z. 2008. Gastrointestinal distress after creatine supplementation in athletes: Are side effects dose dependent? *Research in Sports Medicine* 16(1):15–22.

Ostojic, S., et al. 2007. Glucosamine administration in athletes: Effects on recovery of acute knee injury. *Research in Sports Medicine* 15:113–24.

Paddon-Jones, D., et al. 2008. Protein, weight management, and satiety. *American Journal of Clinical Nutrition* 1558S–61S.

Parkhouse, W. 1988. Regulation of skeletal muscle myofibrillar protein degradation: Relationships to fatigue and exercise. *International Journal of Biochemistry* 20:769–75.

Parry-Billings, M., et al. 1992. Plasma amino acid concentrations in the overtraining syndrome: Possible effects on the immune system. *Medicine & Science in Sports & Exercise* 24:1353–58.

Pasiakos, S., et al. 2014. Effects of protein supplements on muscle damage, soreness and recovery of muscle function and physical performance: A systematic review. *Sports Medicine* 44:655–70.

Pasiakos, S., et al. 2015. The effects of protein supplements on muscle mass, strength, and aerobic and anaerobic power in healthy adults: A systematic review. *Sports Medicine* 45:111–31.

Pavelka, K., et al. 2002. Glucosamine sulfate use and delay of progression of knee osteoarthritis: A 3-year, randomized, placebo-controlled, double-blind study. *Archives of Internal Medicine* 162: 2113–23.

Persky, A. M., and Rawson, E. S. 2007. Safety of creatine supplementation in health and disease. In *Creatine and Creatine Kinase in Health and Disease,* ed. Gajja J. Salomons and Markus Wyss. Dordrecht, the Netherlands: Springer.

Peyrebrune, M., et al. 2005. Effect of creatine supplementation on training for competition in elite swimmers. *Medicine & Science in Sports & Exercise* 37:2140–47.

Phillips, G. 2007. Glutamine: The nonessential amino acid for performance enhancement. *Current Sports Medicine Reports* 6:265–68.

Phillips, S. 2004. Protein requirements and supplementation in strength sports. *Nutrition* 20:689–95.

Phillips, S. 2006. Dietary protein for athletes: From requirements to metabolic advantage. *Applied Physiology, Nutrition & Metabolism* 31:647–54.

Phillips, S. 2013. Defining optimum protein intake for athletes. In *Sports Nutrition. The Encyclopedia of Sports Medicine,* ed. Ronald J. Maughan. Oxford: Wiley-Blackwell.

Phillips, S. 2014. A brief review of higher dietary protein diets in weight loss: A focus on athletes. *Sports Medicine* 44:S149–53.

Phillips, S., et al. 2007. A critical examination of dietary protein requirements, benefits, and excesses in athletes. *International Journal of Sport Nutrition & Exercise Metabolism* 17:S58–S76.

Poortmans, J. 1993. Protein metabolism. In *Principles of Exercise Biochemistry,* ed. J. Poortmans. Basel, Switzerland: Karger.

Poortmans, J., and Dellalieux, O. 2000. Do regular high protein diets have potential health risks on kidney function in athletes? *International Journal of Sport Nutrition & Exercise Metabolism* 10:28–38.

Poortmans, J., and Francaux, M. 1999. Long-term oral creatine supplementation does not impair renal function in healthy athletes. *Medicine & Science in Sports & Exercise* 31:1108–10.

Poortmans, J., et al. 1997. Evidence of differential renal dysfunctions during exercise in man. *European Journal of Applied Physiology* 76:88–91.

Poortmans, J., et al. 2005. Effect of oral creatine supplementation on urinary methylamine, formaldehyde and formate. *Medicine & Science in Sports & Exercise* 37:1717–20.

Preen, D., et al. 2001. Effect of creatine loading on long-term sprint exercise performance and metabolism. *Medicine & Science in Sports & Exercise* 33:814–21.

Preen, D., et al. 2003. Creatine supplementation: A comparison of loading and maintenance protocols on creatine uptake by human skeletal muscle. *International Journal of Sport Nutrition & Metabolism* 13:97–111.

Quesnele, J., et al. 2014. The effects of beta-alanine supplementation on performance: A systematic review of the literature. *International Journal of Sports Nutrition and Exercise Metabolism* 24:14–27.

Ra, S., et al. 2015. Taurine supplementation reduces eccentric exercise-induced delayed onset muscle soreness in young men. *Advances in Experimental Medicine and Biology* 803:765–72.

Rawson, E. S., and Volek, J. S. 2003. The effects of creatine supplementation and resistance training on muscle strength and weightlifting performance. *Journal of Strength and Conditioning Research* 17(4):822–31.

Rawson, E., and Clarkson, P. 2003. Scientifically debatable: Is creatine worth its weight? *Sports Science Exchange* 16(4):1–6.

Rawson, E., and Venezia, A. 2011. Use of creatine in the elderly and evidence for effects on cognitive function in young and old. *Amino Acids* 40:1349–62.

Rawson, E., et al. 2013. Sport-specific nutrition: Practical issues—Strength and power events. In *Sports Nutrition. The Encyclopedia of Sports Medicine,* ed. Ronald J. Maughan. Oxford: Wiley-Blackwell.

Reginster, J., et al. 2007. Current role of glucosamine in the treatment of osteoarthritis. *Rheumatology* 46:731–5.

Reichenbach, S., et al. 2007. Meta-analysis: Chondroitin for osteoarthritis of the knee or hip. *Annals of Internal Medicine* 146:580–90.

Rennie, M., and Tipton, K. 2000. Protein and amino acid metabolism during and after exercise and the effects of nutrition. *Annual Review of Nutrition* 20:457–83.

Res, P., et al. 2012. Protein ingestion before sleep improves postexercise overnight recovery. *Medicine and Science in Sports and Exercise* 44:1560–9.

Reynolds, K., et al. 2006. A meta-analysis of the effect of soy protein supplementation on serum lipids. *American Journal of Cardiology* 98:633–40.

Rockwell, J., et al. 2001. Creatine supplementation affects muscle creatine during energy restriction. *Medicine & Science in Sports & Exercise* 33:61–68.

Rodriguez, N., et al. 2007. Dietary protein, endurance exercise, and human skeletal-muscle protein turnover. *Current Opinions in Clinical Nutrition & Metabolic Care* 10:40–45.

Romano-Ely, B., et al. 2006. Effect of an iso-caloric carbohydrate-protein-antioxidant drink on cycling performance. *Medicine & Science in Sports & Exercise* 38:1608–16.

Romer, L., et al. 2001. Effects of oral creatine supplementation on high intensity, intermittent exercise performance in competitive squash players. *International Journal of Sports Medicine* 22:546–52.

Rowlands, D., and Thomson, J. 2009. Effects of β-hydroxy-β-methylbutyrate supplementation during resistance training on strength, body composition, and muscle damage in trained and untrained young men: A meta-analysis. *Journal of Strength & Conditioning Research* 23(3): 836–46.

Rowlands, D., et al. 2007. Effect of protein-rich feeding on recovery after intense exercise. *International Journal of Sport Nutrition & Exercise Metabolism* 17: 521–43.

Rutherford, J., et al. 2010. The effect of acute taurine ingestion on endurance performance and metabolism in well-trained cyclists. *International Journal of Sport Nutrition and Exercise Metabolism* 20:322–29.

Sacks, F., et al. 2006. Soy protein, isoflavones, and cardiovascular health: An American Heart Association Science Advisory for professionals from the Nutrition Committee. *Circulation.* 113:1034–44.

Sahlin, K., et al. 1998. Energy supply and muscle fatigue in humans. *Acta Physiologica Scandinavica* 162:261–66.

Sale, C., and Harris, R. 2015. β-alanine and carnosine. In *Nutritional Supplements in Sport, Exercise, and Health. An A–Z Guide,* ed. L. M. Castell, S. J. Stear, and L. M. Burke. New York: Routledge.

Sale, C., et al. 2010. Effect of beta-alanine supplementation on muscle carnosine concentrations and exercise performance. *Amino Acids* 39:321–33.

Sale, C., et al. 2013. Carnosine: From exercise performance to health. *Amino Acids* 44:1477–91.

Santos, R., et al. 2004. The effect of creatine supplementation upon inflammatory and muscle soreness markers after a 30 km race. *Life Sciences* 75:1917–24.

Saunders, M. 2007. Coingestion of carbohydrate-protein during endurance exercise: Influence on performance and recovery. *International Journal of Sport Nutrition & Exercise Metabolism* 17:S87–S103.

Schardt, D. 2001. Sam-e so-so. *Nutrition Action Health Letter* 28(2):10–11.

Schardt, D. 2002. Got soy? *Nutrition Action Health Letter* 29(9):8–11.

Schardt, D. 2006. Do glucosamine & chondroitin work? *Nutrition Action Health Letter* 33(7):9–11.

Schilling, B., et al. 2001. Creatine supplementation and health variables: A retrospective study. *Medicine & Science in Sports & Exercise* 33:183–88.

Schoenfeld, B. ,et al. 2013. The effect of protein timing on muscle strength and hypertrophy: A meta-analysis. *Journal of the International Society of Sports Nutrition* 10:53.

Schroeder, C., et al. 2001. The effects of creatine dietary supplementation on anterior compartment pressure in the lower leg during rest and following exercise. *Clinical Journal of Sport Medicine* 11:87–95.

Segura, R., and Ventura, J. 1988. Effect of L-tryptophan supplementation on exercise performance. *International Journal of Sports Medicine* 9:301–5.

Shing, C. 2015. Colostrum. In *Nutritional Supplements in Sport, Exercise, and Health. An A–Z Guide,* ed. L. M. Castell, S. J. Stear, and L. M. Burke. New York: Routledge.

Shing, C., et al. 2006. The influence of bovine colostrum supplementation on exercise performance in highly trained cyclists. *British Journal of Sports Medicine* 40:797–801.

Siervo, M., et al. 2013. Inorganic nitrate and beetroot juice supplementation reduces blood pressure in adults: A systematic review and meta-analysis. *Journal of Nutrition* 143:818–26.

Skare, O., et al. 2001. Creatine supplementation improves sprint performance in male sprinters. *Scandinavian Journal of Medicine & Science in Sports* 11:96–102.

Skibola, C., and Smith, M. 2000. Potential health impacts of excessive flavonoid intake. *Free Radical Biology & Medicine* 29:375–83.

Slater, G. 2015. β-hydroxy β-methylbutyrate (HMB). *In Nutritional Supplements in Sport, Exercise, and Health. An A-Z Guide,* ed. L. M. Castell, S. J. Stear, and L. M. Burke. New York: Routledge.

Slater, G., and Jenkins, D. 2000. Beta-hydroxy-beta-methylbutyrate (HMB) supplementation and the promotion of muscle growth and strength. *Sports Medicine* 30:105–16.

Slavin, J., et al. 1988. Amino acid supplements: Beneficial or risky? *Physician & Sportsmedicine* 16 (March):221–24.

Snijders, T., et al. 2015. Protein ingestion before sleep increases muscle mass and strength gains during prolonged resistance-type exercise training in healthy young men. *Journal of Nutrition* 145:1178–84.

Snow, R., and Murphy, R. 2003. Factors influencing creatine loading into human skeletal muscle. *Exercise & Sport Sciences Reviews* 31:154–58.

Soeken, K., et al. 2002. Safety and efficacy of S-adenosylmethionine (SAMe) for osteoarthritis. *Journal of Family Practice* 51:425–30.

Spriet, L. 2015. Taurine. In *Nutritional Supplements in Sport, Exercise, and Health. An A–Z Guide,* ed. L. M. Castell, S. J. Stear, and L. M. Burke. New York: Routledge.

Spriet, L., and Whitfield, J. 2015. Taurine and skeletal muscle function. *Current Opinion in Clinical Nutrition and Metabolic Care* 8:96–101.

Starling, R., et al. 1996. Effect of inosine supplementation on aerobic and anaerobic cycling performance. *Medicine & Science in Sports & Exercise* 28:1193–98.

Stensrund, T., et al. 1992. L-tryptophan supplementation does not improve running performance. *International Journal of Sports Medicine* 13:481–85.

Struder, H. K., et al. 1998. Influence of paroxetine, branched-chain amino acids and tyrosine on neuroendocrine system responses and fatigue in humans. *Hormone & Metabolic Research* 30:188–94.

Suminski, R., et al. 1997. Acute effect of amino acid ingestion and resistance exercise on plasma growth hormone concentration in young men. *International Journal of Sport Nutrition* 7:48–60.

Sutton, E., et al. 2005. Ingestion of tyrosine: Effects on endurance, muscle strength, and anaerobic performance. *International Journal of Sport Nutrition & Exercise Metabolism* 15:173–85.

Syrotuik, D., and Bell, G. 2004. Acute creatine monohydrate supplementation: A descriptive physiological profile of responders vs. nonresponders. *Journal of Strength & Conditioning Research* 18:610–17.

Syrotuik, D., et al. 2001. Effects of creatine monohydrate supplementation during combined strength and high intensity rowing training on performance. *Canadian Journal of Applied Physiology* 26:527–42.

Tanaka, H., et al. 1997. Changes in plasma tryptophan/branched-chain amino acid ratio in responses to training volume variation. *International Journal of Sports Medicine* 18:270–5.

Tang, J., et al. 2009. Ingestion of whey hydrolysate, casein, or soy protein isolate: Effects on mixed muscle protein synthesis at rest and following resistance exercise in young men. *Journal of Applied Physiology* 107:987–92.

Tarnopolsky, M. 2004. Protein requirements for endurance athletes. *Nutrition* 20:662–68.

Tarnopolsky, M. 2008. Sex differences in exercise metabolism and the role of 17-beta estradiol. *Medicine & Science in Sports & Exercise* 40:648–54.

Tarnopolsky, M., and Safdar, A. 2008. The potential benefits of creatine and conjugated linoleic acid as adjuncts to resistance training in older adults. *Applied Physiology, Nutrition & Metabolism* 33:213–27.

Tarnopolsky, M., et al. 2001. Creatine-dextrose and protein-dextrose induce similar strength gains during training. *Medicine & Science in Sports & Exercise* 33:2944–52.

Tarnopolsky, M., et al. 2004. Creatine monohydrate enhances strength and body composition in Duchenne muscular dystrophy. *Neurology* 62:1771–77.

Theodorou, A., et al. 2005. Effects of acute creatine loading with or without carbohydrate on repeated bouts of maximal swimming in high-performance swimmers. *Journal of Strength & Conditioning Research* 19:265–69.

Tipton, K. 2007. Role of protein and hydrolysates before exercise. *International Journal of Sport Nutrition & Exercise Metabolism* 17:S77–S86.

Tipton, K., and Witard, O. 2007. Protein requirements and recommendations for athletes: Relevance of ivory tower arguments for practical recommendations. *Clinics in Sports Medicine* 26:17–36.

Tipton, K., and Wolfe, R. 1998. Exercise-induced changes in protein metabolism. *Acta Physiologica Scandinavica* 162:377–87.

Tipton, K., and Wolfe, R. 2004. Protein and amino acids for athletes. *Journal of Sports Sciences* 22:65–79.

Tipton, K., et al. 1999. Postexercise net protein synthesis in human muscle from orally administered amino acids. *American Journal of Physiology* 276:E628–E634.

Trudeau, F. 2008. Aspartate as an ergogenic supplement. *Sports Medicine* 38:9–16.

Tufts University. 2000. A look at glucosamine and chondroitin for easing arthritis pain. *Tufts University Health & Nutrition Letter* 17(11):4–5.

Tuttle, J., et al. 1995. Effect of acute potassium-magnesium aspartate supplementation on ammonia concentrations during and after resistance training. *International Journal of Sport Nutrition* 5:102–9.

Tyler, T., et al. 2004. The effect of creatine supplementation on strength recovery after anterior cruciate ligament (ACL) reconstruction: A randomized, placebo-controlled, double-blind trial. *American Journal of Sports Medicine* 32:383–88.

van Essen, M., and Gibala, M. 2006. Failure of protein to improve time trial performance when added to a sports drink. *Medicine & Science in Sports & Exercise* 38:1476–83.

van Hall, G., et al. 1995. Ingestion of branched-chain amino acids and tryptophan during sustained exercise in man: Failure to affect performance. *Journal of Physiology* 486:789–94.

van Hall, G., et al. 1998. Effect of carbohydrate supplementation on plasma glutamine during prolonged exercise and recovery. *International Journal of Sports Medicine* 19:82–86.

van Loon, L. 2007. Application of protein or protein hydrolysates to improve postexercise recovery. *International Journal of Sport Nutrition & Exercise Metabolism* 17:S104–S117.

van Loon, L., et al. 2003. Effects of creatine loading and prolonged creatine supplementation on body composition, fuel selection, sprint and endurance performance in humans. *Clinical Science* 104:153–62.

van Loon, L., et al. 2013. Dietary protein as a trigger for metabolic adaptations. *In Sports Nutrition. The Encyclopedia of Sports Medicine,* ed. Ronald J. Maughan. Oxford: Wiley-Blackwell.

Vandebuerie, F., et al. 1998. Effect of creatine loading on endurance capacity and sprint power in cyclists. *International Journal of Sports Medicine* 19:490–5.

Vandenberghe, K., et al. 1996. Caffeine counteracts the ergogenic action of muscle creatine loading. *Journal of Applied Physiology* 80:452–57.

Vandenberghe, K., et al. 1997. Inhibition of muscle phosphocreatine resynthesis by caffeine after creatine loading. *Medicine & Science in Sports & Exercise* 29:S249.

Vanhatalo, A., et al. 2010. Acute and chronic effects of dietary nitrate supplementation on blood pressure and the physiological responses to moderate-intensity and incremental exercise. *American Journal of Physiology & Regulatory, Integrative & Comparative Physiology* 299:R1121–31.

Vlad, S., et al. 2007. Glucosamine for pain in osteoarthritis: Why do trial results differ? *Arthritis & Rheumatism* 56:2267–77.

Volek, J., and Rawson, E. 2004. Scientific basis and practical aspects of creatine supplementation for athletes. *Nutrition* 20:609–14.

Volek, J., et al. 2001. Physiological responses to short-term exercise in the heat after creatine loading. *Medicine & Science in Sports & Exercise* 33:1101–8.

Volek, J., et al. 2004. The effects of creatine supplementation on muscular performance and body composition responses to short-term resistance training overreaching. *European Journal of Applied Physiology* 91:628–37.

Volek, J., et al. 2006. Nutritional aspects of women strength athletes. *British Journal of Sports Medicine* 40:742–48.

Wagenmakers, A. 1999. Amino acid supplements to improve athletic performance. *Current Opinion in Clinical Nutrition & Metabolic Care* 2:539–44.

Wagenmakers, A. 2000. Amino acid metabolism in exercise. In *Nutrition in Sport,* ed. R. J. Maughan. Oxford: Blackwell Science.

Wagenmakers, A. 2006. The metabolic systems: Protein and amino acid metabolism in muscle. In *ACSM's Advanced Exercise Physiology,* ed. C. M. Tipton. Philadelphia: Lippincott Williams & Wilkins.

Walberg-Rankin, J. W. 1999. Role of protein in exercise. *Clinics in Sports Medicine* 18:499–511.

Walzem, R., et al. 2002. Whey components: Millennia of evolution create functionalities for mammalian nutrition. What we know and what we may be overlooking. *Critical Reviews in Food Science & Nutrition* 42:353–75.

Watson, P., et al. 2004. The effect of acute branched-chain amino acid supplementation on prolonged exercise capacity in a warm environment. *European Journal of Applied Physiology* 93:306–14.

Weideman, C., et al. 1990. Effects of increased protein intake on muscle hypertrophy and strength following 13 weeks of resistance training. *Medicine & Science in Sports & Exercise* 22:S37.

Wesson, M., et al. 1988. Effects of oral administration of aspartic acid salts on the endurance capacity of trained athletes. *Research Quarterly for Exercise and Sport* 59:234–39.

Wilkinson, D., et al. 2013. Effects of leucine and its metabolite beta-hydroxy-beta-methylbutyrate on human skeletal muscle protein metabolism. *Journal of Physiology* 591:2911–23.

Wilkinson, S., et al. 2007. Consumption of fluid skim milk promotes greater muscle protein accretion after resistance exercise than does consumption of an isonitrogenous and isoenergetic soy-protein beverage. *American Journal of Clinical Nutrition* 85:1031–40.

Williams, M. 1999. Facts and fallacies of purported ergogenic amino acid supplements. *Clinics in Sports Medicine* 18:633–49.

Williams, M., et al. 1990. Effect of oral inosine supplementation on 3-mile treadmill run performance and VO₂ peak. *Medicine & Science in Sports & Exercise* 22:517–22.

Willoughby, D., and Rosene, J. 2001. Effects of oral creatine and resistance training on myosin heavy chain expression. *Medicine & Science in Sports & Exercise* 33:1674–81.

Wilson, A., et al. 2007. L-arginine supplementation in peripheral arterial disease: No benefit and possible harm. *Circulation* 116:188–95.

Wilson, J., et al. 2014. The effects of 12 weeks of beta-hydroxy-beta-methylbutyrate free acid supplementation on muscle mass, strength, and power in resistance-trained individuals: A randomized, double-blind, placebo-controlled study. *European Journal of Applied Physiology* 114:1217–27.

Wolfe, R. 2001. Control of muscle protein breakdown: Effects of activity and nutritional states. *International Journal of Sport Nutrition & Exercise Metabolism* 11:S164–69.

Wolfe, R. 2001. Effects of amino acid intake on anabolic processes. *Canadian Journal of Applied Physiology* 26:S220–27.

Wolfe, R. 2006. Skeletal muscle protein metabolism and resistance exercise. *Journal of Nutrition* 136:525S–28S.

Yaguchi, H., et al. 1998. The effect of triathlon on urinary excretion of enzymes and proteins. *International Urology & Nephrology* 30:107–12.

Yoshimura, H. 1970. Anemia during physical training (sports anemia). *Nutrition Review* 28:251–53.

Yquel, R., et al. 2002. Effect of creatine supplementation on phosphocreatine resynthesis, inorganic phosphate accumulation and pH during intermittent maximal exercise. *Journal of Sports Sciences* 20:427–37.

Zanchi, N., et al. 2011. HMB supplementation: Clinical and athletic performance-related effects and mechanisms of action. *Amino Acids* 40:1015–25.

Zhang, M., et al. 2004. Role of taurine supplementation to prevent exercise-induced oxidative stress in healthy young men. *Amino Acids* 26:203–07.

Zoeller, R., et al. 2007. Effects of 28 days of beta-alanine and creatine monohydrate supplementation on aerobic power, ventilatory and lactate thresholds, and time to exhaustion. *Amino Acids* 33:505–10.

Vitamins: The Organic Regulators

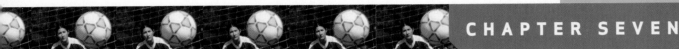

CHAPTER SEVEN

LEARNING OBJECTIVES

After studying this chapter, you should be able to:

1. Describe the various means whereby vitamins may carry out their functions in the human body.

2. Name the essential vitamins, state the RDA or AI for each, and identify several foods rich in each vitamin.

3. Describe the metabolic roles in the human body of each of the 13 essential vitamins and choline.

4. Explain the potential effects on health and sports performance associated with a deficiency of each essential vitamin and choline.

5. Identify those fat-soluble and water-soluble vitamins that are most likely to cause health risks if consumed in excess. Indicate at what doses adverse health effects may be observed, and determine how likely it is that such a dose may be obtained by consuming daily vitamin supplements and fortified foods.

6. Explain the theory as to how supplementation with each vitamin, and choline, may enhance sports performance, and highlight the research findings regarding the ergogenic efficacy of each.

7. Explain the theory as to how vitamin-like compounds may enhance sports performance, and highlight the research findings regarding the ergogenic efficacy of each.

8. Understand why health professionals recommend that we obtain our vitamins through natural foods, such as fruits and vegetables, and why some health professionals recommend that most adults also take a daily multivitamin supplement.

Introduction

Vitamins are a diverse class of 13 known specific nutrients that are involved in almost every metabolic process in the human body. We need only minute amounts of vitamins in our daily diet, so they are classified as micronutrients. Nevertheless, they are one of our most critical nutrients. Noticeable symptoms of a deficiency may appear in 2 to 4 weeks for several of the vitamins, and major debilitating diseases may occur with prolonged deficiencies. Vitamin deficiencies appear to be widespread in many developing countries, and according to Bouis, they affect a greater number of people in the world than does protein-energy malnutrition. Plant breeding of commonly eaten food crops, such as wheat, rice, and corn, to fortify them with vitamins and minerals may help alleviate this major health problem.

Major vitamin deficiencies are rare in industrialized societies because a wide variety of food products are available, many of them fortified with vitamins. Most health professionals recommend that we obtain the vitamins we need from the foods we eat, which is sound advice. However, some also note that certain segments of the population may not be obtaining adequate amounts of vitamins from food alone. Sebastian and others note that many older adults are at risk for vitamin deficiency. According to the 2015 Dietary Guidelines Advisory Committee's Scientific Report to the U.S. Departments of Agriculture and Health and Human Services, vitamins A, D, E, and C; folate; and fiber are consumed by the U.S. population in quantities less than the Estimated Average Requirement or Adequate Intake. The American Institute of Cancer Research (AICR) noted that although vitamin supplements are not recommended to prevent cancer, certain groups may benefit from specific vitamin supplementation, including the elderly, women of childbearing age, and individuals not exposed to sufficient sunlight. Fairfield and Fletcher, in two studies published by the American Medical Association, go a step further

and indicate that it may be *prudent* for *all adults* to take vitamin supplements.

In general, most studies reveal that athletes are obtaining adequate vitamin nutrition, probably because of the additional food energy intake associated with the increased energy expenditure of exercise. Additionally, many athletes take vitamin supplements. For example, Jacobson and others reported that vitamin/mineral pills were the most commonly used dietary supplement by female NCAA Division I collegiate athletes. However, like members of the general population, many athletes may not be obtaining optimal levels of vitamins from the diet. Moreover, certain athletic groups, particularly those who are on weight-reduction programs to qualify for competition or to enhance performance, may not receive adequate vitamin nutrition. Furthermore, individual athletes in generally well-nourished athletic groups may have a suboptimal vitamin intake.

As noted throughout this chapter, adequate vitamin nutrition is essential for both optimal health and athletic performance. But if you do not obtain the RDA for a specific vitamin or vitamins, will your health or physical performance suffer? Will vitamin supplements above

and beyond the RDA improve your health or performance? A major purpose of this chapter is to provide you with factual data, based on the available research, to help answer these two very general questions.

A slightly different approach is used in this chapter and in chapter 8. The first section provides some basic facts about the general role of vitamins in the human body. The next two sections cover the fat-soluble and water-soluble vitamins, respectively, with each individual vitamin discussed in terms of its Dietary Reference Intake (DRI), either its Recommended Dietary Allowance (RDA) or its Adequate Intake (AI); food sources that provide ample amounts; metabolic functions in the body with particular reference to health and the physically active individual; and the findings of research relative to the impact of deficiencies and supplementation. The fourth section focuses on ergogenic aspects of special vitamin or vitamin-like preparations, while the final section highlights some health implications of vitamin supplementation and provides some guidelines for selecting a multivitamin/mineral for those who choose to supplement.

Basic Facts

What are vitamins and how do they work?

Vitamins are a class of complex organic compounds that are found in small amounts in most foods. They are essential for the optimal

functioning of many different physiological processes in the human body. The activity levels of many of these physiological processes are increased greatly during exercise, and an adequate bodily supply of vitamins must be present for these processes to function best.

Coenzyme Functions For the fundamental physiological processes of the body to proceed in an orderly, controlled fashion, a number of complex chemicals known as **enzymes** are necessary to regulate the diverse reactions involved. Hundreds of enzymes have been identified in the human body. Enzymes are necessary to digest our foods, to make our muscles contract, to release the energy stores in our bodies, to help us transport body gases such as carbon dioxide, to help us grow, to help clot our blood, and so on. Enzymes serve as catalysts; that is, they are capable of inducing changes in other substances without changing themselves.

Enzymes are chemicals that generally consist of two parts. One part is a protein molecule and to it is attached the second part, a **coenzyme**. For the enzyme to function properly, both parts must be present. The coenzyme often contains a vitamin or some related compound (figure 7.1). The enzyme is not used up in the chemical process that it initiates or in which it participates, but enzymes may deteriorate with time. Coenzymes also may be degraded through body metabolism. It is now known that the B complex vitamins are essential in human nutrition because of their role in the activation of enzymes, and thus a fresh supply of these water-soluble vitamins is constantly needed.

Antioxidant Functions Various oxidative reactions in the body produce substances called free radicals. **Free radicals** are chemical substances that contain a lone, unpaired electron in the outer orbit. The superoxide radical ($O_2^{\bullet-}$) and hydroxyl radical ($OH^{\bullet}$) are true free radicals. Two other related substances, referred to as non-radical oxygen species, are hydrogen peroxide (H_2O_2) and singlet oxygen ($^1O_2$). These substances are known as reactive oxygen species (ROS) and when nitrogen is involved are known as reactive oxygen/nitrogen species (RONS). The interested reader is referred to the review by Neiss for a detailed discussion. For the purpose of our discussion, we shall refer to them collectively as free radicals.

Free radicals are unstable compounds that possess an unbalanced magnetic field that affects molecular structure and chemical reactions in the body. Free radicals may be very reactive with body tissues.

Linnane notes that formation of free radicals, such as superoxide anion and hydrogen peroxide formation during oxidative processes, is essential to normal cellular function, such as gene expression and muscle contractile force. However, although oxidative processes are essential to life, some oxidations may cause cellular damage by oxidation of unsaturated fats in cellular and subcellular membranes. Free radicals may cause such undesirable oxidations. Halliwell indicated that free radicals may damage DNA, lipids, proteins, and other molecules and may be involved in the development of cancer, cardiovascular disease, and neurodegenerative disease. Fortunately, although free radicals are formed naturally in the body, body cells produce a number of antioxidant enzymes, such as superoxide dismutase, glutathione peroxidase, and catalase, to help neutralize free radicals and prevent cellular damage. To function properly, these enzymes, often referred to as free radical–scavenging enzymes, must contain certain nutrients such as copper, zinc, and selenium. Comparable to these enzymes, as depicted in figure 7.2, vitamins E and C and beta-carotene possess antioxidant properties. These antioxidant vitamins have received much research attention relative to effects on health and physical performance and are discussed at appropriate points later in this chapter.

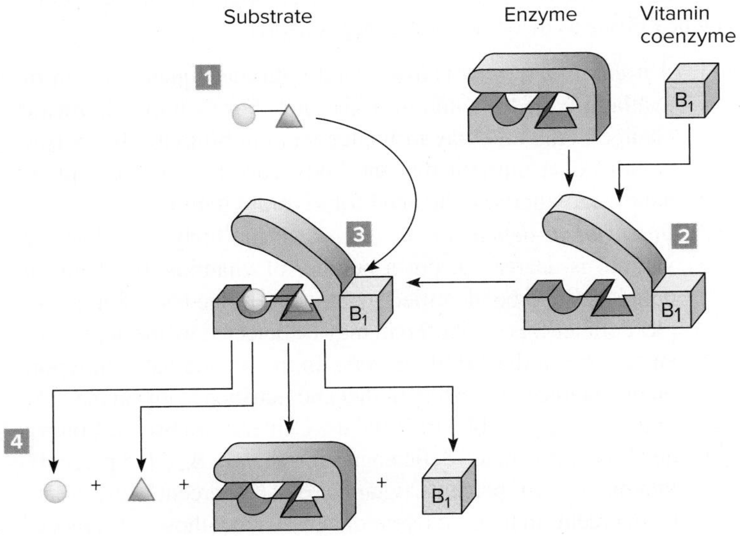

FIGURE 7.1 Role of vitamin as coenzyme. (1) Substrates, such as pyruvate, need enzymes to be converted into more usable compounds. However, many enzymes must be activated before a reaction occurs. Note that the enzyme is in a closed position. (2) An enzyme and a vitamin coenzyme (B_1) combine to form an activated complex, in essence opening up the enzyme. (3) The open, activated enzyme accepts the substrate and (4) splits it into two compounds while releasing the enzyme and coenzyme.

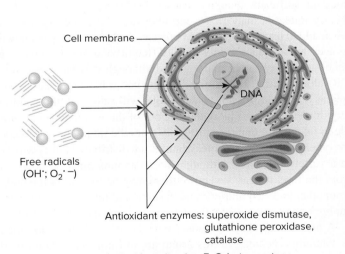

FIGURE 7.2 The antioxidant role of vitamins. To protect against the destructive nature of free radicals, such as hydroxyl radicals and superoxides, the cells contain a number of different enzymes (superoxide dismutase, glutathione peroxidase, catalase) to help neutralize them, thus helping to prevent disintegration of cell membranes or the genetic material within the cell. Additionally, several vitamins (E, C, beta-carotene) may serve as antioxidants. Such vitamins are theorized to be protective against cancer, heart disease, and adverse effects of aging.

Hormone Functions   Although vitamin D exists in vitamin form, it undergoes several conversions in the body and, in its active form, functions as a hormone. After being produced in the kidney, vitamin D circulates in the blood like other hormones and exerts its functions on various tissues to promote bone metabolism. Other vitamins, such as A and K, may be produced in the liver and intestines, respectively, and exert functions in other parts of the body. Although it is normally not referred to as a hormone, Reichrath and others indicated that vitamin A may serve a hormonal function relative to skin health. Some vitamins may be critical in the formation of various hormones—such as the role vitamin C plays in the formation of epinephrine—but are not classified as hormones. Only vitamin D is assigned hormonal status in its active form.

Energy   Although vitamins are indispensable for regulating many body functions and for the maintenance of optimal health, they are not a source of energy. They do not have any caloric value. Moreover, they make no significant contribution to the structure of the body, as do protein and some minerals.

What vitamins are essential to human nutrition?

The existence of vitamins was deduced from their physiological actions before their chemical structures had been identified. In assigning names to vitamins, the alphabet was used in order of their time of discovery. In some cases, a large time gap existed between the discovery of the vitamin and determination of its chemical structure. In others, the chemical nature was discovered rapidly, and the chemical name came into early use.

An *essential vitamin* is one that cannot be synthesized in the body in sufficient quantity, causes deficiency symptoms when dietary intake is inadequate, and alleviates deficiency symptoms when added back to the diet. At present, the human body is known to need an adequate supply of 13 different vitamins. Choline is a water-soluble essential nutrient, and although it is listed with the DRI alongside the B vitamins, at this time it has not been classified as a vitamin. A well-balanced diet will satisfy all the vitamin requirements of most individuals. Four of these vitamins are soluble in fat and are obtained primarily from the fat in our diet, while the other nine, water-soluble, vitamins are distributed rather widely in a variety of foods. Although most vitamins must be obtained from the food we eat, several of them may be formed in the body from other ingested nutrients, by the action of ultraviolet rays from sunlight on our skin, or by the activity of some intestinal bacteria.

A number of other substances have been mistakenly classified as vitamins. Included in this group are inositol, para-amino benzoic acid (PABA), vitamin B_{15} or pangamic acid, and vitamin B_{17} or laetrile. Although it has been suggested that these substances have vitamin activity, their essentiality in the diet has not been established. Other substances have been attributed vitamin-like activity and professed to enhance health or physical performance, such as bee pollen, coenzyme Q_{10} (CoQ_{10}), and ginkgo, but these also are not essential vitamins.

Table 7.1 presents an overview of the 13 essential vitamins and choline with commonly used, interchangeable synonyms, major food sources, major functions in the body, and symptoms associated with deficiencies or excessive consumption. The table also presents the RDA or AI for adults age 19–50, as well as the Daily Value (DV). Note that the DV, which is based on older daily dietary recommendations, may vary considerably with current RDA or AI. The DV was originally set high enough to cover just about anyone but has not been updated to match current recommendations. RDA and AI values for other age groups may be found in DRI tables on the inside front cover, and the UL may be found on the inside back cover. The health and physical performance effects of the essential vitamins and selected vitamin-like substances are covered in the following sections.

Only very small amounts of vitamins are required daily. RDA or AI are usually given in milligrams (mg) or micrograms (mcg). Several vitamins come in various forms and thus the RDA may be given as activity equivalents. For example, vitamin A comes preformed as retinol, or may be derived from the conversion of beta-carotene. Thus, vitamin A requirements are technically known as retinol activity equivalents (RAE). The International Unit (IU) is an older measure of vitamin activity that may still be seen on food labels and vitamin supplements. However, it is gradually being replaced with more appropriate terminology. Because IU is still commonly used, we will include it in our discussion where relevant.

In general, how do deficiencies or excesses of vitamins influence health or physical performance?

Whether or not a vitamin deficiency affects one's health or physical performance may depend on the magnitude of the deficiency. Four stages of vitamin deficiency associated with the duration of undernourishment and inadequate vitamin intake have been described. These same four stages may apply to mineral deficiency diseases discussed in the next chapter.

1. *A preliminary stage* is associated with inadequate amount or availability of the vitamin in the diet. For example, a drastic change in the diet may influence vitamin **bioavailability** (the amount of a nutrient that the body absorbs), whereas pregnancy may increase the need for several vitamins.
2. *Biochemical deficiency.* In this stage, the body's pool of the vitamin is decreased. For a number of vitamins, biochemical deficiency can be identified by blood or tissue tests. For example, deficiencies of riboflavin may be detected by the activity of an enzyme in the red blood cells. In the second national report on biochemical indicators of diet and nutrition status in the U.S. individuals from 2003 to 2006, the Centers for Disease Control and Prevention noted deficiencies for vitamin B_6 (10.5 percent), vitamin D (8.1 percent), vitamin B_{12} (2 percent), and folate (<1 percent) in those ≥1 year of age. Among those ≥6 years of age, deficiency prevalence rates for vitamin C, vitamin A, and vitamin E were 6, <1, and <1 percent, respectively.
3. *Physiological deficiency* is associated with the appearance of unspecific symptoms such as loss of appetite, weakness, or physical fatigue.

   These first three stages are known as latent or marginal vitamin deficiency, or **subclinical malnutrition**. Whether or not these stages impair physical performance may depend

TABLE 7.1   Essential vitamins*

Vitamin name (other terms)	RDA or AI for adults age 19–50*; Daily Value (DV)	Major sources
Fat-soluble vitamins		
Vitamin A (retinol: provitamin carotenoids)	RDA: 900 RAE ♂ 700 RAE ♀ (RAE = retinol activity equivalents) DV = 5,000 IU	Retinol in animal foods: liver, whole milk, fortified milk, cheese; carotenoids in plant foods: carrots, green leafy vegetables, sweet potatoes, fortified margarine from vegetable oils
Vitamin D (cholecalciferol)	RDA: 600 IU or 15 mcg DV = 400 IU	Vitamin D-fortified foods like dairy products and margarine, fish oils; action of sunlight on the skin
Vitamin E (tocopherol)	RDA: 15 mg d-alpha tocopherol DV = 30 IU	Vegetable oils, margarine, green leafy vegetables, wheat germ, vegetable oils, whole-grain products, and egg yolks
Vitamin K (phylloquinone, menoquinone)	RDA: 120 mcg ♂ 90 mcg ♀ DV = 80 mcg	Pork and beef liver, eggs, spinach, and cauliflower; formation in the human intestine by bacteria
Water-soluble vitamins		
Thiamin (vitamin B_1)	RDA: 1.2 mg ♂ 1.1 mg ♀ DV = 1.5 mg	Ham, pork, lean meat, liver, whole-grain products, enriched breads and cereals, and legumes
Riboflavin (vitamin B_2)	RDA: 1.3 mg ♂ 1.1 mg ♀ DV = 1.7 mg	Milk and dairy products, meat, eggs, enriched grain products, green leafy vegetables, beans
Niacin (nicotinamide, nicotinic acid)	RDA: 16 mg ♂ 14 mg ♀ DV = 20 mg	Lean meats, fish, poultry, whole-grain products, beans; may be formed in the body from tryptophan, an essential amino acid
Vitamin B_6 (pyridoxal, pyridoxine, and pyridoxamine)	RDA: 1.3 mg DV = 2 mg	Protein foods: liver, lean meats, fish, poultry, legumes; green leafy vegetables, baked potatoes, bananas
Vitamin B_{12} (cobalamin; cyanocobalamin)	RDA: 2.4 mcg DV = 6 mcg	Animal foods only: meat, fish, poultry, milk, and eggs
Folate (folic acid)	RDA: 400 DFE (DFE = dietary folate equivalents) DV = 400 DFE	Liver, green leafy vegetables, legumes, nuts, and fortified cereals
Biotin	AI: 30 mcg DV = 300 mg	Meats, legumes, milk, egg yolk, whole-grain products, and most vegetables
Pantothenic acid	AI: 5 mg DV = 300 mg	Beef and pork liver, lean meats, milk, eggs, legumes, whole-grain products, and most vegetables
Choline**	AI: 550 mg ♂ 425 mg ♀ DV = none	Milk, liver, eggs, peanuts; found in most foods as part of cell membranes
Vitamin C (ascorbic acid)	RDA: 90 mg ♂ 75 mg ♀ DV = 60 mg	Citrus fruits, green leafy vegetables, broccoli, peppers, strawberries, and potatoes

(Continued)

TABLE 7.1   Essential vitamins*   (Continued)

Major functions in the body	Deficiency symptoms	Symptoms of excessive consumption*
Fat-soluble vitamins		
Maintains epithelial tissue in skin and mucous membranes; forms visual purple for night vision; promotes bone development	Night blindness, intestinal infections, impaired growth, and xerophthalmia	UL is 3 milligrams/day. Nausea, headache, fatigue, liver and spleen damage, skin peeling, and pain in the joints
Acts as a hormone to increase intestinal absorption of calcium and promote bone and tooth formation	Rare; rickets in children and osteomalacia in adults	UL is 4,000 IU, or 100 micrograms/day. Loss of appetite, nausea, irritability, joint pain, calcium deposits in soft tissues such as the kidney
Functions as an antioxidant to protect cell membranes from destruction by oxidation	Extremely rare; disruption of red blood cell membranes; anemia	UL is 1,000 milligrams/day. General lack of toxicity with doses up to 400 mg. Some reports of headache, fatigue, or diarrhea with megadoses
Essential for blood coagulation processes	Increased bleeding and hemorrhage	No UL set. Possible clot formation (thrombosis), vomiting
Water-soluble vitamins		
Serves as a coenzyme for energy production from carbohydrate; essential for normal functioning of the central nervous system	Poor appetite, apathy, mental depression, pain in calf muscles, and beriberi	No UL set. General lack of toxicity
Functions as a coenzyme involved in energy production from carbohydrates and fats; maintenance of healthy skin	Dermatitis, cracks at the corners of the mouth, sores on the tongue, and damage to the cornea	No UL set. General lack of toxicity
Functions as a coenzyme for the aerobic and anaerobic production of energy from carbohydrate; helps synthesize fat and blocks release of FFA; needed for healthy skin	Loss of appetite, weakness, skin lesions, gastrointestinal problems, and pellagra	UL is 35 milligrams/day. Nicotinic acid causes headache, nausea, burning and itching skin, flushing of face, and liver damage
Functions as a coenzyme in protein metabolism; necessary for formation of hemoglobin and red blood cells; needed for glycogenolysis and gluconeogenesis	Nervous irritability, convulsions, dermatitis, sores on tongue, and anemia	UL is 100 milligrams/day. Loss of nerve sensation, impaired gait
Functions as a coenzyme for formation of DNA, RBC development, and maintenance of nerve tissue	Pernicious anemia, nerve damage resulting in paralysis	No UL set. General lack of toxicity
Functions as coenzyme for DNA formation and RBC development	Fatigue, gastrointestinal disorders, diarrhea, anemia, neural tube defects in newborns	UL is 1,000 micrograms/day. May prevent detection of pernicious anemia caused by B$_{12}$ deficiency
Functions as coenzyme in the metabolism of carbohydrates, fats, and protein	Rare; may be caused by excessive intake of raw egg whites: fatigue, nausea, and skin rashes	No UL set. General lack of toxicity
Functions as part of coenzyme A in energy metabolism	Rare; produced only clinically: fatigue, nausea, loss of appetite, and mental depression	No UL set. General lack of toxicity
Functions as a precursor for lecithin, a phospholipid in cell membranes	Rare; liver damage	UL is 3.5 grams/day. May lead to fishy body odor, gastrointestinal distress, and vomiting, low blood pressure
Forms collagen essential for connective tissue development; aids in absorption of iron; helps form epinephrine; serves as antioxidant	Weakness, rough skin, slow wound healing, bleeding gums, anemia, and scurvy	UL is 2,000 milligrams/day. Diarrhea, possible kidney stones, and rebound scurvy

*RDA, AI, and UL values for all age groups may be found on the inside of the front and back covers of this text.
**Not classified as a vitamin.

upon the nature of the sport, but weakness or physical fatigue would certainly be counterproductive to optimal performance.

4. *Clinically manifest vitamin deficiency.* In this final stage, specific clinical symptoms are observed. For example, anemia is a clinical symptom associated with a deficiency of several vitamins, such as folic acid, vitamin B_6, and B_{12}. Both health and performance would be adversely affected with a clinically manifest vitamin deficiency.

In the past, RDA for vitamins have been established to prevent vitamin-deficiency diseases. However, recommendations are beginning to incorporate the role of vitamins in health promotion. For example, as noted later, the new Adequate Intake (AI) for vitamin D has been modified to help prevent osteoporosis, while the folic acid RDA is designed to prevent damage to the nervous system of the unborn child during pregnancy. When scientific evidence is deemed sufficient, vitamin recommendations may be modified to help prevent chronic diseases. If the RDA for some vitamins are increased as a possible means of achieving health promotion objectives, the most likely recommendation will be to obtain the increased amounts from natural foods. However, food fortification or supplementation may be recommended for a few vitamins, such as folic acid.

In general, it is very difficult to obtain excessive amounts of vitamins through the diet to the point that health or physical performance is impaired. Even when supplements are taken, the body may excrete several vitamins, keeping body functions normal. However, overconsumption of some vitamins may induce **hypervitaminosis**, a condition in which a vitamin may function comparable to a drug, not a nutrient, and induce toxic reactions. An excessive intake of vitamin supplements may be a common cause of hypervitaminosis, but some dietary practices may also lead to excessive vitamin intake. As shall be noted later in this chapter, consuming a vitamin supplement and vitamin-fortified foods, such as cereals, on a regular basis could induce vitamin functions that are hypothesized to increase health risks. A Tolerable Upper Intake Level (UL) has been established for 7 of the 13 essential vitamins.

Key Concepts

▶ Vitamins are complex organic compounds that function in the body in a variety of ways. Some act as coenzymes to help regulate metabolic processes; others are antioxidants that protect cell membranes; and one is even classified as a hormone. Vitamins do not contain energy *per se*, such as Calories, but they do help regulate energy processes in the body.

▶ The RDA for vitamins have been established to prevent vitamin-deficiency diseases such as scurvy, but the new DRI may be modified to help prevent chronic diseases, such as osteoporosis, or excessive intake and associated adverse health effects.

▶ There may be four stages in a vitamin deficiency: the preliminary stage, the biochemical deficiency stage, the physiological deficiency stage, and the clinically manifest deficiency stage.

Check for Yourself

▶ Check the food labels for various foods you have in the cupboard to see what vitamins are listed. If the DV is provided, compare the amount of the vitamin provided and its DV with the current RDA or AI. Relate your findings to the text discussion.

Fat-Soluble Vitamins

The four fat-soluble vitamins are A, D, E, and K. Because they are soluble in fat but not in water, dietary sources include foods that have some fat content. The body may contain appreciable stores of each fat-soluble vitamin, and several of them may be manufactured by the body, so deficiencies are relatively rare in industrialized societies. On the other hand, excessive intake may be toxic. With the exception of vitamin E, very little research has been conducted relative to deficiency or supplementation effects upon physical performance.

Vitamin A (retinol)

Vitamin A is a fat-soluble, unsaturated alcohol. The physiologically active form of vitamin A is known as **retinol**. The human body is capable of forming retinol from provitamins known as carotenoids, primarily **beta-carotene**. Both preformed vitamin A, or retinol, and carotenoids are found in the foods we eat.

DRI The RDA for vitamin A may be obtained by consuming preformed retinol, beta-carotene and other carotenoids, or a combination of the two. The RDA may be expressed in several ways, usually as **retinol equivalents (RE)**, **retinol activity equivalents (RAE)** as a combination of retinol and carotenoids, or international units. In brief, 1 RAE equals 1 microgram of retinol, or 12 micrograms of beta-carotene, or about 3.3 IU. The RDA is 900 RAE, or 3,000 IU, for adult males and 700 RAE, or 2,300 IU, for adult females. See the DRI table on the inside cover for more details on vitamin A requirements derived from either retinol or the carotenoids. The Daily Value (DV) for use on food labels is 5,000 IU but should be set at 3,000. The UL for adults is 3 milligrams RAE/day from retinol, or 10,000 IU; no UL has been established for carotenoids. See the UL table on the inside of the back cover for more details.

Food Sources Preformed vitamin A is found in substantial amounts in some animal foods such as liver, butter, cheese, egg yolks, fish liver oils, and fortified milk. Provitamin A, as beta-carotene, is found in dark-green leafy and yellow-orange vegetables, as well as in some fruits such as oranges, limes, pineapples, prunes, and cantaloupes. Fortified margarine also contains beta-carotene. One glass of milk provides about 15 percent of the RDA, while one medium carrot will supply nearly 200 percent and a serving of liver a whopping 1,000 percent or more of the RDA.

Major Functions Vitamin A is essential for maintenance of the epithelial cells, those cells covering the outside of the body and lining the body cavities. It is also essential for proper visual function, such as night vision and peripheral vision. Vitamin A also has a variety of other physiological roles in the body that are not well understood, although it is considered essential in proper bone development and for maintaining optimal function of the immune system. Vitamin A and beta-carotene may function as antioxidants and have been theorized by some scientists to confer some health benefits.

Deficiency: Health and Physical Performance Vitamin A is stored in the body in relatively large amounts. However, an inadequate intake of vitamin A could have serious health implications if prolonged. The gradual loss of night vision is one of the first symptoms of vitamin A deficiency. Other symptoms of mild deficiencies include increased susceptibility to infection and skin lesions. Epidemiological research also has suggested that a deficient intake of beta-carotene could predispose the individual to the development of cancer in the epithelial tissues such as the skin, lungs, breasts, and intestinal lining. Although severe deficiencies are not common in industrialized nations, they do occur in some parts of the world and lead to blindness through destruction of the cornea of the eye, a condition known as **xerophthalmia**. Vitamin A deficiency has been associated with higher mortality rates in children of developing countries, with several million childhood deaths annually. Some, but not all, studies have shown that vitamin A supplementation to such children may decrease the death rate, possibly by strengthening the immune system.

Theoretically, vitamin A deficiency could affect physical performance. Some investigators have suggested that a deficiency may impair the process of gluconeogenesis in the liver, which may be an important consideration for the endurance athlete in the latter stages of competition. Others have implied a reduction in the synthesis of muscle protein and impaired vision, which could negatively affect strength athletes or those involved in sports requiring eye alertness. Very little research is available to support these theoretical views.

Supplementation: Health and Physical Performance Vitamin A in supplements can come from retinol (vitamin A palmitate or acetate) or beta-carotene, or both. Check the label; it may or may not list the separate components. The UL for adults is set at 3,000 RAE, or 10,000 IU. The UL applies only to preformed vitamin A, or retinol, not to carotenoids. In general, supplements of vitamin A as retinol are not recommended unless under the guidance of a health professional. Excessive amounts of vitamin A, generally caused by self-medication with megadoses, can cause a condition known as hypervitaminosis A. Symptoms may include weakness, headache, loss of appetite, nausea, pain in the joints, and peeling of skin. Similar symptoms were reported in a young soccer player who took about 100,000 IU daily for 2 months in an attempt to improve performance. The symptoms were relieved when he stopped taking the supplements.

Excess vitamin A may also weaken the bones. Binkley and Krueger reported that excess vitamin A stimulates bone resorption and inhibits bone formation, leading to bone loss and contributing to osteoporosis. Feskanich and others found that women with the highest intake of vitamin A as retinol, greater than 3,000 micrograms daily, had double the risk of hip fractures compared to women with the lowest intake, less than 1,250 micrograms per day.

As noted by Ross, excessive vitamin A during pregnancy may be teratogenic, causing deformities in the developing embryo or fetus. Research by Rothman and others has indicated that vitamin A doses as low as four times the RDA can markedly increase a pregnant woman's chances of having a baby with birth defects, such as a cleft palate, heart defects, or other problems. Although this amount would not be consumed with a normal diet, it could be obtained by someone who takes a daily supplement, drinks substantial amounts of milk, eats liver, and has several servings of fortified cereals. Additionally, Zachman and Grummer indicated that consuming alcohol during pregnancy may worsen these teratogenic effects of vitamin A. Finally, extremely large doses of vitamin A may lead to severe liver damage, especially with concomitant alcohol intake, and may be fatal.

Beta-carotene supplements are not believed to be toxic but may cause harmless yellowing of the skin when taken in excess because the beta-carotene accumulates in the fat tissues. The supplements may also cause adverse health effects in some individuals, particularly smokers, discussed later in this chapter.

There appears to be little theoretical value in using vitamin A supplementation for ergogenic purposes, and no scientific evidence supports its use as a means to enhance physical performance. However, beta-carotene has been combined with other antioxidants in an attempt to prevent muscle damage during exercise, and this research is discussed later.

Prudent Recommendations In summary, vitamin A supplementation to the diet of the active individual does not have a sound theoretical basis. Moreover, the research conducted with vitamin A and physical performance has shown no beneficial effect. Hence, there appears to be no advantage for the active individual to supplement the diet with vitamin A, particularly not with megadoses that may have undesirable effects. The advisability of beta-carotene supplementation for its antioxidant properties is discussed in the later sections of this chapter dealing with ergogenic and health issues. As shall be noted, individuals should not consume high doses of beta-carotene.

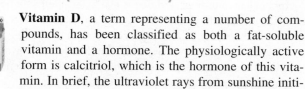

Vitamin D (cholecalciferol)

Vitamin D, a term representing a number of compounds, has been classified as both a fat-soluble vitamin and a hormone. The physiologically active form is calcitriol, which is the hormone of this vitamin. In brief, the ultraviolet rays from sunshine initiate a process that eventually converts a provitamin found in the skin (7-dehydrocholesterol) into **cholecalciferol (vitamin D_3)**, a prohormone, which is released into the blood and is eventually converted by the liver and kidneys into the active hormone, calcitriol (1,25-dihydroxycholecalciferol). Figure 7.3 illustrates the formation of vitamin D from sunlight.

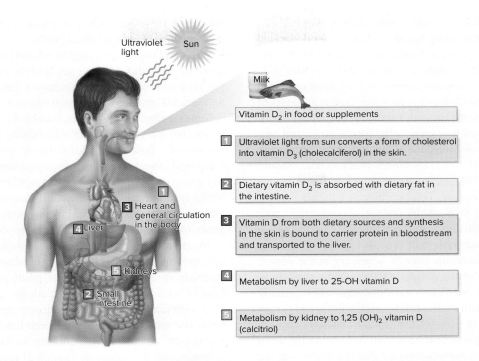

FIGURE 7.3 The many facets of vitamin D metabolism. Whether synthesized in the skin or obtained from dietary sources, vitamin D ultimately functions as a hormone: calcitriol.

Within the figure:

Ultraviolet light — Sun

Milk

Vitamin D₂ in food or supplements

1. Ultraviolet light from sun converts a form of cholesterol into vitamin D₃ (cholecalciferol) in the skin.

2. Dietary vitamin D₂ is absorbed with dietary fat in the intestine.

3. Vitamin D from both dietary sources and synthesis in the skin is bound to carrier protein in bloodstream and transported to the liver.

4. Metabolism by liver to 25-OH vitamin D

5. Metabolism by kidney to 1,25 (OH)₂ vitamin D (calcitriol)

3 Heart and general circulation in the body
4 Liver
5 Kidneys
2 Small intestine

Dietary supplements contain vitamin D_2 (ergocalciferol) and vitamin D_3. For those who take vitamin D supplements, health professionals recommend vitamin D_3 because it is more effective in raising the serum marker (25-hydroxyvitamin D) of vitamin D status. Check supplement labels for "Vitamin D as cholecalciferol" or the ingredients list for vitamin D_3 or cholecalciferol.

DRI The RDA for vitamin D is given in micrograms of cholecalciferol or as IU; 1 microgram of cholecalciferol is the equivalent of 40 IU. Even though sunlight is a major source of vitamin D for some people, the RDA is based on minimal exposure to sunlight. For infants 0–12 months old, the AI is 10 mcg (400 IU); for ages 1 to 70 years, the RDA is 15 mcg (600 IU); and for 70 years and older, the RDA is 20 mcg (800 IU). The DV is 400 IU. The UL for those over age 9 is 100 mcg (4,000 IU). See the DRI tables on the inside front and back covers for more details. Despite the fact that the RDA and UL for vitamin D were recently increased, there is considerable debate as to whether the standards were increased enough to support health. For instance, Hollis and colleagues recommend vitamin D supplementation of 4,000 IU per day for pregnant women, and noted that a supplement of 400 IU per day was comparatively ineffective at raising serum 25-hydroxyvitamin D levels.

Part of the vitamin D controversy is due to the fact that cut points of serum 25-hydroxyvitamin D levels associated with deficiency or insufficiency in terms of bone health, optimal concentration for health or athletic performance, and levels associated with toxicity have not been developed. Larson-Meyer and Willis describe the different thresholds of vitamin D status as follows:

- Deficiency is 25-hydroxyvitamin D <20 ng/mL (ng is nanogram or one-billionth of a gram)

- Insufficiency is <32 ng/mL
- Toxicity is >50 ng/mL when coupled with increased elevated serum calcium

Using 2001–2006 National Health and Nutrition Examination III data, Looker and others reported vitamin D status based on serum 25-hydroxyvitamin D levels in the following Institute of Medicine categories for U.S. citizens ≥1 year of age. IOM categories and prevalence rates are in bold text.

- **Deficiency** <12 ng/ml (<30 nmol/l) leads to rickets in infants and children and osteomalacia in adults **(8 percent)**.
- **Insufficiency** ≥12 to 19 ng/ml (30 to 49 nmol/l) is inadequate for bone and overall health in healthy individuals **(24 percent)**.
- **Adequate** ≥20 to 49 ng/ml (50 to 124 nmol/l) is adequate for bone and overall health in healthy individuals **(67 percent)**.
- **Possibly harmful** ≥50 ng/ml, especially if >60 ng/ml (≥125 nmol/l) is linked to potential adverse effects **(1 percent)**.

Larson-Meyer reports that optimal concentrations may lie between 40 and 70 ng/mL, which is the concentration at which the human genome evolved.

Food Sources Most foods do not contain any vitamin D. Fatty fish, such as wild salmon, mackerel, sardines, and catfish, are good sources and may contain about 200–500 IU in 3 ounces. Shitake mushrooms are also a good source, containing about 250 IU in four mushrooms. Small amounts are found in egg yolks, about 25 IU. Several foods are fortified with vitamin D, such as milk, margarine, and some breakfast cereals. One glass of fortified milk will provide 100 IU, which is 25 percent of the AI for infants and 17 percent of the RDA for children and adults to age 70.

The Consumers Union notes that we normally get about 90 percent of our vitamin D from sunlight and the remaining 10 percent from food. Liebman notes that a light-skinned person out in the sun in a bathing suit, with no sunscreen, can make 20,000 to 30,000 IU in 30 minutes. However, African-Americans may need up to ten times as much sunlight as Caucasians to make similar amounts of vitamin D. Clothes block the action of the sun, but the RDA for vitamin D may be obtained by exposing the hands, arms, and face to 10–20 minutes of summer sunshine about two or three times per week. The ultraviolet-B (UV-B) radiation waves promote vitamin D formation in the skin, but Gilchrest notes that UV-B waves also cause wrinkles and skin cancer. Total sunblocking agents prevent vitamin D formation, but their use by individuals concerned with skin cancer due to sun exposure is still recommended because even very small amounts of sunshine will promote vitamin D formation. Longer periods of exposure may be necessary in the winter, and it may be difficult to obtain adequate vitamin D by sunlight in northern latitudes. Vieth and Fraser indicated this was especially true for the northern latitudes of Canada during winter, and it may also apply to the northern parts of the United States. Formation of vitamin D from sunlight is also decreased in the elderly and in individuals with dark skin. Fortunately, as Gilchrest points out, we can buy vitamin D at the corner store.

Major Functions   Most tissues and cells in the body have receptors for the hormonal form of vitamin D, and between 200 and 2,000 genes are controlled by vitamin D. In particular, vitamin D plays a central role in bone metabolism through its effect on calcium and phosphorus, whose roles in bone metabolism are discussed in the next chapter. It works in conjunction with several other hormones, particularly parathormone secreted by the parathyroid gland. Vitamin D helps to absorb calcium from the intestinal tract and the kidneys, helping to maintain normal serum calcium levels and proper bone metabolism. Vitamin D also helps regulate phosphorus metabolism, another mineral essential in bone formation. Verhaar and others note that besides the classical actions of vitamin D in bone metabolism, it also appears to be important for muscle function. Vitamin D status has been associated with chronic, nonskeletal diseases, including cardiovascular disease, hypertension, multiple sclerosis, arthritis, infection, autism, and certain cancers. A meta-analysis by Autier and Gandini demonstrated that taking vitamin D supplements is associated with decreased mortality. For a detailed review of vitamin D metabolism, the interested reader is referred to the review by Holick.

Deficiency: Health and Physical Performance   Deficiencies of vitamin D are unusual in most temperate climates because the body possesses adequate stores in the liver and can manufacture it through exposure to the sun. Children normally get adequate sun exposure if they play outdoors during daylight. However, deficiencies may occur in individuals who have little exposure to sunshine, such as elderly people who are homebound. Many elderly are more concerned with health and are more likely to wear more clothing and use sunscreen lotions, possibly blocking vitamin D formation. Vegans who avoid sunlight may also be at risk for vitamin D deficiency but may obtain some vitamin D from shiitake mushrooms and fortified products.

Vitamin D deficiency may be related to a variety of health problems. In particular, a deficiency leads to increased serum levels of parathyroid hormone, which removes calcium from bones. Thus, deficiencies may lead to inadequate calcium metabolism and bone deformities known as rickets, especially in children. This was a major concern years ago, but it has nearly been eradicated through the use of vitamin D–fortified foods, primarily milk. However, Calvo and others noted that hypovitaminosis D may occur in various groups, such as those living in northern latitudes. Infants who breast-feed may also be deficient if their mothers have inadequate vitamin D. Thus, Raiten and Picciano noted that there is a reemergence of vitamin D–deficient rickets in young children.

Moreover, in a recent interview, Holick indicated that adults do not drink much milk and many are not getting enough vitamin D to satisfy their body requirements, predisposing them to bone loss. Loss of bone tissue may occur in adults, leading to **osteomalacia**, or a softening of the bones, accompanied by muscular weakness. The muscle weakness has been theoretically linked with an impairment of calcium metabolism in the muscle, possibly due to inadequate activation of vitamin D receptors in muscle. Some research notes a decrease in muscle strength in institutionalized elderly patients who are deficient in vitamin D.

There is increasing evidence that some athletes should be concerned with vitamin D status. Ogan and Pritchett suggest that vitamin D deficiency and insufficiency in athletes likely mirrors what is observed in the general population. In a year-long study of 41 athletes (12 indoor and 29 outdoor), Halliday and others reported that 64 percent of the athletes were vitamin D deficient or insufficient in the winter, 12 percent in the fall, and 20 percent in the spring. Indoor sport athletes (e.g., wrestling and basketball) had lower serum levels of 25-hydroxyvitamin D than did outdoor sport athletes (football, cross-country). Low vitamin D status was correlated with upper respiratory infections, colds, influenza, and gastroenteritis. Shindle and others reported that 80 percent of 89 professional American football players were either vitamin D deficient (<20 ng/ml) or insufficient (20 to 31.9 ng/ml). African-American players and players who suffered muscle injuries had significantly lower vitamin D levels. Larson-Meyer and Willis noted vitamin D deficiency or insufficiency in athletes from all over the world. In a cross-sectional study of 950 ethnically diverse athletes, Allison and others reported that 57 percent were vitamin D deficient or severely deficient. Although Caucasian and African athletes had higher spine, neck, and hip bone mineral density than their Asian or Middle Eastern counterparts, there was no evidence of osteoporosis. In their review, Cannell and others noted that studies from the 1950s showed improved performance following exposure to ultraviolet light; peak performance is seasonal and is related to serum 25-hydroxyvitamin D levels; and vitamin D increases type II fiber size and number and muscle function in older adults. They concluded that vitamin D may improve performance in vitamin D–deficient athletes, and that peak performance may occur when 25-hydroxyvitamin D levels approach 50 ng/ml. Todd and others commented that vitamin D levels below 30 mmol/L (12 ng/ml) are associated with reduced training volume in athletes. Moran and others noted the influence of vitamin D extends beyond calcium metabolism to include proper skeletal and cardiac muscle function, immune function, and cancer prevention. Vitamin D has a recently discovered role in transcription of a binding protein for insulin-like growth factor-1 (IGF-1), an anabolic mediator of human growth hormone, which is discussed in chapter 13. Vitamin D receptors (VDRs) are found in the nuclei of many tissues, including muscle and immune cells. Problems with VDR transcription are thought to play a role in muscle weakness. These mechanisms have implications for athletes. von Hurst and Beck concluded that intervention studies are needed to identify vitamin D levels for optimal performance in athletes.

http://ods.od.nih.gov/factsheets/vitamind/ Find the "Vitamin D Dietary Supplement Fact Sheet" from the NIH Office of Dietary Supplements at this site.

Vitamin D may help inhibit cell proliferation, so a deficiency could lead to increased cell proliferation, a key characteristic in cancer growth. Grant and others reported that solar UVB irradiance and/or vitamin D have been found inversely correlated with incidence, mortality, and/or survival rates for breast, colorectal, ovarian, and prostate cancer and Hodgkin's and non-Hodgkin's lymphoma, and they noted that evidence is emerging that more than 17 different types of cancer are likely to be vitamin D sensitive. Schwartz and Skinner reported that epidemiological studies over the past year lend additional support for important roles for vitamin D in the natural history of several cancers.

Holick and Chen state that vitamin D deficiency is a worldwide problem with serious health consequences. Low levels of serum vitamin D_3 appear to increase health risks. In a large prospective study, Giovannucci and others reported that low levels of vitamin D are associated with higher risk of myocardial infarction in a graded manner, even after controlling for factors known to be associated with coronary artery disease. Dobnig and others reported that low vitamin D levels are independently associated with all-cause and cardiovascular mortality. However, a causal relationship has yet to be proved by intervention trials using vitamin D.

Chiu and others reported that a low level of vitamin D in the blood is associated with insulin resistance and increased risk of diabetes. Additionally, vitamin D deficiency may lead to an increased production of renin by the kidney, which could lead to an increased blood pressure. Low levels of vitamin D may also affect mental health. Balion and others noted that 1,25 dihydroxyvitamin D synthesized in the brain mediates the function of various brain growth factors. In their meta-analysis of 37 studies, they concluded that low vitamin D status (<50 nmol/liter) is associated with poorer cognitive function and greater risk of Alzheimer's disease.

Scientists have hypothesized that vitamin D, obtained either via sunlight or dietary intake, may reduce the risk of various chronic diseases.

Supplementation: Health and Physical Performance Vitamin D supplementation research has focused primarily on bone health and related issues, but the effect on other chronic diseases has also received increased research attention.

Bone health Although some studies have shown that vitamin D and calcium supplementation did not prevent bone fractures, Bischoff-Ferrari and Dawson-Hughes noted such studies had several limitations. In particular, they used the relatively less potent vitamin D_2 or a too low dose of D_3 (400 IU) that may have limited the increase in vitamin D status necessary to prevent bone fractures. More recent extensive reviews indicate that considerable evidence supports the role of both calcium and vitamin D in protecting the skeleton. For example, in the NIH report on multivitamin/mineral supplements and chronic disease prevention, Hyang noted that vitamin D *alone* does not increase bone mineral density or decrease fracture risk, but it does work in combination with calcium to decrease the risk of fractures in postmenopausal women. Each nutrient is necessary to maximize the benefits of the other in bone health. Heaney supports this viewpoint in his review on bone health.

Additionally, research suggests vitamin D supplementation may lower the risk of bone fractures in older people by increasing muscular strength, which helps maintain balance and prevent falls. In a meta-analysis, Jackson and others reported a trend toward a reduction in the risk of falls among patients treated with vitamin D_3 compared with placebo.

Cancer Lips, in a review of vitamin D physiology, indicated that it has an antiproliferative effect that can regulate cell differentiation and function, which may explain how a vitamin D deficiency can play a role in the pathogenesis of certain diseases, such as cancer. Epidemiological studies have shown a reduced risk of colorectal cancer with increased intake of calcium and vitamin D. Some randomized, controlled studies, such as the report by Wactawshi-Wende and others, revealed no effect of supplementation with 1,000 mg of calcium and 400 IU of vitamin D_3, for 7 years, on the development of colorectal cancer in postmenopausal women.

However, Lappe and others, using a supplemental dose of 1,400–1,500 milligrams of calcium plus 1,100 IU of vitamin D_3, did find a substantial reduction in all-cancer risk in postmenopausal women. Moreover, in a meta-analysis, Gorham and others reported that a 50 percent lower risk of colorectal cancer was associated with elevated serum vitamin D levels that could be obtained with a daily intake of 1,000–2,000 IU/day of vitamin D_3. Research is ongoing to clarify the role of vitamin D_3 supplementation as a possible means to help prevent cancer. Dosage may be important.

Diabetes Vitamin D may enhance immune cell functions to help prevent autoimmune diseases, such as type I diabetes. Harris indicated that doses of 2,000 IU and higher daily may have a strong protective effect in children at risk for type I diabetes.

Kidney stones and other adverse health effects In the NIH report, Hyang reported that supplementation with calcium and vitamin D may increase the risk for kidney stones. The elevated serum calcium levels may combine with other substances, such as oxalates or phosphates, to form the kidney stones, which may pass through the urinary tract and cause considerable pain. The calcium may also become incorporated into plaque in the arteries, leading to calcified or hardened plaque. Additionally, hypervitaminosis D may lead to vomiting, diarrhea, weight loss, and loss of muscle tone.

To help promote health, primarily bone health, scientists suggest that a healthy serum D (25-hydroxyvitamin D) concentration should be about 30–60 nanograms per liter (ng/L), which may require 1,000–2,000 IU of vitamin D_3 daily. However, many vitamin D scientists are recommending that the UL be increased. In support of this viewpoint, Hathcock and others recently assessed the risk of vitamin D supplementation and noted the absence of toxicity in trials conducted in healthy adults who used vitamin D_3 doses up to 10,000 IU daily, which supports the selection of this value as the UL.

Heaney indicated that the nutrient status for both vitamin D and calcium tends to be deficient in the adult population of the industrialized nations. Given the health implications of adequate vitamin D and calcium intake, he believes that fortification with both nutrients is appropriate and, given contemporary diets and sun exposure, probably necessary because people normally do not adhere to a regimen of taking supplements daily.

Physical performance Vitamin D supplementation may be related to physical performance. Vitamin D receptors and response elements are located in skeletal muscle and other tissues and regulate over 900 gene variants. In a recent review, Dahlquist and others noted several possible ergogenic mechanisms for vitamin D. Although a specific mechanism remains unclear, the enzymes converting vitamin D_3 to 1,25-dihydroxyvitamin D contain heme iron which may influence oxyhemoglobin affinity and improve aerobic capacity. Vitamin D may also improve post-exercise recovery by inhibiting myostatin; increase force and power production via increased calcium kinetics and cross-bridge cycling; and influence muscle growth by augmenting testosterone production and androgen binding.

Ardestani and colleagues reported that serum 25-hydroxyvitamin D levels are correlated with VO_{2max}. In their meta-analysis of seven studies, Thompson and colleagues observed that vitamin D doses ranging from 4,000–8,500 IU/day for 4 weeks to 6 months significantly increased upper and lower body strength in subjects 18-40 years of age. They also noted that baseline vitamin D levels in three of these studies was below levels deemed adequate (<50 nmol/l or 20 ng/ml) by the Institute of Medicine. Baseline serum vitamin D levels may affect supplementation efficacy. Girgis and others noted that vitamin D supplementation reduces falls risk in susceptible populations such as the elderly and may also affect cell signaling pathways which improve muscle function. Weight training increases the serum concentration of vitamin D, which is theorized to be related to the increased bone mass developed through exercise. Willis and others reported that little is known about the vitamin D status of athletes but suggested sports nutritionists should advise athletes to obtain adequate amounts, either through safe sun exposure or dietary supplementation with 1,000–2,000 IU vitamin D_3 daily. Given data suggesting high prevalence rates of vitamin D deficiency and insufficiency, athletes should consider having their vitamin D levels checked.

There are sound medical reasons for individuals to obtain adequate amounts of both vitamin D and calcium. As noted earlier, they function together. Dietary calcium recommendations are presented in the next chapter.

Prudent Recommendations   Based on the current data, Liebman notes that many health professionals are recommending an intake of 1,000 to 2,000 IU of vitamin D daily for most individuals. Such an amount may be obtained in the diet, but you must select foods rich in vitamin D, such as fatty fish and vitamin D–fortified products such as milk, cereals, and orange juice. Check food labels for vitamin D content, preferably D_3. Remember, the DV is 400 IU, but a food with 100 IU only contains 17 percent of the RDA. Supplements may be recommended for those who do not obtain sufficient vitamin D through sunshine or the diet. In 2007, Canada included the recommendation that people over age 50 should take a daily vitamin D_3 supplement. Liebman also indicates that you take in no more than 2,000 IU daily. Individuals at risk for kidney stones should discuss vitamin D intake with their physician.

Vitamin E (alpha-tocopherol)

Vitamin E is a fat-soluble vitamin. In its natural form, it is a complex family of eight compounds including tocopherols and tocotrienols, both with alpha, beta, gamma, and delta forms. The two major forms are **RRR-alpha-tocopherol** and **RRR-gamma-tocopherol**. Alpha-tocopherol alone is the basis for the RDA and it is the most common form in the bloodstream and dietary supplements. You may see it listed as d-alpha-tocopherol (natural form) or dl-alpha-tocopherol (synthetic form).

DRI   The RDA for vitamin E is 15 mg of natural and other forms of alpha-tocopherol, although you might see the RDA expressed as IU. One mg RRR-alpha-tocopherol is equivalent to about 1.5 IU. The RDA is slightly less for children. See the DRI table on the inside of the front cover for more details. The DV is 30 IU. The UL for adults is 1,000 mg/day, which is equal to 1,500 IU.

Food Sources   Vitamin E is found primarily in the small fat content in various vegetables. The most common dietary sources are polyunsaturated vegetable oils, such as corn, soybean, and safflower oils, and margarines made from these oils; 1 tablespoon contains about 3–5 IU. The amount of the different tocopherols and tocotrienols varies among different oils. Other good sources of vitamin E include fortified, ready-to-eat cereals, whole-grain products, wheat germ oil, and eggs. One ounce of a fortified cereal may include about 10–45 IU of vitamin E, while a tablespoon of wheat germ oil contains about 40 IU. Moderate to small amounts are found in meats, dairy products, fruits, and vegetables, particularly sweet potatoes and dark-green leafy vegetables. Four spears of asparagus contain 2 IU. The fat substitute olestra may retard the absorption of vitamin E found in natural foods, but the FDA has mandated that foods containing olestra be fortified with vitamin E. The RDA for vitamin E actually increases as the amount of polyunsaturated oils in the diet increases. Fish oil supplements may be contraindicated in this regard because they are high in polyunsaturated fatty acids but low in vitamin E unless fortified.

Vitamin E supplements may contain natural or synthetic sources. The form should be listed on the food label. Unlike other vitamins, synthetic vitamin E (dl-alpha-tocopherol) is not the same as the natural source (d-alpha-tocopherol). Synthetic vitamin E is a form of alpha-tocopherol different from that found in natural sources and is less likely to contain other forms of vitamin E, such as gamma-tocopherol. Both forms are appropriate, but you need to take about 40–50 percent more of the synthetic form to get the potency of the natural form.

Major Functions   Traber notes that the total function of vitamin E in human nutrition is unclear, stating that after more than 80 years it is still a vitamin looking for a disease. Its principal role is to serve as an antioxidant in the cell membrane. Vitamin E works in concert with other antioxidants, such as the aqueous vitamin C, to maintain its ability to help prevent the oxidation of unsaturated fatty acids in cell membrane phospholipids, thereby protecting the cell from damage. It may also help prevent the oxidation of vitamin A. Other claims, extrapolated from research with animals, have suggested that vitamin E may also play a key role in the synthesis of hemoglobin or serve a pro-oxidant effect by activating enzymes in the mitochondria to improve cellular oxygen utilization, but these claims are not well documented in humans. Some of the vitamin E antioxidant effects are theorized to help prevent the development of several chronic diseases, or muscle tissue damage during exercise. The related mechanisms are discussed later in this chapter.

Deficiency: Health and Physical Performance   Because vitamin E is rather widely distributed in foods, and because it is also stored in the body, a true vitamin E deficiency in humans is rare. In one experiment, prisoners were fed a vitamin E–deficient diet for 13 months and evidenced no symptoms of a deficiency. However, certain individuals with genetic diseases, such as the inability to absorb fat, do experience a deficiency. Others on very low-fat diets may not obtain enough dietary vitamin E. In such cases, anemia may occur because the membranes of the red blood cells (RBCs) are oxidized and release their hemoglobin. Deficiency symptoms noted in animals include nutritional muscular dystrophy and damage to the heart and blood vessels.

Because of its role in preventing cellular damage from free radical oxidation, a deficiency of vitamin E has been theorized to contribute to the development of heart disease and cancer in humans. For example, vitamin E may help prevent the oxidation of LDL-cholesterol, which, as noted in chapter 5, is associated with atherosclerosis and coronary heart disease. Some studies have suggested that a deficiency will lead to premature aging and decreased fertility.

Although vitamin E deficiency is rare in humans, several authors have used the data from research with animals and those humans with genetic defects to support the need for supplementation by athletes. They suggest that a vitamin E deficiency may lead to impaired oxygen transport due to RBC damage and to reduced oxidative capacity within the muscle cell. These effects would reduce VO_2 max and lead to a decrease in aerobic endurance capacity.

Supplementation: Health and Physical Performance   Vitamin E supplementation, based on the potential antioxidant effects, has been studied extensively as a means of enhancing health and physical performance. Vitamin E has often been combined with other antioxidants to evaluate the effects on disease processes or muscle damage during exercise, and these topics are discussed later in the chapter.

Vitamin E supplementation has also been studied as a means to enhance VO_2 max and aerobic endurance capacity by maintaining red blood cell membrane integrity and polyunsaturated fatty acid content. The resulting improvement in membrane fluidity and deformability could theoretically enhance oxygen delivery. Early studies showed a beneficial effect, particularly at higher altitudes, but the experiments were poorly designed. However, Kobayashi, using a well-designed double-blind, placebo protocol, found that 1,200 IU of vitamin E supplements daily for 6 weeks improved VO_2 max, reduced blood lactic acid during submaximal exercise, and increased aerobic endurance in sedentary subjects at altitudes of 5,000 and 15,000 feet. More recent studies have supported these findings in athletes. Simon-Schnass and Pabst reported that vitamin E (400 mg for 10 weeks) reduced pentane expiration, a marker of lipid peroxidation, and improved anaerobic threshold in high-altitude mountain climbers. Ilavazhagan and others noted that vitamin E maintained RBC deformability and decreased markers of oxidative stress in rats exposed to simulated altitude of 25,000 feet. In their review, Braakhuis and Hopkins noted that vitamin E may protect against altitude-induced red blood cell lysis and oxidative damage. Additional research would appear to be warranted with athletes at altitude.

Exercising in highly polluted areas could also damage the RBC membrane. Since sports competitions often occur in large, urban areas with poor air quality, strategies to prevent RBC damage and peroxidation would be of interest to athletes such as marathon runners. In an old review of animal and human studies, Pryor concluded that vitamin E may attenuate the harmful effects of smog exposure. However, data from animal models do not clearly document an ergogenic effect of supplemented vitamin E above normal values. For ethical reasons, human data are based on short-term exposure instead of chronic long-term exposure. Given the possible effects of vitamin E on preserving RBC membrane integrity and exercise-induced muscle damage (discussed later in this chapter), Simon-Schnass commented that athletes should consume 100–200 IU daily and that it would be bordering on malpractice not to point out the benefits of such supplementation to athletes.

However, the majority of the recent well-designed studies on athletes, using doses from 400 to 1,200 IU, revealed no significant effect on variables such as VO_2 max, aerobic endurance at sea level, or marathon or Ironman-distance triathlon performance. One possible reason for this finding is that the plasma level of vitamin E appears to rise significantly during intense exercise, as reported by Pincemail and others. However, Rokitzki and others found no improvement in VO_2 max and other cycling performance measures in national-class racing cyclists after 5 months of vitamin E supplementation, as compared to a placebo treatment, despite a significant increase in serum vitamin E levels.

The antioxidant effect of vitamin E on exercise-induced oxidative stress has been the subject of several reviews. Nikolaidas and others reviewed the effects of vitamin E or C supplementation on training adaptations and oxidative markers in humans and rat models and concluded that there is no basis for recommendation of vitamin E and/or C supplementation. Although Stepanyan and others found no significant effect of tocopherol supplementation on exercise-induced oxidative stress or muscle damage in their meta-analysis of 20 studies, they noted the complex antioxidant function of tocopherols and that future research should examine additional markers of oxidative stress.

Vitamin K also has an effect on bone health. In their review, Chin and Nirwana concluded that small doses of α-tocopherol have been consistently reported to improve bone health in humans and animals. However, large doses taken for ergogenic purposes may have pro-oxidant effects and interfere with the effects of vitamin K on bone health.

Although the potential ergogenic effect of vitamin E supplementation at altitude warrants additional research, Tiidus and Houston reviewed the scientific literature and concluded that while supplementation may increase tissue or serum vitamin E concentration, there is currently a lack of conclusive evidence that exercise performance or recovery in either elite or recreational athletes would benefit in any significant way.

Prudent Recommendations   Vitamin E is an important antioxidant, and health professionals indicate that diets rich in vitamin E may be beneficial. However, a meta-analysis by Schürks and others noted that vitamin E supplementation in healthy and patient populations increased the risk for hemorrhagic stroke by 22 percent and decreased ischemic stroke by 10 percent. Analyses that have previously looked at total stroke may have missed this important finding. The authors do not encourage vitamin E supplementation. Although vitamin E supplements were once recommended for potential health benefits, caution is now advised, as shall be discussed later in this chapter. Moreover, as a means of enhancing physical performance, vitamin E supplements are not recommended.

Vitamin K (menadione)

Vitamin K is a fat-soluble vitamin. It is often called the blood coagulation vitamin or antihemorrhagic vitamin. Vitamin K was discovered in Denmark, and K is derived from *koagulation,* the Danish word for coagulation. Vitamin K is the generic term for **menadione**, or vitamin K_3.

DRI   The AI is 120 and 90 micrograms/day for adult males and females, respectively. The DV is 80 micrograms. No UL has been established.

Food Sources   Vitamin K is found in a variety of plant and animal foods. *Phylloquinone* (K_1) is the plant form of vitamin K, while *menoquinone* and related compounds (K_2) represent the animal form. Good plant sources include vegetable oils (soybean, olive) and green and leafy vegetables such as kale, peas, broccoli, and spinach; meats and milk contain much lower amounts. Phylloquinone is the major dietary source of vitamin K; 3 ounces of spinach contain 380 micrograms, whereas 3 ounces of meat contain less than 1 microgram. The typical American diet contains about 100–150 micrograms per day. Additionally, vitamin MK (menoquinone) is also formed in the intestines by bacteria, so a

deficiency is unlikely. The AI is usually met easily by a combination of dietary intake and endogenous synthesis.

Major Functions   Vitamin K is needed for the formation of four compounds that are essential in two steps of the blood-clotting process. In addition, vitamin K appears to enhance the function of osteocalcin, a protein that plays an important role in strengthening bones. Suttie has provided a review of the role of vitamin K in human nutrition.

Deficiency: Health and Physical Performance   A deficiency of vitamin K is uncommon in healthy adults but may occur with very low–vitamin K diets and in some individuals when antibiotic medications kill the intestinal bacteria that produce the vitamin. Deficiencies may impair blood clotting and lead to hemorrhage. Zittermann noted that some epidemiological studies have shown an association between low vitamin K intake and increased risk of osteoporotic bone fractures.

There are no data indicating deficiency states in physically active individuals or related effects on physical performance.

Supplementation: Health and Physical Performance   Recent studies have suggested that vitamin K supplementation may have positive effects on bone health. Zittermann indicated that studies with very high pharmacological doses of MK may enhance bone mineralization in individuals with osteoporosis, but the effect of dietary supplements is less clear. However, Weber noted that there is emerging evidence in human intervention studies that vitamin K_1 supplementation may benefit bone health, in particular when coadministered with vitamin D. Moreover, in a meta-analysis of 13 studies, Cockayne and others reported that all studies but one showed an advantage of oral vitamin K supplementation as a means to reduce bone loss. Liebman and Hurley, citing research involving the effect of vitamin K to prevent hip fracture, noted that doses ranging from 150 to 250 micrograms daily were effective.

No supplementation studies are available to evaluate the effect of vitamin K on physical performance because it does not appear to play an important role in this regard. However, as related to bone health, Craciun and others reported an increased index of bone formation markers in female elite athletes following vitamin K supplementation (10 mg/day) for 1 month. Some of the athletes were vitamin K deficient prior to the supplementation protocol. Conversely, in a 2-year clinical study, Braam and others failed to find any effect of supplementary vitamin K on the rate of bone loss in female endurance athletes. The importance of bone health in young female athletes is discussed further in chapter 8.

The National Academy of Sciences has noted that, unlike vitamins A and D, vitamin K as phylloquinone is not very toxic when consumed in large doses. However, Weber notes that individuals taking anticoagulant drugs should consult with their physicians about diet and supplements. As vitamin K promotes clotting, the prescription may have to be adjusted.

Prudent Recommendations   No available evidence supports vitamin K supplementation as a means to improve the health status of the average individual or to improve performance in athletes. Some research suggests that vitamin K supplementation may help promote bone health by increasing bone mineral content. Typical multivitamin tablets may contain about 0–120 micrograms of vitamin K. Individuals desiring to take vitamin K supplements are recommended to do so under the guidance of a physician.

Key Concepts

▶ The fat-soluble vitamins are A, D, E, and K. Although most vitamins must be obtained from the food we eat, several fat-soluble vitamins may be manufactured in the body. Vitamin A may be produced from dietary beta-carotene, vitamin D from exposure to the sun, and vitamin K from intestinal bacterial activity.

▶ Current research suggests that some individuals, particularly the elderly, need to obtain more vitamin D and calcium from their diet. Although obtaining these nutrients through consumption of healthy, nutrient dense foods is ideal, supplements may be recommended for some. Some health professionals recommend daily intake from food and supplements of 1,000–2,000 IU of vitamin D and 1,000–1,300 milligrams of calcium. D_3 is preferable.

▶ Although research is somewhat limited, in general, supplementation with fat-soluble vitamins has not been shown to enhance sports performance.

Water-Soluble Vitamins

There are nine water-soluble vitamins, including eight in the vitamin B complex and vitamin C (ascorbic acid). The B complex vitamins include thiamin, riboflavin, niacin, B_6, B_{12}, folate, biotin, and pantothenic acid. Choline, although included in the DRI for the B vitamins, has not been classified as a vitamin at this time. Being water soluble, they are not, with a few exceptions, stored to any significant extent in the body. The effects of a deficiency may be noted in 2–4 weeks for some of these vitamins, often reducing physical performance capacity. Excess supplements of these vitamins are usually excreted in the urine and are generally considered to be relatively harmless. However, there are some exceptions.

Because several of the B vitamins work closely together in energy metabolism, many studies have investigated the effect of a deficiency or supplementation of multiple vitamins from the *B complex*. A summary of this research follows a discussion of each individual vitamin.

Figure 7.4 provides a broad perspective on the major sites of activity of the water-soluble vitamins, highlighting sites for vitamin E and other antioxidants as well.

Thiamin (vitamin B₁)

Thiamin, also known as **vitamin B₁**, is a water-soluble vitamin and is also known as the antiberiberi or antineuritic vitamin. It was one of the first vitamins discovered.

DRI The RDA for thiamin varies according to the intake of Calories, being approximately 0.5 mg per 1,000 Calories. The average adult male needs approximately 1.2 mg/day, while the adult female needs about 1.1 mg/day. See the DRI table on the inside front cover for more details. The DV is 1.5 mg. No UL has been established.

Food Sources Thiamin is widely distributed in both plant and animal tissues. Excellent sources include whole-grain cereals, beans, and pork. One lean pork chop contains more than 50 percent of the RDA. Several fortified, ready-to-eat cereals contain 100 percent of the RDA for thiamin, as well as most of the other B vitamins.

Major Functions Thiamin has a central role in the metabolism of glucose. It is part of a coenzyme known as thiamin pyrophosphate, which is needed to convert pyruvate into acetyl CoA for entrance into the Krebs cycle. Thiamin is essential for the normal functioning of the nervous system and energy derivation from glycogen in the muscles.

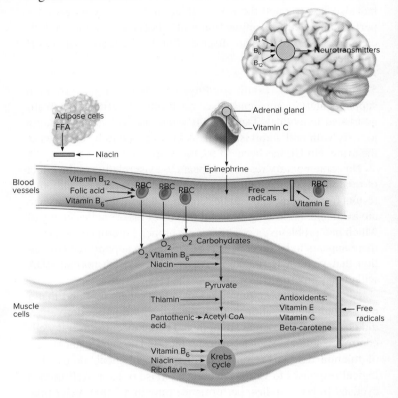

FIGURE 7.4 Roles of vitamins important to sports performance. A number of B vitamins, including thiamin, riboflavin, niacin, B_6, and pantothenic acid, are essential for the conversion of carbohydrate into energy for muscular contraction. Vitamin B_{12} and folic acid are essential for the development of the red blood cells (RBCs), which deliver oxygen to the muscle cell. Vitamin E helps protect the RBC membrane from destruction by free radicals. Vitamin E and other antioxidant vitamins are theorized to prevent free radical damage in muscle cells during exercise. Vitamin C is needed for the formation of epinephrine (adrenaline), a key hormone during strenuous exercise. Niacin may actually block the release of free fatty acids from the adipose tissue, which could be a disadvantage for ultraendurance athletes. Finally, several of the B vitamins are also involved in the formation of neurotransmitters in the brain, which may induce a relaxation effect.

Deficiency: Health and Physical Performance Deficiency symptoms may occur in several weeks and include loss of appetite, mental confusion, muscular weakness, and pain in the calf muscles. Prolonged deficiencies lead to beriberi, a serious disease involving damage to the nervous system and the heart. Fortunately, thiamin deficiency is not very common, although it may be rather prevalent among the homeless, alcoholics, and other special groups.

Of importance to the athlete, two factors that increase the need for thiamin are exercise and high carbohydrate intake. A deficiency of thiamin could prove to be detrimental to the active individual who might rely on high levels of carbohydrate metabolism for aerobic energy production during exercise, such as endurance athletes. Indeed, some well-controlled research conducted during World War II to evaluate military nutrition needs in combat noted decreased endurance capacity after several weeks of a thiamin-deficient diet. More contemporary research has also investigated the role of thiamin deficiency on exercise performance, but in conjunction with riboflavin and niacin deficiencies. These reports are discussed in the section on vitamin B complex.

Supplementation: Health and Physical Performance Thiamin supplementation apparently has no health benefits for a well-nourished individual. Tanphaichitr found no evidence of thiamin toxicity with oral administration, as the excess will be excreted in the urine. No UL has been set for thiamin.

No contemporary research appears to exist relative to the effect of thiamin supplementation upon physical performance, although results from a number of studies conducted more than 50 years ago are available. Following a careful review of these studies, many of which had problems in establishing a proper experimental design, there appears to be no conclusive evidence to support the contention that vitamin B_1 intake above and beyond the normal RDA will enhance performance.

Although not using thiamin, Doyle and others reported that 5 days of supplementation with allithiamine, a thiamin derivative, did not improve muscular strength and endurance. In several well-controlled studies, Michael Webster reported no significant effects of thiamin derivatives on metabolic, physiological, or psychological responses to various cycling exercise tasks in well-trained cyclists. In both studies, performance time in a 2,000-meter time trial (in one study after a 50-kilometer ride) was not affected by the thiamin derivatives.

Thiamin, as indicated, is important for normal neurological functions. In a study from Japan, Suzuki and Itokawa reported that 100 milligrams of thiamin for 3 days increased serum thiamin levels and reduced subjective complaints of fatigue from subjects following a strenuous exercise task. As noted later in the B complex section, thiamin was one of the vitamins proposed to improve neurological function in pistol shooting. These are interesting observations and merit additional research.

As noted previously, physical activity, particularly high-intensity, endurance-type activity, increases the need for thiamin in the diet; this exercise training also increases the need for caloric intake. With proper selection of foods, the increased thiamin

need may be met by the content in the additional foods eaten. An adequate thiamin intake is one of the reasons physically active individuals need to select foods that are dense in nutrients, and in general to avoid foods that provide Calories but few nutrients. Woolf and Manore, in their review of B vitamins and exercise performance, concluded that thiamin intake of most athletes, even those in weight-control sports, appears to be adequate and consistent with recommendations.

Prudent Recommendations Thiamin supplements are not needed by the individual who is consuming an adequate diet, and they do not appear to enhance exercise performance.

Riboflavin (vitamin B₂)

Riboflavin is also known as **vitamin B₂.** It is a water-soluble vitamin and is a component of the B complex.

DRI The RDA for riboflavin is 1.3 mg for the adult male and 1.1 mg for the adult female. The DRI table on the inside front cover contains the RDA for other age groups. The DV is currently 1.7 mg and no UL has been established.

Food Sources Riboflavin is distributed widely in foods. A major source is milk and other dairy products; one glass of milk contains 20 percent of the RDA. Other good sources include liver, eggs, dark-green leafy vegetables, wheat germ, yeast, whole-grain products, and enriched breads and cereals.

Major Functions Riboflavin is important for the formation of several oxidative enzymes known as *flavoproteins,* which are involved in energy production from carbohydrate and fats in the body cells. It is also involved in protein metabolism and maintenance of healthy skin tissue.

Deficiency: Health and Physical Performance Deficiencies are very rare but have been seen in alcoholics and those adhering to various fad diets. Early signs of deficiency include glossitis (an inflammation of the tongue), cracks at the corners of the mouth, and dry, scaly skin at the corners of the nose, symptoms common in individuals who experience multiple nutrient deficits.

Although the effect of a riboflavin deficiency on physical performance has not been studied directly, research from Cornell University suggests that physically untrained women who initiate an aerobic training program may need a higher intake of riboflavin to synthesize more flavoproteins in the muscles. Using a blood test, the investigators determined that the RDA did not maintain proper riboflavin status in the early stages of training, but they suggested that a value of about 1.1 mg per 1,000 Calories would be sufficient. It should be noted that no data were reported relative to the effect of this deficiency on performance. Haralambie also reported a possible deficiency in trained athletes but did not relate it to performance. Most recently, Woolf and Manore reported that although athletes may need more riboflavin than the general population and the current RDA, they can satisfy these increased needs if adequate energy is consumed and they currently appear to be meeting recommendations.

Supplementation: Health and Physical Performance   Riboflavin supplementation apparently has no health benefits for a well-nourished individual. McCormick indicates that toxicity for excess riboflavin intake is doubtful. Excesses will not be stored but will be excreted in the urine. No UL has been set for riboflavin.

Reviews by Keith and van der Beek reveal only one reputable study of the effects of riboflavin supplementation on physical performance. Tremblay and others, studying elite swimmers, reported that 60 mg of riboflavin daily for 16 to 20 days did not improve VO_2 max, anaerobic (lactate) threshold, or swim performance.

Prudent Recommendations   Considering the available research data and the absence of riboflavin deficiency in most individuals, one must conclude that riboflavin supplementation will not enhance health or physical performance.

Niacin

Niacin is also known as nicotinic acid, nicotinamide, or the anti-pellagra vitamin. It is a water-soluble vitamin in the B complex and is sometimes erroneously referred to as vitamin B_3.

DRI   Niacin is found naturally in many foods, but it also may be formed in the body from excess amounts of dietary tryptophan, an essential amino acid. Therefore, the RDA is expressed in **niacin equivalents, or NE.** One NE equals 1 mg of niacin or 60 mg of tryptophan, because 1 mg of niacin can be produced from that amount of tryptophan. The RDA for niacin is 16 NE for adult males and 14 NE for adult females. The requirement is different for other age groups, and specific values may be obtained from the DRI table on the inside front cover. The DV is 20 mg. Because excess niacin intake may cause some health problems, as we will note, an UL of 35 mg/day has been set for adults, and even lower amounts for younger individuals.

Food Sources   Niacin is found in foods that have a high protein content. It is most abundant in lean meats, organ meats, fish, poultry, whole-grain cereal products, legumes such as beans and peanuts, and enriched foods. Milk and eggs contain small amounts of niacin, but they contain sufficient tryptophan. One-half of a chicken breast contains more than 60 percent of the RDA of niacin.

Major Functions   Niacin serves as a component of two coenzymes concerned with energy processes within the cell. One of these coenzymes (nicotinamide adenine dinucleotide, NAD^+) is important in the process of glycolysis, which is the means by which muscle glycogen produces energy both aerobically and anaerobically. The other coenzyme is involved in fat metabolism by promoting fat synthesis in the body, which may block release of free fatty acids from adipose cells.

Deficiency: Health and Physical Performance   Although niacin deficiency was prevalent in the past, the enrichment of foods with niacin has nearly eliminated this problem. Deficiency symptoms include loss of appetite, skin rashes, mental confusion, lack of energy, and muscular weakness. Serious deficiencies lead to pellagra, a disease characterized by severe dermatitis, diarrhea, and symptoms of mental illness.

In theory, physical performance would be impaired by a niacin deficiency because the production of energy from carbohydrate could be impaired. Both aerobic- and anaerobic-type performances could be affected. However, no research has been uncovered that has directly studied the effects of niacin deficiency alone on exercise performance.

Supplementation: Health and Physical Performance   Megadoses of niacin may function as drugs and have been used in attempts to treat several health problems, being relatively ineffective in the treatment of mental disease and somewhat successful in reducing high serum lipid levels. McKenney noted that niacin favorably affects all components of the lipid profile to a significant degree, as it has consistently been shown to significantly reduce levels of total cholesterol, LDL-cholesterol, triglycerides, and lipoprotein (a). In particular, niacin has a very potent effect to increase HDL-cholesterol by blocking the uptake of apolipoprotein A1 by the liver; some indicate that it is the best drug for this purpose. Niacin may be useful as a therapeutic treatment of dyslipidemia. In several reviews of clinical studies, Hunninghake and Bourgeois revealed that niacin, either alone or combined with other agents, can result in regression of atherosclerosis and reduce patient mortality. However, results from the AIM-HIGH trial showed that niacin did not provide any additional protection against heart attacks when taken with the cholesterol-lowering drug Zocor®, also known as simvastatin, but it did increase risk of stroke. Surprisingly, patients ingesting niacin and Zocor® had increased HDL levels and decreased triglycerides, but there was no benefit in terms of disease outcomes. Although medications that reduce LDL are clearly beneficial, there is less evidence that nutrients and medications that increase HDL and decrease triglycerides are as effective at reducing heart disease risk. Given these rather contradictory research findings, individuals with cardiovascular disease should adhere to their physician's recommendations.

Although niacin is generally considered to be nontoxic, large doses in the form of nicotinic acid may cause flushing, with burning and tingling sensations around the face, neck, and hands occurring within 15 to 20 minutes after ingestion (i.e., the histamine-like effect). Taken over long periods, niacin may contribute to liver problems such as hepatitis and peptic ulcers. Pieper noted that niacin comes in three formulations: immediate-release, sustained-release, and extended-release. Niaspan, an extended-release niacin preparation, appears to minimize the flushing effects seen with the immediate-release form and the hepatotoxic effects seen with the sustained-release form. In their review, Guyton and Bays concluded that, overall, the perception of niacin side effects is often greater than the reality and thus, as a result, a valuable medication for cardiovascular risk is underused. Nevertheless, the American Heart Association and the National Institutes of Health recommend that no one take niacin to lower blood cholesterol without guidance from a physician.

Because of the role of niacin in energy metabolism, a number of experiments have been conducted relative to niacin supplementation and physical performance capacity. However, several reviews concluded that niacin supplementation has not been shown to be an effective ergogenic aid for well-nourished athletes, having no effect on various exercise endeavors, including performance in a 10-mile run and in a 3.5-mile cycle time trial following 2 hours of cycling.

As a matter of fact, niacin supplementation is not recommended for most athletes, particularly those involved in endurance-type exercise such as marathon running, because excessive niacin intake (3–9 grams/day) influences fat metabolism, blocking the release of FFA from the adipose tissue. This will decrease the supply of FFA to the muscle, which may lead to an increased dependence on carbohydrate as an energy source during exercise, as shown by Heath and others. This could lead to a more rapid depletion of muscle glycogen, an important energy source during exercise. As noted by Bulow, niacin supplements may reduce endurance capacity.

Niacin supplements may also increase blood flow to the skin due to a histamine-like effect. In one experiment, Kolka and Stephenson found that such an effect could lower the sweat rate and decrease body heat storage during exercise. These effects could be ergogenic to athletes exercising in the heat, but further investigation is needed.

Prudent Recommendations   Unless recommended under the treatment of a physician, niacin supplements are not recommended for a physically active individual on a balanced diet. Excessive intake may actually impair certain types of athletic performance and elicit adverse health effects.

Vitamin B₆ (pyridoxine)

Vitamin B₆ is a collective term for three naturally occurring substances that are all metabolically and functionally related: pyridoxine, pyridoxal, and pyridoxamine. *Pyridoxine* is most often used as a synonym. Vitamin B₆ is water soluble.

DRI   The adult RDA for vitamin B₆ is 1.3 mg/day for ages 19 to 50, and then increases to 1.7 mg for males and 1.5 for females above age 51. Slightly different amounts are needed at different age levels. Consult the DRI table on the inside front cover for specific RDA. Actually, the RDA for vitamin B₆ is based on protein intake, so requirements may increase with high-protein diets. The DV is 2 mg. As excess B₆ intake may cause some health problems, as noted in this section, a UL of 100 mg/day has been set for adults, and even lower amounts for younger individuals.

Food Sources   Vitamin B₆ is widely distributed in foods. The most reliable sources are protein foods such as meats, poultry, fish, wheat germ, whole-grain products, brown rice, and eggs. One-half of a chicken breast contains more than 25 percent of the RDA.

Major Functions   In its coenzyme form (primarily pyridoxal phosphate, PLP), vitamin B₆ is critically involved in the metabolism of protein, but it is also involved in carbohydrate and fat metabolism. It functions with more than 60 enzymes in such processes as the synthesis of dispensable amino acids, the conversion of tryptophan to niacin, the formation of neurotransmitters in the nervous system, and the incorporation of amino acids into body proteins such as hemoglobin, myoglobin, and oxidative enzymes. It is also involved in the breakdown of muscle glycogen, as well as gluconeogenesis in the liver. Interested readers are directed to the review by Woolf and Manore for more details on the metabolic functions of vitamin B₆.

Deficiency: Health and Physical Performance   Vitamin B₆ deficiency is not considered to be a major health problem. The average American diet appears to provide an adequate amount of the vitamin, but poor diets do not. The use of diuretics and oral contraceptives has been associated with deficiencies. Woolf and Manore reported that studies have found poor vitamin B₆ status in some athletes, particularly in endurance athletes. Female athletes on low-energy diets may also have low vitamin B₆ intakes. Deficiency symptoms include nausea, impaired immune function, skin disorders, mouth sores, weakness, mental depression, anemia, and epileptic-like convulsions.

Theoretically, a B₆ deficiency could adversely affect endurance activities dependent on oxygen, for it is involved in the formation of protein compounds, such as hemoglobin, that are essential to oxidative processes. Its role in carbohydrate metabolism, particularly muscle glycogen utilization, is also important to the endurance athlete. Its role in the formation of neurotransmitters could be important to athletes engaged in fine motor control sports, such as archery and riflery. In addition, the requirement for B₆ increases with protein intake, which may have some implications for athletes who may be on high-protein diets. However, because B₆ is found in protein products, it should be easily obtainable in such a diet.

No research has been uncovered that has directly studied the effect of a B₆ deficiency on physical performance. One report did suggest that runners who covered 5 to 10 miles per day appear to use more B₆ than their sedentary counterparts, but these investigators also noted that exercise may actually promote storage of the vitamin in the athlete, thus helping to prevent a deficiency state. Serum levels of B₆ actually increase during exercise. Woolf and Manore indicate that exercise increases plasma levels of PLP, which can be converted into an acid and lost in the urine during exercise; thus, exercise may increase the turnover and loss of vitamin B₆ from the body.

In general, exercise does not appear to cause excessive losses of vitamin B₆ from the body. However, prolonged aerobic endurance exercise tasks may lead to increased B₆ losses. Rokitzki reported loss of 1 milligram from running a marathon, which approximates the daily RDA. In contrast, Leonard and Leklem found that plasma pyridoxal phosphate levels fell following a 50-kilometer ultramarathon, results that are not consistent with those reported in previous studies involving shorter length endurance tasks. However, whether or not ultraendurance athletes are at risk for vitamin B₆ deficiency has not been determined. These vitamin B_6 losses could easily be replaced during recovery from endurance exercise with consumption of meals rich in protein and carbohydrate.

Supplementation: Health and Physical Performance   Vitamin B_6 supplementation has been used to treat the nausea of pregnancy, mental depression associated with the use of oral contraceptives, and premenstrual syndrome (PMS), but its effectiveness for these purposes has received mixed reviews. For example, in a systematic review, Wyatt and others found that conclusions are limited due to the poor quality of most studies, but doses of 100 mg/day of B_6 (which coincides with the UL) are likely to yield benefits in the treatment of PMS symptoms.

As discussed later, folate supplementation may decrease plasma homocysteine levels, which has been studied as a risk factor for CHD. McKinley and others noted that although not as effective as folate, low doses of B_6 (1.6 mg/day) may provide additional homocysteine-lowering benefits to elderly individuals who have adequate intake of the other B vitamins. Vitamin B_6 has also been studied as part of B complex supplementation for prevention of CHD, and the results are presented later in this chapter.

Woolf and Manore suggest that some active individuals, depending on training level, may require 1.5 to 2.5 times the current RDA for B_6 to maintain good B_6 status. Several reports relative to the effect of B_6 supplementation on physical performance are available. Although the muscle may store B_6, Coburn and others noted that B_6 supplementation did not markedly increase muscle stores. Moreover, in general, the studies reveal no significant effect on metabolic functions during exercise or the capacity to do more work. One investigator suggested that B_6 may actually be detrimental to endurance athletes because it may facilitate the use of muscle glycogen and lead to earlier depletion in prolonged events. However, in a study from the laboratory at Oregon State University, Virk and others reported that B_6 supplementation (20 g/day for 9 days) did not influence, either positively or negatively, performance of trained males in an exhaustive aerobic endurance exercise task just under 2 hours in duration.

There appears to be little or no toxicity associated with moderate doses, but Bender noted that at high levels, B_6 supplementation can cause peripheral nerve damage, evidenced by problems such as loss of natural sensation from the limbs and an impaired gait. The National Research Council noted neurological symptoms with smaller dosages, averaging 117 mg/day for 6 months to 5 years.

Prudent Recommendations   Vitamin B_6 supplementation does not appear to be warranted for the physically active individual and may be associated with some health risks if consumed in large doses for prolonged periods.

Vitamin B_{12} (cobalamin)

Vitamin B_{12} (cobalamin) is a water-soluble vitamin. It is part of the B complex and is the latest vitamin to be discovered.

DRI   The adult RDA for B_{12} is 2.4 micrograms (mcg) per day. The average diet contains about 5–15 mcg. Slightly different allowances are made for other age groups; see the DRI table on the inside front cover. Note that recommendations for individuals over age 50 are to obtain the RDA from fortified foods or supplements. The DV is 6 mcg. No UL is available.

Food Sources   Vitamin B_{12} is found in good supply only in animal foods such as meat, fish, poultry, cheese, eggs, and milk. One glass of milk contains nearly 30 percent of the RDA. It is not found in natural plant foods such as fruits, vegetables, beans, and grains, but vitamin-fortified cereals may be an excellent source. It is present in microorganisms such as bacteria and yeast, which may be found in some plant foods, but the bioavailability of B_{12} from these sources is uncertain. Although B_{12} may be produced by microorganisms in the human bowel, the site of production is below the point of absorption.

Major Functions   Vitamin B_{12} is a part of coenzymes present in all body cells and is essential in the synthesis of DNA. It works closely with folic acid, and both have important roles in the development of red blood cells. Vitamin B_{12} is also essential for the formation of the protective sheath around nerve fibers (the myelin sheath) and for the metabolism of homocysteine.

Deficiency: Health and Physical Performance   Deficiency of vitamin B_{12} in humans due to inadequate dietary intake is rare. Even strict vegetarians appear to receive enough in their diet, through either the consumption of microorganisms or the use of fortified products. The body also stores a considerable amount in the liver, which may last for years; the body contains about 2,500 micrograms but loses only about 1 microgram daily. A deficiency normally is caused by the inability to release cobalamin from food or a deficiency of intestinal absorption due to decreased transport proteins. The major symptoms are a severe form of anemia, known as megaloblastic (pernicious) anemia, and nerve damage that may cause paralysis. Pregnant women, particularly vegans, need to obtain adequate B_{12} because a deficit may impair myelination and cause birth defects in the newborn. Aging affects the absorption of B_{12} when it is present in food and bound to protein. The use of certain medications (proton pump inhibitors, histamine 2 receptor antagonists) to decrease the production of gastric acid may adversely affect the absorption of vitamin B_{12}. Lam and others compared almost 26,000 patients with vitamin B_{12} deficiency with almost 125,000 controls and reported an association between previous or current use of gastric acid inhibitors and vitamin B_{12} deficiency.

Because of its role in the formation of RBCs, a deficiency of B_{12} resulting in pernicious anemia would be theorized to decrease aerobic endurance capacity. No research is available relative to the effect of a vitamin B_{12} deficiency on performance, but other types of anemia have been shown to impair exercise performance.

Supplementation: Health and Physical Performance B_{12} megadoses may be an effective medical treatment for pernicious anemia but do not appear to benefit the active individual who eats a balanced diet. However, as noted below, lower-dose supplements may be recommended for some individuals.

Relative to sports, vitamin B_{12} has been one of the most abused vitamins in the athletic world, with some reports of athletes receiving large amounts by injection just prior to competition. The belief probably exists that if a little vitamin B_{12} can prevent anemia, then a lot of it will do something magical to increase performance capacity. However, several well-controlled studies conducted with B_{12} supplementation reached the general conclusion that it will not help to increase metabolic functions, such as VO_2 max or endurance performance. B_{12} supplements appear to be safe, but do not appear to benefit the active individual on a balanced diet.

Prudent Recommendations Individuals who consume animal products normally do not need vitamin B_{12} supplements, and there are no sound data that supplementation will enhance sports performance. However, vegans should consume food products fortified with vitamin B_{12}. Additionally, individuals over age 50, including senior athletes, may have decreased intrinsic factor and limited B_{12} absorption from natural B_{12} food sources, so they are advised to get about 2.4 mcg of B_{12} from fortified food products, such as cereals, or supplements. One serving of B_{12}-fortified cereal contains about 1.5 mcg, whereas a senior multivitamin usually contains 25 mcg.

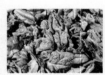

Folate (folic acid)

Folate, or folic acid, is a water-soluble vitamin. It is part of the B complex. Folate is found naturally in some foods, but folic acid is a synthetic form found in fortified foods and dietary supplements; collectively they are called *folacin*.

DRI The RDA for folate is given as micrograms (mcg) of **dietary folate equivalents (DFE)**. One DFE equals 1 mcg of food folate, 0.6 mcg of folic acid in fortified foods, or 0.5 mcg of folic acid supplements taken on an empty stomach. One mcg of folic acid in fortified foods equals 1.7 DFE, while 1 mcg folic acid in a supplement equals 2 DFE, because these forms are better absorbed. The RDA for folate is 400 mcg of DFE/day. During pregnancy, the RDA is increased to 600 mcg of DFE per day, and it is 500 mcg DFE during the early stages of lactation. The DV is 400 mcg of DFE. An UL of 1,000 mcg DFE/day has been set for adults, and even lower amounts for younger individuals.

Food Sources Folate derives its name from *foliage* because it is found in green leafy vegetables such as spinach. Other good sources include organ meats such as liver and kidney, dry beans, whole-grain products, and some fruits such as oranges and bananas. One cup of cooked black or navy beans contains about 60–75 percent of the folate RDA. One banana provides almost 10 percent of the RDA. Currently, all cereal and grain products in the United States are fortified with folic acid to reduce the occurrence of neural tube defects. The average fortification is 140 mcg per 100 grams of food product. Studies indicate that such fortification has increased daily dietary folic acid intake by 100 mcg or more.

Major Functions Folate serves as part of a coenzyme that plays a critical role in the metabolism of methionine, an essential amino

acid. In this regard, folic acid is critical to the formation of DNA, the genetic material that regulates cell division. It is essential for maintaining normal production of RBCs, one of the most rapidly dividing cells in the body. Folate is also critical during the very early stages of pregnancy when cells in the fetus divide rapidly. Researchers indicate during periods of rapid cell division large amounts of folate are needed to make DNA.

Folate is also involved in the metabolism of **homocysteine**, an amino acid derived in a conversion from methionine and considered by some experts to be a possible risk factor for cardiovascular disease. Folate is necessary for the reformation of methionine from homocysteine.

Deficiency: Health and Physical Performance One national survey has reported folate intakes below the RDA for some Americans. Individuals who consume large quantities of alcohol and women who take oral contraceptives may experience deficiencies in folic acid, as these drugs may impair absorption of the vitamin. A folic acid deficiency may impair DNA formation, or lead to an increase in homocysteine.

Due to its effect on DNA synthesis, one of the major effects of folate deficiency is pernicious anemia, attributed to inadequate RBC regeneration. Anemia could impair delivery of oxygen and significantly impair performance in aerobic endurance events.

DNA and chromosomal damage caused by folic acid deficiency has been suggested to increase the risk of cancer. For example, in a Tufts University review, a low level of folate in large intestine cells was associated with an increased risk of colon cancer, a finding one of the authors reported to be consistent with the results of 20 other epidemiological studies, which have found that people who eat the most folic acid are the least likely to get colon cancer. Zhang and others also reported that for women who consume alcohol, those with the lowest dietary folic acid intake were at the highest risk for developing breast cancer.

Due to either DNA damage or the adverse neural effects of homocysteine, women who are folate deficient and become pregnant may give birth to children with neural tube defects (NTD) such as spina bifida, an incomplete closure of the tissue surrounding the spinal cord. Such defects may cause paralysis and severe disabling conditions in the child. Approximately 2,500 infants in the United States are affected each year.

Elevated plasma levels of homocysteine are thought to damage the lining of the blood vessels or initiate growth of cells that form the framework of plaque, increasing the risk for several vascular diseases, including coronary heart disease (CHD), stroke, peripheral vascular disease (PVD), and Alzheimer's disease. However, Wierzbicki contended that it is simply a marker for CHD, not a cause. As an aside, Joubert and Manore, in a review of exercise, nutrition, and homocysteine, noted that no consistent relationship exists between physical activity and plasma homocysteine concentrations. The American Heart Association has not yet classified a high blood level of homocysteine as a major risk factor for CHD.

Supplementation: Health and Physical Performance In a review, Eichholzer and others reported irrefutable evidence that adequate folic acid helps prevent neural tube defects. In countries mandating fortification of flour with folic acid, the incidence of neural tube defects decreased by 31 to 78 percent. The NIH report on vitamin supplementation also noted that multiple studies have supported the effectiveness of folic acid use by women of childbearing age to prevent neural tube defects in offspring. All women who have the potential to become pregnant should consume 400 mcg of synthetic folic acid daily. The 400 mcg should be consumed as folic acid in fortified foods or dietary supplements, in addition to normal food folate intake. When pregnancy is confirmed, the RDA is increased to 600 mcg DFE. Currently, only 1 in 3 women consume 400 mcg DFE daily, so many women need to increase their intake of folic acid-fortified foods or dietary supplements, a recommendation of many health professionals. Some researchers suggest that women at high risk for neural tube defects should take 4,000 mcg daily, but only in consultation with their physicians.

Although folic acid supplementation is effective in preventing neural tube defects, there is ongoing debate relative to beneficial vascular effects associated with homocysteine lowering by folic acid supplementation. For example, Wang and others conducted a meta-analysis of eight studies and found that folic acid supplementation significantly reduced the risk of a first stroke by 18 percent, particularly when supplemented over the course of 3 years and reducing homocysteine levels by more than 20 percent. Conversely, Bazzano and others did a meta-analysis of 12 randomized, controlled studies and reported that folic acid supplementation has not been shown to reduce risk of cardiovascular diseases or all-cause mortality among participants with prior history of vascular disease. Most recently, Clarke and others, based on a meta-analysis of 37,485 individuals, reported that although folic acid supplementation reduces homocysteine, it has no effects on cardiovascular disease, cancer, or mortality in those with increased cardiovascular disease risk.

Research suggests caution with excessive folic acid supplementation. Cole and others conducted a double-blind, placebo-controlled study over 10 years to study the effects of supplementation with folic acid (1 mg/day) or placebo on the development of colorectal adenoma. Folic acid supplementation did not reduce colorectal adenoma risk but was associated with higher risks of having more adenomas and noncolorectal cancers. In their meta-analysis of 15 RCTs, however, Qin and others reported no effect of folate supplementation (mean supplementation = 4.7 mg/day for 48 months) on the incidence of colorectal, prostate, lung, breast, hematological, or total cancer and a decrease in melanoma cancer risk.

A UL of 1,000 mcg/day has been established for folic acid from fortified foods or supplements because megadoses could mask a vitamin B_{12} deficiency by preventing the development of anemia that would otherwise be discovered by a blood test. Unfortunately, folic acid does not prevent nerve damage, so the B_{12} deficiency may lead to paralysis if not detected. Rothenberg indicated that this may be a problem associated with the mandatory folic acid fortification of grain products. Thus, individuals who may be prone to a vitamin B_{12} deficiency are advised to take a B_{12} supplement or consume B_{12}-fortified foods.

One advocate of vitamin supplementation to athletes has reported that runners need additional folic acid to replace RBCs that may be destroyed in heavy training programs. Unfortunately, no evidence is available to support this theory, nor are there any data showing that folic acid supplements will benefit physical performance. Only one study has been uncovered related to folate supplementation to athletes. Matter and her colleagues provided folate therapy (5 mg/day for 11 weeks) to female marathon runners who were diagnosed as being folate deficient. Although the folate therapy restored serum folate levels to normal, no improvements were noted in VO_2 max, maximum treadmill running time, peak lactate levels, or running speed at the lactate anaerobic threshold.

To be sure, anemia resulting from a folate deficiency could have serious consequences for endurance performance, but a balanced diet including fortified grain products should prevent this condition from developing.

Prudent Recommendations All individuals should increase their intake of folate-rich foods, particularly vegetable sources, to obtain not only adequate folate but other healthful nutrients as well. Women in their childbearing years should obtain 400 mcg DFE daily from a supplement to complement natural dietary sources, a recommendation approved by the American Academy of Pediatrics. Given the importance of adequate DFE, the National Academy of Sciences, in establishing the new RDA, indicated that women should get folic acid from fortified foods or supplements. Relative to the theoretical risk of vascular diseases, 400 mcg DFE again appears to be a reasonable amount that may be obtained through the diet, particularly with folic acid-fortified cereals, or with the use of a daily supplement. However, because several studies have linked daily intake of 1,000 mcg of folic acid with increased risk for cancer, Liebman and Schardt suggested that although women of childbearing age are recommended to obtain 400 mcg of folic acid daily, males and postmenopausal women who take multivitamins might be advised to take one every other day and to try to avoid cereals, such as Total, that are fortified with 100 percent of the Daily Value for folic acid.

Folic acid has been combined with other B vitamins to evaluate health benefits of supplementation, which is covered in the section on the vitamin B complex.

Pantothenic acid

Pantothenic acid is a water-soluble vitamin. It is a factor in the B complex. Pantothenate is a salt of pantothenic acid.

DRI The adult AI for pantothenic acid is 5 mg, with lower amounts for younger age groups and greater amounts during pregnancy and lactation. The DV is 10 mg and no UL has been established.

Food Sources Pantothenic acid is distributed widely in foods. It is found in all natural animal and plant products, but best sources include organ meats, eggs, legumes, yeasts, and whole grains. It should also be noted that highly refined, processed foods have lost most of the pantothenate content.

Major Functions   Pantothenic acid is an essential component of coenzyme A (CoA), which plays a central role in energy metabolism. You may recall that acetyl CoA, which may be derived from carbohydrate, fat, and protein metabolism, is the principal substrate for the Krebs cycle. Pantothenic acid is also involved in gluconeogenesis, the synthesis and breakdown of fatty acids, the modification of proteins, and the synthesis of acetylcholine, a chemical released by the motor neuron to initiate muscle contraction.

Deficiency: Health and Physical Performance   Except under experimentally induced conditions, deficiencies are not seen in humans. In such cases, deficiencies have been reported to cause a variety of symptoms, including fatigue, muscle cramping, and impairment of motor coordination.

On a theoretical basis, pantothenic acid appears crucial to the active individual because it has an important function at the center of energy pathways. Several investigators have suggested that a deficiency would decrease the availability of acetyl CoA for the Krebs cycle and thus shift energy production to anaerobic glycolysis, which is less efficient. Because deficiencies of pantothenic acid have not been observed, such effects upon physical performance have not been studied.

Supplementation: Health and Physical Performance   Pantothenic acid supplementation apparently has no health benefits for a well-nourished individual. Liebman, in her review on how to select a multivitamin, indicated that you can ignore it on the label.

Published research findings do not support an effect of pantothenic acid supplementation on coenzyme A levels or physical performance. Webster reported no significant effects of pantothenic acid supplementation (1.8 grams per day for 7 days, combined with allithiamin) on 2,000-meter time trial following a 50-kilometer steady-state ride in highly trained cyclists. There were no significant metabolic, physiological, or psychological effects. Wall and others compared 1 week of supplementation with d-pantothenic acid (1.5 mg/day) combined with l-cysteine (1.5 mg/day) with placebo and found no effect on resting coenzyme A levels; similar declines in postexercise coenzyme A, lactate levels, and energy substrate use; and no difference in work output.

Supplements of pantothenic acid appear to be relatively nontoxic. However, large doses of 10 to 20 grams have been known to cause diarrhea.

Prudent Recommendations   Given the fact that pantothenic acid deficiency is rather nonexistent and there is little research to support a beneficial effect on health or physical performance at this time, supplementation is not recommended. A balanced diet should provide adequate pantothenic acid for the healthy, physically active individual.

Biotin

Biotin is a water-soluble vitamin in the B complex.

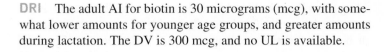

DRI   The adult AI for biotin is 30 micrograms (mcg), with somewhat lower amounts for younger age groups, and greater amounts during lactation. The DV is 300 mcg, and no UL is available.

Food Sources   Good dietary sources of biotin include organ meats such as liver, egg yolk, legumes such as peas and beans, and dark-green leafy vegetables. It is also synthesized in significant amounts in the intestines by bacteria.

Major Functions   McMahon noted recent research suggests that biotin may be involved in the regulation of gene expression, which may be related to its role as a coenzyme for a variety of enzymes involved in amino acid metabolism. Biotin is also involved in the synthesis of glucose and fatty acids. Because biotin is an important coenzyme for gluconeogenesis, it may have some implications relative to endurance performance.

Deficiency: Health and Physical Performance   Deficiency states are rare but may occur when the diet contains large amounts of raw egg whites; a protein in the raw egg white binds biotin and prevents its absorption into the body. In such cases, symptoms include loss of appetite, mental depression, dermatitis, and muscle pain. For athletes who consume eggs for their protein content, it may be important to know that cooking the egg white eliminates this problem while providing the same amount of high-quality protein. It should also be mentioned in passing that raw eggs pose a risk of salmonella, a type of bacteria associated with food poisoning.

Although a biotin deficiency could impair physical performance, no data are available to support this hypothesis.

Supplementation: Health and Physical Performance   No research into the effects of biotin supplementation on health or physical performance has been uncovered. Thus, there is no evidence that biotin supplementation improves health or increases physical performance capacity. Supplements of biotin appear to be harmless, as Mock reports no adverse effects in doses ranging up to 200 mg daily.

Prudent Recommendations   It would appear that biotin supplements are unnecessary for the physically active individual.

Choline

Choline, an amine, is a water-soluble essential nutrient listed in the DRI report with the B vitamins, but it has not been classified as a vitamin. Commercial choline products are available as lecithin or choline salts, but the actual choline content may vary. Check the labels for actual choline content. Choline is also marketed as a powder with carbohydrate and electrolytes to make a sports drink for athletes.

DRI   An AI has recently been set at 550 and 425 mg/day for male and female adults, respectively. Lower amounts have been established for adolescents and children. No DV has been established. The UL is 3.5 grams/day.

Food Sources Choline is found in most foods, particularly as lecithin (phosphotidylcholine) in animal foods and free choline in plants. Milk, liver, and eggs are good animal sources, while good plant sources include vegetables, legumes, nuts, seeds, and wheat germ. Zeisel and Niculescu note that normal diets deliver sufficient choline.

Major Functions Choline functions as a precursor for lecithin, a phospholipid in cell membranes. Choline is also involved in the formation of acetylcholine, an important neurotransmitter in the central nervous system.

Deficiency: Health and Physical Performance As choline is found in most foods as part of cell membranes, choline deficiency is very rare. The only research available, involving individuals fed a choline-deficient solution, revealed the development of fatty livers and liver damage. Plasma choline levels have been reported to be significantly reduced following exhaustive exercise such as marathon running, and thus a possible reduction in acetylcholine levels in the nervous system may be theorized to be a contributing factor to the development of fatigue. However, exercise performance was not evaluated in these reports. Penry and Manore suggested that choline supplementation might only increase endurance performance in activities that reduce circulating choline levels below normal.

Supplementation: Health and Physical Performance As choline deficiency is very rare, the effect of choline supplementation on health status has received little research attention. However, its effect on exercise performance has been the focus of several studies in recent years. According to Zeisel and Niculescu, several reports indicate that choline administration accelerated synthesis and release of acetylcholine by neurons.

Research has shown that choline supplementation, either as choline salts or as lecithin preparations, will increase blood choline levels at rest and during prolonged exercise. Some preliminary field and laboratory research has suggested that increased plasma choline levels are associated with a significantly decreased time to run 20 miles and improved mood states of cyclists 40 minutes after completion of a cycle ergometer ride to exhaustion. In contrast, well-controlled laboratory research has revealed that choline supplementation, although increasing plasma choline levels, exerted no effect on either brief, high-intensity anaerobic cycling tests lasting about 2 minutes or more prolonged aerobic exercise tasks lasting about 70 minutes.

Several reviewers have recommended more research with choline supplementation, particularly controlled laboratory research involving prolonged aerobic endurance exercise tasks greater than 2 hours' duration. Warber and others provided choline (6 g total free choline) to United States Army Rangers during and after 4 hours of strenuous exercise. Although choline supplementation increased plasma choline levels by 128 percent, there were no significant effects on any exercise performance measure, including a treadmill run to exhaustion following the 4-hour treadmill exercise protocol. In a short-term supplementation field study, Buchman and others observed similar results in runners who consumed either a lecithin supplement (2.2 grams total) or placebo 1 day prior to a marathon. The lecithin supplementation increased plasma choline concentration, while the placebo group experienced a significant decrease, but there were no significant differences between marathon running times. In their review, Jäger and others commented that supplementation with phosphatidylcholine (0.2 gram/kg) is more effective than choline in increasing plasma choline levels and may improve performance in activities that have decreased plasma choline concentrations.

Excessive choline intake may lead to a fishy body odor, gastrointestinal distress, vomiting, and low blood pressure. A UL of 3.5 grams/day has been set for adults, and smaller amounts have been set for adolescents and children.

Prudent Recommendations Given the evidence that choline deficiency states are very rare and that supplementation does not appear to enhance health or exercise performance, choline supplementation is not recommended. A balanced diet will provide adequate choline.

Vitamin B complex

There are eight vitamins in the B complex, and because several of the vitamins in the B complex work together in energy metabolism, a number of studies have investigated the effect of either a deficiency or supplement of more than one vitamin upon health or physical performance.

Deficiency: Health and Physical Performance As noted previously, a deficiency of folate has been associated with elevated homocysteine levels. Deficiencies in vitamin B_6 and B_{12} have also been associated with increased plasma homocysteine. The Consumers Union cited an analysis of 72 studies concluding that very high levels of homocysteine can predict heart attack and stroke. As noted previously, elevated levels of homocysteine may be a marker, or result, of disease, but not a cause.

As might be expected from evidence presented on deficiencies of individual vitamins, a deficiency of several B vitamins together would negatively affect physical performance. This theory has been supported by studies in which daily intake was reduced to less than 50 percent of the RDA, such as well-controlled starvation experiments conducted during World War II. van der Beek and others compared a deficient group consuming about one-third of the Dutch DRA for thiamin, riboflavin, B_6, and vitamin C with another group consuming twice the RDA. After 8 weeks, aerobic power and onset of blood lactate accumulation (OBLA) declined by 9.8 and 19.6 percent, respectively, in the deficient group. In a later study, van der Beek and others compared 11 weeks of restricted (≤ 55 percent of the Dutch RDA) and nonrestricted levels of thiamin, riboflavin, and B_6. Vitamin-deficient subjects had decreases in VO_2 max, VO_2 at OBLA, and peak and mean anaerobic power, but there were no vitamin-specific deficiency effects on performance. The findings support earlier research showing a significant decrease in endurance capacity with a B complex deficiency.

2004, the Consumers Union noted a growing body of research involving the role of various B vitamins as a means to help prevent heart disease and other serious cardiovascular problems. At that time, some research had reported cardiovascular health benefits, such as a reduction in blood pressure, associated with folic acid and vitamin B_6 supplementation. However, subsequent research findings were not as promising. In the largest clinical trial, the Vitamin Intervention for Stroke Prevention (VISP) study, B vitamin supplementation (folic acid, 2 mg; vitamin B_6, 400 mcg; vitamin B_{12}, 400 mcg) modestly lowered serum homocysteine levels but had no effect on recurrent stroke, coronary events, or death. Furthermore, in a study with heart attack survivors, those taking a combination of folic acid (800 mcg) and vitamin B_6 (40 mg) actually had an increased risk of heart attack and stroke. However, Schwammenthal and Tanne noted that the VISP study had some limitations, and both studies involved individuals with cardiovascular disease.

Similar studies with healthy individuals are limited but indicate no cardiovascular health benefits of vitamin B supplementation. McMahon and others studied the effects of folate (1 mg), vitamin B_{12} (500 mcg), and vitamin B_6 (10 mg) or a placebo on the blood pressure responses over the course of 2 years in healthy older individuals with elevated homocysteine levels. Although the vitamin B supplementation lowered plasma homocysteine levels, there was no effect on blood pressure. Bleys and others, in a meta-analysis, reported no effect of B vitamin supplements on the progression of atherosclerosis, which is one of the theoretical means whereby vitamin B supplementation may help prevent cardiovascular diseases. Based on the available evidence, the American Heart Association does not recommend widespread use of folic acid and B vitamin supplements to reduce the risk of heart disease and stroke.

In their review of B vitamins and exercise, Woolf and Manore cite several reasons athletes may need more vitamin B. First, the metabolic pathways that produce energy are stressed during physical activity, and thus requirements for several vitamins may increase; second, biochemical adaptations that occur with training in the tissues may increase requirements; third, strenuous exercise may also increase the turnover or loss of a particular micronutrient in sweat, urine, or feces; and finally, additional micronutrients may be required to repair and maintain the higher lean tissue mass of some athletes and active individuals. A diet rich in healthy carbohydrates and protein will provide an adequate amount of the B vitamins.

In general, research supports the idea that individuals who obtain adequate vitamins through a balanced diet will not improve performance through the use of B complex supplements. However, a number of earlier studies, several with children, have shown that when a deficiency state is corrected by vitamin supplements, physical performance is restored to normal. Moreover, some research with large dosages of B_1, B_6, and B_{12} (about 60–200 times the RDA) has shown increases in fine motor control and performance in pistol shooting. Bonke suggested that the beneficial effect was related to the role of these vitamins in promoting the development of neurotransmitters that induce relaxation. Additional research is needed to confirm this finding.

Several of the principal Dutch investigators in this area, such as van Erp-Baart and Saris, suggest that B complex supplementation may be useful in sports with a high energy expenditure if these athletes consume large amounts of foods with empty Calories—high-sugar and high-fat foods. This again stresses the importance of eating foods that are high in nutrient value.

Vitamin B complex supplementation does not appear to be needed for the individual consuming a balanced diet of wholesome, natural foods. However, consuming fortified foods or supplements to provide adequate amounts of all B vitamins for potential health benefits may be prudent. In particular, women of childbearing age should obtain adequate amounts of folic acid. Moreover, athletes involved in intensive training for endurance-type sports and consuming highly processed foods may benefit from a B complex supplement.

Vitamin C (ascorbic acid)

Vitamin C, or **ascorbic acid**, is a water-soluble vitamin. Its alleged effects upon health and physical performance have been the subject of much controversy.

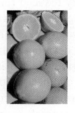

DRI The vitamin C RDA for adult males is 90 mg/day and 75 mg/day for adult females. Slightly lower amounts are recommended for children, whereas somewhat larger amounts are recommended during pregnancy and lactation. The DV is only 60 mg, but the UL has been set at 2,000 mg/day for adults and lower amounts for children and adolescents. For current DRI, see the tables on the inside front and back covers.

Food Sources The best food sources of vitamin C are fruits and vegetables, primarily the citrus fruits and the leafy parts of green vegetables. Excellent sources include oranges, grapefruit, broccoli, and salad greens. Other good sources are green peppers, potatoes, strawberries, and tomatoes. One orange contains the RDA. Milk, meats, and grain products are low in vitamin C. Some products are fortified with vitamin C. Keep in mind when reading food labels that the DV is only 60 milligrams, while the RDA is 75 and 90 for adult females and males, respectively. A food label indicating that 1 serving is 100 percent of the vitamin C RDA would contain only about 67 percent of the current RDA for males.

Major Functions Although vitamin C does not directly participate in enzyme-catalyzed conversions of substrate to product, Jacob suggests that it modifies mineral ions in the enzymes to make them active. Vitamin C has a number of different functions in the body, some of which have important implications for the physically active individual. Its principal role is in the synthesis of collagen, which is necessary for the formation and maintenance of the connective tissues of the body, such as cartilage, tendon, and bone. Vitamin C is also involved in the formation of certain hormones and neurotransmitters, such as epinephrine (adrenaline), which are secreted during stressful situations such as exercise. It helps absorb some forms of iron from the intestinal tract—about a two to fourfold increased absorption—and is involved in the synthesis of RBCs. Vitamin C helps regulate the metabolism of folic acid, cholesterol, and amino acids. It is also important in the healing of wounds through the development of scar tissue. Finally, vitamin C is a powerful antioxidant, which helps it contribute to normal function of the immune system.

Deficiency: Health and Physical Performance   Serious deficiencies of vitamin C are rare in industrialized societies because fresh or frozen fruits and vegetables are abundant. Also, the human body has a pool of vitamin C ranging from 1.5 to 3.0 grams. However, smoking, aspirin, oral contraceptives, and stress may increase the need for this vitamin, and a study by Johnston and others reported marginal vitamin C status in 12–16 percent of college students. The major deficiency disease is scurvy, a disintegration of the connective tissue in the gums, skin, tendons, and cartilage that may develop in a month on a vitamin C–free diet. Typical symptoms include bleeding gums, rupture of blood vessels in the skin, impaired wound healing, muscle cramps, and weakness. Anemia also may develop.

Observations by Ness and others indicate that adequate vitamin C intake is associated with increased serum HDL-cholesterol levels, reduced serum triglycerides, and lower blood pressure. Adequate vitamin C is also needed to maintain optimal antioxidant functions. Thus, inadequate vitamin C may increase the risk for various chronic diseases. Some epidemiological research has indicated that individuals with low plasma levels of vitamin C, most often associated with a vitamin deficiency, had a higher incidence of CHD and stroke. For example, Kurl and others evaluated the effect of serum levels of vitamin C on the incidence of stroke over a 12-year period and found that those with the lowest levels had a 2.4-fold greater risk of stroke than those with the highest levels, especially among hypertensive and overweight men. Additionally, the Consumers Union noted that men with the lowest levels of plasma vitamin C had a 57 percent higher risk of dying from any cause, and a 62 percent higher risk of cancer death, than men with the highest levels. The effects were not seen in women, possibly because they had far more hormone-sensitive cancers, which seem to be unaffected by the vitamin. However, other research from Japan has shown similar benefits, and the vitamin C was consumed mainly from foods, not supplements. Thus, the Consumers Union indicated that the health benefits may be from other substances in foods that accompany vitamin C.

It is obvious that many of the symptoms of a vitamin C deficiency we have cited would impair physical performance. Sensations of weakness could adversely affect all types of performance, whereas anemia would hamper aerobic endurance. Data available from several studies with vitamin C–deficient subjects do suggest such an effect, particularly the widely known Minnesota starvation experiments during World War II, directed by Ancel Keys.

Supplementation: Health and Physical Performance   Vitamin C supplementation has been claimed to have significant health benefits, most notably the prevention of CHD and cancer. Because

vitamin C is an antioxidant, and because many related supplementation studies have included other antioxidant vitamins (beta-carotene and vitamin E), we will discuss its effects on chronic disease and prevention of muscle tissue damage in physically active individuals later in this chapter.

There is some debate regarding the safety of megadoses of vitamin C. Several investigators have found that excessive amounts of vitamin C, such as 5–10 grams daily, may produce some undesirable side effects such as diarrhea; destruction of vitamin B_{12} in the diet; excessive excretion of vitamin B_6; decreased copper bioavailability; predisposition to gout, creating pain in the joints; and formation of kidney stones from oxalate salts, one of the breakdown products of vitamin C. Although for some individuals increased iron absorption is a beneficial effect of vitamin C, it may be a major health problem for individuals prone to iron-storage disease, discussed in the next chapter. Moreover, one study reported increased markers of oxidative DNA damage in some subjects when vitamin C and iron supplements were taken together. Excess vitamin C may potentiate the oxidative effects of iron. Excessive amounts of vitamin C also may interfere with the correct interpretation of certain blood and urine tests. Finally, several case studies revealed the development of a condition known as rebound scurvy when the individual stopped taking the supplements. The researchers suggested a mechanism whereby the increased activity of an enzyme in the body that destroys excess vitamin C during the supplement stages continued after the supplements were stopped, leading to a deficiency and symptoms of scurvy.

Conversely, others have reported megadoses to be relatively harmless because excessive amounts are excreted by the kidneys. They criticize the research upon which claims of adverse effects are based, noting that some of the conclusions rest on isolated case studies. Others support a middle viewpoint, noting that larger doses may be harmless to many, but certain individuals may be prone to problems, such as those who have a family history of kidney stones. For example, a highly controlled supplementation study by Massey and others reported that large daily intakes of vitamin C (2,000 mg) increased the excretion of urinary oxalate and increased the risk for calcium oxalate kidney stones in 40 percent of study participants, both stoneformers and non-stoneformers. Levine and others reported evidence of oxalates appearing in the urine when subjects were supplemented with only 1,000 milligrams of vitamin C per day. These were short-term studies and no observations of kidney stones were detected, but increased oxalates could lead to stone formation over time in those at risk. However, in a longer prospective study involving men between the ages of 40 and 75 with no history of kidney stones, Curhan and others found that after 6 years of follow-up there was no association between vitamin C intake—up to levels of 250–1,500 milligrams per day—and kidney stone formation. Nevertheless, Gerster notes that those at risk for kidney stones should restrict daily vitamin C intake to about 100 mg. The National Academy of Sciences recommends against the routine use of large supplements. Megadose supplementation with vitamin C remains controversial, and the interested reader is referred to the opposing viewpoints presented by Herbert and Enstrom.

The effect of vitamin C supplementation on physical performance has received considerable attention, mainly because it is one of the vitamins that athletes consume in rather substantial quantities. Both early and contemporary research have shown that vitamin C supplementation improves physical performance in subjects who were vitamin C deficient, but a thorough analysis of these studies supports the general conclusion that vitamin C supplementation does not increase physical performance capacity in subjects who are not vitamin deficient. Bell and others found that vitamin C supplementation of 500 mg daily for 30 days did not increase VO_2 max or cardiac output in either young or older men. No solid experimental evidence supports the use of megadoses of 5–10 grams that some athletes take. The interested reader may consult the reviews by Gerster, Keith, and Peake.

Because exercise is a stressor, some investigators have recommended that the active individual may need slightly more vitamin C than the RDA, for example, 200–300 mg per day. Some research with runners doing 5–10 miles a day does not support this viewpoint; in any case, this amount could easily be obtained by wise selection of foods high in vitamin C content. Keith also suggests that vitamin C supplementation may be beneficial to heat acclimation, a topic that merits additional research with trained athletes.

Although exercise normally promotes health benefits, Nieman notes that in contrast to moderate levels of physical activity, prolonged and intensive exertion, such as running an ultramarathon, causes numerous changes in the human immune system that may predispose to certain illnesses, such as upper respiratory tract infection (URTI). Large doses of vitamin C have been claimed to strengthen the immune system and prevent URTI. Some early research suggests that the antihistamine effects of vitamin C may decrease the severity of some symptoms of a cold. For example, Peters and others reported that 600 mg of vitamin C supplementation for 21 days prior to an ultramarathon reduced symptoms of respiratory tract infections, while Douglas and others reported that doses greater than 200 mg may also help prevent URTI in heavy physical exercise in cold environments, such as soldiers in subartic weather conditions. However, more recent research revealed that 200 mg of vitamin C daily will lead to full saturation of plasma and white blood cells, which should optimize immune functions associated with vitamin C. It may be possible that smaller amounts of vitamin C, such as 200 mg, provide effects comparable to those seen with larger doses.

In general, although the duration of the symptoms may be reduced slightly, a review and meta-analysis by Douglas and others indicated that vitamin C (>200 mg per day) supplementation had no effect on developing a cold or its severity. Moreover, vitamin C supplementation does not appear to benefit immune function, even in ultraendurance athletes. David Nieman, an international expert in exercise and immune function, along with his colleagues, reported no effect of 7 days of vitamin C supplementation (1,500 mg/day) on oxidative and immune responses in runners both during and after a competitive ultramarathon race. Two studies by Davison and Gleeson also reported no beneficial effects of vitamin C supplementation, either alone or with carbohydrate, on immune functions following 2.5 hours of cycling at 60 percent

VO_2 max. In a review of his own and other research, Nieman indicated that vitamin C supplementation, as well as combined antioxidant vitamin supplementation, is not an effective countermeasure to exercise-induced immunosuppression.

Prudent Recommendations   A review by Weber and others suggests that adequate vitamin C intake may be associated with various health benefits for certain individuals. The amounts recommended approximate 200 mg per day, an amount easily obtained in the diet. Currently, the Consumers Union indicates that it is premature to recommend vitamin C supplements, but it does recommend a diet rich in fruits and vegetables, which (as previously noted) contain not only substantial amounts of vitamin C but also other healthful substances as well. Eating the recommended five to nine fruits and vegetables daily should supply about 200–350 mg of vitamin C. This is a solid recommendation for both the sedentary and physically active individual.

Key Concepts

▶ The water-soluble vitamins consist of those in the B complex and vitamin C. Choline is also a water-soluble nutrient for which DRI have been established.

▶ In general, water-soluble vitamins are not toxic in excess. However, excess niacin may interfere with proper liver function and excess vitamin B_6 has been associated with neurological problems.

▶ Water-soluble vitamin deficiencies are rare in developed countries. However, supplements may be advised for some individuals. Women of childbearing age should consume 400 mcg of folic acid daily to prevent the possibility of birth defects in the newborn. Elderly individuals should obtain adequate vitamin B_{12} through fortified foods or vitamin supplements.

▶ A water-soluble vitamin deficiency may impair physical performance, usually by interfering with some phase of the energy-producing process. In some cases, impairment may be seen in 2–4 weeks on a deficient diet.

▶ Supplementation with water-soluble vitamins has not been shown to enhance sports performance.

Vitamin Supplements: Ergogenic Aspects

Like the general population, the vast majority of athletes receive the RDA for most vitamins in their daily diet. It is true that some studies report that certain groups of athletes receive less than the RDA for some vitamins or even have indicators of a biochemical deficiency, but other studies, such as that by Ziegler and others involving athletes in weight-control sports with low energy intake, find that biochemical indices of nutritional status are usually within normal limits. Sarah Short of Syracuse University, in her exhaustive review of dietary surveys with athletes, and Larry

Armstrong and Carl Maresh in their review, found that vitamin deficiency symptoms rarely are reported. Moreover, in his review, Michael Fogelholm reported that, at least in developed countries, dietary vitamin intake by athletes is more than required for maximal exercise performance. Nevertheless, elite endurance athletes, such as Tour de France cyclists, and the majority of both high school and college athletes believe that vitamins are essential for success, and it is a matter of fact that many consume vitamin supplements either as nutritional insurance or in the hope of improving performance. For example, in a review of more than 51 studies involving data on more than 10,000 male and female athletes in 15 sports, Sobol and Marquart reported that the overall mean prevalence of athletes' supplement use was 46 percent, a finding supported in a survey by Krumbach and others. Elite athletes use supplements more than college or high school athletes, and women more often than men. Athletes appear to use supplements more than the general population, and some take high doses that may lead to nutritional problems.

In recent years, some vitamin manufacturers have turned their attention to the physically active individual, including older athletes, suggesting through advertisements that their special product enhances athletic performance. In her review, Priscilla Clarkson of the University of Massachusetts suggested that such advertisements were a major reason for the use of vitamin supplements by athletes.

> www.acsm.org/docs/current-comments/vitaminandmine ralsupplementsandexercise.pdf Current comment from the American College of Sports Medicine regarding the use of vitamin and mineral supplements by physically active individuals.

Should physically active individuals take vitamin supplements?

In her review, Volpe commented that the vitamin and mineral needs of athletes have always been a topic of discussion. Although Volpe notes that researchers disagree as to whether athletes need more micronutrients, she indicates that the intensity, duration, and frequency of the sport or exercise training and the overall energy and nutrient intakes of the individual all have an impact on whether micronutrients are required in greater amounts.

There may be some good reasons for physically active individuals to take vitamin supplements. For example, in certain types of athletic activity, such as wrestling, gymnastics, and ballet, participants may undertake prolonged semi-starvation or starvation diets. As discussed in chapter 10, this is not a recommended procedure, but some athletes may do it to obtain or maintain an optimal body weight for competition. In such cases, when the energy intake may be well below 1,200–1,600 Calories per day, many surveys have shown that the athlete may not be receiving enough vitamins. Research suggests that vitamin depletion, mainly the water-soluble vitamins, can occur rapidly in humans on low-Calorie diets and that these vitamins should be replaced daily. Athletes may also need vitamin supplementation if they are subsisting on poor diets, as discussed in the next section. Moreover, some vitamin

requirements are increased in pregnant women and the elderly, so those who exercise need to consume vitamin-rich diets. In a recent review, Brisswalter and Louis noted that antioxidant vitamin supplementation may benefit masters athletes because of the age-related reduction in oxidative stress defenses. They advocate for an antioxidant complex but against high doses in order to avoid blunting training adaptations that are induced by normal oxidative stress-related cell signaling. Active individuals should consult appropriate health professionals before self-prescribing vitamin supplements, particularly megadoses of individual vitamins.

As is obvious from the evidence presented in this chapter, the athlete who is on a balanced diet has no need for vitamin supplementation to improve performance. Nevertheless, some interesting hypotheses suggest that antioxidant vitamin supplements may help prevent muscle tissue damage during training, and a variety of special vitamin-like compounds have been marketed specifically for athletes.

Can the antioxidant vitamins prevent fatigue or muscle damage during training?

Aerobic exercise induces oxidative stress in the body, increasing the production of free radicals. Finaud and others indicate that the effects of the free radicals may be positive or negative. On the positive side, Neiss indicates growing evidence that regular aerobic exercise training enhances the functional capacity of the antioxidant network, upgrading the capacity of the natural antioxidant enzymes in the muscles. Reviews by Ji and Powers noted that *chronic* exercise training increased the activity of superoxide dismutase and glutathione peroxidase in response to free radical generation. These enzymes are important to muscle cell survival during increased oxidative stress. In particular, Knez and others reported that the volumes and intensities of exercise associated with ultraendurance training, such as for Ironman-type triathlon competition, induce favorable changes in innate antioxidant defenses against free radical damage, resulting in improved oxidative balance. One possible benefit is improved immune functions. On the negative side, excessive exercise-induced oxidative stress may occur if the generation of free radicals overwhelms tissue antioxidative defenses, which may disturb cellular homeostasis and cause fatigue or lipid peroxidation and muscle tissue damage.

Antioxidant supplements have been studied as a means to enhance physical performance. However, as noted previously, individual supplementation with either vitamin C or vitamin E has not been shown to enhance exercise performance, with the possible exception of vitamin E at altitude. Moreover, reviews by Powers and Sen and their colleagues concluded that antioxidants, including antioxidant cocktails containing several vitamins, have not been shown to reliably improve physical performance. For example, Zoppi and others found that supplementation with vitamins C (1000 mg/day) and E (800 mg/day) to professional soccer players over the course of 3 months of training had no effect on strength, speed, and aerobic capacity.

Atalay and others suggested that performance should not be the only criterion to evaluate the success of antioxidant supplementation. Faster recovery and minimization of injury time could also be affected by antioxidant therapy. Although Zoppi and others found no performance enhancement with antioxidant supplementation to the soccer players, supplementation was associated with reduced levels of blood markers for muscle tissue damage.

It has been known for years that certain forms of physical training for sports, particularly intense training, can induce muscle damage and soreness. Eccentric muscle contractions, such as those incurred in the quadriceps muscle when running downhill, may cause mechanical trauma to the muscle and connective tissue, resulting in soreness during the following days. Neiss indicates that although an *acute* bout of exercise increases the activity of antioxidant enzymes in the body, strenuous exercise may generate reactive oxygen species to a level to overwhelm tissue antioxidant defense systems. The result is oxidative stress. The magnitude of the stress depends on the ability of the tissues to detoxify ROS. Excessive production of free radicals may induce lipid peroxidation, possibly damaging the integrity of cellular and subcellular membranes in the muscles, leading to muscle injury and muscle soreness.

Most of the research with antioxidant supplements to athletes has focused on prevention of muscle tissue damage and soreness. Theoretically, prevention of muscle tissue damage may enable the athlete to train more effectively, the desired result being improvement in competition. Some endurance athletes will train at altitude in attempts to enhance their oxygen-delivery ability, and as noted earlier in this chapter, vitamin E supplements may convey some benefits when exercising at altitude. Additionally, older individuals may be more susceptible to oxidative stress during exercise, for optimal functioning of the free radical–scavenging enzymes appears to decline with the aging process. Millions of older individuals perform aerobic exercise for the related health benefits and often become involved in various forms of athletic competition, including local, national, and international competition for athletes over age 40. Companies are now marketing *super antioxidants* to speed recovery in athletes during sport training. Do they help?

Numerous studies have been conducted to evaluate the effect of antioxidant supplements on exercise-induced muscle damage and, in some studies, on performance. The designs of these studies have varied, including differences in subjects (animals versus humans, young and old), methods to induce muscle soreness (e.g., downhill running versus level running, resistance exercise), the type and amount of supplement given, and the biochemical markers used to assess muscle damage. The most common supplements used were vitamins E and C and beta-carotene, but coenzyme Q_{10}, selenium, and other substances have also been used. Some studies used "antioxidant cocktails" consisting of approximately 800 IU of vitamin E, 1,000 mg of vitamin C, and 10–30 mg of beta-carotene. The markers of muscle tissue damage include serum enzymes that may leak from the muscle, such as creatine kinase (CK) and lactic acid dehydrogenase (LDH); end products of lipid peroxidation, such as malondialdehyde (MDA); myoglobin leakage from the muscle tissue; and others.

Overall, the results of these studies may be regarded as promising. A number of studies, such as the report by Itoh and others, have shown some beneficial effects of antioxidant supplementation, that is, reduced markers of muscle tissue damage when compared to the placebo treatment. Benefits have been reported for both young and old physically active individuals. Most studies used multiple markers of muscle tissue damage, and in some cases, one marker of muscle damage would be improved by the antioxidant supplements but another would be unaffected. Some studies compared different antioxidants, for example, C versus E, reporting a beneficial effect of one but not the other.

In contrast, more recent studies have reported no significant benefits of antioxidant supplementation to prevent muscle tissue damage during exercise. For example, Mastaloudis and others reported that supplementation with vitamin C (1,000 mg) and vitamin E (300 mg alpha-tocopheryl acetate) before a 50-kilometer ultramarathon had no effect on leg muscle damage or recovery following the race and up to 6 days afterwards. Machefer and others investigated the effect of moderate supplementation with vitamin C, vitamin E, and beta-carotene on muscle tissue damage during and following the Marathon des Sables, a 6-day, 156-mile (254-kilometer) ultramarathon race across the Sahara Desert. The supplement elevated serum vitamin levels but had no effect on markers of muscle tissue damage. Bryer and Goldfarb found that prolonged vitamin C supplementation (3 grams) both before and after eccentric exercise designed to induce muscle soreness produced divergent results on markers of muscle damage and measures of muscle soreness. In general, there were lower levels of creatine kinase 48 hours after testing, but no effect on muscle soreness.

Some studies actually reported adverse effects of supplementation. Nieman and others found that vitamin E supplementation actually promoted lipid peroxidation and inflammation during an Ironman-distance triathlon. Close and others also reported that consuming 1 gram of ascorbic acid 2 hours before and 14 days after completing a downhill run did not prevent delayed onset of muscle soreness (DOMS). Muscle function was impaired in both the vitamin C and placebo groups, but more so in the supplement group, suggesting that vitamin C supplementation may actually inhibit the recovery of muscle function.

Antioxidant supplementation may adversely affect cellular adaptations to chronic training. Gomez-Cabrera and others reported that vitamin C supplementation during training may impair training adaptations, possibly by decreasing production of mitochondria. Similar results were observed by Paulsen and others, who assigned subjects to supplementation (1,000 mg vitamin C/day; 345 mg vitamin E/day) and placebo groups followed by 11 weeks of high-intensity interval training. Although VO_2 max improved by 8 percent in both groups, the supplemented group had decreased activity in cell signaling pathways, which normally stimulate increases in mitochondrial respiration and biogenesis. The endurance athlete may wish to exercise caution in consuming high doses of antioxidants.

The role of antioxidants to prevent exercise-induced muscle tissue damage was the subject of several recent reviews, and the opinions are mixed regarding their efficacy. Adams and Best indicated that although animal studies have shown some promising effects of antioxidant supplementation to lessen exercise-induced oxidative stress damage, studies with humans are less convincing. Relative to vitamin E, Jackson and others concluded that supplements are unlikely to reliably reduce the severity of muscle damage. Viitala and Newhouse also concluded that vitamin E supplementation does not appear to decrease exercise-induced lipid peroxidation in humans. Clarkson and Thompson noted that whether the body's own natural antioxidant defense system is sufficient to combat oxidative stress during prolonged exercise or whether antioxidant supplements are needed is unknown, but trained athletes who received antioxidant supplements have shown evidence of reduced oxidative stress. Ji notes that the aging process lessens the exercise training–induced improvement in natural antioxidant enzymes and suggests that exercise training in older athletes might be assisted with antioxidant supplementation in attempts to optimize antioxidant defense. Sacheck and Blumberg concluded that the use of dietary antioxidants such as vitamin E to reduce exercise-induced muscle injury have met with mixed success, which seems to be the prevailing viewpoint. All reviewers agree that more research is needed to address this issue and to provide guidelines for recommendations to athletes.

Prudent Recommendations   In a review, McGinley and colleagues report that there is little evidence to suggest that high doses of antioxidants, and in particular vitamin E, can reduce muscle damage. For this reason, and because of the potential dangers of long-term antioxidant supplement use, the authors do not suggest the use of high-dose antioxidant supplements for athletes. The meta-analysis of antioxidant supplements by Bjelakovic and others showed that supplementation with beta-carotene, vitamin A, and vitamin E may increase mortality, while the effects of vitamin C and selenium on longevity required more research. However, others note that the prudent use of antioxidant supplementation can provide insurance against a suboptimal diet and/or the elevated demands of intense physical activity and thus may be recommended to limit the effects of oxidative stress in individuals performing regular, heavy exercise. For example, Takanami and others are convinced that vitamin E contributes to preventing exercise-induced lipid peroxidation and possible muscle tissue damage, and they recommend that athletes supplement with 100–200 mg of vitamin E daily to help prevent exercise-induced oxidative damage.

Most experts in this area recommend that physically active individuals obtain antioxidant vitamins naturally from food. Increasing the consumption of fruits, fruit juices, and vegetables will enable athletes to obtain the proposed beneficial amounts of beta-carotene (10–30 mg) and vitamin C (250–1,000 mg) but it would be difficult to obtain 100–200 IU of vitamin E through natural dietary sources. Watson and others indicate that there seems no valid reason to recommend antioxidant supplements to most athletes, except in those known to be consuming a low-antioxidant diet for prolonged periods. For the athlete who wants to supplement vitamin E, inexpensive over-the-counter preparations are available in 100 and 200 IU capsules. For health benefits, remember that most research documents beneficial effects when these vitamins, along with other phytochemicals, are obtained through natural foods, primarily fruits and vegetables.

How effective are the special vitamin supplements marketed for athletes?

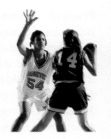

Special athletic vitamin packs have been appearing on the market—even in single packets at your local convenience store—that have been advertised as a means for the athlete to increase energy and reach peak performance. Many of these have simply been multivitamin-mineral supplements, while others have been special concoctions that contain ingredients such as bee pollen and ginseng. Three such products will be highlighted.

Multivitamin-Mineral Supplements   Because in human metabolism vitamins often work together, and often in conjunction with minerals, the ergogenic potential of multivitamin-mineral compounds has been studied for half a century. In a review of the older research, Williams reported that although results of a number of studies suggested ergogenic effects, the experimental designs were usually poorly controlled. In contrast, contemporary research indicates that such supplements, consumed for substantial periods, are not ergogenic for the athlete on a balanced diet. From Timothy Noakes's laboratory in South Africa, Weight conducted a thorough 9-month double-blind, placebo, crossover study. Although multivitamin-mineral supplements did raise blood levels of some vitamins, the authors reported that 3 months of supplementation did not improve maximal oxygen uptake, the anaerobic (lactate) threshold, treadmill run time to exhaustion, or running performance in a 15-kilometer time trial. Anita Singh and her colleagues provided either a high-potency multivitamin-mineral supplement or a placebo to 22 healthy, physically active males for 90 days. The vitamin dosages ranged from 300 to 6,000 percent of the RDA. Although serum levels of many of the vitamins increased, there were no significant effects on physiological variables during a 90-minute run, nor were there any effects on maximal heart rate, VO_2 max, or time to exhaustion. Finally, Richard Telford and his colleagues matched 82 nationally ranked Australian athletes in training at the Australian Institute of Sport and assigned them to either a supplement or placebo treatment. The supplement contained an assortment of vitamins and minerals, ranging from about 100 to 5,000 percent of the RDA. The supplement was taken for approximately 7–8 months, and the subjects were tested on a variety of sport-specific tests (e.g., swim bench) as well as common tests of strength (torque), anaerobic power (400-meter run), and aerobic endurance (12-minute run and VO_2 max). These investigators reported no significant effect of the supplement on any measure of physical performance when compared with athletes whose vitamin and mineral RDA were met by dietary intake.

Vitamins and minerals recently have also been marketed to physically active individuals in liquid forms, such as sports drinks. Although research is limited, Fry and others reported no significant improvement in two tests of anaerobic exercise performance (30-second cycle sprint and one set of squats) following 8 weeks of supplementation with a multivitamin/mineral liquid. Thus, all of the current reputable research refutes an ergogenic effect of multivitamin-mineral supplements in adequately nourished athletes.

Prudent recommendations Although multivitamin-mineral supplements may not enhance athletic performance in well-nourished athletes, those involved in weight-control sports with limited caloric intake might consider taking a simple one-a-day supplement with no more than 100 percent of the RDA for the essential vitamins and minerals. Moreover, the U.S. Anti-Doping Agency, in its booklet on optimal dietary intake, indicated that an athlete who takes a simple one-a-day type of vitamin or mineral that does not exceed the nutrient levels of the RDA/DRI is probably not doing any harm.

Bee Pollen **Bee pollen** has been marketed almost specifically for athletes, primarily runners, as a means to improve performance. Chemical analysis of bee pollen reveals that it is a mixture of vitamins, minerals, amino acids, and other nutrients. Although no specific physiological effects of bee pollen have been documented, theoretical ergogenic effects are based on some of the roles that vitamins have in the body. Advertising claims for bee pollen cite questionable research: a field study showing faster recovery rates in athletes who took pollen supplements. However, six well-designed studies using double-blind placebo protocols revealed that supplementation with bee pollen had no significant effect upon VO_2 max, other physiological responses to exercise, endurance capacity, or rate of recovery from exhausting exercise.

Prudent recommendations Bee pollen supplements are not recommended for physically active individuals. Moreover, caution is necessary, as some individuals may experience an allergic reaction.

CoQ10 The compound **CoQ$_{10}$**, also known as coenzyme Q$_{10}$ and ubiquinone, is actually a lipid but has characteristics common to vitamins; its chemical structure is similar to vitamin K. CoQ$_{10}$ is found in the mitochondria of all mammalian tissues, but concentrations are relatively high in the heart and other organs in humans. It plays an important role in oxidative metabolism within the mitochondria, facilitating the aerobic generation of ATP as part of the electron transfer system. According to Schmelzer and Döring, the reduced form of CoQ$_{10}$ (CoQ$_{10}$H$_2$) also functions as an antioxidant and may protect against oxidative damage to cell membranes and DNA. Onur and colleagues reported that CoQ$_{10}$H$_2$ decreases the activity of gamma glutamyltransferase, an enzyme indicator of oxidative stress. It has been used therapeutically for treatment of cardiovascular disease since 1965 because it may protect heart tissue from damage associated with inadequate oxygen, although Webb noted that not all scientists agree it has shown beneficial applications. Tran and others noted that if used therapeutically, CoQ$_{10}$ should be used only in conjunction with other drugs and not relied on by itself for the treatment of any cardiovascular health problem.

CoQ$_{10}$ has also been theorized to be ergogenic for athletes based on evidence of improved heart function, maximal oxygen uptake, and exercise performance in cardiac patients. In his book, Bucci described several studies indicating that CoQ$_{10}$ levels are lower in trained athletes compared to sedentary controls and that oral supplementation with CoQ$_{10}$ will increase tissue levels. These

two observations lend theoretical support for an ergogenic effect of CoQ$_{10}$ on aerobic endurance performance. Studies described by Bucci report improved VO_2 max, exercise performance, indicators of enhanced aerobic capacity, and antioxidant function in such diverse population as sedentary young men, sedentary middle-aged women, aerobically trained volleyball players, male professional basketball players, and endurance runners. However, these studies do not appear to have been published in peer-reviewed journals. Each study also has one or more major flaws in experimental design, such as no control group, no placebo, no randomization of order for CoQ$_{10}$ or placebo treatments, and prediction of VO_2 max based on submaximal heart rate.

CoQ$_{10}$ must leave the blood and enter the muscle and mitochondria in order to have an ergogenic effect. However, studies by Svensson and Zhou and their associates reported that although CoQ$_{10}$ supplementation significantly increased CoQ$_{10}$ plasma concentrations, there was no corresponding increase in the skeletal muscle or mitochondria. More recently, Bloomer and others reported an increase in plasma CoQ$_{10}$ levels in trained males and females following 4 weeks of supplementation (300 mg/day), but there was no effect on graded treadmill, interval sprint cycle exercise, or markers of oxidative stress compared to placebo.

There are several published studies regarding the effect of CoQ$_{10}$ on exercise performance, but most do not support its ergogenic effectiveness. Weston and others reported no beneficial effects of 1 mg/kg/day of CoQ$_{10}$ for 28 days on oxygen uptake, substrate use, or cycle ergometer exercise time to exhaustion in trained male cyclists and triathletes. Although serum CoQ$_{10}$ levels were increased, Braun and others reported no effect of 100 mg daily for 8 weeks on submaximal physiological indicators of enhanced aerobic capacity, VO_2 max, time to exhaustion on a bicycle ergometer, or lipid peroxidation, indicating no effect on either aerobic metabolism or antioxidant function. Bonetti and others also found no effect of CoQ$_{10}$ supplementation for 8 weeks on VO_2 peak and anaerobic threshold of trained middle-aged cyclists. Laaksonen and others supplemented both young and old physically trained males with 120 mg of CoQ$_{10}$ per day for 6 weeks and reported no significant effect on maximal oxygen uptake or on time to exhaustion in a progressive cycling task following 60 minutes of submaximal cycling. Performance time in the placebo trial was significantly greater than in the CoQ$_{10}$ trial. Additionally, there were no effects of the CoQ$_{10}$ supplement on malondialdehyde (MDA), a marker of lipid peroxidation. Malm and others reported that 120 mg CoQ$_{10}$ per day for 20 days exerted no effect on 15 high-intensity, anaerobic 10-second sprint tests on a cycle ergometer with 50 seconds recovery between each sprint. They noted that, compared to the placebo groups, subjects taking the CoQ$_{10}$ supplement showed evidence of muscle tissue damage. The placebo group improved their performance in the cycle sprints, but the supplement group did not. The findings of Laaksonen and Malm and their colleagues suggest that CoQ$_{10}$ might actually be ergolytic. In contrast, Ylikoski and others reported that CoQ$_{10}$ supplementation (90 mg/day) improved VO_2 max in Finnish cross-country skiers, but they did not evaluate its effect on actual exercise performance. Gül and Gökbel and colleagues showed that 8 weeks of CoQ$_{10}$ supplementation (100 mg/d) resulted in small reductions in MDA and increases in mean cycling power. Alf and others observed a significantly greater increase in cycle ergometer power output in Watts/kg at a lactate threshold of 4.0 mmol/liter following 6 weeks of CoQ_{10} supplementation (300 mg/day) compared to placebo.

CoQ_{10} is also one of the ingredients in a supplement (also containing vitamin E, inosine, and cytochrome C) that has been widely advertised for endurance athletes, particularly triathletes. In a double-blind, placebo, crossover study, Snider and others reported that 4 weeks of supplementation with this commercial product had no ergogenic effect on an endurance task that consisted of a 90-minute treadmill run at 70 percent of VO_2 max followed by a cycling test to exhaustion at 70 percent of VO_2 max. Zhou and others reported no effect of 4 weeks of CoQ_{10} supplementation (150 mg/day), either separately or combined with vitamin E (1,000 IU/day), on VO_2 max. Using the same supplements, Kaikkonen and others found that supplementation with both CoQ_{10} and vitamin E to marathon runners for 3 weeks had no beneficial effects on lipid peroxidation or muscle damage induced by running the marathon. At present, the most contemporary published, well-designed studies do not support an ergogenic effect of CoQ_{10} supplementation.

Prudent recommendations Although promising, the majority of research studies still suggest that CoQ_{10} is not an effective ergogenic aid, and thus it is not recommended as a supplement for physically active individuals.

Quercetin Quercetin is a dietary polyphenolic flavonol that functions as an antioxidant and may also be an anti-inflammatory agent. Some energy drinks marketed to physically active individuals contain quercetin. Nieman and colleagues conducted four studies on the effects of quercetin supplementation (1 gram/day) on immune responses and inflammation. Although several studies revealed that 3 weeks of quercetin supplementation could favorably affect immune responses after exercise or reduce the incidence of upper respiratory tract infections (URTI) during a 2-week recovery from 3 days of intense cycling, quercetin supplementation for 3 weeks before and 2 weeks after a 160-km mountain run did not favorably affect immune responses or illness rates in ultraendurance runners. Another study reported no protection from exercise-induced oxidative stress and inflammation. In a comprehensive review of six studies, Williams concluded that quercetin does not improve performance in various endurance tasks, metabolic outcomes, or decrease perceived exertion in trained individuals. Williams also identified four studies of quercetin supplementation on exercise performance in untrained individuals and noted that the findings were equivocal. In a meta-analysis of ten studies of quercetin supplementation of 600 to 1,000 mg/day for 7 to 72 days, Pelletier and colleagues reported greater efficacy in untrained subjects compared to trained subjects, a minimal overall performance improvement of 0.09 percent, and no dose-dependent effect on endurance performance. Kressler and others reported a statistically significant but trivial meta-analysis effect of quercetin supplementation on VO_2 max and endurance exercise performance. Future studies are needed to determine if quercetin

is effective in untrained persons or those just starting a training program, but quercetin does not appear to perform as claimed, especially in trained individuals.

Prudent Recommendations
At this point, quercetin is not recommended as a supplement to improve exercise performance, although data on the prevention of URTI are promising. More data are needed on the effects of quercetin in untrained individuals and those beginning an endurance training program. Williams suggests that, in the future, researchers focus on flavonoid "cocktails," as flavonoids such as kaempferol, hesperidin, and others may have synergistic effects. Quercetin may interact with medications, such as aspirin, so a health-care practitioner should be consulted before taking this supplement.

What's the bottom line regarding vitamin supplements for athletes?

Given the available scientific data, there does not appear to be a very strong case supporting an ergogenic effect of any single vitamin, vitamin-mineral combinations, or the various vitamin-like compounds. As noted, additional research is warranted for those that have some limited support as an ergogenic, for example, the effect of vitamin E on performance at altitude.

At present, the recommended advice is to obtain adequate vitamin nutrition through a well-planned diet. For example, Melinda Manore noted that athletes involved in heavy training may need more of several vitamins, such as thiamin, riboflavin, and B_6, because they are involved in energy production, but the amount needed is only about twice the RDA and that may be easily obtained through the increased food intake associated with heavy training.

Dan Benardot and other sports nutrition experts indicate that some athletes, such as those in weight-control sports, those who do not have adequate exposure to sunlight, and those who do not eat a well-balanced diet, may be at risk for vitamin deficiency. Thus, some health professionals recommend vitamin supplementation, not only to prevent a deficiency that may impair sport performance but also for beneficial health reasons, as noted in the next section.

Key Concepts

▶ Although research findings regarding the ability of antioxidant vitamin supplements to prevent muscle tissue damage following intense exercise are somewhat equivocal, in general the benefits are minor. Antioxidant vitamin supplementation has not been shown to enhance sports or exercise performance.

▶ Results from well-controlled research generally indicate that multivitamin/mineral supplements and vitamin-like compounds, such as coenzyme Q_{10}, are not effective ergogenic aids.

Vitamin Supplements: Health Aspects

Vitamins are big business, being the most popular of all the dietary supplements. They are marketed to all segments of the population, from infant formulas to geriatric preparations, and for a wide variety of health reasons, ranging from combating the stress of everyday life to helping prevent heart disease and cancer. Surveys indicate that vitamin-supplement users have strong beliefs about their effectiveness, and this is evident in the multibillion-dollar sales annually by the vitamin industry.

In the preceding sections, we have already covered each individual vitamin and the possible effects of deficiencies and supplementation upon health (review table 7.1 for a broad overview). This section summarizes prudent dietary recommendations for overall optimal vitamin nutrition, including the possible use of supplements, relative to health.

Can I obtain the vitamins I need through my diet?

Some advertisements for vitamin supplements may leave you with the impression that it is difficult, if not impossible, to obtain adequate vitamin nutrition through the typical American diet. In contrast, most health professional organizations focusing on nutrition, such as the Academy of Nutrition and Dietetics (AND), support the view that a balanced diet will satisfy all nutrient needs of the healthy individual. There is some truth to both positions, for the typical diet of some individuals may not be a balanced diet. Our selection, storage, and preparation of food may lead to poor vitamin intake.

Vitamin intake may be inadequate for several reasons. First, the refining process of many foods removes vitamins. For example, the preparation of flour for white bread removes many of the vitamins found in the outer parts of the grain. Although some of these vitamins are returned by an enrichment process, not all are restored. Thus, many processed foods may be lower in total vitamin content than their natural counterparts. In some cases, however, processing actually increases the vitamin content of foods. Examples include the fortification of milk with vitamins A and D, grain products with folic acid, and the use of vitamin C as an antioxidant preservative in some foods. Second, improper storage of foods may lead to vitamin losses. Once fruits and vegetables are harvested, the vitamin content begins to diminish. In general, such foods should be refrigerated or frozen in airtight containers as applicable and stored in dark places to minimize vitamin losses caused by exposure to air, heat, and light. Third, improper preparation may also lead to significant vitamin losses from foods.

Prolonged cooking, excessive heat, and cooking vegetables in water should be avoided. Steaming, microwave cooking, and the use of boiling bags and waterless cookware will help retain the natural vitamin content of foods. Thus, the individual who consumes a diet high in processed foods with empty Calories and does not store or prepare foods properly may receive less than the RDA for several vitamins.

The key to adequate vitamin nutrition is to consume a balanced diet of natural foods that have a high nutrient density. Buy foods in their natural state and store them properly as soon as possible. Prepare them to eat so as to minimize vitamin losses.

The position of the AND is that the best nutritional strategy for promoting optimal health and reducing the risk of chronic disease is to obtain essential nutrients through a wide variety of foods. In this way, other nutrients, particularly minerals and other phytonutrients, will be obtained at the same time, as they also are natural constituents of the food we eat. Vitamins often work in conjunction with minerals, such as vitamin D and calcium, vitamin B_6 and magnesium, and vitamin E and selenium. By obtaining vitamins through the selection of a balanced diet containing wholesome, natural foods, we may be assured of receiving sufficient amounts of other nutrients necessary for optimal physiological functioning, in addition to various phytochemicals that may also confer some health benefits. The Consumers Union estimates there are about 5,000 phytochemicals in plant foods.

Moreover, it is recommended that the active individual be selective in choosing foods. The stress of exercise can increase the utilization of some water-soluble and antioxidant vitamins, but these can be replaced easily if the extra Calories expended during exercise are replaced by foods with high nutrient density, that is, foods rich in vitamins and minerals. Table 7.2 presents a quick overview of foods containing substantial amounts of the major vitamins, while table 7.3 presents a list of ten foods, totaling approximately 1,200 Calories, that will provide at least 100 percent of the RDA for every vitamin, assuming adequate sunlight for vitamin D and intestinal synthesis of biotin and vitamin K.

Why are vitamin supplements often recommended?

Several reviews, most notably those by Fairfield and Fletcher, have indicated that there are many bona fide reasons for vitamin supplementation. In her review, Manore also indicated that vitamin supplementation may be important for various groups of physically active individuals. Moreover, although still supporting the view that we should obtain our vitamins through healthful foods, the AND in its position statement noted that additional vitamins and minerals from fortified foods and/or supplements can help some people meet their nutritional needs as specified by such standards as the DRI. Based on these and other reviews, the following groups of individuals may possibly benefit from supplementation.

• Women who are pregnant or lactating have an increased RDA or AI for most vitamins, so many physicians recommend a general vitamin supplement, particularly one containing adequate folic acid. Folic acid supplements are also recommended for all women of childbearing age.

TABLE 7.2　High-vitamin-content foods

Vitamin A	Folate
Beef liver, fish liver oils, egg yolks Milk, butter, cheese, fortified margarine Orange vegetables (carrots, sweet potatoes) Green vegetables (spinach, collards)	Meats, liver, eggs Milk Legumes Whole wheat products Green leafy vegetables

Thiamin (vitamin B_1)	Vitamin B_{12} (cobalamin)
Pork, legumes (dried peas and beans) Milk Nuts Whole-grain and enriched cereal products (bread) All vegetables Fruits	Meats, poultry, fish, eggs Milk, cheese, butter Not found in plant foods

Riboflavin (vitamin B_2)	Biotin
Meats, liver, kidneys, eggs Milk, cheese Whole-grain and enriched cereal products Wheat germ Green leafy vegetables	Meats, liver, egg yolks Legumes, nuts Vegetables

Niacin	Vitamin C
Lean meats, organ meats (liver), poultry Legumes, peanuts, peanut butter Whole-grain and enriched cereal products	Citrus fruits, oranges, grapefruit, melons, berries, tomatoes Broccoli, brussels sprouts, cabbage, salad greens, green peppers, cauliflower

Vitamin B_6 (pyridoxine)	Vitamin D
Meat, poultry, fish Whole-grain cereals, seeds Vegetables	Tuna, salmon, sardines, eggs, shitake mushrooms Fortified milk and margarine

Pantothenic acid	Vitamin E
Meats, poultry, fish Milk, cheese Legumes Whole-grain products	Legumes, nuts, seeds Salad oils, wheat germ oil, margarine Green leafy vegetables

	Vitamin K
	Pork, liver, meats Green leafy vegetables, cauliflower, spinach, cabbage

- Individuals with certain diseases or disorders may have an increased need for a specific vitamin supplement. For example, an impaired ability to absorb fat decreases the availability of the fat-soluble vitamins, while a lack of the intrinsic factor necessitates provision of B_{12}.
- Individuals taking drugs to prevent various illnesses may experience a vitamin deficiency. For example, antibiotics kill intestinal bacteria and decrease the production of vitamin K. In such cases, specific vitamins are prescribed by physicians. Use of social drugs, such as smoking nicotine cigarettes and drinking alcohol, may also increase vitamin needs.
- Elderly individuals have a greater RDA or AI for certain vitamins, such as B_6 and D, and may benefit from the synthetic form of vitamin B_{12} because of difficulty in absorbing the natural form.
- Vegans who abstain from foods fortified with vitamin B_{12} may need to take this specific vitamin supplement.

- Individuals who restrict energy intake for weight loss or maintenance of a low body weight, particularly under 1,200 Calories daily, may need a supplement to obtain the RDA.
- Physically active individuals who do not eat enough to maintain body weight during periods of high-energy expenditure may also benefit from supplementation.
- Individuals who are intolerant to or purposely avoid certain foods, such as dairy products, may limit the intake of certain vitamins, such as riboflavin and vitamin D.
- Individuals who consume enough energy but, because of poor dietary choices, do not obtain the needed vitamins and minerals, will benefit from vitamin-mineral supplementation. This is the case if one eats mainly highly processed foods or if one restricts one or more food groups (such as dairy products) in the diet.

Based on these viewpoints, Fletcher and Fairfield noted that most people do not consume an optimal amount of vitamins by

TABLE 7.3	1,200-Calorie diet containing at least 100 percent of the RDA or AI for each vitamin	
Food	**Amount**
Milk, skim, fortified with vitamins A and D	2 cups
Carrot	1 medium
Orange	1 average
Bread, whole wheat	4 slices
Chicken breast, roasted	3 ounces
Broccoli	1 stalk
Margarine	1 tablespoon
Cereal, Grape-Nuts	2 ounces
Tuna fish, in water	3 ounces
Cauliflower	1/2 cup

diet alone. Pending strong evidence of effectiveness from randomized trials, they indicate that it appears *prudent* for all adults to take vitamin supplements. However, such a recommendation would apply to a general multivitamin supplement, not large amounts of specific vitamins, which may be harmful to some individuals.

If an individual feels he or she is not receiving a balanced diet for some reason, most medical authorities agree that a simple, balanced vitamin supplement containing 50–100 percent of the RDA or AI will not do any harm, and some guidelines for selecting a multivitamin/mineral supplement are presented later in this chapter. There are a number of preparations on the market that contain the daily RDA or AI of most vitamins. However, the Academy of Nutrition and Dietetics recommends low levels that do not exceed the RDA or AI for those who choose to use supplements, and the American Medical Association suggests that use of larger amounts be under medical supervision. Nevertheless, millions of Americans consume vitamin megadoses without such supervision.

Why do individuals take vitamin megadoses?

We have all heard the adage "if a little bit is good, more is better." As already noted, vitamin nutrition for optimal health can be obtained from a proper diet, but foods must be selected wisely. Excluding choline, the adult male RDA or AI for all 13 vitamins only totals approximately 130 milligrams, yet some individuals are consuming prodigious amounts of vitamins—thousands of milligrams—via supplements, for a variety of health reasons, particularly to help deter the effects of aging and the development of various chronic diseases. In a review of data from the National Health and Nutrition Examination Survey (NHANES), Rock reported that about 50 percent of adults take dietary supplements, mainly vitamins and minerals. Individuals with a history of chronic diseases, such as cancer, are more likely to take supplements and more likely to use single vitamin and mineral supplements. Individuals may begin to think of vitamin supplements as drugs, not nutrients. In general, however,

Kamanger and Emadi reported no overall benefit to the majority of vitamin and mineral supplement users in the United States.

Nevertheless, vitamin supplements are actively marketed as a means to prevent aging and chronic diseases. Browse the vitamin supplement section of your local health food, drug, or online supplement store, and you will find numerous products purported to enhance health. In particular, several of the B vitamins and antioxidants, such as vitamins C and E, may be marketed for their putative health benefits. Although most authorities indicate that much needs to be learned about the role of vitamins in prevention of chronic diseases, recent research findings provide a perspective on the potential roles of vitamins as found naturally in food or consumed as dietary supplements.

Do foods rich in vitamins, particularly antioxidant vitamins, help deter chronic disease?

Epidemiological research, although not as objective as experimental research, is an important tool to evaluate the role of diet in the development of chronic diseases over the course of many years. For example, comparing the vegan diet to the typical American diet provides some dietary guidance for the prevention of CHD. In recent years, the vitamin content of the diet, particularly antioxidant vitamins, has been studied as a means to prevent chronic diseases by reducing oxidative damage in the body.

As discussed earlier in this chapter, free radicals may be very reactive with body tissues, causing cellular damage by oxidation of unsaturated fats in cellular and subcellular membranes. Free radicals are theorized to contribute to the aging process and to the development of more than 60 diseases, including cardiovascular disease and cancer. Discussing the free radical theory of aging, Koltover estimated that our life span could be 250 years but for the damage caused by free radicals. Various antioxidant enzymes in the cells counteract undesirable effects of free radicals, but there is increasing evidence that what we eat may also help to prevent certain adverse health effects associated with free radicals.

Fruits and vegetables, along with whole grains, nuts, and seeds, are rich in antioxidants, including vitamins C and E and carotenoids (beta-carotene, lycopene, lutein, and zeaxanthin), as well as other micronutrients and phytochemicals. Mehta indicated that there is no doubt that antioxidants and other micronutrients, taken in their proper form in vegetables and fruits, confer a number of overall health benefits. Prevention of cancer and cardiovascular disease appear to be the two major health benefits. Several reviews, including those by Lee, Gaziano and Hennekens, and Steinmetz and Potter, indicated that the evidence for a protective effect of increased consumption of vegetables and fruits, foods rich in antioxidant vitamins, is consistent for cancers of the stomach, esophagus, lung, endometrium, pancreas, and colon and that the most effective are raw vegetables. The precise mechanism underlying this possible protective effect is not known, although phytochemicals found in some vegetables may block tumor formation. Other investigators believe the antioxidant vitamins (vitamin C, vitamin E, beta-carotene) found naturally in vegetables and fruits may confer the protective effect, for various epidemiological studies have shown that high serum levels of some antioxidant vitamins are associated with a decreased risk of cancer. In a review, Gladys Block presented biochemical data suggesting that optimal antioxidant intake may protect against environmental factors, such as cigarette smoke and polluted air, that may generate free radicals and subsequent cancer. Antioxidant vitamins may also strengthen the immune system, a major defense against cancer, particularly as we grow older. Meydani indicated that cells of the immune system have a very high content of polyunsaturated fatty acids, which makes them susceptible to oxidative damage. When oxidized, polyunsaturated fats may produce PGE_2, an eicosanoid that may suppress immune function by interfering with several major functions, such as the activity of T cells. Dietary antioxidant vitamins may help prevent this undesirable oxidation.

Universally, all reviewers recommend diets rich in fruits, vegetables, whole grains, and other vitamin-rich foods as the best means of obtaining the antioxidant vitamins, and along with other potential health-promoting phytochemicals, as the most effective dietary strategy to promote health and prevent disease. In this regard, the National Cancer Institute has sponsored a campaign called "Five a Day for Better Health," meaning to eat at least 5 servings of fruits and vegetables daily. The point is stressed that 5 is the minimum number of servings and more should be consumed, hopefully 5 servings *each* of fruits and vegetables.

> http://www.heart.org/HEARTORG/ From this link, click Getting Healthy, then Nutrition Center, then Healthy Eating, then Nutrition Basics, then Fruits and Vegetables, then How to Eat More Fruits and Vegetables for tips on how to incorporate more fruits and vegetables into your daily diet.

However, the health benefits of a diet rich in antioxidant-containing nutrients presented here are based on epidemiological studies. Such diets appear to protect against CHD and other chronic diseases, but the underlying mechanism is not known. Fruits and vegetables are rich in various vitamins that may exert beneficial health effects, such as the antioxidant vitamins, folate, and vitamins B_6, and these vitamins may individually or collectively account for such positive health effects. As noted, these foods also contain other micronutrients and phytochemicals, and vitamins may interact with them, either individually or collectively, to provide the apparent health benefits. Thus, controlled, randomized studies have been conducted in attempts to determine whether vitamins are the health-promoting nutrient.

> www.ars.usda.gov/nutrientdata/ORAC Check foods for antioxidant content. The database presents amount of antioxidants, as measured by Oxygen Radical Absorbance Capacity (ORAC), per 100 grams of food, about 3 ounces.

Do vitamin supplements help deter disease?

If the epidemiological evidence suggests that diets rich in vitamins, particularly antioxidant vitamins, may provide some protection against the development of chronic diseases, such as cancer and heart disease, will supplements provide any additional benefit?

Scientists have used a variety of research techniques to evaluate the effect of antioxidant supplementation to prevent disease.

Basic research studies, using *in vitro* techniques or animal models, have evaluated the effects of antioxidants on underlying mechanisms of disease. These studies provide evidence in relation to the theory underlying the beneficial effects of supplementation.

Both retrospective and prospective epidemiological studies of various populations have compared differences in the incidence of disease between supplement users and nonusers. These studies provide evidence of a relationship between supplement use and disease but do not establish a cause-and-effect relationship. Moreover, as Patterson and others have noted, vitamin supplement users are more likely to engage in other healthy behaviors, such as exercising regularly, that may confound the relationship.

Randomized, clinical intervention studies with humans, providing antioxidant supplements to some and placebos to others for years, have evaluated the effect of supplementation on disease. These trials provide cause-and-effect evidence and are considered to be the gold standard in diet-health research.

Nevertheless, as mentioned previously, results from a single study are insufficient to support or refute a theory. The totality of evidence must be considered. In 2006, the National Institutes of Health (NIH) convened a state-of-the-science conference on vitamin and mineral supplements and chronic disease prevention. The conference planning committee chose to focus the evidence report on nutrients for which the potential for impact had been most strongly suggested and on conditions for which supplements were thought to have the most potential influence. The planning committee also limited the scope of the evidence report to consideration of randomized controlled trials (RCTs). The following sections contain some data from basic and epidemiological studies with vitamin supplements, some of the key conclusions of the 2006 NIH conference, and some other relevant and subsequent research findings.

> www.ahrq.gov/clinic/tp/multivittp.htm Check the full report of the National Institutes of Health state-of-the-science conference on vitamin and mineral supplements and chronic disease prevention.

Cardiovascular Disease and Stroke Basic research using *in vitro* techniques and biomarkers of oxidation appears to support the theoretical mechanisms underlying the beneficial effects of antioxidant supplementation on cardiovascular disease. Two early reviews by Diplick and by Devaraj and Jialal note that vitamin E may prevent LDL oxidation by free radicals and, by being incorporated in the cell membrane, may also prevent platelet adhesion and improve endothelial function. Singh and Devaraj note that the anti-inflammatory effects of vitamin E may combat inflammation in atherogenesis. Ashor and others reported small but significant effects of vitamin C, vitamin E, and beta-carotene in reducing arterial stiffness. Although antioxidants were more effective in primary prevention and in those with low vitamin C and E, they noted a trend for reduced arterial stiffness in those with vascular disease. However, Meagher and others reported no significant effect of 8 weeks of vitamin E weeks supplementation (200, 400, 600, 800, or 1,000 IU/day) on three indices of lipid peroxidation. Moreover, in a meta-analysis, Bleys and others found no evidence of a protective effect of antioxidant, or B vitamin, supplements on the progression of atherosclerosis, suggesting that such supplements may not prevent CHD via this mechanism.

The effects of vitamin E on antioxidant activity appear to be more pronounced than for beta-carotene or vitamin C. Rimm and Stampfer noted that several large prospective studies reported reduced CVD risk in subjects taking vitamin E supplements in doses greater than 100 IU/day, but no epidemiological evidence for decreased CVD risk from vitamin C. Mayne reported that beta-carotene supplementation did not reduce CDV risk. In their meta-analysis, Ashor and others found a dose-response in decreased arterial stiffness for vitamin E but not for vitamin C.

Other B complex vitamins may improve heart function in CVD patients. Dhalla and others reported that pyridoxal 5′-phosphate, a vitamin B_6 metabolite, may improve calcium transport and heart rhythm in damaged heart tissue. Kaya and colleagues noted that lipid peroxidation and DNA damage occur in heart disease and that CoEnzyme Q_{10} supplementation may exert an antioxidant cardioprotective effect.

The effects of antioxidant and vitamin B complex supplementation on cerebrovascular disease has also been the focus of recent research. Paganini-Hill and Perez Barreto reported that individuals who took antioxidant vitamin supplements decreased the risk of cerebral occlusion. Huo and others found that an angiotensin-converting enzyme (ACE) inhibitor (10 mg) combined with folate supplementation (0.8 mg/day) significantly reduced the risk of first stroke in hypertensive Chinese adults compared to ACE inhibitor alone. In their meta-analysis of 14 studies, Ji and others reported a small but significant decrease in homocysteine levels and stroke risk following vitamin B supplementation. Reduced risk was greater in subjects with systolic blood pressure greater than 130 mmHg and in those with low folate-fortified diets. There was no effect of vitamin B_{12} on reduced stroke risk. Zeng and others also reported that folate supplementation may elicit a modest homocysteine-lowering effect and decreased stroke risk, especially in areas without folate-fortified foods. Not all epidemiological studies have revealed positive findings. For example, in their eight-year study, Ascherio and others found no significant effect of vitamin C, vitamin E, or beta-carotene on stroke prevention. Genetic modifications may also affect the efficacy of vitamin supplementation on stroke prevention. Using data from the Vitamin Intervention for Stroke Prevention (VISP) trial, Keene and others reported several associations between single nucleotide polymorphisms and vitamin B measurements.

The NIH report of RCTs concluded that the effects of multivitamin/mineral supplementation on cardiovascular disease are inconsistent and indicated that there is insufficient evidence to make any recommendations. More recently, Fortmann and others reported no effect of multivitamin/mineral supplementation on decreased CVD risk in either men or women. In reviews related to physically active individuals, Hamilton also concluded that studies with humans relative to the cardioprotective effects of antioxidant supplements are conflicting, and more research

is needed to determine if various antioxidant supplements may help prevent oxidative damage to the heart following exercise when oxygen radical formation is accelerated. Williams also reported that there is currently insufficient evidence to recommend antioxidant supplements for endurance athletes because the types of long-term studies needed to more adequately assess the health benefits of antioxidant supplements in athletes have not been done.

However, some research suggests that antioxidant supplementation to heart disease patients may be harmful. In a meta-analysis of 19 clinical trials involving vitamin E alone or combined with other antioxidants, Miller and others reported an increased risk of all-cause mortality with dosages greater than 150 IU/day and concluded that high-dosage vitamin E supplements (equal to or greater than 400 IU daily) may increase all-cause mortality and should be avoided. The increased mortality may be due to heart failure, as reported in a recent study by Lonn and others. Bjelakovic and others conducted a meta-analysis of 68 RCTs and reported no effect of antioxidant supplementation on overall mortality. However, when the data from only the best-designed studies were analyzed, the investigators concluded that supplementation with antioxidants might actually increase mortality by 4–16 percent, dependent on the specific antioxidant.

Although most recent RCTs and meta-analyses do not support a protective effect of vitamin supplementation against the development of CHD, Rodrigo and others questioned the methodology of the studies. One criticism was the selection of subjects. Tufts University noted that most of the studies analyzed in the meta-analysis by Bjelakovic and others dealt with people who already have a disease, so the conclusions do not apply to a healthy population. Miller and others noted this limitation in their meta-analysis of vitamin E suggesting an increased all-cause mortality and indicated that the generalizability of their findings to healthy adults is uncertain. Another criticism by Rodrigo and others was the nature of the antioxidant sources of vitamins. For example, supplementation studies with vitamin E have mostly involved alpha-tocopherol. Most recently, however, Sen and Das, along with their associates, have indicated that other forms of vitamin E, particularly the tocotrienols, may have specific health benefits independent of alpha-tocopherol, such as powerful cholesterol-lowering properties.

Tufts University noted that a considerable number of large epidemiological studies have supported the efficacy of diets high in antioxidants, vitamin E in particular, in reducing CVD risk. However, recall from chapter 1 that epidemiological studies examine associations between aspects of diet and disease outcomes and do not establish cause and effect. In their review, Futterman and Lemberg note that even if antioxidants prove to be effective, their place on the therapeutic ladder of cardiovascular disease prevention should be low. Modifying other risk factors, such as treating hypertension and achieving a normal body weight, should have a higher priority. Given the overall evidence currently available, the American Heart Association does not recommend widespread use of B vitamin supplements to reduce the risk of heart disease and stroke. The Consumers Union also notes that the AHA now recommends *against* taking antioxidant supplements.

Cancer Antioxidants are theorized to prevent cancer in several ways, primarily by preventing DNA damage and strengthening the immune system, as noted previously.

In a review, Prasad and others noted that extensive *in vitro* studies and some *in vivo* studies have revealed that individual antioxidants may affect animal and human cancer cells by complex mechanisms and that multiple antioxidant-vitamin supplementation, together with other lifestyle modifications, may improve the efficacy of cancer therapies.

Epidemiological data suggest that antioxidant supplementation, particularly vitamin E, may help in the fight against cancer. Gridley and others indicated that individuals who took supplements of individual vitamins, such as C and E, had a significantly lower risk of oral and pharyngeal cancer, whereas Losonczy and others reported that vitamin E supplementation was associated with about a 50 percent reduction in overall cancer mortality. However, in a review of the relationship between vitamin E and breast cancer, Kimmick and others noted that the epidemiological study results have been inconsistent. In their review of studies for the United States Preventive Services Task Force, Fortmann and colleagues reported that vitamin E did not reduce cancer risk and that beta-carotene actually increased lung cancer in smokers. They concluded that multivitamin/mineral supplements are neither helpful nor harmful in cancer prevention.

Experimental studies do not appear to support a cancer-protective effect of antioxidant supplementation. The NIH concluded that the effects of multivitamin/mineral supplementation on cancer are inconsistent and claimed that there were not enough data to recommend for or against multivitamins based on cancer data. In another major report dealing with nutrition and prevention of cancer, the American Institute of Cancer Research (AICR) indicated that although high-dose dietary supplements can modify the risk of some cancers, usually in high-risk groups, these findings may not apply to the general population. Greenwald and others noted that several large randomized clinical trials are under way, including the Physicians' Health Study II, to help clarify the health effects of multivitamin supplements. The Selenium and Vitamin E Cancer Prevention Trial (SELECT) to detect possible prevention of prostate cancer was scheduled to end in 2012, but the National Cancer Institute stopped the study prematurely in 2008. Data analysis indicated that the supplements did not prevent prostate cancer; moreover, there was a small increase, but not statistically significant, in the number of prostate cancer cases in the men taking vitamin E. The antioxidant effects of selenium are discussed in chapter 8.

The AICR noted that there may be some adverse effects, possibly an increased risk of some cancers, associated with vitamin supplementation. In the NIH report, Hyang and others noted that two large trials designed to test lung cancer prevention with beta-carotene found a surprising increase in lung cancer incidence and deaths in smokers and recommend that smokers avoid beta-carotene supplementation. Cole and others, in a 10-year study with the effects of folic acid supplementation on the development of colorectal adenoma, reported a higher risk of having three or more adenomas and of noncolorectal cancers, and indicated that research is needed to investigate the possibility that folic acid supplementation might increase cancer risk. Lawson and others

reported that although taking more than one multivitamin daily was not associated with an increased risk of developing localized prostate cancer, excessive multivitamin intake did increase the risk of developing advanced prostate cancer, suggesting that such supplementation may promote tumor growth in men who already have the disease.

Fairfield and Stampfer, in a review of issues and evidence relative to vitamin and mineral supplements for cancer prevention, highlighted the numerous difficulties in studying the effects of vitamin and mineral supplementation on cancer development. For example, given the length of time that it takes cancer to develop, existing studies may not have been long enough. They recommended long-term prospective cohort studies, especially with repeated measures and high follow-up, to help provide useful data as the basis for rational recommendations.

Given the overall evidence currently available, the NIH does not provide a recommendation for or against vitamin supplementation to prevent cancer. Based on its worldwide report on nutrition and prevention of cancer, the AICR indicated that individuals should aim to meet nutritional needs through diet alone and concluded that dietary supplements are not recommended for cancer prevention.

Eye Health According to Christen, basic research studies suggest that oxidative mechanisms may play an important role in the pathogenesis of cataract and age-related macular degeneration (ARMD), the two most important causes of visual impairment in older adults. In the United States, almost 1,100 cataract surgeries are performed per 100,000 individuals. Jacques theorized that these eye problems may be prevented by optimal antioxidant nutrition, particularly vitamin E. Johnson notes that the carotenoids lutein and zeaxanthin may protect against eye disease by absorbing blue light. These carotenoids also exert antioxidant and anti-inflammatory effects on brain tissue and may be important in cognitive function. Christen notes that findings from several epidemiological studies are generally compatible with a possible protective effect of antioxidant vitamins, but the data are inconsistent.

The NIH indicated that results from trials investigating the effects of multivitamin/ mineral supplementation on ARMD are inconsistent. However, Evans and Lawrenson concluded that although no evidence exists for nutritional supplementation to affect primary prevention of ARMD, antioxidant vitamins may benefit those with the disease. Evidence from the Age-Related Eye Disease Study might support use of antioxidants and zinc in adults with intermediate-stage ARMD. Evans indicates that data from this single well-designed study provides the main support for such use and that more research is needed. Coleman and Chew indicated that a multivitamin/mineral supplement with a combination of vitamin C, vitamin E, beta-carotene, and zinc (with cupric oxide) may be recommended for ARMD but not cataracts. However, in their review of 14 studies, Zhao and colleagues concluded that multivitamin/mineral supplementation may decrease the risk of nuclear and cortical cataracts.

The Consumers Union recommends that those who are in the intermediate stages of the disease take 400 IU vitamin E daily, along with 500 milligrams of vitamin C, 15 milligrams of beta-carotene, 80 milligrams of zinc, and 2 milligrams of copper. Note that this recommendation is for those who already have ARMD, not for the general public. The Consumers Union recommends that individuals taking such supplements do so under a doctor's supervision. As shall be noted in the next chapter, the recommended zinc intake exceeds the UL.

Seddon indicates that other antioxidants, particularly lutein and zeaxanthin, may be beneficial for ARMD and possibly cataracts. However, Trumbo and Ellwood noted that the FDA, in an evidence-based review, concluded that no credible evidence exists for a health claim about the intake of lutein or zeaxanthin and the risk of ARMD or cataracts. The Age-Related Eye Disease Study II is currently evaluating the role of these supplements in ARMD.

Mental Health   Oxidative damage may contribute to neurological disease such as Alzheimer's disease (AD), a devastating disease developing primarily in the elderly. Early epidemiological studies by Morris and Englehart and their respective colleagues reported decreased AD risk in older individuals who used vitamin C or vitamin E supplements. In a later study, Morris and others reported that reduced AD risk may be associated with vitamin E from food rather than supplements.

Results from RCTs are mixed. Petersen and others reported that 2,000 IU daily for 3 years did not affect the rate of development of AD in older people with mild cognitive impairment. In a 12-year study of male physicians 65 or more years of age, Grodstein and others found no effect of a daily multivitamin containing vitamins C and E on cognitive function compared to placebo. However, Dyksen and others observed slower cognitive decline in patients with mild to moderate AD receiving 20 mg/day of memantine (a drug treating memory loss) plus 2,000 IU of vitamin E/day compared to memantine plus placebo.

Several reviews suggest that vitamin E supplementation may be useful in the prevention and treatment of AD. Munoz and others indicate that vitamin E may decrease the vascular damage caused by peptides involved in development of AD. La Fata and others also note that, based on the results of RCTs to date and in the absence of pharmacological interventions for AD and cognitive decline, vitamin E may be a safe and cost-effective way to promote healthy brain ageing and delay a decline in cognitive function. Berman and Brodaty suggest current clinical practice favors its use during treatment. In their meta-analysis, Rafnsson and others commented that the rates of global cognitive decline were slowest in the highest quartile of vitamin C, vitamin E, and beta-carotene intake. Harrison and others note that although the role of vitamin C in cognitive function is equivocal, a vitamin C deficiency is associated with oxidative stress, which is related to AD. Genetic mutations may affect vitamin C bioavailability and increase demand in the elderly and those with AD.

Vitamin D may also play a role in healthy brain aging. 1,25-Dihydroxyvitamin D is synthesized in the brain and modulates various brain growth factors. In their meta-analysis, Balion and others reported that low vitamin D blood levels (< 50 nmol/L) were associated with poorer cognitive function and greater AD risk.

General Health   The theory of a health-protective effect of vitamin supplementation is enticing, but the available scientific data are somewhat indecisive. The NIH, in its summarization, concluded that the present evidence is insufficient to recommend either for or against the use of multivitamins/minerals by the American public to prevent chronic disease. The resolution of this important issue will require, among other things, advances in research and improved communication and collaboration among scientists. As noted earlier, several large-scale clinical trials are currently under way and, hopefully, will provide us with some findings to provide more specific recommendations. Keep in mind, given possible gene-nutrient interactions, recommendations may become specific to the individual as human genome research advances with the possible individualization of nutrient requirements.

In the meantime, as noted previously, most health professionals recommend that we obtain our antioxidants from healthful foods. Traber makes the point that, in hindsight, clinical trials of a single nutrient, such as vitamin E, have been overly optimistic in their expectation that a vitamin could reverse poor dietary habits and a sedentary lifestyle in treating heart disease. Again, it may be the whole food and its array of nutrients, rather than a single isolated nutrient, that provides health benefits. In an American Heart Association scientific advisory based on its analysis of clinical trials, Kris-Etherton and others concluded that vitamin supplements do not have the same heart-protective effects as a healthy diet rich in fruits, vegetables, whole grains, and legumes.

How much of a vitamin supplement is too much?

As noted throughout this chapter, vitamins play some very important roles in helping us maintain our health. They are the most popular of all the dietary supplements. However, can we get too much of a good thing? Based on possible adverse health effects of excess vitamin intake, the National Academy of Sciences has established the UL, which is the highest level of a vitamin that can be safely taken without any risk of adverse effects. In general, the higher above the UL, the greater the risk. Exceeding the UL on an occasional basis may not pose any significant health risks, but doing so on a daily basis eventually will. A UL has been set for choline and for 7 of the 13 vitamins for which DRI have been developed. These data can be found on the inside of the back cover of this book. For some vitamins, such as niacin and folate, the UL is only about twice the RDA, whereas for others, such as vitamins C and E, the UL is about 20–60 times greater than the RDA.

In general, it is difficult to exceed the UL for any given vitamin by eating natural, wholesome foods. However, in its report, the NIH noted that this can occur not only in individuals consuming high-potency single-nutrient supplements but also in individuals who consume a healthy diet rich in fortified foods in combination with multivitamin/mineral supplements. For example, the adult UL for niacin is 35 milligrams for synthetic niacin derived from fortified foods or supplements and not from niacin in nonfortified foods. Some breakfast cereals may be fortified with 100 percent of the DV for various vitamins, which for niacin would be 20 milligrams, or nearly half the UL. Consumption of a vitamin supplement or other fortified foods could easily lead to excess niacin intake.

If the vitamin content of the body is adequate, excessive vitamin intake serves no useful purpose and may even be harmful in certain situations. As noted previously, vitamins function primarily as coenzymes. When a vitamin enters the body, it travels through the bloodstream to a particular body cell and then forms part of the enzyme complex within that cell. The cell has a limited capacity to produce these enzymes, and when that capacity is reached, the vitamin cannot be used for its basic purpose. It may now have other fates. It may be excreted from the body if in excess, particularly if it is a water-soluble vitamin; it may be stored in some body tissue, particularly if it is a fat-soluble vitamin; or it may begin to function in uncharacteristic ways, as a drug instead of a nutrient.

Mulholland and Benford indicated that the risk of harm occurring from taking vitamin and mineral supplements will depend on the safe intake range of the nutrient concerned, the susceptibility of the individual, and the likely intake of the same nutrient from other supplements or the rest of the diet, such as fortified foods. The NIH panel expressed concern that with the strong trends of increasing multivitamin/mineral and other dietary supplement consumption, and the increasing fortification of the U.S. diet, a growing proportion of the population may be consuming levels considerably above the UL, thus increasing the possibility of adverse effects. Adverse events from multivitamin/minerals appear with some frequency in both the reports of the American Association of Poison Control Centers and the FDA's MedWatch system.

As noted throughout this chapter, megadoses of several vitamins may be pathological, particularly A, D, niacin, and B_6, when not taken under medical supervision. There are more than 4,000 cases of vitamin/mineral overdose in the United States each year, resulting in about 30 fatalities. Although most of these cases occur in children, the literature contains some case reports of serious health problems with adults, including athletes taking vitamin megadoses in attempts to improve athletic performance. A good review of possible adverse effects of excessive vitamin supplementation is presented by Hathcock.

www.fda.gov/medwatch/ Check the safety of specific vitamin or other supplements. Type in the name of the supplement in the search box.

If I want to take a vitamin-mineral supplement, what are some prudent guidelines?

Unfortunately, scientific data are not available to provide specific guidelines relative to the amounts of each particular vitamin or mineral needed to promote optimal health. Although individual vitamin and mineral supplements are available, health professionals do not generally recommend their use. To reiterate, excess amounts of some vitamins (A, D, niacin, and B_6) can be toxic, as can excess amounts of some minerals (calcium, phosphorus, iron, chromium, selenium, and zinc), as discussed in the next chapter. Although antioxidant supplements are hot sellers, the Consumers Union states that there is currently no reason for the average person to take supplements of nutrients such as vitamin A, C, or E or

beta-carotene because of their antioxidant potential. Nor is there any reason to eat concentrated, antioxidant-rich foods. As noted previously, the American Heart Association now recommends *against* taking antioxidant supplements.

In general, health professionals who do recommend vitamin and mineral supplements suggest multivitamin/mineral combinations. Minerals are covered in detail in the next chapter, but because they are found in most multivitamin/mineral preparations, it was deemed appropriate to include them in this discussion. For those who desire to take vitamin supplements, the Academy of Nutrition and Dietetics recommends low levels that do not exceed the RDA or AI. The Center for Science in the Public Interest (CSPI), an organization promoting healthful nutrition, used an educated-guess approach to offer some prudent guidelines. The following are the highlights of the CSPI recommendations, as reported in an article written by Bonnie Liebman, with some modifications based on advice from the Consumers Union, publishers of *Consumer Reports on Health,* and other nutrition health professionals.

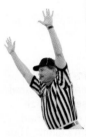

General Points

1. Check the Daily Value (DV). The amounts of vitamins and minerals listed on food and dietary supplement labels are based on the Daily Value (DV) for each nutrient, a value based on the RDA that has not been changed since the 1970s. For example, the DV for vitamin C is 60 milligrams, and yet the new RDA for adult males is 90 milligrams. For zinc, the DV is set at 15 milligrams, yet the new RDA for adult males is 11 milligrams. Thus, supplements that contain 100 percent of the DV may contain less than the current RDA, as in the case of vitamin C, or more than the current RDA, as in the case of zinc. In general, these differences are not substantial, but may be for certain vitamins. For example, the DV for vitamin A is 5,000 IU, while the UL is only twice this amount, or 10,000 IU. A Supplement Facts label is presented in figure 7.5.

2. Buy the inexpensive house brand of vitamins that contains about 100 percent of the DV for most vitamins and minerals. There usually is no need to buy special brands, such as those labeled with catchy terms, such as *high potency*. However, as Yetley notes, multivitamin/mineral products may have widely varied compositions and characteristics. Actual vitamin and mineral amounts often deviate from label values. The Consumers Union warned that you should be leery of bargain-basement brands, such as those found in dollar stores, as tests revealed that more than half did not contain the labeled amount of at least one nutrient. The best buys may be at major drug stores and warehouse stores, which are more likely to carry higher-quality products. Most companies that market vitamins buy their vitamins from the same manufacturers, so the contents in national brands and house brands are similar. Look for labels with USP (United States Pharmacopeia) or better yet, USP-Verified, which means that the product meets standards for quality and purity.

   In an evaluation of vitamin supplements, the Consumers Union and CSPI recommended that if you decide to take

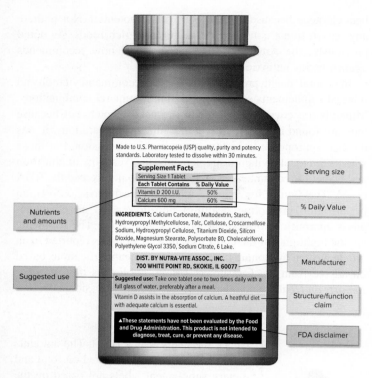

Made to U.S. Pharmacopeia (USP) quality, purity and potency standards. Laboratory tested to dissolve within 30 minutes.

Supplement Facts	
Serving Size 1 Tablet	
Each Tablet Contains	**% Daily Value**
Vitamin D 200 I.U.	50%
Calcium 600 mg	60%

INGREDIENTS: Calcium Carbonate, Maltodextrin, Starch, Hydroxypropyl Methylcellulose, Talc, Cellulose, Croscarmellose Sodium, Hydroxypropyl Cellulose, Titanium Dioxide, Silicon Dioxide, Magnesium Stearate, Polysorbate 80, Cholecalciferol, Polyethylene Glycol 3350, Sodium Citrate, 6 Lake.

DIST. BY NUTRA-VITE ASSOC., INC.
700 WHITE POINT RD, SKOKIE, IL 60077

Suggested use: Take one tablet one to two times daily with a full glass of water, preferably after a meal.

Vitamin D assists in the absorption of calcium. A heathful diet with adequate calcium is essential.

▲These statements have not been evaluated by the Food and Drug Administration. This product is not intended to diagnose, treat, cure, or prevent any disease.

Serving size

% Daily Value

Nutrients and amounts

Manufacturer

Suggested use

Structure/function claim

FDA disclaimer

FIGURE 7.5 Nutrient supplements display a nutrition label that is different from that of foods. This Supplement Facts label must list the ingredient(s), amount(s) per serving, serving size, suggested use, and % Daily Value if one has been established. Note that this label also includes structure/function claims. Thus, it also must include the FDA warning that these claims have not been evaluated by the agency.

vitamins, including antioxidants, avoid high-priced products. In particular, Schardt recommends against purchasing vitamin supplements endorsed by celebrities on television infomercials and on the Internet. The Center for Science in the Public Interest (CSPI) went to one celebrity's Website and clicked on "Vitamin Advisor" to get advice on vitamin supplements. The CSPI answered the questionnaire in a variety of ways, representing individuals whose diets ranged from very poor to individuals in top health consuming a stellar diet rich in fruits and vegetables, dairy, and fish. Even the healthiest individuals received recommendations to buy vitamins sold at the Website, to the tune of about $45–$50 a month.

3. Stick with the basics. The Consumers Union indicates that all most people need is a pill containing 18 nutrients, about 11 vitamins and 7 minerals, in amounts approximating the RDA.

Fat-Soluble Vitamins

1. Buy a supplement low in vitamin A, particularly one with preformed retinol. The CSPI recommends limiting vitamin A to no more than 3,000 IU of retinol, preferably less. Select supplements containing vitamin A from beta-carotene. If the supplement is beta-carotene, 15,000 IU is a recommended limit.

Obtain most of your vitamin A as beta-carotene in fruits and vegetables, a recommendation especially important to smokers. Smokers should not take beta-carotene supplements.

2. Buy a supplement with 400–600 IU of vitamin D if you are elderly, a vegan, or a postmenopausal woman, particularly if you do not drink adequate amounts of vitamin D–fortified milk or do not get enough sunshine. Look for supplements with vitamin D_3, which is more effective than D_2.

3. Buy a supplement containing at least the DV for vitamin E, which is 30 IU. The Consumers Union states you should not take vitamin E to prevent chronic disease; doses of 400 IU or more per day may cause harm. Daily intake of 100–200 IU would appear to pose little risk to most healthy adults. Given the current research data, it may be prudent to limit intake of high-dose vitamin E supplements.

4. Buy a supplement that contains vitamin K. Not all supplements include vitamin K, so check the label. The AI for an adult male is 120 mcg, but the DV is only 80 mcg. Multivitamins contain about 25 mcg of vitamin K.

Water-Soluble Vitamins

1. Buy a supplement that contains 100–200 percent of thiamin, riboflavin, niacin, folic acid, B_6, and B_{12}. You can ignore biotin and pantothenic acid. Check the label to ensure that the supplement contains at least 200–400 mcg of folic acid, which should complement the diet to provide about 400–600 mcg per day.

2. Buy a B_{12} supplement that contains 6 mcg of vitamin B_{12} if you are a vegan, and 25 mcg if you are elderly. The DV for B_{12} is 6 mcg, so many supplements contain this amount. Some preparations for seniors may contain the 25 mcg.

3. Buy a supplement that contains 100–200 percent of vitamin C. The RDA for an adult male is 90 mg, yet the DV is only 60 mg. The supplement should complement vitamin C intake from a variety of fruits and vegetables.

Minerals

1. Buy a supplement with calcium if you are female or elderly and do not consume adequate dietary calcium. Most multivitamin/ mineral tablets contain about 200–300 mg of calcium, which can substitute for a serving of low-fat milk. If you consume no dairy products and few calcium-rich foods, you may consider buying a separate calcium supplement.

2. Buy a supplement limited in iron, copper, and zinc, with no more than 100 percent of the RDA for each. The DV for iron is 18 mg, while the RDA for young women is 15–18 mg. The RDA for adult males and women over age 50 is only 8 mg, so men and postmenopausal women may want to select supplements without iron, since the diet should provide ample amounts.

3. Buy a supplement that provides no more than 100 mg of magnesium and is limited in phosphorus. Magnesium should be obtained primarily from foods, and we normally consume too much phosphorus from foods already.

4. Buy a supplement containing 100 percent of the RDA for chromium and selenium. Selenium is one of the supplements in the SELECT study, mentioned previously, and selenium supplement intake should be limited as suggested in the next chapter.

Food Vitamins and Minerals   Think food first! Although the CSPI published some of these recommendations, they, along with most investigators researching the health implications of vitamin supplementation, note that there is no guarantee of improved health. Almost all health professionals agree we should obtain our vitamin nutrition through consumption of a wide variety of healthful, natural foods, particularly fruits and vegetables. Remember, vitamin supplements do not supply all of the nutrients and other substances, such as phytochemicals, present in foods that are believed to be important to health. For more detailed information on vitamins, the interested reader is referred to the text edited by Ross and others.

through their natural sources—fruits, vegetables, and other wholesome, natural foods. Such foods also provide other nonessential nutrients that may possess health benefits. Epidemiological data strongly suggest that diets rich in fruits and vegetables are associated with lower risks of certain chronic diseases, such as heart disease and cancer.
▶ Megadoses of some vitamins are potentially harmful.
▶ In general, health professionals indicate that vitamin supplements are not necessary for the individual on a well-balanced diet, but they may be recommended for certain individuals, such as the elderly, vegans, and women of child-bearing age. Moreover, some health professionals note that most people do not consume an optimal amount of vitamins by diet alone and indicate that it appears prudent for all adults to take a vitamin supplement. For most individuals who desire to take vitamin or mineral supplements, a basic multivitamin/mineral tablet should suffice.

Key Concepts

▶ Although several national surveys have reported that some Americans and Canadians are receiving less than the RDA for several vitamins, actual vitamin deficiencies resulting in disease are rare.
▶ Vitamins certainly are essential for good health, but most health professionals recommend that vitamins be obtained

Check for Yourself

▶ Use a search engine on the Internet, such as www.google.com, and search for "antioxidant vitamins health." Check out the advertisements and claims, and compare to the text discussion.

APPLICATION EXERCISES

Construct a brief, one-page survey regarding vitamin supplements, and other supplements as well, if you like. For example, you might use some of the following questions:

1. Do you take a vitamin supplement?
   _____ Yes _____ No
2. What type of supplement do you take?
   _____ Multivitamin
   _____ Multivitamin/mineral
   _____ Vitamin B complex
   _____ Vitamin E
   _____ Other

3. How often do you take the supplement?
   _____ Two or more times a day
   _____ Daily
   _____ Several times a week
   _____ Once a week
   _____ Several times a month
   _____ Once a month
   _____ Never
4. Why do you take the vitamin supplement?
   _____ To help guarantee good health
   _____ To enhance my sports or exercise performance
   _____ Other

Once your survey is developed, get permission to administer it to some physically active individuals or athletes, such as participants in recreational sports activities or sports at your school, members of a local cycling or running club, or members of a commercial fitness facility. Share the findings with your class.

Review Questions—Multiple Choice

1. Vitamin A toxicity is most likely to occur from
   a. consuming too many dark green and deep orange vegetables.
   b. eating liver more than once per week.
   c. consuming high-dosage vitamin A supplements.

   d. drinking too much vitamin A–fortified milk.
   e. eating rabbit meat 2 days per week.
2. The task of acquiring enough vitamin B_{12} may pose a problem to vegans who do not eat fortified foods because

   a. fibers in vegetables inhibit its absorption.
   b. vegans lack the intrinsic factor.
   c. B_{12} is found only in animal products.
   d. a deficiency may occur from excess intake of soy products.
   e. folacin retards its absorption.

3. Which of the following statements is not true about vitamin B_6?
   a. The term *vitamin B_6* refers to a family of compounds: pyridoxine, pyridoxal, and pyridoxamine.
   b. As a coenzyme, it acts in the conversion of the amino acid tryptophan into one of the essential vitamins.
   c. It is fat soluble and therefore can be stored in the body.
   d. Foods containing it should be included in the diet daily.
   e. The richest food sources are meats, liver, vegetables, and whole grains.

4. A deficiency of either of these two vitamins produces a similar anemia:
   a. thiamin and riboflavin
   b. riboflavin and niacin
   c. thiamin and vitamin B_2
   d. pantothenic acid and biotin
   e. vitamin B_{12} and folate

5. If an individual is on a well-balanced diet, which of the following vitamin supplements will increase physical performance at sea level competition?
   a. thiamin
   b. niacin
   c. vitamin C
   d. vitamin E
   e. none will

6. Most of the B vitamins function in human metabolism as
   a. coenzymes.
   b. hormones.
   c. antioxidants.
   d. a source of Calories.
   e. activators of mineral metabolism.

7. Although athletes on weight-reduction diets normally may not need vitamin supplementation, which athletes, based on the nature of their sport, may be best advised to take a supplement?
   a. swimmers
   b. wrestlers
   c. baseball players
   d. field hockey players
   e. sprinters

8. Which of the following are fat-soluble vitamins?
   a. vitamins B, C, D, niacin
   b. vitamin E, niacin, thiamin, riboflavin
   c. vitamins A, D, E, K
   d. vitamins A, B, C, D
   e. vitamins B_1, B_2, B_6, C

9. Which of the following are true B vitamins? (1) inositol (2) choline (3) biotin (4) lipoic acid (5) PABA (6) niacin (7) bioflavinoids (8) ubiquinone (9) vitamin B_6 (10) thiamin (11) laetrile (12) pantothenic acid (13) vitamin B_{15} (14) vitamin P (15) vitamin B_{17}
   a. 1, 2, 3, 5, 7
   b. 2, 4, 7, 8, 9
   c. 3, 6, 9, 10, 12
   d. 5, 9, 11, 13, 15
   e. 7, 11, 12, 14, 15

10. The main function of vitamin E in the body is to act as a(n)
    a. antioxidant.
    b. superoxide.
    c. free radical.
    d. hormone.
    e. source of energy.

Answers to multiple choice questions:
1. c; 2. c; 3. c; 4. e; 5. e; 6. a; 7. b; 8. c; 9. c; 10. a

Review Questions—Essay

1. Explain at least three ways whereby vitamins function in metabolic processes in the human body.
2. Name the four fat-soluble vitamins and describe the metabolic function of each in the human body.
3. Name the nine water-soluble vitamins and, along with choline, describe their major metabolic functions in the human body.
4. What is coenzyme Q_{10}, why is it purported to be an ergogenic aid, and does research support its efficacy as an ergogenic?
5. Would you consider taking antioxidant vitamin supplements, such as beta-carotene, E, and C? If so, why so? If not, why not?

References

Books

American Institute of Cancer Research. 2007. *Food, Nutrition, Physical Activity, and the Prevention of Cancer: A Global Perspective.* Washington, DC: AICR.

Bucci, L. 1993. *Nutrients as Ergogenic Aids for Sports and Exercise.* Boca Raton, FL: CRC Press.

Centers for Disease Control and Prevention. 2012. *Second National Report on Biochemical Indicators of Diet and Nutrition in the U.S. Population.*

Washington, DC: United States Department of Health and Human Services.

Keys, A. 1950. *Human Starvation.* Minneapolis, MN: West.

National Academies of Sciences. 1999. *Dietary Reference Intakes for Calcium, Phosphorus, Magnesium, Vitamin D, and Fluoride.* Washington, DC: National Academies Press.

National Academies of Sciences. 2000. *Dietary Reference Intakes for Thiamin, Riboflavin, Niacin, Vitamin B6, Folate,*

Vitamin B12, Pantothenic Acid, Biotin, and Choline. Washington, DC: National Academies Press.

National Academies of Sciences. 2000. *Dietary Reference Intakes for Vitamin C, Vitamin E, Selenium, and Carotenoids.* Washington, DC: National Academies Press.

National Academies of Sciences. Institute of Medicine, Food, and Nutrition Board. 2010. *Dietary Reference Intakes for Calcium and Vitamin D.* Washington, DC: National Academies Press.

National Academy of Sciences. 2002. *Dietary Reference Intakes for Vitamin A, Vitamin K, Arsenic, Boron, Chromium, Copper, Iodine, Iron, Manganese, Molybdenum, Nickel, Silicon, Vanadium, and Zinc.* Washington, DC: National Academies Press.

Ross, A. C., et al., eds. 2014. *Modern Nutrition in Health and Disease,* 11th ed. Philadelphia: Wolters Kluwer, Lippincott, Williams & Wilkins.

Scientific Report of the 2015 Dietary Guidelines Advisory Committee. 2015. United States Department of Agriculture and United States Department of Health and Human Services.

United States Anti-Doping Agency. 2005. *Optimal Dietary Intake.* Colorado Springs, CO: USADA.

Reviews and Specific Studies

Adams, A., and Best, T. 2002. The role of antioxidants in exercise and disease prevention. *Physician and Sportsmedicine* 30 (5):37–44.

AIM-HIGH Investigators. 2011. The role of niacin in raising high-density lipoprotein cholesterol to reduce cardiovascular events in patients with atherosclerotic cardiovascular disease and optimally treated low-density lipoprotein cholesterol: Rationale and study design. The Atherothrombosis Intervention in Metabolic syndrome with low HDL/high triglycerides: Impact on global health outcomes (AIM-HIGH). *American Heart Journal* 161:471–77.

Alf, D., et al. 2013. Ubiquinol supplementation enhances peak power production in trained athletes: A double-blind placebo controlled study. *Journal of the International Society of Sports Nutrition* 10:24 doi: 10.1186/1550-2783-10-24.

Allison, R. J., et al. 2015. No association between vitamin D deficiency and markers of bone health in athletes. *Medicine and Science in Sports and Exercise* 47 (4):782–88.

American Academies of Pediatrics. 1999. Folic acid for the prevention of neural tube defects. *Pediatrics* 104:325–27.

American Dietetic Association. 1996. Position of the American Dietetic Association: Vitamin and mineral supplementation. *Journal of the American Dietetic Association* 96:73–77.

American Dietetic Association. 2001. Position of the American Dietetic Association: Food fortification and dietary supplements. *Journal of the American Dietetic Association* 101:115–25.

Ardestani, A., et al. 2011. Relation of vitamin D level to maximal oxygen uptake in adults. *American Journal of Cardiology* 107:1246–9.

Armstrong, L., and Maresh, C. 1996. Vitamin and mineral supplements as nutritional aids to exercise performance and health. *Nutrition Reviews* 54:S148–S58.

Ascherio, A., et al. 1999. Relation of consumption of vitamin E, vitamin C, and carotenoids to risk for stroke among men in the United States. *Annals of Internal Medicine* 130:963–70.

Ashor, A. W., et al. 2014. Antioxidant vitamin supplementation reduces arterial stiffness in adults: A systematic review and meta-analysis of randomized controlled trials. *Journal of Nutrition* 144 (1):1594–602.

Atalay, M., et al. 2006. Dietary antioxidants for the athlete. *Current Sports Medicine Reports* 5:182–86.

Autier, P., and Gandini, S. 2007. Vitamin D supplementation and total mortality: A meta-analysis of randomized controlled trials. *Archives of Internal Medicine* 167:1730–7.

Balion, C. 2012. Vitamin D, cognition, and dementia: A systematic review and meta-analysis. *Neurology* 79(13):1397–405.

Bazzano, L., et al. 2006. Effect of folic acid supplementation on risk of cardiovascular diseases: A meta-analysis of randomized controlled trials. *Journal of the American Medical Association* 296:2720–26.

Bell, C., et al. 2005. Ascorbic acid does not affect the age-associated reduction in maximal cardiac output and oxygen consumption in healthy adults. *Journal of Applied Physiology* 98:845–49.

Benardot, D., et al. 2001. Can vitamin supplements improve sport performance? *Sports Science Exchange Roundtable* 12 (3):1–4.

Bender, D. 1999. Non-nutritional uses of vitamin B6. *British Journal of Nutrition* 81:7–20.

Berman, K., and Brodaty, H. 2004. Tocopherol (vitamin E) in Alzheimer's disease and other neurodegenerative disorders. *CNS Drugs* 18:807–25.

Binkley, N., and Krueger, D. 2000. Hypervitaminosis A and bone. *Nutrition Reviews* 58:138–44.

Bischoff-Ferrari, H., and Dawson-Hughes, B. 2007. Where do we stand on vitamin D? *Bone* 41:S13–S19.

Bjelakovic, G., et al. 2007. Mortality in randomized trials of antioxidant supplements for primary and secondary prevention: Systematic review and meta-analysis. *Journal of the American Medical Association* 297:842–57.

Bleys, J., et al. 2006. Vitamin-mineral supplementation and the progression of atherosclerosis: A meta-analysis of randomized controlled trials. *American Journal of Clinical Nutrition* 84:880–87.

Block, G. 1992. The data support: A role for antioxidants in reducing cancer risk. *Nutrition Reviews* 50:207–13.

Bloomer, R. J., et al. 2012. Impact of oral ubiquinol on blood oxidative stress and exercise performance. *Oxidative Medicine and Cellular Longevity* 465020. doi: 10.1155/2012/465020.

Bonetti, A., et al. 2000. Effect of ubidecarenone oral treatment on aerobic power in middle-aged trained subjects. *Journal of Sports Medicine and Physical Fitness* 40:51–57.

Bonke, D. 1986. Influence of vitamin B_1, B_6 and B_{12} on the control of fine motoric movements. *Bibliotheca Nutritio et Dieta* 38:104–9.

Bouis, H. 1996. Enrichment of food staples through plant breeding: A new strategy for fighting micronutrient malnutrition. *Nutrition Reviews* 54:131–37.

Bourgeois, C., et al. 2006. Niacin. In *Modern Nutrition in Health and Disease,* ed. M. Shils, et al. Philadelphia: Lippincott Williams & Wilkins.

Braakhuis, A. J., and Hopkins, W. G. 2015. Impact of dietary antioxidants in sport performance: A review. *Sports Medicine* (March 20). [Epub ahead of print]

Braam, L., et al. 2003. Factors affecting bone loss in female endurance athletes: A two-year follow-up study. *American Journal of Sports Medicine* 31:889–95.

Braun, B., et al. 1991. The effect of coenzyme Q_{10} supplementation on exercise performance, VO_2 max, and lipid peroxidation in trained cyclists. *International Journal of Sport Nutrition* 1:353–65.

Brisswalter, J., and Louis, J. 2014. Vitamin supplementation benefits in master athletes. *Sports Medicine* 44 (3):311–18.

Bryer, S., and Goldfarb, A. 2006. Effect of high dose vitamin C supplementation on muscle soreness, damage, function, and oxidative stress to eccentric exercise. *International Journal of Sport Nutrition and Exercise Metabolism* 16:270–80.

Buchman, A., et al. 2000. The effect of lecithin supplementation on plasma choline concentrations during a marathon. *Journal of the American College of Nutrition* 19:768–70.

Bulow, J. 1993. Lipid metabolism and utilization. In *Principles of Exercise Biochemistry,* ed. J. Poortmans. Basel, Switzerland: Karger.

Calvo, M., et al. 2004. Vitamin D fortification in the United States and Canada: Current status and data needs. *American Journal of Clinical Nutrition* 80:1710S–16S.

Cannell, J., et al. 2009. Athletic performance and vitamin D. *Medicine and Science in Sports and Exercise* 41:1102–10.

Chin, K. Y., and Ima-Nirwana, S. 2014. The effects of α-tocopherol on bone: A double-edged sword? *Nutrients* 6(4):1424–41.

Chiu, K., et al. 2004. Hypovitaminosis D is associated with insulin resistance and β cell dysfunction. *American Journal of Clinical Nutrition* 79:820–25.

Christen, W. 1999. Antioxidant vitamins and age-related eye disease. *Proceedings of the Association of American Physicians* 111:16–21.

Clarke, R., et al. 2010. Effects of lowering homocysteine levels with B vitamins on cardiovascular disease, cancer, and cause-specific mortality: Meta-analysis of 8 randomized trials involving 37,485 individuals. *Archives of Internal Medicine* 170:1622–31.

Clarkson, P. 1991. Vitamins, iron and trace minerals. In *Perspectives in Exercise Science and Sports Medicine. Ergogenics: The Enhancement of Sports Performance,* ed. D. Lamb and M. Williams. Indianapolis, IN: Benchmark.

Clarkson, P., and Thompson, H. 2000. Antioxidants: What role do they play in physical activity and health? *American Journal of Clinical Nutrition* 72:637S–46S.

Close, G., et al. 2006. Ascorbic acid supplementation does not attenuate post-exercise muscle soreness following muscle-damaging exercise but may delay the recovery process. *British Journal of Nutrition* 95:976–81.

Coburn, S., et al. 1990. Effect of vitamin B_6 intake on the vitamin content of human muscle. *FASEB Journal* 4:A365.

Cockayne, S., et al. 2006. Vitamin K and the prevention of fractures: Systematic review and meta-analysis of randomized controlled trials. *Archives of Internal Medicine* 166:1256–61.

Cole, B., et al. 2007. Folic acid for the prevention of colorectal adenomas: A randomized clinical trial. *Journal of the American Medical Association* 297:2351–59.

Coleman, H., and Chew, E. 2007. Nutritional supplementation in age-related macular degeneration. *Current Opinion in Ophthalmology* 18:220–23.

Consumers Union. 2001. Surprising health risk from low vitamin C? *Consumer Reports on Health* 13 (5):7.

Consumers Union. 2001. Vitamin A: How much is too much? *Consumer Reports on Health* 13 (10):1, 4–5.

Consumers Union. 2002. Do you need more vitamin D? *Consumer Reports on Health* 14 (11):1, 4–5.

Consumers Union. 2004. Disease-fighting B vitamins. *Consumer Reports on Health* 16 (1):10.

Consumers Union. 2005. Vitamin E pills: What to do now? *Consumer Reports on Health* 17 (7):3.

Consumers Union. 2006. Multivitamins: What to avoid, how to choose. *Consumer Reports* 71 (2):19–20.

Consumers Union. 2007. Antioxidant reality check. *Consumer Reports on Health* 19 (9):1, 4–5.

Craciun, A., et al. 1998. Improved bone metabolism in female elite athletes after vitamin K supplementation. *International Journal of Sports Medicine* 19:479–84.

Curhan, G., et al. 1996. A prospective study of the intake of vitamin C and B_6, and the risk of kidney stones in men. *Journal of Urology* 155:1847–51.

Dahlquist, D.T., et al. 2015. Plausible ergogenic effects of vitamin D on athletic performance and recovery. *Journal of the International Society of Sports Nutrition* 12:33 doi:10.1186/s12970-015-0093-8.

Das, S., et al. 2007. Tocotrienols in cardioprotection. *Vitamins and Hormones* 76:419–33.

Davison, G., and Gleeson, M. 2005. Influence of acute vitamin C and/or carbohydrate ingestion on hormonal, cytokine, and immune responses to prolonged exercise. *International Journal of Sport Nutrition and Exercise Metabolism* 15:465–79.

Davison, G., and Gleeson, M. 2006. The effect of 2 weeks vitamin C supplementation on immunoendocrine responses to 2.5 h cycling exercise in man. *European Journal of Applied Physiology* 97:454–61.

Devaraj, S., and Jialal, I. 1998. The effects of alpha-tocopherol on critical cells in atherogenesis. *Current Opinion in Lipidology* 9:11–15.

Dhalla, N. S., et al. 2013. Mechanisms of the beneficial effects of vitamin B6 and pyridoxal 5-phosphate on cardiac performance in ischemic heart disease. *Clinical Chemistry and Laboratory Medicine* 51 (3):535–43.

Diplock, A. 1997. Will the 'good fairies' please prove to us that vitamin E lessens human degenerative disease? *Free Radical Research* 26:565–83.

Dobnig, H., et al. 2008. Independent association of low serum 25-hydroxyvitamin D and 1,25-dihydroxyvitamin D levels with all-cause and cardiovascular mortality. *Archives of International Medicine* 168:1340–9.

Douglas, R., et al. 2007. Vitamin C for preventing and treating the common cold. *Cochrane Database of Systematic Reviews* 18 (3):CD000980.

Doyle, M., et al. 1997. Allithiamine ingestion does not enhance isokinetic parameters of muscle performance. *International Journal of Sport Nutrition* 7:39–47.

Dysken, M. W., et al. 2014. Effect of vitamin E and memantine on functional decline in Alzheimer disease: The TEAM-AD VA cooperative randomized trial. *Journal of the American Medical Association* 31 (1):33–44.

Eichholzer, M., et al. 2006. Folic acid: A public-health challenge. *Lancet* 367:1352–61.

Englehart, M., et al. 2002. Dietary intake of antioxidants and risk of Alzheimer disease. *Journal of the American Medical Association* 287:3223–29.

Enstrom, J. 1993. Counterpoint: Vitamin C and mortality. *Nutrition Today* 28 (May/June):39–42.

Evans, J. 2006. Antioxidant vitamin and mineral supplements for slowing the progression of age-related macular degeneration. *Cochrane Database of Systematic Reviews* (2):CD000254.

Evans, J. R., and Lawrenson, J. G. 2014. A review of the evidence for dietary interventions in preventing or slowing the progression of age-related macular degeneration. *Ophthalmic and Physiological Optics* 34 (4):390–96.

Fairfield, K., and Fletcher, R. 2002. Vitamins for chronic disease prevention in adults: Scientific review. *Journal of the American Medical Association* 287:3116–26.

Fairfield, K., and Stampfer, M. 2007. Vitamin and mineral supplements for cancer prevention: Issues and evidence. *American Journal of Clinical Nutrition* 85:289S–92S.

Feskanich, D., et al. 2002. Vitamin A intake and hip fractures among postmenopausal women. *Journal of the American Medical Association* 287:47–54.

Finaud, J., et al. 2006. Oxidative stress: Relationship with exercise and training. *Sports Medicine* 36:327–48.

Fletcher, R., and Fairfield, K. 2002. Vitamins for chronic disease prevention in adults: Clinical applications. *Journal of the American Medical Association* 287:3127–29.

Fogelholm, M. 2000. Vitamins: Metabolic functions. In *Nutrition in Sport,* ed. R. J. Maughan. Oxford: Blackwell Science.

Fortmann, S. P., et al. 2013. Vitamin and mineral supplements in the primary prevention of cardiovascular disease and cancer: An updated systematic evidence review for the U.S. Preventive Services Task Force. *Annals of Internal Medicine* 159:824–34.

Fry, A., et al. 2006. Effect of a liquid multi-vitamin/mineral supplement on anaerobic exercise performance. *Research in Sports Medicine* 14:53–64.

Futterman, L., and Lemberg, L. 1999. The use of antioxidants in retarding atherosclerosis: Fact or fiction? *American Journal of Critical Care* 8:130–33.

Gaziano, J., and Hennekens, C. 1996. Update on dietary antioxidants and cancer. *Pathological Biology* 44:42–45.

Gerster, H. 1989. Review: The role of vitamin C in athletic performance. *Journal of the American College of Nutrition* 8:636–43.

Gerster, H. 1997. No contribution of ascorbic acid to renal calcium oxalate stones. *Annals of Nutrition and Metabolism* 41:269–82.

Gilchrest, B. 2007. Sun protection and vitamin D: Three dimensions of obfuscation. *Journal of Steroid Biochemistry and Molecular Biology* 103:655–63.

Giovannucci, E., et al. 2008. 25-hydroxyvitamin D and risk of myocardial infarction in men: A prospective study. *Archives of Internal Medicine* 168:1174–80.

Girgis, C. M., et al. Effects of vitamin D in skeletal muscle: Falls, strength, athletic performance and insulin sensitivity. *Clinical Endocrinology* 80(2):169–81.

Gomez-Cabrera, M., et al. 2008. Oral administration of vitamin C decreases muscle mitochondrial biogenesis and hampers training-induced adaptions in endurance performance. *American Journal of Clinical Nutrition* 87:142–49.

Gorham, E., et al. 2007. Optimal vitamin D status for colorectal cancer prevention: A quantitative meta-analysis. *American Journal of Preventive Medicine* 32:210–6.

Grant, W., et al. 2007. An estimate of cancer mortality rate reductions in Europe and the US with 1,000 IU of oral vitamin D per day. *Recent Results in Cancer Research* 174:225–34.

Greenwald, P., et al. 2007. Clinical trials of vitamin and mineral supplements for cancer prevention. *American Journal of Clinical Nutrition* 85:314S–17S.

Gökbel, H., et al. 2010. The effects of coenzyme Q_{10} supplementation on performance during repeated bouts of supramaximal exercise in sedentary men. *Journal of Strength and Conditioning Research* 24:97–102.

Gridley, G., et al. 1992. Vitamin supplement use and reduced risk of oral and pharyngeal cancer. *American Journal of Epidemiology* 135:1083–92.

Grodstein, F., et al. 2013. A randomized trial of long-term multivitamin supplementation and cognitive function in men: The Physicians' Health Study II. *Annals of Internal Medicine* 159 (12):806–14.

Guyton, J., and Bays, H. 2007. Safety considerations with niacin therapy. *American Journal of Cardiology* 99:22C–31C.

Gül, I., et al. 2011. Oxidative stress and antioxidant defense in plasma after repeated bouts of supramaximal exercise: The effect of coenzyme Q_{10}. *Journal of Sports Medicine and Physical Fitness* 51:305–12.

Halliday, T., et al. 2011. Vitamin D status relative to diet, lifestyle, injury, and illness in college athletes. *Medicine and Science in Sports and Exercise* 43:335–43.

Halliwell, B. 1996. Oxidative stress, nutrition and health: Experimental strategies for optimization of nutritional antioxidant intake in humans. *Free Radical Research* 25:57–74.

Hamilton, K. 2007. Antioxidants and cardioprotection. *Medicine and Science in Sports and Exercise* 39:1544–53.

Haralambie, G. 1976. Vitamin B_2 status in athletes and the influence of riboflavin administration on neuromuscular irritability. *Nutrition and Metabolism* 20:1–8.

Harris, S. 2005. Vitamin D in type 1 diabetes prevention. *Journal of Nutrition* 135:323–25.

Harrison, F. E., et al. 2014. Ascorbic acid and the brain: Rationale for the use against cognitive decline. *Nutrients* 6:1752–81.

Hathcock, J. 1997. Vitamins and minerals: Efficacy and safety. *American Journal of Clinical Nutrition* 66:427–37.

Hathcock, J., et al. 2007. Risk assessment for vitamin D. *American Journal of Clinical Nutrition* 85:6–18.

Heaney, R. 2005. The vitamin D requirement in health and disease. *Journal of Steroid Biochemistry and Molecular Biology* 97:13–19.

Heaney, R., 2007. Bone health. *American Journal of Clinical Nutrition* 85:300S–303S.

Heath, E., et al. 1993. Effect of nicotinic acid on respiratory exchange ratio and substrate levels during exercise. *Medicine and Science in Sport and Exercise* 25:1018–23.

Herbert, V. 1993. Viewpoint: Does mega-C do more good than harm, or more harm than good? *Nutrition Today* 28 (January/February):28–32.

Holick, M. 2006. Vitamin D. In *Modern Nutrition in Health and Disease,* ed. M. Shils, et al. Philadelphia: Lippincott Williams & Wilkins.

Holick, M., and Chen, T. 2008. Vitamin D deficiency: A worldwide problem with health consequences. *American Journal of Clinical Nutrition* 87:1080S–86S.

Hollis, B., et al. 2011. Vitamin D supplementation during pregnancy: Double-blind, randomized clinical trial of safety and effectiveness. *Journal of Bone Mineral Research* Epub June 27.

Hunninghake, D. 1999. Pharmacologic management of triglycerides. *Clinical Cardiology* 22(6 Suppl):II44–II48.

Huo, Y., et al. 2015. Efficacy of folic acid therapy in primary prevention of stroke among adults with hypertension in China. *Journal of the American Medical Association* doi:10.1001/jama.2274.

Hyang, H., et al. 2006. The efficacy and safety of multivitamin and mineral supplement use to prevent cancer and chronic disease in adults: A systematic review for a National Institutes of Health state-of-the-science conferences. *Annals of Internal Medicine* 145:372–85.

Ilavazhagan, G., et al. 2001. Effect of vitamin E supplementation on hypoxia-induced oxidative damage in male albino rats. *Aviation Space and Environmental Medicine* 72 (10):899–903.

Itoh, H., et al. 2000. Vitamin E supplementation attenuates leakage of enzymes following 6 successive days of running training. *International Journal of Sport Medicine* 21:369–74.

Jackson, C., et al. 2007. The effect of cholecalciferol (vitamin D3) on the risk of fall and fracture: A meta-analysis. *Quarterly Journal of Medicine* 100:185–92.

Jackson, M., et al. 2004. Vitamin E and the oxidative stress of exercise. *Annals of the New York Academies of Sciences* 1031:158–68.

Jacobson, B., et al. 2001. Nutrition practices and knowledge of college varsity athletes: A follow-up. *Journal of Strength and Conditioning Research* 15:63–68.

Jacob, R. 1999. Vitamin C. In *Modern Nutrition in Health and Disease,* ed. M. Shils et al. Baltimore: Williams & Wilkins.

Jacques, P. 1999. The potential preventive effects of vitamins for cataract and age-related macular degeneration. *International Journal of Vitamin and Nutrition Research* 69:198–205.

Jäger, R., et al. 2007. Phospholipids and sports performance. *Journal of the International Society of Sports Nutrition* 25 (4):5 doi:10.1186/1550-2783-4-5.

Ji, L. 2000. Free radicals and antioxidants in exercise and sports. In *Exercise and Sport Science,* ed. W. Garrett and D. Kirkendall. Philadelphia: Lippincott Williams & Wilkins.

Ji, L. 2002. Exercise-induced modulation of antioxidant defense. *New York Academies of Sciences* 959:82–92.

Ji, L. 2008. Modulation of skeletal muscle antioxidant defense by exercise: Role of redox signaling. *Free Radicals in Biology and Medicine* 44:142–52.

Ji, Y., et al. 2013. Vitamin B supplementation, homocysteine levels, and the risk of cerebrovascular disease: A meta-analysis. Neurology 81 (15):1298–307.

Johnston, C., et al. 1998. Vitamin C status of a campus population: College students get a C minus. *Journal of the American College of Health* 46:209–13.

Johnson, E.J. 2014. Role of lutein and zeaxanthin in visual and cognitive function throughout the lifespan. *Nutrition Reviews* 72(9):605–12.

Joubert, L., and Manore, M. 2006. Exercise, nutrition, and homocysteine. *International Journal of Sport Nutrition and Exercise Metabolism* 16:341–61.

Kaikkonen, J., et al. 1998. Effect of combined coenzyme Q_{10} and d-alpha-tocopheryl acetate supplementation on exercise-induced lipid peroxidation and muscular damage: A placebo-controlled double-blind study in marathon runners. *Free Radical Research* 29:85–92.

Kamangar, F., and Emadi, A. 2012. Vitamin and mineral supplements: Do we really need them? *International Journal of Preventive Medicine* 3 (3):221–26.

Kaya, Y., et al. 2012. Correlations between oxidative DNA damage, oxidative stress and coenzyme Q_{10} in patients with coronary artery disease. *International Journal of Medical Sciences* 9 (8):621–26.

Keene, K. L., et al. 2014. Genetic associations with plasma B_{12}, B_6, and folate levels in an ischemic stroke population from the Vitamin Intervention for Stroke Prevention (VISP) trial. *Frontiers in Public Health* 2:112. doi: 10.3389/fpubh.2014.00112.

Keith, R. 1994. Vitamins and physical activity. In *Nutrition in Exercise and Sport,* ed. I. Wolinsky and J. Hickson. Boca Raton, FL: CRC Press.

Kimmick, G., et al. 1997. Vitamin E and breast cancer: A review. *Nutrition and Cancer* 27:109–17.

Knez, W., et al. 2007. Oxidative stress in half and full Ironman triathletes. *Medicine and Science in Sports and Exercise* 39:283–88.

Kobayashi, Y. 1974. Effect of vitamin E on aerobic work performance in man during acute exposure to hypoxic hypoxia. Unpublished doctoral dissertation. University of New Mexico.

Kolka, M., and Stephenson, L. 1990. Skin blood flow during exercise after niacin ingestion. *FASEB Journal* 4:A279.

Koltover, V. 1992. Free radical theory of aging: View against the reliability theory. *Experientia Supplementum* 62:11–19.

Kressier, J., et al. 2011. Quercetin and endurance exercise capacity: A systematic review and meta-analysis. *Medicine and Science in Sports and Exercise* 43 (12):2396–404.

Kris-Etherton, P., et al. 2004. Antioxidant vitamin supplements and cardiovascular disease. *Circulation* 110:637–41.

Krumbach, C., et al. 1999. A report of vitamin and mineral supplement use among university athletes in a Division I institution. *International Journal of Sport Nutrition* 9:416–25.

Kurl, S., et al. 2002. Plasma vitamin C modifies the association between hypertension and risk of stroke. *Stroke* 33:1568–73.

La Fata, G., et al. 2014. Effects of vitamin E on cognitive performance during ageing and in Alzheimer's Disease. *Nutrients* 6:5453–72.

Laaksonen, R., et al. 1995. Ubiquinone supplementation and exercise capacity in trained young and older men. *European Journal of Applied Physiology* 72:95–100.

Lam, J. R., et al. 2013. Proton pump inhibitor and histamine 2 receptor antagonist use and vitamin B_{12} deficiency. *Journal of the American Medical Association* 310(22):2435–42.

Lappe, J., et al. 2007. Vitamin D and calcium supplementation reduces cancer risk: Results of a randomized trial. *American Journal of Clinical Nutrition* 85:1586–91.

Larson-Meyer, D., and Willis, K. 2010. Vitamin D and athletes. *Current Sports Medicine Reports* 9:220–6.

Lawson, K., et al. 2007. Multivitamin use and risk of prostate cancer in the National Institutes of Health-AARP Diet and Health Study. *Journal of the National Cancer Institute* 99:754–64.

Lee, I. 1999. Antioxidant vitamins in the prevention of cancer. *Proceedings of the American Association of Physicians* 111:10–15.

Lee, I., et al. 2005. Vitamin E in the primary prevention of cardiovascular disease and cancer: The Women's Health Study: A randomized controlled trial. *Journal of the American Medical Association* 294:56–65.

Leonard, S., and Leklem, J. 2000. Plasma B-6 vitamer changes following a 50-km ultra-marathon. *International Journal of Sport Nutrition and Exercise Metabolism* 10:302–14.

Levine, M., et al. 2006. Vitamin C. In *Modern Nutrition in Health and Disease,* ed. M. Shils et al. Philadelphia: Lippincott Williams & Wilkins.

Liebman, B. 2003. Spin the bottle: How to pick a multivitamin. *Nutrition Action Health Letter* 30 (1):1–9.

Liebman, B. 2006. Are you deficient? *Nutrition Action Health Letter* 33 (9):1–7.

Liebman, B., and Hurley, J. 2002. Vegetables: Vitamin K weighs in. *Nutrition Action Health Letter* 29 (6):13–15.

Liebman, B., and Schardt, D. 2008. Multi-complex: Picking a multivitamin gets tricky. *Nutrition Action Health Letter* 35 (5):1–9.

Linnane, A., et al. 2007. The essential requirement for superoxide radical and nitric oxide formation for normal physiological function and healthy aging. *Mitochondrion* 7:1–5.

Lonn, E., et al. 2005. Effects of long-term vitamin E supplementation on cardiovascular events and cancer: A randomized controlled trial. *Journal of the American Medical Association* 293:1338–47.

Looker, A. C., et al. 2011. Vitamin D status: United States, 2001–2006. NCHS data brief, no 59. Hyattsville, MD: National Center for Health Statistics.

Losonczy, K., et al. 1996. Vitamin E and vitamin C supplement use and risk of all cause and coronary heart disease mortality in older persons: The Established Populations for Epidemiologic Studies of the Elderly. *American Journal of Clinical Nutrition* 64:190–96.

Machefer, G., et al. 2007. Multivitamin-mineral supplementation prevents lipid peroxidation during "the Marathon des Sables." *Journal of the American College of Nutrition* 26:111–20.

Malm, C., et al. 1996. Supplementation with ubiquinone-10 causes cellular damage during intense exercise. *Acta Physiologica Scandinavica* 157:511–12.

Manore, M. 1994. Vitamin B_6 and exercise. *International Journal of Sport Nutrition* 4:89–103.

Manore, M. 2001. Vitamins and minerals: Part I. How much do I need? *ACSM's Health and Fitness Journal* 5 (3):33–35.

Manore, M. 2001. Vitamins and minerals: Part II. Who needs to supplement? *ACSM's Health and Fitness Journal* 5 (4):30–34.

Manore, M. 2001. Vitamins and minerals: Part III. Can you get too much? *ACSM's Health and Fitness Journal* 5 (5):26–28.

Massey, L., et al. 2005. Ascorbate increases human oxaluria and kidney stone risk. *Journal of Nutrition* 135:1673–77.

Mastaloudis, A., et al. 2006. Antioxidants did not prevent muscle damage in response to an ultramarathon run. *Medicine and Science in Sports and Exercise* 38:72–80.

Matter, M., et al. 1987. The effect of iron and folate therapy on maximal exercise performance in female marathon runners with iron and folate deficiency. *Clinical Science* 72:415–22.

Mayne, S. 1996. Beta-carotene, carotenoids, and disease prevention in humans. *FASEB Journal* 10:690–701.

McCormick, D. 2006. Riboflavin. In *Modern Nutrition in Health and Disease,* ed. M. Shils et al. Philadelphia: Lippincott Williams & Wilkins.

McGinley, C., et al. 2009. Does antioxidant vitamin supplementation protect against muscle damage? *Sports Medicine* 39:1011–32.

McKenney, J. 2004. New perspectives on the use of niacin in the treatment of lipid disorders. *Archives of Internal Medicine* 164:697–705.

McKinley, M., et al. 2001. Low-dose vitamin B-6 effectively lowers fasting plasma homocysteine in healthy elderly persons who are folate and riboflavin replete. *American Journal of Clinical Nutrition* 73:759–64.

McMahon, J., et al. 2007. Lowering homocysteine with B vitamins has no effect on blood pressure in older adults. *Journal of Nutrition* 137:1183–87.

McMahon, R. 2002. Biotin in metabolism and molecular biology. *Annual Review of Nutrition* 22:221–39.

Meagher, E., et al. 2001. Effects of vitamin E on lipid peroxidation in healthy persons. *Journal of the American Medical Association* 285:1178–82.

Mehta, J. 1999. Antioxidants are useful in preventing cardiovascular disease: A debate. Con antioxidants. *Canadian Journal of Cardiology* 15:26B–28B.

Meydani, S. 1995. Vitamin E enhancement of T cell-mediated function in healthy elderly: Mechanisms of action. *Nutrition Reviews* 53:S52–S58.

Miller, E., et al. 2005. Meta-analysis: High-dosage vitamin E supplementation may increase all-cause mortality. *Annals of Internal Medicine* 142:37–46.

Mock, D. 2006. Biotin. In *Modern Nutrition in Health and Disease,* ed. M. Shils, et al. Philadelphia: Lippincott Williams & Wilkins.

Moran, D. S., et al. 2013. Vitamin D and physical performance. *Sports Medicine* 43:601–11.

Morris, M., et al. 1998. Vitamin E and vitamin C supplement use and risk of incident Alzheimer disease. *Alzheimer Disease and Associated Disorders* 12:121–26.

Morris, M., et al. 2002. Dietary intake of antioxidant nutrients and the risk of incident Alzheimer disease in a biracial community study. *Journal of the American Medical Association* 287:3230–37.

Mulholland, C., and Benford, D. 2007. What is known about the safety of multivitamin-multimineral supplements for the generally healthy population? Theoretical basis for harm. *American Journal of Clinical Nutrition* 85:318S–22S.

Munoz, F., et al. 2005. The protective effect of vitamin E in vascular amyloid beta-mediated damage. *Subcellular Biochemestry* 38:147–65.

National Institutes of Health. 2006. National Institutes of Health State-of-the-Science conference statement: Multivitamin/mineral supplements and chronic disease prevention. *Annals of Internal Medicine* 145:364–71.

Neiss, A. 2005. Generation and disposal of reactive oxygen and nitrogen species. In *Molecular and Cellular Exercise Physiology,* ed. F. Mooren and K. Völker. Champaign, IL: Human Kinetics.

Ness, A., et al. 1997. Vitamin C and blood pressure: An overview. *Journal of Human Hypertension* 11:342–50.

Nieman, D. 2001. Exercise immunology: Nutritional countermeasures. *Canadian Journal of Applied Physiology* 26:S45–55.

Nieman, D., et al. 2002. Influence of vitamin C supplementation on oxidative and immune changes after an ultramarathon. *Journal of Applied Physiology* 92:1970–77.

Nieman, D., et al. 2004. Vitamin E and immunity after the Kona Triathlon World Championship. *Medicine and Science in Sports and Exercise* 36:1328–35.

Nieman, D., et al. 2007. Quercetin ingestion does not alter cytokine changes in athletes competing in the Western States Endurance Run. *Journal of Interferon and Cyokine Research* 27:1003–11.

Nieman, D., et al. 2007. Quercetin reduces illness, but not immune perturbations after intensive exercise. *Medicine and Science in Sports and Exercise* 39:1561–69.

Nieman, D., et al. 2007. Quercetin's influence on exercise-induced changes in plasma cytokines and muscle and leukocyte cytokine mRNA. *Journal of Applied Physiology* 103:1728–35.

Nikolaidis, M. G., et al. 2012. Does vitamin C and E supplementation impair the favorable adaptations of regular exercise? *Oxidative Medicine and Cellular Longevity* 2012:707941 doi:10.1155/2012/707941.

Office of Dietary Supplements, National Institutes of Health. 2011. Dietary supplement fact sheet: Vitamin D. http://ods.od.nih.gov/factsheets/vitamind/.

Ogan, D., and Pritchett, K. 2013. Vitamin D and the athlete: Risks, recommendations, and benefits. *Nutrients* 5 (6):1856–68.

Onur, S., et al. 2014. Ubiquinol reduces gamma glutamyltransferase as a marker of oxidative stress in humans. *Biomedical Central Research Notes* 7:427. doi: 10.1186/1756-0500-7-427.

Paganini-Hill, A., and Perez Barreto, M. 2001. Stroke risk in older men and women: Aspirin, estrogen, exercise, vitamins, and other factors. *Journal of Gender-Specific Medicine* 4:18–28.

Patterson, R., et al. 1998. Cancer-related behavior of vitamin supplement users. *Cancer Epidemiology, Biomarkers and Prevention* 7:79–81.

Paulsen, G., et al. 2014. Vitamin C and E supplementation hampers cellular adaptation to endurance training in humans: A double-blind, randomized, controlled trial. *Journal of Physiology* 592 (8):1887–901.

Peake, J. 2003. Vitamin C: Effects of exercise and requirements with training. *International Journal of Sport Nutrition and Exercise Metabolism* 13:125–51.

Pelletier, D. M., et al. 2013. Effects of quercetin supplementation on endurance performance and maximal oxygen consumption: A meta-analysis. *International Journal of Sport Nutrition and Exercise Metabolism* 23 (1):73–82.

Penry, J., and Manore, M. 2008. Choline: An important micronutrient for maximal endurance-exercise performance. *International Journal of Sport Nutrition and Exercise Metabolism* 18:191–203.

Peters, E., et al. 1993. Vitamin C supplementation reduces the incidence of postrace symptoms of upper-respiratory-tract infection in ultramarathon runners. *American Journal of Clinical Nutrition* 57:170–74.

Petersen, R., et al. 2005. Vitamin E and donepezil for the treatment of mild cognitive impairment. *New England Journal of Medicine* 352:2379–88.

Pieper, J. 2002. Understanding niacin formulations. *American Journal of Management Care* 8:S308–14.

Pincemail, J., et al. 1988. Tocopherol mobilization during intensive exercise. *European Journal of Applied Physiology* 57:188–91.

Powers, S., et al. 2004. Dietary antioxidants and exercise. *Journal of Sports Sciences* 22:81–94.

Prasad, K., et al. 1999. High doses of multiple antioxidant vitamins: Essential ingredients in improving the efficacy of standard cancer therapy. *Journal of the American College of Nutrition* 18:13–25.

Pryor, W. A. 1991. Can vitamin E protect humans against the pathological effects of ozone in smog? *American Journal of Clinical Nutrition* 53:702–22.

Qin, X., et al. 2013. Folic acid supplementation and cancer risk: A meta-analysis of randomized controlled trials. *International Journal of Cancer* 133:1033–42.

Rafnsson, S., et al. 2013. Antioxidant nutrients and age-related cognitive decline: A systematic review of population-based cohort studies. *European Journal of Nutrition* 52:1553–67.

Raiten, D., and Picciano, M. 2004. Vitamin D and health in the 21st century: Bone and beyond. *American Journal of Clinical Nutrition* 80:1673S–77S.

Reichrath, J., et al. 2007. Vitamins as hormones. *Hormone and Metabolic Research* 39:71–84.

Rimm, E., and Stampfer, M. 1997. The role of antioxidants in preventive cardiology. *Current Opinion in Cardiology* 12:188–94.

Rock, C. 2007. Multivitamin-multimineral supplements: Who uses them? *American Journal of Clinical Nutrition* 85:277S–79S.

Rodrigo, R., et al. 2007. Clinical pharmacology and therapeutic use of antioxidant vitamins. *Fundamental and Clinical Pharmacology* 21:111–27.

Rokitzki, L., et al. 1994. α-tocopherol supplementation in racing cyclists during extreme endurance training. *International Journal of Sport Nutrition* 4:253–64.

Rokitzki, L., et al. 1994. Acute changes in vitamin B_6 status in endurance athletes before and after a marathon. *International Journal of Sport Nutrition* 4:154–65.

Ross, A. 2006. Vitamin A and retinoids. In *Modern Nutrition in Health and Disease,* ed. M. Shils et al. Philadelphia: Lippincott Williams & Wilkins.

Rothenberg, S. 1999. Increasing the dietary intake of folate: Pros and cons. *Seminars in Hematology* 36:65–74.

Rothman, K., et al. 1995. Teratogenicity of high vitamin A intake. *New England Journal of Medicine* 333:1369–73.

Sacheck, J., and Blumberg, J. 2001. Role of vitamin E and oxidative stress in exercise. *Nutrition* 17:809–14.

Schardt, D. 2006. Supplementing their income: How celebrities turn trust into cash. *Nutrition Action Health Letter* 33 (1):1–6.

Schmelzer, C., and Döring, F. 2012. Micronutrient special issue: Coenzyme Q_{10} requirements for DNA damage prevention. *Mutation Research/ Fundamental and Molecular Mechanisms of Mutagenesis* 733:61–68.

Schwammenthal, Y., and Tanne, D. 2004. Homocysteine B-vitamin supplementation, and stroke prevention: From observational to interventional trials. *Lancet Neurology* 3:493–95.

Schwartz, B., and Skinner, H. 2007. Vitamin D status and cancer: New insights. *Current Opinion in Clinical Nutrition and Metabolic Care* 10:6–11.

Schürks, M., et al. 2010. Effects of vitamin E on stroke subtypes: Meta-analysis of randomised controlled trials. *British Medical Journal* 341:c5702.

Sebastian, R., et al. 2007. Older adults who use vitamin/mineral supplements differ from nonusers in nutrient intake adequacy and dietary attitudes. *Journal of the American Dietetic Association* 107:1322–32.

Seddon, J. 2007. Multivitamin-multimineral supplements and eye disease: Age-related macular degeneration and cataract. *American Journal of Clinical Nutrition* 85:304S–7S.

Sen, C., et al. 2000. Exercise-induced oxidative stress and antioxidant nutrients. In *Nutrition in Sport,* ed. R. Maughan. Oxford: Blackwell Science.

Sen, C., et al. 2006. Tocotrienols: Vitamin E beyond tocopherols. *Life Sciences* 78:2088–98.

Sen, C., et al. 2007. Tocotrienols: The emerging face of natural vitamin E. *Vitamins and Hormones* 76:203–61.

Short, S. 1994. Surveys of dietary intake and nutrition knowledge of athletes and their coaches. In *Nutrition in Exercise and Sport,* ed. I. Wolinsky and J. Hickson. Boca Raton, FL: CRC Press.

Shindle, M., et al. 2011. Vitamin D status in a professional American football team. *Proceedings from the AOSSM Annual Meeting* ID 46-9849.

Simon-Schnass, I. 1993. Vitamin requirements for increased physical activity: Vitamin E. In *Nutrition and Fitness for Athletes,* ed. A. Simopoulos and K. Pavlou. Basel, Switzerland: Karger.

Simon-Schnass, I., and Pabst, H. 1988. Influence of vitamin E on physical performance. *International Journal for Vitamin and Nutrition Research* 58:49–54.

Singh, A., et al. 1992. Chronic multivitamin-mineral supplementation does not enhance physical performance. *Medicine and Science in Sport and Exercise* 24:726–32.

Singh, U., and Devaraj, S. 2007. Vitamin E: Inflammation and atherosclerosis. *Vitamins and Hormones* 76:519–49.

Snider, I., et al. 1992. Effects of coenzyme athletic performance system as an ergogenic aid on endurance performance to exhaustion. *International Journal of Sport Nutrition* 2:272–86.

Sobol, J., and Marquart, L. 1994. Vitamin/ mineral supplement use among athletes: A review of the literature. *International Journal of Sport Nutrition* 4:320–34.

Steinmetz, K., and Potter, J. 1996. Vegetables, fruit, and cancer prevention: A review. *Journal of the American Dietetic Association* 96:1027–39.

Stepanyan, V., et al. 2014. Effects of vitamin E supplementation on exercise-induced oxidative stress: A meta-analysis. *Applied Physiology, Nutrition, and Metabolism* 39 (9):1029–37.

Suttie, J. 2006. Vitamin K. In *Modern Nutrition in Health and Disease,* ed. M. Shils et al. Philadelphia: Lippincott Williams & Wilkins.

Suzuki, M., and Itokawa, Y. 1996. Effects of thiamine supplementation on exercise-induced fatigue. *Metabolism in Brain Diseases* 11:95–106.

Svensson, M., et al. 1999. Effect of Q_{10} supplementation on tissue Q_{10} levels and adenine nucleotide catabolism during high-intensity exercise. *International Journal of Sport Nutrition* 9:166–80.

Takanami, Y., et al. 2000. Vitamin E supplementation and endurance exercise: Are there benefits? *Sports Medicine* 29:73–83.

Tanphaichitr, V. 1999. Thiamin. In *Modern Nutrition in Health and Disease,* ed.

M. Shils et al. Philadelphia: Lippincott Williams & Wilkins.

Telford, R., et al. 1992. The effect of 7 to 8 months of vitamin/mineral supplementation on athletic performance. *International Journal of Sport Nutrition* 2:135–53.

Telford, R., et al. 1992. The effect of 7 to 8 months of vitamin/mineral supplementation on the vitamin and mineral status of athletes. *International Journal of Sport Nutrition* 2:123–34.

Tiidus, P., and Houston, M. 1995. Vitamin E status and response to exercise training. *Sports Medicine* 20:12–23.

Todd, J. J., et al. 2015. Vitamin D: Recent advances and implications for athletes. *Sports Medicine* 45:213–29.

Tomlinson, P. B., et al. 2014. Effects of vitamin D supplementation on upper and lower body muscle strength levels in healthy individuals. A systematic review with meta-analysis. *Journal of Science and Medicine in Sport* doi: 10.1016/j.jsams.2014.07.022. [Epub ahead of print]

Traber, M. 2006. Vitamin E. In *Modern Nutrition in Health and Disease,* ed. M. Shils et al. Philadelphia: Lippincott Williams & Wilkins.

Traber, M. 2007. Heart disease and single-vitamin supplementation. *American Journal of Clinical Nutrition* 85:293S–99S.

Tran, M., et al. 2001. Role of coenzyme Q_{10} in chronic heart failure, angina, and hypertension. *Pharmacotherapy* 21:797–806.

Tremblay, A., et al. 1984. The effects of a riboflavin supplementation on the nutritional status and performance of elite swimmers. *Nutrition Research* 4:201.

Trumbo, P., and Ellwood, K. 2006. Lutein and zeaxanthin intakes and risk of age-related macular degeneration and cataracts: An evaluation using the Food and Drug Administration's evidence-based review system for health claims. *American Journal of Clinical Nutrition* 84:971–74.

Tufts University. 2002. Antioxidant supplements lose promise as disease preventers. *Tufts University Health and Nutrition Letter* 20 (1):4–5.

Tufts University. 2007. Antioxidant supplements—Now what? *Tufts University Health and Nutrition Letter* 25 (4):4–5.

van der Beek, E., et al. 1988. Thiamin, riboflavin, and vitamins B_6 and C: Impact of combined restricted intake on functional performance in man. *American Journal of Clinical Nutrition* 48:1451–62.

van der Beek, E. 1991. Vitamin supplementation and physical exercise performance. *Journal of Sports Sciences* 92:77–79.

van der Beek, E. J., et al. 1994. Thiamin, riboflavin and vitamin B_6: Impact of restricted intake on physical performance in man. *Journal of the American College of Nutrition* 13 (6):629–40.

van Erp-Baart, A., et al. 1989. Nationwide survey on nutritional habits in elite athletes. *International Journal of Sports Medicine* 10 (Suppl 1):S11–S16.

Verhaar, H., et al. 2000. Muscle strength, functional mobility and vitamin D in older women. *Aging* 12:455–60.

Vieth, R., and Fraser, D. 2002. Vitamin D insufficiency: No recommended dietary allowance exists for this nutrient. *Canadian Medical Association Journal* 166:1541–42.

Viitala, P., and Newhouse, I. 2004. Vitamin E supplementation, exercise and lipid peroxidation in human participants. *European Journal of Applied Physiology* 93:108–15.

Virk, R., et al. 1999. Effect of vitamin B-6 supplementation on fuels, catecholamines, and amino acids during exercise in men. *Medicine and Science in Sports and Exercise* 31:400–8.

Volpe, S. 2007. Micronutrient requirements for athletes. *Clinics in Sports Medicine* 26:119–30.

von Hurst, P. R., and Beck, K. L. 2014. Vitamin D and skeletal muscle function in athletes. *Current Opinion in Clinical Nutrition and Metabolic Care* 17 (6):539–45.

Wactawshi-Wende, J., et al. 2006. Calcium plus vitamin D supplementation and the risk of colorectal cancer. *New England Journal of Medicine* 354:684–96.

Wall, B. T., et al. 2012. Acute pantothenic acid and cysteine supplementation does not affect muscle coenzyme A content, fuel selection, or exercise performance in healthy humans. *Journal of Applied Physiology* 112 (2):272–78.

Wang, X., et al. 2007. Efficacy of folic acid supplementation in stroke prevention: A meta-analysis. *Lancet* 369:1876–82.

Warber, J., et al. 2000. The effects of choline supplementation on physical performance. *International Journal of Sport Nutrition and Exercise Metabolism* 10:170–81.

Watson, T., et al. 2005. Antioxidant restriction and oxidative stress in short-duration exhaustive exercise. *Medicine and Science in Sports and Exercise* 37:63–71.

Webb, D. 1997. Coenzyme Q_{10}: Miracle nutrient or merely promising? *Environmental Nutrition* 20 (11):1, 4.

Weber, P. 1996. Vitamin C and human health: A review of recent data relevant to human requirements. *International Journal of Vitamin and Nutrition Research* 66:19–30.

Weber, P. 2001. Vitamin K and bone health. *Nutrition* 17:880–87.

Webster, M. 1998. Physiological and performance responses to supplementation with thiamin and pantothenic acid derivatives. *European Journal of Applied Physiology* 77:486–91.

Webster, M., et al. 1997. The effect of a thiamin derivative on exercise performance. *European Journal of Applied Physiology* 75:520–24.

Weight, L., et al. 1988. Vitamin and mineral supplementation: Effect on the running performance of trained athletes. *American Journal of Clinical Nutrition* 47:192–95.

Weston, S., et al. 1997. Does exogenous coenzyme Q_{10} affect aerobic capacity in endurance athletes? *International Journal of Sport Nutrition* 7:197–206.

Wierzbicki, A. 2007. Homocysteine and cardiovascular disease: A review of the evidence. *Diabetes and Vascular Disease Research* 4:143–50.

Williams, M. 1989. Vitamin supplementation and athletic performance. *International Journal for Vitamin and Nutrition Research,* Supplement 30:161–91.

Williams, M. 2011. Sports supplements: Quercetin. *ACSM Health & Fitness Journal.* 15(5):17–20.

Williams, S., et al. 2006. Antioxidant requirements of endurance athletes: Implications for health. *Nutrition Reviews* 64:93–108.

Willis, K., et al. 2008. Should we be concerned about the vitamin D status of athletes? *International Journal of Sport Nutrition and Exercise Metabolism* 18:204–24.

Woolf, K., and Manore, M. 2006. B-vitamins and exercise: Does exercise alter requirements? *International Journal of Sport Nutrition and Exercise Metabolism* 16:453–84.

Wyatt, K., et al. 1999. Efficacy of vitamin B-6 in the treatment of premenstrual syndrome: Systematic review. *British Medical Journal* 318:1375–81.

Yetley, E. 2007. Multivitamin and multimineral dietary supplements: Definitions, characterization, bioavailability, and drug interactions. *American Journal of Clinical Nutrition* 85:269S–76S.

Ylikoski, T., et al. 1997. The effect of coenzyme Q_{10} on the exercise performance of cross-country skiers. *Molecular Aspects of Medicine* 18:S283–90.

Zachman, R., and Grummer, M. 1998. The interaction of ethanol and vitamin A as a potential mechanism for the pathogenesis of fetal alcohol syndrome. *Alcoholism,*

Clinical and Experimental Research 22:1544–56.

Zeisel, S., and Niculescu, M. 2006. Choline and phosphatidylcholine. In *Modern Nutrition in Health and Disease,* ed. M. Shils et al. Philadelphia: Lippincott Williams & Wilkins.

Zeng, R., et al. 2014. The effect of folate fortification on folic acid-based homocysteine-lowering intervention and stroke risk: A meta-analysis. *Public Health Nutrition* 17:1–8.

Zhang, S., et al. 1999. A prospective study of folate intake and the risk of breast cancer. *Journal of the American Medical Association* 281:1632–37.

Zhao, L. Q., et al. 2014. The effect of multivitamin/mineral supplements on age-related cataracts: A systematic review and meta-analysis. *Nutrients* 6 (3):931–49.

Zhou, S., et al. 2005. Muscle and plasma coenzyme Q_{10} concentration, aerobic power and exercise economy of healthy men in response to four weeks of supplementation. *Journal of Sports Medicine and Physical Fitness* 45:337–46.

Ziegler, P., et al. 2002. Nutritional status of teenage female competitive figure skaters. *Journal of the American Dietetic Association* 102:374–79.

Zittermann, A. 2001. Effects of vitamin K on calcium and bone metabolism. *Current Opinion in Clinical Nutrition and Metabolic Care* 4:483–87.

Zoppi, C., et al. 2006. Vitamin C and E supplementation effects in professional soccer players under regular training. *Journal of the International Society of Sports Nutrition* 3:37–44.

Minerals: The Inorganic Regulators

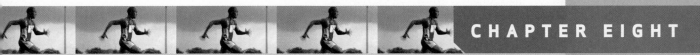

CHAPTER EIGHT

LEARNING OBJECTIVES

After studying this chapter, you should be able to:

1. Describe the various means whereby minerals may carry out their functions in the human body.

2. Name the essential minerals, state the RDA or AI for each, and identify several foods rich in each mineral.

3. Describe the metabolic roles in the human body of calcium, phosphorus, magnesium, iron, copper, zinc, chromium, selenium, manganese, fluoride, and iodine.

4. Explain the role of calcium in bone metabolism and identify the factors that may contribute to bone health and those that may contribute to osteoporosis.

5. Explain the theory as to how phosphate salt supplementation may enhance sports performance and highlight the research findings regarding its ergogenic efficacy.

6. Explain the potential effects on health and sports performance associated with a deficiency of each trace mineral.

7. Explain the theory as to how iron, zinc, chromium, selenium, boron, and vanadium may enhance sports performance and highlight the research findings regarding the ergogenic efficacy of each.

8. Understand why health professionals may recommend mineral supplements under certain circumstances to improve the health of some individuals.

You may recall the periodic table of the elements hanging on the wall in your high school or college chemistry class. At latest count there were 118 known elements, 78 of them occurring naturally and the remainder being synthetic. Many of the natural elements, including a wide variety of minerals, are essential to human bodily structure and function. For example, calcium and phosphorus are main constituents of bone, while iron, magnesium, zinc and other minerals are cofactors of hundreds of enzymes regulating numerous body functions.

Much research attention is currently being devoted to the role of mineral nutrition in health and disease, including both epidemiological and laboratory research. For example, using the RDA as a basis for comparison, national surveys among the general population have revealed that either an inadequate dietary intake of some minerals or an excessive dietary intake of others in certain small segments of the population may be contributing to several health problems. Laboratory studies using either animals or humans as subjects have explored the roles of both deficiencies and excesses of various minerals, including both essential and nonessential elements, on human health and disease processes.

An increasing number of research studies have been conducted with athletes to evaluate the effect of mineral nutrition on physical performance and the converse—the effect of exercise on mineral metabolism. Because some minerals function similarly to vitamins, a deficiency state could adversely affect performance. Moreover, exercise in itself may be a contributing factor to mineral deficiencies or impaired mineral metabolism in some types of athletes. Additionally, several mineral supplements have been marketed specifically for physically active individuals.

This chapter is especially important to all females and young athletes because it addresses two of their major dietary concerns: obtaining sufficient calcium and obtaining sufficient iron. These key minerals are of particular interest to females who participate in sports or are otherwise physically active. The female athlete triad—disordered eating, amenorrhea, and osteoporosis— is introduced in this chapter with the major focus on osteoporosis because of its relationship to calcium metabolism. An expanded discussion of eating disorders is presented in chapter 10. Female endurance athletes also need to obtain adequate dietary iron intake because of its important role in the oxygen energy system.

The major purpose of this chapter is to analyze the available data relative to the effect of mineral nutrition on physical performance and health. The first section discusses some basic facts about the general role of those minerals that are essential to human nutrition. The second and third sections cover, respectively, the major minerals and the trace minerals. In these two sections, each of the minerals is discussed in terms of its Dietary Reference Intake (DRI), good dietary sources, metabolic functions in the body with particular reference to the physically active individual, an evaluation of the research pertaining to the effects of deficiencies or supplementation on health or exercise performance, and prudent recommendations. The last section summarizes dietary mineral nutrition guidelines for those who exercise for health or sport.

Basic Facts

What are minerals, and what is their importance to humans?

A **mineral** is an inorganic element found in nature, and the term is usually reserved for those elements that are solid. Hence, a mineral is an element, but an element is not necessarily a mineral. For example, oxygen is an element, but it is not classified as a mineral. In nutrition, the term *mineral* is usually used to classify those dietary elements essential to life processes.

Minerals are found in the soil and are eventually incorporated in growing plants. Most animals get their mineral nutrition from the plants they eat, whereas humans obtain their supply from both plant and animal food. Drinking water may also be a good source of several minerals. As minerals are excreted daily from the body in sweat, urine, or feces, they must be replaced.

Minerals serve two of the three basic functions of nutrients in foods.

Growth and Development Many minerals are used as the building blocks for body tissues, such as bones, teeth, muscles, and other organic structures. In particular, calcium and phosphorus are important to bone health. Iron is an important component of hemoglobin, which is needed for optimal oxygen transport during aerobic endurance exercise.

Metabolic Regulation A number of minerals are involved in regulation of metabolic processes. Many are components of enzymes known as **metalloenzymes**, such as the cytochrome enzymes in the mitochondria that facilitate ATP production. Others, such as zinc and copper, are part of the natural antioxidant enzymes discussed in chapter 7. Still others exist as **ions**, or **electrolytes**, which are small particles carrying electrical charges. They are important components or activators of several enzymes and hormones. Speich and others reviewed the physiological roles of minerals important to athletes, noting that minerals are involved in muscle contraction, normal heart rhythm, nerve impulse conduction, oxygen transport, oxidative phosphorylation, enzyme activation, immune functions, antioxidant activity, bone health, acid-base balance of the blood, and maintenance of body water supplies. Figure 8.1 provides a broad overview of mineral function in the body.

Energy Minerals are comparable to vitamins relative to energy production in humans. Although minerals may play a significant role in the generation of energy via their metabolic functions, they do not provide a source of calorie energy.

Inadequate mineral nutrition has been associated with impairment of normal physiological functions, as well as with a variety of human diseases, including anemia, high blood pressure, obesity, diabetes, cancer, tooth decay, and osteoporosis. However, excessive intake of minerals may also contribute to significant health risks. Thus, proper dietary intake of essential minerals is necessary for optimal health and physical performance.

What minerals are essential to human nutrition?

Of all the elements in the periodic table, only 25 are currently known to be, or presumed to be, essential in humans. Five of these elements (hydrogen, oxygen, carbon, sulfur, nitrogen) make up the carbohydrate, fat, and protein that we eat and the water we drink. They are the elements of the body water, protein, fat, and carbohydrates stores, which constitute slightly more than 96 percent of the body weight. The remaining 20 minerals compose less than 4 percent of the body weight but are equally important.

Table 8.1 lists those minerals for which the National Academy of Sciences (NAS) has established a DRI or other recommendation. The DRIs include the Recommended Dietary Allowance (RDA), the Adequate Intake (AI), and the Tolerable Upper Intake Level (UL). The NAS has established the RDA or AI for most minerals discussed in this chapter, and for sodium, chloride, and potassium, elements that are discussed in the next chapter. Sulfur is found in the diet mainly as a component of the sulfur-containing amino acids (methionine and cysteine), and body needs are satisfied by the RDA for these amino acids.

Other minerals, such as boron, nickel, silicon, and vanadium, among others, are found in animal tissues and may be important to human nutrition, but their roles have not yet been completely elucidated, and thus no RDA or AI have yet been established. However, UL have been set for boron, nickel, and vanadium.

In general, how do deficiencies or excesses of minerals influence health or physical performance?

Similar to vitamin deficiencies, mineral deficiencies may occur in several stages. The first three stages (preliminary, biochemical deficiency, and physiological deficiency) may be termed subclinical malnutrition and may or may not have significant effects on health or physical performance. In the clinically manifest deficiency state, however, health and performance most likely will suffer.

The interaction of exercise and mineral nutrition may pose some special health problems, as we shall see in later sections of this chapter. In regard to the preliminary stage of a deficiency, some athletes may reduce their mineral intake as they shift toward

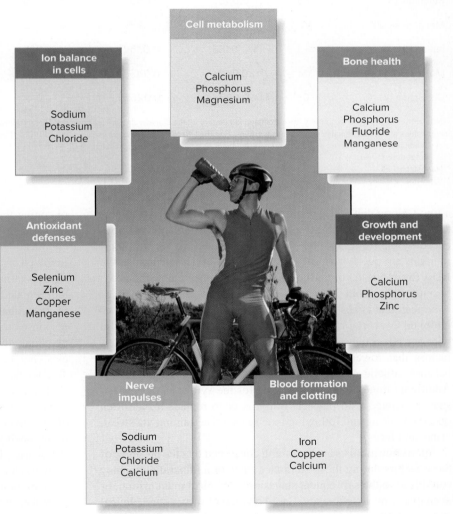

FIGURE 8.1 Minerals contribute to many functions in the body. Mineral deficiencies therefore lead to a variety of health problems and may impair physical performance.

Cell metabolism
Calcium
Phosphorus
Magnesium

Ion balance in cells
Sodium
Potassium
Chloride

Bone health
Calcium
Phosphorus
Fluoride
Manganese

Antioxidant defenses
Selenium
Zinc
Copper
Manganese

Growth and development
Calcium
Phosphorus
Zinc

Nerve impulses
Sodium
Potassium
Chloride
Calcium

Blood formation and clotting
Iron
Copper
Calcium

Mineral	Symbol	RDA or AI (mg)		Daily Value (mg)	UL (mg)	Amount in adult body (g)
Calcium (2)	Ca	1,000♂	1,000♀	1,000	2,500	1,500
Phosphorus (1)	P	700♂	700♀	1,000	4,000	850
Potassium (2)	K	4,700♂	4,700♀	3,500	ND	180
Chloride (2)	Cl	2,300♂	2,300♀	3,400	3,500	75
Sodium (2)	Na	1,500♂	1,500♀	<2,400	2,300	65
Magnesium (1)	Mg	420♂	320♀	400	350***	25
Iron (1)	Fe	8♂	18♀	18	45	5
Fluoride (2)	F	4♂	3.0♀	**	10	2.5
Zinc (1)	Zn	11♂	8♀	15	40	2
Copper (1)	Cu	0.9♂	0.9♀	2	10	0.1
Selenium (1)	Se	0.055♂	0.055♀	0.70	0.4	0.013
Manganese (2)	Mn	2.3♂	1.8♀	2	11	0.012
Iodine (1)	I	0.15♂	0.15♀	0.15	1.1	0.011
Molybdenum (1)	Mo	0.045♂	0.045♀	0.075	2	0.009
Chromium (2)	Cr	0.035♂	0.025♀	0.12	ND	0.006

*Different terms are used to quantify the recommended dietary intake of minerals: (1) Recommended Dietary Allowance (RDA); (2) Adequate Intake (AI). The UL listed is for adult males; lower values are set for females and other age groups. See the DRI tables at www.nal.usda.gov/fnic/DRI/DRI_Tables/DRI_Elements.pdf for more details. Arsenic, boron, nickel, silicon, and vanadium are also covered in the DRI reports, but no RDA or AI have been established. A UL has been set for boron, nickel, and vanadium.
ND = not determined.
**Not established.
***Only pharmacological form.

a low-Calorie diet. Changes in food selection may also be important, for the bioavailability of many minerals is markedly influenced by the form in which they are consumed. In general, most minerals are poorly absorbed from the intestine. For example, the RDA for iron is ten times the amount actually needed by the body, because only about 10 percent of dietary iron from the average American diet is absorbed. Moreover, mineral absorption may be inhibited by certain compounds in foods, and supplementation with one mineral may impair the absorption of another. In athletes, factors that lower intake and absorption may be compounded because athletic activity may raise some mineral requirements. Additional minerals may be needed for the synthesis of new tissues associated with physical training, or to replace losses often observed during and following intense exercise training via sweat, urine, and feces.

Sports nutritionists are becoming concerned that the presence of these factors during the preliminary stage of a mineral deficiency could lead to the subsequent stages of subclinical malnutrition, or even to a clinical deficiency. Based on dietary surveys and clinical studies with biochemical measures of mineral status, Pennington reported there is some concern for adequate calcium, iron, and zinc nutrition in some segments of the United States population. Most dietary surveys indicate that athletes, particularly males, are

obtaining the RDA for all minerals. However, a number of studies have reported athletes with inadequate dietary intake and biochemical deficiencies of several minerals, predominately athletes involved in weight-control sports such as gymnastics, dancing, figure skating, and wrestling. McClung and others recently noted that female athletes could be at risk for mineral insufficiency due to inadequate dietary intake, menstruation, and inflammatory responses to heavy physical activity. Experts disagree about the potential adverse effects of such dietary or biochemical deficiencies, but certain physiological and clinically manifest mineral deficiencies are known to have impaired physical performance.

The human body possesses a very effective control system for some minerals. When a deficiency occurs, the body absorbs more of the mineral from the food in the intestine and excretes less via routes such as the urine. When an excess is consumed, the opposite is true; less is absorbed and more is excreted. However, the body has a limited ability to excrete certain minerals, so excessive consumption may override these natural control systems and cause a number of health problems, even in relatively small dosages.

Additionally, a few minerals not important to human nutrition, such as lead, mercury, cadmium, and arsenic as well as some industrial forms of silicon and chromium, may be extremely toxic to the human body. For example, as discussed in chapter 5, mercury in polluted waterways may accumulate in fish, which if eaten may damage the nervous system of unborn or young children.

Let us now detail the role of various macrominerals and trace minerals in health and exercise performance.

Macrominerals

The seven **macrominerals** (major minerals) are calcium, phosphorus, magnesium, potassium, sodium, chloride, and sulfur. Minerals are classified as macrominerals if the RDA or AI is greater than 100 mg per day or the body contains more than 5 grams. In general, the human body maintains a proper balance of these minerals through precise hormonal control mechanisms, but deficiencies or excesses may occur and disturb normal physiological functions, thus impairing health or physical performance. Sulfur, an integral component of several amino acids and vitamins, is not discussed here because its functions are associated with those nutrients. Because potassium, sodium, and chloride are the major electrolytes in sweat, and in some sports drinks, they are covered in the following chapter dealing with water and temperature regulation.

Calcium (Ca)

Calcium, a silver-white metallic element, is the most abundant mineral in the body, representing almost 2 percent of the body weight.

DRI   The AI for calcium is intended to replace daily losses in the urine, feces, and sweat and provide optimal amounts for health, particularly for bone health and the prevention of osteoporosis. The daily recommendations, in parentheses, are given for several selected age groups: children 1 to 3 years (700 mg); youths 4 to 8 years (1,000 mg); youths and adolescents 9 to 18 years (1,300 mg); adults 19 to 50 (1,000 mg); adults 51 to 70 (1,000 mg for men and 1,200 mg for women); adults over 71 (1,200 mg). Pregnant and breastfeeding women should get the amount recommended for their age group. The DV is 1,000 mg. The UL, for adults 19 to 50 is 2,500 mg.

Food Sources   Calcium content is highest in dairy products. One 8-ounce glass of skim milk, which contains about 300 mg of calcium, supplies about one-third of the RDA for adults and men over 50 and about one-quarter of the RDA for adolescents and women over 50. It is used as the basis of comparison for other foods. Other equivalent dairy foods are 1½ ounces of cheese, 1 cup of yogurt, and 1¾ cups of ice cream. Dairy products supply more than 70 percent of daily calcium intake for adults. Other good sources are fish with small bones, such as sardines and canned salmon, dark-green leafy vegetables (particularly broccoli, kale, and turnip greens), calcium-set tofu, legumes, and nuts. Incorporation of milk or cheese into foods such as soups, pasta dishes, and pizza is an excellent way to obtain dietary calcium. For individuals with lactose intolerance, the use of yogurt, lactase enzymes, or smaller portions of milk may be helpful. Calcium is also used as a preservative in some foods, such as breads, which may provide small amounts. Additionally, some food products such as fruit juice and cereals are now being fortified with calcium; 1 serving of orange juice may contain 300–350 milligrams, while one brand of cereal contains 100 percent of the calcium DV. Some foods high in calcium are listed in table 8.2.

Calcium is one of the key nutrients listed on food labels, and although the food label does not indicate the milligrams of calcium per serving, you can calculate the amount fairly easily. The Daily Value (DV) for calcium is 1,000 milligrams, and the label will provide you with the percentage of the calcium DV contained in 1 serving. All you need to do is multiply the percentage, as a decimal, times 1,000 milligrams. For example, if a glass of calcium-fortified orange juice provides you with 30 percent of the DV, then it contains 300 milligrams of calcium (0.30 × 1,000 milligrams = 300 milligrams). Both the United States and Canada have approved food label health claims for calcium if 1 serving contains 20 percent of the Daily Value, or 200 milligrams.

Titchenal and Dobbs developed a system to assess the quality of food sources for calcium. The system is based on two criteria: the amount of calcium per serving, including nutrient density, and its absorbability.

Substances found in some foods may enhance or impair calcium absorption in the gastrointestinal tract. Calcium in milk appears to be absorbed more readily because vitamin D and lactose in milk facilitate absorption. Straub indicates that absorption from calcium-fortified beverages varies and in general is not equal to that of milk. Phytates (phytic acid compounds) found in legumes and oxalates in spinach may diminish somewhat the absorption of calcium from those foods. Thus, Titchenal and Dobbs indicated that foods such as beans are poor sources of calcium because of poor absorption, while Weaver and Heaney note calcium absorption from spinach is only 5 percent. Dietary fiber may reduce calcium absorption, although the effect is rather variable and

TABLE 8.2 Major minerals: calcium, phosphorus, and magnesium

Major mineral	Major food sources	Major body functions	Deficiency symptoms	Symptoms of excessive consumption
Calcium (Ca)	All dairy products: milk, cheese, ice cream, yogurt; egg yolk; dried beans and peas; dark-green leafy vegetables; soy milk; calcium-fortified food products	Bone formation; enzyme activation; nerve impulse transmission; muscle contraction; cell membrane potential	Osteoporosis; rickets; impaired muscle contraction; muscle cramps	Constipation; inhibition of trace mineral absorption. In susceptible individuals: heart arrhythmias; kidney stones; calcification of soft tissues
Phosphorus (P)	All protein products: meat, poultry, fish, eggs, milk, cheese, dried beans and peas; whole-grain products; soft drinks	Bone formation; acid-base balance; cell membrane structure; B vitamin activation; organic compound component, e.g., ATP-PCr, 2, 3-DPG	Rare. Deficiency symptoms parallel calcium deficiency. Muscular weakness	Rare. Impaired calcium metabolism; gastrointestinal distress from phosphate salts
Magnesium (Mg)	Milk and yogurt; dried beans; nuts; whole-grain products; fruits and vegetables, especially green leafy vegetables	Protein synthesis; metalloenzyme; 2, 3-DPG formation; glucose metabolism; smooth muscle contraction; bone component	Rare. Muscle weakness; apathy; muscle twitching; muscle cramps; cardiac arrhythmias	Nausea; vomiting; diarrhea

presumably small. Dietary phosphorus may also decrease calcium absorption, but decreases its excretion by the kidney as well, so its effect on calcium balance is somewhat neutral. Excess sodium intake increases calcium excretion. Dawson-Hughes indicates that for every 500-mg increase in urinary sodium excretion, there is about a 10-mg increase in urinary calcium loss. Excess dietary protein, as mentioned in chapter 6, may lead to calcium excretion, an estimate cited by the National Dairy Council being 1 milligram of calcium lost for every gram of protein consumed. However, as also noted, adequate protein intake is needed to optimize calcium bone metabolism. High intakes of coffee and alcohol may increase calcium loss from the body, although studies have shown that up to five cups of coffee and moderate alcohol consumption appear to have little effect on calcium balance.

Overall, however, calcium balance in the body is attributed mostly to adequate calcium intake. Although certain food constituents may impair the absorption of calcium, the effect is not as great as once believed. In general, the amounts of protein, phosphorus, fiber, phytates, and oxalates found in the average North American diet do not appear to pose a problem for calcium absorption. For example, research has revealed that vegetarian diets provide adequate calcium nutrition as measured by body stores. Nevertheless, non-lactovegetarian females, as well as females engaged in sports-associated dieting for weight control, should be sure to include calcium-rich foods in their diet.

As we shall see, the major factor underlying calcium deficiency is inadequate calcium intake, and although some of these other dietary factors may adversely influence calcium balance if taken to excess, their effect is lessened if calcium intake is adequate.

Major Functions   The vast majority of body calcium, 98 percent, is found in the skeleton, where it gives strength by the formation of salts such as calcium phosphate. One percent is used for tooth formation. The remainder, which exists in an ionic state

or in combination with certain proteins, exerts considerable influence over human metabolism. Intracellular calcium ions (Ca^{2+}) are involved in all types of muscle contraction, including that of the heart, skeletal muscle, and smooth muscle found in blood vessels such as the arteries. Calcium activates a number of enzymes; in this capacity it plays a central role in both the synthesis and breakdown of muscle glycogen and liver glycogen. Calcium also helps regulate nerve impulse transmission, blood clotting, and secretion of hormones. It should be noted that the skeletal content of calcium is not inert. The physiological functions of calcium, such as nerve cell transmission, take precedence over formation of bone tissue. If the diet is low in calcium for a short time, the body can mobilize some from the skeleton through the action of hormones, such as parathormone and calcitriol (hormonal form of vitamin D), to maintain an adequate amount in ionic form. Weaver and Heaney note that, given the large skeletal reserves, impaired metabolic processes associated with calcium deficiency are almost nonexistent.

Deficiency: Health and Physical Performance   Calcium balance in the human body is rather complex. Figure 8.2 depicts the fate of an intake of 1,000 mg. Only 300 mg (about 30 percent) is absorbed, while the remaining 700 mg is excreted in the feces. The calcium that is absorbed into the blood interacts with the current body stores, the net result being the excretion of 300 mg through the intestines, kidneys, and sweat to balance the amount originally absorbed. Calcium deficiency may develop from inadequate dietary intake or increased excretion.

Inadequate dietary intake of calcium is the major cause of calcium deficiency. The National Health and Nutrition Examination Survey (NHANES) is designed to analyze the nutrient content of the diets of Americans. In a recent NHANES report, *What We Eat in America,* Hoy and Goldman indicated that 42 percent of Americans, mainly females, did not meet the recommendations for daily intake

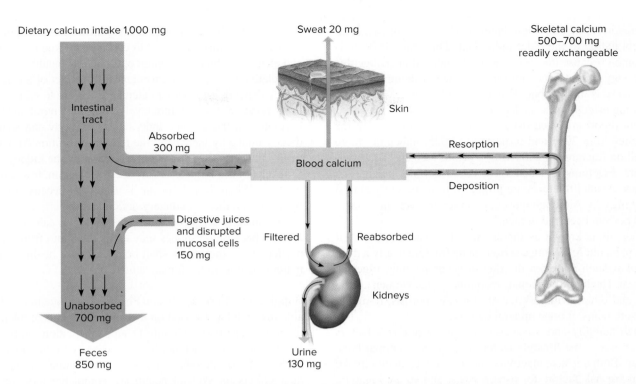

FIGURE 8.2 Calcium balance in an adult who requires 1,000 mg daily. On an intake of 1,000 mg, only about 30 percent, or 300 mg, are absorbed into the body, the remaining 700 mg being excreted in the feces. To maintain calcium balance, 300 mg are excreted, including an additional 150 mg in the feces, 130 mg through the kidneys to the urine, and 20 mg in sweat. See text for further discussion.

of calcium. In particular, older females obtained substantially less calcium than recommended. However, the report provided some good news, indicating that dietary calcium intake has shown an increasing trend since the mid-1990s, with approximately 85 to 190 milligrams more calcium consumed daily across age groups.

The National Institutes of Health (NIH) also indicated that females older than 50 years do not get the recommended amount of calcium, but it also noted other age groups are at risk, including boys (9–13 years), girls (9–18 years), and men (over age 70). The NIH indicated that other than these specific age groups, some other groups of people may be at risk of calcium inadequacy:

- Individuals with lactose intolerance or cow's milk allergy. Such conditions may eliminate milk from the diet, a major source of dietary calcium.
- Women with anorexia nervosa, an eating disorder. Eating disorders, which may interfere with calcium metabolism, are discussed in chapter 10.
- Some vegetarians. Those who consume no dairy produvts, particularly vegans, are at risk.
- Female athletes in weight-control sports. Such athletes may be predisposed to the female athlete triad, discussed later in this section, which may disrupt calcium metabolism.
- Additionally, studies indicate that strenuous exercise may increase calcium losses in the sweat.

The major health problems associated with impaired calcium metabolism involve diseases of the bones. A number of factors are involved in the formation, or mineralization, of bone tissue,

including mechanical stresses such as exercise; hormones such as parathormone, calcitonin, vitamin D (calcitriol), and estrogen; and dietary calcium. An imbalance in any one of these factors could lead to bone demineralization, resulting in the development of rickets in children and osteoporosis in adults. Rickets is most often associated with vitamin D deficiency and is discussed in chapter 7.

Osteoporosis (thinning and weakening of the bones related to loss of calcium stores) is a debilitating disease that affects more than 200 million people worldwide. Aaseth and others described osteoporosis as a multi-factorial disease with potential contributions from genetic, endocrine, exercise, and nutritional factors, with the last including calcium, vitamin D, fluoride, magnesium, and other trace elements. Osteoporosis is age- and gender-related, being prevalent in white, postmenopausal women. However, a National Institutes of Health (NIH) panel noted that osteoporosis occurs in all populations and at all ages and has significant physical, psycho-social, and financial consequences.

A positive family history, or heredity, and low levels of estrogen are the two primary risk factors in women. Caucasian and Asian women are at higher risk for osteoporosis than women of African ancestry. Following menopause, estrogen production is diminished. Estrogen is a hormone essential for optimal calcium balance in women. Bone receptors for estrogen have been identified, indicating an active role in bone metabolism. In general, reduced levels of estrogen lead to negative calcium balance and a rapid onset of bone demineralization. This softening of the bones predisposes to fractures, particularly in the spine, the end of the radius in the forearm, and the neck of the femur at the hip joint, as illustrated in figure 8.3. These latter two fractures may be completely debilitating to the older individual. The spinal fracture is more common because the vertebrae are composed of **trabecular bone**, a spongy type of bone more susceptible to calcium loss than the more dense compact bone. However, both types of bone may be lost during osteoporosis, as depicted in figure 8.4.

A recent report analyzed osteoporosis-related fractures in the United States from 2005 and projected to 2025, indicating more than 2 million fractures in 2005 with a health-care cost of 17 billion dollars. Fractures included vertebral, wrist, hip, pelvic, and other bones. Annual fractures are projected to increase by almost 50 percent in 2025. Although most of the fractures were in women, almost 30 percent occurred in men.

Osteoporosis is known as the silent killer. The disease itself causes no pain, but following a serious bone fracture nearly a third or more of women and men die due to accompanying illnesses within a year. Health professionals recommend that women age 65 and over, and others with risk factors for osteoporosis, routinely have measurements of bone mineral density.

Although heredity and estrogen status are strong risk factors for osteoporosis, some lifestyle factors may impair optimal bone metabolism. Both physical inactivity and inadequate dietary intake of calcium are risk factors for osteoporosis, and so are cigarette smoking, stress, and various medications. Table 8.3 highlights the risk factors for osteoporosis. All these factors may influence **peak bone mass** (the highest bone mass in young adulthood). Modifying your lifestyle to increase your peak bone mass is like putting money in the bank for later in life. However, Modlesky and Lewis note that although the idea that the growing years are an opportune time to optimize bone mass and strength certainly

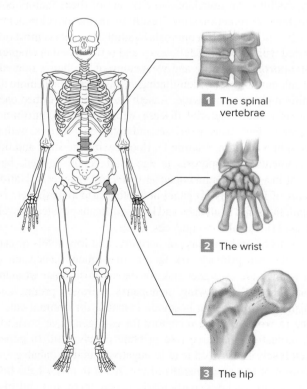

1 The spinal vertebrae

2 The wrist

3 The hip

FIGURE 8.3 Three principal sites of osteoporosis fractures.

has merit, the importance of these gains depends largely on their permanence. Thus, you need to continue to practice good dietary and exercise habits to maintain optimal bone health.

Relative to physical performance, the effect of a calcium deficiency depends on whether calcium levels are low in the blood or in the bones. Serum calcium levels are usually regulated by several hormones in the average individual. The body can adapt to low dietary intake by increasing the rate of absorption from the intestines and decreasing the rate of excretion by the kidneys. Because the skeleton is a large reservoir of body calcium, low serum levels are rare. When they do occur, it usually is because of hormonal imbalances rather than dietary deficiencies.

Fortunately, serious deficiencies of serum calcium are rare in athletes because hormones may extract calcium from the bone as needed. Nevertheless, as shall be noted, bone health is one of the major concerns in the female athlete triad.

Supplementation: Health and Physical Performance Considerable research has focused on the role of calcium supplementation, often in concert with vitamin D supplementation, on bone health. Heaney notes that each nutrient is necessary for the full expression of the effect of the other, and while their actions are independent, their effects on skeletal health are complementary. In addition, exercise may play a role in enhancing bone health.

Bone health As noted above, bone health is an important consideration, particularly for the aged. Although genetic factors are involved in optimal bone health, so are lifestyle factors, particularly diet and exercise. The following discussion focuses on the role of supplements, particularly calcium along with vitamin D, exercise, and drug therapy, as well as a brief discussion of osteoporosis in sports.

Calcium supplements Calcium supplements come in a variety of forms, such as calcium carbonate, calcium citrate, calcium lactate, and calcium gluconate and are found in certain antacids, such as Tums. Weaver and Heaney note that calcium from most supplements is absorbed as well as from milk, but a few calcium salts, including calcium citrate/malate and calcium ascorbate, have superior absorbability. Be sure to check the label for the calcium content per tablet, which may range from 50 to 600 mg depending on the brand. Be aware that some forms of calcium supplements may be contaminated with lead.

In a consensus conference on multivitamin/mineral supplementation, the NIH indicated that supplementation with calcium, along with vitamin D, may be necessary in persons not achieving the recommended dietary intake. Specifically, the NIH panel concluded that calcium and vitamin D supplements could protect and even improve bone mineral density as well as reduce fracture risk in postmenopausal women. However, three more recent reviews by Reid, Aggarwal and Nityanand, and Uusi-Rasi and colleagues concluded that although calcium may have some small beneficial effects in the prevention of bone loss, particularly in postmenopausal women, reviews and meta-analyses suggest no significant prevention of fractures. Reid suggests there is little substantive evidence of benefit to bone health from the use of calcium supplements, and such use needs to be balanced against the likelihood

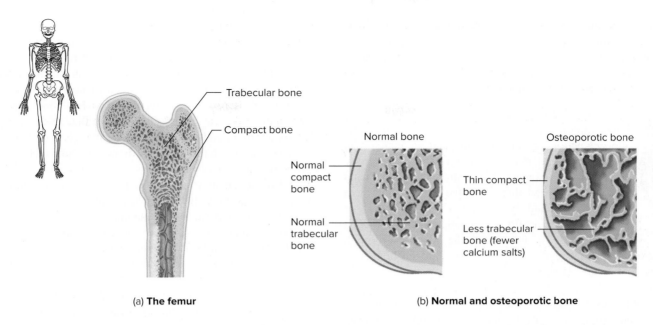

Trabecular bone

Compact bone

(a) **The femur**

Normal bone

Normal compact bone

Normal trabecular bone

Osteoporotic bone

Thin compact bone

Less trabecular bone (fewer calcium salts)

(b) **Normal and osteoporotic bone**

FIGURE 8.4 In osteoporosis, impaired calcium metabolism may decrease the external compact bone thickness and the strength of the internal trabecular bone lattice network.

TABLE 8.3	Risk factors for osteoporosis
Heredity	Positive family history
Race	White or Asian
Gender	Female
Menstrual status	Postmenopausal; amenorrheic
Age	Advanced age
Exercise	Physical inactivity; bed rest
Diet	Inadequate calcium; inadequate vitamin D; excessive coffee; excessive alcohol
Tobacco	Cigarette smoking
Alcohol	Excessive use
Stress	Excessive stress; anxiety
Medications	Certain medications increase calcium losses
Hormonal status	Low estrogen; low testosterone

that calcium supplement use may increase cardiovascular events, kidney stones, and other health problems.

However, based on results from the Women's Health Initiative study, which included a calcium/vitamin D trial, Cauley concluded that, overall, the common practice of taking calcium and vitamin D supplementation with possible benefits for the hip and positive evidence for increased bone mineral density and with few risks is reasonable.

For those who desire to take a calcium supplement, it may be wise to take a tablet with about 200 mg with snacks and small meals three times a day, rather than one tablet with 600 mg, as it appears that more calcium is absorbed when the intake is spread throughout the day. Moreover, when the supplement is combined with meals, gastric acidity and slower transit time in the gut promote calcium absorption. A daily total supplement of 600 mg calcium, combined with a dietary intake of 500–600 mg, should provide adequate calcium nutrition for most individuals. Multivitamin/mineral tablets normally contain about 200 milligrams of calcium, or 20 percent of the AI. However, three tablets are needed to provide 600 milligrams of calcium and may not be the best means to obtain calcium, because the three tablets may provide excess amounts of other nutrients, such as vitamin A.

However, the point should be stressed that careful selection of foods will provide all of the calcium you need from the daily diet, thus eliminating the need for supplements. Nevertheless, as Straub points out, most Americans do not meet the AI for calcium, and supplements can help meet requirements.

Weaver and Heaney note that hypercalcemia essentially never occurs from ingestion of natural food sources, but only with supplements. Although supplements up to 600 mg per day do not appear to pose much danger, excessive amounts may contribute to various health problems, as discussed below. Moreover, excessive dietary calcium or calcium supplements may interfere with the absorption of other key minerals, notably iron and zinc. The calcium AI for some age groups (1,000–1,300 milligrams) may require supplementation for some individuals, but the National Academy of Sciences recommends against supplementation to a total much above the AI. The UL is 2,500 mg, which may be exceeded if one takes supplements and consumes too many calcium-fortified foods. Meal replacement powders and food bars, popular dietary supplements in strength-power athletes, often have 1,000 mg of calcium per serving. A large athlete who consumes three of these products per day for extra Calories and protein can very easily exceed the UL for calcium.

Exercise Exercise places a mechanical stress on the bone, stimulating mechanical receptors that facilitate the deposition of calcium salts and an increase in bone mass and density. In a review of exercise regimens to increase bone strength, Turner and Robling indicated that mechanical loading through exercise will add bone, and a small amount of added new bone results in dramatic increases in bone strength because the location of the new bone through exercise is where mechanical stresses in the bone will cause fracture. However, they note that not all exercises are equally effective. Dynamic exercise, as compared to static exercise, creates a unique stress on the bone to stimulate bone strength gains. Dynamic, high-impact exercise, such as running and jumping, may stimulate bone growth more than low-impact exercise. Kato and others found that young college women who did ten maximal vertical jumps for 3 days a week over the course of 6 months increased bone mineral density in the hip and spinal bones. Studies find that female athletes in high-impact sports have greater bone mineral density than athletes in low-impact sports.

Age is an important consideration in optimizing bone mass with exercise, and youth is the age of opportunity. Turner and Robling also indicate that although exercise has clear benefits for the skeleton, engaging in exercise during skeletal growth is clearly more osteogenic than exercise during skeletal maturity. Periosteal expansion occurs predominantly during growth, and consequently, the childhood and adolescent years provide a window of opportunity to enhance periosteal growth with exercise. As Bloomfield notes, you should get bone in your bone bank by age 30. Exercise is an important means of doing so, and Bloomfield also notes that you should engage in multiple, brief bouts of activity during the day, focusing on weight-bearing activities and a variety of movements.

Although adult bone health is dependent on maximal attainment of peak bone mass in youth and the prevention of bone loss during young adulthood, whether or not exercise prevents bone loss after menopause appears to be debatable. Miller and others, in a review of 13 studies, concluded that the findings provide support for regular aerobic activity in postmenopausal women as a means to offset age-related declines in bone mineral density. Additionally, in a meta-analysis of 18 randomized, controlled trials, Bonaiuti and others concluded that aerobics, weight-bearing, and resistance exercises are all effective in increasing the bone mineral density of the spine in postmenopausal women, and walking is also effective on the hip.

However, others suggest that exercise provides minimal, if any, benefits. The American College of Sports Medicine (ACSM), in a position statement on physical activity and bone health, indicated that although physical activity for optimal bone health is important across the age spectrum, currently there is no strong evidence that even vigorous physical activity attenuates the menopause-related loss of bone mineral in women. These findings were recently confirmed in a review by Fonseca and others, noting that most exercise intervention studies reveal either no effect or only minor benefits of exercise programs in improving bone mineral density in osteoporotic patients. However, they note that exercise interventions in patients with osteoporosis may be beneficial by improving other determinants of bone strength, such as collagen properties and osteocyte density.

Adequate calcium intake may be the answer to these varying viewpoints, as it may be needed to complement the effects of exercise. Zernicke and others indicate that exercise produces increases in bone mineral density only when calcium intake exceeds 1,000 mg daily, and it is generally accepted that chronic exercise and dietary calcium can improve bone mass to a greater extent than calcium intake alone.

The current position statement by the ACSM, complemented by recent reviews, offers the following points relative to exercise and prevention of osteoporosis.

1. Dynamic exercises, such as resistance training through a range of motion and high-impact, weight-bearing aerobic exercise, are effective means to stimulate development of bone.
2. Development of peak bone mass through exercise is best achieved during the developmental years of youth; high-impact exercises are more effective.
3. Exercise may increase bone mass slightly in adulthood, but the primary benefit of exercise at this time of life may be the avoidance of further loss of bone that occurs with inactivity.
4. The optimal program for older women would include moderate- to high-impact activities that improve strength, flexibility, and coordination that may increase postural stability and decrease the incidence of osteoporotic fractures by lessening the likelihood of falling.
5. Exercise will stimulate bone development, but optimal calcium intake approximating 1,000 milligrams or more daily appears to be equally important.

Although the ACSM does recommend exercise throughout the life span for bone health, it also indicates that pharmacological therapy for the prevention of osteoporosis may be indicated even for those postmenopausal women who are habitually physically active.

Hormone replacement or nonhormonal drug therapy In the past, hormone replacement therapy (HRT) involving estrogen, possibly combined with progesterone, was commonly used for prevention and treatment of osteoporosis and, as noted by the Consumers Union, a host of other health benefits. However, in a report from the NIH Women's Health Initiative, the biggest hormone study ever done, women on estrogen-progestin therapy were at increased risk for breast cancer, heart attacks, and strokes as compared to women not taking these hormones. Following this report, Bern highlighted the updated FDA recommendations for postmenopausal women and the use of estrogen-containing drugs. The recommendations vary depending on the health condition, and if a woman and her health-care provider decide that estrogen-containing products are appropriate, they should be used at the lowest doses for the shortest duration to reach treatment goals. In a recent review, Cauley noted that the use of hormone therapy solely for the prevention of osteoporosis is not recommended.

Various non-estrogen drugs are available to help treat or prevent osteoporosis. In 2006, the Consumers Union indicated that bisphosphonates remain the optimal treatment for osteoporosis, and a recent review by Aaseth and others note bisphosphonates are still the drugs of choice. Bisphosphonates represent a class of drugs that inhibit the osteoclasts, thereby decreasing resorption of bone, but they do not inhibit bone mineralization. Thus, they prevent bone loss and possibly increase bone mineral density. Brand names for bisphosphonates include Fosamax, Boniva, and Reclast. Some forms, such as Boniva, may need to be taken orally only once a month. The FDA approved Reclast (zoledronic acid), which requires only a yearly 15-minute infusion, which may help women who do not adhere to other regimens where pills must be taken on a regular basis. However, in 2008 the FDA reported various adverse side effects associated with bisphosphanate use. The hormone testosterone has also been used, particularly with males, as have other nonhormonal drugs, for the prevention and treatment of osteoporosis, but they also may have adverse side effects. Individuals who wish to seek medical treatment for osteoporosis should consult with a medical specialist who treats the disease. Your family doctor may treat you or refer you to a doctor with expertise in osteoporosis.

Osteoporosis in sports   Although osteoporosis occurs primarily in older individuals, investigators are expressing serious concern regarding disturbed calcium metabolism in young female athletes, particularly endurance athletes and those involved in weight-control sports. The **female athlete triad**—*disordered eating, amenorrhea, osteoporosis*—has been reported in numerous studies.

Although the exact cause has not been identified, the underlying behavior appears to be disordered eating, as will be discussed in chapter 10. Females who attempt to lose body weight in order to improve their appearance or competitive ability in sports may modify their diets, decreasing energy and protein intake. They may also exercise excessively to burn Calories. Restrictive diets and excessive exercise regimens may affect hormone status in various ways, including disturbed functioning of the hypothalamus and pituitary gland, two glands that significantly influence overall hormone status in the body including female reproductive hormones, and decreased levels of body fat, which may lead to a reduced production of estrone, a form of estrogen. **Secondary amenorrhea** (cessation of menses for prolonged periods) is a classic sign of disturbed hormonal status associated with disordered eating in postpubertal females, as seen in patients with anorexia nervosa. When observed in athletic females, secondary amenorrhea is often referred to as **athletic amenorrhea** and it may involve oligomenorrhea, or intermittent periods of amenorrhea. In young female athletes, athletic amenorrhea is often associated with osteoporosis. Most recently, the International Olympic Committee updated its consensus statement on the female athlete triad and now refers to

it as relative energy deficiency in sport (RED-S). Mountjoy and others note that RED-S is more comprehensive than the female athlete triad, but some debate this classification. This topic is discussed in more detail in chapter 10.

The medical treatment suggested for this condition depends on the point of view of the individual endocrinologist and may include individualized hormone/drug therapy. An appropriate physician, such as a sports-oriented gynecologist, should be consulted.

Males are at less risk for developing osteoporosis than females; however, reviews by Seeman and by Bennell and others noted that low calcium intake, weight loss, low body fat, and excess alcohol intake, along with other risk factors, may adversely affect bone density in males. Depressed hormone levels, such as testosterone and insulin-like growth factor (IGF-1), may also be associated with decreased bone density.

As discussed in chapter 10, The American College of Sports Medicine indicates that medical attention is mandatory for athletes with disordered eating or amenorrhea, noting that treatment of the triad often requires intervention via a team approach, including a physician, a nutritionist, a psychologist, and the support of family, friends, teammates, and coaches.

Cardiovascular disease   Some scientists have expressed concern about the potential adverse effects of excess calcium intake, particularly from supplements, on cardiovascular health. According to Rautiainen and others, laboratory studies suggest that calcium may be involved in cardiovascular disease development through multiple pathways. One concern is calcification of blood vessels, which could impair blood flow in the coronary arteries. A 2013 meta-analysis of calcium supplements by Reid found a 27–31 percent increase in the risk of myocardial infarction and a 12–20 percent increase in the risk of stroke, and concluded that the health risks of calcium supplements appear to outweigh any skeletal benefits. However, in 2013 Downing and others indicated that in general the studies of calcium use and cardiovascular disease published to date have had important limitations, such as small sample size, and the findings should be interpreted with caution. In their review, Heaney and others noted a number of issues in studies that could interfere with the interpretation of the results. Lewis and others also noted that the design of the meta-analyses showing increased risk of myocardial infarction with calcium supplements has raised some concerns.

Studies and reviews by other scientists suggest calcium supplementation has no adverse effects on cardiovascular health. Paik and others, in the Nurse's Health Study over the course of 24 years, reported that their findings do not support the hypothesis that calcium supplement intake increases cardiovascular disease risk in women. Lewis and others conducted their own meta-analysis using only randomized, controlled trials. They concluded that the current evidence does not support the hypothesis that calcium supplementation with or without vitamin D increases cardiovascular disease risk in elderly women. Heaney and others concluded that the current evidence regarding the hypothesized relationship between calcium supplement use and increased cardiovascular disease risk is insufficient to warrant a change in the Institute of

Medicine recommendations, which advocate use of supplements to promote optimal bone health in individuals.

The current state of affairs relative to the role of calcium supplementation in the development of cardiovascular disease is probably best expressed by Rautiainen and others. In their review, they note the results of research trials suggest calcium supplementation has no effect on cardiovascular disease development, but current research findings also do not allow a definitive conclusion to be drawn. They conclude that only large-scale, randomized trials designed to investigate the effects of calcium supplementation on cardiovascular disease events as the primary end point, as well as short-term trials investigating the effect on coronary disease biomarkers, can provide a definitive answer.

Cancer   The role dietary calcium plays in cancer development appears to be complex. Abid and others cite research suggesting that dietary calcium probably decreases the risk of colorectal cancer but diets high in calcium probably increase the risk of prostate cancer.

On the beneficial side, calcium may bind with carcinogenic compounds in the intestines, which may inhibit their effect on cells in the colon and rectum. The National Cancer Institute noted that the most authoritative review of existing evidence relating nutrition to cancer risk, a 2007 report by the World Cancer Research Foundation and American Institute of Cancer Research, concluded that calcium possibly has a protective effect against colorectal cancer. In a recent meta-analysis, Heine-Bröring and others observed inverse associations for colorectal cancer risk and calcium supplements, suggesting a beneficial role for calcium supplements in the prevention of colorectal cancer.

On the negative side, men with high serum calcium levels may be more at risk for prostate cancer. One theory is that calcium may interact with parathyroid hormone to promote prostate cancer. The National Cancer Institute indicates some studies suggest that a high calcium intake may increase the risk of prostate cancer, but results of more recent systematic reviews and meta-analyses are somewhat conflicting. Aune and others reported an increased risk, Uusi-Rasi and others reported a slightly increased risk, whereas Bristow and others, although noting that their meta-analysis lacked power to detect effects with a long latency, indicated a reduced risk.

In their review, Uusi-Rasi and others noted there was a lot of heterogeneity in the study protocols, which made it difficult to draw any strong conclusions regarding the effect of calcium intake on the development of various diseases, including cancer. Other constituents of the diet may be associated with prostate cancer risk. For example, a recent 24-year study by Wilson and others reported that calcium intakes greater than 2,000 milligrams per day were associated with greater risk of prostate cancer, but the risk was attenuated when phosphorus intake was considered, at least on a short-term basis. Nevertheless, Wilson and others concluded that prolonged (12–16 years), excess calcium intake was associated with an increased risk of prostate cancer.

Obesity and weight control   Calcium supplementation has been theorized to promote weight loss. Zemel indicated that low-calcium diets cause an increase in calcitriol, the vitamin D

hormone, which can stimulate adipose cell calcium influx, promoting fat accumulation; he also notes the converse, that higher-calcium diets inhibit the formation of body fat.

Zemel and others, in several studies, have shown that supplementing a reduced-Calorie diet with calcium—in particular, calcium-rich dairy products—led to greater weight loss compared to placebo groups. However, most other studies comparable to the design of those of Zemel reported no beneficial effects of high-calcium diets or supplements on weight loss.

The results of two recent reviews are somewhat contradictory. De Oliveira Freitas and others indicated the results of most studies suggested that calcium ingestion may improve body composition. Conversely, Soares and others analyzed the effects of 15 randomized, controlled trials on calcium with or without vitamin D and indicated the evidence does not consistently support the contention that calcium accelerates weight or fat loss in obesity.

However, Tremblay and Gilbert suggest dairy calcium may play a role in body weight control, possibly accentuating the impact of a weight-reducing program. They suggest that calcium/dairy supplementation may promote weight loss in several ways: (1) by promoting fecal fat loss and oxidation, (2) by favoring a decrease in energy intake, and (3) by facilitating appetite control. More details on weight-control programs are presented in chapter 11.

Kidney stones   Kidney stones can form in the urine and cause pain in the urinary tract if they are too large to pass. There are several forms of kidney stones, the most common being calcium oxalate formed from calcium and oxalate in the urine.

Possible causes of kidney stones include inadequate fluid intake, too much protein intake, too much salt, or too much sugar, especially fructose. However, Weaver and Heaney note that kidney stones are not caused by *dietary* calcium. They note that although kidney stones contain calcium oxalate, it is the oxalate that may be the problem. They also note that actually increasing calcium intake to about 1,200 milligrams daily may reduce the risk of kidney stones, as the calcium can bind oxalate in the intestines and lead to its excretion, thus decreasing the amount of oxalate in the body.

Sports performance   Research regarding the effect of calcium supplementation on physical performance is almost nonexistent. Given its theoretical role in fat metabolism in weight-loss programs, White and others investigated the acute effect of calcium on fat metabolism and exercise performance in trained female runners. The subjects consumed either a high-calcium (500 mg) or low-calcium (80 mg) drink 60 minutes prior to a 90-minute run at 70 percent VO_2 max, which was followed by a 10-kilometer treadmill time trial. The high-calcium drink did not affect carbohydrate or fat metabolism during the 90-minute run or 10-kilometer run time. In a similar study, Gonzalez and others investigated the effect of 2 weeks of calcium supplementation (1,400 milligrams daily) on carbohydrate and lipid metabolism during a cycling-based exercise test. However, the supplement did not affect either carbohydrate or fat utilization rates during the exercise task.

Calcium may be combined with other salts, such as lactate, to form calcium lactate, which could be used to buffer lactic acid during exercise. Painelli Vde and others recently studied the effect of calcium lactate on intense anaerobic exercise, and although there were increases in bicarbonate and the alkalinity of the blood, performance on intense Wingate cycling tests was not improved. Detailed coverage of the use of buffering agents, such as sodium bicarbonate, are presented in chapter 13.

Low serum calcium levels may impair neuromuscular functions, but such conditions are rare because the body will draw from calcium reserves in the skeleton to restore serum levels. In a review, Kunstel concluded that increased physical activity alone does not necessarily demand an increased intake of dietary calcium. Thus, acute or chronic calcium supplementation is not recommended as a means to enhance sports performance. However, calcium supplementation may be useful to help maintain bone mass in some female and male athletes, particularly those who do not consume adequate calcium from foods.

Prudent Recommendations Adequate daily calcium intake and weight-bearing exercise are very important during the developmental years of childhood and adolescence to maximize peak bone mass, and such practices should be continued throughout adult life. Weaver, an expert in calcium metabolism, recently indicated that the current RDA for calcium appear to be a good target, and potential risks for chronic diseases may occur if intakes fall too short or greatly exceed these recommendations. Calcium supplementation may be recommended to attain the RDA in individuals who do not obtain a sufficient amount through their normal diet. In recent reviews, Cauley, as well as Downing and Islam, notes that overall the possible positive benefits of calcium supplementation on bone health appear to outweigh the few risks.

To help prevent osteoporosis, postmenopausal women and elderly men should obtain about 1,200 milligrams of calcium per day, along with adequate vitamin D (200–600 IU). Both weight-bearing aerobic and resistance strength-training exercises are recommended. Postmenopausal women should consult with their physicians relative to hormone replacement or drug therapy. Older men should also obtain adequate calcium, exercise, and consult their physicians for appropriate drug therapy if warranted.

For younger, premenopausal women, the nonpharmacological approach is recommended. The key with younger women, and men as well, is prevention. They need to develop peak bone mass, the optimal amount within genetic limitations, prior to age 25–30, and attempt to keep the bone mass high in the advancing years. Health professionals note that because evidence suggests that osteoporosis is easier to prevent than to treat, initiating sound health behaviors early in life and continuing them throughout life is the best approach. As the venerable Fred Astaire once noted, "Old age is like everything else. To make a success of it, you've got to start young." Thus, it would appear prudent for young women to develop a lifetime exercise program and obtain the AI of 1,000–1,300 milligrams for calcium in the diet. The earlier the better, for research has suggested a greater increase in bone mass when calcium supplements are given to prepubertal children, but adequate calcium intake is critical for adolescents as well. Weight-bearing exercises, such as walking or jogging, promote bone mineralization by stressing the hips and spine, while resistance strength training and modified push-ups are also excellent for the spine and for the radial bone at the wrist joint.

Dairy products often are not consumed because they are believed to be high in fat and Calories. However, research with young girls has shown that a low-Calorie, calcium-rich diet mainly from dairy products can promote bone health and is not necessarily associated with excess weight gain. Although some dairy products may contain significant amounts of fat, four glasses of skim milk provide 1,200 mg of calcium. In addition, the milk (or its equivalent) would provide 32 grams of protein, which is about 80 percent of the protein RDA for the average woman, and a variety of other vitamins and minerals, in less than 400 Calories.

It should also be noted that a balanced intake of multiple nutrients is needed for optimal bone health. Ilich and Kerstetter note that although approximately 80–90 percent of bone is comprised of calcium and phosphorus, other nutrients such as protein, magnesium, zinc, copper, iron, fluoride, and vitamins A, C, D, and K are also required for bone metabolism. Bonjour stresses the importance of adequate dietary protein, indicating that it is as essential as calcium and vitamin D for bone health and osteoporosis prevention.

Because coffee, alcohol, and tobacco use are secondary risk factors associated with the development of osteoporosis, moderation or abstinence is advocated.

The Consumers Union recommends a bone density test for women at risk, indicating that women over age 65 should be tested every 2 years. For younger women, whether or not to be tested depends on individual risks, such as a family history, being underweight, low calcium intake, little weight-bearing physical activity, and cigarette smoking. Amenorrheic athletes may also be at risk. Men over age 65 should also be tested. A dual energy X-ray absorptiometry (DEXA) test is recommended, not the ultrasound of the heel at your local drugstore.

Phosphorus (P)

Phosphorus is a nonmetallic element and is the second most abundant mineral in the body after calcium.

DRI The adult RDA is 700 mg for both men and women. Higher amounts are needed between ages 9 and 18. Specific values for different age groups may be found in the DRI table at the Website noted in the legend to table 8.1. The DV is 1,000 mg. The UL for adults is 4 grams, but only 3 grams between ages 1–8 and over 70.

Food Sources As noted earlier in table 8.2, phosphorus is distributed widely in foods. Anderson notes that practically all natural foods contain phosphorus as inorganic phosphate salts or organic molecules. Excellent sources include seafood, meat, eggs, milk, cheese, nuts, dried beans and peas, grain products, and a wide variety of vegetables. Phosphate also is a common food additive, and soft drinks have a relatively high phosphate content. In some foods, phosphorus is also a part of phytate, which may diminish the absorption of minerals like calcium, iron, zinc, and copper by forming insoluble phosphate salts in the intestine. However, as noted previously, this is not a major problem with the typical North American diet.

Most Americans consume about twice the amount of the RDA for phosphorus and as noted previously, too little calcium. The recommended calcium:phosphorus ratio is about 1:1, that is, equal amounts of each. In a review, Anderson and Barrett indicated that too much dietary phosphorus, which may occur because of phosphate additives in food, may impair calcium metabolism and predispose to osteoporosis. Too much phosphorus may also stimulate the release of parathyroid hormone. Anderson and Barrett noted that a ratio of up to 1:1.6 may be compatible with bone health, but ratios of 1:4 may be associated with osteoporosis. Studies indicate the daily dietary intake of calcium approximates 900 milligrams while phosphorus is 1,400 milligrams, about a 1:1.6 ratio. Conversely, Heaney and Nordin found that high intakes of dietary calcium may impair phosphorus absorption and eventually lead to phosphorus insufficiency and osteoporosis. A high dietary calcium:phosphorus ratio can occur with the use of calcium supplements and calcium-fortified foods.

Phosphates are regulated in the body by three hormones: parathyroid hormone, calcitriol, and fibroblast growth factor-23 (FGF-23). O'Brien and others indicate that these three hormones work in concert to ensure that serum phosphate concentrations and whole-body phosphate stores remain within a normal range.

Major Functions
O'Brien and others note that phosphorus is a critically important element in every cell in the body. In the human body, phosphorus occurs only as the salt phosphate, which exists as inorganic phosphate or is coupled with other minerals or organic compounds. Phosphates are extremely important in human metabolism. About 80–90 percent of the phosphorus in the body combines to form calcium phosphate, which is used for the development of bones and teeth. As with calcium, the bones represent a sizable store of phosphate salts. Other phosphate salts, such as sodium phosphate, are involved in acid-base balance.

The remainder of the body phosphates are found in a variety of organic forms, including the phospholipids, which help form cell membranes, and DNA. Several other organic phosphates are of prime importance to the active individual. For example, organic phosphates are essential to the normal function of most of the B vitamins involved in the energy processes within the cell. They are also part of the high-energy compounds found in the muscle cell, such as ATP and PCr, which are needed for muscle contraction. Glucose also must be phosphorylated in order to proceed through glycolysis. Organic phosphates also are a part of a compound in the RBC known as 2,3-BPG (2,3-biphosphoglycerate), which facilitates the release of oxygen to the muscle tissues.

Deficiency: Health and Physical Performance
Because phosphorus is distributed so widely in foods and because hormonal control is very effective, O'Brien and others note deficiency states are rare. They have been known to occur in hospital patients with serious illnesses such as diabetic ketoacidosis and severe starvation, in recovering alcoholics, and in those who use antacid compounds for long periods, as the antacid decreases the absorption of phosphorus. Symptoms parallel those of calcium deficiency, such as loss of bone material, resulting in rickets or osteomalacia. Other symptoms include muscular weakness. Extreme muscular exercise may increase phosphorus excretion in the urine but has not been reported to cause a deficiency state. Phosphorus deficiency could theoretically impair physical performance, but it has not been the subject of study because such deficiencies are rare.

Supplementation: Health and Physical Performance
Although various health problems, most notably osteoporosis, could occur with a phosphate deficiency, supplementation for health-related benefits has not received research attention because deficiency states are rare.

Phosphate supplementation for possible health benefits does not appear to be warranted, as there may be some adverse effects. As noted, Americans now consume approximately 1,400 milligrams of phosphorus per day, more than twice the RDA. In a recent review, Anderson suggested several potential health concerns with excess dietary phosphorus, including cancer, obesity, hypertension, diabetes, and an increased mortality. Anderson speculates that even a brief exposure of body cells to high serum phosphate concentrations could interfere with cell metabolism that could adversely affect health, such as promotion of tumor formation and calcification of arterial walls. Anderson notes that although research relative to the potential adverse effects of high-phosphate diets is emerging, it seems pragmatic that steps be taken to reduce the total phosphorus content of processed foods.

However, phosphate salts supplementation has been studied as a means of enhancing exercise performance. Sodium phosphate and potassium phosphate were reported to relieve fatigue in German soldiers during World War I. Other research in Germany during the 1930s suggested that phosphate salts could improve physical performance. More than 60 years ago, one reviewer discredited much of this early research, but he did note that phosphates probably could increase human work output when consumed in quantities exceeding the amounts found in the normal diet. Indeed, they are still marketed on the Internet, one such product being PhosFuel. Although phosphate salt supplementation may influence various physiological processes associated with physical performance, its effects to increase 2,3-BPG and related oxygen dynamics during aerobic endurance exercise have received most research attention. Bremner and others found that a 7-day phosphate loading protocol would increase erythrocyte phosphate pools and 2,3-BPG.

Over the course of the past 30 years the results of contemporary research relative to the ergogenic effect of phosphate supplementation are somewhat equivocal, some showing positive performance-enhancing effects and others reporting no significant improvement in performance.

The following studies, using appropriate experimental methods and the recommended phosphate dosages, have shown performance-enhancing effects of phosphate supplementation on a variety of exercise tasks.

- Cade and others studied the effect of 4 grams (1 gram four times daily) on the performance of highly trained runners. The phosphate salts increased the serum 2,3-BPG, which related closely to an increase in VO_2 max. The amount of lactate produce at a standard exercise workload decreased and was accompanied by a lower rating of perceived exertion (RPE), suggestive of lower psychological stress.
- Kreider and others, using highly trained cross-country runners as subjects, found that 4 grams of trisodium phosphate for

6 days produced a significant increase in VO_2 max, approximately 10 percent. However, the 2,3-BPG did not increase.

- In another study, Kreider and others reported that consuming 4 grams daily for 3–4 days reported a 9 percent increase in VO_2 max, a significantly faster 40-kilometer cycling time trial, and enhanced myocardial efficiency as monitored by echocardiographic techniques.
- Stewart and others, using trained cyclists, reported 3.6 grams of sodium phosphate for 3 days increased 2,3-BPG levels and increased VO_2 max by 11 percent. Exercise time to exhaustion in a cycling test protocol increased by nearly 16 percent.
- Goss and others examined the effect of potassium phosphate supplementation (4 grams per day for 2 days) and reported beneficial effects on ratings of perceived exertion (RPE) during treadmill running at about 70–80 percent VO_2 max.
- Brewer and others reported that trained male cyclists who consumed 50 milligrams per kilogram body mass of tribasic sodium phosphate for 6 days increased VO_2 peak values and possibly cycling time-trial performance. Performance in the 1,000-kilojoule time trial was about 60 to 70 seconds faster but was not significantly different from the placebo trial.
- In another study, Brewer and others, using a similar supplementation protocol with trained male cyclists, reported significant improvements in a cycle ergometer test measuring work and mean power output in both sprint (4 sets of 6 × 15 seconds) and time-trial (2 × 5 minutes) cycling efforts. The beneficial effects were seen both 1 and 4 days after the loading protocol.

In contrast, the results of other well-designed studies have not shown any performance-enhancing effects of phosphate salt supplementation.

- Kreider and others, using highly trained cross-country runners as subjects, found that 4 grams of trisodium phosphate for 6 days had no effect on a 5-mile competitive run on a treadmill.
- Mannix and others reported that although phosphate supplementation did increase 2,3-BPG levels, it did not improve cardiovascular function or oxygen efficiency in subjects exercising at 60 percent of VO_2 max.
- Goss and others reported no effect of potassium phosphate supplementation (4 grams per day for 2 days) on physiological responses to a maximal graded exercise test in highly trained endurance runners.
- Galloway and others provided an acute dose (22.2 grams) of calcium phosphate to trained cyclists and untrained subjects 90 minutes prior to a submaximal cycle test, followed by a maximal exercise test, and reported no significant effects on heart rate, ventilation, oxygen uptake, and time to exhaustion.
- Kramer and others found no effect of 3.5 days of supplementation with a commercial product (PhosFuel) on anaerobic performance in four 30-second Wingate tests with 2 minutes rest between.
- West and others reported that 6 days of supplementation with sodium phosphate (50 milligrams per kilogram body weight) exerted no effect on VO_2 peak in trained men and women.
- Using a supplementation protocol similar to the two studies noted above that reported beneficial performance-enhancing effects of phosphate supplementation, Brewer and others reported no significant effects on two cycling time-trial performances either 1 or 8 days following supplementation. The cycling time trials approximated 3–4 and 10–12 minutes' duration. In addition, no significant differences were found for heart rate, RPE, and postexercise blood lactate.
- Buck and others investigated the effects of three doses of trisodium phosphate supplementation on cycling time-trial performance in female cyclists. The time trials were done on a cycle ergometer and involved 500 kilojoules of work and approximated 40 minutes' duration. No significant differences were noted for time-trial performance between any of the supplementation protocols. Peak power output also was unchanged among trials.

In a review 20 years ago, Tremblay and others addressed methodological differences between studies that could contribute to the equivocal results reported at that time. In a more recent review, Buck and others, although suggesting sodium phosphate may have positive benefits for sporting performance, also indicated not all studies are supportive. Possible differences between study protocols may explain the difference, including the type of phosphate used, the dose, the dosing protocol, and the fitness level of the subjects. Additional research may be warranted.

Adenosine triphosphate (ATP), as you may recall, is the immediate source of energy for muscle contraction. Although some entrepreneurs have marketed ATP supplements for athletes, there is no available evidence that they enhance physical performance. Several studies have evaluated the effect of ATP supplementation on exercise performance but reported no significant effects. Arts and others studied the bioavailability of oral ATP supplements and found they do not appear in the blood, suggesting that such preparations are not bioavailable to the tissues and may help explain why studies show no ergogenic effect.

Creatine phosphate is used to replenish ATP rapidly as a component of the ATP-PCr energy system. As noted in chapter 6, research with oral creatine supplementation has suggested some ergogenic effects on muscular strength and muscle mass with resistance training. Although creatine phosphate has been studied in a medical case study and has shown some beneficial effects on muscle mass during rehabilitation, creatine supplementation also will suffice as there is an adequate amount of phosphate available in the body to form creatine phosphate.

Excesses of phosphorus in the body are excreted by the kidneys. Phosphorus excess *per se* does not appear to pose any problems, with the exception of individuals who have limited kidney function. Subjects consuming phosphate supplements may experience gastrointestinal distress, which may be alleviated by mixing the salts in a liquid and consuming with a meal. Excessive amounts of phosphate over time may impair calcium metabolism and balance.

Prudent Recommendations Given that the average daily intake of phosphorus is approximately twice the RDA, it may be reasonable to reduce intake of dietary sources high in phosphates, many of which are found in highly processed foods that usually contain food additives. Check the food label for terms that contain the word *phosphate,* such as dicalcium phosphate, hexametaphosphate, and sodium tripolyphosphate. Eating a diet rich in wholesome, natural foods, as recommended, may help reduce dietary phosphate intake.

For athletes, some evidence suggests that sodium phosphate salt supplementation may enhance aerobic endurance performance. An accepted protocol appears to be a total of 4 grams of trisodium phosphate per day, consumed in 1-gram portions with food and drink, for 5–6 days. If you decide to experiment with phosphate supplementation, do so in training before using it in conjunction with competition. Given the association with possible adverse health effects, this procedure should be used sparingly. Currently, use of phosphate salts for sports competition is not prohibited.

Magnesium (Mg)

Magnesium is the sixth most abundant mineral found in the body; it is a positive ion and is related to calcium and phosphorus.

DRI The adult RDA for magnesium is 400–420 mg for men and 310–320 mg for women. Slightly different amounts, found in the DRI table at the Website noted in the legend to table 8.1, are required by children and adolescents. The DV is 400 mg. The UL of 350 mg for magnesium, which is greater than the RDA for females, applies only to pharmacological forms of magnesium, as in supplements and fortified foods. There are no restrictions in obtaining magnesium via natural food sources.

Food Sources Magnesium is widely distributed in foods, particularly nuts, seafood, green leafy vegetables, other fruits and vegetables, black beans, and whole-grain products. One-half cup of shrimp or cooked spinach contains about 20 percent of the RDA, and a glass of skim milk has 10 percent. Many other foods contain about 2–10 percent of the RDA per serving. Areas with hard water may contain up to 20 mg of magnesium per liter, and some bottled waters may contain more than 100 mg per liter. About 25–60 percent of dietary magnesium is absorbed in the small intestine, depending on the amount consumed. See table 8.2.

Major Functions The body stores about 50–60 percent of its magnesium in the skeletal system, which may serve as a reserve during short periods of dietary deficiency. Sojka and Weaver indicate that magnesium influences bone metabolism and helps prevent bone fragility. Only about 1 percent is in the extracellular fluid, but the remainder is found in soft tissues such as muscle, where it is a component of numerous enzymes. Rude indicates that magnesium is involved in more than 300 essential metabolic reactions, many of which are important to the physically active individual, including neuromuscular, cardiovascular, and hormonal functions. For example, magnesium is involved in metabolic processes related to ATP production and use, including the glycolytic cycle, the citric acid cycle, and ATPase. As you recall, ATP is the primary source of energy for muscle contraction and numerous other metabolic processes. Magnesium helps regulate the synthesis

of protein and other compounds, such as 2,3-BPG, which may be essential for optimal oxygen metabolism. Magnesium also helps block some of the actions of calcium in the body, such as contraction in both the skeletal and smooth muscles.

Deficiency: Health and Physical Performance In a recent review, Rude noted several conditions that may cause a magnesium deficiency, including inadequate dietary intake, gastrointestinal disorders such as chronic diarrhea, renal losses in urine, endocrine and metabolic disorders such as diabetes mellitus, and cutaneous loss such as excess sweating. Relative to dietary intake, Rosanoff and others reported that almost half of the United States population consumed less than the required amount of magnesium from food. They also noted increases in calcium intake could increase the calcium:magnesium ratio in the body, possibly eliciting a calcium-activated inflammatory cascade and adverse health effects. Rosanoff and others indicated that low magnesium intakes and blood levels have been associated with a variety of diseases, including type 2 diabetes, metabolic syndrome, hypertension, atherosclerotic vascular disease, sudden cardiac death, osteoporosis, migraine headache, asthma, and colon cancer.

However, much is still unknown about magnesium deficiency and disease, mainly because it has not been a major research priority. Rosanoff and others stated that in comparison with calcium, magnesium is an orphan nutrient, receiving much less research attention. They recommend increased research in order to refine the magnesium requirements and to understand how low magnesium status and rising calcium-to-magnesium ratios influence the incidence of type 2 diabetes, metabolic syndrome, osteoporosis, and other inflammation-related disorders.

Relative to exercise or sports performance, a magnesium deficiency could certainly impair performance, as some symptoms are muscle weakness, tremor, and cramps. In addition, overtraining may lead to a decrease in exercise performance, and in a joint consensus statement on prevention, diagnosis, and treatment of the overtraining syndrome by the European College of Sport Science and the American College of Sports Medicine, Meeusen and others indicated nutrient deficiencies, including magnesium, should be considered.

Dietary magnesium intake in athletes may vary. For example, Lukaski reported that dietary survey findings indicated that most male athletes equaled or exceeded the RDA for magnesium. However, Czaja and others reported that elite male Polish athletes consumed low levels of magnesium and recommended supplementation. Lukaski also reported many female athletes were obtaining only about 60–65 percent of the RDA, while athletes in weight-control sports were getting only 30–35 percent. Over time, athletes with such low intakes may incur a magnesium deficiency.

Exercise appears to influence magnesium metabolism in various ways. Deuster has noted that one of the most common research observations is a decrease in plasma levels of magnesium following exercise. It is thought that magnesium enters the tissues in response to exercise-related requirements, for example, of the muscle tissue for energy metabolism and the adipose tissue for lipolysis. Exercise may also increase magnesium losses via urine and sweat. Although the reported sweat losses of 4–15 mg per liter are relatively small in comparison to body stores and daily intake, Nielsen and Lukaski stated that strenuous exercise apparently increases urinary and sweat losses that may increase magnesium requirements by 10–20 percent. Keep in mind that to replace 15 milligrams of magnesium lost from the body, one would need to consume about 40 milligrams at a 40 percent rate of absorption. That is almost 10 percent of the male RDA. On the basis of some of these findings, several reports have recommended that individuals undergoing prolonged, intensive physical training should increase their daily intake of magnesium, but these recommendations are within range of the RDA. The extra Calories consumed when energy expenditure increases during exercise should provide the additional magnesium.

Supplementation: Health and Physical Performance   Relative to health, some epidemiological research from Europe and the United States has indicated that males who consume hard drinking water, which is high in magnesium, experience fewer deaths from myocardial infarction. Rubenowitz and others reported a 35 percent reduction in death for those who consumed the most magnesium from municipal water supplies. High blood pressure is one of the major risk factors for heart disease. Several reviews have suggested that magnesium supplementation may help reduce blood pressure. Kass and others, in a meta-analysis of 22 studies, concluded that magnesium supplementation, with an average dose of 410 milligrams daily, appears to achieve a small but clinically significant reduction in both systolic (3–4 mmHg) and diastolic (2–3 mmHg) blood pressure. In addition, Houston reported that magnesium intake of 500 to 1,000 milligrams per day may reduce both systolic (5.6 mmHg) and diastolic (2.8 mmHg) blood pressure, but clinical studies show a wide range of reduction, with some showing no reduction. However, Houston suggests the combination of increased intake of magnesium and potassium, coupled with reduced sodium intake, is more effective in reducing blood pressure. The DASH diet, discussed in chapter 9 as a means to lower blood pressure, is rich in magnesium and potassium and low in sodium and is one of the most recommended healthful diets, as noted throughout this text.

The effect of magnesium supplementation on exercise performance has received limited research attention over the years, but several reviews are available. In 1988, McDonald and Keen indicated that they are not aware of any data showing a positive effect of magnesium supplementation on exercise performance in individuals who are in adequate magnesium status. In 2000, Newhouse and Finstad conducted a meta-analysis of human supplementation studies involving magnesium supplementation and exercise performance, and they concluded that the strength of the evidence favors those studies finding no effect of magnesium supplementation on any form of exercise performance, including aerobic, anaerobic-lactic acid, and strength activities. In a 2006 review, Nielsen and Lukaski also concluded that magnesium supplementation of physically active individuals with adequate magnesium status has not been shown to enhance physical performance. However, if a magnesium deficiency is corrected, exercise performance may be improved. For example, Lukaski noted that

some earlier studies have shown that magnesium supplementation improved strength and cardiorespiratory function in healthy persons and athletes but also noted that it is unclear as to whether these observations related to improvement of an impaired nutritional status or a pharmacological effect. In a recent study, Setaro and others investigated the effect of magnesium supplementation (350 milligrams daily for 4 weeks) to volleyball players on a variety of exercise performance variables, including VO$_2$ max, isokinetic strength tests, and plyometric jump tests. They noted significant increases in two of the plyometric tests and suggested that magnesium supplementation may improve alactic anaerobic metabolism, even though the players were not magnesium deficient.

At present the data are too limited to support an ergogenic effect of magnesium supplementation, and additional well-controlled research is justified.

As noted, an UL of 350 mg has been established for magnesium supplements or fortified foods. Mildly excessive intakes of magnesium may cause nausea, vomiting, and diarrhea. In individuals with kidney disorders who cannot excrete the excess, increased serum levels of magnesium may lead to coma and death.

Prudent Recommendations   Physically active individuals should obtain adequate magnesium from a balanced diet containing foods rich in magnesium. The DASH diet is recommended. For those trying to lose body weight for competition, dietary magnesium may be compromised. In particular, Newhouse and Finstad indicate that female athletes are at risk for magnesium deficiency. In cases of suspected dietary insufficiency, magnesium supplementation may be recommended via supplements or fortified foods. The amount of magnesium in such products may vary. Pure magnesium supplements may contain about 200–500 milligrams; multivitamin-mineral supplements contain varying amounts, about 50 milligrams or more; fortified foods also contain varying amounts, usually listed as a percentage of the Daily Value. The DV for magnesium is 400 milligrams, so 20 percent would contain 80 milligrams per serving. Check the Supplement Facts and Nutrition Facts labels for magnesium content. The recommended amount from such sources should not exceed 350 milligrams daily. Much lower amounts are recommended for children. There is no need for larger doses, as they may be associated with some adverse effects.

Key Concepts

▶ Calcium is most prevalent in dairy products, or the milk food group. One glass of low-fat milk provides about 30 percent of the daily AI.

▶ Calcium intake is important for everyone, but in particular, children, adolescents, and all women should obtain adequate dietary calcium. Children and adolescents should obtain adequate calcium to increase their peak bone mass; women need calcium to help prevent losses during aging.

Trace Minerals

The **trace minerals** (trace elements) are those needed in quantities less than 100 mg per day. These minerals are often known as *microminerals*. For several, the body needs only extremely minute amounts, such as a few micrograms (millionth of a gram) per day. The term *ultratrace* is applied to these minerals.

Iron (Fe)

Iron is a metallic element that exists in two general forms, ferrous (Fe^{2+}) and ferric (Fe^{3+}).

DRI Depending upon age and sex, the average individual needs to replace about 1.0–1.5 mg of iron that is lost from the body daily. However, because the bioavailability of iron is very low, with only about 10 percent of food iron being absorbed, the RDA is ten times the need. Currently the RDA is 8 mg for men, 11 mg for males age 14–18, and 15 mg for female teenagers and 18 mg for female adults. Slightly different amounts are needed by other age groups and may be found in the DRI table at the Website noted in the legend to table 8.1. Pregnant women need 27 mg, whereas postmenopausal women need only 8 mg. The current DV is 18 mg. The UL range is 40–45 mg/day.

Food Sources Dietary iron comes in two forms. **Heme iron** is associated with hemoglobin and myoglobin and thus is found only in animal foods, such as meat, chicken, and fish. About 35–55 percent of the iron found in meat is heme iron, the percentage being somewhat higher in beef as compared to chicken and fish. **Nonheme iron** is found in both animal and plant foods. About 20–70 percent of the iron in animal foods and 100 percent in plant foods is in the nonheme form. Heme iron has greater bioavailability: About 15–35 percent of it is absorbed from the intestines compared to only 2–20 percent for nonheme iron. The percent absorbed depends on the iron status of the individual. Those with higher levels of body iron stores will absorb less, whereas those with lower levels will absorb more.

Excellent animal sources of dietary iron include liver, heart, lean meats, oysters, clams, and dark poultry meat. One ounce of lean meat provides about 1 mg of heme iron. Good sources of nonheme iron include dried fruits such as apricots, prunes, and raisins; vegetables such as broccoli and peas; legumes; and whole-grain products. Six dried apricot halves or ½ cup of beans provides about 3 mg of nonheme iron, and some breakfast cereals are fortified with nonheme iron to provide 100 percent of the RDA. Cooking in iron pots or skillets also contributes some iron to the diet. On a balanced diet, about 6 mg of iron is provided in every 1,000 Calories ingested. See table 8.4 for foods high in iron.

Certain factors in food may affect the amount of iron absorbed into the body. A muscle protein factor (MPF) found in meat, fish, and poultry is an unknown agent that facilitates the absorption of both heme and nonheme iron. The existence of such a factor is suggested by the fact that small amounts of meat added to vegetable or grain products enhance nonheme absorption. Certain peptides in meat may cause this increased absorption. For example, iron absorption from beans is almost doubled when mixed with small amounts of meat, as in dishes such as chili. Vitamin C prevents the oxidation of ferrous iron to the ferric form (ferrous iron is more readily absorbed) and thus facilitates nonheme iron absorption, but it has no effect on absorption of heme iron. Thus, for breakfast, drinking orange juice improves the bioavailability of iron in toast.

However, substances found naturally in some foods, such as tannins in tea, phytic acid in grains, oxalic acid in vegetables, and excessive fiber, may decrease the bioavailability of nonheme iron by forming insoluble salts (phytates, oxalates) or by promoting rapid transport and excretion through the intestines. Tea, for example, which is high in tannins, decreases iron absorption by 60 percent. However, if the diet is balanced these factors should not pose a major problem for adequate iron nutrition. Certain mineral supplements, particularly calcium, and even the calcium in milk, when taken with a meal, may impair absorption of nonheme iron. This effect may be lessened by ingestion of vitamin C with the meal. As mentioned previously, calcium supplements may be recommended for some individuals, including youths, who also need more dietary iron. Molgaard and others noted increasing evidence suggesting that high calcium intake does not impair iron status. In a study they found that consuming a 500-mg calcium supplement at the evening meal over the course of a year had no effect on the iron status of adolescent girls.

Major Functions Abbaspour and others indicate that iron is an essential element for almost all living organisms, as it participates in a wide variety of metabolic processes. The major function of iron in the body is the formation of compounds essential to the transportation and utilization of oxygen. The vast majority is used to form hemoglobin, a protein-iron compound in the RBC that transports oxygen from the lungs to the body tissues. Other iron compounds include myoglobin, the cytochromes, and several Krebs-cycle metalloenzymes, which help use oxygen at the cellular level. The remainder of the body iron is stored in the tissues,

TABLE 8.4   Trace minerals: iron, copper, zinc, chromium, selenium

Trace mineral*	Major food sources	Major body functions	Deficiency symptoms	Symptoms of excessive consumption
Iron (Fe) RDA: 8 mg♂ 18 mg♀ DV: 18 mg	Organ meats such as liver; meat, fish, and poultry; shellfish, especially oysters; dried beans and peas; whole-grain products; green leafy vegetables; spinach; broccoli; dried apricots, dates, figs, raisins; iron cookware	Hemoglobin and myoglobin formation; electron transfer; essential in oxidative processes	Fatigue; anemia; impaired temperature regulation; decreased resistance to infection	Hemochromatosis; liver damage
Copper (Cu) RDA: 900 mcg DV: 2 mg	Organ meats such as liver; meat, fish, and poultry; shellfish; nuts; eggs; whole-grain breads; bran cereals; avocado; broccoli; banana	Proper use of iron and hemoglobin in the body; metalloenzyme involved in connective tissue formation and oxidations	Rare; anemia	Rare; nausea; vomiting
Zinc (Zn) RDA: 11 mg♂ 8 mg♀ DV: 15 mg	Organ meats; meat, fish, poultry; shellfish, especially oysters; dairy products; nuts; whole-grain products; vegetables, asparagus, spinach	Cofactor of many enzymes involved in energy metabolism, protein synthesis, immune function, sexual maturation, and sensations of taste and smell	Depressed immune function; impaired wound healing; depressed appetite; failure to grow; skin inflammation	Increased LDL- and decreased HDL- cholesterol; impaired immune system; nausea; vomiting; impaired copper absorption
Chromium (Cr) AI: 35 mcg♂ 25 mcg♀ DV: 120 mcg	Organ meats such as liver; meats; oysters; cheese; whole-grain products; asparagus; beer	Enhances insulin function as glucose tolerance factor	Glucose intolerance; impaired lipid metabolism	Rare from dietary sources
Selenium (Se) RDA: 55 mcg DV: 70 mcg	Meat, fish, poultry; organ meats such as kidney, liver; seafood; whole grains and nuts from selenium-rich soil	Cofactor of glutathione peroxidase, an antioxidant enzyme	Rare; cardiac muscle damage	Nausea; vomiting; abdominal pain; hair loss

*RDA or AI: adults age19–50 DV: Daily Value.

principally as protein compounds called **ferritins**. The iron in the blood, serum ferritin, is used as an index of the body iron stores, as are a number of other markers such as transferrin, protoporphyrin, and hemoglobin. Other major storage sites include the liver, spleen, and bone marrow. When ferritin levels become excessive in the liver, the iron is stored as hemosiderin, an insoluble form. Approximately 30 percent of the body iron is in storage form, while the remaining 70 percent is involved in oxygen metabolism. Because iron is so critical to oxygen use in humans, it is essential that those individuals engaged in aerobic endurance-type exercises have an adequate dietary intake. Figure 8.5 represents a brief outline of iron metabolism in humans. For a comprehensive review of iron metabolism and regulation, the interested reader is referred to the review by Wood and Ronnenberg.

As noted below, both a deficiency and excess of iron in the body may lead to serious health problems. Fortunately, Wessling-Resnick indicates humans have an important iron regulatory hormone, **hepcidin**, that helps regulate body iron stores. According to Zhao and others, the main function of hepcidin is to decrease iron concentrations in the blood by various means. Nemeth and Ganz indicate that when serum iron levels are elevated, the liver will synthesize more hepcidin to help inhibit iron absorption from the intestines and suppress release into the blood. Contrarily, when serum iron stores are depressed, synthesis of hepcidin is decreased, leading to increased iron absorption.

Deficiency: Health and Physical Performance As noted previously, iron deficiency is one of the leading risk factors for disability and death worldwide. Wessling-Resnick indicates iron deficiency is perhaps the most significant worldwide nutritional problem, noting that it affects more than 2 billion people, particularly women and children in developing countries, many of whom develop iron-deficiency anemia. A deficiency in children may alter the energy metabolism of the brain, impairing brain development in early life with associated learning and motor defects. Additionally, Scott and others suggest that approximately 1.8 million deaths in children under age 5 could be avoided each year by increasing their serum hemoglobin levels by 1 gram per deciliter. Iron is one of the few nutrients found to be slightly deficient in the diet of many Americans.

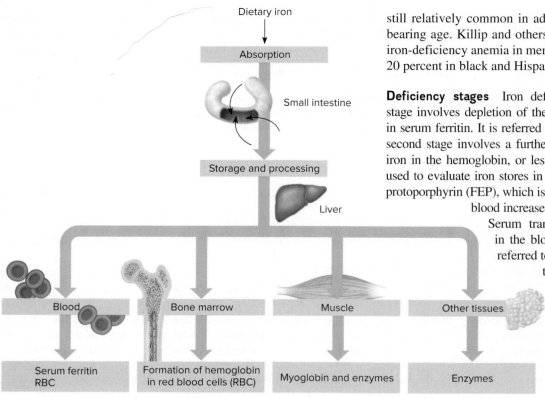

Dietary iron

Absorption

Small intestine

Storage and processing

Liver

Blood

Bone marrow

Muscle

Other tissues

Serum ferritin
RBC

Formation of hemoglobin
in red blood cells (RBC)

Myoglobin and enzymes

Enzymes

FIGURE 8.5 Simplified diagram of iron metabolism in humans. After digestion, iron is used in the formation of hemoglobin, myoglobin, and certain cellular enzymes, all of which are essential for transportation of oxygen in the body.

still relatively common in adolescent girls and women of child-bearing age. Killip and others reported a 2 percent prevalence of iron-deficiency anemia in men, 9–12 percent in white women, and 20 percent in black and Hispanic women.

Deficiency stages Iron deficiency occurs in stages. The first stage involves depletion of the bone marrow stores and a decrease in serum ferritin. It is referred to as the stage of iron depletion. The second stage involves a further decrease in serum ferritin and less iron in the hemoglobin, or less circulating iron. Other markers are used to evaluate iron stores in this stage, including free erythrocyte protoporphyrin (FEP), which is used to form hemoglobin. FEP in the blood increases when adequate iron is not available. Serum transferrin, a protein that carries iron in the blood, also increases. This is the stage referred to as iron-deficiency erythropoiesis. In these first two stages the hemoglobin concentration in the blood is still normal. Collectively, these stages are often alluded to as **iron deficiency without anemia**. Wessling-Resnick notes that reduced serum ferritin is the key indicator of iron depletion, or iron deficiency without anemia, with levels lower than 30 nanograms per milliliter. The third stage consists of a very low level of serum ferritin and decreased hemoglobin concentration, or **iron-deficiency anemia**. Wessling-Resnick indicates the hallmark of iron-deficiency anemia is low hemoglobin levels, with males less than 13 grams per deciliter and females less than 12 grams per deciliter. Symptoms of iron-deficiency anemia include paleness, tiredness, low vitality, and impaired ability to regulate body temperature in a cold environment. Most notably, iron-deficiency anemia impairs muscular performance. In their review of 29 research reports, Haas and Brownlie noted a strong causal effect of iron-deficiency anemia to impaired work capacity in both humans and animals.

Deficiency in athletes Because iron is so critical to the oxygen energy system, it is essential for endurance athletes to have adequate iron in the diet to maintain optimal body supplies. Buratti and others note that low body iron levels can cause anemia and thus limit the delivery of oxygen to exercising muscle, but they also indicate iron deficiency may also have adverse effects on oxidative metabolism within the muscle.

Recent reviews suggest certain groups of athletes may be at risk for iron deficiency. Kong and others indicated that exercise-induced iron-deficiency anemia is notably high in athletic populations, particularly those with heavy training loads. This could include some male athletes, such as gymnasts, wrestlers, and distance runners. Relative to distance runners, Zourdos and others noted that among competitive athletes, marathoners are at greater risk to develop anemia and other clinical syndromes

The body normally loses very little iron through such routes as the skin, gastrointestinal tract, hair, and sweat. About 8 mg of dietary iron daily will replace these losses. Females also lose some additional iron in the blood flow during menstruation. They need about 15–18 mg of dietary iron per day to replace their total losses. Adolescent boys need about 11 mg, as they are increasing muscle tissue and blood volume during this rapid period of growth. With 6 mg of iron per 1,000 Calories, the adult male has no problem meeting his requirement of 8 mg per day. With a normal intake of 2,900 Calories, he will receive 17.4 mg. With 2,200 Calories, the average intake for females, only 13.2 mg iron would be provided. This is somewhat short of the 15–18 mg needed.

The main factor underlying iron deficiency in Western diets is inadequate dietary intake. Fairbanks indicates that the diet has evolved so that many individuals consume iron-poor diets, such as snack foods, white bread, and soft drinks. However, most females have normal hemoglobin and serum ferritin status. Because the normal loss of iron from the body is relatively low, and because excessive amounts in the body may be harmful, as noted previously the intestine limits the amount absorbed from the diet. In contrast, when an individual becomes iron deficient, the intestine may increase the amount of dietary iron absorbed to above 30 percent. Nevertheless, iron deficiency and iron-deficiency anemia are that may be associated with inadequate dietary intake of iron. In particular, McClung and others indicated female athletes are at risk, noting recent studies that have documented poor iron status and associated declines in both cognitive and physical performance. In a study of elite women soccer players 6 months before the FIFA Women's World Cup, Landahl and others reported that 57 percent had iron deficiency and 29 percent had iron-deficiency anemia.

The normal hemoglobin level is 14–16 grams per deciliter (100 mL) of blood for males and 12–14 grams for females. As noted previously, males have been classified as anemic with less than 13 grams, whereas values less than 12 grams have been used as the criterion for anemia in females. Randy Eichner, a hematologist involved in sports medicine, poses the interesting question of whether an athlete whose usual hemoglobin is 16 grams per deciliter is anemic if his level decreases to 14 grams.

Most sport scientists indicate it is important to monitor the diet and iron status of certain athletes. In its position statement relative to nutrition for the athlete, the American College of Sports Medicine (ACSM) and two other professional associations recommended periodic screening of iron status for some athletes. In the United States some, but not all, universities screen for iron deficiency in female athletes.

Causes of deficiency in athletes   There may be a number of causes for the low iron or hemoglobin levels found in some athletes, including inadequate dietary intake, excessive menstruation, and various exercise protocols.

Inadequate dietary intake   Zourdas and others state that inadequate dietary intake of iron has been identified as one key factor underlying decreased performance in athletes, such as marathon runners. In fact, they note that iron is one of the few nutrients recommended as a supplement by the ACSM and other professional associations in their position stand noted above.

Excessive menstruation   McClung and others indicate that increased loss of blood through menstruation could eventually lead to an iron deficiency. In such cases, consultation with a physician could be necessary to determine the cause and appropriate treatment.

Various exercise protocols   Exercise may contribute to iron deficiency in various ways. Hinton indicates that strenuous endurance exercise training may be associated with iron deficiency. Sim and others reported that intense exercise training may induce increases in inflammatory cytokines, such as interleukin-6, which may elevate hepcidin levels, leading to a decrease in iron absorption. They note hepcidin levels have been shown to be significantly elevated after prolonged exercise training, such as for a marathon, in female athletes. Decreased iron absorption and metabolism could lead to anemia.

Some types of exercise may increase iron loss though the urine, feces, and sweat. Distance runners may experience **hematuria**, the presence of hemoglobin or myoglobin in the urine. Repetitive impact of the feet with the ground may rupture blood cells as they pass through the foot vascular system, a process known as **hemolysis**, releasing hemoglobin for circulation to the kidneys and excretion in the urine. Additionally, prolonged running may lead to ruptured muscle cells, releasing iron-containing myoglobin, which may have the same fate.

Intense, prolonged exercise has been shown to cause inflammation and bleeding in the GI tract. Additionally, many athletes may also use aspirin or other anti-inflammatory drugs as a pain reliever during intense training, and use of such medications has been associated with GI bleeding. Bleeding in the gastrointestinal tract leads to a loss of iron in the feces. Additionally, athletes may lose some iron during heavy sweating. Iron sweat losses may vary, one approximation being about 0.18–0.20 milligrams per liter of sweat. Although not a substantial amount of iron loss, copious sweat losses could accumulate to 0.4 milligrams, which would necessitate 4 milligrams of dietary iron to replace based on a 10 percent absorption rate.

Athletes who begin to train at altitude will need to ensure adequate dietary iron intake, because the increased production of red blood cells at altitude will draw upon the body reserves.

Overall, athletes in training may lose more iron than nonathletes. In their review, Weaver and Rajaram noted that when compared to the reference value of sedentary individuals, iron losses in the feces, urine, and sweat may be 75 percent greater in male athletes (1.75 versus 1.0 milligrams) and about 65 percent greater in female athletes (2.3 versus 1.4 milligrams).

Sports anemia   As would be expected, the problem of concern to the endurance athlete is the development of iron-deficiency anemia. A number of studies have shown that anemia causes a significant reduction in the ability to perform prolonged, high-level exercise. The donation of blood causes a drop in hemoglobin, which may also decrease performance capacity. This is, of course, related to the decreased ability to transport and use oxygen in the body.

One form of anemia associated with endurance training is sports anemia, mentioned in chapter 6. Sports anemia is not a true anemia. Although the hemoglobin concentration is toward the lower end of the normal range, the other indices of iron status are normal. Whether sports anemia is a beneficial physiological response to endurance exercise or a condition that will hinder performance is not known. Short-term sports anemia appears to develop in some individuals during the early phases of training or when the magnitude of training increases drastically. One of the effects of endurance training is to increase both the plasma volume and the number of RBC. However, the plasma expansion appears to be greater, so there is a dilution of the RBC and a lowering of the hemoglobin concentration. This effect is believed to be beneficial to the athlete, however, because it reduces the viscosity, or thickness, of the blood and allows it to flow more easily. In many athletes the hemoglobin concentration returns to normal after the first month or so of training. Long-term sports anemia is often seen in highly trained endurance athletes. One theory proposes that the production of RBC by the bone marrow is decreased in endurance athletes because the RBC become so efficient in releasing oxygen to the tissues. The authors of this theory suggest that sports anemia is not due to poor iron status. Moreover, in a review relating hematological factors to aerobic power, Gledhill and his associates indicated that an increase in blood volume can compensate for a moderate reduction in hemoglobin concentration.

Eichner noted that the term *sports anemia* indicates a pseudoanemia, or a false anemia in athletes who are aerobically fit. Weight also indicated that the term is misleading and its use should be discouraged because athletes who develop anemia do so not because of exercise, but for the same reasons that nonathletes do, primarily inadequate dietary iron.

Iron deficiency without anemia As noted above, Buratti and others indicated that an iron deficiency in the tissues may have adverse effects on exercise performance. Thus, an athlete may have an iron deficiency but not to the extent of being anemic. The effect of iron deficiency without anemia on exercise performance has been studied over the course of 25 years. In a recent review, Rowland noted that whether iron deficiency without anemia decreases performance in humans is debatable. He indicated that research evidence in animals is clear cut, indicating that depletion of iron stores without a decrease in hemoglobin diminishes exercise performance. Decreased iron stores in the tissues diminished intracellular metabolic capacity. However, Rowland notes that research in humans has not provided sufficient evidence to support the effect seen in animals, indicating that research with human subjects suffers from numerous methodological weaknesses. From the available data, he concludes that it is difficult to mount a compelling argument that an iron deficiency without anemia impairs endurance performance in athletes.

Supplementation: Health and Physical Performance The importance of iron to oxygen transport and endurance capacity and the possibility that many athletes, particularly females, may be iron deficient have led a number of investigators in the area of sports nutrition to recommend that more athletes take dietary iron or supplements. Others discourage the indiscriminate use of iron supplements by athletes.

Does iron supplementation improve physical performance? Many studies have been conducted in attempts to answer this question, and the answer appears to be dependent upon the iron status of the individual.

Iron-deficiency anemia If the individual suffers from iron-deficiency anemia, iron therapy could help correct this condition and concomitantly improve health status and exercise performance capacity. In a review, Lomango and others reported improvement in various aspects of mood, memory, and intellectual ability after iron supplementation. In a meta-analysis, Avni and others found that iron replacement therapy in cardiac patients improved quality-of-life measures as well as performance in a 6-minute walking test. In their review, Rodenberg and Gustafson concluded that athletes who are found to be anemic secondary to iron deficiency do benefit and show improved performance with appropriate iron supplementation.

Iron deficiency without anemia The effect of iron supplementation in iron-deficient, nonanemic individuals has been studied for possible effects on both health and physical performance.

Relative to health, Lobera-Jáuregu notes that iron deficiency without anemia may cause cognitive disturbances, mainly in attention span, intelligence, and sensory perception, but also notes that despite methodological differences among studies, there is some evidence that iron supplementation improves cognitive functions. Supplementation may have some other health benefits as well, particularly for women during pregnancy, as plasma and red blood cell production increases, possibly causing a deficiency. During pregnancy the RDA for iron increases by 50 percent.

The effect of iron supplementation on physical performance capacity in iron-deficient but nonanemic individuals is somewhat controversial. Although iron supplementation may improve markers of iron status, the effect on exercise performance is debatable. In a previous edition of this text, Williams cited six studies favoring a beneficial effect of iron supplementation on exercise performance, and eight studies showing no effect. Subsequent reviews report conflicting findings. In their review, Rodenberg and Gustafson indicated that supplementation does not appear to be justified solely to improve performance. Conversely, two separate reviews by DellaValle and Burden and others concluded that iron supplementation would improve iron status in female athletes. DellaValle also concluded supplementation may improve measures of physical performance, while Burden and others reported a moderate effect on improving hemoglobin and aerobic capacity as measured by VO_2 max.

Additional research may be recommended to help resolve these contradictory findings.

Iron saturated Iron supplementation offers no benefits to individuals with normal hemoglobin and iron status. Some well-controlled research on highly active, nonanemic females with normal iron status has shown no effect of iron supplementation on hemoglobin concentration or exercise performance.

However, endurance athletes with normal hemoglobin status who attempt to increase their red blood cells (RBC) and hemoglobin levels may benefit from iron supplementation. Increased hemoglobin levels increase the ability to transport oxygen to the muscles, with the goal of enhancing performance. Previously, athletes used blood doping techniques (reinfusion of one's own blood previously drawn or from a blood-matched donor) or injection of recombinant erythropoietin (rEPO), a hormone that stimulates RBC and hemoglobin production. However, both blood doping and rEPO have been prohibited by the International Olympic Committee, not only because they may provide an unfair advantage but also because their use may be lethal.

The technique of "Live high, train low" may be an effective alternative. When one ascends to altitude, such as 2,500 meters (8,225 feet) or so, the atmospheric oxygen pressure decreases, leading to lower oxygen pressure in the blood. The body immediately begins to adapt. The kidneys produce natural EPO, which stimulates the bone marrow to produce more RBC. Over time, the RBC and hemoglobin concentration are elevated. This is the benefit of "Live high." However, given the decreased oxygen pressure, athletes may not train as intensely at altitude, and thus may not train optimally, as they could at sea level, the "Train low" component. Some athletes may reside in locations where it is possible to live high and train low by driving an hour or so to a lower altitude. Such is not the case for most athletes, so scientists have constructed houses at sea level whose inside atmosphere has been manipulated to resemble one of high altitude. Thus, the athlete can "Live high" in the house, and produce EPO naturally, but can also step outside and "Train low" at sea-level atmosphere. Additionally, tents used as sleeping chambers are available commercially.

Research supports the efficacy of a "Live high, train low" protocol to enhance aerobic endurance performance. Wilber and others suggest that the optimal dose is to live at a natural elevation of 2,000–2,500 meters for at least 4 weeks with more than 22 hours a day at that altitude.

Although living at natural altitude is effective, Mazzeo and Fulco contended that the results from using alternative means, such as altitude houses or sleeping tents, are equivocal.

For athletes who use this strategy, iron supplementation may be necessary to provide substrate for hemoglobin synthesis. Mazzeo and Fulco note that this is true particularly for women who come to altitude with inadequate or borderline iron stores. Iron supplementation prior to and during their stay at altitude will increase hematocrit similarly to men. Thus, they recommend that prior to coming to altitude, women (and men) should ensure that they have adequate iron stores, especially for athletes who plan on training or competing at high elevations.

Excess Iron   Iron is both an essential nutrient and a potentially harmful toxicant to cells. If you plan to take iron supplements, you should have your serum ferritin checked, because some danger is associated with iron supplements if they lead to excessive iron in the body. Prolonged consumption of large amounts can cause a disturbance in iron metabolism in susceptible individuals. Iron then tends to accumulate in the liver as hemosiderin, which in excess can cause **hemochromatosis**, the most serious health consequence of excessive iron intake. This condition causes cirrhosis and may lead to the ultimate destruction of the liver. Of every 1,000 Americans, approximately two to three have a genetic predisposition to hemochromatosis, but Wessling-Resnick indicates that the blood disorder may be either genetic or acquired.

The National Institutes of Health indicated that iron overload can contribute to the development of additional health problems. Other than the liver, iron can accumulate in other body organs, such as the heart and pancreas. The NIH indicates that too much iron in the heart can cause irregular heartbeats and contribute to heart failure. Excess iron may also accumulate in the pancreas, possibly leading to diabetes. Additionally, excessive iron may be fatal to young children; more than 30 deaths occur each year from overdoses of iron obtained by eating large amounts of candy-flavored vitamin tablets with iron.

Prudent Recommendations   In summary, it would be wise for developing adolescent males and females to be aware of the iron content in their diets. This concern is especially important to endurance athletes, although it would appear that the extra Calories they eat to meet the additional energy requirements of training would provide the necessary iron. All active males and females should be aware of heme iron–rich foods, such as lean red meat, and be sure to include them in the daily diet, or at least two to three times a week. Mixing small amounts of meat with iron-rich plant foods, such as lean beef and chili beans, will enhance iron nutrition. Eating foods rich in vitamin C with nonheme iron–containing foods and using iron cookware also will increase iron bioavailability.

DellaValle recommended that female athletes most at risk of iron deficiency be screened at the beginning of and during the training season using tests for hemoglobin and serum ferritin, and appropriate dietary and/or supplementation recommendations should be made to those with compromised iron status. Iron supplementation by commercial preparations may be recommended for certain individuals who have or who are at high risk of having low serum ferritin levels, including female distance runners, some vegetarian athletes, those who experience heavy menstrual blood flow, athletes who initiate altitude training, and athletes who are on restricted caloric intake. Over-the-counter multivitamin/mineral preparations vary in iron content. Some contain none, such as those marketed to men and postmenopausal women, while others contain the Daily Value of 18 mg iron, which is 100 percent of the RDA for adult females and 120 percent for adolescent girls. One tablet a day may be advisable for these individuals, and it should be consumed on an empty stomach to minimize adverse effects of some foods on absorption. For women who have iron deficiency without anemia who want a rapid restoration of serum iron, injections may be preferable. Dawson and others had women consume either an iron tablet (105 mg iron) for 30 days or receive five intramuscular injections (100 mg elemental iron) over a 10-day period. The iron injections were significantly more effective (both in time and degree of increase) in improving serum ferritin levels over the course of 30 days. The individual with iron-deficiency anemia should consult a physician for iron therapy, which may consist of 100–200 mg of elemental iron per day until the condition is corrected.

It is important to reemphasize that iron supplementation should not be done indiscriminately, but preferably only after determination of one's iron status. Kong and others reported that increased iron stores are a common finding in elite athletes who have used long-term iron supplementation, putting the athletes at an increased risk of developing iron overload–related diseases. In an investigation of iron status in marathoners, Mettler and Zimmermann showed signs of iron overload in 17 percent of male runners. Health professionals indicate that iron supplements should be given to athletes only by prescription, primarily only in cases of iron-deficiency anemia.

Copper (Cu)

Kim and others have noted that copper is a vital mineral in human metabolism but indicated serious health concerns are associated with its deficiency or excess accumulation in the body.

DRI The RDA for copper is 900 micrograms, or 0.90 mg, for adults age 19–50, but amounts vary for other age groups and may be found in the DRI table at the Website noted in the legend to table 8.1. The DV is 2 mg, or about twice the amount of the RDA. The UL for adults is 10 milligrams/day.

Food Sources Copper is widely distributed in foods and is high in seafoods, meats, nuts, beans, whole-grain products, and foods containing chocolate. One cup of whole-grain cereal contains about 8 percent of the DV, or nearly 18 percent of the adult RDA. Copper also may be found in drinking water, particularly soft water, which leaches it from copper pipes. Some good food sources are listed in table 8.4. Collins indicates copper absorption under normal conditions is approximately 10 percent of dietary intake, and the average intake in the United States is about 1.2 milligrams daily, slightly more than the RDA.

Major Functions Collins indicates that copper serves a prominent role as a cofactor for many enzymes, metalloenzymes known as cuproenzymes, most of which are involved in oxidation processes. Copper works closely with iron in oxygen metabolism. It is needed for the absorption of iron from the intestinal tract, helps in the formation of hemoglobin, and is involved in the activity of a specific cytochrome (cytochromes C oxidase), an oxidative enzyme in the mitochondria. Copper is also a component of ceruloplasmin, a glycoprotein in the plasma, and is in superoxide dismutase (SOD), an enzyme that functions as an antioxidant to quench free radicals. Collins notes that copper is also involved in the normal function of connective and bone tissue, lipid metabolism, and prevention of anemia. Additionally, Gaier and others indicate copper plays an important role in the brain.

Deficiency: Health and Physical Performance Copper deficiency is rare in humans. A genetic disorder, Menkes syndrome, may impair copper metabolism, eliciting deficiency symptoms in the newborn with numerous developmental and neurological defects; affected children live only a few years. Other genetic disorders may impair copper metabolism and cause deficiency-associated health problems in later childhood and adulthood. Other than genetic causes, a deficiency has occurred in some patients receiving prolonged intravenous feeding of a copper-free solution. Collins also indicates that individuals consuming large doses of zinc supplements or antacids may also experience copper deficiency. The major deficiency symptom is anemia, but osteoporosis, neurological defects, and heart disease may also develop.

Available surveys indicate that most athletes consume ample amounts of copper. The effects of exercise or exercise training on serum copper levels are variable, with studies showing increases, decreases, or no changes. Several studies have reported decreases in serum copper in athletes involved in prolonged training or after an endurance exercise task. The authors theorized that the decreased levels were due to sweat or fecal losses. However, no deficiency symptoms were noted. In his review, Lukaski indicated that physical training does increase the copper-containing SOD, and normal body stores of copper are apparently adequate to support the increase of this antioxidant enzyme.

Supplementation: Health and Physical Performance Dietary supplements contain varying amounts of copper, but normally the RDA, which is 0.9 milligram. Fortified foods may also contain copper, usually the Daily Value, which is 2.0 milligrams. Although copper (2 mg) is used in a supplement being studied to help prevent age-related macular degeneration, it is not because it plays a role in eye health but rather to help counter the effect of the high zinc content that could reduce copper absorption. Supplements are not recommended because excessive copper intake, even 5–10 milligrams, may cause nausea and vomiting. The UL is 10 milligrams. The National Academy of Sciences reports that toxicity from dietary sources is rare. However, Turnlund indicates that copper poisoning can result from excess intake via supplements.

In recent years scientists have been exploring the role of copper in the etiology of Alzheimer's disease. Some individuals have a genetic disorder predisposing them to increased concentrations of copper in various body tissues, including the brain. This condition is known as Wilson disease with numerous symptoms, including some comparable to Alzheimer's. Although Wilson disease is hereditary, Squitti and others suggest a diet-gene interplay may be involved. In this regard, Brewer hypothesizes that the dietary factor is inorganic copper in drinking water, leached from copper plumbing, the use of which coincides with the epidemic of Alzheimer's. Kaler reported that symptoms associated with Wilson disease are reduced by copper chelation therapy, a method used to bind and excrete metals from the body.

Prudent Recommendations Consuming a balanced diet should provide adequate amounts of dietary copper. Consumption of numerous servings of fortified foods, such as many breakfast cereals containing the DV of 2 milligrams, may exceed the UL of 10 milligrams. Copper supplements are not recommended for either health or enhancement of sports performance.

Zinc (Zn)

Zinc is a blue-white metal that is an essential nutrient for humans.

DRI The RDA for zinc is 11 mg per day for adult males and 8 mg per day for adult females. The DV is 15 mg per day. The UL for adults is 40 mg per day.

Food Sources King and Cousins note that zinc bioavailability is determined primarily by quantities of zinc and phytate in the diet. Phytate decreases zinc absorption. Good sources of zinc are animal protein, such as meat, milk, and seafood, particularly oysters. Three ounces of meat contain approximately 30–50 percent of the RDA, whereas only one oyster will provide more that 70 percent. Absorption of zinc from animal foods is about twice the amount compared to plant foods; the MPF enhances zinc absorption. Whole-grain products and legumes also contain significant amounts of zinc, but the phytate and fiber content will slightly decrease its bioavailability. Zinc is lost in the milling process of wheat, but some breakfast cereals are fortified to 25–100 percent of the RDA. In general, if you receive enough protein in the diet you will obtain the RDA for zinc. About 20–50 percent of dietary zinc is absorbed. Daily intake of zinc is recommended because the body has no specific zinc storage system. Table 8.4 presents foods high in zinc.

Major Functions   Zinc is found in virtually all tissues in the body, with 95 percent in the cells. Total body zinc approximates 1.5 grams in females and 2.5 grams in males. Livingstone notes that zinc has a large number of physiological functions, which may be related to its key role in the activity of more than 300 enzymes. The following are some of the major functions of zinc in human metabolism:

- Promotion of immune system functions
- Promotion of eye health
- Promotion of wound healing
- Production of energy via the lactic acid energy system
- Synthesis of DNA, protein, and insulin
- Support of cellular and body growth
- Promotion of bone formation
- Promotion of red blood cell production
- Regulation of gene expression
- Promotion of proper sense of taste and smell

In addition, Maret notes that the role of zinc in human metabolism, and disease, may be intertwined with how it interacts with other minerals in the body, particularly copper and iron.

Deficiency: Health and Physical Performance   Plasma zinc concentration is normally used as a marker for zinc status, but it does not reflect zinc status in the cells. According to King and Cousins, nearly half of the world's population is at risk for zinc deficiency, mainly in Asia and Africa. Livingstone notes, in general, that adaptive mechanisms enable the body to maintain normal total body zinc status over a wide range of intakes, but deficiency can occur because of reduced absorption or increased gastrointestinal losses. In less developed countries in Asia and Africa, and other parts of the world, the diet consists primarily of plant-based foods, which are rich in phytates. As you may recall, phytates decrease zinc absorption. Additionally, most daily losses of zinc are via the gastrointestinal tract. Diarrhea may be prevalent in less developed countries, leading to increased gastrointestinal losses of zinc. Other possible mechanisms of zinc loss from the body include menstruation and sweat losses.

Zinc deficiency poses serious health risks, particularly in the young and in pregnant women, as it may lead to impaired growth and development. Penny states that zinc deficiency is responsible for 4 percent of global child morbidity and mortality.

The National Institutes of Health notes that overt zinc deficiency is uncommon in North America. However, certain individuals may be at risk and need to include zinc-rich foods in their diets, including vegetarians, individuals with gastrointestinal disorders such as Crohn's disease, and pregnant and lactating women. Alcoholics may also have low zinc status because alcohol decreases zinc absorption and increases its excretion.

Roohani and others indicate that epidermal, gastrointestinal, central nervous, immune, skeletal, and reproductive systems are the organs most affected clinically by zinc deficiency. Some common symptoms of zinc deficiency include failure to grow properly, impaired wound healing, and depressed appetite, but other symptoms such as weight loss, taste abnormalities, mental depression, and impotence may occur. Such symptoms may be associated with a variety of factors, so authorities indicate a medical examination is necessary to determine the presence of a zinc deficiency.

Most research indicates that athletes who obtain sufficient dietary Calories generally meet the RDA for zinc, but some athletes may be at risk. In particular, young athletes in sports that stress weight loss for optimal performance or competition, such as gymnastics, wrestling, and cross-country running, may adopt very low-Calorie diets, often low in animal protein, and thus may not obtain sufficient dietary zinc. Vegetarian athletes may also be at risk due to decreased zinc absorption associated with the high phytate content of plant foods. Sweat losses of zinc may also contribute a zinc deficiency, with one study reporting zinc losses in sweat accounted for approximately 8 percent to 9 percent of the daily RDA in men and women. However, in reviews by two experts in mineral nutrition, both Lane and Lukaski noted that, in general, there is no evidence that exercise causes a poor zinc status or that a marginal deficiency impairs performance.

Supplementation: Health and Physical Performance   Zinc supplementation has been studied in relation to a number of health conditions. Das and others indicated that food fortification with zinc may be a cost-effective strategy to overcome zinc deficiency in developing countries. In this regard, King and Cousins noted that zinc supplementation has been associated with physical growth of children in various population groups and, in some studies, impressive reductions in childhood morbidity and mortality. Penny recently reported that zinc supplements could reduce diarrhea mortality in children age 12-59 months by an estimated 23 percent. Mayo-Wilson and others, in an analysis of 80 studies, concluded that the benefits of preventive zinc supplementation may outweigh any potentially adverse effects in areas where risk of zinc deficiency is high.

Relative to eye health, zinc is found in high concentrations in the retina, and diets rich in zinc have been theorized to help decrease the risk of age-related macular degeneration (AMD), a major cause of visual problems and blindness in the United States. In their review, Vishwanathan and others concluded that current evidence on zinc intake for the prevention of AMD is inconclusive. However, based on the strength of the results from a major study, the Age-Related Eye Disease Study (AREDS), zinc may be recommended as a supplement when combined with other nutrients, particularly copper and vitamins C and E. The recommended amount of zinc is 80 milligrams in the form of zinc oxide. The National Eye Institute, part of the National Institutes of Health, notes that the AREDS formulation is the only treatment known to reduce the risk of advanced AMD.

As noted previously, Brewer hypothesized that excess intake of copper, mostly from drinking water leached from copper plumbing, may be associated with Alzheimer's disease. Based on some limited research, Brewer suggested zinc supplementation may be linked to reduced risk of Alzheimer's disease mainly by reducing body copper levels. In a subsequent study, Brewer and Kaur reported that in patients 70 years and older, zinc therapy significantly lowered blood copper levels and protected against cognition decline compared to placebo controls, suggesting zinc efficacy could be due to restoring neuronal zinc levels, to lowering blood copper levels, or to both. On the other hand, King and Cousins indicate excess zinc has been implicated in the pathogenesis of Alzheimer's disease, possibly by altering beta-amyloid protein and causing it to aggregate and accumulate as amyloid plaque, a hallmark of Alzheimer's disease. Hopefully, future research will help provide a more definitive explanation relative to the role of zinc, and other dietary metals, in the etiology of Alzheimer's disease.

Zinc supplementation has been advocated as a means of enhancing immune functions, particularly treatment of the common cold, a health problem that could impair exercise training. Nearly a dozen clinical studies have evaluated the effect of zinc lozenges as a means to reduce the duration of symptoms of the common cold, but a review by Nieman and a meta-analysis by Jackson and others concluded that evidence supporting its effectiveness in this regard is still lacking. King and Cousins also note that the results of studies relative to zinc supplementation, mainly zinc lozenges, and the common cold are mixed. Additionally, in a review of nutrition support to maintain proper immune status during intense exercise training written by a prominent exercise immunologist, Gleeson noted that although an adequate intake of dietary zinc is particularly important in the maintenance of immune function, it is safe to say with reasonable confidence that supplementation with zinc is unlikely to boost immunity or reduce infection risk in athletes.

Beletate and others indicated that zinc plays a key role in the synthesis and action of insulin, both physiologically and in diabetes mellitus. Hypothetically, zinc supplementation may help prevent type 2 diabetes. However, in their review, research was very limited and they concluded that there is currently no evidence to suggest the use of zinc supplementation in the prevention of type 2 diabetes mellitus.

Given the many metabolic functions of zinc, it is unusual that only limited research has evaluated its effects on exercise performance. Several studies have been conducted and used several different tests of exercise performance to evaluate the effect of zinc supplementation, but the results revealed significant benefits of supplementation on some exercise tests but not on others. In his review, Lukaski noted that study designs limit our ability to provide recommendations regarding zinc supplementation to athletes. Zinc supplementation studies are needed, particularly using physically trained subjects.

Maret and Sandstead indicated that individuals in affluent countries may experience the problem of chronic zinc toxicity caused by excessive consumption of zinc supplements. Small amounts of zinc supplements do not appear to pose any major problems to the healthy individual, but larger doses may.

The National Eye Institute indicated that zinc toxicity can occur in both acute and chronic forms. The acute adverse effects of high zinc intake (about 500 milligrams) include nausea, vomiting, loss of appetite, abdominal cramps, diarrhea, and headaches. Chronic effects associated with intakes of 150–450 milligrams of

zinc per day include low copper status, altered iron function, and reduced immune functions. The doses of zinc used in the AREDS study (80 milligrams per day for about 6 years) have been associated with a significant increase in hospitalizations for genitourinary causes. Thus, long-term use of zinc doses greater than the UL may increase the risk of adverse health effects. However, the National Eye Institute notes that the UL do not apply to individuals receiving zinc for medical treatment, but such individuals should be under the care of a physician who monitors them for adverse health effects.

Prudent Recommendations   On the basis of available evidence, zinc supplementation is not warranted for most individuals, including athletes. Foods rich in zinc, similar to the animal protein rich in iron, should be selected to replace the increased Calories expended through exercise. However, athletes such as wrestlers and others incurring weight losses, as well as older endurance athletes whose immune system normally declines, should be exceptionally aware of high-zinc foods. Zinc-fortified foods may provide the RDA for zinc. Check the food label. Keep in mind that the current DV used on food labels is 15 milligrams, or nearly twice the RDA for females and almost 40 percent higher than the RDA for males. Eating several servings of fortified foods daily could provide enough zinc to exceed the UL. If a supplement is recommended it should not exceed the RDA.

Chromium (Cr)

Chromium is a very hard metal believed to be essential in human nutrition. Eckhert indicates that chromium exists in various oxidative states, with chromium III and chromium IV being the most important to human health.

DRI   The AI for chromium is 35 and 25 micrograms per day, respectively, for adult males and females. Lower amounts are recommended for children and for older adults. The DV used on food labels is 120 micrograms. Thus, a vitamin pill containing 100 percent of the DV for chromium will provide about three to five times the RDA for adult males and females. No UL is currently available. However, it should be noted that in its review of the role of chromium in human nutrition, the European Food Safety Authority concluded that the setting of an Adequate Intake for chromium is not appropriate, and Vincent suggested chromium should be removed from the list of essential trace elements.

Food Sources   Good sources of chromium include broccoli, brewer's yeast, whole grains, baked beans, nuts, molasses, cheese, mushrooms, and asparagus. Beer also contains some chromium. One-half cup of broccoli provides approximately 25 percent of the AI for chromium. Whole wheat bread is a good source of chromium, but processed white bread contains only about half as much. Cooking acidic foods in stainless steel cookware provides negligible additional chromium. Chromium is poorly absorbed from the intestinal tract, less than 1 percent being absorbed, with intakes in the AI range. At lower dietary intakes, absorption is somewhat increased.

Major Functions Eckhert indicates that chromium is involved in insulin metabolism and notes scientists have suggested that chromium III increases insulin activity. Chromium is considered to be an essential component of the glucose-tolerance factor associated with insulin in the proper metabolism of blood glucose. Hua and others report that the molecular mechanisms of chromium on insulin activity remain elusive. Vincent suggests chromium may act as a second messenger for insulin, which may amplify its effects. Such an effect could help move glucose and amino acids into the cells, maintain blood glucose levels, promote glycogen formation in the muscles, and help promote muscle tissue synthesis.

Deficiency: Health and Physical Performance Eckhert states no cases of chromium deficiency in a healthy population have been reported but have been noted in patients. Abnormally high blood glucose levels have been reported in hospital patients receiving prolonged intravenous nutrition containing no chromium. Adding chromium to the solution reduced the elevated blood glucose levels.

The major problem in assessing the effect of chromium deficiency on health or physical performance is determining if a deficiency exists. In its *Dietary Supplements Fact Sheet,* the National Institutes of Health states that chromium status is difficult to determine because various measures, such as blood and urine tests, do not reflect body stores and no specific biochemical marker to reliably access chromium status in humans has been found.

Nevertheless, given its potential role in human metabolism, a chromium deficiency could impair insulin activity and both health and physical performance could be adversely affected. Impaired insulin sensitivity could lead to diabetes and body weight gain, accompanied by their associated health risks, particularly cardiovascular disease. Impaired insulin sensitivity could also impair physical performance, possibly by interfering with carbohydrate and protein metabolism. Decreased muscle glycogen could impair performance in endurance athletes, while decreased uptake of amino acids into the muscle could impair muscle growth in strength athletes.

Lefavi speculated that athletes may incur a negative chromium balance under three conditions. One, increased intensity and duration of exercise may increase chromium excretion; exercise may increase urinary excretion of chromium. Two, athletes who consume substantial amounts of carbohydrates may need more chromium to process glucose. And three, athletes who lose weight for competition may decrease dietary intake of chromium.

However, to our knowledge, no research has evaluated the effect of chromium deficiency on physical performance.

Supplementation: Health and Physical Performance Given the potential role of chromium in glucose metabolism, supplementation has been studied for possible benefits to blood sugar and glucose tolerance, particularly in individuals with type 2 diabetes. In a meta-analysis of 41 studies, Balk and others noted that although chromium supplementation significantly improved blood glucose control among patients *with* diabetes, they noted that future studies that address the limitations in the current evidence are needed before definitive claims can be made about the effect of chromium supplementation. In a more recent review, Wang and Cefalu indicated the data fail to consistently demonstrate significant improvement in individuals with type 2 diabetes following chromium supplementation. They note that patient selection may be an important factor, suggesting a favorable clinical response (improved insulin sensitivity) in diabetic subjects who are insulin resistant. Hua and others also reported that chromium supplementation has been shown to reduce insulin resistance in some, but not all, studies with type 2 diabetics. In their meta-analysis, Balk and others reported no significant effect of chromium on lipid or glucose metabolism in people *without* diabetes.

Theoretically, chromium supplementation might benefit the endurance athlete by improving insulin sensitivity and carbohydrate metabolism during exercise. Also, because chromium may enhance the anabolic effect of insulin, it may increase amino acid uptake into the muscle and modify the body composition, increasing muscle mass and decreasing body fat. Given the potential commercial application of this latter theoretical possibility to both athletes and the general population, most of the research to date has focused on the effect of chromium supplementation on body composition, but several recent studies have evaluated its effect on strength. Most studies have used chromium picolinate.

Although chromium supplementation may provide beneficial effects for some diabetics, its major popularity was related to marketing to the public as a supplement for body weight control, mainly by promoting fat loss. Chromium supplements were also marketed to physically active individuals as a means to promote gains in muscle mass. Vincent indicated that chromium supplements became so popular that sales were second only to calcium among mineral supplements. In particular, chromium picolinate was a best-selling supplement; picolinate is a natural derivative of tryptophan, an amino acid, and apparently facilitates the absorption of chromium into the body. The popularity of chromium picolinate may have been associated with some research in the late 1980s.

In a review of several of his own studies involving chromium picolinate supplementation to male college athletes and students involved in weight training, Evans suggested chromium picolinate supplementation enhanced body composition by decreasing body fat and increasing lean body mass. Following the publicity associated with this report, chromium picolinate was billed in certain muscle magazines as the alternative to anabolic steroids. The advertisers suggested that chromium's insulin-like effects may elicit significant anabolic hormone effects in the body. Advertisements also appeared in magazines targeted for the general population, suggesting that chromium picolinate would facilitate the loss of body fat.

However, well-controlled research does not support these advertisement claims. Numerous studies have concluded that supplementation with chromium picolinate and other forms of chromium, usually in conjunction with an exercise training program, had no effect on body composition or various measures of physical performance when compared to the placebo condition. Several of the studies used research protocols similar to those of Evans. The following is a summary of those findings:

- No effect on body composition or strength in untrained males after 12 weeks of resistance training
- No effect on lean body mass, body fat percentage, or strength in college football players after 9 weeks of training
- No effect on body weight and composition in nonexercising women over the course of 12 weeks
- No effect on body fat or lean muscle mass in men after 8 weeks of training
- No effects on body fat or lean muscle mass in either men or women engaging in aerobic exercise for 16 weeks
- No effect on body composition, resting metabolic rate, or blood glucose in moderately obese women in a walking exercise program for 12 weeks
- No effect on body composition or strength of older women after 12 weeks of resistance training
- No effect on body composition or neuromuscular or metabolic performance in highly trained NCAA Division I wrestlers during 14 weeks of training
- No effect on body composition and muscular strength in female softball players during 6 weeks of resistance training
- No effect on prolonged, intermittent, high-intensity exercise in physically active men following ingestion of a sports drink with added chromium

Relative to weight loss, recent reviews and meta-analyses do not support claims of major body weight or body fat losses following supplementation with chromium. Onakpoya and others, in a meta-analysis of 11 studies, did show a statistically significant difference in weight loss favoring chromium supplementation over placebo. However, although statistically significant, the effect was very small, only a loss of about 1 pound, which the investigators noted had uncertain clinical significance. In their review, Tian and others found no current, reliable evidence to provide firm decisions about the efficacy of chromium picolinate supplements in reducing body weight in overweight or obese adults. In his review, Vincent has a stronger viewpoint, indicating chromium has been conclusively shown not to have beneficial effects on body mass or composition in human studies.

Overall, these findings indicate chromium supplementation has little to no effect on body composition in sedentary individuals, individuals engaged in various forms of exercise training, or athletes engaged in training for their sport. Chromium supplementation also does not appear to benefit various forms of exercise performance.

Relative to safety the National Institutes of Health, in its *Fact Sheets on Dietary Supplements,* indicates no UL has been established for chromium, mainly because few serious adverse effects have been linked with high intakes of dietary chromium. In its review, the Institute of Medicine reported that no consistent, frequent adverse events were evident from human studies with chromium supplementation but also noted there is a lack of information on the long-term effects of chronic chromium picolinate supplementation at the recommended doses, and does recommend additional research to resolve any uncertainties.

However, Eckhert indicates that chromium VI, an industrial form of chromium used in the metal industry, may be inhaled and is well established as a carcinogen.

Prudent Recommendations   In a review of chromium supplementation by Schardt and Schmidt, the Center for Science in the Public Interest provided a bottom-line recommendation, which appears to be in accord with this presentation of the scientific data. If you are glucose intolerant or a type 2 diabetic, consult your medical advisor about chromium supplementation. In general, chromium supplementation will not help you lose weight or gain muscle. If you insist on taking a chromium supplement, it should not exceed a total of 200 micrograms daily taken in three separate doses. Chromium might best be taken as part of an inexpensive multivitamin-mineral tablet containing the other essential vitamins and minerals. The typical multivitamin/multimineral tablet contains about 120 micrograms of chromium, which is the Daily Value. Keep in mind, however, that the best sources of chromium are whole grains, fruits, and vegetables.

Selenium (Se)

Selenium is a chemical element resembling sulfur. Selenium was initially thought to be a toxin. One such chemical form is selenium sulfide, used in some skin lotions, and is classified as a carcinogen. However, selenium is found naturally in many foods and eventually was identified as an essential nutrient. Nevertheless, Kurokawa and Berry note that although selenium is an essential micronutrient, it is also recognized as toxic in excess.

DRI   The RDA for selenium is 55 micrograms per day for males and females, with lower amounts for children. The DV currently is 70 micrograms. The UL has been set at 400 micrograms/day for adults, but somewhat lower levels for children and adolescents.

Food Sources   Most selenium found in nature is a part of protein, known as selenoproteins. One of the richest sources of dietary selenium is Brazil nuts; a 1-ounce serving contains over 500 micrograms. Other rich sources of selenium are organ meats such as kidney and liver, seafood, and other meats. Plants such as cereals, grains, fruits, and vegetables grown in soil abundant in selenium are also good sources. About 3 ounces of meat contains more than 30 micrograms of selenium, as does 3 ounces of wheat bread.

Major Functions   Selenium is actually part of selenocysteine, an amino acid incorporated in about 25 selenoproteins, many of which are involved in oxidoreductase activity involving the transfer of electrons from one molecule to another. In particular, selenium is involved in the activity of glutathione peroxidase, an antioxidant enzyme that helps protect cells, such as the membranes of red blood cells, from potentially damaging oxidation. Roman and others note selenoproteins may serve as biomarkers of several diseases such as diabetes and several forms of cancer.

Deficiency: Health and Physical Performance   Selenium deficiency is rare in industrialized countries. The National Institutes of Health indicates most Americans consume adequate amounts of selenium, citing a recent national survey reporting the average daily selenium intake from foods is about 108 micrograms and from both foods and supplements is about 120 micrograms. However, deficiency diseases may be noted in geographical areas where the selenium content in the soil is low. Keshan disease, which is associated with impaired heart function, was evident in parts of China because the primary sources of food are plants grown locally in selenium-depleted soil. However, Sunde noted the disease has disappeared from China with improved economic and living conditions. In particular, the government initiated a program of selenium fortification in foods.

Given selenium's role in antioxidant activity in the body, a selenium deficiency has been hypothesized to be related to the development of various diseases. For example, decreased prevention of DNA damage could lead to cancer. A diminished ability to prevent the oxidation of LDL-cholesterol could lead to heart disease. Some researchers indicated a link between selenoproteins and glucose metabolism, possibly associated with type 2 diabetes. Other potential health problems associated with selenium deficiency include cognitive decline with aging and impaired thyroid gland function. However, as noted above, selenium deficiency is rare in developed countries.

For the athlete, selenium deficiency may impair antioxidant functions during intense exercise, possibly leading to muscle tissue or mitochondrial damage, thus impairing physical performance. However, there are no data to support this notion.

Supplementation: Health and Physical Performance   Intervention trials in China have shown that selenium supplementation may help prevent Keshan disease by preventing a deficiency. But can selenium supplementation help prevent cardiovascular disease, cancer, or diabetes in Western populations with better nutritional status?

Relative to cardiovascular disease, selenium supplementation may help prevent LDL oxidation, one of its major risk factors. However, in a recent systematic review of 12 studies, Rees and others evaluated the effects of selenium supplementation relative to primary prevention of cardiovascular disease, including major risk factors and mortality. They concluded the limited evidence that is available does not support the use of selenium supplements in the primary prevention of cardiovascular disease. Additionally, the National Institutes of Health noted that the limited clinical-trial evidence to date does not support the use of selenium supplements for preventing heart disease, particularly in healthy people who already obtain sufficient selenium from food. Additional clinical trials are needed to better understand the contributions of selenium from food and dietary supplements to cardiovascular health.

Some earlier epidemiological studies had indicated that the higher the body selenium levels, the lower the risk of prostate cancer, and at one time the National Institutes of Health concluded there is a suggestion that selenium may reduce risk for prostate cancer. However, Thompson notes that in a major clinical trial, the Selenium and Vitamin E Cancer Prevention Trial (SELECT),

selenium supplementation had no effect on prostate cancer risk. Sunde indicates the study was stopped prematurely because an independent monitoring committee found that both selenium and vitamin E may, independently, have some adverse health effects. In two separate reviews, Vinceti and others concluded selenium supplementation has no beneficial effect on cancer risk, more specifically on risk of prostate cancer. They also indicate some trials suggest harmful effects of selenium exposure.

Some studies have suggested an increased risk of type 2 diabetes with increased selenium supplementation. Zhou and others noted that although selenium was found to act as an insulin mimic and to be antidiabetic in earlier studies, recent research has shown an unexpected risk of prolonged high selenium intake to increase insulin resistance and type 2 diabetes. However, the mechanism remains unclear. Rayman and Stranges also note recent findings from observational cross-sectional studies have raised concern that high selenium exposure may be associated with type 2 diabetes or insulin resistance, at least in well-nourished populations, though trial results have been inconsistent.

Sunde notes that some health food supplements contain more than 700 times the RDA for selenium per serving, and episodes of acute selenium poisoning have occurred mainly by consuming such products. Symptoms may include nausea, diarrhea, fatigue, and peripheral neuropathy.

Vinceti indicates selenium is of considerable interest to humans from a nutritional perspective, with a very narrow safe range of intake. One investigator indicates a complex relationship between selenium intake and health status, suggesting it may be U-shaped, with possible harm occurring both below and above the physiological range for optimal activity of some or all selenoproteins. Sunde supports this viewpoint, stressing the need for additional research to find a good marker of selenium status so that individualized dietary recommendations for health may be developed.

As related to physical performance, the effects of selenium supplementation by itself has received only limited research attention. Although antioxidant supplements have not universally been shown to prevent peroxidation of lipids in cell membranes and other cell structures, some studies by Tessier and his associates have shown that selenium supplementation will enhance glutathione peroxidase status and reduce lipid peroxidation during prolonged aerobic exercise. Although these findings are intriguing, selenium supplementation did not improve actual physical performance, as evaluated by VO_2 max or running performance of an aerobic/anaerobic nature. In a subsequent study, Margaritis and others reported that selenium supplementation (180 micrograms/day) had no effect on muscle antioxidant capacity or exercise performance during 10 weeks of endurance training.

Prudent Recommendations   Adequate selenium may be obtained on a healthful, balanced diet containing substantial amounts of grain products. In the United States and Canada, most grains are produced in the upper Great Plains, where the soil is rich in selenium. Selenium in foods is present in an organic form, which may be more effectively used by the body than inorganic selenium salt supplements. Selenium supplements do not appear to enhance exercise training or performance, but if you decide to take a selenium supplement, note that most experts agree such a supplement, or a multivitamin-mineral supplement, should not exceed 200 micrograms. Larger doses are not recommended at the present time. Moreover, Liebman and Schardt from the Center for Science in the Public Interest recommend caution, possibly limiting selenium to 100 micrograms a day.

Boron (B)

Boron, atomic number 5, is classified as a metalloid, an element with properties associated with both metals and nonmetals.

DRI Although boron is an essential nutrient for plants, no RDA or AI has been established. However, some scientists suggest that it is of nutritional and clinical importance and most likely is an essential nutrient for humans. In a recent review, Nielsen indicated that boron is a bioactive food component that may provide beneficial health effects, and although the science base may not be considered adequate for establishing an AI, he indicates such a classification should be discussed. In one report Nielsen suggested an acceptable safe range for adults could well be 1–3/mg/day. Although no AI has yet been established, a UL of 20 mg/day has been set for adults, with smaller amounts for younger age groups.

Food Sources Eckhert indicates all foods made from plants and their by-products contain boron as an essential structural component of the cell wall. The Mediterranean diet contains ample boron. Excellent plant sources include nuts, legumes, dried fruits, and fresh vegetables, while milk and dairy products, grape juice, and wine also contain good amounts. One ounce of almonds contains about 0.75 milligram of boron. Five servings of fruits and vegetables, along with legumes and some nuts, could easily provide 3 milligrams.

Major Functions Nielsen indicates human experiments have shown that boron may form compounds known as boroesters, which may be incorporated in various biological molecules affecting a variety of body functions, including beneficial effects on bone growth, reduced arthritic symptoms, enhanced central nervous system function, facilitated hormone action, and reduced risk for some types of cancer. Relative to hormone actions, some investigators suggest a role of boron in estrogen metabolism, which could impact bone health. Others note effects on testosterone metabolism, with possible effects on muscle growth.

Deficiency: Health and Physical Performance The National Institutes of Health indicates Americans consume varying amounts of boron depending on their diet. Diets considered to be high in boron provide approximately 3.25 mg of boron per 2,000 Calories per day, whereas diets considered to be low in boron provide 0.25 mg of boron per 2,000 Calories per day. Nielsen notes that both animal and human data indicate that a boron intake of less than 1.0 mg/day inhibits its health benefits and that dietary surveys indicate such an intake is not rare. As noted below, experimental research by Nielsen induced a boron deficiency, which had adverse effects on some markers of bone health. Nielsen also noted that low intakes of boron may be associated with impaired brain function and immune response.

Supplementation: Health and Physical Performance Boron supplementation may not increase body stores. Hunt and others reported that a boron supplement of 3 milligrams did not accumulate in the body. Eckhert noted more than 90 percent of ingested boron is eliminated as boric acid in the urine.

In his review, Nielsen presents an excellent example of how the results of a single study may be distorted by nutritional supplement entrepreneurs to market new products. In their study, Nielsen and his colleagues designed a diet for 12 postmenopausal women to deprive them of adequate dietary boron for nearly 4 months, and then fed them the same diet for 48 days but supplemented with 3 milligrams of boron daily, an amount found in a diet high in fruits and vegetables. The authors reported that the boron supplements reduced the plasma concentration of calcium and the urinary excretion of calcium and magnesium, at the same time elevating the serum concentration of one form of estrogen and testosterone. The authors concluded that correcting a boron deficiency with boron supplements elicits physiological effects associated with the prevention of calcium loss and bone demineralization, suggesting that dietary boron may play an important nutritional role in the prevention of osteoporosis. The major focus of this study was on the effects of boron deprivation and deficiency, not boron supplementation. The authors simply created a boron deficiency to see its physiological effects, then restored normal dietary boron to evaluate its effects.

Nielsen notes that these findings were completely misinterpreted, the media reporting erroneously that boron could end bone disease. Commercial enterprises immediately began marketing boron supplements for prevention of osteoporosis. In his review, Nielsen negates the sensational claims the media propagated but did indicate that boron may be one of a number of nutrients that may play a role in the prevention of osteoporosis.

One of the other findings of this study, the elevated serum testosterone levels in these postmenopausal women, was also sensationalized. Advertisements began to appear in muscle magazines indicating that boron supplements could act pharmacologically as anabolic steroids. However, Nielsen indicated that this was an erroneous extrapolation of the research data, noting that boron supplementation increased serum testosterone only after these postmenopausal women had been deprived of boron for nearly 4 months; continuation of boron supplementation did not further elevate serum testosterone levels. Moreover, Nielsen conducted other studies with males and reported no significant changes in serum testosterone levels when dietary boron intake was modified.

Limited research data are available relative to the ergogenic efficacy of boron supplementation. Ferrando and Green randomly assigned 19 nonsteroid-using, male bodybuilders to receive either a placebo or 2.5 milligrams of a commercial boron supplement daily for 7 weeks. The bodybuilders maintained their normal diets and consumed no other supplements. The authors found that although boron supplements increased serum boron levels, there were no significant effects on total and free testosterone, lean body mass, or strength. In his review, Kreider concluded that currently there is no evidence that boron supplementation promotes muscle growth during resistance training. These limited findings indicate that boron supplements are not ergogenic.

Nielsen notes that 10 milligrams per day may be obtained in the diet, and that this amount is probably not too high. As noted, a UL of 20 milligrams per day has been set for adults, which could serve as a marker for maximal intake.

Prudent Recommendations Based on the available scientific evidence, boron may play a role in maintaining a healthy body, especially bone health. A balanced diet containing adequate amounts of plant foods will provide sufficient dietary boron. Physically active individuals who consume a typical diet should have no problem with boron deprivation. Boron supplements have not been shown to enhance exercise performance.

For those who insist on taking a boron supplement, they are available in various forms, including boron only and boron combined with other minerals. The usual dosage is 3 milligrams, which matches the average daily upper intake of Americans. However, others may contain 10 milligrams, which if consumed in excess could exceed the UL. In general, boron supplements are not recommended.

Obtain your boron from food. The Mediterranean diet would provide substantial amounts of boron, as well as other nutrients associated with good health.

Vanadium (V)

Vanadium is a light gray metallic element. It is found in food as vanadyl sulfate. However, vanadium also exists in other forms, such as vanadium pentoxide, a toxic industrial pollutant that may cause cancer.

DRI No RDA or AI has been established for vanadium. The average human body contains about 1 milligram. A UL of 1.8 mg/day has been set for adults.

Food Sources Good sources of vanadium include shellfish, grain products, parsley, mushrooms, and black pepper. The average North American diet supplies 15–30 micrograms of vanadium daily, with grains providing about 15–30 percent. About 5 percent of dietary vanadium is absorbed into the body.

Major Functions Eckhert notes that a functional role for vanadium has not been identified in humans. Research with animals suggests that vanadium may be involved in several enzymatic reactions in the body, including the metabolism of carbohydrate and lipids. Eckhert indicates vanadyl complexes potentiate the effect of insulin, but the underlying mechanism remains unknown.

Deficiency: Health and Physical Performance As noted, a vanadium deficiency has not been detected in humans. However, if vanadium does induce an insulin-like effect, a deficiency could impair glucose metabolism, which could have negative effects on both health and physical performance.

Supplementation: Health and Physical Performance Vanadium supplements are available as vanadyl salts, primarily vanadyl sulfate. The amount of vanadium in pure vanadium supplements may vary, approximating 5 to 10 milligrams. Multimineral supplements may contain about 50 micrograms. Check the supplement label.

Given its potentiating effect on insulin, vanadium has been studied in vitro and in vivo with animals. In their review, Clark and others reported that careful administration of vanadium in a variety of forms has produced impressive long-lasting control of blood glucose levels in both type 1 and type 2 diabetes in animals. Heart problems are often associated with diabetes, and Clark and others noted also a complete correction of the diabetic cardiomyopathy following vanadium supplementation. Rehder reported that in clinical trials with humans, one vanadium complex has revealed encouraging results in phase IIa trials, which are specifically designed to assess how much of a drug should be used. Rehder notes that vanadium compounds have not yet found approval for medicinal applications, but current research suggests some potential for the future. Clark and others also recommend additional research to help uncover any unknown long-term effects of vanadium accumulation in the heart and other organs of the body.

Vanadyl salts have been marketed to athletes as a means to favorably modify body composition, comparable to the proposed effects of chromium supplementation. However, there are very limited research data with vanadium supplementation. In a well-controlled study, Fawcett and others found that supplementation with about 40 milligrams daily of vanadyl sulfate to subjects undertaking strength training for 12 weeks had no effect on body fat or lean muscle mass. The investigators also studied strength gains in four power and endurance strength tests but reported no effect in three of the tests. The investigators concluded that vanadyl sulfate supplementation was ineffective in changing body composition, and any modest performance-enhancing effect requires further investigation.

As noted, inhalation of vanadium in one of its gas forms may cause cancer. Excess intake of vanadium salts, found in supplements, may also cause some health problems in humans, including stomach cramps, diarrhea, fatigue, increased blood pressure, decreased number of red blood cells, and mild neurological effects. Some of these effects were associated with dosages of about 13 milligrams per day.

Prudent Recommendations Type 2 diabetics should consult with their physicians regarding the use of vanadyl salt as a therapeutic agent to control blood glucose. Vanadyl salt supplementation is not recommended for the average individual, or for the physically active individual, because it has not been found to enhance either body composition or physical performance. Moreover, excess amounts may be toxic.

Manganese (Mn)

Manganese is a silver/gray metal found in nature in various oxidized states. Buchman indicates manganese (2^+) is the only form absorbed by humans, and it is oxidized to manganese (3^+). Manganese is used in industry for a variety of purposes.

DRI   The AI for manganese is 1.8 milligrams for female adults age 19–50 and 2.3 milligrams for male adults of the same age. The AI is somewhat less for children and adolescents, and slightly increased during pregnancy and lactation. The UL is 11 milligrams per day for adults, and somewhat less for children and adolescents. The current DV for manganese is 2 milligrams.

Food sources   Manganese is found in the soil and is essential for plant growth. Thus, rich sources include nuts, seeds, whole grains, and green leafy vegetables. Some seafood, such as clams and mussels, are excellent sources; 3 ounces of cooked mussels contain about 6 milligrams of manganese. A vegetarian diet contains substantial manganese. However, food processing may reduce the amount of manganese. Whole grains contain almost twice as much manganese as refined grains, so choosing whole wheat over processed white bread helps increase manganese intake.

Major functions   Manganese is considered to be essential for human health, as it is involved as a cofactor in many metalloenzymes essential to metabolism, including formation of bone and connective tissue, carbohydrate and fat metabolism, and sex hormone activity. As a cofactor for superoxide dismutase it plays an important role in the antioxidant defense system. Of particular interest, manganese is necessary for normal brain function.

Deficiency   Buchman notes that except for a few case studies, human manganese deficiency has not been well documented. Some reports indicated reduced magnesium levels in the body may lead to impaired bone metabolism, muscular weakness, and infertility. In a recent study, Eum and others reported a low level of serum manganese was associated with low birth weight, but so were excessive levels.

Supplementation   Manganese may be found in some dietary supplements, including multivitamin/multimineral supplements. Given their potential role in bone metabolism, manganese supplements have been used primarily as a means to prevent osteoporosis. In such supplements, manganese is usually coupled with other nutrients, including calcium and glucosamine. The amount of manganese in supplements may vary, but ranges from 1 to 5 milligrams have been observed. Five milligrams would be 250 percent of the DV. Users of manganese supplements should use caution, as it may be easy to exceed the UL of 11 milligrams.

Excessive manganese intake, either via industrial exposure, dietary sources, or supplements, may cause some harmful side effects. Tuschl and others note that when first observed, the condition associated with excess manganese intake was labeled *manganism*. Excessive manganese intake may lead to accumulation in various parts of the brain, such as the basal ganglia, globus pallidus, and subthalamic area, impairing the function of the neurotransmitter dopamine. Symptoms resemble those of Parkinson's disease, such as hypokinesia, a partial or complete loss of muscle movement. Treatment involves chelation therapy to help reduce body manganese levels.

No research has been uncovered regarding the effect of manganese supplementation on exercise or sports performance.

Prudent Recommendations   As with many other nutrients, obtaining adequate manganese may be assured by consuming a healthy diet rich in plant foods, such as the Mediterranean diet. Individuals susceptible to osteoporosis should consult with their medical advisors regarding the use of dietary supplements. Given the potential adverse health effects of excess manganese intake, use of such supplements should be limited. Check supplement labels for manganese content.

Other Trace Minerals

A number of other trace minerals have physiological roles that may have important implications for health or physical performance. Food sources, RDA or AI, major physiological functions, and the effects of deficiencies and excesses are summarized in table 8.5. Only trace minerals for which an RDA or AI have been developed are included. Other elements, such as nickel, tin, silicon, and arsenic, may prove to be essential. It should be noted that deficiencies and excesses due to dietary sources for most of these nutrients are extremely rare. However, to help prevent a deficiency it is important to consume unprocessed foods, because many of the trace elements that are removed during processing are not returned. For example, as already noted, one slice of whole wheat bread provides about 15 percent of the daily requirement of chromium, whereas a slice of white bread contains only 1 percent. Excesses may occur with use of supplements or through industrial exposure, and a UL has been set for nickel.

Two of these trace elements deserve mention because they have been shown to prevent health problems in humans.

Fluoride   Fluoride appears to benefit dental health and may influence bone health. A fluoride AI has been established, ranging from about 1 to 4 mg/day from childhood through adulthood.

Fluoride is found in some natural waterways and may be added to water supplies via fluoridation. Harding and O'Mullane indicate current estimates suggest that approximately 370 million people in 27 countries consume fluoridated water, with an additional 50 million consuming water in which fluoride is naturally occurring. Since the early 1980s, fluoride, mainly sodium fluoride, has been added to toothpaste and mouthwash solutions for dental health purposes.

Clark and Slayton indicate that dental caries remains the most common chronic disease of childhood in the United States, but it is a largely preventable condition with use of various fluoride modalities. Fluoride may prevent dental caries, possibly by inhibiting bacterial enzymes and demineralization of the tooth.

Water supplies of fluoride, either naturally or artificially fluoridated, appear to be an effective means to supply communities with adequate amounts. However, Peckham and Awofeso indicate water fluoridation remains a controversial public health measure. They conclude that available evidence suggests that fluoride has a potential to cause major adverse human health problems, while having only a modest dental caries prevention effect. However, a large number of studies conducted worldwide demonstrate the effectiveness and safety of water fluoridation. In their review, Harding and O'Mullane,

TABLE 8.5   Trace minerals: cobalt, fluoride, iodine, molybdenum

Trace mineral	RDA or AI*	Major food sources	Major body functions	Deficiency symptons	Symptons of excessive consumption	Recommended as dietary supplement
Cobalt (Co)	**	Meat, liver, milk	Component of vitamin B_{12}; promotes development of red blood cells	Not found in humans	Nausea, vomiting, death	No
Fluoride (F)	3.0–4.0 mg	Milk, egg yolks, drinking water, seafood	Helps form bones and teeth	Higher incidence of dental cavities	Discolored teeth	No
Iodine (I)	150 micrograms	Iodized salt, seafood, vegetables	Helps in formation of thyroid hormones	Goiter, an enlarged thyroid gland	Depressed thyroid gland activity	No
Molybdenum (Mo)	45 micrograms	Liver, organ meats, whole-grain products, dried beans and peas	Works with riboflavin in enzymes involved in carbohydrate and fat metabolism	Not found in humans	Rare	No

*For adults. RDA or AI for other age groups may be found on the website listed in the legend to Table 8.1.
**Essential as part of vitamin B_{12}.

reported objections to water fluoridation have been raised since its inception and center mainly on safety. However, they note systematic reviews of water fluoridation attest to its safety and efficacy, with dental fluorosis identified as the only adverse outcome. Fluorosis is a condition of varying shades of whiteness (known as mottling) in the outer tooth enamel and may be caused when fluoride interferes in some way with the maturation of dental enamel.

Other effective methods are available to obtain the dental health benefits of fluoride. Topical application of fluoride, either by dentists or self-applied, is also effective in prevention of dental caries. In a review associated with American Dental Association clinical recommendations, Maguire noted one of the recommendations indicated that for all age groups, except children under 6 years, the use of professionally applied and prescription strength, home-use topical fluoride agents conferred benefits that outweighed potential harm. Additionally, fluoride in toothpaste and mouthwashes is beneficial. Rugg-Gunn and Bánóczy reviewed the efficacy of fluoride-containing toothpastes and mouthwashes and concluded extensive testing has demonstrated that they are effective and their use should be encouraged.

Fluoride supplements are also available as tablets, lozenges, and drops. However, they are not available over the counter, but only by prescription. Individuals should use such fluoride supplements only under the medical guidance of their dental health professional.

Fluoride may possess other health benefits, as it is believed to work with calcium and other minerals in bone mineralization. Comparable to the advice relative to using fluoride supplements for dental health, osteoporotic patients should consult with their physicians regarding use of fluoride supplements.

Iodine   According to Laurberg, the only established role of iodine in humans is to be a component of thyroid hormones. The RDA for iodine is 320 and 420 milligrams for adult females and males, respectively. Smaller amounts are recommended for children, with somewhat larger amounts for women who are pregnant or lactating.

Decreased production of the thyroid hormones thyroxine and triiodothyronine would lower the body's metabolism, a possible contributing factor to the development of obesity. Zimmermann and Boelaert indicate iodine deficiency early in life may have significant adverse effects, including impaired cognition and growth. Laurberg notes that the clinical consequence of severe iodine deficiency in pregnancy and fetal life and during the first years is cretinism. However, the use of iodized salt has nearly eliminated iodine deficiency in the United States and has thereby greatly reduced the incidence of goiter, a serious iodine-deficiency disease. Nevertheless, some health professionals are concerned that individuals who restrict salt intake in attempts to prevent the development of high blood pressure may be at risk for iodine deficiency and thus recommend that such individuals use dietary supplements containing iodine.

However, Weng and others note that in some parts of the world people are still suffering from iodine deficiency. One estimate is nearly 750 million people suffer from goiter. Although iodized salt may be used, such countries have also used iodine-rich, plant-based foods as a supplement to help increase iodine intake.

Research literature relative to the effect of exercise on the metabolic fates of iodine as well as fluoride is almost nonexistent, and no research has been uncovered regarding the effect of iodine or fluoride supplementation on exercise performance. One study by Smyth and Duntas indicated that athletes or those participating in vigorous exercise can lose a considerable amount of iodine in sweat, depending on environmental factors, such as temperature and humidity, and suggested sustained iodine loss may have implications for thyroid status and possibly consequences for athletic performance. However, they concluded there is no case as yet for iodine supplementation in those who engage in vigorous exercise. Nevertheless, as noted in chapter 9, sodium losses may be considerable in exercise-induced sweating. Using iodized salt with meals would appear to be a sound recommendation.

Mineral Supplements: Exercise and Health

Perusal of the Internet reveals numerous advertisements for mineral supplements and their effects on health or sports performance. For example, various mineral supplements are marketed to improve bone health, brain health, and sexual health, and one company markets a mineral supplement designed to provide anabolic mineral support for elite-level athletes. As the foregoing discussion indicates, individuals who have a mineral deficiency may experience improved health or physical performance if that deficiency is corrected. In general, however, supplementation has little effect on the individual whose mineral status is adequate. This last section summarizes some key points relative to mineral nutrition, focusing on the need for supplementation.

Does exercise increase my need for minerals?

Exercise may induce mineral losses from the body by several mechanisms. Many minerals appear to be mobilized into the circulation during exercise, probably being released from body stores in the muscles or elsewhere. As they circulate, some may be removed by the kidneys and excreted in the urine, whereas others may appear in the sweat, particularly in a warm environment. Losses from the gastrointestinal tract may also occur during exercise, although the mechanism is not totally understood.

Other body changes mediated by exercise may influence mineral requirements. The female athlete who develops secondary amenorrhea may need additional calcium, as might the male endurance athlete in whom trabecular bone mass is decreased. The need for iron in the female athlete may decrease somewhat with the cessation of menses in secondary amenorrhea.

Because of potential mineral losses, some sports nutritionists have suggested that mineral supplementation be considered for athletes, particularly those with poor dietary habits. However, although supplementation may be helpful for some, the first concern should be to educate the athlete about obtaining adequate mineral nutrition through dietary means.

Can I obtain the minerals I need through my diet?

As many dietary surveys have shown, many Americans are not obtaining the RDA or AI for a variety of minerals, including iron, zinc, calcium, and chromium. Similar dietary deficiencies have been noted in surveys with athletes, but mainly with athletes who participate in activities such as wrestling, distance running, ballet, and gymnastics, where weight control is a concern. Let us briefly highlight the dietary recommendations that will help ensure adequate amounts of nutrients in the diet.

In general, as with all other nutrients, a balanced diet is essential. Select a wide variety of foods from all the food groups and within each group. Table 8.6 presents the percentage of the DV provided by servings of different foods from several food groups. Keep in mind that the DV, the value used on food labels, may vary with the RDA and AI, being higher for some minerals and lower for others. But the purpose of this table is simply to support the value of eating a wide variety of foods to obtain adequate mineral nutrition.

Note that the percentage values for the minerals differ not only between food groups but also for some minerals in foods within the same group. For example, note that calcium is high in dairy foods but low in meats. Conversely, iron is high in meats but low in dairy products. Also, in the meat group, an oyster is high in copper, but lean beef is relatively low, even more so if you consider the caloric value of each. It is also important to eat foods in their natural state as much as possible. The milling of flour removes many minerals, but some may be replaced in the enrichment process. Note the differences between whole wheat and enriched white bread in table 8.6. These figures are based on one nutrient analysis database. Some white breads may be fortified, so check the food label. Also, there is a whole wheat white bread, made from a special white whole wheat, which contains the same

TABLE 8.6   Approximate percentages of the DV in various foods for selected minerals

Food	Serving	Calories	Ca (1,000 mg)	P (1,000 mg)	Mg (400 mg)	Fe (18 mg)	Cu (2 mg)	Zn (15 mg)
Milk, skim	1 glass	90	30	25	7	1	2	7
Cheese, cheddar	1 ounce	114	21	15	2	1	0	6
Oyster	1 ounce	20	1	4	4	11	40	166
Liver, beef	3 ounces	150	1	34	4	32	150	35
Beef, lean sirloin	3 ounces	230	1	18	6	13	7	33
Potato, baked	medium	220	2	11	14	15	15	4
Beans, kidney, cooked	1/2 cup	110	4	12	9	14	12	5
Broccoli	1/2 cup	25	4	5	5	4	2	2
Bread, whole wheat	1 slice	70	2	5	5	4	14	3
Bread, enriched white	1 slice	70	2	2	2	4	6	1

nutrient value as the traditionally brown whole wheat bread. Some food products rich in other healthful nutrients, such as orange juice and whole-grain cereal, are fortified with minerals and may be an effective means to ensure adequate mineral nutrition.

A basic principle of mineral nutrition is to eat natural foods that are rich in calcium and iron, two of the key nutrients. If you select a diet to provide your RDA for these two minerals, you should receive adequate amounts of the other major and trace minerals at the same time. Dairy products and meats are excellent sources of these minerals, but other foods such as legumes and dark-green leafy vegetables also may provide significant amounts if selected wisely. Note the foods rich in calcium and iron in table 8.2 and 8.4, and compare the similarity to the foods listed for the other minerals in these two tables and table 8.5. As noted previously, the Mediterranean diet may be rich in minerals.

Are mineral megadoses or some nonessential minerals harmful?

One of the generally accepted facts relative to mineral nutrition in the healthy individual is that the levels associated with toxicity can normally be obtained only through the use of supplements or fortified foods, not through natural dietary sources. Because they hope to improve health or physical performance, many individuals purchase supplements containing minerals. However, surveys indicate that the most common preparations purchased contain the RDA or DV, or less, which should pose no health problems to the healthy individual. Unfortunately, as indicated in the last chapter, many individuals self-prescribe and may consume more than the recommended daily dosage. Although the toxicity and possible health problems associated with excessive intake of several

minerals, such as calcium, iron, zinc, and copper, are fairly well documented, the level of safety for intake of a variety of other minerals, particularly some of the trace minerals suggested to be therapeutic in nature, has been more difficult to document. Nevertheless, the National Academy of Sciences has noted that all trace minerals are toxic if consumed at high doses for a long enough time.

Of increasing concern is the potential role of several metals in the etiology of Alzheimer's disease. Ayton and others have proposed a metal hypothesis relative to the development of Alzheimer's disease, primarily involving iron, copper, and zinc. Such minerals may affect brain proteins, possibly leading to neurodegeneration, the hallmark of Alzheimer's. Ayton and others suggest targeting these metals might be an alternative approach to treat the disease. Obtaining adequate amounts of iron and zinc and avoiding excess intake of copper may be important.

Several nonessential minerals may be consumed inadvertently and cause significant health problems, even in small amounts. Lead can displace other minerals, such as calcium and zinc, in various enzymes and thus interfere with intracellular processes involving protein and gene expression. Industrial chromium is regarded as a carcinogen. Of recent concern is mercury, which may be found in foods that we normally think of as healthy: fish!

Methylmercury, an industrial waste product, has been dumped into the seas, where it may be consumed by fish. As noted in chapter 5, high levels of mercury may accumulate more in larger, older, predatory fish, such as shark, swordfish, king mackerel, and tilefish. Tuna may contain somewhat less mercury. However, the Consumers Union cites FDA data indicating that some light tuna, which normally has lower levels of mercury than white (Albacore) tuna, may have as much as or more.

Houston indicates that mercury may displace other minerals, such as zinc and copper, thus reducing the effectiveness of various metalloenzymes, including antioxidant enzymes, inducing numerous pathological effects. In particular, too much mercury may damage the nervous system, especially the brain during its formative years prior to birth and the first 7 years of life. Thus, the FDA advises women who are or who can become pregnant and small children not to eat any shark, swordfish, king mackerel, or tilefish. Additional information is presented on pages 209–210.

Should physically active individuals take mineral supplements?

In general, the answer to this question for most athletes is *no*—for several reasons.

- First, contrary to advertising claims of mineral-supplement manufacturers, you can obtain adequate mineral nutrition from the diet if you adhere to some of the guidelines presented throughout this chapter.
- Second, although some athletes may not be obtaining the recommended amounts of several minerals, such as zinc and calcium, mineral deficiencies to the point of impairing physical performance are rare. Very few data are available on this topic, but the evidence that is available with most minerals suggests that though serum levels may be low, physical performance is not affected. An exception may be low levels of serum iron, for, as noted previously, supplementation, although controversial, has been helpful to some athletes.
- Third, many minerals may be harmful when taken in excess. As noted throughout this chapter, the absorption rate for most minerals is relatively low. Only 40 percent of calcium is absorbed from the intestinal tract, while the percentages for iron and chromium are, respectively, 10 and 1–2 percent. Also, a high dietary intake of several minerals that are easily absorbed increases their excretion rate by the kidney. Thus, a low absorption or high excretion rate prevents the accumulation of excess amounts of minerals in the body, which may interfere with normal metabolism. However, large supplemental doses may overload the body and cause numerous health problems and, as noted for several minerals, may be fatal.

Nevertheless, it is recognized that certain athletes may not be obtaining adequate mineral nutrition from their diets and may benefit from supplementation. As noted previously, athletes who are attempting to lose weight for performance are at most risk for developing a mineral deficiency. Because many of the dietary surveys of these athletes have reported intakes lower than the RDA for iron and calcium, it may be assumed that their diets are also low in other trace minerals.

If there is concern for the nutritional status of the athlete, the ideal situation would be to consult a sports nutritionist or nutritionally oriented physician. Unfortunately, this approach does not appear to be common among athletes who may be in need of nutritional counseling, although the situation is improving. For example, many professional sports teams as well as athletes in many colleges and universities now have access to sport dietitians with expertise in sport physiology, many of whom are members of the College and Professional Sport Dietitians Association.

For athletes who cannot or will not seek professional advice, it may be prudent to recommend a one-a-day vitamin-mineral supplement to those who are known to have poor nutritional habits. The tablet should contain no more than 50–100 percent of the RDA or DV for any mineral. Additionally, the point should be made to the athlete that the supplement is being recommended to help prevent a deficiency, not for any ergogenic purposes. As noted in chapter 7, large doses of multivitamin-mineral supplements taken over prolonged periods of time have not been shown to enhance physical performance. In the meantime, efforts should be undertaken to educate the athlete concerning sound nutritional practices.

For those considering mineral supplementation for health reasons, the DRI developed by the National Academy of Sciences reflect a paradigm in which the determination of nutrient requirements includes consideration of the total health effects of nutrients, not just their roles in preventing deficiency pathology. For example, the AI for calcium and vitamin D as a possible means to prevent osteoporosis reflect this paradigm. Although much research is needed before concrete recommendations may be made relative to mineral supplementation and purported health benefits, the recommendations presented on pages 315–317 may be useful guidelines for healthy sedentary and physically active individuals to use in the meantime.

Key Concepts

▶ Health professionals recommend that individuals obtain their mineral needs from healthful foods. A diet that provides the RDA for iron and the AI for calcium, as well as Calories from a balanced selection of foods throughout the different food groups, will provide adequate amounts of both the major and trace minerals.

▶ Mineral supplements may be recommended for some individuals as a means to improve health or sports performance, but excessive intake is not recommended because of potential health problems.

Check for Yourself

▶ Calcium and iron are two of our key nutrients for health and sports performance. If you obtain adequate amounts of each through natural dietary sources, you should obtain adequate amounts of most other essential minerals. Using food labels or computerized dietary analyses, calculate the calcium and iron intake of your typical daily diet to determine if you are obtaining the RDA for your gender and age.

Your municipal water supply may contain a variety of minerals, such as calcium, magnesium, fluoride, and sodium. Contact the appropriate governmental authorities in your community to see if you may obtain a detailed water quality report highlighting the mineral content of city drinking water. Calculate the amount of various minerals you consume with each quart of water.

Mineral Content of Municipal Drinking Water

Minerals	Calcium	Magnesium	Fluoride	Sodium	Other	Other
Mineral content in 1 quart of water						

Review Questions—Multiple Choice

1. Which statement does *not* describe the role of major minerals in the body?
   a. They give teeth and bone their rigidity and strength.
   b. They help to regulate body processes.
   c. They are constituents of soft tissues.
   d. They provide a source of caloric energy.
   e. They help to maintain the acid-base balance.

2. Which of the following groups needs iron the least, as specified by the RDA?
   a. adolescent boys
   b. adolescent girls
   c. young adult females
   d. adult males
   e. female distance runners

3. To help prevent the development of osteoporosis in later life, females should consume adequate quantities of which nutrient during the years in which they are developing peak bone mass?
   a. calcium
   b. iron
   c. retinol
   d. vitamin E
   e. ascorbic acid

4. Which mineral is theorized to be an effective ergogenic aid for runners, because it may increase the delivery of oxygen to the muscle cell by facilitating its release from hemoglobin?
   a. calcium
   b. phosphorus
   c. zinc
   d. magnesium
   e. chromium

5. Excessive intake of iron can lead to a condition called hemachromatosis, which damages which organ in the body?
   a. arterial walls
   b. kidney
   c. heart
   d. liver
   e. lungs

6. Approximately how much calcium is found in one glass (8 ounces) of skim milk?
   a. 50 milligrams
   b. 100 milligrams
   c. 300 milligrams
   d. 800 milligrams
   e. 1,200 milligrams

7. Which of the following would not contain heme iron?
   a. liver
   b. dried beans
   c. fish
   d. chicken
   e. beef

8. Which of the following contains the least amount of calcium?
   a. milk
   b. meat
   c. dried beans
   d. dark-green leafy vegetables
   e. cheese

9. Which Food Exchange is the best source of zinc, iron, and copper in regard to the concept of bioavailability?
   a. milk
   b. meat
   c. starch/bread
   d. fruit
   e. vegetable

10. Which of the following statements concerning trace minerals is false?
    a. Copper and iron are needed for optimal functioning of the red blood cell.
    b. Selenium works as an antioxidant with one of the vitamins.
    c. Chromium appears to be essential in the use of blood glucose.
    d. Zinc is a part of numerous metalloenzymes.
    e. Mercury is essential for carbohydrate metabolism.

Answers to multiple choice questions:
1. d; 2. d; 3. a; 4. b; 5. d; 6. c; 7. b; 8. b; 9. b; 10. e

Review Questions—Essay

1. Explain several ways whereby minerals function in metabolic processes in the human body.
2. Name three macrominerals and at least five trace minerals and describe the metabolic function of each in the human body.
3. Osteoporosis is a significant health problem in the United States and Canada. Discuss the risk factors for osteoporosis and provide specifics as to how life-style behaviors may help prevent its development.
4. Discuss the role that iron supplementation may play if provided to an athlete under three conditions: (a) normal iron and hemoglobin status; (b) iron deficiency without anemia; (c) iron-deficiency anemia.
5. Several minerals have been alleged to possess ergogenic potential. Select two of the following, explain the theoretical rationale underlying their purported ergogenic effects, and highlight the current research findings regarding their efficacy: chromium, phosphate salts, boron, vanadium

References

Books

American Institute of Cancer Research. 2007. *Food, Nutrition, Physical Activity, and the Prevention of Cancer: A Global Perspective.* Washington, DC: AICR.

Institute of Medicine. 2005. *Dietary Supplements: A Framework for Evaluating Safety.* Washington, DC: National Academies Press.

National Academy of Sciences. 1999. *Dietary Reference Intakes for Calcium, Phosphorus, Magnesium, Vitamin D, and Fluoride.* Washington, DC: National Academies Press.

National Academy of Sciences. 2000. *Dietary Reference Intakes for Vitamin C, Vitamin E, Selenium and Carotenoids.* Washington, DC: National Academies Press.

National Academy of Sciences. 2002. *Dietary Reference Intakes for Vitamin A, Vitamin K, Arsenic, Boron, Chromium, Copper, Iodine, Iron, Manganese, Molybdenum, Nickel, Silicon, Vanadium, and Zinc.* Washington, DC: National Academies Press.

National Academy of Sciences. 2010. *Dietary Reference Intakes for Calcium and Vitamin D.* Washington, DC: National Academies Press.

Nelson, M. 2005. *Strong Women, Strong Bones.* New York: Penguin Putnam.

Reviews and Specific Studies

Aaseth, J., et al. 2012. Osteoporosis and trace elements—An overview. *Journal of Trace Elements in Medicine and Biology* 26:149–52.

Abbaspour, N., et al. 2014. Review on iron and its importance for human health. *Journal of Research in Medical Sciences* 19:164–74.

Abid, Z., et al. 2014. Meat, dairy, and cancer. *American Journal of Clinical Nutrition* 100:386S–93S.

Aggarwal, S., and Nityanand, S. 2013. Calcium and vitamin D in post menopausal women. *Indian Journal of Endocrinology and Metabolism* 17:S618–20.

American College of Sports Medicine. 2004. Physical activity and bone health. *Medicine & Science in Sports & Exercise* 36:1985–96.

Anderson, J., and Barrett, C. 1994. Dietary phosphorus: The benefits and the problems. *Nutrition Today* 29 (2):29–34.

Anderson, J. 2013. Potential health concerns of dietary phosphorus: Cancer, obesity, and hypertension. *Annals of the New York Academy of Sciences* 1301:1–8.

Arts, J., et al. 2012. Adenosine 5′-triphosphate (ATP) supplements are not orally bioavailable: A randomized, placebo-controlled cross-over trial in healthy humans. *Journal of the International Society of Sports Nutrition* 9 (1):16. doi: 10.1186/1550-2783-9-16.

Aune, D., et al. 2015. Dairy products, calcium, and prostate cancer risk: A systematic review and meta-analysis of cohort studies. *American Journal of Clinical Nutrition* 101:87–117.

Avni, T., et al. 2012. Iron supplementation for the treatment of chronic heart failure and iron deficiency: Systematic review and meta-analysis. *European Journal of Heart Failure* 14:423–9.

Ayton, S., et al. 2015. Biometals and their therapeutic implications in Alzheimer's disease. *Neurotherapeutics* 12:109–20.

Balk, E., et al. 2007. Effect of chromium supplementation on glucose metabolism and lipids: A systematic review of randomized controlled trials. *Diabetes Care* 30:2154–63.

Beletate, V., et al. 2007. Zinc supplementation for the prevention of type 2 diabetes mellitus. *Cochrane Database of Systematic Reviews* 24:CD005525.

Bennell, K., et al. 1996. Effect of altered reproductive function and lowered testosterone levels on bone density in male endurance athletes. *British Journal of Sports Medicine* 30:205–8.

Bern, L. 2003. The estrogen and progestin dilemma: New advice, labeling guidelines. *FDA Consumer* 37 (2):10–11.

Blaszczykm, U., and Duda-Chodak, A. 2013. Magnesium: Its role in nutrition and carcinogenesis. *Roczniki Państwowego Zaktadu Higieny* 64:165–71.

Bloomfield, S. 2001. Optimizing bone health: Impact of nutrition, exercise, and hormones. *Sports Science Exchange* 14 (3):1–4.

Bonaiuti, D., et al. 2002. Exercise for preventing and treating osteoporosis in postmenopausal women. *Cochrane Database of System Reviews* 3:CD000333.

Bonjour, J. 2005. Dietary protein: An essential nutrient for bone health. *Journal of the American College of Nutrition* 24:526S–36S.

Bremner, K., et al. 2002. The effect of phosphate loading on erythrocyte 2,3-bisphophoglycerate levels. *Clinical Chimica Acta* 323:111–14.

Brewer, C., et al. 2013. Effect of repeated sodium phosphate loading on cycling time-trial performance and VO$_2$ peak. *International Journal of Sport Nutrition and Exercise Metabolism* 23:187–94.

Brewer, C., et al. 2014. Effect of sodium phosphate supplementation on cycling time trial performance and VO$_2$ 1 and 8 days post loading. *Journal of Sports Science & Medicine* 13:529–34.

Brewer, C., et al. 2014. Effect of sodium phosphate supplementation on repeated high-intensity cycling efforts. *Journal of Sport Science* 10:1–8.

Brewer, G. 2012. Copper excess, zinc deficiency, and cognition loss in Alzheimer's disease. *Biofactors* 38:107–13.

Brewer, G., and Kaur, S. 2013. Zinc deficiency and zinc therapy efficacy with reduction of serum free copper in Alzheimer's disease. *International Journal of Alzheimers Disease* 2013:586365.

Bristow, S., et al. 2013. Calcium supplements and cancer risk: A meta-analysis of randomised controlled trials. *British Journal of Nutrition* 110:1384–93.

Buchman, A., et al. 1998. The effect of a marathon run on plasma and urine mineral and metal concentrations. *Journal of the American College of Nutrition* 17:124–27.

Buck, C., et al. 2013. Sodium phosphate as an ergogenic aid. *Sports Medicine* 43:425–35.

Buck, C., et al. 2014. Sodium phosphate supplementation and time trial performance in female cyclists. *Journal of Sports Science & Medicine* 13:469–75.

Buratti, P., et al. 2015. Recent advances in iron metabolism: Relevance for health, exercise, and performance. *Medicine & Science in Sports & Exercise* 47:1596–604. [Epub ahead of print]

Burden, R., et al. 2014. Is iron treatment beneficial in iron-deficient but non-anaemic (IDNA) endurance athletes? A meta-analysis. *British Journal of Sports Medicine.* doi:10.1136/bjsports-2014-093624.

Burk, R. 2002. Selenium, an antioxidant nutrient. *Nutrition in Clinical Care* 5:75–79.

Cade, R., et al. 1984. Effects of phosphate loading on 2,3-diphosphoglycerate and maximal oxygen uptake. *Medicine & Science in Sports & Exercise* 16:263–68.

Cauley, J. 2013. The Women's Health Initiative: Hormone therapy and calcium/vitamin D supplementation trials. *Current Osteoporosis Reports* 11:171–8.

Clark, K., and Slayton, R. 2014. Fluoride use in caries prevention in the primary care setting. *Pediatrics* 134:626–33.

Clark, T., et al. 2014. Alternative therapies for diabetes and its cardiac complications: Role of vanadium. *Heart Failure Reviews* 19:123–32.

Collins, J. 2014. Copper. In *Modern Nutrition in Health and Disease,* ed. A. C. Ross et al. Philadelphia: Wolters Kluwer/Lippincott Williams & Wilkins.

Consumers Union. 2004. Stronger bones without the hype. *Consumer Reports on Health* 16 (5):1, 4–5.

Consumers Union. 2006. Bone-building drugs. *Consumer Reports on Health* 18 (5):3.

Consumers Union. 2006. Mercury in tuna. *Consumer Reports on Health* 71 (7):20–21.

Consumers Union. 2008. Dew concerns for bone-building drugs. Consumer Reports on Health. 20(4):3.

Czaja, J., et al. 2011. Evaluation for magnesium and vitamin B6 supplementation among Polish elite athletes. *Roczniki Państwowego Zaktadu Higieny* 62:413–8.

Das, J., et al. 2013. Systematic review of zinc fortification trials. *Annals of Nutrition & Metabolism* 62 (Supplement 1):44 –56.

Dawson, B., et al. 2006. Iron supplementation: Oral tablets versus intramuscular injection. *International Journal of Sport Nutrition and Exercise Metabolism* 16:180–86.

Dawson-Hughes, B. 2006. Osteoporosis. In *Modern Nutrition in Health and Disease,* ed. M. Shils et al. Philadelphia: Lippincott Williams & Wilkins.

de Oliveira Freitas, D., et al. 2012. Calcium ingestion and obesity control. *Nutricion Hospitalaria* 27:1758–71.

DellaValle, D. 2013. Iron supplementation for female athletes: Effects on iron status and performance outcomes. *Current Sports Medicine Reports* 12:234–9.

Derom, M., et al. 2013. Magnesium and depression: A systematic review. *Nutritional Neuroscience* 16:191–206.

Desbrow, B., et al. 2014. Sports Dietitians Australia position statement: Sports nutrition for the adolescent athlete. *International Journal of Sport Nutrition and Exercise Metabolism* 24:570–84.

Deuster, P. 1989. Magnesium in sports medicine. *Journal of the American College of Nutrition* 8:462.

Downing, L., and Islam, M. 2013. Influence of calcium supplements on the occurrence of cardiovascular events. *American Journal of Health-System Pharmacy* 70:1132–9.

Eckhert, C. 2014. Trace elements. In *Modern Nutrition in Health and Disease,* ed. A. C. Ross et al. Philadelphia: Wolters Kluwer/Lippincott Williams & Wilkins.

Eichner, E. 1992. Sports anemia, iron supplements, and blood doping. *Medicine & Science in Sports & Exercise* 24:S315–S18.

Eichner, E. 2001. Anemia and blood boosting. *Sports Science Exchange* 14 (2):1–4.

Eum, J., et al. 2014. Maternal blood manganese level and birth weight: A MOCEH birth cohort study. *Environmental Health* (April 29) 13(1):31.

European Food Safety Authority. 2014. Scientific opinion on Dietary Reference Values of chromium. *EFSA Journal* 12:3845–70.

Evans, G. 1989. The effect of chromium picolinate on insulin controlled parameters in humans. *International Journal of Biosocial and Medical Research* 11:163–80.

Fairbanks, V. 1999. Iron in medicine and nutrition. In *Modern Nutrition in Health and Disease,* ed. M. Shils et al. Baltimore: Williams & Wilkins.

Fawcett, J., et al. 1996. The effect of oral vanadyl sulfate on body composition and performance in weight-training athletes. *International Journal of Sport Nutrition* 6:382–90.

Ferrando, A., and Green, N. 1993. The effect of boron supplementation on lean body mass, plasma testosterone levels, and strength in male bodybuilders. *International Journal of Sport Nutrition* 3:140–49.

Fonseca, H., et al. 2014. Bone quality: The determinants of bone strength and fragility. *Sports Medicine* 44:37–53.

Gaier, E., et al. 2013. Copper signaling in the mammalian nervous system: Synaptic effects. *Journal of Neuroscience Research* 91:2–19.

Galloway, S., et al. 1996. The effects of acute phosphate supplementation in subjects of different aerobic fitness levels. *European Journal of Applied Physiology* 72:224–30.

Gledhill, N., et al. 1999. Haemoglobin, blood volume, cardiac function, and aerobic power. *Canadian Journal of Applied Physiology* 24:54–65.

Gleeson, M. 2013. Nutritional support to maintain proper immune status during intense training. *Nestle Nutrition Institute Workshop Series* 75:85–97.

Gonzalez, J., et al. 2014. The influence of calcium supplementation on substrate metabolism during exercise in humans: A randomized controlled trial. *European Journal of Clinical Nutrition* 68:712–8.

Goss, F., et al. 2001. Effect of potassium phosphate supplementation on perceptual and physiological responses to maximal graded exercise. *International Journal of Sport Nutrition and Exercise Metabolism* 11:53–62.

Haas, J., and Brownlie, T. 2001. Iron deficiency and reduced work capacity: A critical review of the research to determine a causal relationship. *Journal of Nutrition* 131: 676S–88S.

Hansen, K., and Tho, S. 1998. Androgens and bone health. *Seminars in Reproductive Endocrinology* 16:129–34.

Harding, M., and O'Mullane, D. 2013. Water fluoridation and oral health. *Acta Medica Academica* 42:131–9.

Heaney, R. 2007. Bone health. *American Journal of Clinical Nutrition* 85:300S–3S.

Heaney, R., and Nordin, B. 2002. Calcium effects on phosphorus absorption: Implications for the prevention and co-therapy of osteoporosis. *Journal of the American College of Nutrition* 21:239–44.

Heaney, R., et al. 2012. A review of calcium supplements and cardiovascular disease risk. *Advances in Nutrition* 3:763–71.

Heine-Bröring, R., et al. 2015. Dietary supplement use and colorectal cancer risk: A systematic review and meta-analysis of prospective cohort studies. *International Journal of Cancer* 136: z388–401.

Hinton, P. 2014. Iron and the endurance athlete. *Applied Physiology, Nutrition, and Metabolism* 39:1012–8.

Houston, M. 2007. The role of mercury and cadmium heavy metals in vascular disease, hypertension, coronary heart disease, and myocardial infarction. *Alternative Therapies in Health and Medicine* 13:S128–S33.

Houston, M. 2011. The role of magnesium in hypertension and cardiovascular disease. *Journal of Clinical Hypertension* 13:843–7.

Hoy, M., and Goldman, J. 2014. Calcium intake in the U.S. population. *What We Eat in America.* NHANES 2009–2010. Food Surveys Research Group Dietary Data Brief No. 13. September.

Hua, Y., et al. 2012. Molecular mechanisms of chromium in alleviating insulin resistance. *Journal of Nutritional Biochemistry* 23:313–9.

Hunt, C., et al. 1997. Metabolic responses of postmenopausal women to supplemental dietary boron and aluminum during usual and low magnesium intake: Boron, calcium, and magnesium absorption and retention and blood mineral concentrations. *American Journal of Clinical Nutrition* 65:808–13.

Ilich, J., and Kerstetter, J. 2000. Nutrition in bone health revisited: A story beyond calcium. *Journal of the American College of Nutrition* 19:715–37.

Jackson, J., et al. 2000. Zinc and the common cold: A meta-analysis revisited. *Journal of Nutrition* 130:1512S–5S.

Kaler, S. 2013. Inborn errors of copper metabolism. *Handbook of Clinical Neurology* 113:1745–54.

Kass, L., et al. 2012. Effect of magnesium supplementation on blood pressure: A meta-analysis. *European Journal of Clinical Nutrition* 66:411–8.

Killip, S., et al. 2007. Iron deficiency anemia. *American Family Physician* 75:671–8.

Kim, H., et al. 2013. SLC31 (CTR) family of copper transporters in health and disease. *Molecular Aspects of Medicine* 34:561–70.

King, J., and Cousins, R. 2014. Zinc. In *Modern Nutrition in Health and Disease,* ed. A. C. Ross, et al. Philadelphia:Wolters Kluwer/Lippincott Williams & Wilkins.

Kong, W., et al. 2014. Hepcidin and sports anemia. *Cell & Bioscience* 4:19.

Kraemer, W., et al. 1995. Effects of multibuffer supplementation on acid-base balance and 2,3-diphosphoglycerate following repetitive anaerobic exercise. *International Journal of Sport Nutrition* 5:300–14.

Kreider, R., et al. 1990. Effects of phosphate loading on oxygen uptake, ventilatory anaerobic threshold, and run performance. *Medicine & Science in Sports & Exercise* 22:250–56.

Kreider, R., et al. 1992. Effects of phosphate loading on metabolic and myocardial responses to maximal and endurance exercise. *International Journal of Sport Nutrition* 2:20–47.

Kreider, R. 1999. Dietary supplements and the promotion of muscle growth with resistance exercise. *Sports Medicine* 27:97–110.

Kunstel, K. 2005. Calcium requirements for the athlete. *Current Sports Medicine Reports* 4:203–6.

Kurokawa, S., and Berry, M. 2013. Selenium. Role of the essential metalloid in health. *Metal Ions in Life Sciences* 13:499–534.

Landahl, G., et al. 2005. Iron deficiency and anemia: A common problem in female elite soccer players. *International Journal of Sport Nutrition and Exercise Metabolism* 15:689–94.

Lane, H. 1989. Some trace elements related to physical activity: Zinc, copper, selenium, chromium, and iodine. In *Nutrition in Exercise and Sport,* ed. J. Hickson and I. Wolinsky. Boca Raton, FL: CRC Press.

Laurberg, P. 2014. Iodine. In *Modern Nutrition in Health and Disease,* ed. A. C. Ross et al. Philadelphia: Wolters Kluwer/Lippincott, Williams & Wilkins.

Lefavi, R. 1992. Efficacy of chromium supplementation in athletes: Emphasis on anabolism. *International Journal of Sport Nutrition* 2:111–22.

Lewis, J., et al. 2015. The effects of calcium supplementation on verified coronary heart disease hospitalization and death in postmenopausal women: A collaborative meta-analysis of randomized controlled trials. *Journal of Bone Mineral Research* 30:165–75.

Liebman, B., and Schardt, D. 2008. MultiComplex: Picking a multivitamin gets tricky. *Nutrition Action Health Letter* 35 (5):1–9.

Livingstone, C. 2015. Zinc: Physiology, deficiency, and parenteral nutrition. *Nutrition in Clinical Practice* 30: 371–82. [Epub ahead of print]

Lobera-Jáuregu, J. 2014. Iron deficiency and cognitive functions. *Journal of Neuropsychiatric Disease and Treatment* 10:2087–95.

Lomagno, K., et al. 2014. Increasing iron and zinc in pre-menopausal women and its effects on mood and cognition: A systematic review. *Nutrients* 14:5117–41.

Lukaski, H. 1995. Micronutrients (magnesium, zinc, and copper): Are mineral supplements needed for athletes? *International Journal of Sport Nutrition* 5:S74–S83.

Lukaski, H. 1999. Chromium as a supplement. *Annual Reviews in Nutrition* 19:279–302.

Lukaski, H. 2001. Magnesium, zinc, and chromium nutrition and athletic performance. *Canadian Journal of Applied Physiology* 26:S13–22.

Lukaski, H. 2004. Vitamin and mineral status: Effects on physical performance. *Nutrition* 20:632–44.

Lukaski, H., et al. 1991. Altered metabolic response of iron deficient women during graded, maximal exercises. *European Journal of Applied Physiology* 63:140–45.

Lukaski, H., et al. 1996. Chromium supplementation and resistance training: Effects on body composition, strength, and trace element status of men. *American Journal of Clinical Nutrition* 63:954–65.

Lukaski, H., et al. 2007. Chromium picolinate supplementation in women: Effects on body weight, composition, and iron status. *Nutrition* 23:187–95.

Maguire, A. 2014. ADA clinical recommendations on topical fluoride for caries prevention. *Evidence-Based Dentistry* 15:38–9.

Mannix, E., et al. 1990. Oxygen delivery and cardiac output during exercise following oral phosphate-glucose. *Medicine & Science in Sports & Exercise* 22:341–47.

Maret, W. 2013. Zinc and human disease. *Metal Ions in Life Sciences* 13:389–414.

Maret, W., and Sandstead, H. 2006. Zinc requirements and the risks and benefits of zinc supplementation. *Journal of Trace Elements in Medicine and Biology* 20:3–18.

Margaritis, I., et al. 1997. Effects of endurance training on skeletal muscle oxidative capacities with and without selenium supplementation. *Journal of Trace Elements in Medicine and Biology* 11:37–43.

Mayo-Wilson, E., et al. 2014. Preventive zinc supplementation for children, and the effect of additional iron: A systematic review and meta-analysis. *BMJ Open* 4 (6):e004647.

Mazzeo, R., and Fulco, C. 2006. Physiological systems and their responses to conditions of hypoxia. In *ACSM's Advanced Exercise Physiology,* ed. C. Tipton. Philadelphia: Lippincott Williams & Wilkins.

McClung, J., et al. 2014. Female athletes: A population at risk of vitamin and mineral deficiencies affecting health and performance. *Journal of Trace Elements in Medicine and Biology* 28:388–92.

McDonald, R., and Keen, C. 1988. Iron, zinc and magnesium nutrition and athletic performance. *Sports Medicine* 5:171–84.

Meeusen, R., et al. 2013. Prevention, diagnosis, and treatment of the overtraining syndrome: Joint consensus statement of the European College of Sport Science and the American College of Sports Medicine. *Medicine & Science in Sports & Exercise* 45:186–205.

Mettler, S., and Zimmermann, M. 2010. Iron excess in recreational marathon runners. *European Journal of Clinical Nutrition* 64:490–4.

Micheletti, A., et al. 2001. Zinc status in athletes: Relation to diet and exercise. *Sports Medicine* 31:577–82.

Miller, L., et al. 2004. Bone mineral density in postmenopausal women. *Physician and Sportsmedicine* 32 (2):18–24.

Modlesky, C., and Lewis, R. 2002. Does exercise during growth have a long-term effect on bone health? *Exercise and Sport Sciences Reviews* 30:171–76.

Molgaard, C., et al. 2005. Long-term calcium supplementation does not affect the iron status of 12–14-y-old girls. *American Journal of Clinical Nutrition* 82:98–102.

Mountjoy, M., et al. 2014. The IOC consensus statement: Beyond the Female Athlete triad—Relative energy deficiency in sport (RED-S). *British Journal of Sports Medicine* 48:491–7.

Naghii, M. 1999. The significance of dietary boron, with particular reference to athletes. *Nutrition and Health* 13:31–37.

National Cancer Institute. 2009. Calcium and cancer prevention: Strengths and limits of the evidence. www.cancer.gov/cancertopics/causes-prevention/risk-factors/diet/calcium-fact-sheet.

National Institutes of Health. 2006. National Institutes of Health State-of-the-Science conference statement: Multivitamin/mineral supplements and chronic disease prevention. *Annals of Internal Medicine* 145:364–71.

Nemeth, E., and Ganz, T. 2006. Regulation of iron metabolism by hepcidin. *Annual Review of Nutrition* 26:323–42.

Newhouse, I., and Finstad, E. 2000. The effects of magnesium supplementation on exercise performance. *Clinical Journal of Sport Medicine* 10:195–200.

Nielsen, F. 1992. Facts and fallacies about boron. *Nutrition Today* 27:6–12.

Nielsen, F. 1998. The justification for providing dietary guidance for the nutritional intake of boron. *Biological Trace Element Research* 66:319–30.

Nielsen, F. 2008. Is boron nutritionally relevant? *Nutrition Reviews* 66:183–91.

Nielsen, F. 2014. Should bioactive trace elements not recognized as essential, but with beneficial health effects, have intake recommendations. *Journal of Trace Elements in Medicine and Biology* 28:406–8.

Nielsen, F. 2014. Update on human health effects of boron. *Journal of Trace Elements in Medicine and Biology* 28:383–9.

Nielsen, F., and Lukaski, H. 2006. Update on the relationship between magnesium and exercise. *Magnesium Research* 19:180–89.

Nieman, D. 2001. Exercise immunology: Nutritional countermeasures. *Canadian Journal of Applied Physiology* 26:S45–S55.

O'Brien, K., et al. 2014. Phosphorus. In *Modern Nutrition in Health and Disease,* ed. A. C. Ross et al. Philadelphia: Wolters Kluwer/Lippincott Williams & Wilkins.

Onakpoya, I., et al. 2013. Chromium supplementation in overweight and obesity: A systematic review and meta-analysis of randomized clinical trials. *Obesity Reviews* 14:496–507.

Paik, J., et al. 2014. Calcium supplement intake and risk of cardiovascular disease in women. *Osteoporosis International* 25:2047–56.

Painelli Vde, S., et al. 2014. The effects of two different doses of calcium lactate on blood pH, bicarbonate, and repeated high-intensity exercise performance. *International Journal of Sport Nutrition and Exercise Metabolism* 24:286–95.

Peckham, S., and Awofeso, N. 2014. Water fluoridation: A critical review of the physiological effects of ingested fluoride as a public health intervention. *Scientific World Journal* (February 26);293019.

Pennington, J. 1996. Intakes of minerals from diets and foods: Is there a need for concern? *Journal of Nutrition* 126:2304S–8S.

Penny, M. 2013. Zinc supplementation in public health. *Annals of Nutrition and Metabolism* 62 (Supplement 1):31–42.

Rautiainen, S., et al. 2013. The role of calcium in the prevention of cardiovascular disease—A review of observational studies and randomized clinical trials. *Current Atherosclerosis Reports* 15(11):362.

Rayman, M., and Stranges, S. 2013. Epidemiology of selenium and type 2 diabetes: Can we make sense of it? *Free Radicals in Biology & Medicine* 65:1557–64.

Rees, K., et al. 2013. Selenium supplementation for the primary prevention of cardiovascular disease. *Cochrane Database of Systematic Reviews* (January 31) 1:CD009671.

Rehder, D. 2013. Vanadium. Its role for humans. *Metal Ions in Life Sciences* 13:139–69.

Reid, I. 2013. Cardiovascular effects of calcium supplements. *Nutrients* 5:2522–9.

Reid, I. 2014. Should we prescribe calcium supplements for osteoporosis prevention? *Journal of Bone Metabolism* 21:21–8.

Rodenberg, R., and Gustafson, S. 2007. Iron as an ergogenic aid: Ironclad evidence? *Current Sports Medicine Reports* 6:258–64.

Roman, M., et al. 2014. Selenium biochemistry and its role for human health. *Metallomics* 6:25–54.

Roohani, N., et al. 2013. Zinc and its importance for human health: An integrative review. *Journal of Research in Medical Sciences* 18:144–57.

Rosanoff, A., et al. 2012. Suboptimal magnesium status in the United States: Are the health consequences underestimated? *Nutrition Reviews* 70:153–64.

Rowland, T. 2012. Iron deficiency in athletes. *American Journal of Lifestyle Medicine* 6:319–27.

Rowland, T., et al. 1988. The effect of iron therapy on the exercise capacity of non-anemic iron-deficient adolescent runners. *American Journal of Diseases in Children* 142:165–69.

Rubenowitz, E., et al. 1996. Magnesium in drinking water and death from acute myocardial infarction. *American Journal of Epidemiology* 143:456–62.

Rude, R. 2014. Magnesium. In *Modern Nutrition in Health and Disease,* ed. A. C. Ross et al. Philadelphia: Wolters Kluwer/Lippincott Williams & Wilkins.

Rugg-Gunn, A., and Bánóczy, J. 2013. Fluoride toothpastes and fluoride mouthrinses for home use. *Acta Medica Academica* 42:168–78.

Schardt, D., and Schmidt, S. 1996. Chromium. *Nutrition Action Healthletter* 23 (4):10–11.

Scott, S., et al. 2014. The impact of anemia on child mortality: An updated review. *Nutrients* 6:5915–32.

Seeman, E. 1999. The structural basis of bone fragility in men. *Bone* 25:143–47.

Setaro, L., et al. 2014. Magnesium status and the physical performance of volleyball players: Effects of magnesium supplementation. *Journal of Sport Sciences* 32:438–45.

Sim, M., et al. 2014. Iron regulation in athletes: Exploring the menstrual cycle and effects of different exercise modalities on hepcidin production. *International Journal of Sport Nutrition and Exercise Metabolism* 24:177–87.

Smyth, P., and Duntas, L. 2005. Iodine uptake and loss—Can frequent strenuous exercise induce iodine deficiency? *Hormone and Metabolic Research* 37:555–8.

Soares, M., et al. 2011. Calcium and vitamin D for obesity: A review of randomized controlled trials. *European Journal of Clinical Nutrition* 65:994–1004.

Sojka, J., and Weaver, C. 1995. Magnesium supplementation and osteoporosis. *Nutrition Reviews* 53:71–80.

Speich, M., et al. 2001. Minerals, trace elements and related biological variables in athletes and during physical activity. *Clinical Chimica Acta* 312:1–11.

Squitti, R., et al. 2014. Low-copper diet as a preventive strategy for Alzheimer's disease. *Neurobiology of Aging* 34:S40–S50.

Stewart, I., et al. 1990. Phosphate loading and the effects on VO_2 max in trained cyclists. *Research Quarterly for Exercise and Sport* 61:80–84.

Straub, D. 2007. Calcium supplementation in clinical practice: A review of forms, doses, and indications. *Nutrition in Clinical Practice* 22:286–96.

Sunde, R. 2014. Selenium. In *Modern Nutrition in Health and Disease,* ed. A. C. Ross et al. Philadelphia: Wolters Kluwer/Lippincott Williams & Wilkins.

Tessier, F., et al. 1995. Selenium and training effects on the glutathione system and aerobic performance. *Medicine & Science in Sports & Exercise* 27:390–96.

Thompson, I., et al. 2014. Prevention of prostate cancer: Outcomes of clinical trials and future opportunities. *American Society of Clinical Oncology Educational Book* e76–e80.

Tian, H., et al. 2013. Chromium picolinate supplementation for overweight or obese adults. *Cochrane Database of Systematic Reviews* (November 29) 11:CD010063.

Titchenal, C., and Dobbs, J. 2007. A system to assess the quality of food sources of calcium. *Journal of Food Composition and Analysis* 20:717–24.

Tremblay, A., and Gilbert, J. 2011. Human obesity: Is insufficient calcium/dairy intake part of the problem? *Journal of the American College of Nutrition* 30:449S–53S.

Tremblay, M., et al. 1994. Ergogenic effects of phosphate loading: Physiological fact or methodological fiction? *Canadian Journal of Applied Physiology* 19:1–11.

Turner, C., and Robling, A. 2003. Designing exercise regimens to increase bone strength. *Exercise and Sport Sciences Reviews* 31:45–50.

Turnlund, J. 2006. Copper. In *Modern Nutrition in Health and Disease,* ed. M. Shils et al. Philadelphia: Lippincott Williams & Wilkins.

Tuschl, K., et al. 2013. Manganese and the brain. *International Review of Neurobiology* 110:277–312.

Uusi-Rasi, K., et al. 2013. Calcium intake in health maintenance—A systematic review. *Food & Nutrition Research* (May 16) 57.

Vincent, J. 2014. Is chromium pharmacologically relevant? *Journal of Trace Elements in Medicine and Biology* 28:397–405.

Vincent, J. 2015. Is the pharmacological mode of action of chromium(iii) as a second messenger? *Biological Trace Element Research* 166: 7–12. [Epub ahead of print]

Vinceti, M., et al. 2001. Adverse effects of selenium in humans. *Reviews on Environmental Health* 16:233–51.

Vinceti, M., et al. 2013. Friend or foe? The current epidemiologic evidence on selenium and human cancer risk. *Journal of Environmental Science and Health. Part C, Environmental Carcinogenesis & Ecotoxicology Reviews* 31:305–41.

Vinceti, M., et al. 2014. Selenium for preventing cancer. *Cochrane Database of Systematic Reviews* (March 30) 3:CD005195.

Vinceti, M., et al. 2014. Selenium neurotoxicity in humans: Bridging laboratory and epidemiologic studies. *Toxicology Letters* 230:295–303.

Vishwanathan, R., et al. 2013. A systematic review on zinc for the prevention and treatment of age-related macular degeneration. *Investigative Ophthalmology & Visual Science* 54:3985–98.

Wang, Z., and Cefalu, W. 2010. Current concepts about chromium supplementation in type 2 diabetes and insulin resistance. *Current Diabetes Reports* 10:145–51.

Weaver, C. 2014. Calcium supplementation: Is protecting against osteoporosis counter to protecting against cardiovascular disease? *Current Osteoporosis Reports* 12:211–8.

Weaver, C., and Heaney, R. 2014. Calcium. In *Modern Nutrition in Health and Disease,* ed. A. C. Ross et al. Philadelphia: Wolters Kluwer/Lippincott Williams & Wilkins.

Weaver, C., and Rajaram, S. 1992. Exercise and iron status. *Journal of Nutrition* 122:782–87.

Weng, H., et al. 2014. An innovative approach for iodine supplementation using iodine-rich phytogenic food. *Environmental Geochemistry and Health* 36:815–28.

Wessling-Resnick, M. 2014. Iron. In *Modern Nutrition in Health and Disease,* ed. A. C. Ross et al. Philadelphia: Wolters Kluwer/Lippincott Williams & Wilkins.

West, J., et al. 2012. The effect of 6 days of sodium phosphate supplementation on appetite, energy intake, and aerobic capacity in trained men and women. *International Journal of Sport*

Nutrition and Exercise Metabolism 22:422–9.

White, K., et al. 2006. The acute effects of dietary calcium intake on fat metabolism during exercise and endurance exercise performance. *International Journal of Sport Nutrition and Exercise Metabolism* 16:565–79.

Wilber, R., et al. 2007. Effect of hypoxic "dose" on physiological responses and sea-level performance. *Medicine & Science in Sports & Exercise* 39:1590–99.

Williams, M. 2010. *Nutrition for Health, Fitness, & Sport.* New York: McGraw-Hill.

Wilson, K., et al. 2015. Calcium and phosphorus intake and prostate cancer risk: A 24-y follow-up study. *American Journal of Clinical Nutrition* 101:173–83.

Wood, R., and Ronnenberg, A. 2006. Iron. In *Modern Nutrition in Health and Disease,* ed. M. Shils et al. Philadelphia: Lippincott Williams & Wilkins.

Zemel, M. 2005. Dairy augmentation of total and central fat loss in obese subjects. *International Journal of Obesity and Related Metabolic Disorders* 29:391–97.

Zemel, M. 2005. The role of dairy in weight management. *Journal of the American College of Nutrition* 24:537S–46S.

Zemel, M., et al. 2005. Effects of calcium and dairy on body composition and weight loss in African-American adults. *Obesity Research* 13:1218–25.

Zernicke, R., et al. 2006. The skeletal-articular system. In *ACSM's Advanced Exercise Physiology,* ed. C. Tipton. Philadelphia: Lippincott Williams & Wilkins.

Zhao, N., et al. 2013. Iron regulation by hepcidin. *Journal of Clinical Investigations* 123:2337–43.

Zhou, J., et al. 2013. Selenium and diabetes—Evidence from animal studies. *Free Radicals in Biology & Medicine* 65:1548–56.

Zimmermann, M., and Boelaert, K. 2015. Iodine deficiency and thyroid disorders. *The Lancet Diabetes and Endocrinology* 3:286–95.

Zourdos, M., et al. 2015. A brief review: The implications of iron supplementation for marathon runners on health and performance. *Journal of Strength & Conditioning Research* 29:559–65.

Water, Electrolytes, and Temperature Regulation

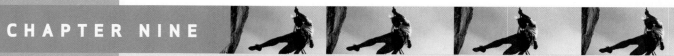

LEARNING OBJECTIVES

After studying this chapter, you should be able to:

1. Identify the principal water compartments in the body, describe the general function of each, and explain how your body maintains overall water balance.

2. Identify foods that are high or low in sodium and potassium, and explain the physiological responses of your body to restore normal serum sodium levels following a high salt intake.

3. List the four components of environmental heat stress recorded by the wet-bulb globe temperature (WBGT), and explain how each may affect the heat balance equation during exercise under hot, humid environmental conditions.

4. Describe how exercise in the heat may impair endurance performance as compared to exercise in a cooler environment, and explain the physiological responses your body would make to promote heat loss.

5. Outline the key guidelines for consuming water, electrolytes, and carbohydrate before, during, and after exercise under warm or hot environmental conditions, and offer general recommendations to athletes participating in such events.

6. Describe the theory underlying the use of glycerol as an ergogenic aid, and understand the current research findings regarding its efficacy in enhancing exercise performance.

7. Learn various strategies to reduce the risk of heat illness while exercising in a hot environment, but also be able to identify the various heat illnesses along with their causes, clinical findings, and appropriate treatment.

8. Understand the meaning of high blood pressure and associated health risks, and describe the role that diet and exercise may play in its prevention and treatment.

Water (H_2O) is the most important nutrient and, except for minerals, the simplest nutrient. The average individual can survive several weeks without food but only a week without water. Rapid losses of water and electrolytes through dehydration or diarrhea can be fatal in an even shorter period of time. The essence of water to life was keenly understood by primitive humankind many centuries prior to our current (and evolving) understanding of the nutrients described in chapters 4–8. Smith describes the historical contribution of John Snow, a British physician considered one of the fathers of modern epidemiology, in the importance of clean drinking water. In 1855, Snow debunked the prevailing "miasma" (i.e., "bad air") etiology of cholera by observing a death rate in London households that were supplied by the Southwark and Vauxhall Company (downstream from fecal waste discharge into the Thames River) that was 8.5 times that of households supplied by the Lambeth Company (upstream of waste discharge). Clean drinking water is described by Rush as being taken for granted in developed countries. Water is the solvent for the body's chemical processes and accounts for most of our body mass. Our ability to derive energy from nutrients in food requires water for the chemical reaction known as hydrolysis. In separate reviews, Kenefick and Cheuvront and Maughan note the importance of water intake, availability, and adequate hydration for regulation of body temperature in both physically active and vulnerable populations, respectively.

Electrolytes, part of the mineral class of nutrients discussed in the previous chapter, have a myriad of physiological roles, some of which are muscle contraction, neural action potentials, cofactors in energy metabolism, and activation of enzymes. Although electrolyte balance is normally tightly regulated by the body and adequate electrolyte intake is available in a healthy diet, a significant loss of electrolytes accompanies the loss of water by profuse sweating, vomiting, or diarrhea. Deaths in children less than 5 years of age have dropped 47 percent since 1990 due in part to the standard WHO oral rehydration therapy (ORT) solution (sodium, potassium, chloride, and glucose) to rapidly replace lost fluid and electrolytes. However, diarrhea still accounts for 9 percent of all deaths in this age group and is the fourth leading cause of death of young children in certain regions of Africa and Southeast Asia.

In addition to health, proper fluid replacement and electrolyte balance are important for performance in recreational/competitive sports and in the workplace. Since the early 1960s, the United States Army Research Institute of Environmental Medicine has focused on research preparing military personnel to function in extreme environmental conditions. Much of this research has focused on risk factors associated with exercise under warm or hot conditions, strategies to acclimatize personnel, and the development of policies to reduce morbidity and mortality from heat illness. Scientists and coaches also recognized the need for sports ORT to offset impaired performance and fatigue from fluid and electrolyte losses through sweating in runners, cyclists, football players, and other athletes. The formulation of Gatorade® in 1965 by the University of Florida's Dr. Robert Cade was the first entry in the "sports drink" (**carbohydrate electrolyte solution**, or CES) industry, which thrives today. Optimal CES composition, palatability,

and factors promoting absorption continue to receive research attention.

Physically active individuals are aware that a hot and/or humid environment can impair performance. Environmental and metabolic heat results in loss of body water and electrolytes, which compromises the body's ability to dissipate heat and regulate core temperature. At best, loss of fluid and electrolytes will impair performance. Inability to regulate core temperature can lead to heat illness, the most extreme form of which can be fatal. This chapter will discuss the roles of water and the key electrolytes sodium, chloride, and potassium in fluid regulation and performance; the effects of water and electrolyte loss on performance; strategies for proper hydration before exercise and proper rehydration during and after exercise; the recognition and prevention of heat illnesses; and the role of fluid/electrolyte balance, diet, and exercise in high blood pressure (hypertension) prevention and management.

Water

How much water do you need per day?

Daily AI values for water intake have been established as 3.7 liters and 2.7 liters (3.9 and 2.9 quarts) for average males and females, respectively, based on 2005–2010 National Health and Nutrition Examination Survey (NHANES) data. Drewnowski and colleagues reported that large percentages of older (75+ years) adults and children age 4–13 fail to meet recommended AI water intakes. Adults, but not children, generally exceed the 1 liter/1,000 Calories water intake recommendation. Somewhat lower AI have been established for teenagers and children. The actual requirement for a given individual depends on factors such as body mass, health status, age, environmental conditions, and physical activity. Water requirements may be increased substantially during exercise, particularly under warm environmental conditions, and will be discussed later in this chapter. Heinz Valtin, an expert on body water balance, in general noted that thirst is a good guide to help maintain normal body water balance. In his 2002 review, Valtin questioned the anecdotal recommendation to drink at least eight 8-oz (237-mL) glasses of water per day. More recently, Vivanti also identified problems with generalized equations for estimating water intake in a health-care setting. As will become apparent in this chapter, water requirements are highly variable between and within individuals as a result of a variety of factors such as health status, environmental conditions, physical activity, acclimatization, and diet.

Body water balance is maintained when the output of body fluids is matched by the input of water. Drewnowski and others note that water, soda, alcohol, caffeinated beverages, milk, fruit juices, and sports drinks contribute 75–84 percent of water intake, with the remainder coming from food. A small amount of water is lost in the feces and through the exhaled air in breathing. **Insensible perspiration** on the skin, which is not visible, is almost pure water and accounts for about 30 percent of body-water losses. Perspiration, or sweat, losses may be increased considerably during exercise and/or hot environmental conditions. Urinary output is the main avenue for water loss. It may increase somewhat through the use of diuretics, including alcohol and caffeine. Stookey indicates that we lose about 1 milliliter of water for every milligram of caffeine, and 10 milliliters for every gram of alcohol. Recent research has challenged the assumption that caffeine is a significant diuretic, however. In his review, Armstrong found no evidence of fluid-electrolyte imbalances after caffeine ingestion in the 100- to 680-mg range. Armstrong and others reported no differences in hydration status in subjects following 0, 3, and 6 mg/kg doses of caffeine each day for 4 days. More recently, Silva and colleagues used a crossover design to examine the effect of caffeine ingestion (5 mg/kg/day for 4 days) on water volume and distribution in 30 nonsmoking males who were low users of caffeine. Compared to placebo, caffeine ingestion did not alter total body water regardless of body composition, physical activity, or daily water ingestion. Consumption of a high-protein diet produces urea, which has to be excreted by the kidneys and may increase urine output.

Fluid intake of beverages, such as water, soda, milk, juice, coffee, and tea, provides about 80 percent of total water needed to replenish losses. Valtin notes that we obtain significant amounts of fluid from caffeinated and alcoholic beverages, such as coffee and beer. Although both beverages contain diuretics, the Consumers Union noted that if you are used to drinking caffeinated or alcoholic beverages, the diuretic effect of each may be offset by the amount of fluid in the beverage and you probably gain more fluid from beverages, such as colas, coffee and beer, than you lose. About 20 percent of our daily total water intake comes from the foods we eat. Solid foods also contribute as a water source in two different ways. First, food contains water in varying amounts; certain foods such as lettuce, celery, melons, and most fruits contain about 80–90 percent water; meats and seafood contain about 60–70 percent water; even bread, an apparently dry food, contains 36 percent water. Second, the metabolism of carbohydrate, fat, and protein for energy produces water. Fat, carbohydrate, and protein all produce water when broken down for energy. You may recall the reaction when glucose is metabolized to produce energy, with one of the by-products being **metabolic water**:

$$C_6H_{12}O_6 + 6O_2 \rightarrow Energy + 6CO_2 + 6H_2O$$

Figure 9.1 summarizes the daily water loss and intake for the maintenance of water balance for an adult female. Amounts would be greater for an adult male. As shall be seen later, however, these amounts may change drastically under certain conditions.

What else is in the water we drink?

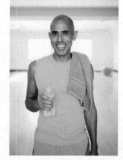

The tap water we drink, although generally safe, is not pure. Solutes entering drinking water from natural geological formations include minerals such as calcium, magnesium, fluoride, iron, sodium, and zinc. Calcium and magnesium may be beneficial. Fluoride is beneficial in preventing dental caries and is added to the municipal water supply, but too much can stain teeth and adversely affect bone health. Some minerals, such as excess sodium, arsenic, and lead, may lead to various health problems, whereas others, such as calcium and magnesium, may be beneficial. Brown and Margolis stress that all sources of lead should be controlled or eliminated because lead accumulates in the body and there is no "safe" blood lead level in children. Of greater concern to public health in economically developed nations are humanmade solutes in the water supply. Murray and others identified three broad classes of "emerging contaminants" as industrial chemicals, pesticides, and pharmaceuticals/personal care products. Under the Safe Drinking Water Act, the Environmental Protection Agency (EPA) provides a list of contaminants and their maximum contaminant level (MCL) at water.epa.gov/drink/contaminants/basicinformation/index.cfm. Most, but not all, municipal water treatment facilities conform to these standards. The EPA also provides guidance for special populations such as pregnant women, infants and children, and the elderly regarding exposure to contaminants in drinking water.

If you are concerned about your tap water, know that some health professionals suggest a water filter as the best alternative. Water filters added to your tap may help remove unwanted substances, such as chlorine or chlorinated by-products; some water filters are designed to eliminate lead and mercury, and others can even trap parasites. Many types of water filters are on the market, so, if interested, have your water analyzed and then seek an appropriate filter to help purify your tap water. To get information on the quality of your water supply, you may contact your local water utility and ask for the latest water quality or Consumer Confidence Report, or contact the EPA Website.

http://water.epa.gov/drink/local/ The Environmental Protection Agency provides information on the quality of local drinking water.
www.fda.gov/food/foodborneillnesscontaminants/buys-toreservesafefood/ucm077079.htm The Food and Drug Administration provides information on bottled water.
www.bottledwater.org/ The International Bottled Water Association Website.

Bottled water is the current rage. The International Bottled Water Association (IBWA) reported sales of 11.8 billion dollars in 2012. A 2013 *New York Times* article by Stephanie Strom reported that bottled water sales are projected to overtake carbonated beverage sales by 2020. The Food and Drug Administration (FDA) regulates bottled water as stringently as the EPA regulates tap water. Artesian water is drawn from a well that taps a confined aquifer; mineral water comes from a protected underground source and must contain ≥225 parts per million in minerals from a geological underground source; spring water flows naturally from an underground source; purified water is produced by distillation, deionization, or some comparable process; and sparking water contains carbon dioxide in the same concentration after treatment as before. Vitamin, herbal, nutraceutical, fitness, and oxygen waters, the last of which will be discussed later in this

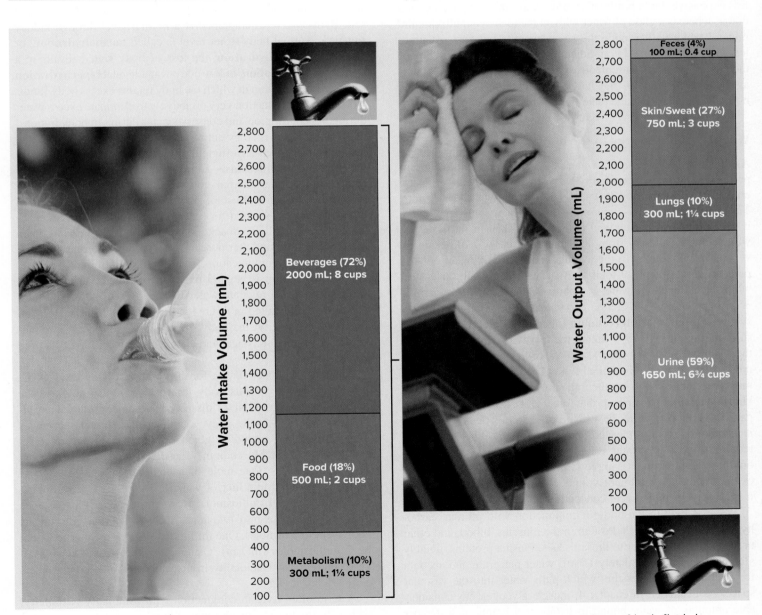

FIGURE 9.1 Estimate of water balance—intake versus output—in a woman. We primarily maintain our volume of body fluids by adjusting water output to intake. As you can see, most water comes from the liquids we consume. Some comes from the moisture in more solid foods, and the remainder is manufactured during metabolism. Water output includes losses from the lungs, urine, skin, and feces.

chapter, are also in the marketplace. About 85 percent of bottled water manufacturers belong to the IBWA, which sets even tougher standards for its members than the FDA. Individuals who drink bottled water should be aware that approximately 25 percent is simply tap water that has undergone a purification process. The nation's two best-selling bottled waters, Aquafina and Dasani, are purified municipal water. Also, surveys have shown that most bottled waters do not contain fluoride. For example, Lalumandier and Ayers reported that only 5 percent of 57 samples of bottled water contained fluoride within the recommended range. Check bottled water labels for mineral content. The FDA is also seeking legislation requiring that bottled water manufacturers list contaminant levels on bottle labels.

Bottled water isn't cheap. One *gourmet* bottled water, Bling, is marketed at $55 or more per bottle. Other specialty waters are less expensive, but a bottle of vitamin water may cost well over a dollar, whereas a glass of water with an inexpensive multivitamin/mineral tablet will provide the same benefits but cost ten times less. The Consumers Union indicates that you do not need any of the specialty waters to replenish fluids, but if their taste encourages you to drink more, they may be worthwhile, especially if you normally do not drink adequate fluids.

Where is water stored in the body?

As illustrated in Figure 9.2, water is stored in several body compartments but moves constantly between compartments. The reference 70-kilogram (154-lb) man is 60 percent water, or 42 liters. The average female is approximately 50 percent water. More water is found in muscle and nonfat tissue than in fat tissue, so water content can vary from 40 percent in obese to 70 percent in very lean individuals. In the average male, approximately 60–65 percent (25–28 liters) of total body water is **intracellular water**, while the extracellular water compartment makes up the remaining 35–40 percent (14–17 liters). The **extracellular water** is further subdivided into the **intercellular** (interstitial) **water** between or surrounding the cells (8–9 liters), the **intravascular water** within the blood vessels (3–4 liters), and miscellaneous water compartments such as the cerebrospinal fluid (1–3 liters). Water compartments are measured using the indicator dilution method, where a known quantity of an appropriate tracer that cannot leave the compartment is injected into the space. For example, deuterium oxide is a common tracer to measure total body water. Other tracers are required to measure water volume in specific areas. After equilibration, a compartment sample is analyzed for the concentration of the tracer. Compartment volume (mL) is calculated as tracer mass (mg) ÷ sample tracer concentration (mg/mL).

Water is held in the body in conjunction with protein, carbohydrate, and electrolytes. Protein in the muscles, blood, and other tissues helps bind water to those tissues. Plasma proteins, notably albumin, bind approximately 15 mL water per gram and account for colloid oncotic pressure, which pulls water into the vascular space. As discussed in chapter 4, muscle glycogen has considerable amounts of water bound to it (about 3 grams of water per gram of glycogen), which may prove to be an advantage when exercising in the heat. In essence, the metabolism of 350 grams of carbohydrate during exercise will provide nearly 1 liter of water for body functions, as documented by Rogers and others. The sodium in the extracellular fluid, including sodium in the vascular system, also attracts water.

Proper water and electrolyte balance within these compartments is of extreme importance to the athletic individual. Fluid shifts such as decreases in blood volume and cellular dehydration, both of which may develop during exercise in the heat, could contribute to the onset of fatigue or heat illness.

How is body water regulated?

Johnson notes that maintaining body water and sodium balance is so critical to health that the central nervous system has developed specific neural patterns fostering an appetite for both water and salt. Body water is maintained at a normal level through kidney function. Normal body-water level is called **normohydration**, or **euhydration**. **Dehydration**, the loss of body water, results in a state of **hypohydration**, or low body-water level. **Hyperhydration** represents a condition in which the body retains excess body fluids. Normal kidneys function very effectively to eliminate excess water during hyperhydration and conserve water during hypohydration.

Because water is so essential to life, it is indeed fortunate that the body possesses an efficient mechanism to maintain proper water balance. **Homeostasis** is the term used to describe the maintenance of a normal internal environment so that the body has the proper distribution and use of water, electrolytes, hormones, and other substances essential for life processes. Homeostatic mechanisms are essentially feedback loops consisting of commands from the CNS to fluid and thermoregulatory organs (efferent outflow) in response to communication from the tissue (afferent input). A detailed discussion is beyond the scope of this text, but several feedback loops to regulate water balance, electrolytes, and temperature are illustrated in figure 9.4. If these feedback devices are functioning properly, the body usually has no problem in maintaining the normal physical and chemical composition of its fluid compartments.

The main feedback device for the control of body water is the osmolality of the various body fluids. **Osmolality** refers to the amount, or concentration, of dissolved substances, known as *solute*, in a solution. In the body, a number of different substances affect osmolality, including glucose, protein, and several electrolytes, most notably sodium. These substances are dissolved in the body water. One mole of a nonionic substance, such as glucose, dissolved in a liter of water is 1 osmole. One millimole (1/1,000 mole) is 1 milliosmole. However, a mole of a substance that can dissociate into two ions, such as sodium chloride, is equivalent to 2 osmoles. One millimole of sodium chloride would be 2 milliosmoles (mOsm). Osmolality is expressed in mOsm/kg of body mass. Osmolality in normally hydrated conditions is 275–295 mOsm/kg.

A term often used in conjunction with osmolality is **tonicity**, which means tension or pressure. When two solutions have the same osmotic pressure they are said to be *isosmotic* or, more

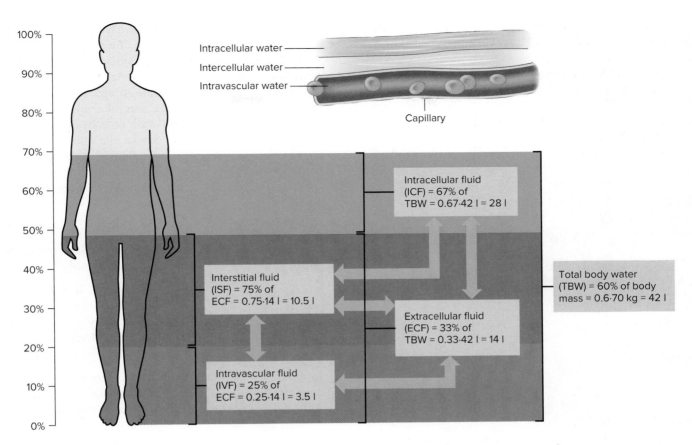

FIGURE 9.2 Body-water compartments in the 70-kg reference male. As illustrated by the blue arrows, there is a constant interchange among the different body-water compartments. The water inside the body cells, the intracellular water, is important for cell functions. The extracellular space includes intercellular, intravascular, and miscellaneous (e.g., cerebrospinal fluid). The intracellular water constitutes about 60–65 percent of the total body water, while the extracellular water constitutes the remaining 35–40 percent. In the blood, some of the water is intracellular in the blood cells, while the remainder is extracellular in the plasma. Decreases in blood volume (intravascular water) may adversely affect endurance capacity.

commonly, *isotonic. Iso* means "same." When two solutions with different solute concentrations are compared, the one with the higher osmotic pressure is called hypertonic and the other is hypotonic.

When two solutions with different solute concentrations are separated by a permeable membrane, as in the human body between the fluid compartments, a potential pressure difference may develop between the solutions that will allow for water movement. This pressure is known as *osmotic pressure.* Water moves through cell membrane proteins, known as aquaporin water channels, from the hypotonic solution (low solute concentration and high water content) to the hypertonic solution (high solute concentration and low water content). In essence, high solute concentrations create high osmotic pressures and tend to draw water into their compartments. Figure 9.3 depicts this mechanism between the blood and the body cells.

To briefly illustrate the feedback mechanism for control of body water, let us look at what happens when you become dehydrated owing to excessive body-water losses or lowered water intake. The blood then becomes more concentrated, or hypertonic. Because maintenance of a normal blood volume is of prime importance, the blood tends to draw water from the body cells. Certain cells in the hypothalamus, called *osmoreceptors,* are sensitive to changes in osmotic pressure. These cells react to the more concentrated body fluids by stimulating the release of a hormone from the pituitary gland, the so-called master gland of the body. This hormone is called the **antidiuretic hormone (ADH)**, also known as arginine vasopressin. The ADH travels by the blood to the kidneys and directs them to reabsorb more water. Hence, urinary output of water is diminished considerably. Figure 9.4 illustrates several feedback loops that regulate body water and blood volume. During hyperhydration, which would produce a hypotonic condition in the body fluids, a reverse process would occur, leading to increased water excretion.

Because maintenance of euhydration is critical for health and physical performance, it is important to note that ADH is only one of several hormones that help to regulate body-water balance. Other hormones are involved in the maintenance of sodium and

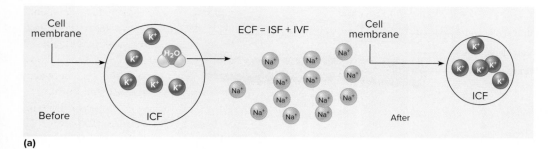

(a)

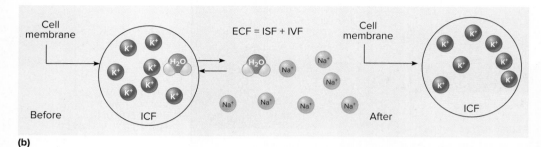

(b)

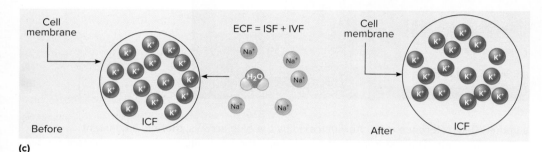

(c)

FIGURE 9.3 Osmosis and tonicity. (a) When the extracellular fluid (ECF) contains more electrolytes or other osmotic substances, it is hypertonic to the intracellular fluid (ICF) and water will flow from the ICF space to the ECF space (interstitial fluid [ISF] + intravascular fluid [IVF]) and the cell decreases in volume. In other words, water flows to the area of greater osmotic pressure. (b) When the solute concentration is the same in the cell and outside the cell, there is no net gain or loss of water from either space; therefore, there is no change in cell volume. (c) When the ICF contains more electrolytes or higher osmotic pressure than the ECF, water will flow into the ICF space from the ECF space, and the cell increases in volume.

potassium, which also affect body-water levels, and the role of one is discussed in the next section on electrolytes.

How do I know if I am adequately hydrated?

Osmoreceptors and other mechanisms also may stimulate the sensation of thirst, which is usually a good guide to body-water needs and is effective in restoring body water to normal on a day-to-day basis. Some sports scientists contend that thirst may also be a good guide to hydration status during exercise. For example, Fudge and others studied elite Kenyan runners during a 5-day training period and found that they remained well hydrated day-to-day with *ad libitum* fluid intake. However, as shall be noted later, it may be advisable to start consuming fluids during exercise under warm conditions before you become thirsty. One of the best guides to indicate a state of normohydration is the color of your urine. In general, it should be a clear, pale yellow. A deeply colored urine,

usually excreted in small amounts, is indicative of a state of hypohydration. However, vitamin supplements containing riboflavin (B_2) may also cause the urine to appear yellow and suggest a state of dehydration when the individual is euhydrated. Cheuvront and Sawka indicate that change in body weight is also a reliable and easy method to evaluate hydration status. Some guidelines are presented later in this chapter.

What are the major functions of water in the body?

Water is essential if the other nutrients are to function properly within the human body; it is the solvent for life. It has a number of diverse functions that may be summarized as follows:

1. Water provides the essential building material for cell protoplasm, the fundamental component of all living matter.
2. Because water cannot be compressed, it protects key body tissues such as the spinal cord and brain.
3. Water is essential in the control of the osmotic pressure in the body, or the maintenance of a proper balance between water, interstitial and intravascular proteins, and the electrolytes. Any major changes in the electrolyte concentration may adversely affect cellular function. A serious departure from normal osmotic pressure cannot be tolerated by the body for long.
4. Water is the main constituent of blood, the major transportation mechanism in the body for conveying oxygen, nutrients, hormones, and other compounds to the cells for their use, and for carrying waste products of metabolism away from the cells to organs such as the lungs and kidneys for excretion from the body.
5. Water is essential for the proper functioning of our senses. Hearing waves are transmitted by fluid in the inner ear. Fluid in the eye is involved in the reflection of light for proper vision. For the taste and smelling senses to function, the foods and odors must be dissolved in water.
6. Of primary importance to the active individual is the role that water plays in the regulation of body temperature. Water is the major constituent of sweat, and through its evaporation from the surface of the skin, it can help dissipate excess body heat. Of all the nutrients, water is the most important to the physically active person and is one of several that may have

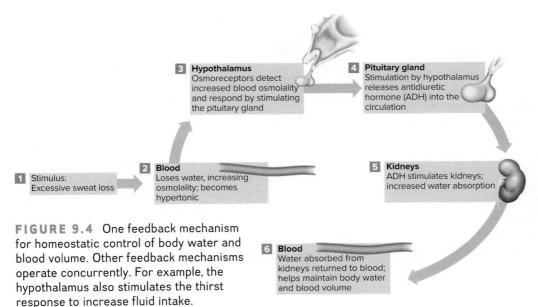

3 Hypothalamus
Osmoreceptors detect increased blood osmolality and respond by stimulating the pituitary gland

4 Pituitary gland
Stimulation by hypothalamus releases antidiuretic hormone (ADH) into the circulation

1 Stimulus:
Excessive sweat loss

2 Blood
Loses water, increasing osmolality; becomes hypertonic

5 Kidneys
ADH stimulates kidneys; increased water absorption

6 Blood
Water absorbed from kidneys returned to blood; helps maintain body water and blood volume

FIGURE 9.4 One feedback mechanism for homeostatic control of body water and blood volume. Other feedback mechanisms operate concurrently. For example, the hypothalamus also stimulates the thirst response to increase fluid intake.

beneficial effects on performance when used in supplemental amounts before or during exercise. Hence, the athletic individual should know what is necessary to help maintain proper fluid balance, a topic covered in detail later in this chapter.

Can drinking more water or fluids confer any health benefits?

Although the major functions of water have been long known, nutrition scientists now theorize that drinking enough water may have specific health benefits. In their review of available literature, Lotan and others suggest that low fluid intake may be associated with urinary system diseases. Drewnowski and colleagues reported plain water accounts for only 30–37 percent of total dietary water of U.S. adults. Coffee, tea, and other beverages contributing to total water intake may also have potential positive or negative effects on health. Caffeine will be discussed in chapter 13. The Consumers Union indicated a similar relationship between water intake and colon cancer. Theoretically, increased water intake could flush carcinogens from the urinary tract and colon. Some dietitians indicated that increased water intake may help one reduce excess fat in a weight-control program by increasing the sensation of fullness and suppressing hunger. Research suggests that this may be the case: de Castro reported that subjects consumed fewer Calories, at least on a short-term basis, when eating foods with high water content; as discussed in chapter 11, high-volume, low-energy foods may be an integral part of a weight-control diet. Other benefits might include less chance of kidney stones, fewer asthma attacks, and better oral health, all of which are attributed to better hydration. Although you can consume water in a variety of beverages, such as juices, soda, or coffee, scientists recommend water itself. It is cheap and Calorie free.

However, most of us do obtain our daily water needs from beverages other than water. Some beverages, such as pure fruit juices, may provide some health benefits associated with their vitamin,

mineral, and phytonutrients content. Other beverages have been suggested to pose health threats, such as alcoholic beverages, which are discussed in chapter 13. In response to a link between overweight and obesity and consumption of high-Calorie beverages, Popkin and other health professionals formed a Beverage Guidance Panel in 2006 to provide guidance to consumers on the relative health and nutritional benefits and risks of various beverage categories. In general, the panel recommends that the consumption of beverages with no or few Calories should take precedence over the consumption of beverages with more Calories and concluded that drinking water was ranked as the preferred beverage to fulfill daily water needs. In their case study of 2000–2010 Coca-Cola and PepsiCo corporate sales in U.S., Brazil, and China markets, Kleiman and others reported a possible shift to lower-Calorie products suggested by increased total revenue and energy per capita but decreased energy density (kjoules per 100 milliliters). This trend was more pronounced in the United States while the total energy per capita increased in the Brazil and China markets. As this issue deals with weight control, additional information will be presented in the next two chapters.

Key Concepts

▶ The average adult, who needs 2 to 3 quarts of water per day, maintains fluid balance primarily by drinking liquids, but substantial amounts of water are also obtained from solid foods in the diet. Caffeine is not as potent a diuretic as once thought, and beverages containing caffeine, such as coffee and cola sodas, may augment daily fluid intake.

▶ Normal water levels in the various body-fluid compartments are maintained by a feedback mechanism involving specific receptors for osmotic pressure, the antidiuretic hormone (ADH), and the kidneys.

▶ Water has a number of functions in the body. One of its most important benefits for people who exercise is the control of body temperature.

▶ Plain water is an effective and inexpensive means to help maintain fluid balance in the body. Some beverages, such as pure fruit juices, may provide healthful nutrients, whereas others, such as alcoholic beverages, may pose a health risk.

Check for Yourself

▶ Use a measuring cup and accurately measure the amount of fluids you drink for a day.

Electrolytes

What is an electrolyte?

An **electrolyte** is defined as a substance that, in solution, conducts an electrical current. The solution itself may be referred to as an electrolyte solution. Acids, bases, and salts are common electrolytes, and they usually dissociate into ions, particles carrying either a positive (cation) or a negative (anion) electrical charge. The major electrolytes in the body fluids are sodium, potassium, chloride, bicarbonate, sulfate, magnesium, and calcium. Electrolytes can act at the cell membrane and generate electrical current, such as in a nerve impulse. Electrolytes can also function in other ways, activating enzymes to control a variety of metabolic activities in the cell. In chapter 8 we covered some of the important metabolic functions of calcium, phosphorus, and magnesium; in this chapter the focus is on sodium, chloride, and potassium because of their presence in sports drinks, popular beverages used to replace fluid losses in physically active people.

The concentration of all elements in the body may be expressed in a variety of ways, such as milligrams per unit volume, millimoles, and milliequivalents. The equivalencies for sodium, chloride, and potassium will be provided, as you may often see these various terms in the literature.

In later sections we shall look at the interaction of these electrolytes with exercise in warm environmental conditions and their role in the etiology of high blood pressure. But first, let us briefly cover the function of each of these electrolytes in the human body.

Sodium (Na)

Sodium is a mineral element also known as natrium, from which the symbol *Na* is derived. It is one of the principal positive ions, or electrolytes, in the body fluids. The gram atomic weight of sodium is 23 grams, so the milligram atomic weight for sodium is 23 milligrams. One millimole of sodium is 23 milligrams, as is 1 milliequivalent. One millimole of sodium chloride (salt) is 58.5 milligrams, as is 1 milliequivalent, containing 23 milligrams of sodium and 35.5 milligrams of chloride.

DRI The National Academy of Sciences (NAS) set an AI for sodium at 1.5 grams (1,500 milligrams) for males and females age 9 to 50, and somewhat lower amounts for young children and older adults. There is no evidence that higher intakes confer any additional health benefits. In fact, a recent study by He and associates documented an association between reduced sodium intake and reduced blood pressure and mortality from stroke and coronary heart disease. However, this AI contains no allowance for large sodium losses through exercise-induced sweating. Common table salt (sodium chloride) is about 40 percent sodium, so only about 3.8 grams (3,800 milligrams) are needed to supply the minimum requirement. The NAS also established a UL at 2.3 grams, or the equivalent of about 5.8 grams of salt. Currently, the amount used as the Daily Value for food labels is 2.4 grams (2,400 milligrams), which is higher than the UL. Keep this in mind when purchasing foods if you are attempting to limit sodium intake. According to the National Health and Nutritional Examination Survey (NHANES) 2007–2010 baseline data for *Healthy People 2020,* the average intake of sodium for all Americans age 2 years and older was 3,586 milligrams daily, or more than twice the recommended amount. Powles and associates estimated average global sodium intake in 2010 as 3,950 milligrams/day.

Food Sources Sodium is distributed widely in nature but is found in rather small amounts in most natural foods. However, significant amounts of salt, and hence sodium, are usually added from the salt shaker for flavor. One teaspoon of salt contains about 2,000 milligrams of sodium. Moreover, processing techniques add significant amounts of salt to the foods we buy. For example, a serving of fresh or frozen green peas contains only 2 milligrams of sodium but increases to 240 milligrams in the canning process. In general, natural foods are low in sodium, whereas processed foods are relatively high.

The Center for Science in the Public Interest has indicated that the FDA is investigating means to lower sodium content in food, and some companies are being proactive and decreasing sodium content. In 2008, the FDA prepared voluntary labeling guidelines for restaurants and other retail establishments to reduce salt intake. For example, canned soups may contain more than 1,300 milligrams of sodium per serving, but some brands are available that contain much less, only 40–60 milligrams of sodium per serving. Nevertheless, most Americans obtain about 75–80 percent of their sodium intake from processed and restaurant foods. Table 9.1 highlights the sodium content in several foods within the major food groups and some restaurant fast foods. Note the difference in sodium content between fresh and processed foods. Checking food labels is the best means to control sodium intake. Food labels must list the sodium content, both in milligrams and in percent of the Daily Value, and may carry claims such as "sodium free" if the product meets certain restrictions (see table 9.2). For a more extensive list of sodium in foods, visit the following U.S. Department of Agriculture Website: www.lmra.org/content/Facility/2/downloads/11-09-USDA-Sodium-Content.pdf

Cooking your own food can help reduce salt intake. With some canned vegetables, draining and rinsing the product with fresh water removes some of the sodium. Herbs and other spices can add flavor and be used to replace salt added to home-prepared meals. Salt substitutes are available, such as Morton Salt Substitute, which is 100 percent sodium free, containing only potassium. Light salts are also available, such as Morton's Lite Salt, that contain less than 50 percent sodium.

Major Functions Sodium is an important element in a number of body functions. As the principal electrolyte in the extracellular fluids, it primarily helps maintain normal body-fluid balance and osmotic pressure. In this regard it is essential in the control of normal blood pressure through its effect on the blood volume. The role of sodium in the etiology of high blood pressure is discussed in a later section.

In conjunction with several other electrolytes, sodium is critical for nerve impulse transmission and muscle contraction. It is also

TABLE 9.1	Sodium content of common foods	
Food Exchange item	**Amount**	**Sodium (mg)**
Milk		
Low-fat milk	1 c	120
Cottage cheese		
Creamed	1/2 c	320
Unsalted	1/2 c	30
Cheese, American	1 oz	445
Vegetables		
Beans, cooked fresh	1 oz	5
Beans, canned	1 oz	150
Pickles, dill	1 medium	900
Potato, baked	1 medium	6
Fruits		
Banana	1 medium	1
Orange	1 medium	1
Starch		
Bread, whole wheat	1 slice	130
Bran flakes	3/4 c	340
Oatmeal, cooked	1 c	175
Pretzels	1 oz	890
Meat		
Luncheon meats	1 oz	450
Chicken	3 oz	40
Beef, steak	3 oz	70
Tuna, low sodium	3 oz	35
Tuna, in oil	3 oz	800
Fats		
Butter, salted	1 tsp	50
Margarine, salted	1 tsp	50
Canned foods and prepared entrees		
Spaghetti, canned	1 c	1,220
Turkey dinner, frozen	1	1,735
Chicken noodle soup	5 oz	655
Chicken noodle soup, low sodium	5 oz	120
Restaurant fast foods		
Arby's chicken breast fillet sandwich	1	1,220
McDonald's Big Mac	1	1,010
Subway club (6 inches)	1	1,310
Taco Bell bean burrito	1	1,220
Condiments		
Mustard	1 tbsp	195
Tomato catsup	1 tbsp	155
Soy sauce	1 tbsp	1,320

As you can see in this table, the sodium content of foods can vary greatly. In general, canned and processed foods have a much higher sodium content than do fresh foods. Eat fresh meats, fruits, vegetables, and bread products whenever possible and prepare them with little or no salt. Avoid highly salted foods such as pickles, pretzels, and soy sauce. Look for "sodium free" or "low sodium" labels when shopping for canned foods.

Source: U.S. Department of Agriculture. See www.lmra.org/content/Facility/2/downloads/ 11-09-USDA-Sodium-Content.pdf for a more complete listing of sodium in foods.

TABLE 9.2	Nutrition Facts label terms for sodium*
Sodium-Free or Salt-Free Less than 5 milligrams per serving	
Very Low Sodium 35 milligrams or less per serving	
Low Sodium 140 milligrams or less per serving	
Reduced-Sodium or Less Sodium At least 25 percent less than the regular product	
No Salt Added Amount of sodium per serving must be listed	

*Food labels must list the milligrams of sodium and the percent of the Daily Value, which is 2,400 mg.

a component of several compounds, such as sodium bicarbonate, that help maintain normal acid-base balance and, as noted in chapter 13, may be an effective ergogenic aid. An overview of sodium is presented in table 9.3.

Deficiency and Excess Because the maintenance of normal blood pressure is critical to life, and because sodium is critical to maintenance of blood volume and pressure, Geerling and Loewy indicate that humans have developed a sodium appetite, a behavioral drive to ingest salt. The human body has developed an effective regulatory feedback mechanism allowing for a wide range of dietary sodium intake. The hypothalamus helps regulate sodium as well as water balance in the body. If the sodium concentration decreases in the blood, a series of complex reactions leads to the secretion of **aldosterone**, a hormone produced in the adrenal gland, which stimulates the kidneys to retain more sodium. In contrast, excesses of serum sodium will lead to decreased aldosterone secretion and increased excretion of sodium by the kidneys in the urine. Other hormones, notably ADH via its effect on water absorption in the kidneys, help maintain normal sodium equilibrium in the body fluids. During exercise, particularly intense exercise, sodium concentration increases in the blood, which helps to maintain blood volume. Exercise also leads to increased secretion of ADH and aldosterone, which helps conserve body water and sodium supplies.

Because this regulatory mechanism is so effective, deficiency states due to inadequate dietary intake of sodium are not common. Indeed, humans even have a natural appetite for salt, assuring adequate sodium intake and sodium balance over time. Nevertheless, excessive losses of sodium from the body, usually induced by prolonged sweating while exercising in the heat, may lead to short-term deficiencies that may be debilitating to the athletic individual. The importance of sodium in thirst stimulation and complete volume replacement in all water compartments following exercise is described by Stachenfeld in her review. These problems are discussed later in this chapter in the sections on fluid and electrolyte replacement and health aspects.

TABLE 9.3 Major electrolytes: sodium, chloride, and potassium*

Major electrolyte	Adequate intake	Major functions in the body	Deficiency symptoms	Symptoms of excess consumption
Sodium	1,500 milligrams	Primary positive ion in extracellular fluid; nerve impulse conduction; muscle contraction; acid-base balance; blood volume homeostasis	Hyponatremia; muscle cramps; nausea; vomiting; loss of appetite; dizziness; seizures; shock; coma	Hypertension (high blood pressure) in susceptible individuals
Chloride	2,300 milligrams	Primary negative ion in extracellular fluid; nerve impulse conduction; hydrochloric acid formation in stomach	Rare; may be caused by excess vomiting and loss of hydrochloric acid; convulsions	Hypertension, in conjunction with excess sodium
Potassium	4,700 milligrams	Primary positive ion in intracellular fluid; same functions as sodium, but intracellular; glucose transport into cell	Hypokalemia; loss of appetite; muscle cramps; apathy; irregular heartbeat	Hyperkalemia; inhibited heart function

*Food sources for sodium and potassium may be found in tables 9.2 and 9.4, respectively; food sources for chloride are similar to those for sodium.

Chloride (Cl)

Chloride is the major negative ion in the extracellular fluids. The gram atomic weight of chloride is 35.5 grams, so the milligram atomic weight for chloride is 35.5 milligrams. One millimole of chloride is 35.5 milligrams, as is 1 milliequivalent.

DRI The chloride AI for individuals age 9–50 is 2.3 grams, or the equivalent of about 3.8 grams of salt. The UL is 3.5 grams, or 5.8 grams of salt. The DV for food label use is 3,500 milligrams, which is the UL.

Food Sources Chloride is distributed in a variety of foods. Its dietary intake is closely associated with that of sodium, notably in the form of common table salt, which is 60 percent chloride.

Major Functions Chloride ions have a variety of functions in the human body. They work with sodium in the regulation of body-water balance and electrical potentials across cell membranes. They also are involved in the formation of hydrochloric acid in the stomach, which is necessary for certain digestive processes.

Deficiency Under normal circumstances chloride deficiency is rather rare. However, because the losses of sodium and chloride in sweat are directly proportional, the symptoms of chloride loss during excessive dehydration through sweating parallel those of sodium loss. The effects of sweat electrolyte losses and replacement on physical performance and health are covered in later sections of this chapter. An overview of chloride is presented in table 9.3.

Potassium (K)

Potassium is a mineral element also known as kalium, from which the symbol K is derived. It is a positive ion. The gram atomic weight of potassium is 39 grams, so the milligram atomic weight for potassium is 39 milligrams. One millimole of potassium is 39 milligrams, as is 1 milliequivalent.

DRI The potassium AI for individuals age 14 and above is 4.7 grams (4,700 milligrams), and somewhat less for children. No UL has been established for potassium from foods. Supplements are not recommended. The DV used for food labels is 3.5 grams, which is less than the AI. American adults take in much less, only about 2,500 milligrams a day.

Food Sources Potassium is found in most foods and is especially abundant in bananas, citrus fruits, fresh vegetables, milk, meat, and fish. Table 9.4 provides some data on the potassium content of several common foods in the major food groups. Additional information on foods with high, moderate, and low potassium content can be found at the United States Department of Agriculture link http://ndb.nal.usda.gov/ndb/nutrients/index and selecting potassium in the first nutrient dropdown window

Major Functions As the major electrolyte inside the body cells, potassium works in close association with sodium and chloride in the maintenance of body fluids and in the generation of electrical impulses in the nerves and the muscles, including the heart muscle. Potassium also plays an important role in the energy processes in the muscle; it helps in the transport of glucose into the muscle cells, the storage of glycogen, and the production of high-energy compounds.

Deficiency and Excess Potassium balance, like sodium balance, is regulated by aldosterone but in a reverse way. A high serum potassium level stimulates the release of aldosterone from the adrenal cortex, leading to an increased excretion of potassium by the kidneys into the urine. A decrease in serum potassium levels elicits a drop in aldosterone secretion and hence a greater conservation of potassium by the kidneys. Because a potassium imbalance in the body may have serious health consequences, potassium regulation is quite precise. Deficiencies or excessive accumulation is extremely rare under normal circumstances.

Although potassium deficiencies are rare, they may occur under certain conditions such as during fasting, diarrhea, and the use of diuretics. In such cases **hypokalemia**, or low serum potassium

TABLE 9.4	Potassium content in some common foods in the major Food Exchanges	
Food	**Amount**	**Milligrams of potassium**
Milk		
Skim milk	8 oz glass	410
Yogurt, low-fat	1 c	530
Cheese, cheddar	1 oz	28
Meat		
Chicken breast	1 oz	70
Beef, lean	1 oz	100
Fish, flounder	1 oz	160
Starch		
Bread, whole wheat	1 slice	65
Cereal, Cheerios	1 oz	110
Fruit		
Banana	1 medium	460
Orange	1 avg	260
Apple	1 avg	35
Vegetables		
Potato, baked	1 avg	780
Broccoli	1 stalk	270
Carrot	1 medium	275

Key Concepts

▸ The recommended Adequate Intake (AI) for sodium is 1,500 milligrams. The recommended Upper Limit (UL) for sodium is 2,300 milligrams. However, the Daily Value (DV) for sodium on food labels is 2,400 milligrams, an amount that is greater than the UL. The percentage of the DV for sodium listed on a food label should actually be 60 percent higher, given that the DV is 60 percent greater than the AI.

▸ Sodium and chloride perform vital functions such as generating electrical impulses for contraction of muscles, including the heart. Sodium is also very important in the regulation of blood pressure.

▸ Potassium works with sodium and chloride in the regulation of blood pressure and normal neural functions, and it participates in other metabolic functions such as storage of muscle glycogen.

▸ Sodium, chloride, and potassium concentrations in the body are precisely regulated. Deficiencies or excesses are rare but can and do occur without replacement of daily losses or excessive supplementation, respectively. Electrolyte deficiencies or excess may contribute to serious health problems.

Check for Yourself

▸ Go to the supermarket and compare the cost of a serving of various bottled waters, the sodium content of various brands of soup, and the contents of various sports drinks.

levels, could lead to muscular weakness and even cardiac arrest due to a decreased ability to generate nerve impulses and an irregular heartbeat. Several deaths of individuals on unbalanced liquid-protein fasting diets several years ago were associated with potassium deficiencies.

Excessive body potassium stores also are not very common, occurring mainly in conjunction with several disease states or in individuals who overdose on potassium supplements. **Hyperkalemia**, or excessive potassium in the blood, may disturb electrical impulses, causing cardiac arrhythmias and possible death. Hyperkalemia may result when potassium ingestion overwhelms the aldosterone regulatory system discussed above and in the previous chapter. John and associates reported two case studies of near-fatal hyperkalemia, one from a salt substitute and the other from a muscle-building supplement. More than 18,000 milligrams may cause a heart attack. For this reason, individuals should never take potassium supplements in large doses without the consent of a physician. An overview of potassium is presented in table 9.3.

In theory, a potassium deficiency could adversely affect physical performance capacity. However, given the potential risks associated with excess potassium supplementation, there is very little research evaluating its ergogenic effects. The role of potassium in the etiology of high blood pressure has also been studied. The results of this research are presented in later sections of this chapter.

Regulation of Body Temperature

What is the normal body temperature?

The temperature of different body parts may vary considerably. The skin may be very cold but the body internally is much warmer. When we speak of body temperature, we mean the internal, or **core**, or **temperature**, and not the external shell temperature. **Shell temperature**, which represents the temperature of the skin and the tissues directly under it, varies considerably depending upon the surrounding environmental temperature. A recent review by Sawka, Cheuvront, and Kenefick describes the importance of a wide gradient between core and shell temperature for optimal regulation of body temperature and the adverse effect of dehydration on heat dissipation and performance.

In humans, normal body temperature is approximately 98.6°F (37°C). This core temperature may be measured in a variety of ways. The two most common methods are orally and rectally. For research purposes, a thermocouple is inserted through the nose down into the esophagus to provide a more precise measure of core temperature. Capsules, containing miniature electronic thermometers, may be swallowed and use wireless telemetry to transmit core temperatures during rest or exercise, an excellent means to study temperature responses in athletes during actual sports competition. Normal body temperature at rest varies and may range from 97 to 99°F (36.1 to 37.2°C). At rest, the rectal temperature is normally about 0.5–1.0°F higher than the oral temperature; however, assessing temperature following a road race, one study reported that the rectal temperature was 5.5°F higher than the oral temperature, suggesting that an oral reading may not be an accurate reflection of the true body temperature in an assessment of heat injury. Shell temperatures may be measured by adhesive thermometer pads attached to the skin.

Humans can survive a range of core temperatures for a short time, but optimal physiological functioning usually occurs within a range of 97–104°F (36.1–40.0°C). A variety of factors may affect body temperature. Here we are concerned with the effect exercise has on the core temperature and how the body adjusts to help maintain heat balance.

What are the major factors that influence body temperature?

Humans are warm-blooded animals and are able to maintain a constant body temperature under varying environmental temperatures. To do this, the body must constantly make adjustments to either gain or lose heat.

Approximately 80 percent of metabolism is in the form of thermal (heat) energy. The basal metabolic heat production is provided through normal burning (oxidation) of the three basic foodstuffs in the body—carbohydrate, fat, and protein. A higher basal metabolic rate, infectious diseases, shivering, and exercise are several factors that might increase heat production.

The human body also has a variety of means to lose heat. Heat loss is governed by four physical means—conduction, convection, radiation, and evaporation.

Conduction—heat is transferred from the body by direct physical contact, as when you sit on a cold seat.
Convection—heat is transferred by movement of air or water over the body.
Radiation—heat energy radiates from the body into the surrounding air.
Evaporation—heat is lost from the body when it is used to convert sweat to a vapor, known as the heat of vaporization. Sweating is the body's most important heat loss mechanism during hot weather exercise. The lungs also help to dissipate heat through evaporation.

During rest and under normal environmental temperatures, body heat is transported from the core to the shell by way of conduction and convection, the blood being the main carrier of the heat. The vast majority of the heat escapes from the body by radiation and convection, with a smaller amount being carried away by the evaporation of insensible perspiration. A cooler environment, increased air movement such as a cool wind, increased blood circulation to the skin, or an increased radiation surface would facilitate heat loss.

In contrast, under certain environmental conditions, such as exercising in the sunlight on a hot day, some of these processes may be reversed, with the body gaining heat instead of losing it. For example, radiant energy from the sun could add heat to the body.

The well-known **heat-balance equation** may be used to illustrate these interrelationships:

$$H = M \pm W \pm C \pm R - E$$

where H = heat balance, M = resting metabolic rate, W = work done (exercise), C = conduction and convection, R = radiation, E = evaporation. Note that C and R are means by which the body can either gain or lose heat, while E is a heat loss mechanism.

If any of these factors governing heat production or heat loss is not balanced by an opposite reaction, heat balance will be lost and the body will deviate from its normal value. During exercise, W increases heat production. Hence, compensating adjustments in C, R, and E must be made to dissipate the extra heat. Figure 9.5 illustrates heat stress factors and mechanisms of heat loss during exercise.

How does the body regulate its own temperature?

Body temperature is controlled by the autonomic division of the central nervous system. The hypothalamus is an important structure in the brain that is involved in the control of a wide variety of physiological functions, including body temperature. The hypothalamus is thought to function pretty much as the thermostat does in your house. If your house gets too cold, the heat comes on; if it gets too warm, the air conditioning system starts. The human body makes similar adjustments.

The temperature-regulating center in the hypothalamus receives input from several sources. First, receptors in the skin can detect temperature changes and send impulses to the hypothalamus. Second, the temperature of the blood can directly affect the hypothalamus as it flows through that structure.

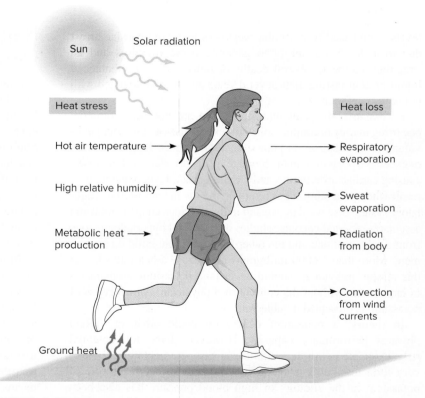

FIGURE 9.5 Sources of heat gain and heat loss to the body during exercise. See text for details.

In general, if the skin receptors detect a warmer temperature or the blood temperature rises, the body will make adjustments in an attempt to lose heat. Two major adjustments may occur. First, the blood will be channeled closer to the skin so that the heat from within may get closer to the outside and radiate away more easily. Second, sweating will begin and evaporation of the sweat will carry heat away from the body.

If the skin receptors detect a colder temperature or the blood temperature is lowered, then the body will react to conserve heat or increase heat production. First, the blood will be shunted away from the skin to the central core of the body. This decreases heat loss by radiation and helps keep the vital organs at the proper temperature. Second, shivering may begin. Shivering is nothing more than the contraction of muscles, which produces extra heat by increasing the metabolic rate. Thermoregulatory feedback loops are illustrated in figure 9.4. Figure 9.6 is a simplified schematic of body temperature control.

The hypothalamus is usually very effective in controlling body temperature. However, certain conditions may threaten temperature control. For example, an individual who falls into cold water will lose body heat rapidly, for water is an excellent conductor of heat. Such a situation may lead to **hypothermia** (low body temperature) and a rapid loss of temperature control. Hypothermia may also develop in slower runners during the latter part of a road race under cold, wet, and windy environmental conditions, when heat is lost more rapidly than it is produced through exercise. Muscular incoordination and mental confusion are early signs of hypothermia.

On the other hand, the most prevalent threat to the athletic individual is **hyperthermia**, or the increased body temperature that occurs with exercise in a warm or hot environment. Hyperthermia is one of the major factors limiting physical performance and one of the most dangerous.

What environmental conditions may predispose an athletic individual to hyperthermia?

Four environmental factors interact to determine the heat stress imposed on an active individual:

1. Air temperature. Caution should be advised when the air temperature is 80°F (27°C) or above. However, if the relative humidity and solar radiation are high, lower air temperatures, even 70°F, may pose a risk of heat stress during exercise.
2. Relative humidity. Evaporation of sweat is the body's main cooling system during exercise. As the water content in the air increases, the relative humidity rises, which impairs the ability of sweat on the skin to vaporize and cool the body. Baker and Kenney note that with a high relative humidity, 70 percent and above, sweat evaporation is decreased. With humidity levels from 90 to 100 percent, heat loss via evaporation nears

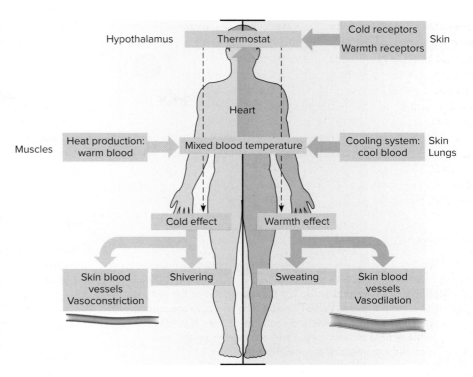

FIGURE 9.6 Simplified schematic of body temperature control. The temperature of the blood returning from the muscles and the skin stimulates the temperature regulation center (thermostat) in the hypothalamus, as do nerve impulses from the warmth and cold receptors in the skin. An overall cold effect will elicit a constriction of the blood vessels near the body surface and muscular shivering, thus helping to conserve body heat. An overall warmth effect will elicit a dilation of blood vessels near the skin and sweating, thus increasing the loss of body heat.

zero. Some note that caution should be used when the relative humidity exceeds 50–60 percent, especially when accompanied by warmer temperatures.

3. Air movement. Still air limits heat carried away by convection. Even a small breeze may help keep body temperature near normal by moving heat away from the skin surface.
4. Radiation. Radiant heat from the sun may create an additional heat load.

Some useful guidelines have been developed taking these four factors into consideration. The wet-bulb globe temperature (WBGT) thermometer, illustrated in figure 9.7, measures all four. Small hand-held WBGT thermometers are available. The dry-bulb thermometer (DB) measures air temperature, the globe thermometer (G) measures radiant heat, and the wet-bulb thermometer (WB) evaluates relative humidity and air movement as they influence air temperature. The **WBGT index** is computed as follows:

$$\text{WBGT index} = 0.7 \text{ WB} + 0.2 \text{ G} + 0.1 \text{ DB}$$

For example, if the WB reads 70, the G is 100, and the DB is 80, then the WBGT = $(0.7 \times 70) + (0.2 \times 100) + (0.1 \times 80) = 77°F$. It is important to note that 70 percent of the heat stress is associated with the effects of humidity to decrease heat loss from the body.

Another indicator of heat stress is the **heat index** (figure 9.8), which combines the air temperature and relative humidity to determine the apparent temperature, or how hot it feels. Figure 9.8

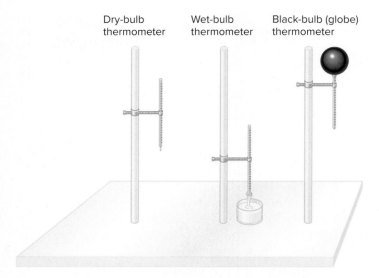

FIGURE 9.7 A typical setup for measurement of the wet-bulb globe temperature (WBGT) index. The dry bulb measures air temperature, the wet bulb indirectly measures humidity, and the black bulb measures the radiant heat from the sun. Computerized commercial devices that measure the WBGT rapidly are also available.

Dry-bulb thermometer   Wet-bulb thermometer   Black-bulb (globe) thermometer

also contains some temperature levels predisposing to heat disorders based on the heat index. Other models incorporate physiological variables of interest to assess heat stress. For example, the Predicted Heat Strain model incorporates core temperature, skin temperature, and sweat rate and may take into consideration the effect of movement and clothing.

The American College of Sports Medicine (ACSM) has published a position statement with guidelines for the prevention of heat illness during distance exercise training and competition. These guidelines are incorporated into the last section of this chapter.

How does exercise affect body temperature?

As noted in chapter 3, exercise increases the metabolic rate and the production of energy. Under a normal mechanical efficiency ratio of 20–25 percent, the remaining 75–80 percent of energy is released as heat. The total amount of heat produced in the body depends on the intensity and duration of the exercise. A more intense exercise will produce heat faster, while the longer the exercise lasts, the more total heat is produced.

Specific heat is defined as the heat in Calories required to raise the temperature of 1 kilogram of a substance by 1 degree Celsius. As a hypothetical example, consider the following 70-kg

Heat index

Relative humidity (%)	70°	75°	80°	85°	90°	95°	100°	105°	110°
100	72°	80°	91°	108°					
90	71°	79°	88°	102°	122°				
80	71°	78°	86°	97°	113°	136°			
70	70°	77°	85°	93°	106°	124°	144°		
60	69°	76°	82°	90°	100°	114°	132°	149°	
50	70°	75°	81°	88°	96°	107°	120°	135°	150°
40	68°	74°	79°	86°	93°	101°	110°	123°	137°
30	67°	73°	78°	84°	90°	96°	104°	113°	123°
20	66°	72°	77°	82°	87°	93°	99°	105°	112°
10	65°	70°	75°	80°	85°	90°	95°	100°	105°
0	64°	69°	73°	78°	83°	87°	91°	95°	99°

Air temperature (°F)

Heat index	Heat disorders possible with prolonged exposure and/or physical activity
80° – 89°	Fatigue
90° – 104°	Sunstroke, heat cramps, and heat exhaustion
105° – 129°	Sunstroke, heat cramps, or heat exhaustion likely and heat stroke possible
130° or higher	Heat stroke/sunstroke highly likely

NOTE: Direct sunshine increases the heat index by up to 15°F.

FIGURE 9.8 Possible heat disorders in runners and other high-risk groups based on the heat index (air temperature and relative humidity versus apparent temperature).

(154-lb) runner. At rest, he expends approximately 80 Calories per hour. Eighty percent of these Calories, or 64 Calories (80 × 0.8) are released as heat. The specific heat (heat storage or capacitance) would be 58 Calories/hr (0.83 × 70). If there were no way to dissipate metabolic heat, his resting body temperature would increase by 1.1°C (or 2°F, 64 Calories ÷ 58 Calories = 1.1°C). Thus, if no heat is lost, body temperature would increase to 38.1°C (100.6°F).

Our runner expends 900 Calories during a 7.5-mile training run in 1 hour. Eighty percent of these Calories, or 720 Calories, are released as heat. As calculated above, the storage of 58 Calories would raise body temperature by 1°C, but this run would increase his body temperature by 12.4°C (22°F) if the heat were not dissipated (720 Calories ÷ 58 Calories = 12.4°C). A body temperature of 49.4°C (120°F) is fatal. Although the core temperature does rise during exercise, it rarely hits these extreme levels. The average core temperature during exercise, even during moderately warm temperatures, may reach about 102.2–104.0°F (39–40°C). This is because of the body's cooling system.

How is body heat dissipated during exercise?

During exercise in a cold or cool environment, body heat is lost mainly through radiation and convection via the air movement around the body. Some evaporation of sweat and evaporative heat loss from the lungs may also contribute to maintenance of heat balance.

However, when the environmental temperature rises, the evaporation of sweat becomes the main means of controlling an excessive rise in the core temperature. For example, evaporation of sweat may account for about 20 percent of total heat loss when exercising in an ambient temperature of 50°F (10°C) but increases to about 45 percent at 68°F (20°C) and 70 percent at 86°F (30°C). Although variable, the maximal evaporation rate is about 30 milliliters of sweat per minute, or 1.8 liters per hour. However, greater sweat rates may occur when sweat drops off the skin without vaporizing. Only sweat that evaporates has a cooling effect. One liter of sweat, if perfectly evaporated, will dissipate about 580 Calories of heat. In the previous example, the evaporation of 1.24 liters of sweat (720/580) would prevent a dangerous rise in the core temperature. However, the evaporation of sweat from the body is not perfect, as sweat can drip off the body and not carry away body heat, so more than 1.24 liters may be lost. If we assume that 2.0 liters were lost, then this individual would have lost 4.4 lbs of body fluids during the 1-hour run; 1 liter of sweat weighs 1 kg, or 2.2 lbs. It should be noted that sweat rates may vary considerably between individuals. Ron Maughan, an environmental physiologist from England, studied two marathoners who completed a race in the same time and had the same fluid intake; one lost only 1 percent of his body weight, while the other lost 6 percent.

Under most warm environmental circumstances, the evaporative mechanisms and the body's natural warning signals are able to keep the core temperature during exercise below 104°F (40°C) and prevent heat injuries. However, an excessive rise in the core temperature, above 104°F, or excessive fluid and electrolyte losses may lead to diminished performance or serious thermal injury in some individuals. Heat illnesses will be discussed in the last section of this chapter.

Key Concepts

▶ Our core temperature is about 98.6°F (37°C). One degree Celsius (C) equals 1.8 degrees Fahrenheit (F). The freezing points of F and C, respectively, are 32° and 0°. Convert C to F by the formula [(C × 1.8°) + 32°]. Convert F to C by the formula [(F − 32°)/1.8°].

▶ Humans are heat producers and their body temperature, regulated by the brain's hypothalamus, is dependent upon the amount of heat they produce and how much they gain or lose from the environment.

▶ High environmental temperatures, high relative humidity, or radiant heat from the sun can impose a severe heat stress on those who exercise under such conditions.

▶ Exercise can produce significant amounts of heat, but the body temperature usually can be regulated quite effectively by activation of heat-loss mechanisms. Body heat is lost mainly by radiation, conduction, and convection, but evaporation of sweat is a major avenue of heat loss during exercise in the heat.

Check for Yourself

▶ Calculate how much heat you would generate if you ran for 60 minutes. Assume that you were running at 20 percent mechanical efficiency. How much sweat would you have to evaporate to keep your body temperature at the same level? Assume that you do not lose any heat from other avenues such as radiation and convection.

Exercise Performance in the Heat: Effect of Environmental Temperature and Fluid and Electrolyte Losses

Athletes train and compete in all types of weather conditions, as do many individuals who exercise for fitness and health. Not all types of physical performance are impaired when performed under warm or hot environmental conditions, but some are. In their recent review, Cheuvront and Kennefick commented that a dehydration threshold of >2 percent is supported by the literature for impaired aerobic performance, but no such criterion or mechanism exists for dehydration-related impaired performance in strength, power, and speed events. The major concern is performance in prolonged exercise and whether or not the core body temperature is maintained. Sawka and Young noted that with **compensated heat stress**, a condition in which heat loss balances heat production, a set body temperature is maintained and the individuals can continue to exercise. In contrast, if heat loss is insufficient to offset heat production, a condition known as **uncompensated heat stress**, the body temperature continues to rise and exhaustion eventually occurs. Sawka and others point out that impaired aerobic performance during exercise in the heat is due to dehydration and the resulting inability to maintain a significant core-skin temperature gradient to dissipate body heat. Environmental heat stress itself may contribute to impaired performance, but so can fluid and electrolyte losses over time.

How does environmental heat affect physical performance?

Performance in more prolonged aerobic endurance activities is normally worse when compared to performance in cooler temperatures. In their respective reviews, Marino, Febbraio, Hargreaves and Febbraio, and Maughan noted that the cause of fatigue during prolonged exercise in the heat has not been clearly established, but changes in brain function, blood circulation, skeletal muscle function, hyperthermia, and dehydration, either separately or collectively, could impair performance. Much of the research evaluating the effect of heat on endurance performance has been conducted with runners. In this regard, McCann and Adams reported a significant linear relationship between the WBGT and decreased performance in endurance events such as the 10,000-meter run. Montain and others analyzed data of elite runners from 140 race-years of major marathons and found that as environmental temperature increased, so did finishing times. Slower runners suffered even greater performance decrements in warmer weather. In general, Sawka and Young note that marathon running performance declines by about 1 minute for each 1°C increase in air temperature beyond 8–15°C (each 1.8°F increase in air temperature beyond 46–59°F).

Environmental heat may affect exercise performance in various ways:

- Central neural fatigue caused by increased brain temperature
- Cardiovascular strain caused by changes in blood circulation
- Muscle metabolism changes caused by increased muscle temperature
- Dehydration caused by excessive sweat losses

Central Neural Fatigue   The brain appears to play an important role in the development of fatigue during exercise in the heat. Cheung and Sleivert suggest that fatigue occurs when the brain reaches a critical core temperature. In his latest review on heat stress and central nervous system (CNS) fatigue, Nybo indicated that the main factor adversely affecting muscle tissue activation appears to be elevated brain temperature. Subjects exercising in the heat seem to reach the point of voluntary fatigue at similar and consistent core body temperatures despite various experimental manipulations. In essence, the elevated brain temperature impairs central arousal of voluntary activation of muscle. In his review, Marino compares two neuroprotective mechanisms of CNS protection during exercise in the heat. The key feature of the "critical limiting temperature" mechanism is a decrease in voluntary activation of exercising muscles due to elevated brain temperature, leading to termination of exercise. The "selective brain cooling" mechanism features countercurrent heat exchange between blood entering and leaving the brain as a means to attenuate brain temperature during hot weather exercise. Although environmental heat normally does not affect muscle power production, Tucker and others reported reductions in both neuromuscular stimulation

and power output during exercise in the heat before there was any abnormal increase in rectal temperature, heart rate, or perception of effort. In other words, the brain apparently anticipates heat stress and reduces heat production (by decreasing muscle contraction) accordingly. Theoretically, this may be the reason Drust and others reported a decrease in mean power output during five 15-second maximal cycle ergometer sprints when exercising in the heat as compared to exercising in normal temperature. These investigators note that an elevated muscle temperature normally is expected to improve sprint performance. In contrast, Périard and colleagues found no difference in 20-sec maximal voluntary contraction activation and force production following 40-km time trials under cool and hot conditions, despite a significantly greater rectal temperature in the hot condition. Central fatigue is discussed in more detail in chapter 3.

Cardiovascular Strain   Cheung and Sleivert noted that other factors may also inhibit performance in the heat, such as high levels of cardiovascular strain. For example, in a 5-kilometer race the runner will be performing at a rather high metabolic rate and thus will be producing heat rapidly. To prevent hyperthermia, blood flow to the skin will increase so as to dissipate heat to the environment. This shifting of blood to the skin will result in a smaller proportion of blood, and hence oxygen, being delivered to the active musculature. As illustrated in figure 9.9, decreased plasma volume from sweating will decrease central blood volume. The inability of increased heart rate to offset decreases in diastolic filling and stroke volume will ultimately result in decreased cardiac output and delivery of oxygen to exercising muscle. Young found that under these conditions cellular metabolism changes somewhat, with greater accumulation of lactic acid if the athlete attempts to maintain the pace normally done in a cooler environment. Yaspelkis and others reported similar lactate findings but found no increase in muscle glycogen utilization. They speculated that the increased lactic acid could be associated with decreased clearance by the liver. Nevertheless, increased lactic acid could be associated with a greater sensation of stress. In some individuals, the circulatory adjustments may not be adequate and the body temperature will rise rapidly, leading to hyperthermia and symptoms of weakness. Because of these changes, and possibly others not yet identified, the runner normally must slow the pace.

Muscle Metabolism   In two reviews, Febbraio indicated that exercise in the heat may adversely affect muscle metabolism with possible reduction in physical performance. He indicated that exercising in the heat appears to shift energy metabolism toward increased carbohydrate use and decreased fat use. In particular, muscle glycogen use is accelerated, possibly due to an augmented sympatho-adrenal response and intramuscular temperature increases. A more rapid depletion of muscle glycogen could impair prolonged endurance performance. Depletion of muscle glycogen as a cause of fatigue is discussed in chapter 4. The loss of intracellular water due to dehydration stimulates glycogenolysis. Regulation of intracellular volume is critical to homeostasis. As discussed by Lang, increases in the concentration of intracellular molecules such as glucose-6-phosphate (a metabolite in

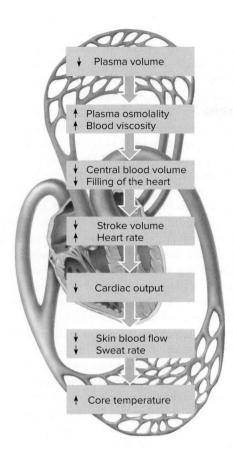

FIGURE 9.9 Some physiological effects of dehydration. The decreased blood volume and increased core temperature may contribute to premature fatigue and heat illness.

Within the figure:
- ↓ Plasma volume
- ↑ Plasma osmolality / ↑ Blood viscosity
- ↓ Central blood volume / ↓ Filling of the heart
- ↓ Stroke volume / ↑ Heart rate
- ↓ Cardiac output
- ↓ Skin blood flow / ↓ Sweat rate
- ↑ Core temperature

glycogenolysis) is an attempt to attract water into the cell (see figure 9.3). Febbraio also indicated that increased intramuscular temperature may in some way lead to dysfunction of skeletal muscle contraction, which could decrease performance capacity. Supportive of this viewpoint is the review by Marino, who notes that precooling the body prior to exercise, such as by taking a cold shower or bath to lower the body temperature, may be beneficial for endurance exercise tasks up to 30–40 minutes. Body cooling techniques as an ergogenic aid are discussed later in this chapter.

Dehydration   Dehydration may also impair exercise performance. In their review, Cheuvront and Kenefick report a dehydration threshold of 2 percent for impaired endurance exercise performance due to volume loss. Although the 5-kilometer runner will sweat heavily, the duration of the event is usually short, so an excessive loss of body fluids does not occur. However, in more prolonged events, athletes may suffer the problems noted previously plus the adverse effects of dehydration. Marathoners may lose 5 percent or more of their body weight (mostly water) during a race, which may not only deteriorate performance but have serious health consequences as well. Goulet recommends fluid intake during prolonged (>1 hour) exercise according to the dictates of thirst in order to maintain exercise-induced weight loss at no more than 3 percent.

How do dehydration and hypohydration affect physical performance?

The dehydration literature consists largely of studies conducted under tightly controlled laboratory conditions, but the ultimate application of control of water balance during exercise is in the field (i.e., the actual practices of athletes in training and in competition). In her review, Stachenfeld notes that field research provides fundamental questions to be examined in the laboratory. The effect of dehydration on physical performance has been studied from two different viewpoints. Voluntary dehydration is often used by athletes such as wrestlers and boxers to qualify for lower weight classes prior to competition. In other athletes, dehydration occurs involuntarily during training or competition as the body attempts to maintain temperature homeostasis. Dehydration leads to hypohydration.

Hypohydration may affect numerous physiological processes that may impair physical performance. In several reviews, Sawka and others noted that hypohydration may lead to decreases in both intracellular and extracellular fluid volumes (particularly blood volume) with associated decreases in stroke volume and cardiac output. Body heat storage may increase by reducing sweating rate and skin blood flow responses. Kenefick and others found that hypohydration induced an earlier onset of the lactate threshold during exercise, an adverse effect relative to aerobic endurance performance. Hypohydration could also lead to electrolyte imbalances in the muscle, with subsequent adverse effects. Despite these well-documented adverse effects on performance, Cheuvront and others, in separate reviews, acknowledge the difficulty in quantitative assessment of dehydration due to volemic and/or osmotic regulatory mechanisms.

Voluntary Dehydration   Voluntary dehydration techniques used by wrestlers have included exercise-induced sweating, thermal-induced sweating such as the use of saunas, diuretics to increase urine losses, and decreased intake of fluids and food.

Much of the research with voluntary dehydration has been conducted with wrestlers. Evaluation criteria have emphasized factors such as strength, power, local muscular endurance, and performance of anaerobic exercise tasks designed to mimic wrestling. In one review, Barr noted that the effects of hypohydration on muscle strength and endurance are not consistent and require further study. Many studies conducted in this area suggest that hypohydration, even up to levels of 8 percent of the body weight, will not affect these physical performance factors in events involving brief, intense muscular effort. For example, Greiwe and others reported that 4 percent reduction in body weight had no effect on isometric muscle strength or endurance. In its position stand on fluid replacement, the ACSM indicated that dehydration of 3–5 percent of body weight does not degrade either anaerobic performance or muscular strength.

In contrast, Schoffstall and others reported that passive dehydration resulting in approximately 1.5 percent loss of body mass adversely affected bench press 1-repetition maximal performance, but these adverse effects seem to be overcome by a 2-hour rest period and water consumption. Judelson and others reported that dehydration by 5 percent significantly decreased total work during four of six sets of a back-squat protocol, but dehydration by 2.5 percent diminished total work in only one set. Neither level of dehydration affected performance in vertical jump height or peak lower-body power. Other studies have reported significant impairments in such tasks with body weight losses of 4 percent or higher. The adverse effects on strength are not consistent, but anaerobic muscular endurance tasks lasting longer than 20–30 seconds have been impaired when subjects were hypohydrated. For example, Montain and others recently reported that a 4 percent decrease in body weight decreased knee-extension endurance by 15 percent. Suggested mechanisms of impairment include loss of potassium from the muscle, higher muscle temperatures during exercise, and decreased central drive, or the ability of the central nervous system to stimulate the musculature. It should also be noted that there is no evidence that hypohydration improves performance in these exercise tasks. Investigators recommend more research.

Involuntary Dehydration Involuntary dehydration is most common during prolonged physical activity. Dehydration may occur during exercise in cold or temperate environments, but the ACSM, in its position stand on fluid replacement, indicated that dehydration (3 percent body weight) has marginal influence on degrading aerobic exercise performance when exercising in colder environments. However, the adverse effects of involuntary dehydration are most severe on aerobic endurance performance when exercising in warm, humid environmental conditions. The following represent the major highlights of the ACSM position stand on fluid replacement relative to dehydration and prolonged endurance exercise performance.

- Dehydration increases physiological strain and perceived effort to perform the same exercise task and is accentuated in warm-hot weather.
- Dehydration can degrade aerobic exercise performance, especially in warm-hot weather.
- The greater the dehydration level, the greater the physiological strain and aerobic exercise performance impairment.
- The critical water deficit and magnitude of exercise performance degradation are related to the heat stress, exercise task, and the individual's unique biological characteristics.

In several major reviews, Michael Sawka, Kent Pandolf, and John Greenleaf have suggested that the deterioration in aerobic endurance performance appears to be related to adverse effects on cardiovascular functions and temperature regulation. Reduction in the plasma volume may reduce cardiac output and blood flow to the skin and the muscles. Reductions in skin blood flow have been shown to lower the sweat rate and raise the core temperature. In his review, Coyle reported some of the effects of dehydration in endurance-trained cyclists. In general, he reported that skin blood flow decreased with dehydration and that the greater the level of dehydration, the greater the rise in the core temperature and heart rate and the greater the decrease in the stroke volume (amount of blood pumped by the heart per beat). In a meta-analysis of

literature including a cycling time-trial performance, Goulet reported no difference in performance between euhydration and up to 4 percent dehydration. Furthermore, optimal time-trial performance was related to reliance on thirst for fluid replacement, a notion espoused by Noakes. Montain and others noted that hypohydration decreased cardiac output, and the greater the intensity of the exercise, the greater the decrease. The effects of dehydration on cardiovascular dynamics are depicted in figure 9.9.

One of the key points of the ACSM position stand is the effect an individual's unique biological characteristics and the exercise task may play regarding hydration status and exercise performance, and some research suggests that highly trained endurance runners may be able to better tolerate some, but not all, of the adverse effects of dehydration. In an article on marathon runners, Noakes contends that there is no evidence that athletes who drink according to thirst are at any significant disadvantage from the 3–5 percent level of dehydration that they may develop. In support of this viewpoint, Armstrong and others found that dehydration up to 5.7 percent had no adverse effect on running economy in highly trained collegiate distance runners during 10 minutes of running at 70 or 85 percent VO_2 max. Further, Byrne and others suggested that the effects of body weight loss (used as the measure for dehydration via sweat loss) on temperature regulation may vary in actual outdoor race competition under warm conditions, as compared to controlled laboratory conditions. They reported that core temperature after running a half-marathon was not affected by level of dehydration, which ranged from 1.62 to 4.0 liters in 18 nonelite runners. However, the authors did not appear to evaluate the effect of weight loss on performance time, as they had no measures of running speed during the race. Although, as noted previously, Armstrong and others reported that dehydration did not affect running economy, but did result in increased heart rate and rectal temperature, concurrent with reduced stroke volume and cardiac output. Over time, these physiological responses would lead to impaired performance. As noted previously, there is a strong relationship between higher environmental temperatures and slower running times in elite and slower runners. As one champion commented years ago at the start of the Olympic marathon on a hot day, "Men, today we die a little."

The ACSM also noted that dehydration might degrade mental/cognitive performance, which may be caused by adverse effects of hyperthermia on mental processes. In several reports, Baker and others reported that dehydration may impair vigilance in dynamic sports environments, such as basketball, leading to increased errors of omission and commission and impaired reaction time. In one study, skilled basketball players were dehydrated by 1, 2, 3, and 4 percent prior to taking a test mimicking basketball skills in a fast-paced game. The players experienced a progressive deterioration in performance as dehydration progressed from 1 to 4 percent, but performance was not significantly impaired until dehydration reached 2 percent. Dougherty and others also reported impaired basketball skill performance, including sprint times and shooting percentage, in young (12–15 years), skilled basketball players who were dehydrated by 2 percent prior to a simulated

48-minute basketball game. Edwards and colleagues studied the impact of dehydration on sport-specific activities in male soccer players. The athletes performed the protocol in a random order with no fluid intake, fluid intake, and a mouth rinse. The protocol included 45 minutes of pre-match cycling, a 45-minute soccer match, followed by a sport-specific test (Yo-Yo Intermittent Recovery Test) and a mental concentration test. After the soccer match, body mass was reduced by 2.14 percent in the mouth-rinse trial, 2.4 percent in the no-fluid trial, and only 0.7% in the fluid trial. Although dehydration had no impact on the mental concentration tests, sport-specific performance was decreased by 13–15 percent when fluid was not ingested. Adan reported that 2 percent dehydration adversely affects attention, psychomotor skills, and immediate memory, but not long-term/working memory and executive functions. Cheuvront and Kennedick comment that impaired cognition as related to dehydration is relatively small, primarily related to discomfort, and is task dependent. Additional research would appear to be warranted to explore the effects of dehydration on other mental aspects of sports performance.

Dehydration may also be a major factor in the onset of gastrointestinal (GI) distress, according to Rehrer and her associates. GI symptoms include nausea, vomiting, bloating, GI cramps, flatulence, diarrhea, and GI bleeding, many of which could impair performance if severe enough. In their review, de Oliveira and others reported that 30 to 50 percent of athletes experience gastrointestinal distress that is physiological, mechanical, and/or nutritional in nature and that our understanding of the underlying etiology and efficacy of possible intervention strategies is far from complete.

The ACSM indicated that dehydration is also a risk factor for various heat illnesses, which are covered in a later section of this chapter.

How fast may an individual dehydrate while exercising?

In his review, Mack indicated that sweat rates as high as 3–4 liters per hour, or a loss of about 6.5 to 9.0 pounds, have been reported. Most athletes may lose somewhat less, maybe 2–3 liters, when exercising strenuously in the heat, but even then it will not take long to incur a 2–3 percent decrease in body weight. Two liters of sweat is the equivalent of 4.4 pounds (1 liter = 1 kg = 2.2 pounds), so a 150-pound runner could experience a loss of 3 percent body weight in 1 hour (4.4/150 = 0.03; 0.03 × 100 = 3 percent), which could cause premature fatigue. Research has shown that some athletes, such as football players, may lose up to 10 kg (22 pounds) over a day with multiple daily workouts. Training intensity also plays a role in rate of dehydration. Duffield and colleagues reported greater sweat rates and electrolyte losses in professional male soccer players following "high-intensity" and "game simulation" conditions compared to "low-intensity" conditions. They concluded that individualized rehydration strategies should be employed based on training intensity and other factors. Eijsvogels and colleagues reported lower fluid intake, higher fluid losses, and higher blood sodium levels in males compared to females in response to prolonged exercise of the same duration and intensity.

There may be some gender and age differences in sweating. Smith and Havenith reported greater regional and gross sweat rates of aerobically trained males compared to females at both 60 and 75 percent of VO_2 max. Meyer and Bar-Or indicate that while children may sweat somewhat less than adults, they still may reach hypohydration levels comparable to adults. Young tennis players may lose 1–2 liters of sweat per hour in tournament play, and some older adolescents as much as 3 liters per hour. Excessive dehydration may impair not only one's physical performance but possibly also one's health, as discussed later in this chapter.

How can I determine my sweat rate?

The rate of sweating varies among different individuals, so some may be more prone to dehydration than others. As Cheuvront and others state, dehydration can be difficult to assess and the average individual will not have access to clinical markers such as plasma and urine osmolality and indicator dilution techniques to measure volumes of different water compartments. Nevertheless, Cheuvront and Sawka indicated that there are a number of methods to evaluate your sweat loss and hydration status, but body weight change is reliable and easy to do. However, Maughan and others note that although sweat rate and hydration status are often estimated from body weight loss, several sources of error may give rise to misleading results. For example, respiratory water losses can be substantial during hard work in dry environments and body mass loss also results from substrate oxidation, such as fat. Additionally, water produced as a by-product of oxidation, and possible water released from muscle glycogen, may add to the body-water pool. Mack notes that burning 100 grams of glycogen per hour could liberate about 0.3 to 0.4 liter of water into the total body-water pool. Other factors may also be involved so that an individual may lose body weight but maintain total body water. Nevertheless, although body weight loss may not always be a reliable marker of changes in hydration status, when adjusted for fluid intake and urine losses, Cheuvront and Sawka indicate that it is primarily a function of sweat losses. Urine is darker in the dehydrated state. Another test of possible volume depletion as described by Cheuvront and others is a simple 20+ beats/min increase in heart rate from the sitting to the standing position.

The Gatorade Sports Science Institute has presented a method to calculate the sweat rate during exercise. To do so, one must accurately measure body weight before and after exercise, measure the amount of fluid consumed during exercise, and measure the amount of urine excreted, if any, during exercise. You may use the following examples as a guide to calculate your own sweat rate during exercise (see the Application Exercise at the end of this chapter). The sweat rate for athlete A is calculated in the metric measurement system and for athlete B in the English system. Remember, 1 gram equals about 1 milliliter, and 1 pound equals 16 ounces.

	Athlete A	Athlete B
A. Body weight before exercise	70.5 kg	180 lbs
B. Body weight after exercise	68.9 kg	174 lbs
C. Change in body weight	−1.6 kg	−6 lbs
	1,600 g	96 oz
D. Drink volume	+300 mL	16 oz
E. Urine volume	−100 mL	0 oz
F. Sweat loss (C + D − E)	1,800 mL	112 oz
G. Exercise time	60 min	90 min
H. Sweat rate (F ÷ G)	30 mL/min	1.25 oz/min

What is the composition of sweat?

The human body contains two different types of sweat glands. Apocrine sweat glands, located in hairy areas of the body such as the armpits, secrete an oily mixture to decrease friction and are the source of odor associated with sweating. Eccrine sweat glands, about 2–3 million over the surface of the body, are primarily involved in temperature regulation.

Sweat is mostly water (about 99 percent), but a number of major electrolytes and other nutrients may be found in varying amounts. Sweat is hypotonic in comparison to the fluids in the body. This means that the concentration of electrolytes is lower in sweat than in the body fluids.

The composition of sweat may vary somewhat from individual to individual and will even be different in the same individual when acclimatized to the heat, as contrasted to the unacclimatized state. The major differences are the concentrations of the solid matter in the sweat, the electrolytes or salts. Meyer and colleagues reported higher sweat lactate and ammonia concentrations and lower sweat pH in boys and girls compared to adults following two 20-min bouts of exercise at 50 percent of VO_2 max.

The major electrolytes found in sweat are sodium and chloride, as sweat is derived from the extracellular fluids, such as the plasma and intercellular fluids, which are high in these electrolytes. You may actually note the formation of dried salt on your skin or clothing after prolonged sweating. Mack has reported that the concentration of salt in sweat is variable but averages about 55 mEq (3.2 grams) per liter of sweat during exercise with sweat losses of about 1–1.5 liters per hour.

Other minerals lost in small amounts include potassium, magnesium, calcium, iron, copper, and zinc. As noted in chapter 8, certain athletes, especially those who lose large amounts of sweat, may need to increase their dietary intake of certain trace minerals, such as iron and zinc, to replace losses during exercise.

Small quantities of nitrogen (N), amino acids, and some of the water-soluble vitamins also are present in sweat, but these amounts are easily restored by consuming a balanced diet.

Is excessive sweating likely to create an electrolyte deficiency?

There are two ways to look at this question. What happens to electrolyte balance during exercise? And what happens during the recovery period on a day-to-day basis?

The concentration of electrolytes in the blood during exercise with excessive sweating has been studied under laboratory conditions, as well as immediately after endurance events such as the Ironman triathlon and a marathon run. In general, exercise raises the concentration of several electrolytes in the blood. Sodium and potassium concentrations are elevated; the sodium increase may be due to greater body-water loss than sodium loss, so a concentration effect occurs. The potassium may leak from the muscle tissue to the blood, thereby increasing the blood concentration of this ion. Calcium ion concentration remains relatively unchanged during exercise. Magnesium levels usually fall, possibly because the active muscle cells and other tissues need this ion during exercise and it passes from the blood into the tissues. Thus, during acute, prolonged bouts of exercise, even in marathon running, it appears that an electrolyte deficiency will not occur. Meyer and colleagues found increased sodium and chloride and decreased potassium in the sweat of young adult males and females compared to pubescent and prepubescent boys and girls. There were no gender differences between age groups. They concluded that maturation may be a factor in selecting an "optimal" fluid-electrolyte replacement beverage.

This is not to say that electrolyte replacement is not important. As we shall see in the next section, an electrolyte imbalance may occur in the body during extremely prolonged endurance events, such as ultramarathoning and Ironman-type triathlons, if proper fluid replacement techniques are not used. Moreover, what happens during the recovery period after excessive sweating may contribute to an electrolyte deficiency. Prolonged sweating has been shown to decrease the body content of sodium and chloride by 5–7 percent and potassium by about 1 percent. If these electrolytes are not replaced daily, an electrolyte deficiency may occur over time. The next section deals with the need for water and electrolyte replacement.

Key Concepts

▶ Both hyperthermia and dehydration may impair endurance capacity.
▶ Sweat consists mainly of water and some minerals, primarily sodium and chloride. It is hypotonic compared to the body fluids.

Exercise in the Heat: Fluid, Carbohydrate, and Electrolyte Replacement

Evidence-based guidelines for maintaining hydration and electrolyte balance before, during, and following exercise have evolved as the body of literature on fluid and electrolyte replacement has grown in recent years. Earlier (1996) American College of Sports Medicine (ACSM) and International Olympic Committee

(IOC) guidelines were criticized by Noakes because the ACSM recommendation to drink "as much as tolerable" during exercise may contribute to excess fluid intake and hyponatremia (a serious condition to be discussed later in the chapter) and because of the dearth of appropriately controlled, randomized, prospective studies providing the foundation for the IOC recommendations. Updated ACSM guidelines in 2007 represent a synthesis of the best research available, provide recommendations that are considered to be prudent, are more likely to help delay the onset of premature fatigue during prolonged exercise in the heat, may help in the prevention of exercise-associated heat illness, and are less likely to cause other exercise-associated health problems.

Which is most important to replace during exercise in the heat—water, carbohydrate, or electrolytes?

In the 1960s Robert Cade, a scientist-physician working at the University of Florida, developed an oral fluid replacement for athletes that was designed to restore some of the nutrients lost in sweat. This product was eventually marketed as Gatorade (Gator is the nickname for University of Florida athletes) and was the first glucose-electrolyte solution (GES, now referred to as **carbohydrate-electrolyte solutions, or CES**) to appear as a sports drink in the athletic marketplace. The three main ingredients in sports drinks are water, carbohydrates of various sources and concentrations, and electrolytes.

CES were the first commercial fluid-replacement preparations designed to replace both fluid and carbohydrate. Today, Gatorade has many competitors in the CES market. Other than water, the major ingredients in these solutions are carbohydrates, usually in various combinations of glucose, glucose polymers, sucrose, or fructose and some of the major electrolytes. As noted in chapter 4, sports drinks containing multiple carbohydrates, such as glucose, fructose, sucrose, and maltodextrins (glucose polymer), may be a good choice. In a 2014 review, Jeukendrup recommended that carbohydrate intake be individualized based on the intensity and duration of the exercise task and stated that multiple carbohydrates increase intestinal absorption and oxidation. The sugar content ranges from about 5 to 10 percent depending on the brand. The caloric values range from about 6 to 12 Calories per ounce. The major electrolytes include sodium, chloride, potassium, and phosphorus. These ions are found in varying amounts in different brands. Some brands may also include a variety of other substances, including vitamins (B vitamins and C), minerals (calcium and magnesium), amino acids (BCAA), drugs (caffeine), herbals (ginseng), and artificial coloring and flavoring. Do not confuse the standard sports drinks with the newer "Energy," "Sports Energy," or "sports shots" drinks in the marketplace, which contain considerably more carbohydrate and numerous other ingredients. Other beverages that appear to be sports drinks may contain minimal carbohydrate content. Nutrition Facts labels on sports drinks will provide you with the actual content, including source of carbohydrates. The contents of selected ingredients for several CES are presented in table 9.5. The European Food Safety Authority issued a consensus statement on CES efficacy and safety in 2011. As noted in a recent review by Baker and Jeukendrup, fluid-electrolyte replacement is important to individuals dehydrated from diarrheal disease as well as individuals exposed to exercise and/or environmental stress. Therefore, the optimal content of fluid-electrolyte replacement beverages depends on many factors, not the least of which is the reason for fluid and/or electrolyte loss.

Each of the components of CES may be important to the athlete, depending on the circumstances. When dehydration or hyperthermia is the major threat to performance, water replacement is the primary consideration. In prolonged endurance events, where muscle glycogen and blood glucose are the primary energy sources, carbohydrate replacement, as noted in chapter 4, may help improve performance. In very prolonged exercise in the heat with heavy sweat losses, such as ultramarathons, electrolyte replacement may be essential to prevent heat injury. Although the beneficial effects of carbohydrate intake during exercise were covered in chapter 4, the role of carbohydrate as a component of the CES is stressed in this chapter.

The following questions focus on the importance and mechanisms of water, carbohydrate, and electrolyte replacement for the individual incurring sweat losses while exercising under heat stress conditions.

What are some sound guidelines for maintaining water (fluid) balance during exercise?

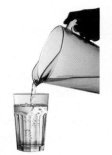

Proper hydration is probably the most important nutritional strategy an athlete can use in training and competition. As compared to hypohydration, adequate hydration will help decrease fluid loss, reduce cardiovascular strain, enhance performance, and prevent some heat illnesses. Athletes have used several strategies to help prevent hypohydration and excessive increases in body temperature associated with certain types of sports competition. Depending on the sport, three commonly used practices are skin wetting, hyperhydration, and rehydration. Another procedure, body cooling, is discussed in the section on ergogenic aids.

Skin Wetting Skin wetting techniques, such as sponging the head and torso with cold water or using a water spray, have been shown to decrease sweat loss. This could be an important consideration in a long run, as body-water supplies may be depleted less rapidly. These techniques also cool the skin and offer an immediate sense of psychological relief from the heat stress, which may help to improve performance. However, skin wetting techniques as they may be used in athletic competition have not been shown to cause any major reductions in core temperature or cardiovascular responses. Bassett and others reported no change in rectal temperature, heart rate, perceived exertion, sweat loss, or plasma volume change following skin wetting in runners completing 120-minute treadmill runs under two humidity conditions. Decreases in skin temperature and skin blood flow were observed, presumably due to vasoconstriction. Some researchers have theorized that skin wetting techniques may be potentially harmful: The psychological sense of relief may encourage athletes to accelerate their pace,

TABLE 9.5 Fluid-replacement and high-carbohydrate* beverage comparison chart per 8-oz serving

Beverage	Carbohydrate ingredient	Carbohydrate (% concentration)	Carbohydrate (grams)	Sodium (mg)	Potassium (mg)
Gatorade Thirst Quencher (Gatorade Company)	Sucrose, glucose, fructose	6	14	110	30
Gatorade Endurance Formula	Sucrose, glucose, fructose	6	14	200	90
Accelerade (Pacific Health Laboratories)	Sucrose, trehalose (disaccharide), fructose	6	14	127	43
PowerAde (The Coca-Cola Company)	High-fructose corn syrup	6	14	100	25
Lucozade Sport (GlaxoSmithKline)	Glucose; maltodextrin	6	15	Trace	Trace
Ultima (Ultima Replenisher)	Maltodextrin	1.5	3	37	75
Cytomax Performance Plus (Cytosport)	alpha-l-polylactate	9	13	55	30
Coca-Cola	High-fructose corn syrup, sucrose	11	27	30	0
Diet soft drinks	None	0	0	0–25	Low
Orange juice (100% juice)	Fructose, sucrose	11	26	0	450
Water	None	0	0	Low	Low
Gatorade Carb Energy Drink (Gatorade Company)	Maltodextrin, glucose, fructose	24	55	147	0

*Compiled from product labels and sources provided by the Gatorade Company; some products are in powdered form to be mixed with water.

increasing heat production without providing for control of the body temperature. If the core temperature increases, heat illness may occur. Although some scientists suggest that skin wetting is not beneficial, many endurance athletes claim that it helps. There is little research on skin wetting. Bassett's study is almost 30 years old. Additional research appears to be warranted.

Hyperhydration Hyperhydration, also known as superhydration, is simply an increase in body fluids by the voluntary ingestion of water or other beverages. It is an attempt to ensure that the body-water level is high before exercising in a hot environment. In a review of hyperhydration strategies, Lamb and Shehata noted that increasing body water above normal by drinking fluids before exercise is likely to improve cardiovascular functions and temperature regulation when it is impossible to ingest sufficient fluids during exercise. Although these effects would appear to help prevent fatigue, Lamb and Shehata also indicated that there was insufficient evidence to support the claim that preexercise hyperhydration improves exercise performance. Sawka and others support this viewpoint, noting that hyperhydration provides no advantages over euhydration regarding thermoregulation and exercise performance in the heat.

However, given hyperhydration's potential benefits, the American College of Sports Medicine recommends that it be used prior to exercise in heat stress environments. Either cold water or a CES may be used to hyperhydrate, although the CES will provide some carbohydrate and sodium that may be helpful. The ACSM guidelines relative to hyperhydration are presented later in this section.

Glycerol supplementation may help retain more water with hyperhydration, an effect that has been theorized to improve endurance performance. The proposed ergogenic effects of glycerol-induced hyperhydration are discussed later in this chapter.

Rehydration Of the various techniques used, research has shown that rehydration is the most effective to enhance performance. Rehydration techniques have been used to replenish fluid loss associated with both voluntary and involuntary dehydration in sports such as wrestling and distance running, respectively.

One laboratory research approach to evaluate the effects of rehydration is related to the sport of wrestling, in which athletes dehydrate to qualify for a weight class and then attempt to rehydrate rapidly prior to competition. In this approach, subjects performed some exercise or mental task, such as a measure of strength, power, anaerobic endurance, or cognitive function, were then dehydrated and tested again, and finally were rehydrated and tested one more time to see if rehydration could improve performance back to the predehydration level. The results of such research are mixed. In some studies, no effect of rehydration was found, probably because as some studies have shown, dehydration may not impair strength, power, or local muscular endurance. Thus, rehydration would not improve performance as measured by these criteria beyond that usually seen in normohydration. However, some studies reported a partial improvement in endurance performance after rehydration, but usually not all the way back to normal. In one study rehydration returned cognitive functions to normal. Because rehydration may bring about performance improvements beyond the dehydrated level, it is therefore recommended for wrestlers when feasible.

A second approach in studying rehydration is to have subjects ingest fluids during prolonged endurance exercise, particularly in warm environments. Rehydration has been shown to minimize the rise in core temperature, to reduce stress on the cardiovascular system by minimizing the decrease in blood volume, and to help maintain an optimal race pace for a longer period. This beneficial effect is usually attributed to decreased dehydration and the maintenance of a better water balance in the blood and other fluid compartments. Rehydration techniques, both with water alone or with CES solutions, have been shown to improve performance in exercise tasks of 1 hour or more in the heat. Although not all studies have shown improved performance with rehydration, Jeukendrup and Martin, in their review of techniques to improve cycling performance, indicate that carbohydrate-electrolyte drinks may decrease 40-kilometer (25-mile) cycling time by 32–42 seconds. Hargreaves and others also reported that water intake may help reduce muscle glycogen use in prolonged exercise, another benefit.

If fluid replacement is to be effective, water has to be absorbed into the circulating blood so that the reduction in blood volume and sweat production that occurs during prolonged endurance exercise will be minimized. Research in which water was labeled with radionuclides showed that water ingested during exercise may appear in plasma and sweat within 10–20 minutes. However, the amount of the ingested fluid that enters the circulation to benefit the athlete depends on two factors: gastric emptying and intestinal absorption.

The ACSM position stand on fluid replacement during exercise focuses mainly on replacing fluid losses during exercise in the heat, and the related recommendations are presented later in this section.

What factors influence gastric emptying and intestinal absorption?

In a later section we will discuss factors, such as palatability, that may influence how much fluid you drink during exercise. For any fluid to be of benefit during exercise, it must first empty from the stomach and then be absorbed into the bloodstream from the intestines.

Gastric Emptying   A number of factors may influence the gastric emptying rate, including volume, solute or caloric density, osmolality, drink temperature, exercise intensity, mode of exercise, and dehydration.

Volume is one of the most important factors affecting gastric emptying. In a review, Gisolfi noted that the larger the volume of fluid ingested, up to approximately 700 milliliters, the greater the rate of gastric emptying. However, large volumes consumed during exercise may cause discomfort to the athlete because of abdominal distention.

Although some preliminary data by Murray and others indicated that an 8 percent CES, as compared to 0, 4, and 6 percent CES, decreased gastric emptying, the decrease was only 6 ounces over 90 minutes. Gant and others compared a CES (6.2 percent) with flavored water during repetitive sprint performance of male soccer players over 60 minutes and reported no differences in gastric emptying. Other studies have shown that CES up to 8 percent carbohydrate had no adverse effect on gastric emptying of fluids, a finding in accord with the ACSM position stand on fluid replacement during exercise. Thus, 6 to 8 percent carbohydrate solutions may provide the athlete with the best of both worlds, water and carbohydrate. However, solutions with higher concentrations, particularly above 10 percent, may impair gastric emptying. The mechanism is not known but may be related to the effects of carbohydrate on osmolality.

Fluids with a higher osmolality generally inhibit gastric emptying. Adding electrolytes and carbohydrates to fluids increases their osmolality, and Gisolfi indicated that this effect may be attributed mostly to the carbohydrate content. Although glucose polymers have less effect on osmolality than glucose, some investigators have observed little difference in gastric emptying of fluids that had marked differences in osmotic pressure created by adding electrolytes, glucose, or glucose polymers. Nevertheless, more recent research has found that some hypotonic glucose polymers emptied from the stomach more rapidly than hypertonic solutions, about 80 percent faster in the first 10 minutes. Rowlands and others reported significantly faster fluid absorption (measured by uptake of deuterium oxide tracer) following consumption of a hypotonic sports drink compared to isotonic and hypertonic sports drinks and a noncaloric control drink in cyclists consuming these drinks (2 liters: 250 mL each 15 minutes) over a over 2-hour period, followed by an incremental test to exhaustion. In general, cold fluids empty rapidly and may help cool the body core. In their meta-analysis, Burdon and colleagues reported increased subject preference for, greater consumption of, and attenuated dehydration following consumption of cold (0–10°C) or cool (10–22°C) beverages compared to warmer beverages.

Moderate exercise intensity facilitates emptying, whereas intense exercise greater than 70–75 percent VO_2 max has been reported to exert an inhibitory effect. Little difference is noted in gastric emptying between cycling and running during the first hour even at an exercise intensity of 75 percent VO_2 max, but some research suggests that more fluids appear to be emptied during the later stages of prolonged cycling.

Ryan and others noted that hypohydration to approximately 3 percent of body weight does not impair gastric emptying. However, excessive dehydration may inhibit gastric emptying and may be associated with gastric discomfort experienced by some athletes who consume large amounts of fluids during prolonged exercise in warm environmental conditions.

Intestinal Absorption Factors affecting intestinal absorption of ingested fluids during exercise have not been studied as extensively as gastric emptying, but several important findings have been presented by key investigators in this area, particularly Carl Gisolfi. Murray and Shi present a detailed review of gastrointestinal system functions during exercise and fluid intake.

Gisolfi indicated that the absorptive capacity of the intestines is not likely to limit the effectiveness of an oral rehydration solution. Water is absorbed fairly readily by passive diffusion, and theoretically water absorption may actually be helped by concurrent absorption of glucose and sodium. As highlighted in figure 9.10(a), glucose and sodium interact in the intestinal wall; glucose stimulates sodium absorption, and sodium is necessary for glucose absorption. When glucose and sodium are absorbed, these solutes tend to pull fluid with them via an osmotic effect, thus facilitating the absorption of water from the intestine into the circulation. However, research by Hargreaves and others noted that beverage sodium content of either 0, 25, or 50 mmol per liter had no effect on plasma glucose levels during exercise. Gisolfi indicated that the intestines themselves contain enough sodium from body fluids, so adding sodium to the rehydration solution

provides no additional benefits. Gisolfi and others also noted no difference in intestinal fluid absorption or plasma volume changes during exercise when consuming either a hypotonic or an isotonic 6 percent carbohydrate beverage with or without sodium. Murray and Shi noted that when compared to a single form of carbohydrate, using multiple, different forms, such as glucose, fructose, and polymers, enhanced intestinal absorption of water. Each form of carbohydrate may have its own receptor for absorption and pull water with it.

However, as discussed in chapter 4, excess carbohydrate in the intestine may cause a reverse osmotic effect, as depicted in figure 9.10(b). Highly concentrated sugars in the intestine draw water from the blood, leading to gastrointestinal distress with symptoms such as abdominal cramping and diarrhea. In her review, Leslie Bonci notes that this may be one of the problems associated with some of the "energy" drinks available, as they may be too highly concentrated with simple sugars. Distance runners have coined the term *runner's trots* to characterize one of the adverse effects.

Whether exercise impairs intestinal absorption is controversial. High-intensity exercise may compromise blood flow to the intestine, which might impair absorption. Gisolfi, in his review, noted

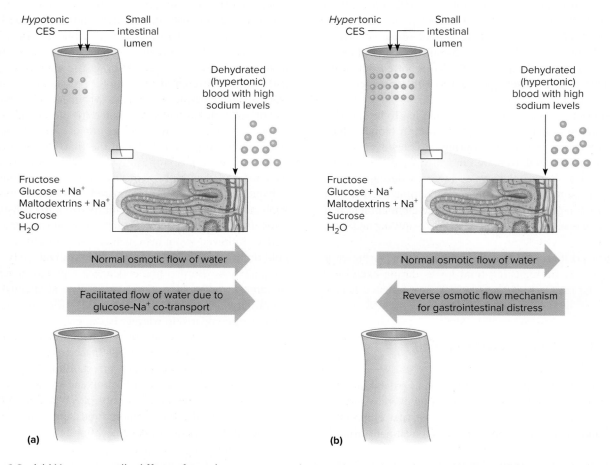

(a)

(b)

FIGURE 9.10 (a) Water normally diffuses from the intestine to the circulation via osmosis. Glucose and sodium in a CES enhance osmosis, as shown by the larger arrow. Rehydration + exogenous CHO absorption = adequate thermoregulation + sustained performance. (b) A hypertonic solution may actually reverse osmosis, moving fluid from the circulatory system to the intestines, possibly leading to gastrointestinal distress symptoms such as diarrhea. Reverse osmosis impairing rehydration + less exogenous CHO absorption = suboptimal thermoregulation + impaired performance.

some of the methodological difficulties in studying this problem, citing studies showing that exercise either reduced or had no effect on intestinal absorption.

It should be noted that individual differences in both gastric emptying and intestinal absorption may be significant. In reviewing studies of gastric emptying, Costill noted some subjects could empty 80–90 percent of the ingested solution in 15–20 minutes, whereas others emptied only 10 percent. As noted previously, some subjects may also develop diarrhea caused by ineffective intestinal absorption of fluids. Training to drink during exercise is recommended as a possible means of enhancing tolerance to consuming larger amounts of fluids. As suggested by Maughan and Meyer, endurance athletes should ingest fluids during training in order to "train" the stomach to handle fluids during competition.

How should carbohydrate be replaced during exercise in the heat?

The value of carbohydrate intake during exercise as a means to improve performance was detailed in chapter 4, primarily in relation to performance in a cool environment. Keep in mind that carbohydrate intake may be useful primarily in prolonged exercise, under conditions where one is exercising at a high level of intensity for an hour or more. Carbohydrate is the primary fuel during such exercise tasks, and research suggests that warm environmental conditions and cellular dehydration may accelerate the use of muscle glycogen. Thus, carbohydrate intake may also improve performance during exercise in the heat, but if temperature regulation is of prime importance, water replacement should receive top priority. Hence, one of the goals of researchers has been to develop a fluid that will help replace carbohydrate during exercise in the heat without affecting water absorption. As discussed previously, carbohydrate-electrolyte solutions have been developed for this purpose.

Research indicates that an appropriate amount of carbohydrate in solution may maintain body temperature as effectively as water and may enhance performance during prolonged exercise. Water and carbohydrate complement each other to improve physical performance. In a unique study, Fritzsche and others, from Coyle's laboratory at the University of Texas, investigated the individual and combined effects of water and carbohydrate intake on power, thermoregulation, cardiovascular function, and metabolism in endurance-trained cyclists exercising for 2 hours in a hot environment. They found that although water alone attenuated the decline in power, ingestion of water with carbohydrate was even more effective. Similar findings have been reported for exercise tests of about an hour duration. Below and others found that water alone and carbohydrate alone improved 1-hour cycling performance in the heat, but the beneficial effects were additive when both were consumed. Millard-Stafford reported that a carbohydrate solution, in comparison to water alone, improved performance in highly trained runners in a 15-kilometer run.

Scores of studies have compared the effectiveness of different carbohydrate combinations and concentrations in enhancing physical performance during prolonged endurance tasks. Most of this research is discussed in chapter 4. The following are the pertinent general findings relative to CES intake during prolonged exercise under warm environmental conditions.

In general, CES between 5 and 10 percent seem to empty from the stomach as effectively as water during prolonged exercise in a hot environment, a finding supported by Rogers and others. They may also be absorbed more readily from the intestinal tract. No significant adverse effects of these solutions upon plasma volume, sweat rate, or temperature regulation, when compared to water ingestion, have been observed. Actually, they may help maintain plasma volume, liver glycogen, and blood glucose levels during prolonged exercise, and, as noted, most investigators report that carbohydrate intake during exercise enhances endurance capacity in a variety of prolonged tasks in the heat.

Several studies by Jeukendrup's research group at the University of Birmingham have shown that using a mixture of carbohydrates may be the best choice. Jentjens and others reported that ingestion of a glucose/fructose drink (1.0 g/0.5 g per minute), as compared to a glucose drink (1.5 g per minute) increased exogenous carbohydrate oxidation rates approximately 36 percent. Other studies from Jeukendrup's laboratory suggest that about 1.5–1.7 grams of carbohydrate per minute may be oxidized if a mixture of carbohydrates, such as glucose, fructose and sucrose, is used.

Although higher concentrations of carbohydrates deliver more glucose to the intestine, solutions higher than 10–12 percent may significantly delay gastric emptying, decrease intestinal absorption, and cause gastrointestinal distress, as noted previously. High concentrations of fructose in some fruit juices or juice blends may be particularly debilitating. However, ultraendurance athletes may experiment with higher concentrations of carbohydrate in training and may adapt to such concentrated solutions for use during competition. In a case study, Alice Lindeman noted that one cyclist involved in the Race Across America (RAAM) consumed a 23 percent carbohydrate solution with no gastrointestinal problems. In such competitions, where cyclists may ride 20 hours or more a day, such high carbohydrate concentrations may be necessary to meet the high energy demands.

In brief, Louise Burke concludes that although carbohydrate ingestion may not enhance the performance of all events undertaken in hot weather, there are no disadvantages to the consumption of beverages containing recommended amounts of carbohydrate and electrolytes.

The ACSM position stand on fluid replacement during exercise includes some guidelines on the composition of fluids to be consumed, including carbohydrate concentration.

Table 9.6 calculates the amount of fluid you must consume, for a given concentration, to obtain 30–100 grams of carbohydrate. As an example, how much of an 8 percent CHO-electrolyte solution does a 70-kg (154-lb) marathon runner need to consume in order to ingest 1.5 g exogenous CHO/kr/hr?

Total exogenous CHO/hr = 1.5 g/kg/hr × 70 kg = 105 g/hr
8 percent CHO-electrolyte solution = 8 grams/100 mL = 80 g/ liter 105 g/80 g = 1.313 liters/hr (44.4 oz/hr)

Additional strategies for carbohydrate intake before and after exercise are presented in chapter 4.

TABLE 9.6 Fluid consumption (milliliters) at a given percent carbohydrate concentration to obtain desired grams of carbohydrate

Percent concentration	Grams of carbohydrate delivered							
	30	40	50	60	70	80	90	100
2%	1,500	2,000	2,500	3,000	3,500	4,000	4,500	5,000
4%	750	1,000	1,250	1,500	1,750	2,000	2,250	2,500
6%	500	666	833	1,000	1,166	1,333	1,500	1,666
8%	375	500	625	750	875	1,000	1,125	1,250
10%	300	400	500	600	700	800	900	1,000
12%	250	333	417	500	583	667	750	833
15%	225	300	375	450	525	600	675	750
20%	150	200	250	300	350	400	450	500

How should electrolytes be replaced during or following exercise?

Because the major solid component of sweat consists of electrolytes, considerable research has been conducted relative to the need for replacement of these lost nutrients, primarily sodium and potassium. We shall look at this question from two points of view, one dealing with the need for replacement during exercise and the other involving daily replacement.

During Exercise   Because sweat is hypotonic to the body fluids, the concentration of electrolytes in the blood and other body fluids actually increases during exercise and makes the body fluids hypertonic. Thus, electrolyte replacement during moderately prolonged exercise is not necessary. In a study of cyclists who exercised 90 minutes at 60 percent VO_2 max, Sanders and others concluded that a 40-millimole sodium solution (Gatorade is about 20-millimole), compared to plain water, may not be of much advantage to athletes who practice normal fluid replacement during such exercise tasks. Several studies have reported that even during strenuous prolonged exercise with high levels of sweat losses, like marathon running for several hours, water alone is the recommended fluid replacement to help maintain electrolyte balance, although added carbohydrate may provide some needed energy.

However, electrolyte replacement, particularly sodium, may be necessary for some athletes participating in very prolonged bouts of physical activity, such as marathons, ultramarathons, Ironman-type triathlons, or tennis tournaments where one might play off and on all day. A number of medical case studies following such events have reported complications resulting from an electrolyte imbalance in the blood, which is the topic of a subsequent question.

Daily Replacement   In general, heavy daily sweat losses do not lead to an electrolyte deficiency. If body levels of sodium and potassium begin to decrease, the kidneys begin to reabsorb more of these minerals and less are excreted in the urine. Research has shown that water alone, in combination with a balanced diet, will adequately maintain proper body electrolyte levels from day to day, even when an individual is exercising and is losing large amounts of sweat.

However, if electrolytes are not adequately replaced because of poor dietary intake, a deficit may occur over 4–7 days of very hard training, especially in hot environmental conditions where fluid losses will tend to be high. Thus, in a review, Maughan noted that exercising individuals who experience heavy daily sweat losses need both adequate fluids and sodium to ensure adequate rehydration. For such individuals, adding salt to meals and drinks may help. Ray and others reported that consuming high-sodium foods, such as chicken broth or chicken noodle soup, improved fluid retention following dehydration. The sodium is needed in the body to help retain water and maintain normal osmotic pressures. In her review, Stachenfeld states that plain water preferentially hydrates plasma volume over interstitial and intracellular volumes and that sodium ingestion during and after exercise maintains the dipsogenic (thirst) drive for more complete rehydration.

A good method of checking on the adequacy of fluid replenishment on a day-to-day basis is to check your body weight in the morning; it should be nearly the same every day. If you weigh several pounds less from one day to the next, it is likely that you are hypohydrated. Conversely, if you weigh several pounds more, you may be overhydrated.

What is hyponatremia and what causes it during exercise?

Hyponatremia is a condition of subnormal levels of sodium in the blood. Also known as *water intoxication,* it can occur at rest simply by consuming too much water. Hyponatremia can also occur following prolonged exercise, in which case it may be known as *exercise-associated hyponatremia (EAH)*. The Second International Exercise-Associated Hyponatremia Consensus Development Conference in 2007 defined EAH as a serum sodium concentration below the normal reference range, or less than 135 mmol/liter (135 mEq/liter). Milder forms are 130–134 mmol/liter and may be asymptomatic, but not always. Signs and symptoms of mild hyponatremia usually occur when serum sodium goes below 130 mmol/liter and may include the following:

- Bloating
- Puffiness of hands and feet
- Nausea
- Vomiting
- Headache

Severe cases, below 120 mmol/liter, may cause massive brain swelling, which may be associated with the following:

- Seizures
- Coma
- Respiratory arrest
- Permanent brain damage
- Death

In a study from the 2002 Boston marathon, Almond and others tested 488 runners following the race; 13 percent, or one in eight, had a serious fluid and salt imbalance from drinking too much water or sports drinks, and one 28-year-old woman died from hyponatremia. In addition to affecting endurance athletes exercising in the heat, according to Rogers and Hew-Butler, EAH has been documented in hikers, climbers, trekkers, and cold-climate endurance athletes. Treatment of individuals with symptomatic hyponatremia is a medical emergency, and transportation to a hospital is essential. Infusion of hypertonic solutions may be necessary.

Various risk factors have been identified that predispose individuals to development of EAH in marathons and other endurance events, including the following:

- Excessive drinking of fluids before, during, and after the event
- Considerable weight gain over the course of the event
- Slower finishers
- Females
- Low body weight
- Heat-unacclimatized, poorly trained competitors
- High sweat sodium losses
- Race inexperience
- Nonsteroidal anti-inflammatory drug (NSAID) use, altered kidney functions to excrete fluids

Hyponatremia may be caused by water dilution, excess sodium losses, or both. The EAH consensus conference committee indicated that dilutional hyponatremia, caused by an increase in total body water relative to the amount of total body sodium, is the current etiology of EAH. The ACSM, in its position stand on fluid replacement, indicates that fluid consumption that exceeds sweating rate is the primary factor leading to exercise-associated hyponatraemia. Additionally, factors that normally control body water balance, mainly hormones such as arginine vasopressin

and the kidney, may malfunction. NSAIDs interfere with normal kidney function. Wharam and others reported that 2004 New Zealand Ironman triathletes using NSAIDs experienced significantly lower serum sodium levels upon completion of an Ironman triathlon.

Many of these factors may interact to contribute to the development of EAH. For example, females may be of lower body weight; generally run slower marathon times than males, may be more conscientious about consuming fluids, given the old adage *to drink as much as you can;* and thus have more time to consume more fluids and gain proportionately more weight. The weight gain is water, which dilutes the serum sodium concentration. The ACSM advises athletes to not excessively overhydrate during and after exercise, the main contributing factor to hyponatremia.

Although sports drinks do contain some sodium, the EAH consensus committee notes that ingesting sports drinks does not prevent the development of EAH in athletes who drink to excess, because all such drinks are hypotonic. Indeed, sports drinks are constituted to be palatable so that athletes will drink more. Passe and others reported that exercising individuals consumed more fluid as sports drinks as compared to water and orange juice. Peacock and colleagues reported a 46 percent greater *ad libitum* fluid ingestion with CES compared to water. However, the EAH consensus committee did note some studies showing that consuming sports drinks can decrease the severity of EAH.

Twenty milliequivalents (20 mEq, 20 mmol/liter) of sodium may be found in some commercial sports drinks, but research by Barr and others suggests that this amount may be inadequate to prevent a decrease in plasma sodium during prolonged exercise in the heat. Higher amounts approaching the salt content of sweat (about 30–50 mEq per liter) have been suggested by Nancy Rehrer. In their study, Twerenbold and others reported that consuming sodium, in a solution approximating 30 mEq (680 milligrams/liter), minimized hyponatremia in female endurance athletes running for 4 hours; two athletes in the water control trial developed hyponatremia (<130 mmol serum sodium). Anatasiou and colleagues investigated the effectiveness of sports drinks with different sodium content to prevent hyponatremia. They found that if sports drinks were consumed at a rate equal to body mass change, a relatively small amount of sodium (19.9 mmol/l) was effective in preventing the decrease in plasma sodium frequently seen when sodium-free beverages are consumed during exercise in the heat. Some commercial sports drinks may contain higher amounts of sodium. For example, the Gatorade Endurance Hydration Formula contains more than 800 milligrams of sodium per liter, or about 35 mEq. The point should be stressed, however, that although sports drinks may help replace some lost sodium, drinking to excess may still lead to hyponatremia.

Treatment for hyponatremia varies. Chorley recommends that for mild symptomatic hyponatremia, drinking of hypotonic fluids should be restricted until the athlete is urinating. Hypertonic solutions may be provided if the athlete can drink fluids. For severe hyponatremia, intravenous hypertonic (e.g., 3 percent) sodium chloride solutions will speed recovery and improve outcomes. Athletes who do not recover rapidly should be sent to the nearest medical emergency facility.

Individual differences may dictate who may be prone to developing hyponatremia during prolonged exercise, but given the current evidence, it appears that athletes involved in ultraendurance events should consume adequate salt in their diet the days before competition to help assure normal serum sodium levels and consume fluids with added sodium during the event. More research is needed to help refine current recommendations. In the meantime, experiment with salty solutions during practice. You can carry some fluids with you in competition, and in others you may have personal beverages located at specific aid stations on the course.

http://www.medscape.com/viewarticle/847443 This link contains educational materials on EAH and preventative strategies for those engaged in endurance exercise. From this link, the interested reader can access the Statement of the Third International Exercise-Associated Hyponatremia Consensus Development Conference held in February 2015.

Are salt tablets or potassium supplements necessary?

In general, the use of salt tablets to replace lost electrolytes, primarily sodium, is not necessary. As noted, an adequate diet will replace, on a daily basis, electrolytes lost in sweat.

The concentrations of salt in sweat may vary. Some individuals who have a high amount of salt in their sweat are sometimes referred to as "salty sweaters." According to Maughan and Shirreffs, a rough self-assessment may be done by wearing a black t-shirt during exercise and looking for salt stains when the sweat has evaporated. We have noted previously that the average sweat salt concentration may be about 3.2 grams of salt per liter, although there are reports as high as 4.5 grams per liter in unacclimatized individuals, and as low as 1.75 grams per liter in the heat-acclimatized individual. Because salt is 40 percent sodium and 60 percent chloride, the sodium content in 3.2 grams of salt is 1.3 grams, in 4.5 grams of salt is 1.8 grams, and in 1.75 grams of salt is 0.7 gram. If an athlete lost about 8–9 pounds of body fluids during an exercise period, a total of 4 liters of fluid (about 4 quarts) would be lost because a liter weighs 2.2 pounds. Four liters of sweat would contain, at the most, 7.2 grams of sodium in the unacclimatized individual, but less than 3 grams in one who was acclimatized. Because the average meal contains about 2–3 grams of sodium if well salted, three meals a day would offer 6–9 grams, about enough to just cover the losses in the sweat. However, sodium is lost through other means, primarily in the urine; thus, a slight increase in sodium intake may be reasonable for the unacclimatized athlete. Doug Hiller, a physician who has worked extensively with endurance athletes, suggests that during the week or two of acclimatization to exercising in the heat, athletes should consume about 10–25 grams of salt daily, or 4–10 grams of sodium. Consuming more high-sodium foods or a more liberal salting of the food should provide an adequate amount; 1 teaspoon of salt contains about 5 grams of salt, or 2 grams of sodium. Although this sodium intake is much greater than the UL of 2.3 grams recommended by the National Academy of Sciences, that recommendation is based on the sedentary individual, not an athlete losing copious amounts of sodium during a period of acclimatization. Stachenfeld notes

that acute high sodium intake following exercise may cause a transient increase in blood pressure, but not sustained hypertension in healthy individuals. However, once an athlete is acclimatized to the heat, sodium intake may be reduced to normal.

Common salt tablets contain only sodium and chloride. They are not necessary to replace lost sodium but may be recommended for unacclimatized athletes who do not replace sodium through normal dietary means in the early stages of an acclimatization program. Salt tablets should be taken only if the athlete loses substantial amounts of weight via sweat losses during a workout. Checking the body weight before and after a workout provides a good estimate of sweat loss. If we switch to the English system, 1 quart of sweat equals 2 pounds; 1/2 quart, or a pint, is 1 pound. One recommendation is that salt tablets should be taken only if the athlete needs to drink more than 4 quarts of fluid per day to replace that lost during sweating: that is, an 8-pound weight loss. The general rule is to take two salt tablets with each additional quart of fluid beyond the 4 quarts; this would be equal to 1 gram of sodium (the average tablet has 1/2 gram of sodium) per quart. Another way to look at it is to take 1 pint of water with every salt tablet. The use of salt tablets should be discontinued after the athlete is acclimatized, usually about 6–9 days.

Potassium supplements are not recommended—for several reasons. First, research by David Costill and his associates has revealed that a deficiency of potassium is rare, even with large sweat losses and a diet low in potassium. Second, as noted previously, excessive potassium may be lethal, as it can disturb the electrical rhythm of the heart. The moderate use of substitutes, such as potassium chloride for common table salt, may be helpful in assuring potassium replacement, but investigators recommended particular attention to the diet, citing citrus fruits and bananas as two of the many foods high in potassium. For example, a large glass of orange juice will replace the potassium lost in 2 liters of sweat.

What are some prudent guidelines relative to fluid replacement while exercising under warm or hot environmental conditions?

In sports nutrition, no other area has received as much research attention as the objective of determining the optimal formulation of an oral rehydration solution (sports drink) for individuals doing prolonged exercise under warm or hot environmental conditions. This may be because water and carbohydrates are two nutrients that may enhance performance in such events, and water and electrolytes may also help to prevent heat-related illnesses. As discussed previously in relation to the need for fluid, carbohydrate, or electrolytes, a number of factors—in particular, the intensity and duration of the exercise task, the prevailing environmental conditions, and individual differences in sweat rate, gastric emptying, and intestinal absorption—may influence the desired composition of the sports drink. Given these considerations, many of the leading investigators in exercise-hydration research indicate that there is no agreement on the optimal formulation of an oral rehydration solution that would suit the needs of all individuals who engage in a variety of prolonged exercise tasks. Indeed, as noted previously, the ACSM identified the individual's unique biological characteristics as a factor affecting hydration status and exercise performance. As noted by Baker and Jeukendrup, the source of fluid loss (e.g., sweat, diarrhea, vomiting, other) is a factor in determining the optimal composition of a fluid-replacement solution.

Through their concerted research efforts over the years, sports scientists such as Louise Burke, Edward Coyle, Ronald Maughan, Timothy Noakes, Michael Sawka, and Scott Montain have provided a sound basis to promote prudent recommendations regarding fluid replacement before, during, and after exercise. The latest guidelines on fluid replacement for exercise have been published by the ACSM, which serve as the basis for these prudent recommendations.

http://journals.lww.com/acsm-msse Access the American College of Sports Medicine 2007 position stand on fluid replacement by clicking on the link for ACSM Position Stands and Joint Position Statements on the right-hand side of the page.

Before Competition and Practice The goal of the ACSM guidelines is to start in a state of euhydration with normal plasma electrolyte levels. Unfortunately, not all athletes come to practice adequately hydrated. Osterberg and colleagues examined pregame hydration in players from five teams in the National Basketball Association and found that 52 percent began the game dehydrated. National Collegiate Athletic Association Division I athletes were assessed for their prepractice hydration status by Volpe and others. They found that 66 percent of the college athletes hypohydrated prior to practice, with a greater percentage of men in a hypohydrated state compared to women. Here are some key points:

1. Be sure you are adequately hydrated the day before competition. Minimize consumption of alcoholic beverages the night before competition, for they may lead to hypohydration in the morning.
2. Drink slowly about 5–7 milliliters/kilogram (0.08–0.11 ounce/pound) body weight at least 4 hours prior to exercise.
   - Fluid palatability (temperature, sodium, flavoring) will enhance fluid intake. Peacock and others reported that CES ingestion significantly increased pleasure ratings, ingested volume, and plasma glucose concentrations compared to water.
   - If the exercise task is to be prolonged, carbohydrate may be added. A concentration of 6–8 percent is advisable, but concentrations of 20 percent and higher have been used by some individuals without adverse effects.
   - Beverages with sodium (20–50 mEq/l) and/or salty foods or snacks will help stimulate thirst and retain fluids.
3. If no urine is produced, or urine is dark or highly concentrated, drink another 3–5 mL/kg body weight about 2 hours prior to exercise. Your urine should be a clear, pale yellow before competition or practice.

4. Do not excessively overhydrate, which may increase the risk of dilutional hyponatremia if fluids are aggressively replaced during and after exercise.

www.urinecolors.com/dehydration.php Provides a Dehydration Urine Color Chart to help estimate your level of dehydration.

During Competition and Practice A review of the literature by Garth and Burke revealed little information about self-selected hydration by elite and nonelite athletes during practice and competition. There are varied practices across and within competitive events and many factors, some beyond the athlete's control, that call into question the existence of true *ad libitum* fluid intake during competition. The goal of the ACSM guidelines is to prevent excessive dehydration (>2 percent body weight loss from water deficit). The amount and rate of fluid replacement depend on individual sweating rate, exercise duration, and opportunities to rehydrate. Here are some key considerations:

1. Individuals should monitor body weight changes during training/competition sessions to estimate fluid losses during a particular exercise task.
2. Although some believe that thirst is the best stimulus for fluid ingestion in situations where fluid is readily available, the ACSM believes it is important to start rehydrating early in endurance events because thirst does not develop until about 1–2 percent of body weight has been lost. The ACSM guidelines recommend a possible starting point for marathon runners is to drink *ad libitum* about 0.4–0.8 liter of fluids per hour, smaller runners might consume 0.4 liter, while bigger runners consume 0.8 liter. Consuming 0.4 liter (about 14 ounces) per hour could be accomplished by drinking 3–4 ounces every 15 minutes, while drinking about 7 ounces every 15 minutes would provide 0.8 liter per hour. These amounts may be adjusted to individual preferences and to increase carbohydrate content, as discussed later.

   It is important to realize that during periods of heavy sweating, it is very difficult to consume enough fluids to replace those lost. Costill has noted that, per minute, 50 milliliters or more of fluid may be lost though sweating (3 liters per hour), but only 20–30 milliliters per minute may be absorbed from the intestines. The sweating rate in this case simply outweighs the absorption of ingested fluids. Although some dehydration will occur, rehydration will help maintain circulatory stability and heat balance, thereby delaying deterioration of endurance capacity. Cheuvront and Haymes reported that replacing 60–70 percent of sweat losses helps to maintain thermoregulatory responses during hot and warm weather conditions. By calculating your typical sweat losses, as discussed on page 390 and determined in the Application Exercise at the end of this chapter, you may be able to estimate how much fluid you should consume per hour.
3. Cold water is effective when carbohydrate intake is of little or no concern, for example, in endurance events lasting less than

50–60 minutes. Sports drinks with 6–8 percent carbohydrates and normal electrolyte content may also be consumed but, in general, provide no advantages over water alone.

4. The composition of the fluid is considered important for prolonged endurance events. Carbohydrates and electrolytes may provide some advantages, and these components may be in the drink or nonfluid sources such as gels or energy bars. Palatability and the presence of other ingredients may also be important considerations.

- Carbohydrate provides energy for longer-duration events. If carbohydrate is desired in the drink, the concentration should not be excessive. A 6–10 percent concentration is recommended. Concentrations greater than 10–12 percent may retard gastric emptying and contribute to gastrointestinal distress. Use a sports drink containing multiple sources of carbohydrate, including glucose, sucrose, fructose, and maltodextrins. Such a mixture may enhance absorption and utilization of the exogenous carbohydrate, possibly up to 1.2–1.7 grams per minute. Check the food label for ingredients.

  The ACSM recommends that athletes consume enough fluid to provide about 30–80 grams of carbohydrate per hour. Similarly, Bob Murray indicates that the consumption of about 1 gram of carbohydrate per kilogram body weight per hour appears sufficient to improve performance in prolonged exercise. On average, sports drinks containing 6–8 percent carbohydrate provide about 2 grams of carbohydrate for every ounce of fluid consumed. Thus, you need to drink about 15–16 ounces of a sports drink per hour to obtain about 30 grams of carbohydrate, or about 1 liter per hour to obtain 60 grams. See table 9.6 for guidelines.

  It may be difficult for some athletes, such as marathon runners, to consume the amount of fluid during exercise to obtain the recommended grams of carbohydrate. Many runners do not consume a liter per hour, which is needed to provide 60 grams from a 6 percent sports drink. However, consuming other sources of carbohydrate with the sports drink, such as sports gels or sports beans, can provide the additional grams of carbohydrate.

  Athletes in prolonged, intermittent, high-intensity sports, such as soccer, may use various rehydration procedures. Clarke and others provided the same total amount of a CES to soccer players during a 90-minute soccer specific protocol. In one trial, the CES was given at 0 and 45 minutes, while in a second trial it was provided in smaller volumes at 0, 15, 30, 45, 60, and 75 minutes. There were no differences in metabolic responses during the soccer protocol, and sprint power was not different, suggesting that the two methods of providing fluids were equally effective.

- The fluid should contain small amounts of electrolytes, particularly sodium and potassium, to help replace lost electrolytes. The ACSM recommends about 20–30 mEq of sodium and 2–5 mEq of potassium, which are amounts present in many commercial sports drinks. However, for athletes involved in very prolonged endurance events under warm environmental conditions, some recommend a range of about 700–1,150 milligrams of sodium per liter (approximately 30–50

mmol per liter) and 120–225 milligrams of potassium per liter (approximately 3–6 mmol per liter). Some commercial sports drinks contain electrolytes comparable to this range. For example, for each 8-ounce serving, Gatorade Endurance Formula contains 200 milligrams of sodium and 90 milligrams of potassium, which is more than 800 milligrams of sodium (about 36 mmol) and 360 milligrams of potassium (about 10 mmol) per liter.

- The fluid should be palatable and not interfere with normal gastrointestinal functions. Research has shown that the voluntary intake of fluids increases when they are tasty. Being cold and sweet enhances palatability. In their review, Burdon and others noted 50 percent greater consumption by volume of cool/cold versus warm beverages. In contrast, Lambert and others noted that subjects exercising in the heat consumed less fluid when it was carbonated, suggesting a lower palatability compared to noncarbonated beverages. Carbonated beverages do not appear to inhibit gastric emptying, nor does the use of the artificial sweetener aspartame, but Zachwieja and others noted that certain flavorings, such as citric acid, may impair gastric emptying by as much as 25 percent.

- Caffeine is found in some sports drinks and may help sustain performance. Detailed information on caffeine and exercise performance is presented in chapter 13. In brief, however, caffeine supplementation appears to be an effective ergogenic aid for aerobic endurance performance, and its use is currently not prohibited by the World Anti-Doping Agency (WADA). Moreover, caffeinated sports drinks maintain hydration and metabolic and thermoregulatory functions as well as standard sports drinks.

- Some sports drinks include protein, but they do not appear to enhance performance more than typical CESs. Van Essen and Gibala, in a well-designed study, compared the effects of a carbohydrate/protein drink (6 percent with 2 percent protein added) to a carbohydrate drink (6 percent) on performance of well-trained cyclists in a laboratory 80-kilometer time trial. Although performance time was significantly faster with the two sports drinks, as compared to the placebo, there was no difference between them. As noted in chapter 6, other studies have not reported performance enhancement associated with protein-containing CES when compared to typical CES. However, several studies, such as that by Bird and others, did provide evidence suggestive of reduced muscle tissue damage. Review pages 237–238 for details.

After Competition and Practice The goal of the ACSM guidelines is to fully replace any fluid and electrolyte deficit. Replacement may have to be rapid, such as in preparation for a subsequent exercise endeavor on the same day. For example, tennis players may compete in two or more events daily with a short recovery period, while some athletes may also train twice daily. In other situations, fluid replacement may be more leisurely if time permits.

1. If time is short to the next exercise session, aggressive rehydration is important.

- Drink 1.5 liters of fluid for every kilogram of body weight loss, or about 1.5 pints for each pound loss. The additional fluid is needed to compensate for increased urine output.
- Consume adequate carbohydrates and electrolytes as well. Fruit juices and sports drinks are helpful when you need to replenish both fluids and carbohydrates. Pretzels and other salty snacks may provide sodium, as well as carbohydrate. This may be especially important for competition. Osterberg and others found that the inclusion of carbohydrate (3 percent, 6 percent, and 12 percent) to an electrolyte beverage enhanced the retention of fluid following exercise-induced dehydration. Bilzon and others found that, provided adequate hydration status is maintained, inclusion of carbohydrate within an oral rehydration solution will delay the onset of fatigue in subsequent prolonged exercise.
- Some preliminary research suggests that consuming a sports drink with protein may help. Seifert and others reported that a CES with protein, as compared to a CES and water, restored more fluids in a 3-hour recovery period following a 2.5 percent dehydration; the protein solution helped retain 88 percent, the carbohydrate 75 percent, and water only 53 percent.

2. If recovery time permits (24 hours), normal meal and water intake will restore euhydration, provided sodium intake is adequate. In separate reviews, Rehrer and Stachenfeld note that sodium is necessary in the recovery period to restore fluid balance.
   - A diet rich in wholesome, natural foods adhering to healthy eating practices will help replenish needed electrolytes.
   - Sodium replacement is important, particularly if your sweat contains significant amounts. Check your skin and clothing for traces of dried salt after exercise; if white streaks occur, you may be losing substantial amounts of sodium during exercise.
   - Extra salt may be added to meals when sodium losses are high.
   - Drink fluids with added sodium or consume salty foods or snacks.

3. Minimize alcohol intake. Shirreffs and Maughan noted that drinks containing 4 percent alcohol or more, such as beer, tend to delay the recovery process, as measured by restoration of blood and plasma volume.

In Training

1. Maughan and Meyer stress the importance of proper hydration during training in order to maintain high training loads and to "train" the intestinal tract to accommodate hydration during competition. Practice consuming fluids while you train. Use a trial-and-error approach. Some research indicates that consuming CES during training, particularly high-intensity training, may result in a more effective workout, which could lead to better performance in competition. By consuming various formulations while you train, particularly during training comparable to the intensity and duration experienced in competition, you will be able to determine what fluids work specifically for you. Consuming fluids during training may help you overcome some of the factors that inhibit fluid intake during exercise, such as the uncomfortable sensation of fluid in the stomach, and lead to increased fluid intake during competition. This is especially important for older athletes, who tend to drink less than their younger counterparts.

2. If you sip sports drinks throughout the day to stay hydrated, be sure to practice sound dental hygiene. As noted in chapter 4, some research has shown that sports drinks may exert significant eroding effects on dental enamel.

A summary of guidelines for fluid, carbohydrate, and electrolyte replacement during exercise under warm environmental conditions is presented in table 9.7. In brief, the ACSM guidelines present three key points to prevent hypohydration during exercise. Hydrate well before the exercise task; drink according to your personal needs; and rehydrate rapidly in preparation for subsequent exercise bouts on the same day, or more leisurely if recovery time permits. Use of sports drinks may be helpful. In their review, Coombes and Hamilton concluded that in studies where a practical protocol has been used along with a currently available sports beverage (less than 10 percent carbohydrate solutions), there is evidence to suggest that consuming a sports drink will improve performance compared with consuming a placebo beverage.

Key Concepts

▶ Hyperhydration before exercise is important, but rehydration is the most important nutritional consideration when exercising in the heat.

▶ Rehydration with cold water is effective in moderating body temperature during exercise in the heat, but carbohydrate solutions may be equally effective and provide a source of energy for more prolonged endurance exercise.

▶ An effective rehydration solution is one that optimizes gastric emptying and intestinal absorption of fluid.

▶ Electrolyte replacement generally is not needed during exercise but may be helpful during very prolonged exercise tasks. Water alone, in combination with a balanced diet, including adequate sodium and potassium, will adequately restore normal electrolyte levels in the body on a day-to-day basis.

▶ Current research suggests that 6–10 percent solutions of glucose, fructose, sucrose, glucose polymers, or combinations of these different carbohydrates, may be effective for athletes who need carbohydrate replacement during exercise.

▶ Research has shown that combinations of carbohydrates (e.g. glucose and fructose) in CES may increase the oxidation rate of ingested carbohydrates.

▶ Excessive fluid consumption during very prolonged exercise, coupled with inadequate salt intake, may contribute to hyponatremia, a potentially dangerous condition.

▶ One ounce of a typical 6–8 percent carbohydrate-electrolyte solution (CES) contains about 2 grams of carbohydrate. Drinking 20 ounces of a CES per hour during exercise will provide about 40 grams of carbohydrate.

▶ Individuals who desire to rehydrate rapidly following exercise should consume about 120–150 percent of the fluid lost. Added salt will help the body retain the ingested fluids.

Before competition and practice
The goal of the ACSM guidelines is to start in a state of euhydration with normal plasma electrolyte levels.

- Drink slowly about 5–7 milliliters/kilogram (0.08–0.11 ounce/pound) body weight at least 4 hours prior to exercise. For an athlete weighing 70 kg (154 pounds), this would approximate 350–490 milliliters, or 12–17 ounces of fluids. Athletes weighing more or less will drink accordingly.
- Drink another 3–5 mL/kg body weight about 2 hours prior to exercise if no urine is produced or the urine is dark or highly concentrated. Your urine should be a clear, pale yellow before competition or practice.
- Drink water. However, carbohydrate-electrolyte solutions (CES) also may be used if preferred.
- Drink beverages with carbohydrate (6–8 percent) to help increase body stores of glucose and glycogen for use in prolonged exercise bouts.
- Drink beverages with sodium (20–50 mEq/l) and/or consume salty foods or snacks to help increase body stores of sodium and water for prolonged exercise.
- Do not drink excessively, which may increase the risk of dilutional hyponatremia if fluids are aggressively replaced during and after exercise.

During competition and practice
The goal of the ACSM guidelines is to prevent excessive dehydration (>2% body weight loss from water deficit).

- Determine your sweat loss for a given intensity and duration of exercise in the heat. This will provide you with an estimate for fluid intake during exercise. A procedure is presented on page 390.
- Drink about 0.4 to 0.8 liter of fluids per hour, which is about 14 to 28 ounces. Smaller athletes may consume 14 ounces, or about 3–4 ounces every 15 minutes. Larger athletes my consume 28 ounces, or about 7 ounces every 15 minutes. However, the fluids may be consumed at your pleasure, or *ad libitum,* on other time schedules as conditions permit. Athletes can adjust the amounts according to personal needs.
- Drink cold water when carbohydrate intake is of little or no concern, such as in endurance events of less than 50–60 minutes. CES may be consumed during such events if preferred but provide no advantages over water alone.
- Drink fluids with carbohydrates for longer-duration events.
  - Select a CES with a 6–8 percent concentration.
  - Use a CES containing multiple sources of carbohydrate, including glucose, sucrose, fructose, and maltodextrins.
  - Consume enough fluid to provide about 30–80 grams of carbohydrate per hour. One ounce of a CES provides about 2 grams of carbohydrate.
  - Use sports gels or sports beans to provide additional carbohydrate if the necessary fluid intake would be unreasonable. Sports gels and beans may provide about 25–30 grams of carbohydrate per serving.
- Drink fluids with small amounts of electrolytes, particularly sodium and potassium. Many CES contain about 20–30 mEq of sodium and 2–5 mEq of potassium, which amounts to about 110–160 grams of sodium and 19–45 grams of potassium in an 8-ounce serving.

After competition and practice
The goal of the ACSM guidelines is to fully replace any fluid and electrolyte deficit.

- Rapid replacement
  - Drink 1.5 liters of fluid for every kilogram of body weight loss, or about 1.5 pints for each pound loss.
  - Consume about 1.0 to 1.5 grams of carbohydrate per kilogram body weight (about 0.5 to 0.7 gram per pound body weight) each hour for 3–4 hours. For a 60-kg athlete, this would represent about 60–90 grams of carbohydrate per hour.
  - Consume adequate sodium. Salty carbohydrate snacks, such as pretzels, may provide both sodium and carbohydrate.
- Leisurely replacement (24-hour recovery)
  - Eat a diet rich in wholesome, natural foods adhering to healthy eating practices to help replenish needed electrolytes.
  - Extra salt may be added to meals when sodium losses are high.
  - Drink fluids with added sodium or consume salty foods or snacks.

These guidelines have been adapted from the position stand on fluid replacement developed by the American College of Sports Medicine. The guidelines are appropriate for athletes competing or training for endurance or high-intensity, intermittent sports, such as 10-kilometer races, marathons and ultramarathons, endurance cycling races, Olympic- to Ironman-distance triathlons, soccer and field hockey games, and tennis matches. These guidelines are approximations and may be modified based on individual preferences derived through personal experience in both training and competition. See text for additional information.

Ergogenic Aspects

If preventing or correcting a nutrient deficiency is seen as an ergogenic technique, then certainly water could be construed to be an ergogenic aid. Compared to taking in no fluid during exercise, rehydration has been shown to enhance temperature regulation or exercise performance by optimizing hydration status. However, some athletes have attempted to lose body water for ergogenic purposes. Although we have seen that hypohydration generally does not improve performance, and indeed may actually impair performance in endurance-type events, certain athletes such as high jumpers may use drugs like diuretics to lose weight rapidly without losses in power. Research has shown that diuretic-induced weight losses may improve vertical jumping ability because the athlete can develop the same power to move a lower body weight. Detailed coverage of these drugs is beyond the scope of this text.

Moreover, the use of diuretics is banned by most athletic governing bodies, such as the United States Olympic Committee and the National Collegiate Athletic Association.

Over the years, athletes have attempted to modify body water stores or body temperature using various ergogenic techniques, including supplementation with various nutrients, in attempts to enhance sports performance.

Does oxygen water enhance exercise performance?

Oxygen water, or water oxygenated before bottling, has been marketed to physically active individuals. One brand claims to be a *performance water,* suggesting that tests show that it positively affects cardiovascular and muscular performance and endurance. The amount of oxygen dissolved in a bottle of water is about the same amount as found in a single breath. It is unlikely that oxygen is absorbed by the intestine into the bloodstream. Finally, oxygen is relatively insoluble in water. Only 0.3 mL of the normal arterial oxygen content of 20 mL oxygen/100 mL blood is physically dissolved in the blood. Peer-reviewed research does not support marketing claims that oxygen water enhances energy and boosts athletic performance. Hampson and others reported no effect of oxygenated water on oxygen consumption during exercise and noted that the amount of oxygen contained in the bottle would last only about 2 seconds in an individual doing moderate exercise. Wing-Gaia and others reported no differences in blood oxygenation, performance, or other physiological response in recreational cyclists exercising under hypoxic conditions following consumption of oxygen versus regular water.

The available scientific evidence does not support an ergogenic effect of oxygen water.

Do pre-cooling techniques help reduce body temperature and enhance performance during exercise in the heat?

Pre-cooling may be an effective ergogenic strategy for some athletes competing in the heat, and there may be several possible reasons. Sawka and Young indicated that cooling the skin will decrease skin blood flow, so theoretically more blood could be shuttled to the muscles during exercise. According to Quod and others, the main theory is that an increased heat storage capacity will allow an athlete to complete a greater amount of work before a critical body temperature is reached. Research supports this viewpoint. Hunter and others found that female collegiate distance runners wearing an ice-vest during the warm-up period, in comparison to runners not wearing the vest, experienced a significantly lower core temperature prior to the start and a smaller increase in core temperature at the finish.

Yeargin and others reported that cold water immersion following 90 minutes of cross-country running improved performance in a 2-mile run. Uckert and Joch found that 20 minutes of pre-cooling with a vest resulted in lower heart rate, core and skin temperatures, and performance after 30 minutes of treadmill exercise compared to warm-up or no pre-exercise preparation. Webster and others evaluated the effect of a lightweight cooling vest on endurance running performance. The subjects wore the cooling vest during stretching and warm-up, but not during the running tests. The vest cooled the body core temperature by 0.5° Celsius and decreased sweat rate by approximately 10–23 percent during a 30-minute run at 70 percent of VO_2 max, and it improved endurance time by 49 seconds when running at 95 percent of VO_2 max.

According to Hunter and others, ice-vests appeared to be effective in keeping body temperatures down and improving the performance of American and Australian marathon runners at the 2004 Olympic Games in Athens.

Three recent reviews have examined the efficacy of pre-cooling techniques. In their meta-analysis, Wegmann and colleagues reported the greatest effect sizes for pre-cooling in hot conditions, for subjects with high aerobic capacity, and for endurance compared to sprint performance. The best methods were cold drinks and cooling packs. The pre-cooling effect on time trial performance, the most relevant task for an ergogenic effect, was 3.7 percent. In another meta-analysis, Bongers and others reported similar effect sizes on exercise performance for pre-cooling and percooling (during exercise). Pre-cooling resulted in a lower core temperature compared to control conditions. Multiple techniques and ice-vests were the most effective strategies for pre-cooling and percooling, respectively. Ross and colleagues also reported support for multiple pre-cooling strategies for enhancing prolonged exercise under hyperthermic conditions. Additional research is recommended for specific applications to athletes. Castle and others found that leg cooling (ice bags to legs) improved peak power output in cycling more than total body or upper body cooling. The efficacy of cooling techniques in the recovery interval between bouts of exercise was studied by Hausswirth and others. Both cool water immersion and a cooling vest attenuated the thermal strain of the second bout of exercise.

Does sodium loading enhance endurance performance?

An electrolyte deficiency could impair physical performance, but supplements above and beyond normal electrolyte nutrition have not been recommended for ergogenic purposes. However, sodium concentration is one of the main determinants of water retention and blood volume. As Gledhill and others note, an increased blood volume may increase VO_2 max. Luetkemeier and others noted that ingestion, or infusion, of a saline solution before exercise (**sodium loading**) may expand the plasma volume, leading to cardiovascular responses that could benefit exercise performance, but at the time they also noted that such advantages have yet to be reported.

Subsequently, Sims and others studied the effect of sodium loading on the plasma volume and the physiological strain of moderately trained males running in the heat. In a crossover design, subjects consumed either a high-sodium (164 mmol/l) or low-sodium (10 mmol/l) beverage before running to exhaustion at 70 percent VO_2 max in warm conditions (32°C). About 0.75 liter was consumed over the course of 60 minutes, with an additional 45 minutes of rest before testing. The high sodium increased plasma volume before exercise, reduced ratings of perceived exertion during exercise, and involved greater time to exhaustion when stopped because of an ethical end point (core temperature at

39.5°C). The authors concluded that consuming the high-sodium beverage involved less thermoregulatory and perceived strain during exercise and increased exercise capacity in warm conditions. Although exercise was terminated upon attainment of the predetermined core temperature and subjects technically did not run to exhaustion, the data support an ergogenic effect. Using a similar research protocol with trained female cyclists who cycled to exhaustion at 70 percent VO_2 max in warm conditions (32°C), Sims and others reported again that consumption of the high-sodium beverage increased plasma volume, reduced thermoregulatory strain, and increased exercise performance.

These data are supportive of an ergogenic effect of sodium loading *before* exercising in a hot environment. As mentioned in chapter 13, sodium bicarbonate supplementation has been shown to enhance endurance performance in some studies when provided before exercise, which could be related to the sodium content in the bicarbonate preparation. However, consuming sodium tablets *during* exercise does not appear to enhance performance. Hew-Butler and others, in a study of more than 400 triathletes, reported no ergogenic effect from consuming additional sodium in tablet form (a total of 3.6 grams more than the placebo and control groups) on finishing time in Ironman competition.

Does glycerol supplementation enhance endurance performance during exercise under warm environmental conditions?

Glycerol, as noted in chapter 5, is an alcohol that combines with fatty acids to form a triglyceride. Years ago, glycerol had been studied as an ergogenic aid because it may be a source of energy during exercise or used as a substrate for gluconeogenesis. However, Massicotte and others reported that only a small portion, about 4 percent, of glycerol consumed during exercise is converted to glucose for oxidation or directly oxidized for energy. Results of studies have not supported an ergogenic effect of glycerol when used for its energy content.

More recently, glycerol supplementation has been studied in attempts to enhance endurance performance in warm environments. Glycerol has been combined with water during hyperhydration prior to exercise to study its potential ergogenic effects on performance in prolonged endurance events, often under warm environmental conditions. A typical supplementation protocol has been to add approximately 1 g glycerol/kg body mass to approximately 25 mL/kg body mass. Glycerol supplementation has also been based on lean body mass or total body water and combined with carbohydrates. Theoretically, glycerol-induced hyperhydration will increase osmotic pressure in the body fluids, helping to retain more total body water and possibly increase the plasma volume, factors that could enhance temperature regulation and exercise performance. Thus, a 70-kilogram male would consume 70 grams of glycerol in about 1.4–1.75 liters of water or similar fluid. Glycerol-induced hyperhydration protocols were normally compared to water-induced hyperhydration techniques.

Research data are equivocal regarding the effects of glycerol-induced hyperhydration, compared to water-induced hyperhydration, on body-water levels. Freund and his associates from the

U.S. Army Research Institute of Environmental Medicine found that glycerol-induced hyperhydration as compared to water hyperhydration resulted in a greater retention of fluids in the body. The investigators noted that the glycerol helped to maintain the osmolality of the blood, leading to better preservation of serum ADH levels, which they suggested may have contributed to the lower urinary output of water. van Rosendal and colleagues reported the greatest fluid retention following 4 percent dehydration with oral glycerol with intravenous infusion of saline + sports drink compared to either oral sports drink + water, oral glycerol + sports drink + water, or intravenous saline + sports drink + water. Conversely, using similar hyperhydration protocols, two reports by Latzka and others have not shown any advantage of glycerol-induced hyperhydration over water-induced hyperhydration on total body water. Hillman and others reported reduced postexercise oxidative stress in cyclists following glycerol and water preexercise hyperhydration treatments compared to euhydration, but there was no difference between any of the hydration conditions in thermoregulatory response or performance. Overall, however, glycerol hyperhydration does appear to increase body water. Goulet and others conducted a meta-analysis of 14 studies and concluded that glycerol hyperhydration significantly increased body fluid retention compared to water rehydration.

Research data regarding the effects of glycerol-induced hyperhydration on temperature regulation and on performance are also equivocal. Lyons and others found that glycerol-induced hyperhydration was more effective than water-induced hyperhydration in reducing the thermal stress of moderate exercise in the heat. Montner and others, Scheett and others, and Anderson and others reported improved cycling performance and evidence of lower thermal stress such as increased plasma volume, lower rectal temperature, and lower heart rate following glycerol-induced hyperhydration. Kavouras and others have reported improved cycling performance following glycerol-induced hyperhydration and increased plasma volume, but no other thermoregulatory benefit following glycerol-induced hyperhydration. In a field study involving a crossover protocol, Coutts and others studied the effects of glycerol hyperhydration on competitive Olympic distance triathlon performance. The triathlon was conducted outdoors. The weather on the day of the first competitive triathlon was classified as hot (WBGT, 30.5°), while on the day of the second triathlon it was classified as warm (WBGT, 25.4°). The glycerol hyperhydration induced a significantly greater plasma expansion compared to the placebo, and the increase in the triathlon completion time between the hot and warm conditions was significantly less than the placebo trial. Based on this finding, the authors suggested that glycerol hyperhydration prior to triathlon competition in high ambient temperatures may provide some protection against the negative performance effect of competing in the heat. Although competitive field studies such as this one are important, the rather substantial temperature difference on the two days of competition may have confounded the results.

In contrast, Latzka and others reported that glycerol-induced hyperhydration did not affect sweating dynamics, body temperature, or physiological responses during exercise in two studies. In one of these studies, glycerol-induced hyperhydration did improve exercise performance in the heat at 55 percent VO_2 max compared to control conditions, but the improvement was not significantly greater than that noted in the water-induced hyperhydration trial. van Rosendal and colleagues reported no difference in cycle performance in the heat (40-km time trial) between any of the previously described rehydration strategies involving oral glycerol + water and oral or intravenous saline + sports drink. Goulet and others, in a crossover study with a placebo control, found that a standard glycerol-loading protocol did not affect sweat rate, heart rate, or thermal regulation during cycling for 2 hours at 66 percent VO_2 max, nor did it enhance performance in a subsequent cycling test to exhaustion. Magal and others compared the effects of glycerol-induced and water-only hyperhydration on tennis-related performance in highly skilled male tennis players. Each trial consisted of three phases: hyperhydration with or without glycerol over 150 minutes; 120 minutes of exercise-induced dehydration; and rehydration with or without glycerol over 90 minutes. After each phase, subjects performed various tests, including short sprints, repeated agility drills, and tennis skills. Compared to the placebo trial, the glycerol hyperhydration protocol provided a better hydration status and greater plasma volume after both the initial hydration phase and the rehydration phase, but no performance benefits were observed. Wingo and others reported that although glycerol hyperhydration resulted in less dehydration and post-race thirst during a 30-mile mountain-bike race in the heat, there was no significant difference in final race time, even though the cyclists completed the final 10-mile loop 5 minutes faster during the glycerol trial. Compared to water hyperhydration, Marino and others also reported no significant effect of a standard glycerol-hyperhydration protocol on a 60-minute cycling time trial under hot, humid conditions.

The ergogenic effect of glycerol-induced hyperhydration has been the subject of several reviews, and even the conclusions of these reviewers are somewhat equivocal. Some reviewers concluded that glycerol hyperhydration is an effective ergogenic for endurance athletes exercising in the heat, whereas others concluded that it is ineffective and should be avoided. Still others concluded that the research findings are equivocal. For example, in its position stand on fluid replacement, the ACSM indicated that although hyperhydration, including use of glycerol, does not provide any thermoregulatory advantages, it can delay the onset of dehydration, which may be responsible for any small performance benefits that are occasionally reported. A meta-analysis supports this qualified appraisal. Goulet and others analyzed 14 studies comparing glycerol hyperhydration with water hyperhydration. However, only 4 studies met the criteria for comparing the two treatments on endurance performance. The meta-analysis indicated that glycerol hyperhydration significantly improved performance by 2.6 percent, but due to the limited research available, more research is needed before more definitive conclusions can be drawn as to the ergogenic effects of glycerol hyperhydration. Articles in bodybuilding magazines suggest that glycerol-induced hyperhydration may enhance vascularity during judged competition, providing a "cut" appearance for aesthetic purposes. Glycerol-containing products have been marketed to both endurance and strength athletes. GlycerGrow and other such products have been or are advertised on Websites for strength athletes.

There may be several caveats for individuals who use glycerol supplements, including health and performance issues. Although the dosages used in these studies appear to be safe, researchers indicate that if larger doses are used there may be some concern with the possibility of excess fluid being retained in the intracellular spaces, leading to abnormal pressures and possible tissue damage. Some investigators suggest that glycerol-induced hyperhydration may predispose individuals to hyponatremia. Additionally, reviewers indicate that glycerol supplementation may cause nausea, vomiting, and headaches in some subjects, all of which are symptoms of hyponatremia. From a health perspective, van Rosendal and others advise against glycerol supplementation for certain populations, including pregnant females and those with diabetes, renal disease, migraine and headache disorders, cardiovascular disease, and liver disorders. This recommendation is due to the actions of glycerol on liver gluconeogenesis, kidney filtration, cardiovascular homeostasis, and hydration homeostasis.

Glycerol supplementation may be ergolytic, not ergogenic for some athletes. Studies showing ergogenic effects of glycerol-induced hyperhydration have used cycling protocols. Although hyperhydration may be ergogenic for cyclists, who need not be too concerned with the additional body weight associated with water retention, runners may be at a slight disadvantage because the potential benefits of hyperhydration may not counteract the potential adverse effects of the extra weight, which may result in impaired performance. However, a 2003 report in *Runer's World* magazine indicated that several elite U.S. marathon runners used glycerol in some of their best marathons run in the heat.

In 2010 the World Anti-Doping Agency added glycerol to its list of banned substances due to concerns that glycerol-related water retention and subsequent hemodilution might mask evidence of illegal doping. In their review, van Rosendal and Coombes warn that glycerol doses that are much lower than what is required for hyperhydration may be detected through testing.

Key Concepts

► There is no evidence from well-controlled research that oxygen water has an ergogenic effect.

► Various pre-cooling strategies such as wearing an ice vest and cool water immersion have been shown to improve performance.

► Glycerol supplementation appears to enhance hyperhydration, increase blood volume, and produce favorable physiological responses during exercise. However, research findings are equivocal regarding its effects as a means of improving endurance performance. Glycerol hypohydration, if abused, may also be associated with several adverse health effects.

► Athletes in WADA-regulated sports should be aware that glycerol was added to the list of banned substances in 2010. It is thought that levels well below the dose required for hyperhydration may be detected through testing.

Health Aspects: Heat Illness

Heat illness, as the name implies, involves various health problems associated with environmental heat stress. As noted previously, excessive dehydration may impair physical performance, and individuals who overhydrate in attempts to prevent dehydration during exercise may experience exercise-associated hyponatremia, which could have serious health consequences. Dehydration and loss of electrolytes may also cause health problems during exercise, some more serious than others.

However, high environmental heat stress poses one of the most serious health threats to athletes and others who exercise, and such individuals should use caution when exercising in the heat.

Should I exercise in the heat?

Given the potential health threats of exercising in the heat, the American College of Sports Medicine published a position stand on exertional heat illness during training and competition, which is available on the ACSM Website. In general, this position stand presents guidelines targeted to sports medicine personnel, such as athletic trainers, and water sport administrators who should be aware of environmental heat conditions that suggest modification or cancelation of competition or practice. However, individuals may also use these guidelines to determine when to modify exercise protocols in the heat. The guidelines are based on the WBGT, which may not be readily available to most individuals. However, local television stations or various Websites usually can provide a heat index, which is a good approximation of the WBGT when exercising in the shade; exercising in the sun adds to the heat index. Table 9.8 presents a modification of the ACSM guidelines.

http://www.acsm.org/public-information/position-stands The ACSM position stand "Exertional Heat Illness during Training and Competition" can be accessed from the list on this web page.

www.weather.com
www.wunderground.com Various Websites may provide you with the temperature, humidity, wind, and possibility of sunshine. They also generally provide a heat index, indicating that although the air temperature is only 85°F, it may feel like 95°F due to humidity.

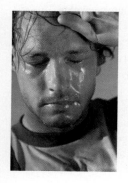

What are the potential health hazards of excessive heat stress imposed on the body?

One of the most serious threats to the performance and health of the physically active individual is heat illness, which is often referred to as exertional heat illness or exercise-associated heat illness when it occurs with exercise. Basu and colleagues reported strong positive associations (percent increased risk per 10°F) between ambient temperature and morbidities such as central and cerebral vascular disease, diabetes, hypotension, renal failure, and intestinal infection in addition to heat illness and dehydration. According to National Center for Health Statistics data from 1999–2010, there was an annual average of 618 deaths related to excessive heat exposure. Any athlete who exercises in a warm environment is susceptible to heat injury, but the increasing popularity of road racing has generated concern for runners who are not prepared for strenuous exercise in the heat, or who participate in races that are poorly organized in regard to preventing and treating heat injuries. Marathon running is becoming increasingly popular, with some major races having tens of thousands of runners. Even well-organized events may experience problems in providing for the needs of runners when the environmental heat stress becomes excessive, as occurred recently during an unexpected heat wave in races that normally have cooler weather.

The individual who exercises unwisely under conditions of environmental heat stress may experience one or several of a variety of heat injuries. Three factors may contribute to these injuries: increased core temperature, loss of body fluids, and loss of electrolytes. However, other factors may also be involved, as Noakes noted that several of the heat illnesses, such as muscle cramps, also occur during exercise in cold environments.

Figure 9.11 represents a simple flow chart of heat disorders. When a combination of exercise and environmental heat stress is imposed on the body, vasodilation and sweating increase as the body tries to cool itself. When these two adjustments begin to falter, problems develop. In essence, the circulation is attempting to regulate both body temperature and blood pressure at the same time, and when stressed excessively, control of blood pressure wins and body temperature regulation is impaired. In addition, if the exercise metabolic load is very great, heat injuries may develop independent of circulatory and sweating inadequacies. In their 2011 review, Sawka and others describe a pathological pathway of heat stress, beginning with lack of gut blood flow and resulting in cell necrosis; the release of endotoxins and mitochondrial DNA fragments; and cascade of vascular and immunological pathologies that result in multi-organ failure and damage.

Heat Syncope Excessive vasodilation may contribute to circulatory instability. The blood vessels expand and have a much greater capacity. Owing to a decreased relative blood volume, cardiac output may decrease and the blood pressure will fall, reducing blood flow to the brain. Dizziness and fainting may occur. This condition is called **heat syncope** and is usually associated with heat exhaustion, as discussed later; a newer term, **exercise-associated collapse,** has been introduced, of which simple fainting may be a mild form, whereas more severe forms may include heat stroke or hyponatremia.

Kenefick and Sawka also note that fainting after a race may be due to the reduced muscle pump activity. When the runner stops, venous pooling in the legs may reduce blood return to the heart and, subsequently, to the brain. Runners are advised to keep the legs moving at the completion of the race. If dizzy, lie down with feet elevated.

Heat Cramps The ACSM indicates that exercise-associated muscle cramping can occur with exhaustive work in any temperature

TABLE 9.8   American College of Sports Medicine guidelines for modifying or canceling competition or training to help prevent heat illness

WBGT (°F)	WBGT (°C)	Continuous activity and competition	Training and noncontinuous activity
<50–65	(10–18.3)	Generally safe	Normal activity
65.1–72.0	(18.4–22.2)	Risk of heat illness begins to rise *High-risk:* Should be monitored or not compete	*Low-risk:* Normal activity *High-risk:* Increase rest: exercise ratio and monitor fluid intake
72.1–78.0	(22.3–25.6)	Risk for all competitors is increased	*Low-risk:* Normal activity and monitor fluid intake *High-risk:* Increase the rest: exercise ratio and decrease total duration of activity
78.1–82.0	(25.7–27.8)	*High-risk:* Risk is high	*Low-risk:* Normal activity and monitor fluid intake *High-risk:* Increase the rest: exercise ratio and decrease intensity and total duration of activity
82.1–86.0	(27.9–30.0)	Cancel for those at risk of exertional heat stroke	*Low-risk:* Plan intense or prolonged exercise with discretion* *High-risk:* Increase the rest:exercise ratio to 1:1 and decrease intensity and total duration of activity*
86.1–90.0	(30.1–32.2)		*Low-risk:* Limit intense exercise and total daily exposure to heat and humidity *High-risk:* Cancel or stop practice and competition
>90	(>32.3)		Cancel exercise when uncompensable heat stress exists for all athletes*

Low-risk: Individuals acclimatized to the heat for 3 weeks; high fitness level.
High-risk: Individuals nonacclimatized to the heat; unfit; using certain medications; dehydrated; recent illness; previous heat illness, particularly exertional heat stroke.
*Differences of local climate and individual heat acclimatization status may allow activity at higher levels than outlined in the table. Athletes and coaches should consult with sports medicine staff and be cautious when exercising in extreme heat conditions.
The WBGT is the wet-bulb globe thermometer temperature. Commercial devices are available to quickly and accurately measure the WBGT and should be used to help assess environmental heat stress and modify training or competition as recommended. For those who wish to construct an inexpensive WBGT device, consult the reference cited by Spickard at the end of this chapter.

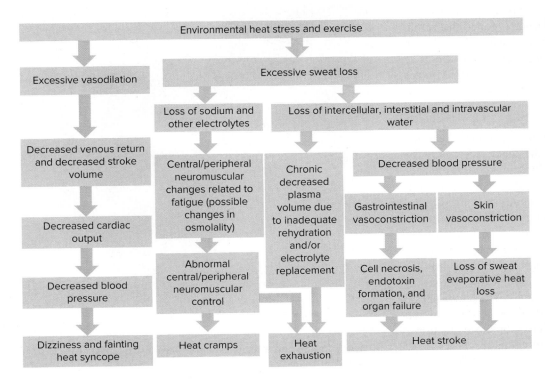

FIGURE 9.11 Basic flow chart for heat illnesses. The combination of environmental heat and exercise may cause an excessive vasodilation or pooling of blood. These conditions may decrease blood return to the heart and brain, causing dizziness and fainting. Excessive loss of sweat may cause significant losses of body water and electrolytes, leading to various heat illnesses. See text for details.

range but appears to be more prevalent in hot and humid conditions (**heat cramps**). As discussed in a review by Minetto and colleagues, a plausible mechanism for cramp formation, first postulated by Schwellnus, is spinal-mediated hyperexcitability of motor neurons resulting from fatigue or other changes in afferent input. Possibly normal neural activity is disturbed by an electrolyte imbalance.

Conversely, Eichner notes that although not all cramps are alike, he indicates three lines of evidence suggesting that heat cramping is caused by "salty sweating," specifically by the triad of salt loss, fluid loss, and muscle fatigue. First, historically, heat cramping in industrial workers is alleviated by salt. Second, field studies of athletes show that heat-crampers tend to be salty sweaters. Stofan and others reported that American football players who were prone to muscle cramps averaged more than twice the amount of sodium loss than those not prone to cramping. Third, intravenous saline can reverse heat cramping, and more salt in the diet and in sports drinks can help prevent heat cramping. Eichner concludes that for heat cramping, the solution is saline.

To help prevent cramps, Bergeron recommends that at the first sign of subtle muscle twitching, which usually is about 20–30 minutes before full-blown cramps, the athlete should consume a salt solution, such as half a teaspoon of salt in 16 ounces of a sports drink. The athlete should then continue to drink small amounts of a similar solution (the same amount of salt in 32 ounces of a sports drink) at regular intervals for the remainder of the exercise session. Several case studies with tennis players who consistently experienced heat cramps have shown that increased intake of either sodium or magnesium, along with adequate fluids, was effective in preventing muscle cramping during exercise.

Several electrolyte products have been developed for athletes who are prone to muscle cramps. Products such as EnduroLyte and GatorLYTES contain sodium, potassium, calcium, and magnesium, all of which may be helpful in the prevention of muscle cramping. However, Sulzer and others, studying triathletes who were either prone to muscle cramping or not, reported that serum electrolytes (sodium, chloride, potassium, and magnesium) did not appear to be associated with muscle cramps. The cause of muscle cramping still remains a mystery. Nevertheless, the ACSM notes that muscle cramping usually responds to rest and replacement of fluid and salt (sodium).

Heat Exhaustion   **Heat exhaustion** is a common heat illness during exercise. Dehydration is the main risk factor for exercise-associated heat exhaustion. Inadequate salt replacement over the course of several days may also be a contributing factor, as blood volume may decrease. A high body mass index (BMI) also increases the risk. Heat exhaustion is a cause of heat syncope. Fatigue and weakness are key signs of heat exhaustion, which may be associated with dizziness and fainting; other signs and symptoms include rapid pulse, headache, nausea, vomiting, unsteady walk, muscle cramps, chills or goose bumps. The rectal temperature is usually less than 104°F (40°C), which the ACSM notes may be the only discernable difference between severe heat exhaustion and exertional heat stroke in on-site evaluations. Heat exhaustion may incapacitate the individual for a few hours but will generally resolve with body cooling and fluid intake.

Heat Stroke   **Heat stroke** may occur under heat stress conditions even when resting, particularly in older individuals. When heat stroke occurs during exercise, it is known as **exertional heat stroke**, as illustrated in figure 9.12. The ACSM indicates that exertional heat stroke can affect seemingly healthy athletes even when the environment is relatively cool. However, it occurs more during exercise in heat stress environments, and dehydration is a major risk factor. Along with dehydration, Eichner indicated that heat stroke in sport is caused by a combination of the following:

- Hot environment
- Strenuous exercise
- Clothing that limits evaporation of sweat
- Inadequate adaptation to the heat
- Too much body fat
- Lack of fitness

Although inconvenient, Ronneberg and others reported that rectal temperature was very effective in diagnosing hyperthermic

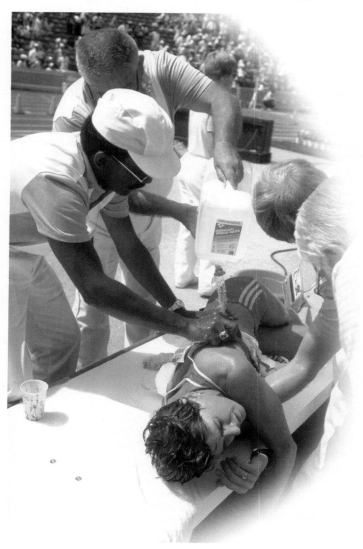

FIGURE 9.12 Proper acclimatization and adequate hydration before, during, and after competition are important factors in preventing heat illness.

runners. As reported in a review by Mazerolle and others, oral temperature is not a valid method to assess changing core temperature because differences in measurement exceeded 0.27°C (0.5°F), with even greater discrepancies at highest rectal temperatures observed in exertional heat illnesses. The ACSM defines exertional heat stroke as a rectal temperature greater than 40°C (104°F) accompanied by symptoms or signs of organ system failure, most frequently central nervous system changes such as confusion, disorientation, agitation, aggressiveness, blank stare, apathy, irrational behavior, staggering gait, delirium, convulsions, unresponsiveness, or coma. Other signs of possible heat stroke include weak and rapid pulse, vomiting, involuntary bowel movement, and hyperventilation. William Roberts, former ACSM president and medical director of the Twin Cities Marathon, stated that the skin appearance is usually ashen and sweaty, can be either warm or cool to touch, and is rarely pink, hot, and dry as described in textbooks.

Heat stroke is the most dangerous heat injury, as it may be fatal. Several deaths of professional and collegiate athletes have been associated with such circumstances, and one involved the use of ephedrine, which as noted in chapter 13 can stimulate metabolism and heat production and predispose to heat stress. Exertional heat stroke may lead to rhabdomyolysis, damaged muscle tissue that leaks its contents into the blood, eventually leading to kidney damage and possible death.

What are the symptoms and treatment of heat injuries?

As noted, the symptoms of impending heat injury are variable. Among those reported are weakness, feeling of chills, pilo-erection (goose pimples) on the chest and upper arms, tingling arms, nausea, headache, faintness, disorientation, muscle cramping, and cessation of sweating. Continuing to exercise in a warm environment when experiencing any of these symptoms may lead to heat injury. Table 9.9 presents the major heat injuries along with principal causes, clinical findings, and treatment. In general, treatment of heat syncope, heat cramps, and heat exhaustion involves resting (preferably lying down), cooling the body if overheated, and drinking fluids, preferably with sodium. Most individuals recover fairly rapidly but should be monitored until in a safe environment.

The ACSM indicates that early recognition and rapid cooling can reduce both the morbidity and mortality associated with exertional heat stroke. Casa and his associates indicate that cold-water immersion is the *gold standard* for exertional heat stroke. In the field, such as at marathon races, Roberts indicates that the optimal treatment of heat stroke is immediate, total-body cooling with ice-water tub immersion. If not available, rapidly rotating ice-water towels to the trunk, extremities, and head, combined with ice packing of the neck, axillae, and groin, may be very effective.

For collapsed athletes, Sallis indicates that it is essential to check vital signs (especially rectal temperature if heat stroke is suspected), assess fluids status (dehydrated versus fluid overload), and perform laboratory tests when needed. He notes that the most common cause of collapse is low blood pressure due to blood pooling in the legs after cessation of exercise, which is benign and resolves upon rest. However, both hyponatremia,

mentioned previously, and heat stroke are serious medical problems and require prompt medical attention. It is critical to differentiate between heat exhaustion or heat stroke and hyponatremia. Providing hypotonic fluids to individuals with hyponatremia will exacerbate the condition because they are already overhydrated.

www.acsm-msse.org For the American College of Sports Medicine position stand on heat illness during exercise and training, click on *Position Stands* on the right side of the page, then on *Exertional Heat Illness during Training and Competition.*

Do some individuals have problems tolerating exercise in the heat?

A number of predisposing factors have been associated with heat injury, including gender, level of physical fitness, age, body composition, previous history of heat injury, and degree of acclimatization.

Poor Physical Fitness One of the major factors contributing to exertional heat illness is poor physical fitness. For example, in a study of Marine Corps recruits in training, Gardner and others found that one of the major predictors of exertional heat illness was poor aerobic fitness as measured by 1.5-mile run performance. In general, the better the physical fitness, the better tolerance to a given heat stress. However, even highly trained athletes may experience heat illnesses when using unsafe training practices. NCAA Division I wrestlers have died from heat stroke or related causes in attempts to reduce body weight for competition through exercise-induced sweating in a hot environment. For example, one of the wrestlers was wearing a rubber suit while riding a stationary bicycle in a steam-filled shower.

Gender In earlier studies, investigators found that female subjects tolerated exercise in the heat less well than males. These findings may have been related to the higher percentage of body fat and the generally lower level of physical fitness of women in those studies. However, in their review, Baker and Kenney reported that when women and men are matched for fitness, acclimatization state, adiposity, and body size, there do not appear to be gender-related differences in thermoregulatory function other than a lower sweating rate in women as compared to men. They note that the latter may be a disadvantage in hot-dry environments, but an advantage in hot-humid conditions, because they are less likely to dehydrate. Previous studies have also suggested that increased progesterone levels during the luteal phase of the menstrual cycle could alter the core temperature at which sweating begins, but Baker and Kenney indicated that the menstrual cycle has minimal effects on tolerance to exercise-heat stress. They also noted that while hyponatremia occurs more in women than men, it is not because of gender but mainly behaviors associated with overconsumption of fluids.

Age Individuals at both ends of the age spectrum may have problems exercising in the heat. The American Academy of Pediatrics (AAP) recognizes that when children and adolescents are engaging in sports and physical activity in the heat, special considerations, preparations, modifications, and monitoring are

TABLE 9.9   Heat injuries: causes, clinical findings, and treatment

Heat injury	Causes	Clinical findings	Treatment*
Heat syncope (exercise-associated collapse)	Excessive vasodilation: pooling of blood in the skin	Fainting Weakness Fatigue	Place on back in cool environment; give cool fluids
Heat cramps	Excessive loss of electrolytes in sweat; inadequate salt intake	Muscle cramps	Rest in cool environment; oral ingestion of salt drinks; salt foods daily; medical treatment in severe cases
Heat exhaustion	Excessive loss of water and salt; inadequate fluid and salt intake	Fatigue Nausea Cool, pale, moist skin Weakness Dizziness Chills Rectal temperature lower than 104°F (40°C)	Rest in cool environment; replace fluids and salt by mouth; medical treatment if serious
Heat stroke (exercise-associated heat stroke)	Excessive body temperature	Headache Confusion Blank stare Disorientation Unconsciousness Rectal temperature greater than 104°F (40°C)	Cool body immediately to 102°F (38.9°C), preferably with cold-water immersion; if not, cool body areas with ice packs, ice, or cold water; give cool drinks with glucose if conscious; administer intravenous fluids if available; get medical help immediately
Hyponatremia (exercise-associated hyponatremia)	Excessive fluid intake	Confusion Lethargy Agitation Coma ** Need to determine by serum sodium level lower than 135 mmol/l	Mild cases may be treated with hypertonic fluids; more severe cases may need intravenous fluids and possible hospitalization

*Begin treatment as soon as possible. In cases of heat stroke, begin immediately.
**Symptoms of hyponatremia may be similar to other heat illnesses; determination must be made by measurement of serum sodium levels less than 135 mmol/l. Providing hypotonic fluids to individuals with hyponatremia could exacerbate the condition.

essential. In their review, Gomes and others state that young children have a lower release of catecholamines and androgens during exercise, providing a partial explanation of "sweat gland immaturity," and thus a lower sweat rate compared to adults. Lower sweat rates in children have been consistently reported in the literature and were discussed earlier in the chapter. Combined with lower body surface area to mass ratios favoring heat storage, young children are at greater risk for heat illness. However, according to the most recent policy statement from the AAP "youth do not have less effective thermoregulatory ability, insufficient cardiovascular capacity or lower physical exertion tolerance compared with adults during exercise in the heat when adequate hydration is maintained." The American College of Sports Medicine, in a consensus statement, indicated that sports such as youth football may pose increased risks. Using 2005/06 to 2010/11 data from the National High School Sports-related Injury Surveillance System, Kerr and others reported an incidence rate of exertional heat illness of 1.2 per 100,000 athlete exposures, affecting approximately 9,000 annually. The rate for football players was 11.4 times that of all other sports combined. The AAP recently outlined new recommendations for preventing heat illnesses in children, which are

in accord with the recommendations provided in the next section. The ACSM also developed some guidelines that may be used to restrain physical activities for children under conditions of heat stress, which are presented in table 9.10.

At high levels of heat stress, tolerance to the heat is decreased in older individuals, possibly because they experience decreased blood flow to the skin and sweat less. Reduced heat toleration in the elderly may also be related to fitness levels. However, more and more people have become and remain physically active throughout middle age and advanced years. Larry Kenney, an expert in temperature regulation at Penn State University, has studied thermoregulation in the elderly. In a review, Baker and Kenney note that well-trained and heat-acclimated older athletes' regulation of body temperature is comparable to that of younger athletes. They also indicate that for healthy older men and women who maintain a high degree of aerobic fitness, the risk of heat-related illness is not significantly greater than that of young adults. However, they do report a decreased thirst sensation when exercising and therefore a need to focus on consuming adequate fluid intake when exercising in the heat. Sports drinks may help. Baker found that when exercising intermittently in the heat, older men

TABLE 9.10 WBGT temperature guidelines to modify practice sessions for exercising children

WBGT (°F)	WBGT (°C)	Restraints on activities
<75.0	<24.0	All activities allowed, but watch for symptoms of heat illnesses in prolonged events
75.0–78.6	24.0–25.9	Have longer rest periods in the shade; enforce fluid intake every 15 minutes
79.0–84.0	26.0–29.0	Stop activity for unacclimatized and high-risk children; limit activities of others; cancel long-distance races and cut the duration of other activities
>85.0	>29.0	Cancel all athletic activities

Modifications of the recommendations on climatic heat stress in exercising children and adolescents proposed by the American Academy of Pediatrics Committee on Sports Medicine and Fitness.

and women consumed adequate fluids to rehydrate and consumed more when sports drinks were available compared to water.

Obesity Obese individuals not only have high amounts of body fat to deter heat losses but also generate more heat during exercise because of a low level of fitness; thus, they are more susceptible to heat injuries. In the Marine Corps study cited previously, another major predictor of exertional heat illness was a higher body weight in relation to height.

Previous Heat Illness Individuals who have experienced previous heat injury may be less tolerant of exercise in the heat. Many individuals do regain heat tolerance 8–12 weeks after heat injury. Others lose some of the ability for the circulatory system to adjust to heat stress, possibly because temperature-regulating centers in the brain are irreversibly damaged. The transfer of heat from the core to the skin becomes impaired and the body temperature rises faster.

Acclimatization One of the more important factors determining an individual's response to exercise in the heat is degree of acclimatization, which is discussed on the following pages. Although some individuals may be susceptible to heat illnesses, all individuals who exercise under warm or hot environmental conditions may benefit from the following recommendations.

How can I reduce the hazards associated with exercise in a hot environment?

In his review, Eichner indicated that the best treatment for heat illness is prevention. The following list represents a number of guidelines which, if followed, will reduce considerably your chances of suffering heat injury.

1. Check the temperature and humidity conditions before exercising. Even if the dry temperature is only 65–75°F, high humidity will increase the heat stress. Warm, humid conditions cause fatigue sooner, so slow your pace or shorten your exercise session. As noted previously, local news stations and several Websites may provide information on heat stress conditions.
2. Exercise in the cool of the morning or evening to avoid the heat of the day.
3. Exercise in the shade, if possible, to avoid radiation from the sun. If you run in the sun, wear an appropriate sunscreen to prevent sun damage to the skin.
4. Wear sports clothing designed for exercise in the heat, such as CoolMax-type material. Clothing should be loose to allow air circulation, white or a light color to reflect radiant heat, and porous to permit evaporation. Do not wear a hat if running in the shade, but wear a loose hat if running in the sun.
5. If you are running and there is a breeze, plan your route so that you are running into the wind during the last part of your run. The breeze will help cool you more effectively at the time you need it most.
6. Hyperhydrate if you plan to perform prolonged, strenuous exercise in the heat. In general, drink about 16 ounces of fluid 30–60 minutes prior to exercising.
7. Drink cold fluids periodically. For a long training run, plan your route so that it passes some watering holes, such as gas stations or other sources of water. Alternatively, you may purchase a water-bottle belt or backpack that will help you carry your own water supply. Take frequent water breaks, consuming about 6–8 ounces of water every 15 minutes or so. As a rough gauge, one mouthful of water is approximately 1 ounce of fluid.
8. Replenish your water daily. Keep a record of your body weight. For each pound you lose, drink about 20–24 ounces of fluid. Your body weight should be back to normal before your next workout.
9. Replenish lost electrolytes (salt) if you have sweated excessively. Put a little extra salt on your meals and eat foods high in potassium, such as bananas and citrus fruits.
10. Avoid excessive intake of protein, as extra heat is produced in the body when protein is metabolized. This may contribute slightly to the heat stress.
11. Avoid dietary supplements containing ephedrine. Ephedrine is a potent stimulant that can increase metabolism and heat production, leading to an increased body temperature during exercise in warm environmental conditions and predisposing to heat illness.
12. If you drink caffeinated beverages, check your responses. Current research indicates that caffeinated beverages may not affect hydration status or temperature regulation during exercise. However, some individuals may respond differently to caffeine intake. Caffeine can increase heat production at rest, which could raise the body temperature before exercise.
13. Because alcohol is a diuretic, excess amounts should be avoided the night before competition or prolonged exercise in the heat.
14. If you are sedentary, overweight, or aged, you are less likely to tolerate exercise in the heat and should therefore use extra caution.

15. Be aware of the signs and symptoms of heat exhaustion and heat stroke, as well as the treatment for each. Chills, goose pimples, tingling arms, dizziness, weakness, fatigue, mental disorientation, nausea, and headaches are some symptoms that may signify the onset of heat illness. Stop activity, get to a cool place, and consume some cool fluids.

16. Do not exercise if you have been ill or have had a fever within the last few days.

17. Check your medications. Some medications, such as antihistamines used to treat cold symptoms, may block sweat production. Drugs used to treat high blood pressure, such as beta-blockers and calcium-channel blockers, may impair skin blood flow and decrease heat loss from the body.

18. If you plan to compete in a sport held under hot environmental conditions, you must become acclimatized to exercise in the heat.

> **www.gssiweb.com** The Gatorade Sports Science Institute (GSSI) provides very useful information on a wide variety of topics in sports nutrition, especially information relative to proper hydration practices to help enhance performance and prevent heat illness when exercising in the heat. Under the Sport Science Exchange tab, relevant information can be located under the Thermoregulation, Heat, Hyponatremia,, and Hydration options.

How can I become acclimatized to exercise in the heat?

It is a well-established fact that **acclimatization** to the heat will help increase performance in warm environments as compared with an unacclimatized state. Simply living in a hot environment confers a small amount of acclimatization. Physical training, in and of itself, provides a significant amount of acclimatization, possibly up to 50 percent of that which can be expected and increases body-water levels. However, neither of these two adjustments, either singly or together, can prevent the deterioration of exercise performance in the heat by an unacclimatized individual. Thus, a period of active acclimatization is necessary to optimize performance when exercising in the heat.

The technique of acclimatization is relatively simple. Simply cut back on the intensity or duration of your normal activity when the hot weather begins. Do not avoid exercise in the heat completely, but after an initial reduction in your activity level, increase it gradually. For example, if you were running 5 miles a day, cut your distance back to 2 to 3 miles in the heat; if you need to do 5 a day, do the remaining miles in the evening. Eventually build up to 3, 4, and 5 miles. As illustrated in figure 9.13, the acclimatization process usually takes about 10 to 14 days to complete. Bar-Or notes that heat acclimatization in children takes several weeks. However, even when acclimatized, an athlete's endurance capacity in the heat, particularly with high humidity, still will be less than under cooler conditions.

If you live in a cool climate, like New England, and want to compete in a marathon in Florida in January, how do you become acclimatized? Exercising indoors at a warmer temperature will help.

Extra layers of clothes can help prevent evaporation and build a hot, humid microclimate around your body. Research has shown that this technique can provide a degree of acclimatization. However, this is advisable only in cool weather and should not be attempted under hot conditions. Wearing a sweat suit or rubberized suit while exercising in the heat may precipitate heat illness. Moreover, even in a cool environment this technique may cause heat injury. Again, be wary of the symptoms of impending heat illness.

Repeated exposure to a high core temperature during exercise helps the body make the following important adjustments during acclimatization to the heat. Here are some of the benefits of heat acclimatization that will help improve performance and reduce the risk of heat stroke and heat exhaustion.

1. Total body water increases considerably, which usually includes increased plasma volume. Blood vessels may conserve more sodium, which tends to hold plasma water. This occurs because the blood vessels conserve more protein and sodium, which tend to hold water.

2. The increased blood volume allows the heart to pump more blood per beat, so the stress on the heart is reduced.

3. When volume increases, more blood flows to the muscles and skin. The muscles receive more oxygen and skin cooling increases, improving endurance performance.

4. Less muscle glycogen may be used as an energy source at a given rate of exercise, sparing this energy source in endurance events.

5. The sweat glands hypertrophy and secrete about 30 percent more sweat, allowing for greater evaporative heat loss.

6. Body salt losses decrease. The amount of salt in the sweat decreases considerably; evaporation becomes more efficient and electrolytes are conserved. Sweat losses of calcium, magnesium, copper, zinc, and iron also decrease with acclimatization.

7. Sweating starts at a lower core temperature, leading to earlier cooling.

8. The core temperature will not rise as high or as rapidly as in the unacclimatized state.

9. The psychological feeling of stress is reduced at a given exercise rate.

In essence, as illustrated in figure 9.13, these changes increase the ability of the body to dissipate heat with less stress on the cardiovascular system. The end result is a more effective body-temperature control and improved performance when exercising in the heat. These adaptations may be maintained by exercising in the heat several days per week but are lost in about 7–10 days in a cool environment. If you are interested in learning more about acclimatization, consult the reviews by Sawka and others, Cheuvront and others, Goulet, and Stachenfeld.

Key Concepts

▶ Heat injuries, of which heat stroke is potentially the most dangerous, may be due to increased body core temperature, loss of body fluids, or loss of electrolytes. Some individuals, such as the obese, are more susceptible to heat injury.

- The general treatment for heat-stress illnesses is to rest, drink cool liquids, and cool the body. Rapid body cooling is essential in cases of heat stroke.
- If you exercise in the heat, you should be aware of signs of impending heat injury, such as chills, dizziness, and weakness. You should also be aware of methods to reduce heat gain to the body and methods to facilitate heat loss.
- Acclimatization to exercise in the heat takes about 10–14 days, but endurance capacity in the heat is still limited somewhat even when one is fully acclimated.

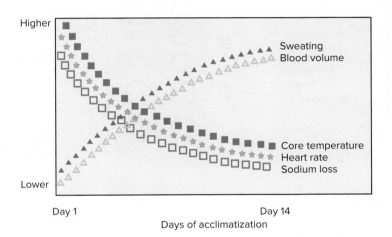

FIGURE 9.13 Changes with acclimatization. Acclimatization to the heat for 7 to 14 days will lead to an increase in the blood volume and the ability to sweat. For a standardized exercise task in the heat, these changes will lead to a lower heart rate, less sodium loss, and a lower core temperature. These changes will lead to improved exercise performance in the heat.

Health Aspects: High Blood Pressure

What is high blood pressure, or hypertension?

Arterial blood pressure is the product of cardiac output (flow) and the resistance to blood flow, or total peripheral resistance. It is the force that is exerted by the blood against the arterial wall. Blood pressure is an important variable in physiology and overall health. Blood pressure is usually measured by a sphygmomanometer, which records the pressure in millimeters of mercury (mmHg) (see figure 9.14). Blood pressure is variable relative to the working and resting phases of the cardiac cycle. Blood pressure readings are given in two numbers. The higher number (e.g., 120 mmHg) represents the *systolic* phase, when the heart is pumping blood through the arteries. The lower number (e.g., 80 mmHg) represents the *diastolic* phase, when the heart is resting between beats and blood is flowing back into it. A blood pressure measurement of 120/80 mmHg would be considered "normal" blood pressure, or "normotensive."

High blood pressure, also known as **hypertension** (hyper = high; tension = pressure), is known as a silent disease. According to the World Health Organization, over 1 billion people are hypertensive, with a prevalence rate of 40 percent for adults ≥25 years of age. In a 2013 American Heart Association report, Go and others reported that 78 million U.S. adults ≥20 years of age are hypertensive. Only 82 percent of hypertensive adults are aware they are hypertensive, mainly because there no outstanding symptoms. Surprisingly, Hansen and others estimated that about 2 million American youths have high blood pressure, which they associated with rising levels of obesity in children. Aglony and others estimate that approximately 75 percent of the cases of hypertension and 90 percent of the prehypertensive cases in children and adolescents are not yet diagnosed. Some general symptoms include headaches, dizziness, and fatigue, but because they can be caused by a multitude of other factors, they may not be recognized as symptoms of high blood pressure. Although a great deal of research about the cause of high blood pressure has been conducted, the exact cause is unknown in about 90 percent of all cases. In these cases, the condition is known as **essential hypertension**, which cannot be cured. According to Go and others, only 53 percent of hypertensive individuals have their blood pressure under complete control.

High blood pressure is dangerous for several reasons. The heart must work much harder to pump the extra blood volume or to overcome the peripheral vascular resistance. This normally leads to an enlarged heart. Over time the increase in heart size becomes excessive and the efficiency of the heart actually decreases, making it more prone to a heart attack. Second, high blood pressure may directly damage the arterial walls. It is thought to be a major contributing factor in the development of atherosclerosis and a predisposing factor to coronary disease and stroke. High blood pressure is itself a disease and is involved in the etiology of other diseases. It is one of the primary risk factors for heart disease and stroke.

The National Research Council has noted that any definition of high blood pressure is arbitrary. Traditionally, physicians have used elevations in diastolic blood pressure as the basis for their diagnosis, but the Joint National Committee on Detection, Evaluation, and Treatment of High Blood Pressure (JNCDET) of the National Institutes of Health, in its classification of blood pressure for adults age 18 years and older, includes both systolic and diastolic pressures. The classification system is presented in table 9.11.

http://www.heart.org/beatyourrisk/en_US/hbpRiskCalc.html Consult the American Heart Association Website for your personal risk factor assessment for high blood pressure.

How is high blood pressure treated?

Although essential hypertension is incurable, Israili and others suggest that gene therapy or the use of vaccines may be feasible to prevent its development but are not likely to be available in the near future. Currently, many individuals with essential hypertension need to take medications to control their blood pressure.

1. No sound is heard because there is no blood flow when the cuff pressure is high enough to keep the brachial artery closed.

2. **Systolic pressure** is the pressure at which a Korotkoff sound is first heard. When cuff pressure decreases and is no longer able to keep the brachial artery closed during systole, blood is pushed through the partially opened brachial artery to produce turbulent blood flow and a sound. The brachial artery remains closed during diastole.

3. As cuff pressure continues to decrease, the brachial artery opens even more during systole. At first, the artery is closed during diastole, but, as cuff pressure continues to decrease, the brachial artery partially opens during diastole. Turbulent blood flow during systole produces Korotkoff sounds, although the pitch of the sounds changes as the artery becomes more open.

4. **Diastolic pressure** is the pressure at which the sound disappears. Eventually, cuff pressure decreases below the pressure in the brachial artery and it remains open during systole and diastole. Nonturbulent flow is reestablished and no sounds are heard.

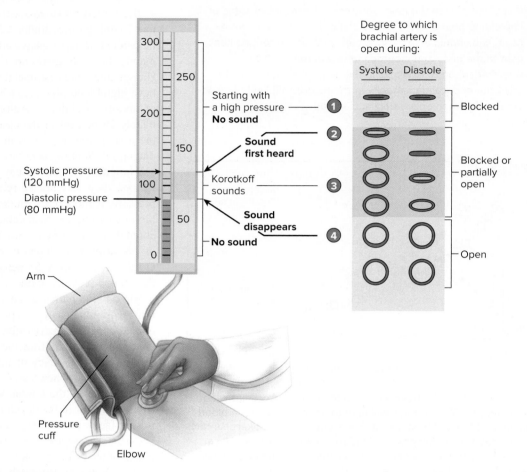

FIGURE 9.14 Blood pressure measurement.

TABLE 9.11	Classification of blood pressure for adults age 18 years and older	
Category	**Systolic (mmHg)**	**Diastolic (mmHg)**
Normal	<120	<80
Prehypertension	120–139	80–89
Hypertension		
Stage 1	140–159	90–99
Stage 2	>160	>100

Source: National Heart, Lung, and Blood Institute.

A variety of drugs are available to treat hypertension, including diuretics, beta-blockers, angiotensin-converting enzyme (ACE) inhibitors, and calcium-channel blockers. If your blood pressure is elevated, you and your doctor need to take aggressive action. If drug therapy is recommended, you may need to experiment, with your physician, as to type and dose of medicine to use. This is especially important for athletic individuals. Oliveira and Lawless suggest using drugs that are less likely to have adverse effects on exercise performance. For example, diuretics and beta-blockers may impair aerobic endurance performance. Physicians should also be aware that use of beta-blockers is prohibited for competition in some sports. The 2004 American College of Sports Medicine position stand on exercise and hypertension suggests angiotensin-converting enzyme (ACE) inhibitors, angiotensin II receptor blockers, or calcium-channel blockers as antihypertensive medications with the lowest adverse impact on exercise capacity.

Other than impairment of aerobic endurance capacity, blood pressure drugs may cause other adverse health effects. Thus, a nonpharmacological approach is often a first choice of treatment in cases of mild to moderate hypertension. The Canadian Hypertension Education Program emphasizes the point that lifestyle modifications are the cornerstone of antihypertensive therapy.

What dietary modifications may help reduce or prevent hypertension?

How much and what you eat may influence your blood pressure. The following are the key points to help reduce or prevent hypertension.

1. *Achieve and maintain a healthy body weight.* Numerous studies have shown that reducing body weight, even as little as 10 pounds, will reduce blood pressure in overweight, hypertensive individuals. Maintaining a healthy body weight may be one of the most effective preventive measures. Thus, restriction of caloric intake to either lose or maintain body weight may be a helpful dietary strategy. According to a review by Savica and others, obesity in adolescents seems to increase the sensitivity of blood pressure to salt intake. However, weight loss appears to decrease the sensitivity to salt in this younger population. Healthful methods of losing excess body fat are presented in chapter 11.

2. *Reduce or moderate sodium intake.* This remains one of the most controversial recommendations, but it may be a prudent behavior for most individuals. A recent review of the dietary sodium literature by the Institute of Medicine (IOM) and a 2014 meta-analysis offer support for Alderman's opinion that the available data provide no support for any universal recommendation for a particular level of sodium intake. The IOM report stated there was insufficient evidence to conclude that dietary sodium intake of <2,300 mg/day either increases or decreases disease risk. In their meta-analysis, Graudal and others reported a U-shaped association between sodium intake and all-cause and cardiovascular disease mortality, with a lower mortality in "low-usual" (115–165 mmol/day = 2,645–3,795 mg/day) and "high-usual" sodium intake 166–215 mmol/day = 3,818–4,945 mg/day) compared to low (<115 mmol/day) and high sodium intake (>215 mmol/day). The IOM reported considerable methodological variations in the literature regarding the measurement of sodium intake or estimation from urinary excretion, which make it difficult to compare studies. Graudal's meta-analysis did not include any randomized, controlled trials.

In contrast, others recommend a significant reduction in current sodium intake in industrialized and developing societies. Powles and others reported 2010 global mean per capita sodium intake, estimated through urinary excretion, at 3.95 g/day, almost twice the World Health Organization recommendation of 2.0 g/day. Cappuccio has noted that most prospective studies have shown that higher salt intake predicts the incidence of cardiovascular events, but the lack of large and long, randomized trials on the effects of salt reduction has encouraged some people to argue against a policy of salt reduction in populations. However, Cook and others conducted such a study, the long-term Trials of Hypertension Prevention (TOHP) study. Adults with prehypertension reduced sodium intake by about 800 to 1,000 milligrams daily for 18 months and up to 4 years. In a follow-up assessment of 10–15 years, the sodium reduction resulted in a 25 percent lower risk of experiencing a cardiovascular event, such as a heart attack, stroke, or cardiovascular death. The investigators concluded that sodium reduction, previously shown to lower blood pressure, may also reduce long-term risk of cardiovascular events. Using three modeling approaches over 10 years involving, respectively, a gradual 40 percent reduction in sodium intake, an immediate 40 percent reduction to a population mean intake of 2,200 mg/day, and an immediate decrease in mean intake to 1,500 mg/day, Coxson and others projected that 28,000–500,000 deaths might be averted. He and others attributed significant decreases in stroke and ischemic heart disease mortality, decreased blood pressure, and decreased serum cholesterol in part to a 1.4 g/day decrease in sodium intake in England from 2003 to 2011.

Most health governmental agencies and professional groups promote dietary sodium restriction. Penner and others noted that one in four Canadians have hypertension, and with the lifetime risk of developing hypertension being more than 90 percent in an average life span, the need for a population-based approach to reducing hypertension is clear. Thus, the 2010 Canadian Hypertension Education Program, as documented by Hackman and others, recommended restricting sodium intake to 1,500 milligrams/day for adults younger than 50 years of age, to 1,300 milligrams/day for adults 51–70 years of age, and to 1,200 milligrams/day for adults older than 70 years of age. The AI for Americans is 1,500 milligrams/day, whereas the UL is 2,300 milligrams/day. The American Medical Association (AMA) has developed a campaign to reduce sodium intake nationwide. The AMA has urged the FDA to remove salt from the GRAS (generally recognized as safe) list and require high-salt foods to carry a distinctive label, such as pictures of salt shakers bearing the word *High.* Although some question the wisdom in recommending salt restriction in all individuals, many health professionals suggest that this is a good policy.

An effort by most normotensive individuals to reduce salt intake is seen by many experts as good public health policy. Although most individuals possess physiological control systems that effectively maintain a proper balance of sodium in the body, many individuals are sodium-sensitive and their blood pressure may increase with excessive consumption of salt. Sodium may accumulate in the body, possibly due to a defect in aldosterone-mediated excretion, and hold fluids, particularly blood, which could increase blood pressure. In their review, McCarron and Reusser report that salt sensitivity is present in about 30 percent of normotensive and 50 percent of hypertensive persons and is more prevalent among African-Americans and older individuals. As discussed in a review by Richardson and others, low renin-aldosterone response, reduced potassium intake, and other humoral and genetic perturbations may predispose certain individuals (e.g., non-Hispanic blacks and Hispanics) to salt sensitivity, requiring individualized dietary and pharmacological intervention. Franco and Oparil also note that salt sensitivity in both normotensive and hypertensive persons has been associated with increased cardiovascular disease events. That being so, and because many individuals do not know their blood pressure, millions of Americans may benefit from the recommendation to moderate salt intake. Moreover, the American Institute for Cancer Research report on nutrition and cancer indicates that high salt intake may damage the stomach lining and may have a synergistic interaction with gastric carcinogens. The research panel concluded that salted and salty foods are a probable cause of stomach cancer.

The current prudent medical recommendation for dietary prevention or treatment of hypertension is to decrease sodium consumption simply by eating a wide variety of foods in their natural state. Avoid highly salted foods, restrict intake of processed foods, and hide your salt shakers. The recommended upper limit is somewhat less than 6 grams of salt per day, just a little over 1 teaspoon, the equivalent of about 2.3 grams of sodium. The AI, based on potential healthful effects on blood pressure, is only 1.5 grams, or less than 4 grams of salt daily. Individuals who sweat during training most likely do not need to be concerned with the sodium content in sports drinks. Over the course of a month, Roberts reported no change in blood pressure in normotensive individuals who worked strenuously outside and consumed about 4.5 liters of a typical CES daily.

It should be noted that decreasing salt and sodium intake poses some practical difficulties. Most salt we eat comes from the packaged foods we buy. Even minimally processed foods, such as milk and bread, may contain significant amounts of sodium. Salt is also high in most restaurant foods; some single servings of fast food have more than 1,000 milligrams of sodium, some up to nearly 5,000 milligrams. Thus, one might have to buy most foods in their natural state and prepare and cook them at home, from scratch. For those with hypertension, it may be a challenge—but worth it.

3. *Consume a diet rich in fruits, vegetables, and low-fat, protein-rich foods and with reduced saturated and total fat.* McCarron and Reusser note that large-scale studies have shown that whereas manipulation of single nutrients may have beneficial health effects for some individuals, it is improving the total dietary profile that will consistently provide health benefits, such as reducing high blood pressure. The **DASH** (Dietary Approaches to Stop Hypertension) **diet** emphasizes fruits and vegetables, nuts, low-fat dairy foods, fish, and chicken instead of red meat, low-sugar and low-refined carbohydrate foods, and reduced saturated and total fat. The DASH eating plan for a 2,000-Calorie diet is presented in table 9.12. The number of servings may be modified to meet other caloric requirements. The DASH diet is rich in potassium, magnesium, calcium, and fiber, which have been suggested to help prevent high blood pressure. The JNCDET, in its seventh report, particularly recommends increased consumption of potassium, which is abundant in fruits and vegetables. According to Brill, foods that are high in potassium (e.g., raisins); nitrates, which are converted to nitrous oxide, a vasodilator (e.g., beets); omega-3 fatty acids and magnesium (e.g., walnuts); and low-fat fluid dairy products can help lower blood pressure.

www.nhlbi.nih.gov For a detailed DASH eating plan, visit this Website and type DASH Eating Plan in the search box. This site also provides other detailed information on high blood pressure.

As noted in earlier chapters, Appel and others modified the DASH diet by replacing about 10 percent of the DASH's carbohydrates (mostly desserts and fruits) with either *good* proteins (fish, poultry, beans, tofu) or *good* fats (olive oil, canola oil, nuts). They found that such replacements resulted in additional decreases in blood pressure, and they called it the OmniHeart diet. However, in a meta-analysis of randomized, controlled trials, Shah and others concluded that although diets rich in carbohydrate may be associated with slightly higher blood pressure than diets rich in monounsaturated fat, the magnitude of the difference may not justify making recommendations to alter the carbohydrate and monounsaturated fat content of the diet to manage blood pressure. In a prospective study, Chen and others found that a reduction in sugar-sweetened beverage intake over an 18-month period resulted in reductions in both systolic and diastolic blood pressures. A reduction in sugar-sweetened beverage intake is one of the goals of the *Dietary Guidelines for Americans 2010*.

Both the DASH and OmniHeart diets are based on healthy concepts, being rich in fruits and vegetables, healthy protein, and phytonutrients and low in bad fats, sweets, and salt. Both diet plans may help reduce blood pressure and help reduce the risks of other risk factors associated with heart disease and stroke. For example, Azadbakht and others indicated that the DASH diet can likely produce multiple health benefits other than reduced blood pressure, including higher HDL-cholesterol and lower triglycerides, fasting blood glucose, and body weight. In a prospective, cohort study, Fung and others assessed the association between adherence to a DASH-style diet and risk of coronary heart disease (CHD) and stroke in middle-aged women. They found, over the course of 24 years, that adherence to a DASH-style diet was associated with a lower risk of CHD and stroke.

For those with hypertension, and even normotensive individuals, some health professionals recommend the DASH or OmniHeart diet and the extra effort to cut back to 1,500 milligrams of sodium per day. In a randomized, controlled trial, Sacks and others found that the DASH diet for 30 days resulted in significant reductions in both systolic and diastolic blood pressure. All individuals in this study were also randomly assigned to three different levels of salt intake for a 30-day period, and the decrease in blood pressure was greatest when subjects consumed the diet with the lowest amount of salt, only 1,500 milligrams per day.

4. *Moderate alcohol consumption.* As noted in chapter 4, and discussed extensively in chapter 13 moderate alcohol consumption may actually confer some health benefits, particularly the prevention of cardiovascular disease. However, excess alcohol intake may increase the heart disease risk, possibly because it is linked to high blood pressure.

TABLE 9.12   The DASH eating plan

Food group	Servings	Serving sizes	Examples and notes	Significance to the DASH eating plan
Grains	6–7 per day	1 slice bread 1 oz dry cereal ½ cup cooked rice, pasta, or cereal	Whole wheat bread, English muffin, pita bread, bagel, cereals, oatmeal, unsalted pretzels, popcorn	Major sources of energy and fiber
Vegetables	4–5 per day	1 cup raw leafy vegetable ½ cup cooked vegetable ½ cup vegetable juice	Tomatoes, potatoes, carrots, green peas, broccoli, kale, spinach, lima beans, sweet potatoes	Rich sources of potassium, magnesium, and fiber
Fruits	4–5 per day	½ cup fruit juice 1 medium fruit ¼ cup dried fruit	Apricots, bananas, dates, grapes, oranges, orange juice, melons, peaches pineapples, raisins, strawberries	Important sources of potassium, magnesium, and fiber
Low-fat or fat-free dairy foods	2–3 per day	1 cup milk 1 cup yogurt 1½ oz cheese	Fat-free (skim) milk, fat-free or low-fat regular or frozen yogurt, low-fat and fat-free cheese	Major sources of calcium and protein
Lean meats, poultry, and fish	6 or less per day	1 oz cooked meats, poultry, or fish 1 egg	Select only lean; trim away visible fats; broil, roast, or boil, instead of frying; remove skin from poultry	Rich sources of protein and magnesium
Nuts, seeds, and dry beans	4–5 per week	⅓ cup or 1½ oz nuts 2 Tbsp or ½ oz seeds ½ cup cooked dry beans or peas 2 Tbsp peanut butter	Almonds, mixed nuts, peanuts, walnuts, sunflower seeds, kidney beans	Rich sources of energy, magnesium, potassium, protein, and fiber
Fats and oils	2–3 per day	1 tsp soft margarine 1 Tbsp low-fat mayonnaise 2 Tbsp light salad dressing 1 tsp vegetable oil	Soft margarine, low-fat mayonnaise, light salad dressing, vegetable oil (olive, corn, canola)	DASH has 27 percent of Calories as fat, including fat in or added to foods 1 Tbsp fat-free dressing equals 0 servings
Sweets and added sugars	5 or less per week	1 Tbsp sugar 1 Tbsp jelly or jam ½ cup sorbet, gelatin 1 cup lemonade	Sugar, jelly, jam, jelly beans, hard candy, sorbet, ices	

Adapted from The DASH Eating Plan. National Heart, Lung, and Blood Institute. For more details, go to www.nhlbi.nih.gov/health/public/heart/hbp/dash/new_dash.pdf.

5. *Be cautious with dietary supplements.* Haddy and others report that potassium serves as a vasodilating substance, and they indicate that potassium supplementation can lower blood pressure, but it is slow to appear, taking about 4 weeks. In a meta-analysis, Dickinson and others analyzed six randomly controlled trials and found that potassium supplementation resulted in a large but statistically nonsignificant reduction in both systolic and diastolic blood pressure. They noted that, given the data from these studies, the evidence about the effect of potassium supplementation on blood pressure is not conclusive, and additional research is needed. In their review, Savica and others concluded that there is significant controversy in the literature concerning whether high calcium and magnesium intakes lower blood pressure.

Given the potential health risks of potassium supplementation, as noted earlier, individuals considering such supplementation should do so only under the guidance of their physician.

As you probably noticed, all of these recommendations are in accord with the Prudent Healthy Diet. The more of these recommendations you follow, the better. In one study, subjects who lost weight, increased physical activity, and reduced sodium and alcohol intake experienced significant reductions in blood pressure, but subjects who also adhered to the DASH diet experienced the greatest reduction.

Can exercise help prevent or treat hypertension?

Regular mild- to moderate-intensity aerobic exercise, such as jogging, brisk walking, swimming, cycling, and aerobic dancing, has also been recommended to reduce high blood pressure. The exercise need not be continuous. Elley and others found that four 10-minute *exercise snacks* consisting of brisk walking, as compared to a single 40-minute continuous bout of brisk walking, done over the course of a day elicited similar reductions in both systolic and diastolic blood pressure. Individuals can work these exercise *snacks* into their daily schedule when they can't find a large block of free time.

Because exercise may be an effective means of losing excess body fat, it may exert a beneficial effect on blood pressure through this avenue. However, the exact role or mechanism of exercise as an independent factor in lowering blood pressure has not been totally resolved. Kramer and others theorize that exercise may exert favorable effects on the hypothalamus, inducing the sympathetic nervous system to decrease constriction of blood vessels and reduce vascular resistance, which is one factor contributing to elevated blood pressure.

Some individuals, called nonresponders, will not experience a decrease in blood pressure with exercise training. Nevertheless, most health professionals find the available information sufficient to justify an aerobic exercise program as a useful adjunct for the treatment of high blood pressure.

Most research has focused on the chronic effect of exercise training on blood pressure. Most recent reviews and meta-analyses report significant reductions in both diastolic and systolic blood pressure, more so in hypertensive than normotensive individuals. In a meta-analysis of 72 studies, Fagard concluded that aerobic endurance exercise training reduced blood pressure by about 3 mmHg, and the reduction was greater in subjects with hypertension (-6.9 mmHg) than those who were normotensive (-1.9 mmHg). Although the number of studies was limited, Fagard also noted that resistance training was able to reduce blood pressure. Artero and colleagues examined the effect of isotonic muscle strength (sum of leg and bench press 1-repetition max) and aerobic fitness on all-cause mortality in 1,506 hypertensive men over an average 18.3 years of follow-up. There was a significant dose response in age-adjusted death rates per 10,000 man-years across strength tertiles (81.8, 65.5, 52.0). After adjustment for aerobic fitness, the strongest third of the subjects had the lowest risk of death. In a more recent meta-analysis of 93 randomized, controlled exercise training trials, Cornelissen and Smart reported reductions in systolic and diastolic pressures after endurance ($-3.5/-2.5$ mmHg); dynamic resistance ($-1.8/-3.2$); and isometric ($-10.9/-6.2$) training regimens. Interestingly, across all studies, combined training elicited a significant decrease in diastolic (-2.2), but not systolic, blood pressure. Endurance exercise elicited the greatest blood pressure changes in hypertensive subjects ($-8.3/-5.2$) compared to normotensive subjects ($-0.75/-1.1$), whereas dynamic resistance training was most effective among prehypertensive subjects ($-4.0/-5.2$) compared to hyper- or normotensive subjects. These overall reductions in blood pressure appear to be small, but

Israili and others note that even small reductions in systolic blood pressure (for example, 3–5 mmHg) produce dramatic reduction in adverse cardiac events and stroke.

The American College of Sports Medicine, in its position stand on exercise and hypertension, stated that exercise is the cornerstone therapy for the primary prevention, treatment, and control of hypertension. These are some of the major points of the position stand:

- Exercise programs that involve endurance activities, such as walking, jogging, running, or cycling, coupled with resistance training, help to prevent the development of hypertension and to lower blood pressure in adults.
- Exercise should be done daily for 30 minutes or more at a moderate level.
- A higher level of physical activity and fitness resulting from long-term exercise training has a protective effect against hypertension; fitter people with hypertension will have lower blood pressure than those who are less fit.
- Even a single-session (acute) exercise bout provides an immediate reduction in blood pressure, which can last for a major portion of the day. Promoting the benefits of lowering blood pressure through single bouts of exercise may help motivate people to exercise. In a review comparing 27 acute aerobic and 5 acute resistance exercise studies, Anunciação and Polito reported that aerobic exercise elicited postexercise hypotension of greater magnitude and of longer duration.

Special considerations for exercise with hypertension include the following:

- Individuals with controlled hypertension and no cardiovascular or kidney disease may participate in an exercise program.
- Overweight adults should use exercise to lose weight.
- People on medications, such as beta-blockers, should be cautious of developing heat illness when exercising. As noted by the ACSM, calcium-channel blockers, ACE inhibitors, and angiotensin II receptor blockers are less likely to affect exercise tolerance.
- Adults with hypertension should extend the cool-down period of the workout; some medications may cause blood pressure to lower too much after abruptly ending exercise.

Individuals who have high blood pressure and who have concerns about exercising should consult with their physicians about mode and intensity of exercise. Although aerobic exercise may help reduce blood pressure at rest and may evoke a lessened blood pressure rise during exercise, a protective effect, other exercises may be harmful. For example, high-intensity anaerobic exercise and activities that require intense straining, lifting, or hanging, such as isometric exercises, weight lifting, or pull-ups might be inappropriate for some individuals. In it interesting to note, however, that Cornelissen and Smart reported a significantly larger decrease in systolic blood pressure in five isometric studies compared to endurance, dynamic resistance, or combined training studies. The use of handheld weights might be contraindicated for some hypertensive individuals due to the pressor (elevated blood pressure and heart rate) response that can occur with upper-body exercise. Thus, hypertensive individuals need to consult with their physicians regarding exercise indications and contraindications.

In summary, the more healthful behaviors one adopts, the greater will be the reduction in blood pressure. The JNCDET noted that a healthy lifestyle may be sufficient to avoid pharmacological therapy for some patients and is a valuable adjunct to drug therapy for most. The JNCDET quantified the potential blood pressure–lowering effects of various health behaviors, as follows:

- Weight reduction (5–20 mmHg/10 kg)
- DASH eating plan (8–14 mmHg)
- Dietary sodium reduction (2–8 mmHg)
- Increased physical activity (4–9 mmHg)
- Moderation of alcohol consumption (2–4 mmHg)

APPLICATION EXERCISES

Determine your body temperature response and sweating rate.

First, measure your body temperature accurately before exercise. An oral thermometer is acceptable, but keep your mouth closed tightly during all measurements. Also, weigh yourself exactly in dry, light clothes.

Second, exercise for about 30–60 minutes, preferably under warm environmental conditions, either indoors or outdoors. Record exactly the amount of fluid you consume during exercise.

Third, immediately after exercise, record your body temperature. Then, immediately towel dry and weigh yourself in the same dry set of clothes. Calculate your body temperature increase from the difference between the pre-exercise and postexercise recordings. Calculate your sweat loss by subtracting your postexercise weight from your initial weight and adding to this amount the number of ounces of fluid you consumed. This will provide you with your sweat rate for the time you exercised, which you can then calculate to sweat rate per hour.

If feasible, conduct this little self-experiment before and after acclimatization to exercise in the heat and compare the responses. What might you expect to find?

Body Temperature Response and Sweating Rate

Step 1		Step 2	Step 3	
Pre-exercise temperature		Fluid consumed during exercise	Postexercise temperature	
Pre-exercise weight			Postexercise weight	

Determination of body temperature response and sweating rate to exercise

Sweating rate

A. Enter your pre-exercise body weight (nearest 0.25 pound). _____

B. Enter your postexercise body weight in pounds (nearest 0.25 pound). _____

C. Subtract B from A. _____

D. Convert C to ounces (1 pound = 16 fluid ounces). _____

E. Enter the amount of fluid (in ounces) you consumed during the run. _____

F. Add E to D. _____

G. Divide F by the number of minutes of exercise to calculate sweat rate per minute. _____

H. Multiply G by 60 to obtain sweat rate per hour. _____

The final figure provides you with a guide to replenish fluids per hour. You need not fully replenish what you lose per hour, but replacing about 60 percent or more will help you prevent excessive dehydration.

Body temperature response

A. Enter your pre-exercise body temperature in degrees Fahrenheit or Celsius. _____

B. Enter your postexercise body temperature in degrees Fahrenheit or Celsius. _____

C. Subtract B from A. _____

The final figure represents your core body temperature increase for the intensity and duration of exercise and for the given environmental conditions (air temperature, humidity, solar radiation).

1. Which of the following blood pressure values for adults 18 years of age and older represents the minimal blood pressure for the first stage of hypertension (mild)? The values listed are systolic and diastolic, in that order.
   a. 130 and 80
   b. 130 and 90
   c. 140 and 90
   d. 160 and 100
   e. 210 and 120

2. Which of the following does *not* occur in acclimatization to exercise in the heat?
   a. increased sweat production during exercise
   b. increased blood volume
   c. a lower rise in the core temperature during exercise
   d. a lower rise in the heart rate response to exercise
   e. an increased sodium loss in each liter of sweat

3. Which of the following statements is false?
   a. The maximal sweat rate appears to be about 2–3 liters per hour.
   b. Dehydration as low as 2 percent of the body weight may lead to a decrease in aerobic endurance performance.
   c. Sweat is mainly water.
   d. The major electrolytes found in sweat are calcium and potassium.

4. Which of the following is most limited in the DASH diet?
   a. calcium
   b. fiber
   c. magnesium
   d. sodium
   e. potassium
   f. phytonutrients

5. Excessive loss of sweat during exercise in the heat will lead to a condition in the body known as
   a. hyperhydration.
   b. hypohydration.
   c. homeostasis.
   d. normohydration.
   e. euhydration.

6. Which of the following is not one of the physical means whereby heat is lost from the human body?
   a. condensation
   b. conduction
   c. evaporation
   d. convection
   e. radiation

7. A high relative humidity and sunshine impose a heat stress during exercise by their adverse effects on the body, respectively, as
   a. increased condensation of sweat and decreased radiant heat to the body.
   b. increased convection heat loss and decreased radiant heat to the body.
   c. decreased evaporation of sweat and increased radiant heat to the body.
   d. decreased condensation of sweat and decreased convection of heat to the body.
   e. increased evaporation of sweat and increased convection of heat to the body.

8. Calculate the increase in the body temperature, in degrees Celsius, that would occur if an individual was unable to dissipate heat and were exercising at an intensity of 3 liters of oxygen per minute for 20 minutes. The athlete weighs 60 kg, her mechanical efficiency is 20 percent, and the specific heat of her body is 0.83.
   a. 2.2
   b. 4.8
   c. 10.2
   d. 6.0
   e. 9.4

9. Which of the following statements regarding bottled water is false?
   a. Bottled water is normally much more expensive than municipal water supplies.
   b. Bottled water must conform to the same safety standards as municipal water supplies.
   c. Some bottled waters are simply municipal water that has undergone purification.
   d. Bottled water normally contains more fluoride than fluoridated municipal water supplies.

10. During prolonged endurance exercise in the heat, excessive intake of water and inadequate intake of salt may lead to a dangerous health condition known as
    a. hypercalcemia.
    b. hypotension.
    c. hypohydration.
    d. hyponatremia.
    e. hyperkalemia.

Answers to multiple choice questions:
1. c; 2. e; 3. d; 4. d; 5. b; 6. a; 7. c; 8. b; 9. d; 10. d

1. Discuss the means whereby your body maintains normal water balance. Include in your discussion the role of the blood, hypothalamus, pituitary gland, antidiuretic hormone, and kidney.

2. Name the four components of heat stress that are recorded by the wet-bulb globe temperature (WBGT) thermometer, and discuss how each factor may contribute to heat stress during exercise under warm environmental conditions.

3. Your friend is going to run a marathon. The projected weather forecast is sunny, warm, and humid. What advice would you offer regarding consumption of fluids, including carbohydrate and electrolytes, before and during the race?

4. List and discuss five strategies to help reduce the hazards associated with exercise in a hot environment.

5. What is high blood pressure? Why is it dangerous to your health? What lifestyle behaviors may help in its prevention or treatment?

Books

American Institute of Cancer Research. 2007. *Food, Nutrition, Physical Activity, and the Prevention of Cancer: A Global Perspective.* Washington, DC: AICR.

National Academy of Sciences, Institute of Medicine, Food and Nutrition Board. 2004. *Dietary Reference Intake for Water, Potassium, Sodium, Chloride, and Sulfate.* Washington, DC: National Academies Press.

Reviews and Specific Studies

Adan, A. 2012. Cognitive performance and dehydration. *Journal of the American College of Nutrition* 31(2):71–78.

Aglony, M., et al. 2009. Hypertension in adolescents. *Expert Review of Cardiovascular Therapy* 7:1595–1603.

Alderman, M. 2006. Evidence relating dietary sodium to cardiovascular disease. *Journal of the American College of Nutrition* 25:256S–61S.

Almond, C., et al. 2005. Hyponatremia among runners in the Boston Marathon. *New England Journal of Medicine* 352:1550–56.

American Academy of Pediatrics. 2000. Climatic heat stress and the exercising child and adolescent. *Pediatrics* 106:158–59.

American College of Sports Medicine. 2004. American College of Sports Medicine position stand: Exercise and hypertension. *Medicine & Science in Sports & Exercise* 36:533–53.

American College of Sports Medicine. 2005. Youth football: Heat stress and injury risk. *Medicine & Science in Sports & Exercise* 37:1421–30.

American College of Sports Medicine. 2007. American College of Sports Medicine Position Stand: Exertional heat illness during training and competition. *Medicine & Science in Sports & Exercise* 39:556–72.

American College of Sports Medicine. 2007. Exercise and fluid replacement. *Medicine & Science in Sports & Exercise* 39:377–90.

American Running and Fitness Association. 1996. Glycerol helps fluid balance. *FitNews* 14 (6):1.

Anastasiou, C., et al. 2009. Sodium replacement and plasma sodium drop during exercise in the heat when fluid intake matches fluid loss. *Journal of Athletic Training* 44:117–23.

Anderson, M., et al. 2001. Effect of glycerol-induced hyperhydration on thermoregulation and metabolism during exercise in heat. *International Journal of Sport Nutrition and Exercise Metabolism* 11:315–33.

Anunciação, P. G., and Polito, M. D. 2011. Review on post-exercise hypotension in hypertensive individuals. *Arquivos Brasileiros de Cardiologia* 96 (5):e100–9.

Appel, L., et al. 2005. Effects of protein, monounsaturated fat, and carbohydrate intake on blood pressure and serum lipids: Results of the OmniHeart randomized trial. *Journal of the American Medical Association* 294:2455–64.

Armstrong, L. E. 2002. Caffeine, body fluid-electrolyte balance, and exercise performance. *International Journal of Sport Nutrition and Exercise Metabolism* 12 (2):189–206.

Armstrong, L., et al. 2005. Fluid, electrolyte, and renal indices of hydration during 11 days of controlled caffeine consumption. *International Journal of Sport Nutrition and Exercise Metabolism* 15:252–65.

Armstrong, L., et al. 2006. No effect of 5% hypohydration on running economy of competitive runners at 23 degrees C. *Medicine & Science in Sports & Exercise* 38:1762–69.

Artero, E. G., et al. 2011. A prospective study of muscular strength and all-cause mortality in men with hypertension. *Journal of the American College of Cardiology* 57 (18):1831–37.

Azadbakht, L., et al. 2005. Beneficial effects of a Dietary Approaches to Stop Hypertension eating plan on features of the metabolic syndrome. *Diabetes Care* 28:2823–31.

Baker, L. B., and Jeukendrup, A. E. 2014. Optimal composition of fluid-replacement beverages. *Comprehensive Physiology* 4 (2):575–620. doi: 10.1002/cphy.c130014.

Baker, L., and Kenney, W. 2007. Exercising in the heat and sun. *President's Council on Physical Fitness and Sports Research Digest* 8 (2):1–8.

Baker, L., et al. 2005. Sex differences in voluntary fluid intake by older adults during exercise. *Medicine & Science in Sports & Exercise* 37:789–96.

Baker, L., et al. 2007. Dehydration impairs vigilance-related attention in male basketball players. *Medicine & Science in Sports & Exercise* 39:976–83.

Baker, L., et al. 2007. Progressive dehydration causes a progressive decline in basketball skill performance. *Medicine & Science in Sports & Exercise* 39:1114–23.

Bar-Or, O. 1994. Children's responses to exercise in hot climates: Implications for performance and health. *Sports Science Exchange* 7 (2):1–4.

Barr, S. I. 1999. Effects of dehydration on exercise performance. *Canadian Journal of Applied Physiology* 24:164–72.

Barr, S., et al. 1991. Fluid replacement during prolonged exercise: Effects of water, saline, and no fluid. *Medicine & Science in Sports & Exercise* 23:811–17.

Bassett, D. R., et al. 1987. Thermoregulatory responses to skin wetting during prolonged treadmill running. *Medicine and Science in Sport and Exercise* 19 (1):28–32.

Basu, R., et al. 2012. The effect of high ambient temperature on emergency room visits. *Epidemiology* 23 (6):813–20.

Below, P., et al. 1995. Fluid and carbohydrate ingestion independently improve performance during 1 h of intense exercise. *Medicine & Science in Sports & Exercise* 27:200–210.

Bergeron, M. 2002. Averting muscle cramps. *Physician and Sportsmedicine* 30 (11):14.

Bilzon, J., et al. 2000. Short-term recovery from prolonged constant pace running in a warm environment: The effectiveness of a carbohydrate-electrolyte solution. *European Journal of Applied Physiology* 82:305–12.

Bird, S., et al. 2006. Liquid carbohydrate/protein amino acid ingestion during a short-term bout of resistance exercise suppresses myofibrillar protein degradation. *Metabolism* 55:570–77.

Bonci, L. 2002. "Energy" drinks: Help, harm, or hype? *Sports Science Exchange* 15 (1):1–4.

Bongers, C. C. W. G., et al. 2014. Precooling and precooling (cooling during exercise) both improve performance in the heat: A meta-analytical review. *British Journal of Sports Medicine Online First* (April 19). doi: 10.1136/bjsports-2013-092928.

Brill, J. f 2014. 5 Foods that fight high blood pressure. *Bottom Line* 35(11):7–8.

Brown, M. J., and Margolis, A. 2012. Lead in drinking water and human blood lead levels in the United States. *Morbidity and Mortality Weekly Report Centers for Disease Control Surveillance Summaries* (August 10) 61:S1–S9.

Burdon, C. A., et al. 2012. Influence of beverage temperature on palatability and fluid ingestion during endurance exercise: A systematic review. *International Journal of Sport Nutrition and Exercise Metabolism* 22:199–211.

Burke, L. 2001. Nutritional needs for exercise in the heat. *Comparative Biochemistry and Physiology. Part A. Molecular & Integrative Physiology* 128:735–48.

Byrne, C., et al. 2006. Continuous thermoregulatory responses to mass-participation distance running in heat. *Medicine & Science in Sports & Exercise* 38:803–10.

Cappuccio, F. 2007. Salt and cardiovascular disease. *British Medical Journal* 334:859–60.

Casa, D., et al. 2007. Cold water immersion: The gold standard for exertional heatstroke treatment. *Exercise and Sport Sciences Reviews* 35:141–49.

Castle, P., et al. 2006. Precooling leg muscle improves intermittent sprint exercise in hot, humid conditions. *Journal of Applied Physiology* 100:1377–84.

Center for Science in the Public Interest. 2007. *CSPI year-end report.* Washington, DC: CSPI.

Chen, L., et al. 2010. Reducing consumption of sugar-sweetened beverages is associated with reduced blood pressure: A prospective study among United States adults. *Circulation* 121:2398–406.

Cheung, S., and Sleivert, G. 2004. Multiple triggers for hyperthermic fatigue and exhaustion. *Exercise and Sports Sciences Reviews* 32:100–6.

Cheuvront, S. N., and Kenefick, R. W. 2014. Dehydration: Physiology, assessment and performance effects. *Comprehensive Physiology* 4 (1):257–85. doi: 10.1002/cphy.c130017.

Cheuvront, S. N., et al. 2013. Physiologic basis for understanding quantitative dehydration assessment. *American Journal of Clinical Nutrition* 97:455462.

Cheuvront, S., and Haymes, E. 2001. *Ad libitum* fluid intakes and thermoregulatory responses of female distance runners in three environments. *Journal of Sport Sciences* 19:845–54.

Cheuvront, S., and Sawka, M. 2005. Hydration assessment of athletes. *Sports Science Exchange* 18 (2):1–6.

Chorley, J. 2007. Hyponatremia: Identification and evaluation in the marathon medical area. *Sports Medicine* 37:451–54.

Clarke, N., et al. 2005. Strategies for hydration and energy provision during soccer-specific exercise. *International Journal of Sport Nutrition and Exercise Metabolism* 15:625–40.

Consumers Union. 1999. Do you drink enough water? *Consumer Reports on Health* 11 (11):8–10.

Consumers Union. 2003. Clear choices for clean drinking water. *Consumers Reports* 68 (1):33–38.

Consumers Union. 2006. A guide to the best and worst drinks. *Consumer Reports on Health* 18 (7):8–9.

Cook, N., et al. 2007. Long term effects of dietary sodium reduction on cardiovascular disease outcomes: Observational follow-up of the trials of hypertension prevention (TOHP). *British Medical Journal* 334:885.

Coombes, J., and Hamilton, K. 2000. The effectiveness of commercially available sports drinks. *Sports Medicine* 29:181–209.

Cornelissen, V. A., and Smart, N .A. 2013. Exercise training for blood pressure: A systematic review and meta-analysis. *Journal of the American Heart Association* 2:e004473. doi: 10.1161/jaha.112.004473.

Costill, D. 1977. Sweating: Its composition and effects on body fluids. *Annals of the New York Academy of Sciences* 301:160–74.

Costill, D. 1990. Gastric emptying of fluids during exercise. In *Perspectives in Exercise Science and Sports Medicine. Fluid Homeostasis during Exercise,* ed. C. Gisolfi and D. Lamb. Indianapolis, IN: Benchmark.

Costill, D., et al. 1982. Dietary potassium and heavy exercise: Effects on muscle water and electrolytes. *American Journal of Clinical Nutrition* 36:266–75.

Coutts, A., et al. 2002. The effect of glycerol hyperhydration on Olympic distance triathlon performance in high ambient temperatures. *International Journal of Sport Nutrition and Exercise Metabolism* 12:105–19.

Coxson, P. G., et al. 2013. Mortality benefits from US population-wide reduction in sodium consumption. Projections from 3 modeling approaches. *Hypertension* 61:564–70.

Coyle, E. 2004. Fluid and fuel intake during exercise. *Journal of Sports Sciences* 22:39–55.

de Castro, J. 2005. Stomach filling may mediate the influence of dietary energy density on the food intake of free-living humans. *Physiology & Behavior* 86:32–45.

de Oliveira, E. P., et al. 2014. Gastrointestinal complaints during exercise: Prevalence, etiology, and nutritional recommendations. *Sports Medicine* 44 (Supplement 1):S79–S85.

Dickinson, H. O., et al. 2006. Potassium supplementation for the management of primary hypertension in adults. *Cochrane Database of Systematic Reviews* 19 (3):CD004641.

Dougherty, K., et al. 2006. Two percent dehydration impairs and six percent carbohydrate drink improves boy's basketball skills. *Medicine & Science in Sports & Exercise* 38:1650–58.

Drewnowski, A., et al. 2013. Water and beverage consumption among adults in the United States: Cross-sectional study using data from NHANES 2005-2010. *BMC Public Health* 13:1068–76.

Drewnowski, A., et al. 2013. Water and beverage consumption among children age 4–13 y in the United States: Analysis of 2005–2010 NHANES data. *Nutrition Journal* 12:85–93.

Drust, B., et al. 2005. Elevations in core and muscle temperature impairs repeated sprint performance. *Acta Physiologica Scandinavica* 183:181–90.

Duffield, R., et al. 2012. Hydration, sweat and thermoregulatory responses to professional football training in the heat. *Journal of Sports Science* 30 (10):957–65.

Edwards, A., et al. 2007. Influence of moderate dehydration on soccer performance: Physiological responses to 45 min of outdoor match-play and the immediate subsequent performance of sport-specific and mental concentration tests. *British Journal of Sports Medicine* 41:385–91.

Eichner, E. 1998. Treatment of suspected heat illness. *International Journal of Sports Medicine* 19:S150–S53.

Eichner, E. 2002. Heat stroke in sports: Causes, prevention, and treatment. *Sports Science Exchange* 15 (3):1–4.

Eichner, R. 2007. The role of sodium in "heat cramping." *Sports Medicine* 37:368–70.

Eijsvogels, T. M., et al. 2013. Sex differences in fluid balance responses during prolonged exercise. *Scandinavian Journal of Medicine and Science in Sports* 23 (2):198–206.

Elley, R., et al. 2006. Do snacks of exercise lower blood pressure? A randomized crossover trial. *New Zealand Medical Journal* 113:2642–50.

European Food Safety Authority. 2011. Scientific opinion on the substantiation of health claims related to carbohydrate-electrolyte solutions and reduction in rated perceived exertion/effort during exercise, enhancement of water absorption during exercise, and maintenance of endurance performance pursuant to Article 13(1) of Regulation (EC) No 1924/20061. *European Food Safety Authority Journal* 9 (6):2211–40.

Fagard, R. 2006. Exercise is good for your blood pressure: Effects of endurance training and resistance training. *Clinical and Experimental Pharmacology & Physiology* 33:853–56.

Febbraio, M. 2000. Does muscle function and metabolism affect exercise performance in the heat? *Exercise and Sport Sciences Reviews* 28:171–76.

Febbraio, M. 2001. Alterations in energy metabolism during exercise and heat stress. *Sports Medicine* 31:47–59.

Food and Drug Administration. 2008. Guidance for industry: A labeling guide for restaurants and other retail establishments selling away-from-home foods. (April).

Franco, V., and Oparil, S. 2006. Salt sensitivity: A determinant of blood pressure, cardiovascular disease and survival. *Journal of the American College of Nutrition* 25:247S–55S.

Freund, B., et al. 1995. Glycerol hyperhydration: Hormonal, renal, and vascular fluid responses. *Journal of Applied Physiology* 79:2069–77.

Fritzsche, R., et al. 2000. Water and carbohydrate ingestion during prolonged exercise increase maximal neuromuscular power. *Journal of Applied Physiology* 88:730–37.

Fudge, B., et al. 2008. Elite Kenyan endurance runners are hydrated day-to-day with *ad libitum* fluid intake. *Medicine & Science in Sports & Exercise* 40:1171–79.

Fung, T., et al. 2008. Adherence to a DASH-style diet and risk of coronary heart disease and stroke in women. *Archives of Internal Medicine* 168:713–20.

Gant, N., et al. 2007. Gastric emptying of fluids during variable-intensity running in the heat. *International Journal of Sport Nutrition and Exercise Metabolism* 17:270–83.

Gardner, J., et al. 1996. Risk factors predicting exertional heat illness in male Marine Corps recruits. *Medicine & Science in Sports & Exercise* 28:939–44.

Garth, A. K., and Burke, L. M. 2013. What do athletes drink during competitive sporting activities? *Sports Medicine* 43 (7):539–64.

Geerling, J., and Loewy, A. 2008. Central regulation of sodium appetite. *Experimental Physiology* 93:177–209.

Gillespie, C. D., and Hurvitz, K. A. 2013. Prevalence of hypertension and controlled hypertension—United States, 2007–2010. *Morbidity and Mortality Weekly Report* 62(03):144–48. www.cdc.gov/mmwr/.

Gisolfi, C. 1996. Fluid balance for optimal performance. *Nutrition Reviews* 54: S159–S68.

Gisolfi, C., et al. 1998. Effect of beverage osmolality on intestinal fluid absorption during exercise. *Journal of Applied Physiology* 85:1941–48.

Gisolfi, C., et al. 2001. Intestinal fluid absorption during exercise: Role of sport drink osmolality and [Na$^+$]. *Medicine & Science in Sports & Exercise* 33:907–15.

Gledhill, N. 1999. Haemoglobin, blood volume, cardiac function, and aerobic power. *Canadian Journal of Applied Physiology* 24:54–65.

Go, A. S., et al. 2013. Heart disease and stroke statistics—2013 update: A report from the American Heart Association. *Circulation* 127:e6-e245. doi: 10.1161/CIR.0b013e31828124ad.

Gomes, L. H. L. S., et al. 2013. Thermoregulatory responses of children exercising in a hot environment. *Revista Paulista de Pediatria* 31 (1):104–10.

Goulet, E. D. 2011. Effect of exercise-induced dehydration on time-trial exercise performance: A meta-analysis. *British Journal of Sports Medicine* 45 (14):1149–56.

Goulet, E. D. 2012. Dehydration and endurance performance in competitive athletes. *Nutrition Reviews* 70 (S2):S132–36.

Goulet, E., et al. 2006. Effect of glycerol-induced hyperhydration on thermoregulatory and cardiovascular functions and endurance performance during prolonged cycling in a 25 degrees C environment. *Applied Physiology, Nutrition and Metabolism* 31:101–9.

Goulet, E., et al. 2007. A meta-analysis of the effects of glycerol-induced hyperhydration on fluid retention and endurance performance. *International Journal of Sport Nutrition and Exercise Metabolism* 17:391–410.

Graudal, N., et al. 2014. Compared with usual sodium intake, low- and excessive-sodium diets are associated with increased mortality: A meta-analysis. *American Journal of Hypertension* (April 26). [Epub ahead of print] doi:10.1093/ajh/hpu028

Greiwe, J., et al. 1998. Effect of dehydration on isometric muscular strength and endurance. *Medicine & Science in Sports & Exercise* 30:284–88.

Hackman, D., et al. 2010. The 2010 Canadian hypertension education program recommendations for the management of hypertension: Part 2—Therapy. *Canadian Journal of Cardiology* 26:249–58.

Haddy, F., et al. 2006. Role of potassium in regulating blood flow and blood pressure. *American Journal of Physiology. Regulatory, Integrative and Comparative Physiology* 290:R546–52.

Hampson, N., et al. 2003. Oxygenated water and athletic performance. *Journal of the American Medical Association* 290:2408–9.

Hansen, M., et al. 2007. Underdiagnosis of hypertension in children and adolescents. *Journal of the American Medical Association* 298:874–79.

Hargreaves, M., and Febbraio, M. 1998. Limits to exercise performance in the heat. *International Journal of Sports Medicine* 19:S115–16.

Hargreaves, M., et al. 1994. Influence of sodium on glucose bioavailability during exercise. *Medicine & Science in Sports & Exercise* 26:365–68.

Hargreaves, M., et al. 1996. Effect of fluid ingestion on muscle metabolism during prolonged exercise. *Journal of Applied Physiology* 80:363–66.

Hausswirth, C. et al. 2012. Post-exercise cooling interventions and the effects on exercise-induced heat stress in a temperate environment. *Applied Physiology Nutrition and Metabolism* 37:965–975.

He, F. J., et al. 2014. Salt reduction in England from 2003 to 2011: Its relationship to blood pressure, stroke, and ischaemic heart disease mortality. *British Medical Journal Open* 4 (4):e004549. doi: 10.1136/bmjopen-2013-004549.

Hew-Butler, T., et al. 2005. Consensus statement of the 1st International Exercise-Associated Hyponatremia Consensus Development Conference. *Clinical Journal of Sports Medicine* 15:208–13.

Hew-Butler, T., et al. 2006. Sodium supplementation is not required to maintain serum sodium concentrations during an Ironman triathlon. *British Journal of Sports Medicine* 40:255–59.

Hiller, D. 1989. Dehydration and hyponatremia during triathlons. *Medicine & Science in Sports & Exercise* 21:S219–21.

Hillman, A. R., et al. 2013. A comparison of hyperhydration versus ad libitum fluid intake strategies on measures of oxidative stress, thermoregulation, and performance. *Research in Sports Medicine* 21 (4):305–17. doi: 10.1080/15438627.2013.825796.

Hunter, I., et al. 2006. Warming up with an ice vest: Core body temperature before and after cross-country racing. *Journal of Athletic Training* 41:371–74.

Institute of Medicine. 2013. *Sodium Intake in Populations: Assessment of Evidence.* Washington, DC: National Academies Press.

Israili, Z., et al. 2007. The future of antihypertensive treatment. *American Journal of Therapeutics* 14:121–34.

Jentjens, R., et al. 2006. Exogenous carbohydrate oxidation rates are elevated after combined ingestion of glucose and fructose during exercise in the heat. *Journal of Applied Physiology* 100:807–16.

Jeukendrup, A. E. 2007. Fueling during exercise. www.nestlenutrition-institute. org/resources/library/Secured/sportFocus/Documents/Publication00266/6_ Fueling%20During%20Exercise.pdf.

Jeukendrup, A. E. 2014. A step towards personalized sports nutrition: Carbohydrate intake during exercise. *Sports Medicine* 44 (Suppl 1):S25–33. doi: 10.1007/ s40279-014-0148-z.

Jeukendrup, A., and Martin, J. 2001. Improving cycling performance: How should we spend our time and money? *Sports Medicine* 31:559–69.

John, S. K., et al. 2011. Life-threatening hyperkalemia from nutritional supplements: Uncommon or undiagnosed? *American Journal of Emergency Medicine* 29 (9):1237.e1-2. doi: 1016/j,ajem.2010.08.029.

Johnson, A. 2007. The sensory psychobiology of thirst and salt appetite. *Medicine & Science in Sports & Exercise* 39:1388–400.

Joint National Committee on Prevention, Detection, Evaluation and Treatment of High Blood Pressure. 2003. The Seventh Report of the Joint National Committee on Prevention, Detection, Evaluation and Treatment of High Blood Pressure. *Hypertension* 42:1206–52.

Judelson, D., et al. 2007. Effect of hydration state on strength, power, and resistance exercise performance. *Medicine & Science in Exercise & Sports* 39:1817–24.

Kavouras, S., et al. 2006. Rehydration with glycerol: Endocrine, cardiovascular, and thermoregulatory responses during exercise in the heat. *Journal of Applied Physiology* 100:442–50.

Kenefick, R. W., and Cheuvront, S. N. 2012. Hydration for recreational sport and physical activity. *Nutrition Reviews* 70:S137–42.

Kenefick, R., and Sawka, M. 2007. Heat exhaustion and dehydration as causes of marathon collapse. *Sports Medicine* 37:378–81.

Kenefick, R., et al. 2002. Hypohydration adversely affects lactate threshold in endurance athletes. *Journal of Strength and Conditioning Research* 16:38–43.

Kerr, Z. Y., et al. 2013. Epidemiology of exertional heat illness among U.S. high school athletes. *American Journal of Preventive Medicine* 44 (1):8–14.

Khan, N., et al. 2007. The 2007 Canadian Hypertension Education Program recommendations for the management of hypertension: Part 2—Therapy. *Canadian Journal of Cardiology* 23:539–50.

Kleiman, S., et al. 2012. Drinking to our health: Can beverage companies cut calories while maintaining profits? *Obesity Research* 13 (3):258–74.

Kramer, J., et al. 2002. Exercise and hypertension: A model for central neural plasticity. *Clinical and Experimental Pharmacology & Physiology* 29:122–26.

Lalumandier, J., and Ayers, L. 2000. Flouride and bacterial content of bottled water vs tap water. *Archives of Family Medicine* 9:246–50.

Lamb, D., and Shehata, A. 1999. Benefits and limitations to prehydration. *Sports Science Exchange* 12 (2):1–6.

Lambert, G., et al. 1993. Effects of carbonated and noncarbonated beverages at specific intervals during treadmill running in the heat. *International Journal of Sport Nutrition* 3:177–93.

Lang, F. 2011. Effect of cell hydration on metabolism. Nestlé Nutrition Institute Workshop Series 69:115–26; discussion 126–130. doi: 10.1159/000329290.

Latzka, W., et al. 1997. Hyperhydration: Thermoregulatory effects during compensable exercise-heat stress. *Journal of Applied Physiology* 83:860–66.

Latzka, W., et al. 1998. Hyperhydration: Tolerance and cardiovascular effect during uncompensable exercise-heat stress. *Journal of Applied Physiology* 84:1858–64.

Lefferts, L. 1990. Water: Treat it right. *Nutrition Action Health Letter* 17:5–7.

Lindeman, A. 1991. Nutrient intake of an ultraendurance cyclist. *International Journal of Sport Nutrition* 1:79–85.

Lotan, Y., et al. 2013. Impact of fluid intake in the prevention of urinary system diseases: A brief review. *Current Opinions in Nephrology and Hypertension* (May 22), S1–10.

Luetkemeier, M., et al. 1997. Dietary sodium and plasma volume levels with exercise. *Sports Medicine* 23:279–86.

Lyons, T., et al. 1990. Effects of glycerol-induced hyperhydration prior to exercise in the heat on sweating and core temperature. *Medicine & Science in Sports & Exercise* 22:477–83.

Mack, G. 2006. The body fluid and hemopoietic systems. In *ACSM's Advanced Exercise Physiology,* ed. C. Tipton. Philadelphia: Lippincott Williams & Wilkins.

Magal, M., et al. 2003. Comparison of glycerol and water hydration regimens on tennis-related performance. *Medicine & Science in Sports & Exercise* 35:150–56.

Marino, F. 2002. Methods, advantages, and limitations of body cooling for exercise performance. *British Journal of Sports Medicine* 36:89–94.

Marino, F., et al. 2003. Glycerol hyperhydration fails to improve endurance performance and thermoregulation in humans in a warm humid environment. *Pflugers Archiv* 446:455–62.

Marino, F. E. 2011. The critical limiting temperature and selective brain cooling: neuroprotection during exercise? *International Journal of Hyperthermia* 27 (6):582–590.

Massicotte, D., et al. 2006. Metabolic fate of a large amount of 13C-glycerol ingested during prolonged exercise. *European Journal of Applied Physiology* 96:322–29.

Maughan, R. 2000. Water and electrolyte loss and replacement in exercise. In *Nutrition in Sport,* ed. R. Maughan. Oxford: Blackwell Science.

Maughan, R. J. 2012. Hydration, morbidity, and mortality in vulnerable populations. *Nutrition Reviews* 70:S152–55.

Maughan, R. J., and Meyer, N. L. 2012. Hydration during intense exercise training. 76th Nestlé Nutrition Institute Workshop, Oxford.

Maughan, R., and Shirreffs, S. 2010. Development of hydration strategies to optimize performance for athletes in high-intensity sports and in sports with repeated intense efforts. *Scandinavian Journal of*

Medicine & Science in Sports 20 (Suppl 2):59–69.

Maughan, R., et al. 2005. Fluid and electrolyte balance in elite male football (soccer) players training in a cool environment. *Journal of Sports Sciences* 23:72–79.

Maughan, R., et al. 2007. Errors in the estimation of hydration status from changes in body mass. *Journal of Sports Sciences* 25:797–804.

Maughan, R., et al. 2007. Water balance and salt losses in competitive football. *International Journal of Sport Nutrition and Exercise Metabolism* 17:583–94.

Mazerolle, S. M., et al. 2011. Is oral temperature an accurate measurement of deep body temperature? A systematic review. *Journal of Athletic Training* 46 (5):566–73.

McCann, D., and Adams, W. C. 1997. Wet bulb globe temperature index and performance in competitive distance runners. *Medicine & Science in Sports & Exercise* 29:955–61.

McCarron, D., and Reusser, M. 2000. The power of food to improve multiple cardiovascular risk factors. *Current Atherosclerosis Reports* 2:482–86.

Meyer F., et al. 1992. Sweat electrolyte loss during exercise in the heat: Effects of gender and maturation. *Medicine and Science in Sports and Exercise* 24 (7):776–81.

Meyer, F., et al. 2007. Effect of age and gender on sweat lactate and ammonia concentrations during exercise in the heat. *Brazilian Journal of Medical and Biological Research* 40:135–43.

Michaud, D., et al. 1999. Fluid intake and the risk of bladder cancer in men. *New England Journal of Medicine* 340:1390–97.

Millard-Stafford, M. 1997. Water versus carbohydrate-electrolyte ingestion before and during a 15-km run in the heat. *International Journal of Sport Nutrition* 7:26–38.

Minetto, M. A., et al. 2013. Origin and development of muscle cramps. *Exercise and Sport Sciences Reviews* 41 (1):3–10.

Montain, S., et al. 1998. Hypohydration effects on skeletal muscle performance and metabolism: A 31P-MRS study. *Journal of Applied Physiology* 84:1889–94.

Montain, S., et al. 1998. Thermal and cardiovascular strain from hypohydration: Influence of exercise intensity. *International Journal of Sports Medicine* 19:87–91.

Montain, S., et al. 2007. Marathon performance in thermally stressing conditions. *Sports Medicine* 37:320–23.

Montner, P., et al. 1996. Pre-exercise glycerol hydration improves cycling endurance time. *International Journal of Sports Medicine* 17:27–33.

Morbidity and Mortality Weekly Report *(MMWR)* QuickStats: Number of Heat-Related Deaths by Sex 1999–2010. National Vital Statistics System, United States 61 (36);729 September 14, 2012. www.cdc.gov/mmwr/.

Murray, K. E., et al. 2010. Prioritizing research for trace pollutants and emerging contaminants in the freshwater environment. *Environmental Pollution* 158:3462–71.

Murray, R. 2007. The role of salt and glucose replacement drinks in the marathon. *Sports Medicine* 37:358–60.

Murray, R., and Shi, X. 2006. The gastrointestinal system. In *ACSM's Advanced Exercise Physiology,* ed. C. Tipton. Philadelphia: Lippincott Williams & Wilkins.

Murray, R., et al. 1999. A comparison of the gastric emptying characteristics of selected sports drinks. *International Journal of Sport Nutrition* 9:263–74.

Nadel, E. R., et al. 1974. Mechanisms of thermal acclimation to exercise and heat. *Journal of Applied Physiology* 37(4):515–20.

Noakes, T. 2007. Drinking guidelines for exercise: What evidence is there that athletes should drink "as much as tolerable," "to replace the weight lost during exercise" or "ad libitum?" *Journal of Sports Sciences* 25:781–96.

Noakes, T. 2007. Hydration in the marathon. *Sports Medicine* 37:463–66.

Nybo, L. 2010. CNS fatigue provoked by prolonged exercise in the heat. *Frontiers in Bioscience* E2:779–92.

Oliveira, L., and Lawless, C. 2010. Hypertension update and cardiovascular risk reduction in physically active individuals and athletes. *Physician and Sportsmedicine* 38:11–20.

Osterberg, K., et al. 2009. Pregame urine specific gravity and fluid intake by National Basketball Association players during competition. *Journal of Athletic Training* 44:53–57.

Osterberg, K., et al. 2010. Carbohydrate exerts a mild influence on fluid retention following exercise-induced dehydration. *Journal of Applied Physiology* 108:245–50.

Pandolf, K. B., et al. 2011. United States Army Research Institute of Environmental Medicine: Warfighter research focusing on the past 25 years. *Advances in Physiology Education* 35:353–60.

Passe, D., et al. 2004. Palatability and voluntary intake of sports beverages, diluted orange juice, and water during exercise. *International Journal of Sport Nutrition and Exercise Metabolism* 14:272–84.

Peacock, O. J., et al. 2012. Voluntary drinking behavior, fluid balance, and psychological affect when ingesting water or a carbohydrate-electrolyte solution during exercise. *Appetite* 58:56–63.

Penner, S., et al. 2007. Dietary sodium and cardiovascular outcomes: a rational approach. *Canadian Journal of Cardiology* 23:567–72.

Popkin, B., et al. 2006. A new proposed guidance system for beverage consumption in the United States. *American Journal of Clinical Nutrition* 83:529–42.

Powles, J., et al. 2013. Global, regional and national sodium intakes in 1990 and 2012; a systematic analysis of 24 h urinary sodium excretion and dietary surveys worldwide. *British Medical Journal Open* 3 (12):e003733. doi: 10.1136/bmjopen-2013-003733.

Périard, J. D., et al. 2011. Neuromuscular function following prolonged intense self-paced exercise in hot climatic conditions. *European Journal of Applied Physiology* 111:1561–69.

Quod, M., et al. 2006. Cooling athletes before competition in the heat: Comparison of techniques and practical considerations. *Sports Medicine* 36:671–82.

Ray, M., et al. 1998. Effect of sodium in a rehydration beverage when consumed as a fluid or meal. *Journal of Applied Physiology* 85:1329–36.

Rehrer, N. 2001. Fluid and electrolyte balance in ultra-endurance sport. *Sports Medicine* 31:701–15.

Rehrer, N., et al. 1992. Gastrointestinal complaints in relation to dietary intake in triathletes. *International Journal of Sport Nutrition* 2:48–59.

Richardson, S. I., et al. 2013. Salt sensitivity: A review with a focus on non-Hispanic blacks and Hispanics. *Journal of the American Society of Hypertension* 7 (2):170–79.

Roberts, D. 2006. Blood pressure response to 1-month electrolyte-carbohydrate beverage consumption. *Journal of Occupational and Environmental Hygiene* 3:131–36.

Roberts, W. 2007. Exercise-associated collapse care matrix in the marathon. *Sports Medicine* 37:431–33.

Roberts, W. 2007. Exertional heat stroke in the marathon. *Sports Medicine* 37:440–43.

Rogers, G., et al. 1997. Water budget during ultra-endurance exercise. *Medicine & Science in Sports & Exercise* 29:1477–81.

Rogers, I., and Hew-Butler, T. 2009. Exercise-associated hyponatremia: Overzealous fluid consumption. *Wilderness and Environmental Medicine* 20:139–43.

Rogers, J., et al. 2005. Gastric emptying and intestinal absorption of a low-carbohydrate sport drink during exercise. *International Journal of Sport Nutrition and Exercise Metabolism* 15:220–35.

Ronneberg, K., et al. 2008. Temporal artery temperature measurements do not detect hyperthermic marathon runners. *Medicine & Science in Sports & Exercise* 40:1373–75.

Ross, M., et al. 2013. Precooling methods and their effects on athletic performance. *Sports Medicine* 43:207–25.

Rowlands, D. S., et al. 2011. Unilateral fluid absorption and effects on peak power after ingestion of commercially available hypotonic, isotonic, and hypertonic sports drinks. *International Journal of Sports Nutrition and Exercise Metabolism* 21 (6):480–91.

Ryan, A., et al. 1998. Effect of hypohydration on gastric emptying and intestinal absorption during exercise. *Journal of Applied Physiology* 84:1581–88.

Sacks, F., et al. 2001. Effects on blood pressure of reduced dietary sodium and the Dietary Approaches to Stop Hypertension (DASH) diet. *New England Journal of Medicine* 344:3–10.

Sallis, R. 2004. Collapse in the endurance athlete. *Sports Science Exchange* 17 (4):1–6.

Sanders, B., et al. 1999. Water and electrolyte shifts with partial fluid replacement during exercise. *European Journal of Applied Physiology* 80:318–23.

Savica, V., et al. 2010. The effect of nutrition on blood pressure. *Annual Review of Nutrition* 30:365–401.

Sawka, M. H., et al. 2011. Integrated physiologic mechanisms of exercise performance, adaptation, and maladaptation to heat stress. *Comprehensive Physiology* 1 (4):1883–928. doi: 10.1002/cphy.c100082.

Sawka, M. N., et al. 2012. High skin temperature and hypohydration impair aerobic performance. *Experimental Physiology* 97 (3):327–32.

Sawka, M., and Greenleaf, J. 1992. Current concepts concerning thirst, dehydration, and fluid replacement: Overview. *Medicine & Science in Sports & Exercise* 24:643–44.

Sawka, M., and Pandolf, K. 1990. Effects of body water loss on physiological function and exercise performance. In *Perspectives in Exercise Science and Sports Medicine. Fluid Homeostasis during Exercise,* ed. C. Gisolfi and D. lamb. Indianapolis, IN: Benchmark.

Sawka, M., and Young, A. 2006. Physiological systems and their responses to conditions of heat and cold. In *ACSM's Advanced Exercise Physiology,* ed. C. Tipton. Philadelphia: Lippincott Williams & Wilkins.

Sawka, M., et al. 2000. Effects of dehydration and rehydration on performance. In *Nutrition in Sport,* ed. R. J. Maughan. Oxford: Blackwell Science.

Sawka, M., et al. 2001. Hydration effects on thermoregulation and performance in the heat. *Comparative Biochemistry and Physiology. Part A. Molecular and Integrative Physiology* 128:679–90.

Scheett, T., et al. 2001. Effectiveness of glycerol as a rehydrating agent. *International Journal of Sport Nutrition and Exercise Metabolism* 11:63–71.

Schoffstall, J., et al. 2001. Effects of dehydration and rehydration on the one-repetition maximum bench press of weight-trained males. *Journal of Strength and Conditioning Research* 15:102–8.

Schwellnus, M., et al. 2008. Muscle cramping in athletes—Risk factors, clinical assessment, and management. *Clinics in Sports Medicine* 27:183–94.

Seifert, J., et al. 2006. Protein added to a sports drink improves fluid retention. *International Journal of Sport Nutrition and Exercise Metabolism* 16:420–29.

Shah, M., et al. 2007. Effect of high-carbohydrate or high-cis-monounsaturated fat diets on blood pressure: A meta-analysis of intervention trials. *American Journal of Clinical Nutrition* 85:1251–56.

Shirreffs, S., and Maughan, R. 2000. Rehydration and recovery of fluid balance after exercise. *Exercise and Sport Sciences Reviews* 28:27–32.

Silva, A. M., et al. 2012. Total body water and its compartments are not affected by ingesting a moderate dose of caffeine in healthy young adult males. *Applied Physiology Nutrition and Metabolism* 36 (6):626–32.

Sims, S., et al. 2007. Preexercise sodium loading aids fluid balance and endurance for women exercising in the heat. *Journal of Applied Physiology* 103:534–41.

Sims, S., et al. 2007. Sodium loading aids fluid balance and reduces physiological strain of trained men exercising in the heat. *Medicine & Science in Sports & Exercise* 39:123–30.

Smith, C. J., and Havenith, G. 2012. Body mapping of sweating patterns in athletes: A sex comparison. *Medicine and Science in Sports and Exercise* 44 (12):2350–61.

Smith, G.D. 2002. Commentary: Behind the Broad Streen pump: aetiology, epidemiology and prevention of cholera in mid-19th century Britain. *International Journal of Epidemiology* 31:920–932.

Sorace, P. et al. 2012. Resistance training for hypertension. Design safe and effective programs. *ACSM's Health and Fitness Journal* 16 (1):13–18.

Spickard, A. 1968. Heat stroke in college football and suggestions for prevention. *Southern Medical Journal* 61:791–96.

Stachenfeld, N. S. 2008. Acute effects of sodium ingestion on thirst and cardiovascular function. *Current Sports Medicine Reports* 74 (4):S7–S13.

Stachenfeld, N. S. 2014. The interrelationship of research in the laboratory and the field to assess hydration status and determine mechanisms involved in water regulation during physical activity. *Sports Medicine* 44(S1):S97–S104.

Stofan, J., et al. 2005. Sweat and sodium losses in NCAA football players: A precursor to heat cramps. *International Journal of Sport Nutrition and Exercise Metabolism* 15:641–52.

Stookey, J. 1999. The diuretic effects of alcohol and caffeine and total water intake misclassification. *European Journal of Epidemiology* 15:181–88.

Strom, S. 2013. Bottled water sales rising as soda ebbs. *New York Times,* October 25.

Suh, J. S., et al. 2010. Recent advances in oral rehydration therapy (ORT). *Electrolyte Blood Press* 8:82–86.

Sulzer, N., et al. 2005. Serum electrolytes in Ironman triathletes with exercise-associated muscle cramping. *Medicine & Science in Sports & Exercise* 37:1081–85.

Tejada, T., et al. 2006. Nonpharmacologic therapy for hypertension: Does it really work? *Current Cardiology Reports* 8:418–24.

Tucker, R., et al. 2004. Impaired exercise performance in the heat is associated with an anticipatory reduction in skeletal muscle recruitment. *Pflugers Archive* 448:422–30.

Twerenbold, R., et al. 2003. Effects of different sodium concentrations in replacement fluids during prolonged exercise in women. *British Journal of Sports Medicine* 37:300–3.

Uckert, S., and Joch, W. 2007. Effects of warm-up and precooling on endurance performance in the heat. *British Journal of Sports Medicine* 41:380–84.

Valtin, H. 2002. "Drink at least eight glasses of water a day." Really? Is there scientific evidence for "8 × 8?" *American Journal of Physiology. Regulatory Integrative and Comparative Physiology* 283:R993–1004.

Van Essen, M., and Gibala, M. 2006. Failure of protein to improve time trial performance when added to a sports drink. *Medicine & Science in Sports & Exercise* 38:1476–83.

van Rosendal, S. P., and Coombes, J. S. 2012. Glycerol use in hyperhydration and rehydration: Scientific update. *Medicine and Sport Science* 59:104–12. doi: 10 1159/000341959.

van Rosendal, S. P., et al. 2012. Performance benefits of rehydration with intravenous fluid and oral glycerol. *Medicine*

and Science in Sports and Exercise 44 (9):1780–90.

van Rosendal, S., et al. 2010. Guidelines for glycerol use in hyperhydration and rehydration associated with exercise. *Sports Medicine* 40:113–39.

Volpe, S., et al. Estimation of prepractice hydration status of National Collegiate Athletic Association Division I athletes. *Journal of Athletic Training* 44:624–29.

von Fraunhofer, J., and Rogers, M. 2005. Effects of sports drinks and other beverages on dental enamel. *General Dentistry* 53:28–31.

Webster, J., et al. 2005. A light-weight vest enhances performance of athletes in the heat. *Ergonomics* 48:821–37.

Wegmann, M., et al. 2012. Pre-cooling and sports performance: A meta-analytic review. *Sports Medicine* 42 (7):545–64.

Wharam, P., et al. 2006. NSAID use increases the risk of developing hyponatremia during an Ironman triathlon. *Medicine & Science in Sports & Exercise* 38:618–22.

White, J., et al. 1998. Fluid replacement needs of well-trained male and female athletes during indoor and outdoor steady state running. *Journal of Science and Medicine in Sport* 1:131–42.

Wing-Gaia, S., et al. 2005. Effects of purified oxygenated water on exercise performance during acute hypoxic exposure. *International Journal of Sport Nutrition and Exercise Metabolism* 15:680–88.

Wingo, J., et al. 2004. Influence of a pre-exercise glycerol hydration beverage on performance and physiologic function during mountain-bike races in the heat. *Journal of Athletic Training* 39:169–75.

Yaspelkis, B., et al. 1993. Carbohydrate metabolism during exercise in hot and thermoneutral environments. *International Journal of Sports Medicine* 14:13–19.

Yeargin, S., et al. 2006. Body cooling between two bouts of exercise in the heat enhances subsequent performance. *Journal of Strength and Conditioning Research* 20:383–89.

Young, A. 1990. Energy substrate utilization during exercise in extreme environments. *Exercise and Sport Sciences Reviews* 18:65–118.

Zachwieja, J., et al. 1992. The effects of a carbonated carbohydrate drink on gastric emptying, gastrointestinal distress, and exercise performance. *International Journal of Sport Nutrition* 2:239–50.

Body Weight and Composition for Health and Sport

CHAPTER TEN

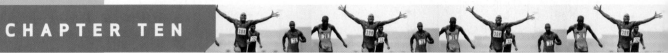

LEARNING OBJECTIVES

After studying this chapter, you should be able to:

1. List the various components that constitute human body composition.

2. Describe the various techniques used to assess body composition and discuss the general uses and limitations of such techniques.

3. Identify body mass index and body fat values associated with underweight, overweight, and degrees of obesity.

4. Explain the mechanisms whereby the human body regulates body weight, including the role of the central nervous system and feedback from peripheral organs and tissues.

5. List and explain the various genetic and environmental factors that may affect the normal regulation of body weight, particularly factors that may predispose to the development of overweight and obesity.

6. Outline the health problems that are associated with obesity in both adults and youth.

7. Describe the health problems associated with excessive weight loss involving the use of drugs, very low-Calorie diets, and various eating disorders.

8. Understand the potential health problems associated with the female athlete triad.

9. Understand how either excess or insufficient body weight may impair sports or physical performance.

The human body is a remarkable machine. Energy systems, which were discussed in chapter 3, capture a portion of the chemical energy primarily in carbohydrates and fats (and protein), as discussed in chapters 4–6, for ATP synthesis. Energy balance reflects, quite literally, a balance between the dietary energy one consumes and the metabolic and thermal energy produced by the body throughout the day. In order to maintain a given body weight, energy input (diet) must balance energy output (metabolism). If there is a long-term imbalance between energy input and energy output, body weight will either increase or decrease. A surplus of 50 Calories per day adds up to 18,250 Calories (over 5 pounds) a year. Conversely, a deficit of 50 Calories per day will result in a 5-pound weight loss over a year.

The term **body image** refers to the mental image we have of our own physical appearance, and it can be influenced by a variety of factors, including how much we weigh and how that weight is distributed. Body weight appears to be a major concern of many Americans. In a survey of U.S. adults, Fallon and others report body image dissatisfaction rates of 13.4–31.8 percent and 9.0–28.4 percent for women and men, respectively, depending on how dissatisfaction was measured. Similar findings have been reported at the high school and even the elementary school level, primarily with female students, and some research has found that 85 percent of both male and female first-year college students desire to change their body weight.

The primary cause of this concern is the value that society, in general, assigns to physical appearance. Males and females alike are bombarded by unrealistic body images in various media. Overweight and obesity are viewed by many as a handicap to both personal and professional fulfillment. The term *fattism* has been coined to reflect society's prejudice toward the obese. Vartanian and others reported greater feelings of disgust in separate samples evaluating obese stereotypes such as laziness/sloppiness. Most individuals who are dissatisfied with their physical appearance feel that they are overweight, and federal surveys have shown that about two-thirds of American adults are trying to lose weight or keep from gaining weight, and they are spending a lot of money to do so. The Federal Trade Commission reported that consumers spent about $2.4 billion annually on weight-loss products and services in 2013, many based on fraudulent or deceptive claims In 2014, the highest court in the European Union ruled that obesity could be considered a disability but did not require protection under antidiscrimination laws for obese individuals. Weight-loss strategies will be discussed in detail in chapter 11.

Obesity, or *globesity,* is a worldwide epidemic in Western and Westernizing countries and is associated with poverty in developing countries. From 1980 to 2013, Ng and others reported increases in overweight and obesity of 27.5 and 47.1 percent for adults and children, respectively. Worldwide, an estimated 2.1 billion people are overweight or obese. According to the Centers for Disease Control and Prevention, the prevalence of overweight and obesity has increased at an alarming rate in the United States over the past three decades. Ogden and others report that 34.9 percent of adults and 17 percent of children in the USA were obese in 2011–2012. In a separate report, Ogden and others note significant relationships among socioeconomic status, gender, and obesity, with higher obesity rates in poorer females with lower education levels and in non-Hispanic blacks and Hispanic groups. According to data from the National Center for Health Statistics, the prevalence of overweight and obesity among U.S. adults age 20 years and older increased from 54.9 percent in 1988–1994 to 69 percent in 2011–2012. In the same time period, the prevalence of obesity increased from 11.3 to 17.7 percent (56 percent) in children 6–11 years and from 10.5 to 20.5 percent (95 percent) in children 12–19 years. Sturm and Hattori report the prevalence of extreme obesity (BMI > 50 kg/m^2) in the United States increased ten-fold from 2000 to 2010, with a decline in the rate of increase since 2005. Based on current time trends, Wang and Lim predict increases in the global prevalence of overweight and obese preschool-aged children from 6.7 percent in 2010 to 7.8 percent in 2015 and 9.1 percent in 2020. This is an alarming trend, since obesity is associated with other comorbidities, most notably diabetes mellitus. Catenacci and others contend that children in this generation might be the first in history to experience a decreased life span due to the health problems associated with excess body weight.

As we shall see, being overweight or obese may contribute to the development of numerous health problems. Catenacci and others note that because of the complexity of obesity, it is likely to be one of the most difficult public health issues our society has faced, mainly because the World Health Organization (WHO) identifies obesity as one of the few risk factors that contribute to the development of the majority of chronic diseases. In the United States, a report from the National Bureau of Economic Research indicated that 16.5 percent of medical costs ($164.8 billion) can be blamed on obesity, and these costs may be expected to increase as the prevalence of obesity also increases. Thus, the Public Health Service has stated in *Healthy People 2020* that one of the major health objectives for the year 2020 is to decrease the proportion of adults and children who are significantly overweight or obese. Some contend that obesity should be targeted for reduction as aggressively as cigarette smoking has been.

Excess body weight may affect physical performance as well. For some athletes, simply being a little overweight may prove to be detrimental to physical performance because it costs energy to move the extra body mass. In contrast, increased body weight, provided it is of the right composition, may be advantageous to other athletes.

At the other end of the body-weight continuum, weight losses leading to excessive thinness also may have an impact upon health and physical performance. Anorexia nervosa and bulimia nervosa are two serious health disorders associated with obsessive concern about body weight. Hudson and colleagues estimate prevalence rates of 0.9 percent (anorexia nervosa), 1.5 percent (bulimia nervosa), and 3.5 percent (binge-eating disorder) in females. Although losing excess body fat may improve performance in some sports, excessive weight losses may have a negative impact on both health and athletic performance.

The preceding discussion has focused on extremes in body *weight*. It is important to stress that body weight is not synonymous with optimal body *composition* for health and performance. The major focus of this chapter is on the basic nature of body composition and its effect on health and physical performance. The following two chapters deal with weight-control methods used to maintain or modify body composition.

Body Weight and Composition

What is the ideal body weight?

Most individuals have a perception of an *"ideal"* body weight for standing height, age, and gender that is usually related to physical appearance. Most research efforts have attempted to find an ideal body weight for good health. Actuarial data collected by life insurance companies during the past century have been compiled into "normal" or "desirable" ranges of body weight for a given height and age. These height-weight charts, such as the Metropolitan Life Height/Weight Charts appearing in many physicians' offices, represent the ideal weights at which Americans can expect to live the longest. Enhanced physical appearance may also improve one's body image and self-esteem, factors important to psychological health. Although society may create a perception of an ideal body weight for appearance, this perceived ideal body weight may or may not be in accord with reality, optimal health, or physical performance. An enhanced physical appearance may also influence performance in certain sports that involve judging of aesthetic movements, such as gymnastics and diving.

There appears to be no sound evidence to suggest a specific ideal weight for a given individual. Instead of *ideal* body weight for health and performance, a more appropriate concept is *healthy* body weight, which is grounded in the concept of healthy body composition. Many factors will influence the body weight for a given individual, not the least of which is the measurement error in various body composition assessment techniques, a topic discussed in this chapter. The major focus of this chapter is to discuss general guidelines that have been proposed for body composition and body weight relative to health and physical performance.

Although height-weight charts have been used to screen for normal body weight in the past, the body mass index (BMI) is the current standard, which is also based on a height-weight relationship. The **body mass index (BMI)**, also known as *Quetelet's Index,* is a weight:height ratio. Using the metric system, the formula is body weight in kilograms ÷ (height in meters)^2. In English units, the formula is [(body weight in pounds) × 705] ÷ (height in inches)^2. The following is an example:

$$200\text{-pound (90.9-kg), 71-inch (1.8-m) male} = 90.9 \div 1.80^2$$
$$= 28 \text{ kg/m}^2$$
$$200 \times 705 \div 71^2 = 28 \text{ kg/m}^2$$

In general, a BMI range of 18.5–25 is considered to be normal for adults. Adult BMI categories for normal weight, overweight, obesity, and disease risk are presented in table 10.1. We will discuss waist circumference, patterns of fat deposition, and risk of disease later in the chapter. You may calculate your BMI using method A in appendix C or at the following Website: http://www.cdc.gov/healthyweight/assessing/bmi/adult_bmi/english_bmi_calculator/bmi_calculator.html

Calculating the BMI for children and teens is somewhat more complex and includes both age and gender. The BMI is used as a screening tool to identify possible weight problems for children, and both the Centers for Disease Control and Prevention (CDC) and the American Academy of Pediatrics (AAP) recommend the use of BMI in children beginning at 2 years old. The CDC has developed BMI-for-age growth charts for girls and boys that can be consulted to provide a percentile for a child's or teen's sex and age. The percentile ranking places the child in one of the following five categories:

Underweight (<5 percentile)
Healthy weight (5−<85 percentile)
Overweight (85−<95 percentile)
Obese (≥95 percentile)
Severely obese (≥120 percent of the 95th percentile)

The following Website provides detailed information on calculation and interpretation of the BMI for children and teens: http://nccd.cdc.gov/dnpabmi/Calculator.aspx

TABLE 10.1 Classification of disease risk based on body mass index and waist circumference

Category	BMI (kg/m^2)	Disease Risk Relative to Normal Weight and Waist Circumference*	
		Normal Risk Visceral Fat Deposition* Men ≤102 cm (40 inches); Female ≤88 cm (35 inches)	**High Risk Visceral Fat Deposition*** Men >102 cm (40 inches); Females >88 cm (35 inches)
Underweight	<18.5	–	–
Normal	18.5–24.9	–	–
Overweight	25.0–29.9	Increased	High
Obesity I	30.0–34.9	High	Very high
Obesity II	35.0–39.9	Very high	Very high
Obesity III	≥40	Extremely high	Extremely high

*Research suggests that waist sizes greater than 37 inches in men and 31.5 inches in women may increase health risks when accompanied by other conditions, such as high blood pressure.

Source: National Heart, Lung, and Blood Institute of the National Institutes of Health www.nhlbi.nih.gov/health/educational/lose_wt/BMI/bmi_dis.htm.

What are the values and limitations of the BMI?

In relation to determining whether an individual possesses normal body weight for a given height, the BMI may be a useful screening device for health problems. As we will discuss in later sections of the chapter, high BMI values may be associated with overweight or obesity and various metabolic diseases such as diabetes mellitus, cardiovascular disease, and metabolic syndrome. At the other end of the continuum, low BMI values may also be the result of hormonal imbalances, malnutrition, or eating disorders. Specific BMI values related to potential health status are presented later. BMI is also used in large epidemiological studies instead of more sophisticated body composition assessment techniques as an apparent indicator of increased prevalence of overweight/obesity in a population over time. Assuming the existence of standardized measurements of body weight and height, such studies can detect associations between apparent increases in body fatness (increased BMI) and health. The use of BMI as an indicator of fatness is based on the assumption that increased BMI over time is due to increased body weight (the numerator), which in most individuals is most likely the result of increased adiposity over time. Since the mid-1980s, the Centers for Disease Control and Prevention has been tracking the prevalence of obesity (operationally defined as BMI ≥30) in the United States through the Behavioral Risk Factor Surveillance Survey. These data can be viewed at the following CDC Website: www.cdc.gov/obesity/data/adult.html

As a caveat, however, BMI actually reveals nothing about body composition. The BMI value does not represent percent body fat, as some mistakenly think. As illustrated in figure 10.1, two individuals may be exactly the same height and weight and have the same BMI, but the distribution of their body weight might be so different that one individual could be considered obese while the other might be considered very muscular. In a comparison of BMI and more sophisticated body composition assessment techniques (discussed later) in college athletes and nonathletes, Ode and others reported that BMI incorrectly classified normal-fat athletes as overweight because of generally larger muscle mass present in male and female athletes. Conversely, many female nonathletes were classified as normal weight by the BMI but actually were overfat. Those who do not exercise, and yet are thin, may have excessive amounts of internal fat and thus may be thin on the outside but fat on the inside. BMI should be used cautiously when classifying fatness in college athletes and other muscular individuals as well as nonathletes.

Although BMI is not perfect and may be inappropriate for use with very muscular individuals, it is a good guide that the average person may use to think about a healthier body weight. However, other methods are needed to evaluate actual body composition.

What is the composition of the body?

The human body contains many of the elements of the earth, 25 of which appear to be essential for normal physiological functioning. Most of the human body, about 96 percent, consists of four elements (carbon, hydrogen, oxygen, and nitrogen) in various combinations. These four elements are the structural basis for body protein, carbohydrate, fat, and water. The remaining 4 percent of the body is composed of minerals, primarily calcium and phosphorus in the bones; other macrominerals such as chlorine, sulfur, sodium, and magnesium; and the microminerals iron, cobalt, zinc, iodine, selenium, fluorine, manganese, molybdenum, chromium, and others that were discussed in chapter 8.

Because body composition may have a significant impact on health and physical performance, scientists have developed a variety of techniques to measure various body components. Wang and others noted that depending on the purpose, body

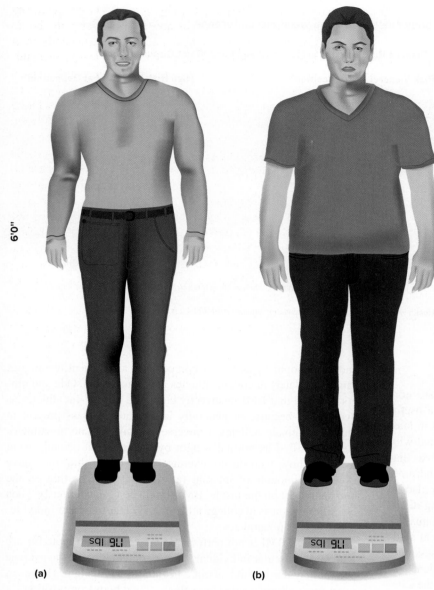

6'0"

175 lbs

(a)

175 lbs

(b)

FIGURE 10.1 Body mass index (BMI), although a good general indicator of overweight and obesity, does not assess body composition in any given individual. Two individuals may have the same height and weight, but one may have excess body fat while the other may be very muscular with a low body-fat percentage.

for comparison is water, which has a density of essentially 1.0, or 1 g/mL, the exact density depending on the water temperature. Corresponding densities for the other components are approximately 1.3–1.4 for bone, 1.1 for fat-free protein tissue, and 0.9 for fat. The total body density value may be used to estimate the body-fat percentage, with a higher density representing a greater amount of fat-free mass and a lower amount of body fat. The total human body density may range from approximately 1.010 g/mL (estimated 40 percent fat) to 1.090 g/mL (estimated 4 percent fat). Although there is little interindividual variance in the densities of fat and water, bone and fat-free densities may vary considerably between individuals and as a function of health status. As a result, the use of constant densities for these components is a source of error in attempts to estimate body-fat percentage from total-body density.

Depending on the purpose, body composition is usually analyzed as two, three, or all four components. The two components most commonly measured are total body fat and fat-free mass; bone mineral content and body water may be measured with more elaborate techniques. Wang and others also introduced a six-component model, which in addition to these four components adds measurement of soft-tissue minerals and glycogen.

Total Body Fat The total body fat in the body consists of both essential fat and storage fat. **Essential fat** is necessary for proper functioning of certain body structures such as the brain, nerve tissue, bone marrow, heart tissue, and cell membranes. Essential fat in adult males represents about 3 percent of the body weight. Adult females also have an additional 9–12 percent of essential fat associated with normal reproductive function. This additional sex-specific fat gives females a total of 12–15 percent essential fat, although this amount may vary considerably among individuals. **Storage fat** is simply a depot for excess energy, the quantity of which may vary considerably between and within individuals due to factors discussed later in this chapter.

composition may be evaluated at five levels: atomic, molecular, cellular, tissue-system, and whole-body levels. Of major interest to body composition scientists are four major body components: total body fat, fat-free mass, bone mineral, and body water. The location of body fat deposits, whether under the skin (subcutaneous) or deep in the body (visceral), is related to health status. As will be discussed later in the chapter, large deposits of visceral fat are associated with diabetes mellitus, cardiovascular disease, and metabolic syndrome. Each of these components has a different density. According to Archimedes' principle, density, also known as specific gravity, equals mass divided by volume. In body composition, density is usually expressed as grams per milliliter (g/mL) or grams per cubic centimeter (g/cc^3). The standard

Some storage fat is found around body organs for protection, but about 70–80 percent of total body fat is found just under the skin and is known as **subcutaneous fat**. **Cellulite** is a certain type of subcutaneous fat more common in females than males. According to Rossi and Katz, cellulite is caused by the sequestration of adipocytes in chambers surrounded by connective tissue. The peripheral adipocytes in these chambers expand with water, stretching and thickening the connective tissue, giving rise to a dimpled surface appearance perceived by many as aesthetically undesirable. Other storage fat is located deep in the body, particularly in the abdominal area. This deep fat is referred to as **visceral fat**, which as noted later is associated with increased health risks.

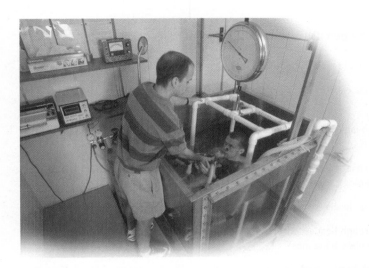

FIGURE 10.2 Underwater weighing is one of the more common laboratory means for determining body composition. However, all current techniques for estimating percent body fat are subject to error. See text for discussion.

Fat-Free Mass   **Fat-free mass** primarily consists of protein and water, with smaller amounts of minerals and glycogen. The tissue of skeletal muscles is the main component of fat-free mass, but the heart, liver, kidneys, and other organs are included also. A more common term often used interchangeably with *fat-free mass* is **lean body mass**; technically, however, lean body mass includes essential fat. In the simplistic two-component model of body composition assessment, total body mass is the sum of fat-free mass (or lean body mass) and fat mass. For example, a 200-pound sedentary person with an estimated 30 percent fat is assumed to have a fat mass of 60 pounds (200 × 0.3) and a corresponding 70 percent, or 140 pounds (200 × 0.7), of fat-free mass.

Bone Mineral   Bone gives structure to the body, but it is also involved in a variety of metabolic processes. Bone consists of about 50 percent water and 50 percent solid matter, including protein (collagen) and minerals, primarily calcium and phosphorus. Although total bone weight, including water and protein, may be 12–15 percent of the total body weight, the mineral content is only 3–4 percent of total body weight.

Body Water   As was discussed in chapter 9, the average adult body weight is approximately 60 percent water, the remaining 40 percent consisting of dry weight materials that exist in this internal water environment. Some tissues, like the blood, have a high water content, whereas others, like adipose tissue, are relatively dry. The fat-free mass is about 70 percent water, while adipose fat tissue is less than 10 percent. Under normal conditions the water concentration of a given tissue is regulated quite nicely relative to its needs. When we look at the percentage of the body weight that may be attributed to a given body tissue, the weight of that tissue includes its normal water content.

Factors Affecting the Components of Body Composition   Body composition may be influenced by a number of factors such as age,

sex, diet, and level of physical activity. Age effects are significant during the developmental years as muscle and other body tissues are being formed. There are some minor differences in body composition between boys and girls up to the age of puberty, but at this age the differences become fairly great. In general, girls deposit more fat beginning with puberty, whereas boys develop more muscle tissue. Factors contributing to a loss of muscle mass during adulthood include a decline in physical activity and **sarcopenia,** the age-related loss of muscle mass. Physical inactivity also contributes to a positive energy balance leading to increased body fat storage. As was discussed in chapter 8, loss of bone mineral content (osteopenia) occurs with age, with high prevalence rates of osteoporosis in some populations. Diet can affect body composition over the short haul, such as during acute water restriction and starvation, but the main effects are seen over the long haul, with chronic overeating leading to increased body fat stores. Physical activity may also be very influential, with a sound exercise program helping to build muscle and lose fat. Strategies to combat increased body fat and weight will be discussed in the next chapter. As a result of these and other factors, the amount of fat, lean tissue, bone, and water can vary significantly between and within individuals. A lean 154-pound male may be compartmentalized into 60 percent (92 pounds) water and 40 percent (62 pounds) solid matter subdivided into fat (14 percent, 22 pounds); protein (22 percent, 34 pounds); and bone minerals (4 percent; 6 pounds).

What techniques are available to measure body composition and how accurate are they?

The measurement of body fat has become very popular in recent years. Many high school and university athletic departments routinely analyze the body composition of their athletes in attempts to predict an optimal weight for competition. In some sports, such as wrestling, measurement of body composition is mandated by various state or national sport associations. Fitness and wellness centers also usually include a body-fat analysis as one of their services. Unfortunately, some of the individuals who analyze body composition in these situations are unaware of the limitations of the tests they employ.

The only direct, accurate method of analyzing body composition is by chemical extraction of all fat from body tissues, which is obviously not appropriate with living humans. Thus, a variety of indirect methods have been developed to assess body composition. Some are relatively simple, such as visual observation by an experienced judge, and others are rather complex, such as nuclear magnetic resonance imaging, using multimillion-dollar machines. Indirect methods are used to measure body fat, lean body mass, bone mineral content, and body water. Some techniques are also used to measure fat in specific locations of the body.

All indirect assessment techniques discussed in this section that are employed *in vivo* (i.e., on the living, breathing individual)— even technologically sophisticated ones—ultimately provide only estimates of various components of body composition, including body fat. These estimates vary in precision and are prone to error depending on the technique. Such errors usually are expressed statistically as standard errors of measurement or estimate, which

TABLE 10.2	Methods used to determine body composition using the two (2)- or three (3)-component models
Anthropometry (2)	Measures body segment girths to predict body fat
Bioelectrical impedance analysis (BIA) (2)	Measures resistance to electrical current to predict body-water content, lean body mass, and body fat
Body plethysmography (2)	Whole-body plethysmograph measures air displacement and calculates body density; comparable to water displacement protocol used in underwater weighing
Computed tomography (CT) (3)	X-ray scanning technique to image body tissues; useful in determining subcutaneous and deep fat to predict body-fat percentage; used to calculate bone mass
Dual energy X-ray absorptiometry (DEXA; DXA) (3)	X-ray technique at two energy levels to image body fat; used to calculate bone mass
Dual photon absorptiometry (DPA) (3)	Beam of photons passes through tissues, differentiating soft tissues and bone tissues; used to predict body fat and calculate bone mass
Infrared interactance (2)	Infrared light passes through tissues, and interaction with tissue components used to predict body fat
Magnetic resonance imaging (MRI) (3)	Magnetic-field and radio-frequency waves are used to image body tissues similar to CT scan; very useful for imaging deep abdominal fat
Neutron activation analysis (3)	Beam of neutrons passes through the tissues, permitting analysis of nitrogen and other mineral content in the body; used to predict lean body mass
Skinfold thicknesses (2)	Measures subcutaneous fat folds to predict body-fat content and lean body mass
Total body potassium (2)	Measures total body potassium, the main intracellular ion, to predict lean body mass and body fat
Total body water (hydrometry) (2)	Measures total body water by isotope dilution techniques to predict lean body mass and body fat
Ultrasound (2)	High-frequency ultrasound waves pass through tissues to image subcutaneous fat and predict body-fat content
Underwater weighing (hydrodensitometry) (2)	Underwater-weighing technique based on Archimedes' principle to predict body density, body fat, and lean body mass

can be used to show the accuracy of the body-fat measurement. For example, a wrestler undergoes preseason body composition assessment. A skinfold technique predicts 7 percent body fat and has a standard error of measurement (SEM) of 3 percent. If the same wrestler is measured repeatedly with no change in body composition, the technique will generate different estimates. Approximately 68 percent of these actual measurements would be within 1 SEM of the average value, so there is a 68 percent level of confidence that the actual body fat percentage of this wrestler is between 4 and 10 percent ($\pm$1 SEM). This is actually an example of a *doubly* indirect technique, since an *estimate* of body density is used to *estimate* body fat percentage. Body composition assessment should only be considered as providing a range, which may include the actual body fat percentage at a certain level of confidence, not as a precise measurement.

Most field methods used, such as skinfolds and bioelectrical impedance analysis (BIA), are two-component models, as are some laboratory methods, such as hydrostatic weighing and air-displacement plethysmography. Going indicates that methods based on two-component models are associated with greater errors than are methods based on multicomponent models, such as dual energy X-ray absorptiometry (DEXA). Three- and four-component models that combine measures of body density with body water and mineral content dramatically reduce the errors associated with the traditional simplistic two-component model. A number of body composition measurement techniques are highlighted in table 10.2, but only the more commonly used or promising techniques will be discussed. In her review, Heyward discusses the validity of various anthropometric techniques and bioelectrical impedance in children, young adults, and older adults. Going and colleagues discuss ten questions summarizing laboratory- and field-based body composition research and pose future questions concerning human growth and development, aging, fitness, health, and disease. Ackland and colleagues provide an excellent review of body composition assessment and application in training for weight-class (e.g., wrestling), aesthetic (e.g., gymnastics), and gravitational (e.g., jumping, cycling, and running) sports. Heyward and Wagner's book provides prediction formulas for various athletic populations. Finally, Fosbøl and Zerahn provide an excellent review of contemporary assessment methods, assumptions underlying the use of each method, sources of error, and variables to consider in selection of a method for a given individual.

The selected body composition technique will depend on the availability of resources, the laboratory-versus field-based nature

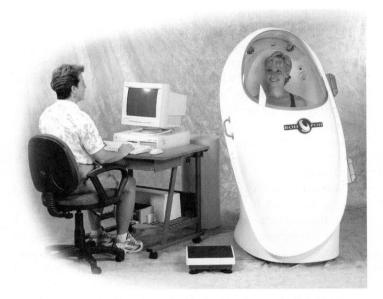

FIGURE 10.3 The Bod Pod. An application of total body plethysmography, an air displacement technique, to evaluate body composition.

Photo courtesy of Life Measurement Instruments.

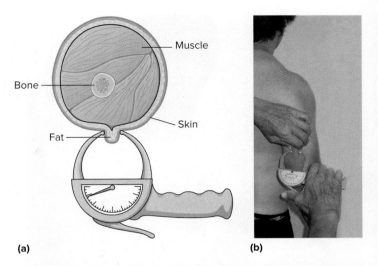

(a)   **(b)**

FIGURE 10.4 (a) Schematic drawing showing the skinfold of fat that is pinched up away from the underlying muscle tissue. (b) Measurement of the triceps skinfold. Precise location: a vertical fold on the posterior aspect of the right arm halfway between the acromial process of the shoulder and olecranon process of the elbow.

of assessment, and other factors. Regardless of the chosen method, the following general guidelines should be followed.

1. The measurement error will be smaller if the same method is used to assess changes in an individual throughout the period of assessment.
2. Skinfold measurements may have a low inter-measurer reliability due to differences in grasping technique and anatomical site location. Measurements should be taken by the same trained technician throughout the assessment period.
3. Population-specific equations have been developed from homogeneous subjects based on characteristics such as gender, age, ethnicity, and athletic group. The individual being assessed should belong to the population upon which the equation was developed. Heyward and Wagner's book provides prediction formulas for various athletic populations.

Hydrostatic Weighing   One of the most common research techniques for determining body density is **hydrostatic weighing**, also known as underwater weighing or *hydrodensitometry*. Hydrostatic weighing is a volumetric technique based on Archimedes' principle that a body immersed in a fluid is acted upon by a buoyancy force that is directly related to the volume of water displaced (see figure 10.2). Because fat is less dense and bone and muscle tissue are more dense than water, a given weight of fat will displace a larger volume of water and exhibit a greater buoyant effect than the corresponding weight of bone and muscle tissue. Different formulas are recommended for determination of body density, depending upon the age and sex of the individual. Although this technique was once referred to as the "gold standard" in body composition analysis, it is an indirect two-component model with associated weaknesses. As previously mentioned, the assumption

that the density of the fat-free protein tissue is 1.10 g/mL may not be valid for all individuals, such as athletes and older persons. The standard error is still about 2–2.5 percent. Thus, Wagner and Heyward noted that underwater weighing should not be regarded as the "gold standard" because of these errors. The hydrostatic-weighing technique is rather time-consuming and difficult for some individuals. For example, the quality of the data is affected by the subject's comfort level with the water medium, so non-swimmers may have difficulty with the technique. Other techniques (e.g., air displacement plethysmography, discussed next) have been developed for either research purposes or practical applications. The interested reader is referred to the review by Going and the book by Heyward and Wagner.

Air Displacement Plethysmography (ADP)   Another volumetric technique is **air displacement plethysmography (ADP)**, sometimes referred to as body plethysmography. Subjects enter a dual-chamber plethysmograph designed to measure the amount of air they displace, somewhat comparable to the water displacement technique of underwater weighing. One commercial product available is called the Bod Pod (see figure 10.3). It is portable, easy to operate, requires little time, and eliminates the necessity of going underwater, several clear advantages compared to underwater weighing. Several reviews, including one by Wagner and Heyward, have noted that it may be more valid and reliable than hydrodensitometry for certain individuals, such as those who fear underwater submersion, but has similar limitations. In this regard, Fields noted that the ADP and underwater weighing agree within 1 percent of body fat for adults and children, but when compared to multicomponent models ADP generally underestimated body fat by 2–3 percent. Several studies compared the Bod Pod to DEXA and reached different conclusions. A study with men reported a 2.2 percent difference in body fat between the two methods,

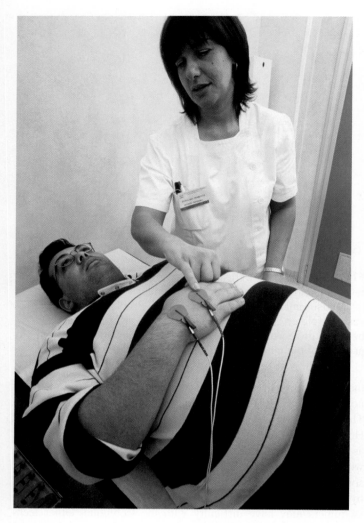

FIGURE 10.5 Bioelectrical impedance analysis. A low-voltage current is optimally conducted through a body with a high fat-free mass (high water content) while high-fat mass (low water content) offers resistance to the current. Electrodes are placed at the hands and feet (not shown).

administered with an acceptable pair of skinfold calipers by an experienced tester. Ultrasound techniques are also available to assess skinfold thicknesses, but these are more expensive than calipers. Orphanidou and others found that measurements of subcutaneous body fat with skinfold techniques were comparable to those obtained by ultrasound and computed tomography, suggesting that the use of skinfold calipers in the clinical setting is appropriate. Utter and Hager reported that ultrasound provided similar estimates of fat-free mass as hydrostatic weighing in high school wrestlers and suggested it could be an alternative field-based method.

Skinfold equations to estimate body density are usually based on total body density measured by hydrostatic weighing. As a result, the standard error for the skinfold technique is about 3–4 percent and reflects error in both measurement of the skinfold thickness and the hydrostatic weighing used to generate the prediction equation. Nevertheless, Lohman and others indicated that the skinfold technique is one of the best practical methods to measure body composition. Wagner and Heyward noted that the technique can provide accurate results for lean subjects, such as athletes. Using a population-specific formula for gender, age, ethnicity, and sport, if available, will help reduce prediction errors. Clark and others validated the NCAA skinfold technique as a means to predict minimal weight classes for wrestlers. Appendix D includes commonly used generalized equations to estimate body density from three gender-specific skinfold sites and age, based on the work of Jackson and Pollock (males), and Jackson, Pollock, and Ward (females), respectively, with subsequent conversion of estimated body density to estimated body fat percentage using the Siri equation. O'Connor and others have developed equations for non-Hispanic White, Hispanic, and African-American adults with standard errors of estimate between 3 and 4 percent.

Bioelectrical Impedance Analysis (BIA)

A more expensive, practical field technique is **bioelectrical impedance analysis (BIA)** illustrated in figure 10.5. BIA is based on the principle of resistance to an electrical current that is applied to the body. The less the recorded resistance, the greater the water content, and hence the greater the body density. Early research with BIA revealed large standard errors in predicting lean body mass, so it was not considered to be very valid. However, Jaffrin, in an update on BIA, reported that it has been compared with medical impedance meters and with dual X-ray absorptiometry measurements and found reasonably accurate, except for individuals with very low or high BMI. The BIA instrument may have preprogrammed prediction equations to use, which ideally should include age, gender, and ethnicity; most do not have athlete-specific equations based on a multicomponent model including total body water, as noted in a review by Moon. In its position stand on nutrition for the athlete, the Academy of Nutrition and Dietetics, Dietitians of Canada, and American College of Sports Medicine indicated that the prediction accuracy of BIA is similar to that of skinfold assessment, but BIA may be preferable because it does not require the technical skill associated with skinfold measurements. Pichard

whereas a study with women reported no significant differences. Overall, Noreen and Lemon indicate that ADP appears to be a reliable method to use in tracking changes in body composition in individuals over time.

Skinfolds

The **skinfold technique** is designed to measure the thickness of subcutaneous fat in millimeters at specific anatomical sites (see figure 10.4). It appears to be the most common procedure for nonresearch purposes. The skinfold thickness values are inserted into an appropriate equation to estimate total body density, which in turn is used in another equation to estimate body fat percentage. Some formulas also have been developed for specific athletic groups. To improve the accuracy of this technique, skinfold measures should be obtained from a variety of body sites because using a single skinfold site may be unrepresentative of total storage fat. The test also should be and others reported valid BIA equations for female runners but recommended research to validate equations for other athletes.

Dual Energy X-Ray Absorptiometry (DXA, DEXA) **Dual energy X-ray absorptiometry (DXA or DEXA)** is a computerized X-ray technique used to image body tissues and has been used to assess bone mineral content, fat-free mass, and body fat concurrently (see figure 10.6). DEXA may also be used to assess regional fat depots such as deep visceral fat, as can other sophisticated techniques, such as magnetic resonance imaging (MRI) and computed tomography (CT). DEXA is also used in clinical settings to detect the presence of osteoporosis.

Going notes that DEXA has emerged as a criterion method used to validate other methods. However, different DEXA manufacturers' scanners and software give different results, which is the main limitation of DEXA. In their study of competitive male and female athletes, Rodriguez-Sanchez and Galloway reported decreases in total body mass (2.3 percent) and lean mass in a dehydrated state compared to euhydration, a reflection of sweat loss. The estimated percent fat increased slightly (0.3 percent) with no change in fat mass. They concluded that subjects should be euhydrated when DEXA is used to monitor body composition changes over time.

Near-Infrared Interactance Another device marketed commercially is based on near-infrared light interactance. In essence, infrared light passes through the tissues, and its interaction with tissue

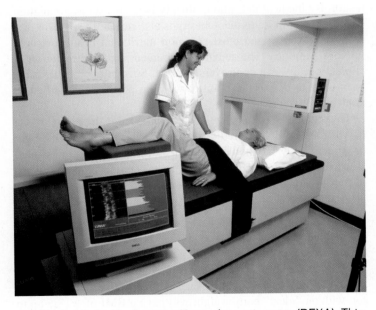

FIGURE 10.6 Dual energy X-ray absorptiometry (DEXA). This method measures body fat by releasing small doses of radiation through the body that a detector then quantifies as fat, lean tissue, or bone. The scanner arm moves from head to toe and in doing so can determine body fat as well as bone density. DEXA is currently considered the most accurate method for determining body fat as long as the person is not too obese to fit on the table and/or under the arm of the instrument. The radiation dose is minimal.

components is used to predict body fat. The Futrex Corporation's 6100® model is one example of such a device. Wagner and Heyward reported somewhat higher standard errors of measurement with near-infrared interactance, greater than 3.5 percent. In separate studies comparing various body composition assessment techniques with a three-component model as the criterion method, Moon and colleagues concluded that near-infrared interactance (Futrex 6100®) was an acceptable field method for college-aged females (SEE = 2.5 percent, r = 0.82) but not for college-aged males (SEE = 4.2 percent, r = 0.49).

Anthropometry Anthropometry, or measurement of body parts, is an inexpensive, practical method to assess body composition. Body measurements include circumferences such as the neck and abdomen, and bone diameters such as the hip, shoulders, elbow, and wrist. Although circumference and/or bone diameter measurements may be incorporated into various equations to predict body fat and lean body mass, Moon and colleagues reported high standard errors of estimate (range = 3.78 to 3.97 percent) for various equations using abdominal and/or neck circumferences generated for use on male United States Army, Navy, Air Force, and Marine Corps personnel.

Circumference measurements of the abdomen, hips, buttocks, thigh, and other body parts may indicate **regional fat distribution**. As discussed later in the chapter, the pattern of fat distribution may be an important indicator of major health problems such as obesity, diabetes, and metabolic syndrome. The principal measure of regional fat distribution is the **waist circumference**, the abdominal or waist girth measured by a flexible tape at the narrowest section of the waist as seen from the front. The waist circumference is a good screening technique for regional fat distribution, but it does not provide an accurate measure of deep visceral fat, such as provided by CT or MRI techniques.

Multicomponent Model The multicomponent model uses several methods, such as hydrodensitometry, total body water, and DEXA to reduce the errors associated with any single method and to provide information on body fat, body water, bone mass, and lean body mass. Lohman and Going recommend use of a multicomponent model when assessing body composition in children and youths, including waist circumference, selected skinfolds, and DEXA. Wagner and Heyward note that the multicomponent model is now regarded as the "gold standard" in body composition assessment and should be used when feasible. Lara and others recently reported that *aggregate* two- (fat mass + fat-free mass based on total body density measurement), three- (water + fat mass + fat-free dry tissue based on total body density and total body water measurements), and four-component (water + bone minerals + fat mass + protein + carbohydrates based on total body density, total body water, and bone mineral mass measurements) improved the accuracy of changes in fat mass in overweight and obese subjects compared to any *single* two-, three-, or four-component approach. Shared variances between the four-component aggregate models and the three- and two-component aggregate models were 0.99 and 0.72, respectively.

What problems may be associated with rigid adherence to body fat percentages in sport?

Table 10.2 lists most of the methods used to estimate body composition. Historically, hydrostatic weighing has been the criterion method by which other techniques have been validated. More recently, DEXA or a four-component model has been used as the criterion. As has been previously discussed, different techniques have sources of error, which contribute to different standard errors of measurement and resulting differences in estimated body fat percentages. Pourhassan and others compared a four-component model (lipids, water, mineral, and protein) to air displacement plethysmography (ADP), total body water (TBW) measurement, DEXA, and magnetic resonance imaging (MRI) in normal-weight and overweight adult subjects over 2 to 4 years. Compared to the four-component model, DEXA and TBW underestimated fat mass gain and overestimated fat-free mass gain in subjects gaining weight, while ADP underestimated fat mass gain and overestimated fat-free mass gain. The researchers attributed this bias to the erroneous assumption in two-component models of a constant hydration state for fat-free mass. Using bioelectrical impedance analysis and six different skinfold equations, Webster and Barr estimated body-fat percentage ranging from 21 to 28.1 percent for female speed skaters and 10.3 to 22.8 percent for female gymnasts. Stout and others cross-validated 16 skinfold equations for prediction of body fat in wrestlers, reported error values of almost 5 percent, and concluded that this level of accuracy is unacceptable. However, Clark and others found that the NCAA skinfold equation is a valid predictor of body fat and support the NCAA method of estimating body fat in college wrestlers for establishment of minimum weight. Oppliger and others developed new infrared interactance equations to predict body fat in high school wrestlers and noted that they are comparable to skinfold equations currently used. Loenneke and colleagues comment that much of the research literature for the NCAA minimum weight (MW) protocol is based on studies of high school wrestlers, which may not accurately represent the body composition status of collegiate wrestlers. Aspects of the policy requiring additional research attention include the effect of overhydration (low urine specific gravity); use of skinfold calipers from different manufacturers; and use of the Brożek equation to estimate fat percentage from estimated body density, which may erroneously increase MW in African-American wrestlers.

Given the problems with assumptions underlying the various methods of body composition determination, body-fat percentage estimates are only approximations. The rigid use of body-fat percentages in weight-control sports, such as gymnastics and wrestling, may lead to excessive weight loss. For example, if a wrestler who has 8 percent fat is required by his coach to reach 5 percent fat, the wrestler may already be at 5 percent fat because the skinfold technique has a 3 to 4 percent standard error of measurement. Losing extra weight may be very difficult for the wrestler because he is already near minimal body-fat levels. In his attempt to heed the coach's mandate, the wrestler may lose lean muscle mass, which will place him at a competitive disadvantage. In young athletes, such practices may also lead to disordered eating and, possibly, clinical eating disorders.

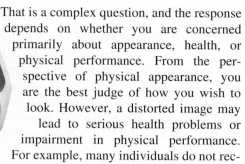

How much should I weigh or how much body fat should I have?

That is a complex question, and the response depends on whether you are concerned primarily about appearance, health, or physical performance. From the perspective of physical appearance, you are the best judge of how you wish to look. However, a distorted image may lead to serious health problems or impairment in physical performance. For example, many individuals do not recognize that they are overweight and may suffer adverse health consequences. Already thin individuals who desire to be even thinner may be prone to eating disorders. Muscular bodybuilders who perceive themselves as not sufficiently muscular may suffer psychologically. In a survey of U.S. adults, Fallon and colleagues reported body dissatisfaction prevalence estimates of 13.4 to 31.8 percent for females and 9 to 28.4 percent for males, with evidence of a plateau or decline in dissatisfaction compared to previous estimates.

The effect of body weight and body fat on physical performance is discussed in a later section, although some general guidelines are presented here. The effect of body weight and fat on health has received considerable research attention. Although being underweight may impair health, most of the focus has been on excess body weight and fat, particularly the relationship of obesity to health. By medical definition, **obesity** is simply an accumulation of fat in the adipose tissue. Obesity is also referred to as a disease or disorder and is the most common nutritional health problem in North America. The actual measurement and determination of clinical obesity is a controversial issue. Several approaches have been used to define the point at which a person is classified as clinically obese.

Unfortunately, our present level of knowledge does not provide us with the ability to predict precisely what the optimal weight or percent body fat should be for health in any given individual. However, some general guidelines have been developed by various professional and health organizations.

Body Mass Index BMI may be used as a crude technique to calculate a target body weight, as shown in appendix C and various Websites (www.nhlbi.nih.gov/health/educational/lose_wt/BMI/bmicalc.htm). According to guidelines from the National Academy of Sciences and the National Institutes of Health, a person with an "ideal" body weight will have a BMI of ≥18.5 up to ≤24.9. The BMI equation can be rearranged to solve for a target weight as follows:

$$\text{weight in kg} = \text{desired BMI, a value from 18.4 to 24.9} \times \text{height measured in meters}^2$$

or

$$\text{weight in lbs} = \text{desired BMI, a value from 18.4 to 24.9} \times \text{height measured in inches}^2 \div 705$$

Higher BMI values are usually, but not always, associated with overweight and obesity, as described in table 10.1. As previously discussed, BMI values are based on height and weight and should not be confused with body-fat percentages. Most Americans are focused on weight maintenance or weight loss, strategies of which are covered in chapter 11. At the other extreme, low BMI values may be indicative of starvation. The Food and Agriculture Organization has proposed the following BMI categories as indicative of use of a BMI less than 18.5 as a criterion for chronic energy deficiency (CED). CED grades and associated BMI values are based on a Physical Activity Level (PAL=measured energy expenditure or intake÷measured basal metabolic rate) of less than 1.4. The PAL concept is discussed in chapters 3 and 11.

BMI	CED Grade
≥18.5	Apparently normal nutritional status
17.0−18.4	Grade I CED
16.0−16.9	Grade II CED
<16.0	Grade III CED

The health and performance of some Americans will actually benefit from weight gain consisting of fat-free mass, strategies of which will be discussed in chapter 12.

Body-Fat Percentage   As noted previously, the use of the BMI height-weight relationship does not evaluate body composition. A low BMI may be a symptom of a serious disease, not a cause. Muscular individuals may have a high BMI and not be obese. For health purposes, the body requires a minimal level of fat, called essential fat, found in cell membranes, bone marrow, and nervous tissue and considered to be approximately 3 percent for males and 12 to 15 percent for females. Several authorities have included additional levels of storage fat and suggested that minimal levels of total body fat for health range from 5 to 10 percent for males and 15 to 18 percent for females. Depending on gender and sport, levels of body fat in the range of 5 to 10 percent may be recommended for distance runners, gymnasts, dancers, and wrestlers. However, some athletes have performed very successfully even though their body-fat percentage was higher than the recommended values.

Although different levels of body-fat percentages have been cited as the criterion for obesity, the Academy of Nutrition and Dietetics and the National Research Council set the value at 25 percent for males and 30 percent for females. The National Academy of Sciences, in its DRI on energy intake, also published criteria for obesity, setting the level at 25 percent body fat for males but 37 percent for females. The NAS noted that over 31 percent and 42 percent body fat in males and females, respectively, was indicative of clinical obesity.

Body-fat percentage categories from essential to very poor (overweight/obese) for males and females by age are presented in table 10.3. Several points should be kept in mind when using such tables. All body-fat prediction methods contain a source of error. The essential, very lean, and excellent categories pertain to athletes competing in weight-control sports or sports where excess body fat may be a disadvantage. As will be discussed later, obesity generally increases health risks, but some individuals with higher body-fat percentages may not develop obesity-related health problems if they are otherwise physically fit and consume a healthful diet. Finally, as will also be discussed later in this chapter, the location of the fat in the body may have significant health consequences.

Waist Circumference   It may not be how much fat you have that affects your health but where that fat is located. The health implications of regional fat distribution are discussed later, but you may use method C in appendix C to calculate your waist circumference and evaluate associated health risks. As a screening measure for deep visceral fat, increased health risks are associated with waist circumferences greater than 35 inches in females and 40 inches in males. However, as discussed later, lower waist circumferences may be associated with increased risks if accompanied by other conditions, such as high blood pressure. Table 10.1 highlights the risk of chronic disease associated with the BMI and waist size.

Key Concepts

▶ Body mass index (BMI) does not measure body composition, but it may be useful as a screening device to determine whether one is overweight or obese. *Overweight* and *obese* are not synonymous terms. It is possible to be overweight but not obese or at a "normal" weight with too much body fat.

▶ The body consists of four components: body fat, protein, minerals, and water. However, for practical purposes, body composition may be classified as consisting of two components: fat-free weight, which is about 70 percent water, and body fat.

▶ All techniques that are currently used to measure body composition, primarily body fat, are indirect and prone to error; even the hydrostatic-weighing technique, once considered to be the most accurate, may be in error by 2.0–2.5 percent.

▶ Our present level of knowledge does not provide us with the ability to predict precisely what the optimal body composition should be for health or physical performance. However, BMI and body-fat levels higher than normal are associated with increased health risks.

Check for Yourself

▶ Using appendix C, calculate both your body mass index (BMI) and your waist circumference. Compare your findings to the rating scale in table 10.1.

TABLE 10.3 Body-Fat Categories by Gender and Age

| Category | Males
Age Group | | | | | |
	20–29	30–39	40–49	50–59	60–69	70+
Essential	3.0					
Very lean	≤6.6	≤10.3	≤12.9	≤14.8	≤16.2	≤15.5
Excellent	7.9–10.5	12.4–14.9	15.0–17.5	17.0–19.4	18.0–20.2	17.5–20.1
Good	11.5–14.8	15.9–18.4	18.5–20.8	20.2–22.3	21.0–23.0	21.0–22.9
Fair	15.8–18.6	19.2–21.6	21.4–23.5	23.0–24.9	23.6–25.6	23.7–25.3
Poor	19.7–23.3	22.4–25.1	24.2–26.6	25.6–28.1	26.4–28.8	25.8–28.4
Very poor	≥24.9	≥26.4	≥27.8	≥29.2	≥29.8	≥29.4
Category	Females					
Essential	12.0–15.0					
Very lean	≤14.0	≤13.9	≤15.2	≤16.9	≤17.7	≤16.4
Excellent	15.1–16.8	15.5–17.5	16.8–19.5	19.1–22.3	20.2–23.3	18.3–22.5
Good	17.6–19.8	18.3–21.0	20.6–23.7	23.6–26.7	24.6–27.5	23.7–26.6
Fair	20.6–23.4	22.0–24.8	24.6–27.5	27.6–30.1	28.3–30.8	27.6–30.5
Poor	24.2–28.2	25.8–29.6	28.4–31.9	30.8–33.9	31.5–34.4	31.0–34.0
Very poor	≥30.5	≥31.5	≥33.4	≥35.0	≥35.6	≥35.3

Modified from *American College of Sports Medicine's Guidelines for Exercise Testing and Prescription*, 9th Edition, and The Cooper Institute, Dallas, TX.

Regulation of Body Weight and Composition

How does the human body normally control its own weight?

An individual may eat more than a ton of food—nearly a million Calories—a year and yet not gain 1 pound of body weight. For this to occur, the body must possess an intricate regulatory system that helps to balance energy intake and output both on a short-term and a long-term basis. The regulation of human energy balance is complex, involving numerous feedback loops to help control energy balance. At the present time, we do not know all the exact physiological mechanisms whereby body weight is maintained relatively constant over short or long periods, but research suggests that a variety of specific interactions between the brain and peripheral tissues may be involved in the control of both energy intake and energy expenditure.

Energy Intake Bray indicates that food intake is a regulated system. The central nervous system, the brain in particular, is the center for appetite control, either creating a sensation of satiety or stimulating food-seeking behavior. However, its activity is dependent upon a complex array of signals from various body systems. The interaction of the brain with these signals helps regulate the appetite on a short-term (daily) basis, or on a long-term basis, as in keeping the body weight constant for a year.

In a detailed review, Rui describes brain structures, neurotransmitters, and neural pathways involved in short-term and long-term regulation of energy intake and body weight. A simplified schematic of these regulatory pathways is presented in figure 10.7. In general, short-term (meal-to-meal) regulation of energy intake is governed by brainstem structures, which receive input from stomach fullness and peptides produced in the gut following a meal. The brainstem also controls the motor aspects of eating, such as chewing and swallowing. The hypothalamus contains neural areas promoting eating and satiety, respectively, to regulate food intake on a long-term basis by modulating brainstem sensitivity to the above-described input. This area of the hypothalamus is called the **appestat**, with certain neurons referred to as a **hunger center** and other neurons referred to as a **satiety center**. Specific neural receptors within the appestat monitor various stimuli that may increase or decrease the appetite to control energy intake. Woods suggests that these brain centers may involve receptors that induce sensations of pleasure, which may increase the desire to consume food. The corticolimbic and mesolimbic neuronal circuits, which secrete dopamine, control "reward" and "pleasure" aspects of food consumption and are subject to modulation by the hypothalamus and brainstem. The hypothalamus also has neural receptors that function as a thermostat to either stimulate energy (heat) production or loss in the regulation of body temperature.

Stimuli influencing the appetite include signals from the stomach, intestine, muscles, fat depots, pancreas, liver, and other body tissues and organs; blood levels of various nutrients; metabolites;

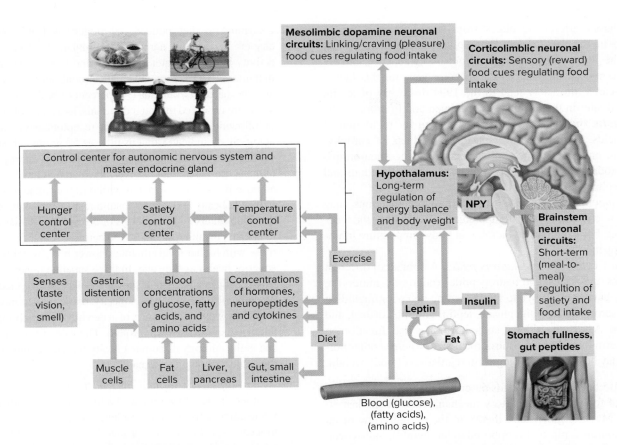

FIGURE 10.7 Simplified schematic for afferent and efferent control of energy balance and body weight. According to the set-point theory, the hypothalamus regulates energy intake and body weight, comparable to its role as a thermostat in regulating body temperature. Increases in the normal body weight would lead to compensations, such as decreased appetite or increased basal metabolic rate, which would lead to weight loss and restoration of normal body weight. The opposite would occur with decreases in the normal body weight. The numerous control centers in the hypothalamus are influenced by feedback from the body, such as the blood concentration of glucose and other nutrients. Such nutrients may also affect the pleasure/reward center in the brain, which may influence the hypothalamus. Exercise may influence the hypothalamus in a variety of ways, such as stimulating the secretion of several hormones by endocrine glands in the body, stimulating the temperature control center, and modifying blood levels of several nutrients, all of which may affect energy intake and output. Detailed coverage of the many brain structures, peptides, neurotransmitters, and stimuli directly or indirectly regulating energy balance is beyond the scope of this text.

hormones; and environmental cues. These stimuli are integrated and interpreted by the hypothalamus and directed to other brain centers and body organs to help maintain energy balance. Some factors may function to control body weight on a short-term basis, while others may exert long-term effects. The following stimuli may be involved in body-weight control in one way or another.

- *Senses.* Stimulation of several senses such as sight, sound, and smell may influence neural or hormonal activity to stimulate or depress our appetites, even before food is ingested. The sense of taste also has a significant impact on appetite and energy intake. Ventura and Worobey describe sensory preference as beginning *in utero* and continuing in infancy with exposure to nutrients in amniotic fluid and breast milk. These early preferences may be modified by psychological and environmental stimuli later in life.
- *Stomach fullness.* An empty or full stomach may influence mechanical stretch receptors in the stomach walls that provide

vagal feedback to the central nervous system. An empty stomach may stimulate the hunger center by various neural pathways, whereas a full stomach may stimulate the satiety center. The stomach may also release hormone-like substances that stimulate or diminish hunger. Although postmeal stretch provides feedback to avoid overeating, Brunstrom stressed the importance of learned decisions about portion/meal size before a meal (i.e., meal planning based on expected satiety) over postmeal stomach stretch as a control mechanism for food intake.
- *Blood nutrient levels.* Receptors in the hypothalamus, liver, or elsewhere may be able to monitor nutrient levels in the blood. In regard to this, three theories center on the three energy nutrients. The **glucostatic theory** originally proposed in the 1950s by Jean Mayer suggests that food intake is related to changes in the levels of blood glucose. Fehm and others indicated that a fall in blood glucose will stimulate glucose-sensitive neurons in the hypothalamus and increase appetite, whereas an increased blood glucose level will decrease appetite. The **lipostatic theory**

of regulatory afferent feedback from stored fat is based on research in the 1950s identifying *ob/ob* obese mice, which lacked the gene expressing a factor controlling appetite, and *db/db* obese mice, which lacked the receptor gene for this factor. This research ultimately lead to the 1994 discovery of leptin, discussed later in this chapter, by Colemen and Friedman. The **aminostatic theory** is a similar mechanism for regulation of amino acids, or protein. In essence, by-products of carbohydrate, fat, and protein metabolism may influence neurotransmitter production influencing appetite, such as serotonin and norepinephrine, in the hypothalamus.

- *Body temperature.* A thermostat in the hypothalamus may respond to changes in body temperature and influence the feeding center. For example, an increase in body temperature inhibits the appetite.

- *Hormones, cytokines, and neuropeptides.* A number of different hormones, cytokines, and neuropeptides (neurotransmitters) in the body have been shown to affect feeding behavior, including insulin, serotonin, norepinephrine, leptin, ghrelin, cortisol, and thyroxine. As discussed later, some hormones may function on a short-term basis to help control meal size, whereas other hormones may be involved in long-term regulation of body weight.

In his 2013 brief review, Woods described the increased knowledge base of food intake regulatory mechanisms over the last 40 years from Mayer's glucostatic theory to the current view of an extremely complex, plastic (as opposed to hardwired), interwoven system of neural circuitry involving many brain areas that receive input from an ever-growing list of recently discovered peptides, neurotransmitters, and hormones. Our understanding of feeding regulatory mechanisms will no doubt increase in the future.

Energy Expenditure The other side of the energy-balance equation is energy expenditure, or metabolism. Although exercise is one way to increase energy expenditure, the vast majority of the energy that is expended by the body on a daily basis is accounted for by the basal energy expenditure (BEE) or resting energy expenditure (REE), as was discussed in chapter 3. Changes in the REE may be involved in the regulation of body weight. Several mechanisms of body-weight regulation have been proposed.

- *Brown adipose tissue.* **Brown adipose tissue (BAT)** is distinct from the white adipose tissue (WAT) that comprises most fat tissue in the body. There are two basic types of BAT cells: constitutive (cBAT), developed during embryogenesis, and recruitable (rBAT), appearing postnatally in WAT and skeletal muscle. BAT differentiation and metabolism are regulated by neuroendocrine signals from the brain, thyroid, skeletal muscle, pancreas, WAT, liver, and heart. Mitochondrial uncoupling proteins (UCP) in BAT are proton pores in the inner mitochondrial membrane that allow hydrogen ions to "leak" from the intermembrane space to the matrix independently of the proton gradient created by the electron transport chain that is harnessed by ATP synthase for ATP formation. BAT has a high rate of metabolism and releases energy in the form of heat without ATP production. This activity is referred to as *nonshivering thermogenesis.* BAT may also

contribute to diet-induced thermogenesis (DIT), discussed in chapter 3, through adrenergic stimulation. BAT thermogenic activity is much greater in rodents and hibernating animals than in humans. BAT is found in small amounts around the neck, back, and chest areas of humans ($\leq$1 percent of body fat). Higher BAT levels are observed in lean individuals, as a result of cold exposure or following stimulation of specific receptors. BAT decreases with aging. Stock indicates that as little as 50 grams (about 2 ounces) could make a contribution of 10–15 percent energy turnover in humans. Research with rats has indicated that low levels of brown adipose tissue are associated with a higher incidence of dietary-induced obesity and greater insulin resistance. Mattson suggested that individuals with low levels of brown adipose tissue are prone to obesity, insulin resistance, and cardiovascular disease, whereas those with higher levels maintain lower body weights and exhibit superior health as they age. In three separate reviews, Townsend, Loyd, Schulz and their respective colleagues discuss the future potential of BAT in battling obesity, diabetes, and metabolic syndrome as well as clearance of triacylglycerol-rich chylomicrons and very-low-density lipoprotein. The role of brown adipose tissue in the etiology of human obesity remains controversial and is the subject of ongoing research.

- *White adipose tissue and muscle tissue.* UCP are also found in other tissues. In a review, Melby and others noted that both white adipose tissue and muscle tissue may also experience thermogenesis without ATP production under conditions of high energy intake, particularly as dietary fat. Such an effect could help prevent weight gain. rBAT can differentiate from progenitor cells and appear in WAT in a process known as "browning."

- *Hormones.* Levels of hormones from the thyroid and adrenal glands may rise or fall and affect energy metabolism accordingly. The thyroid hormones triiodothyronine (T_3) and thyroxine (T_4) may be involved in the stimulation of BAT, which has a high expression of enzymes catalyzing the conversion of T_4 into the more active T_3. Hormones such as epinephrine also may increase the activity of certain enzymes, resulting in increased energy expenditure. Decreases in such hormonal activity may depress energy metabolism. Other hormones may stimulate or depress thermogenesis in adipose or muscle tissues.

- *Nonexercise activity thermogenesis (NEAT).* Varying levels of nonexercise activity thermogenesis (NEAT) could have a significant impact on daily energy expenditure. Levine indicates that NEAT is the energy expended for everything we do that is not sleeping, eating, or sports-like exercise. According to Kotz and colleagues, NEAT can be defined in the strictest sense as unconscious movement and in the broadest sense as any caloric expenditure not associated with formal exercise, otherwise known as activities of daily living. It is unclear at this time if NEAT is the result of "hardwired" homeostatic control in response to nutrition or is instead due to genetics, development, environment, and the interactions between these factors that are unique to the individual. In animal models, various neuropeptides have the potential to increase spontaneous physical activity (SPA) and NEAT. The interested reader is referred to the reviews by Butterick and Teske and their respective colleagues.

Feedback Control of Energy Intake and Expenditure The human body has developed a number of *feedback systems* to regulate most physiological processes. Short-term and long-term feedback systems control energy balance and body weight. Short-term (daily) control mechanisms may either decrease or increase food intake. The stomach expands during a meal, with afferent input from stretch receptors in the stomach wall to the hypothalamus to suppress food intake. Moran notes that ingested nutrients alter the release of a variety of peptides from the stomach, intestines, and pancreas, which regulate energy intake. Cholecystokinen, pancreatic glucagon, obestatin, and amylin are released rapidly with eating and have short actions leading to meal termination. Body stores of carbohydrate, protein, and fat are also regulated on a short-term basis. The human body has a limited capacity to store excess carbohydrate and protein, so changes in blood glucose and amino acid levels help regulate carbohydrate and protein intake. Although the human body possesses a high capacity to store fat, blood lipids and other factors help maintain body-fat balance on a short-term basis. However, Stubbs indicated that although dietary protein and carbohydrate exert potent effects on satiety, dietary fat is less satiating and may lead to excess energy intake. Other short-term mechanisms increase food intake. **Ghrelin** is a peptide hormone released by the stomach, mainly before mealtime when the stomach is relatively empty. Ghrelin acts on the hypothalamus to stimulate the appetite. Abizaid indicates that ghrelin may also affect dopaminergic neurons in the brain, possibly increasing secretion of dopamine, which induces sensations of pleasure that may be involved in long-term regulation of body weight, as discussed later.

The **set-point theory** of weight control is a long-term proposed feedback mechanism primarily developed from rat models and applied to energy intake and expenditure in human behavior. This theory proposes that the body is programmed to be a certain weight, or set point, something comparable to a set body temperature (37°C or 98.6°F). Based on animal studies, Sullivan and others indicate that the maternal nutrition status during the perinatal period, or just before and after birth, may be critical in establishing the offspring's body weight set point. Keesey and Hirvonen indicate the hypothalamus plays a central role as the potential set-point regulator. Fehm indicates that the hippocampus may also be involved in homeostatic weight control. In several reviews, Levin noted that the brain has special sensing neurons that are involved in the control of energy homeostasis. In particular, Levin notes that neuropeptide Y (NPY) neurons in the hypothalamus represent an example of a neuron capable of sensing both glucose and a host of other peripheral metabolic signals, such as leptin, an adipokine secreted by adipose tissue. Deviation from the set point results in metabolic adjustments known as *adaptive thermogenesis,* which either increases or decreases heat production. According to Egecioglu and colleagues, hypothalamic homeostatic control can also be influenced by hedonic (pleasure- and reward-seeking) signals, which stimulate dopamine-secreting neurons in certain areas of the brain, as illustrated in figure 10.7. As a result, homeostatic control may be compromised due to greater reinforcement for food intake associated with hedonic behavior. Over time, less effective feedback control of energy intake and expenditure by peptides would contribute to weight gain and obesity.

Leptin is a regulating peptide hormone encoded and produced by the *OB* gene in the adipose cells. Klok and others note that leptin exerts long-term effects on energy balance by suppressing food intake, decreasing appetite, and inducing weight loss. Leptin production and secretion are greater when fat stores are high; conversely, secretion is lower when fat stores are low. Bloodborne leptin inhibits the production of neuropeptide Y (NPY), which is known to stimulate the appetite, increase energy intake, and reduce resting energy expenditure (REE). Feedback control of NPY by leptin suppresses hunger and voluntary food intake. Greater fat stores result in greater leptin secretion, which exerts an anorexigenic (appetite-inhibiting) effect and inhibits the orexigenic (appetite-stimulating) effect of NPY. A decrease in NPY formation in the hypothalamus may also increase REE by stimulating thermogenesis in adipose tissue and muscle. Likewise, decreased leptin secretion results in increased NPY formation by the hypothalamus. Baile notes that leptin and its receptors provide the molecular basis for the lipostatic theory of energy-balance regulation proposed 40 years ago, namely that circulating factors generated in proportion to body-fat stores act as signals to the brain and elicit changes in energy intake and expenditure.

Ghrelin may also be involved in long-term control of body weight. As noted by separate reviews by Abizaid, Rui, and Egecioglu and colleagues, ghrelin may also affect parts of the brainstem containing neurons secreting dopamine which stimulate the mesolimbic and corticolimbic pleasure and reward brain centers (see figure 10.7). As a result, ghrelin not only stimulates the appetite but may also help establish strong memories between eating certain foods and sensations of pleasure. Kessler and Liebman note that some food ingredients, such as sugar and fat, may stimulate the desire to eat more, possibly because of such stored memories, possibly leading to *hypereating* and long-term weight gain. According to Sclafani and Ackroff, dopamine reward circuits in the brain are involved in the conditioning of carbohydrate and fat intake, but less is known about gut/brain pathways regulating protein intake.

Less research has been conducted relative to feedback control of physical activity, but Rowland proposed an **activity-stat**, a center in the brain that functions as a set point to increase or decrease physical activity. Increasing or decreasing the daily amounts of NEAT may be related to the activity-stat. As previously discussed and illustrated in figure 10.7, several brain structures are thought to regulate NEAT via afferent stimulation by various central and peripheral peptides. If substantiated, a central activity-stat center could also support the set-point theory of body-weight control. Although the set point is a theory, it may help explain why some people maintain a normal body weight throughout life but when disrupted may lead to an excessive gain or loss of body mass. It is important to note that although the set-point theory is based on subconscious control mechanisms underlying energy intake and energy expenditure, the forebrain can consciously override these subconscious mechanisms and increase or decrease body mass if necessary.

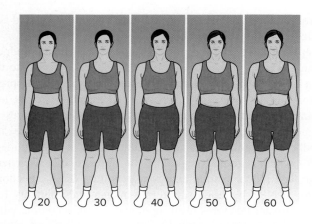

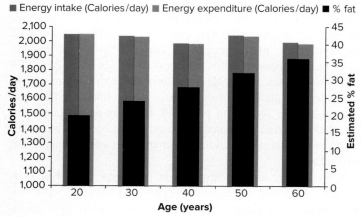

FIGURE 10.8 Adult-onset obesity is often referred to as creeping obesity. Energy balance is the difference between energy intake and energy expenditure. In this hypothetical example, a surplus of as little as ~9 Calories/day through decreased expenditure and/or increased intake can contribute to slow, steady gain in weight and body fat. Note the increases in estimated fat percentage and BMI over the decades of adult life. Of course, a greater surplus results in a greater rate of weight (and fat) gain. If her daily surplus were 200 Calories, she would gain over 20 lbs in 1 year.

How is fat deposited in the body?

The actual deposition of fat in the human body may occur in two ways: **hyperplasia** (an increase in the number of adipocytes, or fat cells) or **hypertrophy** (an increase in the amount of fat in each cell). Earlier research appeared to support the theory that hyperplasia is a major cause of childhood obesity, whereas hypertrophy is the primary cause in adulthood. However, Avram and others noted that the development of obesity is dependent on the coordinated interplay of an increased fat cell size as well as an increased fat cell number, and evidence suggests that adipocyte hyperplasia occurs throughout life, both in response to normal cell turnover and in response to the need for additional fat mass stores that arises when caloric intake exceeds nutritional requirements. Sargeant and Stephens describe adipogenesis as a complex balance between transcription factors, which either promote or inhibit differentiation of precursor stem cells into adipocytes. Existing fat cells apparently have a maximal size potential (about 1 microgram

of fat per cell), which when exceeded stimulates the formation of new fat cells or the accumulation of fat in preadipocytes, small cells in the adipose tissue that have the potential to become adipocytes. Thus, although a genetic predisposition to inherit a greater number of fat cells, thereby facilitating the development of obesity, may exist, individuals without this genetic predisposition may still become obese with a positive energy balance stored as fat. Interestingly, Pi-Sunyer indicated that once fat cells are formed, the number seems to remain fixed even if weight is lost. To lose body fat, one must reduce the amount of fat in the adipose cells to normal, or even below normal. The development of pharmacological agents that inhibit adipogenesis without adversely affecting normal metabolism (fat storage and insulin sensitivity) may be a future strategy in reducing the prevalence of obesity.

What is the cause of obesity?

Energy processes in the human body are governed by the laws of thermodynamics. If the human body consumes less energy in the form of food Calories than it expends in metabolic processes, then a negative energy balance will occur and the individual will lose body weight. Conversely, a greater caloric intake in comparison to energy expenditure will result in a positive energy balance and a gain in body weight. In simple terms, obesity is caused by this latter condition of energy imbalance—more Calories in than out.

Although the first law of thermodynamics provides the basic answer as to how we get fat, it does not provide any insight relative to the specific mechanisms. Bouchard noted that at this time there is no common agreement on the specific determinants of obesity, stressing that numerous factors are correlated with body-fat content. In general, most leading obesity scientists support a multi-causal theory involving the interaction of a number of genetic and environmental factors.

Genetic Factors Heredity appears to be a very important factor in the etiology of obesity, particularly **morbid obesity**. For example, several genetic diseases result in clinical obesity. Studies of adopted children, including both fraternal and identical twins who were separated and adopted by different families, have shown a greater relationship of the body composition between the children and their biological parents as compared to the adoptive parents. Two seminal studies of the genetic role in obesity were conducted by Bouchard and colleagues, who examined long-term overfeeding of identical twins, and Stunkard and others, who examined BMI of twins who were raised apart. According to Bouchard, the available data suggest genetics explains approximately 25–40 percent of the variance in obesity. Heredity may determine those internal factors in the body that may predispose one to gain weight.

Research into the genetics of obesity has been progressing at a rapid pace. Hirsch and Leibel note that several obesity genes have already been identified, which in some persons may maintain an unhealthful set point. Levin suggests that individuals genetically predisposed to obesity may establish neural circuits that are not easily abolished, particularly circuits involving the brain's pleasure center. Ongoing prospective, multi-generational investigations and genome–wide association studies (GRAS) have identified genetic mutations that are associated with obesity. The influence of such mutations on (fat mass and obesity related) FTO and other genes on prevalence of obesity in diverse populations has been the focus of considerable research and reviewers such as Yeo; Fawcett and Barroso; and others. Recently, Claussnitzer and others confirmed the effect of a variant in the FTO gene contributing to obesity by manipulating genetic signaling in humans and mice to inhibit and overexpress genes for specific downstream proteins hypothesized to influence thermogenesis and obesity. Inhibition increased beige adipocyte differentiation and thermogenesis while overexpression decreased beige adipocyte differentiation and thermogenesis and increased white adipocyte differentiation and lipid storage. Chaput and his colleagues in the Quebec Family Study have identified genetic changes affecting intracellular signaling pathways that are associated with fatness as well as inability to control food intake. In their meta-analysis, Tang and colleagues reported significant associations between obesity and a genetic mutation leading to leptin resistance and ineffective feedback regulation of NPY which stimulates the appetite. Mutations of genes expressing thermogenic uncoupling proteins in brown fat (*UCP1*) and white fat and muscle (*UCP2*) may also decrease resting energy expenditure. Altered lipid and carbohydrate metabolism, appetite control, oxidative damage, and thrombolytic (blood clotting) activity are also implicated in obesity-related genetic mutations. In general, researchers indicate that genes affecting energy balance in the body appear to be very efficient as a means to promote energy intake and weight gain, but relatively inefficient to promote energy expenditure and weight loss.

Small and others identified a *master gene* that regulates numerous genes throughout the body associated with obesity. Rankinen and others have developed an annually updated human obesity gene map whose purpose is to identify loci on chromosomes associated with the development of obesity in humans. Genetic factors that have been implicated in the development of obesity include the following:

- a predisposed taste for sweet, high-fat foods
- impaired function of hormones such as insulin and cortisol
- decreased levels of human growth hormone
- low plasma leptin concentrations
- leptin resistance
- inability of nutrients or hormones in the blood to suppress the appetite control center
- a greater number of white fat cells
- lower body levels of brown fat
- an enhanced metabolic efficiency in storing fat
- a lower REE
- a decreased TEF
- low rates of fat oxidation
- lower levels of spontaneous physical activity, or NEAT, during the day
- lower levels of energy expenditure during light exercise

Hetherington and Cecil indicate that common obesity is polygenic, involving complex gene-gene and gene-environment interactions that increase energy intake and involve neural pathways regulating addiction and reward behaviors which contribute to overeating and obesity.

Prehistoric humans conserved energy in times of plenty against the inevitable times of hardship. The term *thrifty gene* has been associated with this efficiency of energy conservation which served our ancestors well. According to Wells, this gene does not serve modern humans who generally have an uninterrupted abundance of food and rely on the same physiology as prehistoric humans to store excess energy. Lutter and Nesler describes the *selfish gene,* a more accurate reflection of contemporary energy balance and the obesity epidemic, as dominance by the dopaminergic pleasure centers in the brain over the hypothalamus in regulating food intake and increasing the desire to consume foods that are highly palatable.

Environmental Factors In addition to genetic heritability, environmental factors also contribute to obesity. Wadden and others commented that the worldwide increase in obesity is attributed to energy imbalance, specifically the widespread availability of large portions of high-fat/high-sugar foods and societal influences that decrease physical activity. Mendoza and others concluded in their review that dietary energy density is a major predictor of obesity. Consuming a high-Calorie diet, either high or low in fat, may lead to excess caloric intake and weight gain. Cohen and Farley contend that eating may be an automatic behavior over which the environment has more control than does the individual. The amount of food eaten is strongly influenced by factors such as portion size, food visibility, and the ease of obtaining food. The following discussion highlights the variety of environmental factors that may contribute to excessive weight gain. The main contributors are excessive caloric intake and decreased physical activity, both of which may be influenced by other environmental factors.

High-fat, high-Calorie Foods Excess caloric intake may lead to obesity. In comparing caloric intake and activity levels of weight-stable and weight-gaining groups, Pearcey and de Castro found the weight-gaining group consumed about 400 more Calories per day during the period of active weight gain. Brownell and Liebman implicate industry marketing of unhealthy, fattening food as one reason most Americans are overweight. A small, unbuttered bag of popcorn at Regal Cinemas contains 400 calories, while the large, buttered order contains 1,640 calories (source: www.myfitnesspal.com/food/calorie-chart-nutrition-facts). Ebbeling and others note that high palatability, high-fat content, high content of sugar in liquid form, and high-energy density of fats in food promote excess energy intake. Fast foods are relatively inexpensive, mainly because fat and sugar are the cheapest source of Calories on earth and thus are generally high in fat and Calories. Lee and colleagues recently reported public housing neighborhoods had more fast-food restaurants with cheaper high-sugar beverages and "super-size" menu items compared to middle-income neighborhoods. Residents in neighborhoods of lower socioeconomic status may be disproportionately targeted with unhealthy food options. Several longitudinal studies have linked fast-food consumption with weight gain. Over a 15-year follow-up, Pereira and others found that those who ate at fast-food restaurants more than two times a week gained about 10 pounds more than their peers who dined at such places less than once a week. Fast-food consumption had strong positive associations with weight gain and insulin resistance, suggesting that fast food increases the risk of obesity and type 2 diabetes. Two recent reviews of large, well-controlled, prospective studies by Nago and Lachat and their respective colleagues reported significant associations of frequent "out-of-home eating," specifically at fast-food restaurants, with overweight/obesity, waist circumference, lower intake of micronutrients (e.g., vitamin C, calcium, and iron), and BMI in women.

Although an excess of caloric input over output will lead to a weight gain, researchers suggest that dietary fat is the main culprit leading to obesity. The National Academy of Sciences concluded that higher fat intakes are accompanied by increased energy intake and therefore increased risk for weight gain in populations already disposed to being overweight and obese, such as North America and other developed/developing countries. Obesity researchers have identified at least three reasons for these associations. First, the high palatability of dietary fat elicits a hedonistic response in many individuals and may encourage overconsumption. Although dietary fat contains more Calories per gram, Gibbs noted that compared to dietary protein and carbohydrates, the body responds more slowly to dietary fat, resulting in the ingestion of too much fat (and Calories) from a high-fat meal. Green and Blundell note that fats, Calorie for Calorie, are less effective in suppressing subsequent food intake than carbohydrates. In a brief review, De Vadder and colleagues describe dietary protein as playing a "satiety role" in regulating energy intake by providing input from the intestine to the brain. Shah and Garg also reported that spontaneous energy intake is higher on an unrestricted high-fat diet compared to a high-carbohydrate diet. Second, dietary fat may be stored as fat more efficiently compared to carbohydrate and protein. Dattilo noted that three to four times more energy is required to convert dietary carbohydrate and protein to body fat compared to dietary fat. Third, it is thought that a chronic high-fat diet may alter hypothalamic response to factors, such as leptin, that normally suppress appetite. For example, as previously discussed, leptin resistance impairs feedback control of NPY, an orexigenic peptide that stimulates energy intake and body-fat deposition. Additional information on the association between fast-food consumption and obesity and macronutrient intake and satiety can be found in the respective reviews of Nago and De Vadder.

Low-fat, large-portion-size, high-calorie foods Dietary fat is not the only explanation for obesity. Walker and others noted that while the prevalence of obesity in the United States has dramatically increased over the past 35 years, daily energy derived from dietary fat has actually decreased. One reason for this apparent inconsistency may be an increased daily Calorie intake from low-fat, high-Calorie foods loaded with simple sugars. "Fat-free" foods are not necessarily "Calorie free." Low-fat, high-Calorie food and in supersize proportions with significantly increased caloric content is aggressively marketed everywhere. Portion sizes have increased dramatically over the years and what was once small is now large.

Most reviews conclude that liquid Calories appear to be involved in weight gain. A 12-ounce sugar-sweetened soda contains the equivalent of 10 teaspoons of table sugar, or about 150 Calories. Today, the average soft drink is more than 50 percent larger than in past years and contains more sugar and Calories. Geier and others note that most individuals consume food on a "unit" instead of a "quantity" or "volume" basis. Consumption of a 20-ounce bottle (unit) of soda will add 100 Calories to energy intake compared to the 12-ounce bottle. Flood and others reported that Americans drink about 22 percent of their total daily caloric intake, many from sweetened high-carbohydrate beverages, and do not compensate by eating less solid food at meals. According to Welsh and colleagues, although United States per capita added sugar consumption decreased from 2000 to 2008, primarily because of a decline in sugar-sweetened beverage consumption, added-sugar consumption still exceeds recommended levels. In a separate review, Welsh and others acknowledge restricting advertising to children, limiting school sales, and increasing availability of smaller portion sizes as contributions of the beverage industry to the reduction in sugar-sweetened beverage consumption. In their review of 32 high-quality prospective longitudinal studies and randomized clinical trials, Malik and others concluded that a greater consumption of sugar-sweetened beverages is associated with weight gain in children and adults. Consuming sugar-sweetened drinks *per se* may not be a cause of obesity, but it may be one avenue to exceeding recommended caloric intake. For example, Johnson and others noted that Americans consume about 22 teaspoons of sugar daily, about 350 Calories, almost 75 more Calories per day than was consumed about 30 years ago. These additional daily Calories would increase body weight by 8 pounds over the course of a year, an example of creeping obesity, as discussed later.

Physical inactivity and NEAT Excess energy intake is not the sole explanation for overweight and obesity. Although technological advances generally improve life, sedentary entertainment/leisure activities and labor-saving devices lower energy expenditure and can contribute to overweight, obesity, and other chronic diseases. According to the laws of thermodynamics, the total energy in a system is constant, consists of potential and kinetic energies, and is neither created nor destroyed. A change in potential energy is matched by a corresponding opposite change in kinetic energy. As discussed in chapter 3, the metabolic pathways conserve some of the potential energy in the macronutrients in the form of ATP, with the remainder lost as metabolic heat. Surplus dietary potential energy not transferred to ATP or dissipated as heat is stored as fat, glycogen, and/or amino acids. As discussed in reviews by Kotz and Teske, obesity resistance observed in animal models and in human research is related to a complex interaction between peripheral and central peptides and neurotransmitters and brain structures to regulate spontaneous physical activity and nonexercise activity thermogenesis (NEAT).

Levine contends that the variability in total daily energy expenditure is attributed mainly to NEAT. Technology has decreased the amount of energy expended via NEAT each day, such as walking, standing, and even fidgeting, which may lead to an energy imbalance and weight gain. Marra and others reported that fidgeting was higher in a group of "constitutionally lean" women compared to anorexic, normal, and obese women. There was evidence of greater fat oxidation in the lean women.

Watching television and other such sedentary, seated behaviors decrease NEAT, which Levine indicates may be of profound importance in the development of obesity. In their review, Levine and others reported that NEAT varies substantially between people, as much as 2,000 Calories per day. In particular, an excessive amount of sitting has been an increasing concern. Owen and others noted that excessive sitting, such as sitting in front of a computer 8 to 9 hours a day or spending 4 hours or more per day in front of the television, may contribute to weight gain and a higher incidence of chronic health problems, even in individuals who exercise regularly. The term *active couch potato* has been used by Owen and others to classify individuals who may have compromised metabolic health if they sit for prolonged periods, even if they meet public health guidelines on physical activity. Swinburn and Shelly note that excessive television viewing may pose a double threat for weight gain, not only because of the prolonged sitting but also because advertisements for energy-dense foods may increase total caloric consumption. In their review, Tremblay and others reported a dose-response relationship between sedentary behavior and adverse health outcomes in children age 5–17 years. Specifically, more than 2 hours/day of TV watching was associated with decreased fitness, increased fatness, lowered self-esteem, and lower academic performance.

Other environmental factors Other environmental factors may predispose to weight gain.

Sleep and Emotional Stress Inadequate sleep may alter hormonal response to energy intake and control. In their review, McNeil and others note significant epidemiological and experimental evidence of a role of sleep restriction in higher BMI, body fat, and insulin resistance. Sleep restriction may not only result in increased energy intake but also alter the hormonal milieu, with higher evening cortisol levels impairing insulin-mediated glucose uptake the next morning. Over time, a greater insulin secretion required for a given glucose load may lead to insulin resistance. Zimberg and others note sleep restriction is associated with increased ghrelin levels and decreased leptin levels, which promotes increased energy intake. Decreased energy expenditure is a plausible result of fatigue associated with sleep restriction.

Physical and psychological stress provokes the "fight-or-flight" response with an up-regulation of the hypothalamic-pituitary-adrenal (HPA) axis. In their review, Lucassen and Cizza describe circular relationships between obesity, sleep, and stress-induced alterations in the HPA axis. During stress, the HPA axis and the sympathetic nervous system synergistically affect each other and adversely affect the quantity and quality of sleep. Cortisol, a glucocorticoid hormone secreted by the adrenal cortex, in response to HPA up-regulation, suppresses immune function, promotes gluconeogenesis, and decreases insulin sensitivity. Obese individuals have elevated levels of the enzyme converting inactive cortisone into active cortisol, which promotes lipogenesis and fat deposition, particularly in the visceral/abdominal area.

Personal relationships Social and family relationships may contribute to weight gain. In one study, Christakis and Fowler studied the role of friendship on weight gain in 12,000 subjects over the course of 32 years. They reported that a person's chances of becoming obese increased by 57 percent if he or she had a friend who became obese in a given interval. Among pairs of adult siblings, if one sibling became obese, the chance that the other would become obese increased by 40 percent. If one spouse became obese, the likelihood that the other spouse would become obese increased by 37 percent. They concluded that obesity appears to be spread through social ties. In a 2013 review of social contagion theory, Christakis and Fowler calculated approximately a 170 percent increase in probability of obesity in a given individual if his or her friend was also obese and if both considered each other "mutual friends." Although not tested in their study, the possibility of a similar relationship may occur among friends or family who maintain a healthy body weight.

Salvy and others reported that overweight youths who ate with an overweight friend or an overweight unfamiliar peer consumed more food than when eating with a nonoverweight friend or unfamiliar peer. The authors suggest that promoting long-term weight-control programs among overweight youths may be difficult because their social network is likely to reinforce overeating. In a later study, Salvy and others reported a significantly greater maternal influence in support of healthy eating by children (5–7 years) compared to peer influence. On the other hand, teenaged (13–15 years) girls but not boys consumed fewer Calories from unhealthy snacks and more calories from healthy snacks when in the presence of friends compared to their mothers. These data suggest age and gender differences in the effect of peer influence of dietary choices.

Drugs and environmental chemicals Certain drugs may increase body weight. Individuals with asthma or pulmonary disease may use corticosteroids containing cortisone, which may be converted to cortisol and cause weight gain, as previously discussed. Two important factors may be the use of social drugs, alcohol and nicotine. Alcohol is rich in Calories. At 7 Calories per gram, it is comparable to a gram of fat, which contains 9 Calories. The National Academy of Sciences has noted that if the energy derived from alcohol is not utilized, the excess is stored as fat. Tremblay and others reported that concurrent alcohol intake does not suppress the appetite, nor does it suppress fat intake. As a result, the Calories in alcohol are additive and may lead to an energy surplus and weight gain.

Nicotine in cigarettes is a stimulant that may inhibit the appetite and increase REE. In a meta-analysis of 62 studies, Aubin and colleagues reported a 4.67-kg (10.3-lb) increase in weight within 12 months after smoking cessation. There is a large 12-month postcessation weight-change variance in this literature, with 16 percent losing weight and 13 percent gaining more than 10 kg (22 lbs). Teenagers and young adults may start smoking to prevent weight gain, but smoking is a well-documented primary risk factor for heart and lung disease and cancer. Healthier and more effective ways to maintain weight will be the focus of chapter 12.

Environmental stress may induce epigenetic modifications, such as DNA methylation, that alter gene transcription. The "Dutch hunger winter studies" described in Inadera's review are the focus of ongoing prospective research. During World War II, the Nazis blockaded food supplies to occupied lands in the Netherlands from October 1944 until the lands were liberated in May 1945. Children exposed *in utero* to maternal caloric deprivation and born with low birth weight (LBW) gained weight at an accelerated rate when exposed to adequate childhood nutrition. Maternal caloric deprivation may promote expression of the "thrifty gene" phenotype, which serves the child well in the caloric-restricted *in utero* condition but not later in life. LBW has been associated with insulin resistance and greater prevalence rates of type 2 diabetes and obesity. Interestingly, there is evidence of a multigenerational effect as the adult daughters of these mothers also have LBW babies.

Emerging evidence implicates certain environmental (endocrine-disrupting) chemicals in the development of obesity, diabetes, and the metabolic syndrome discussed later in this chapter. Phthalates, used to soften polyvinylchloride (PVC) in the manufacture of many products, is a thyroid antagonist and stimulates nuclear receptors that play a role in fat storage. Phthalates have been associated with central obesity. Polybrominated biphenyl esters, a flame retardant used in many products, decrease thyroid function, lipolysis, and insulin-mediated glucose oxidation. Dithiocarbamates found in cosmetics inhibit the enzyme-converting cortisol to cortisone. As previously discussed in up-regulation of the HPA axis, increased cortisol concentrations could increase energy intake and abdominal fat deposition. Other chemicals such as bisphenol A and phytoestrogens are also associated with obesity. The interested reader is referred to the reviews by Newbold and by De Coster and Larebeke for more information on these and other endocrine-disrupting chemicals associated with obesity and other chronic diseases.

Viruses Recent attention has focused on the effect of viruses on obesity. In their studies of the effects of human adenovirus AD-36 on *in vitro* pre-adipocytes and in infected versus noninfected rats, Vangipuram and colleagues observed decreased leptin secretion, increased insulin-mediated glucose uptake by adipocytes, increased fatty acid synthesis, and greater lipid accumulation in infected rats compared to noninfected rats. According to Hur and others, adenovirus infections may decrease immune function, suppress norepinephrine and leptin secretion, and increase leptin resistance, thereby increasing appetite. At present, the link between viral exposure and obesity is stronger in animal models. The relationship of viruses with human obesity is correlational rather than causative. Esposito and colleagues note that while adenovirus AD-36 is associated with childhood obesity, susceptibility to recurring viral infection may also lead to lower activity and obesity. More research is necessary to either confirm or refute a causal link between viral exposure and obesity.

Built environment The *built environment* is defined as all infrastructure designed by humans for use by humans. Availability (or lack thereof) of parks, recreation centers, sidewalks, and trails impacts the perceived convenience of physical activity as a strategy to combat obesity. As will be discussed in chapter 11, convenience is an important factor to consider when developing an exercise program for weight control. Residents of neighborhoods in close proximity to retail, dining, and entertainment venues may find walking or bicycling to be more convenient than residents of large "urban sprawl" developments. In their review, Sallis and others identified recreation/exercise, school/work, transportation, and household as four distinct domains affecting physical activity that receive little to no design input from health professionals as opportunities to promote physical activity. As a result of greater future partnerships between health-care professionals, urban planners, civil engineers and others, the built environments may become more conducive to physical activity.

Another aspect of the built environment is the effect of ambient temperature control on thermogenesis, which was discussed in chapter 9. Hansen and others hypothesize that more body heat is generated in cold weather to help maintain the core temperature, resulting in greater energy expenditure, whereas hot weather increases core temperature and curbs the appetite. Prolonged exposure to cold or hot ambient environments would tend to curb weight gain. However, heating, ventilating, and air conditioning (HVAC) technology has minimized time individuals are exposed to ambient extremes. The thermogenic-neutral environment generated by HVAC climate control does not increase basal energy expenditure or curb appetite and may be an important causal co-factor in the worldwide increase in obesity. The Centers for Disease Control and Prevention has provided ten strategies for communities to increase physical activity to combat weight gain, which may be found at the following Website.

www.cdc.gov/obesity/downloads/PA_2011_WEB.pdf

Interaction of Genetics and Environment Hetherington and Cecil indicate that common obesity involves complex gene-gene and gene-environment interactions. The previously described Dutch winter hunger studies are examples of gene-environment interactions that result in heritable epigenetic modifications. Children of calorically deprived mothers may have developed the "thrifty gene" phenotype, described by Peters and others. Later childhood exposure to what Lee described as an *obesogenic* environment—abundant, inexpensive, energy-dense food and inadequate physical activity—may explain associations between low birth weight, insulin resistance, and obesity observed later in life and from one generation to the next.

Kral and Rauh identify moderate to high heritability for several food consumption behaviors such as eating and sucking rate, neophobia (avoidance of new food), preference for protein, and disinhibition (excess eating due to loss of self-control), which can be modified by environmental influences such as parent modeling and healthy food choices in the home environment. Naukkarinen and colleagues reviewed studies of 14 Finnish discordant (obese, non-obese) monozygotic twin pairs. Such studies provide unique control of genetics, gender, age, and early childhood experiences. Since BMI is highly heritable, the existence of the non-obese individual provides strong support for physical activity in offsetting prediabetic and pre-atherogenic tendencies such as insulin resistance, fatty deposits in the liver, inflammation, and down-regulation of oxidative enzyme activity. The genetically identical but physically inactive and obese mate may risk a "vicious cycle" of worsening pathological changes leading to less activity and greater obesity. Such studies provide valuable insight into beneficial and detrimental environment effects on the genomics of obesity, but as Waterland notes, our understanding of epigenetic regulators of energy balance is far from complete.

Many individuals who have maintained a normal body weight during childhood and adolescence begin to put on weight gradually in young adulthood (ages 20–40). For young college students, the first year may involve increased psychological stress, which may adversely affect various lifestyle behaviors, such as dietary habits and physical activity, and lead to weight gain. A meta-analysis of 24 studies by Vella-Zarb and Elgar concluded that the average weight gain was only 3.86 pounds (1.75 kg). However, the proverbial "freshman 15"—a weight gain of 15 pounds in the freshman year—appears to be an exaggeration by the popular media. Although weight gain during the freshman year is not as extreme as once suggested, it may be the first step in the phenomenon called creeping obesity, illustrated in figure 10.8 and caused by increased caloric intake, decreased levels of physical activity, or a combination of the two over adulthood.

Can the set point change?

Researchers continue to refine models of obesity in order to account for known principles of feedback control, genetic and epigenetic adaptations, and social/environmental influences. Speakman and colleagues compared various models of energy balance regulation and obesity. The set-point (contemporary lipostatic) theory of a defended body weight, is well-grounded in physiological feedback control, but it does not explain social and environmental influences contributing to the obesity epidemic. In the settling-point theory, the set point may be increased (or decreased) in response to a change in fat mass, which is the direct result of increased (or decreased) intake and to increased (or decreased) expenditure. This model accounts for social and environmental changes over time (e.g., creeping obesity) but does not explain genetic factors, brain regulation, or peptides involved in feedback control of energy intake or expenditure. A *general model* combines aspects of the set-point and settling-point theories in describing regulation of intake as functions of "uncompensated" (social/environmental) and "compensated" (genetics and feedback control) factors. The *dual intervention point model* describes "competition" between physiological control factors that defend an upper point of weight or fat mass and environmental factors favoring either weight gain or loss. During weight gain, environmental factors promoting increased intake "win out," with physiological control factors forced to defend a higher upper point. Genetics and epigenetics influence this new equilibrium. As an example, Gibbs compared two groups of the Pima Indian nation, one in the United States consuming a high-fat diet with a high obesity rate and a genetically similar normal-weight group in Mexico consuming a grain- and vegetable-based diet.

A weight-loss diet may lower the set point to help maintain body weight at a lower level. Weinsier and others found that caloric restriction in obese women induced a transient decrease in REE, which would be counterproductive to weight loss. However, metabolism returned to normal at the completion of the weight-loss program when energy intake was then adequate to maintain the reduced body weight, suggesting that the set point may settle to a lower level over time. Changes in environmental conditions, such as the diet, may help change neural circuits involved in weight control. Genetics and environment interact to influence body weight and composition, possibly by their interactive effects in establishing a body weight set point.

Major and others note that the epidemic of obesity is developing faster than the scientific understanding of an efficient way to overcome it. The low success rate of short- and long-term weight-loss interventions suggests that the body tends to defend a higher set point. Therefore, prevention of obesity may be the key strategy.

Why is prevention of childhood obesity so important?

As noted previously, there is an obesity epidemic in the United States, and it is affecting children as well as adults. According to a Centers for Disease Control and Prevention report by Sarafrazi and colleagues, 17 percent of children 8–15 years of age were obese in 2011–2012, with 48 percent of obese boys and 36 percent of obese girls considering themselves to be at about the right weight. Once an individual is obese, treatment is not very effective. In their respective reviews, Levin and Waterford note that neural circuits predisposing to obesity are not easily abolished. Most scientists agree that prevention of obesity is of prime importance, particularly in childhood. In their meta-analysis of 21 studies across various ethnic groups, Liu and others reported significant associations between the fat mass and obesity-associated (FTO) gene mutation and obesity in children. Kral and Rauh discuss heritable traits such as eating/sucking rate, preference/avoidance of certain foods, and disinhibition which predispose a child toward obesity. Epigenetic alterations can occur *in utero,* resulting in transgenerational obesity. Other environmental influences such viruses and chemical exposure may create neural circuits that are not easily altered with interventions later in life. Nader and others, in a longitudinal 12-year study, found that obesity persists from preschool through elementary school and into young adolescence. Children who are overweight at an early age are likely to remain so through childhood and into adolescence. Therefore, prevention at any stage of childhood and adolescence is an important consideration, and as with adults, diet and exercise are two key factors.

The role of diet and physical activity in the development of obesity during childhood is not totally clear. Children have little control over their own dietary choices and are influenced by parental modeling of preference/availability of high-Calorie/low-nutrient-density foods and physical inactivity. Of the two, an improper diet appears to be the major problem. Foods high in sugar and fat are abundant. Lee and others reported disproportionately greater fast-food marketing and availability to youths in low-income compared to middle-class neighborhoods. Challenges and opportunities in the advertisement and marketing of food to children was the topic of a workshop sponsored by the National Academies of Sciences' Institute of Medicine in 2013.

Moreno and Rodríguez found that consumption of sugar-sweetened drinks is associated with obesity in children and adolescents. Bowman reported that fast-food consumption has increased fivefold among children since 1970, noting that children who ate fast food on a regular basis (2 days/week) consumed 187 more daily Calories, which total up to about 6 pounds more per year. In a retrospective clinical chart review of obese children in a pediatric weight-management program, Carvalho and colleagues reported a significantly greater frequency of fast food consumption in the subgroup with three or more obesity-related co-morbidities compared to those with fewer than three co-morbidities. Although some studies have shown that obese children do not consume more Calories than their nonobese peers, the data were not collected during the period when the obese children were gaining weight. Studies in which the investigators actually lived with the children suggest that the obese child does eat more, and eats faster. Kral and Rauh describe eating and sucking rates as traits with high heritability.

Bar-Or has indicated that physical inactivity may be one cause of juvenile obesity. Direct relationships between TV viewing time and childhood obesity have been reported in the literature. According to Andersen and others, children who watch 4 or more hours of television daily have significantly more body fat than those who watch less than 2 hours. Greater amounts of time spent watching TV and playing computer/video games ("screen-based" sedentary behaviors) are considered as surrogates for physical inactivity in the literature. Marshall and others comment that relationships between sedentary behavior and youth obesity are unlikely to be explained using single markers of inactivity. In a cross-sectional study of European children, Ekelund and associates reported TV viewing and physical activity were not associated with each other and emerged as separate independent risk factors for childhood obesity and increased metabolic risk. Compared to TV watching, less is known about the role of prolonged sitting and overall sedentary time as risk factors for obesity. Swinburn and Shelly comment that the relationship between TV viewing time and obesity may be mediated by exposure to marketing of energy-dense foods. Wiecha and others concluded that each hour increase in television viewing was associated with consumption of an additional 167 Calories from energy-dense foods. Saunders and colleagues report that increased total time spent in *any* sedentary activity, including prolonged sitting, is a risk factor for cardio-metabolic disease in children. In a 12-year prospective study, O'Brien and others concluded that children who were more physically active after school spent less time watching television and were less likely to become overweight by age 12.

In a review of prospective studies on obesity in children ages 5 to 18, Pate and associates reported a consistent association with low physical activity but also noted the need for more well-designed, large-scale, long-term prospective studies using appropriate methodology to examine the role of other potential factors such as sedentary behavior; diet/nutrition; and family, peer, and community support in the development of childhood obesity. Many children eat breakfast and lunch, and have access to snacks, at school. Citing a National Institutes of Health study, Strecker noted that healthier meals and increased physical activity reduced obesity and overweight by 21 percent in school children. Nihiser and colleagues stated that school-based BMI surveillance systems, if administered in a nonthreatening manner and according to American Academy of Pediatrics criteria, may prove effective in increasing awareness of obesity in children, parents, school administrators, and community leaders. According to Niemeier and others, parental participation is a significant aspect of interventions to reduce BMI in children. Salvy and others comment that peers can exert a positive influence on overweight/obese friends to increase physical activity. As Hills and others note, habitual physical activity established during the early years may provide the greatest likelihood of impact on health and longevity. It appears that the battle to reduce the prevalence of childhood obesity will be fought on multiple fronts.

Fat is easy to gain, and hard to lose is the key underlying concept cited by scientists who stress the importance of prevention in the battle against obesity. Although prevention of excess weight gain is important at all stages of life, childhood and adolescence are key times to adopt healthier eating and physical activity practices that promote a healthy body weight. Several Websites provide information and program activities to help fight childhood obesity.

http://letsmove.gov A program promoted by First Lady Michelle Obama to help parents, teachers, and kids to eat healthier and get more exercise.

www.newmovesonline.com A school-based physical education program for girls only to promote increased physical activity and healthier eating.

Key Concepts

▶ The brain's hypothalamus appears to be the central control mechanism in appetite regulation, which involves a complex interaction of physiological and psychological factors. Neural and hormonal feedback from the senses, gastrointestinal tract, adipose cells, and other body organs help to drive hunger or signal satiety.

▶ Although the ultimate cause of obesity is a positive energy balance, the underlying cause is not known but probably involves the interaction of many genetic and environmental factors.

▶ Prevention of weight gain in the first place is recommended because once excess body fat accumulates, it is difficult to lose and difficult to maintain the loss over time. Childhood and adolescence are key periods of life for prevention.

Check for Yourself

▶ As you go about your normal activities for a day, pay particular attention to environmental conditions that are conducive to consuming high-Calorie foods and discouraging physical activity. Compare your results with those of your classmates.

Weight Gain, Obesity, and Health

Although the World Health Organization recognized obesity as a disease in 1948, James notes that only within the past 20 years has its global role in disease and escalating medical costs been recognized. From 2002 to 2010, obesity prevalence rates increased in every WHO region.

Increased adipose tissue mass places extra strain on the heart and musculoskeletal system. In their 2013 National Lipid Association position statement, Bays and others describe adipocyte dysfunction as ***adiposopathy (sick fat),*** contributing to various metabolic diseases. Pathogenic mechanisms associated with adiposity include alterations in adipogenesis, which adversely affect fat storage; insulin resistance in liver and muscle tissue; up-regulation of pro-inflammatory and down-regulation of anti-inflammatory adipokines; dyslipidemia; and atherosclerosis directly and indirectly through high associations with hypertension and diabetes. Adipocytes contain aromatase, the rate-limiting enzyme in estrogen synthesis, and other hormones in the estrogen biosynthetic pathway. The conversion of androgens to estrogens may contribute to visceral fat accumulation and metabolic disease. Given these effects, Bays and others suggest that pathogenic adipose tissue is no less a disease than diseases of other body organs.

The literature is not unanimous in reporting obesity as a risk factor for chronic disease or early mortality. Wildman notes that approximately 30 percent of obese individuals may possess what is known as a *healthy obese* phenotype, which does not increase their risk of cardiovascular disease. One reason for this finding may be a genetic predisposition to secrete protective anti-inflammatory adipokines from adipose tissue. Many studies used BMI, which does not distinguish between fat and fat-free mass or consider patterns of fat deposition. Another confounding factor may be that the level of physical activity is not measured. Blüher comments there are no universally accepted criteria to define a healthy obese phenotype. In general, obesity appears to increase health risks and premature death, though the effect may vary in any given individual.

What health problems are associated with overweight and obesity?

Scientific reviews have identified the following list of health problems and risk factors associated with obesity. These health problems may be associated with the strain of the increased body mass, the metabolic effects of adipokines or estrogen, psychological processes, and/or interactions with several of these factors.

Asthma
Cancer
Cardiovascular disease
Cognitive decline, dementia, and Alzheimer's disease
Diabetes (type 2)
Dyslipidemia
Gallstones
Gastrointestinal reflux disease
Gout
Hypertension
Insulin resistance

Low back pain
Low-grade inflammation
Low self-image and self-esteem
Osteoarthritis and knee pain
Respiratory dysfunction
Sleep apnea
Social disabilities
Stroke
Vertebral disk herniation

According to the Centers for Disease Control and Prevention, the health costs of obesity parallel those associated with smoking-related disease. According to Tsai and colleagues, estimated per capita costs of overweight and obesity in 2008 were $266 and $1,723, respectively, with an estimated total cost of $113.9 billion (approximately 5 percent of U.S. health-care spending). The majority of these health-care costs appear to be associated with the two main chronic diseases associated with obesity, namely cardiovascular disease and cancers.

Cardiovascular Disease and Related Health Risks The primary health condition associated with excess body fat is coronary heart disease (CHD). In 1983, Hubert and colleagues were among the first to report obesity as an independent risk factor for CHD in a 26-year follow-up of 5,209 original Framingham cohort members. Obesity is now well recognized as a risk factor for CHD by many professional groups and societies. However, this relationship has recently been complicated by clinical observations that mild-to-moderate obesity may be associated with improved survival in heart failure patients. This phenomenon, discussed in a review by Clark and colleagues, is called the "obesity paradox" and may be explained by genetics, cardiorespiratory fitness, the anti-inflammatory effect of adiponectin, greater mass to counteract catabolic effects of heart failure, or other mechanisms.

Some adipokines may be involved in the etiology of cardiovascular disease, such as the following:

- Adiponectin   Anti-inflammatory
- Resistin   Pro-inflammatory
- Tissue necrosis factor-alpha (TNF-α)   Pro-inflammatory
- Visfatin   Pro-inflammatory

Reviews by Bays and others, Pi-Sunyer, and Fantuzzi and Mazzone indicate that adipokines may directly influence homeostasis in heart blood vessels by influencing the function of endothelial cells, arterial smooth muscle cells, and macrophages in the vessel wall. Some of these effects may be beneficial, while others may be harmful to heart health. For example, Pi-Sunyer has noted that adiponectin has potent anti-inflammatory and anti-atherogenic properties, whereas other adipokines, such as tissue necrosis factor-alpha (TNF-α), may promote inflammation and clotting, two factors contributing to atherosclerosis. Pi-Sunyer notes that adiponectin levels are usually lower in obese individuals, while TNF and other atherogenic adipokines may be elevated.

Excess body fat also increases the risk of developing high blood pressure, hypercholesterolemia, and diabetes, all of which are risk factors leading to the development of CHD. In particular, obesity increases the risk of type 2 diabetes, whose rate has increased dramatically over the past decade in concert with the parallel increase in obesity. *Shape Up America,* a nonprofit organization that promotes a healthy body weight, has coined the term ***Diabesity*** ™ to highlight the relationship between the two. Adipose tissue secretes an adipokine called resistin, which is reported to induce insulin resistance, linking diabetes to obesity. The greater the amount of adipose tissue, the greater potential for diabetes. Bays and others report a strong relationship between BMI and prevalence of type 2 diabetes. Below-normal/normal-weight individuals, overweight, and obese individuals account for 17.5, 31.6, and 50.9 percent of cases, respectively. The detrimental effects of obesity relative to the development of chronic disease occur when it persists for 10 years or more. This may be a serious health problem in the near future, as Peters estimated that given the dramatic rise in overweight children and obesity among children, one in three born in the year 2000 will become diabetic in their lifetime. In a review of 15 studies, Owen and others reported considerable variability in estimates across studies but concluded that BMI was directly related to CHD risk later in life. The future looks bleak, as the Centers for Disease Control and Prevention predicts that obesity rates may triple by 2050.

Cancers   Obesity has been regarded as a risk factor for colorectal, esophageal, pancreatic, liver, kidney, thyroid, postmenopausal breast, prostate, ovarian, and other cancers. Berger notes that obesity has contributed to 14 and 20 percent of cancer deaths in men and women, respectively. According to Calle and others, those with the highest BMI (40 or over) were at greatest risk. Normal BMI (<25 kg/m^2) is projected to prevent 90,000 cancer-related deaths in the USA. Renehan and others reviewed 141 studies with more than 280,000 subjects and reported that over the course of 15 years, men and women who experienced a 5-point increase in their BMI experienced a significant risk of a wide variety of cancers. The 2007 American Institute of Cancer Research worldwide report on nutrition and cancer presents convincing evidence of associations between increased body fatness and cancers of the breast, colorectum, pancreas, esophagus, and kidney. Overall, Wolin and others reported that weight gain and obesity account for approximately 20 percent of all cancer cases.

www.aicr.org/assets/docs/pdf/reports/Second_Expert_Report.pdf   World Cancer Research Fund/American Institute for Cancer Research. Food, Nutrition, Physical Activity, and the Prevention of Cancer: Summary on pages xiv–xvi of the report with panel recommendations following this summary.

Obesity may influence the development of cancers in various ways. Fat tissue leads to an overproduction of estrogen and other steroid hormones. Increased serum estrogen levels are associated with an increased incidence of breast cancer in women. Carmichael and Bates reported most large epidemiological studies found overweight or obese women are at increased risk of developing postmenopausal breast cancer and indicated that all treatment modalities for breast cancer may be adversely affected by the presence of obesity. However, the role of obesity may be modified by other risk factors. Renehan and others re-examined their 2008 meta-analysis data and reported that postmenopausal hormone

therapy significantly lowers associations between BMI and postmenopausal breast, endometrial, and ovarian cancers. Smoking was also found to attenuate the associations between BMI and esophageal, lung, and pancreatic cancers.

According to Riondino and colleagues, increases in secretions from visceral adipose tissue promoting inflammation and/or cell proliferation play a role in the development of colorectal cancer. Obesity increases production of insulin-like growth factor-1 (IGF-1) and decreases IGF-1 receptors and cell signaling pathways, resulting in insulin resiatance. IGF-1 can stimulate cell proliferation, which is a precursor to cancer development. Adipokine imbalances favoring inflammation may also promote tumor growth. Obesity may also have a local effect, contributing to gastrointestinal reflux in which stomach acids irritate cells and induce cancer in the lower esophagus. Other unknown factors may also be involved.

Alzheimer's Disease and Other Dementia   Since 2003, a growing body of research has implicated midlife obesity with mental decline. According to Kiliaan and colleagues, a number of adipokines, hormones, thrombotic factors, and growth factors secreted by adipose tissue could play a role in blood-brain barrier disturbances, changes in white matter, and brain atrophy associated with the cognitive and physical decline observed in Alzheimer's disease and other dementia. Obesity may also exert secondary effects on late-life brain function through its established role as a risk factor for hypertension, peripheral and cerebral vascular disease. In their meta-analysis, Loef and Walach reported significantly increased relative risks for late-life dementia in adults who were overweight and obese in middle age compared to normal weight adults. They also modeled significantly higher dementia prevalence estimates for the years 2030 and 2050 in the United States and China than current forecasts that do not include midlife obesity.

Maternal Health   Women naturally gain weight during pregnancy, but excess maternal weight gain may adversely affect pregnancy outcomes and fetal health. In a meta-analysis of 38 studies, Aune and colleagues reported modest but significant associations between maternal BMI and the following pregnancy outcomes: fetal death, stillbirth, perinatal (5 months pre- to 1 month post-birth) death, neonatal death, and infant death.

In its update on guidelines for weight gain during pregnancy, the National Academies of Sciences Institute of Medicine (IOM) stated that women today are heavier, a greater percentage of them are entering pregnancy overweight or obese, and many are gaining too much weight during pregnancy. The following IOM recommendations for weight gain rate and total weight gain are based on pre-pregnancy BMI:

Underweight (<18.5 kg/m^2; 1 lb/week; 28–40 lbs total)
Normal weight (18.5–24.9 kg/m^2; 1 lb/week; 25–35 lbs total)
Overweight (25.0–29.9 kg/m^2; 0.6 lb/week; 15–25 lbs total)
Obese (≥30.0 kg/m^2; 0.5 lb/week; 11–20 lbs total)

The guidelines have been developed with the welfare of both infant and mother in mind.

Mortality, Morbidity, and Quality of Life Hippocrates recognized that persons who are naturally fat are apt to die sooner than slender individuals. In a meta-analysis of 97 studies of 2.88 million individuals and 270,000 deaths and using normal-weight BMI (18.5–24.9) as the reference group, Flegal and others reported the following hazards ratios between all-cause mortality and BMI categories 0.94 (overweight, lower), 0.95 (grade 1 obesity, no difference), and 1.29 (grades 2 and 3 obesity, higher). In his review, Dixon reported that 300,000 deaths in the USA are related to overweight and obesity, 80 percent of which occur in subjects with a BMI or 30 kg/m^2 or greater. Loss of life for 40-year-old obese nonsmoking males and females is estimated at 5.8 and 7.1 years, respectively. In general, thinner individuals live longer, particularly if physically fit, as discussed later in this chapter.

Being overweight, and in particular being obese, is associated with premature death, but excess fat also contributes to morbidity, or the increase in various diseases such as diabetes and its associated disabilities. Those who are overweight and have such health problems may experience significant impairments in their quality of life.

Epidemiological research clearly indicates that being obese increases one's health risks. The location of the fat in the body is also an important contributing factor underlying these health risks.

How does the location of fat in the body affect health?

Classifications of different types of obesity based on regional fat distribution have been proposed, the most popular differentiation being the android versus the gynoid types. **Android-type** (male-type) **obesity** is characterized by accumulation in the abdominal region—particularly the intraabdominal region—of deep, visceral fat but also of subcutaneous fat. Android-type obesity is also known by other terms, such as abdominal, central, upper body, or lower trunk obesity, and is sometimes referred to as apple-shape obesity. In mice, up-regulation of the enzyme converting cortisone into cortisol results in overproduction of cortisol, which tends to facilitate the deposition of fat in the abdominal region. **Gynoid-type** (female-type) **obesity** is characterized by fat accumulation in the gluteal-femoral region—the hips, buttocks, and thighs. It is also known as lower body obesity and is often referred to as pear-shape obesity (see figure 10.9). In a study of young and old adult monozygotic and dizygotic twins, Malis and others reported high heritability estimates of 0.71 to 0.85 for trunk, lower body, and trunk/lower body fat distribution. Waist circumference measurement may be an appropriate screening technique for android-type or gynoid-type obesity. The procedure for determining waist circumference is described in appendix C and the increase in health risk associated with an

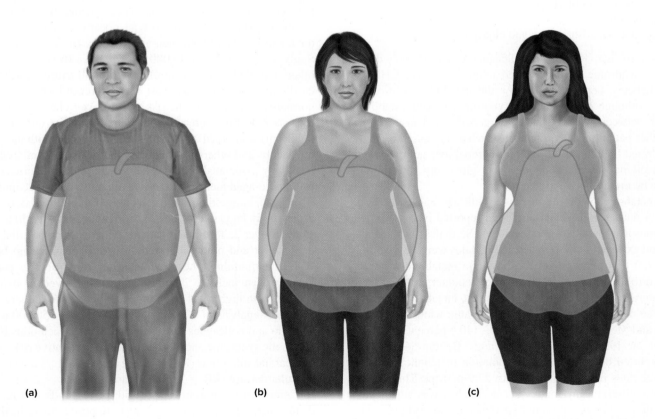

(a) (b) (c)

FIGURE 10.9 Patterns of fat deposition. (a) The android, or "apple-shape," pattern is associated with diabetes, coronary heart disease, hypertension, dyslipidemia, metabolic syndrome, and other chronic diseases. (b) Although more common in males, females can also present with the higher-risk apple-shape pattern. (c) The gynoid, or "pear-shape," pattern, more common in females, is generally associated with a lower risk of chronic disease than the apple shape.

increased circumference and various BMI levels is presented in table 10.1 on page 431.

Android-type obesity is increasingly being recognized as causing a greater health risk than obesity itself. It appears that android-type fat cells, particularly the deep visceral fat cells, possess dissimilar biochemical functions. These visceral fat cells are large and highly metabolically active, possibly due to differences in the activity of lipoprotein lipase and higher cortisol levels. Pi-Sunyer indicates that android-type obesity is a cardiovascular health risk factor associated with a release of pro-inflammatory adipokines such as resistin and TNF-α; a decrease in the anti-inflammatory adipokine adiponectin; and an increase in plasminogen activator inhibitor 1, which impairs fibrinolytic (clot-dissolving) action. Resistin is also theorized to be involved in the development of insulin resistance.

Epidemiological data have shown that android-type obesity is associated with a cluster of metabolic disorders, which Reaven labeled "syndrome X" and later renamed **metabolic syndrome.** As mentioned previously, some have labeled abdominal fat the *sick fat.*

The symptoms of the metabolic syndrome include the following:

- Hyperinsulinemia
- Insulin resistance
- Impaired glucose tolerance
- Hypertriglyceridemia
- Increased small, dense LDL-cholesterol
- Decreased HDL-cholesterol
- Hypertension
- Increased plasma fibrinogen and clotting

In their review, Kassi and colleagues report those with the metabolic syndrome have increased relative risks for CHD and type 2 diabetes, depending on how the metabolic syndrome is defined. Although the metabolic syndrome is well established as a link between visceral fat, atherogenesis, and insulin resistance, other pathological mechanisms such as increased oxidative stress, altered hypothalamic-pituitary-adrenal axis activity, renin-angiotenson-aldosterone function, and glucocorticoid function may also be involved.

The metabolic syndrome increases with age and BMI. Using NHANES data from 2003–2006, Ervin reported increased metabolic syndrome prevalence rates for U.S. males and females. Obese and extremely obese males and females were, respectively, 9.6 and 6.0 times more likely to have the metabolic syndrome compared to their normal or underweight counterparts. Race/ethnicity interacts with gender, as the largest metabolic syndrome prevalence rates are observed in non-Hispanic white males (37.2 percent) and Mexican-American females (40.6 percent).

Based on 1999–2010 NHANES data, Beltrán-Sánchez and others reported declines in total population metabolic syndrome prevalence rates from 25.5 percent to 22.9 percent. This decline, which was observed in females but not males, was attributed to pharmacological intervention in hypertension and dyslipidemia as components of the metabolic syndrome. During the same period, however, there were increases in prevalence rates of visceral fat deposition (waist circumferences >102 cm for males; >88 cm for females; 45.4 to 56.1 percent) and hyperglycemia (12.9 to 19.9

percent). Visceral adiposity continues to be serious public health concern. Reaven stressed the importance of treating the associated cardiovascular risk factors, such as high blood pressure. The metabolic syndrome has stimulated drug research leading to development of single drugs that simultaneously treat multiple components of the metabolic syndrome, such as high blood pressure and cholesterol levels.

In 2009, Alberti and others representing various international societies developed the following consensus clinical criteria for the diagnosis of the metabolic syndrome:

	Men	Women
Elevated waist circumference according to population- and country-specific definitions (inches [cm] for the USA)	>40 [102]	>34.6 [88]
Elevated serum triglycerides (mg/dL)	>150	>150
Subnormal HDL-cholesterol (mg/dL)	<40	<50
Elevated blood pressure (mmHg)	130/85	130/85
Elevated fasting blood sugar (mg/dL)	100	100

As noted in table 10.1, the gender-specific waist circumferences have been associated with increased health risks. Lower waist circumference criteria for males (37 inches, 94 cm) and females (31.5 inches, 80 cm) have been recommended by some experts. Wang and others reported an increased risk for type 2 diabetes in men with waist circumferences greater than 37 inches.

Studies show that android-type obesity is a major risk factor for mortality in both men and women. In the Nurses' Health Study involving nearly 45,000 women over 16 years, Zhang and others reported increased mortality from all causes, cardiovascular disease, and cancer as waist circumference increased. Even in normal-weight women, the risk of cardiovascular disease mortality was 3.02 times greater with increased waist circumferences (>88 cm) compared to normal-weight women without visceral fat. Jacobs and others also reported that waist circumference was positively associated with mortality within all categories of BMI for middle-aged men and women, even those with a recommended BMI level, suggesting that the increased mortality risk related to excess body fat is mainly due to abdominal adiposity. In a clinical study of over 2,200 French patients with acute myocardial infarction, Zeller and others reported an inverse relationship between BMI and mortality (the previously described obesity paradox). However, an increase in mortality was observed in males and females with high waist circumference but low to moderate BMI. In a meta-analysis of 87 studies including over 950,000 patients, Mottillo and colleagues reported significant associations between metabolic syndrome and all-cause mortality (relative risk = 1.58); myocardial infarction (RR = 1.99); stroke (RR = 2.27); cardiovascular disease (RR = 2.35) and mortality (RR = 2.4).

Compared to android fat, gynoid fat responds less readily to diet/exercise intervention but appears to pose a lower health risk. In their review, Lee and others describe several physiological differences between visceral and subcutaneous fat depots, which are consistent with gender- and age-related differences in fat deposition.

Does being obese increase health risks in youth?

According to the World Health Organization, approximately 43 million children in the world are obese. Permanent alterations of neural pathways regulating energy intake and expenditure may result from overconsumption of high-energy foods and physical inactivity during childhood. Pulgarón's review of 79 studies reveals that obese children have adult-like metabolic syndrome co-morbidities such as vascular disease, fatty liver disease, and type 2 diabetes. Obese children are also more susceptible to dental caries, asthma, and sleep apnea.

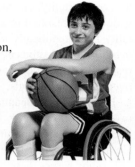

Obese children are often ridiculed and bullied by peers, adults, and even parents. As a result, they may also suffer from a constellation of psychological co-morbidities such as anxiety, depression, low self-esteem, negative self-image, attention deficit hyperactivity disorder, delayed social development, and even serious psychological illness. Since personality traits are established in childhood and adolescence, excessive body fat may contribute more greatly to social-emotional problems at this time than during adult-onset obesity. Stein and colleagues also identify low socioeconomic status, lack of a social support network, and social marginalization as psychosocial factors contributing to childhood obesity. Competences particularly affected are physical competence, appearance, and social functioning. Psychological problems may also be related to the adverse effect of excessive body fat on physical fitness and athletic performance. Southern indicates that obese children respond differently emotionally to exercise than do normal-weight children and thus may experience negative consequences from participation in physical activities. A child who is unsuccessful in play activities probably will not participate, and thus will miss the socializing aspects and physical benefits of play. When used in conjunction with appropriate dietary prescriptions and consistent behavior modification, exercise serves as a promising modality that may reverse obese conditions during childhood and improve psychological health.

Franks and others, in a major study on childhood obesity, indicated that it will have very serious long-term health effects through midlife. Researchers are looking for clues, such as genetic, metabolic, or anthropometric markers, that can predict which children will become obese so that appropriate interventions may be enacted earlier in life, when chances of success to prevent obesity may be greater.

Does losing excess body fat reduce health risks and improve health status?

Numerous studies document the beneficial effects of weight loss by reducing the risk factors for disease, including several major diseases—cardiovascular disease, cancer, and type 2 diabetes. Arena and others list ideal weight (BMI 18.5–24.9) and a DASH-type diet as two of seven key metrics, in an American Heart Association policy statement on worksite health screening. The 2007 World Cancer Research Fund/American Institute of Cancer Research listed proper weight control as one of its key recommendations to help prevent a variety of cancers. Aucott reported that intentional weight loss reduces the risk of developing diabetes in the long term. Individuals with diabetes who lose weight often have reduced clinical symptoms and mortality risk. As noted in chapter 2, the first healthful dietary guideline is to achieve a healthy body weight.

As noted by Beltrán-Sánchez, Lee, and others, visceral fat is a key component of the metabolic syndrome and a logical target for interventions to reduce risk of cardiovascular disease and type 2 diabetes. Several studies in men, women, and adolescents have shown that weight loss via dieting and exercise will preferentially decrease fat from the abdominal area and, concomitantly, reduce several of the metabolic syndrome risk factors, such as high blood pressure and serum levels of glucose and triglycerides. Reducing abdominal fat may reduce the production of pathological adipokines, resulting in decreased inflammation and other factors contributing to disease. For example, Romero-Corral and others note that impaired endothelial function recovers after weight loss.

As shall be noted in chapter 11, lifestyle changes, including adoption of an appropriate diet and exercise program, are appropriate for individuals desiring to attain a healthy weight. A variety of diets are available, containing varying percentages of the three macronutrients—carbohydrate, fat, and protein. For weight loss, caloric balance is the key, so weight loss will occur if the total caloric intake, regardless of the macronutrient content of the diet, is less than caloric expenditure. However, as noted in previous chapters, some overall dietary plans, such as the DASH and OmniHeart diets, as well as certain foods, such as fruits, vegetables, and fish, may provide health benefits beyond those associated with weight loss. Chapters 4, 5, and 6 highlight healthful carbohydrates, fats, and protein, and chapter 9 discusses the DASH and OmniHeart diets.

Does being physically fit negate the adverse health effects associated with being overweight?

In general, research findings documenting increased health risks associated with obesity have been derived from the general population and have been based primarily on BMI values. Although BMI may be useful in determining health risks in the general population because a high value is usually associated with excess body fat, it does not apply to muscular individuals. A high BMI may be associated with the development of various chronic diseases if it does represent obesity and increases various risk factors, such as high serum cholesterol levels and high blood pressure. However, BMI does not evaluate body composition or provide an indication of fatness in all individuals.

The BMI also does not measure fitness, and a physically active lifestyle may be an important moderating factor in the association between fatness and health. However, whether or not fitness counteracts the adverse health effects of fatness is a matter of debate among exercise scientists.

Several studies suggest that fitness counteracts the adverse effects of fatness on heart health. In a study of older (>60 years) adults, Sui and others found that being obese (BMI ≥30) or having a large waist circumference (34 inches, women; 40 inches, men) was significantly associated with increased mortality, but not when cardiorespiratory fitness was considered. High levels of fitness have been shown to be protective against premature mortality. In a cross-sectional study of women, Farrell and others reported that across all levels of adiposity, higher levels of cardiorespiratory fitness were associated with lower incidence rates of all-cause mortality. They concluded that using adiposity measures as predictors of all-cause mortality in women may be misleading unless cardiorespiratory fitness is also considered. Some suggest that being overweight does not increase mortality unless it is associated with adverse effects on blood pressure, glucose tolerance, serum cholesterol levels, and other risk factors for chronic diseases. Physical activity may help to counteract such adverse effects.

The Healthy at Every Size (HAES®, www.sizediversityandhealth.org/) movement began in the 1960s in order to promote weight-neutral dietary and physical activity strategies for health improvement in overweight and obese individuals. In their review, Kim and Park state that exercise without weight loss can improve insulin sensitivity and decrease insulin resistance in obese adults. Although there are reports of similar effects in children and adolescents, more research is needed on the optimal training volumes and modes to reduce insulin resistance in obese youth. According to Buresh, exercise improves muscle glucose uptake by increasing GLUT-4 receptor migration to the muscle cell membrane in an insulin-independent manner and by opposing mechanisms that impair insulin signaling and lead to insulin resistance.

An acute exercise bout can increase insulin sensitivity for up to 16 hours afterwards. Chronic exercise training potentiates the effect of exercise on insulin sensitivity through multiple adaptations in glucose transport and metabolism. Gerson and Braun reported that estimated insulin sensitivity was only slightly lower in overweight but fit women compared to lean women of equal cardiorespiratory fitness. Although exercise training may not help some individuals lose weight, it may result in significant health improvements.

Although fitness is important to counteract some of the adverse health effects of fatness, losing excess body fat may provide additional health benefits. In their meta-analysis of studies with 10 or more years of follow-up, Kramer and colleagues reported that metabolically healthy obese individuals had a slightly higher relative risk for all-cause mortality and cardiovascular events (1.24) compared to metabolically healthy normal-weight individuals.

Carroll and Dudfield indicated that exercise works best when coupled with weight loss. The combination of exercise and weight loss has been shown to produce numerous health effects, including decreased blood pressure, improved serum lipid status, reduced blood glucose, increased self-esteem, and improved psychological health. In their meta-analysis of 26 studies of the effect of weight loss on mortality, Harrington and others reported that intentional weight loss resulted in a small, but significant, reduction in mortality in metabolically *unhealthy* obese, but not in metabolically *healthy* obese, subjects. Mortality actually slightly increased in response to intentional weight loss in healthy normal-weight and overweight individuals.

Barry and colleagues examined ten longitudinal studies (average follow-up = 14.3 ± 2.6 years) on all-cause mortality that included measures of cardiorespiratory fitness and BMI. Compared to normal-weight-fit individuals (1.0), the overall hazards ratios across these studies were 2.42 for normal weight unfit; 2.14 for underweight unfit; 1.13 for overweight fit; 2.46 for obese unfit; and 1.21 for obese fit. Fit subjects had a similar mortality risk regardless of apparent fatness. In a similar study, Kenchaiah and others reported the following hazards ratios for heart failure by BMI and fitness categories: 1.00 for lean, active; 1.19 for lean, inactive; 1.49 for overweight, active; 1.78 for overweight, inactive; 2.68 for obese, active; and 3.93 for obese, inactive. Heart failure risk increased with weight gain, but the risk was reduced somewhat by being physically active.

Weinstein and others, in a prospective study of nearly 39,000 women over the course of nearly 11 years, evaluated the interaction of physical activity and body mass index on the risk of coronary heart disease (CHD). They found that the lowest risk for CHD was in women who were of normal weight and physically active. Being overweight and physically inactive increased the risk, and women who were obese and inactive had the highest risk. The authors concluded that although the risk of CHD associated with elevated body mass index is considerably reduced by increased physical activity levels, the risk is not completely eliminated, reinforcing the importance of being lean and physically active. These investigators concluded that being fit does not reverse all of the increased health risks associated with excess adiposity. The results of these studies in part support the HAES® position of weight neutrality in health improvement. Although being *fit and fat* appears to be better healthwise than being *unfit and fat,* losing weight to become *fit and unfat* may confer some additional health benefits.

It is important to note that a normal BMI does not automatically connote good health. One may have a normal BMI but have relatively high amounts of abdominal fat and associated health risk.

Prevention of obesity is the key because once individuals become obese, treatment is difficult. When used in conjunction with appropriate dietary prescriptions and consistent behavior modification, exercise serves as a promising modality not only to prevent obesity in the first place but perhaps also to help reverse it both during childhood and adulthood.

http://www.niddk.nih.gov/health-information/health-topics/weight-control/active-at-any-size/Pages/active-at-any-size.aspx. **Access the Weight Control Information Network to access *Active at Any Size*.**

Excessive Weight Loss and Health

Losing excess body fat, even only 5–10 percent of body weight, and attaining a desirable body weight may confer some significant health benefits by counteracting the adverse effects of obesity. However, many individuals attempt to lose weight for other reasons. Slimness is currently very fashionable, particularly among females of all ages. It is desired not only for attractiveness but also for psychological undertones of independence, achievement, and self-control. Male and female athletes, such as distance runners, gymnasts, wrestlers, jockeys, and dancers, practice weight control to improve their performance. Losing body weight for improved performance may also provide some health benefits. For example, Williams theorized that the elevated HDL-cholesterol concentrations of long-distance runners are primarily a result of reduced adiposity. However, excessive weight loss may actually lead to deterioration of health.

What health problems are associated with improper weight-loss programs and practices?

As shall be noted in chapter 11, a well-designed diet and proper exercise are the cornerstones of a sound weight-control program. However, some individuals may establish unrealistically low body-weight goals, which may lead to pathogenic weight-control behaviors. Such techniques as complete starvation, self-induced vomiting, or the improper or excessive use of drugs, diet pills, laxatives, and diuretics may initially be employed to achieve rapid weight losses but may evolve into serious medical disorders, even death, if prolonged. The following discussion highlights some of the areas of concern in which weight-loss practices may be harmful if abused. The use, efficacy, and potential health risks of dietary supplements for weight loss are discussed in chapter 11.

Dehydration Dehydration may be induced by exercise, exposure to the heat (as with a sauna), or the use of diuretics and laxatives. The effect of dehydration on health, particularly in relation to heat illnesses, was discussed in chapter 9. Laxatives and diuretics, which are illegally used by some athletes to lose weight and to mask the use of illegal supplements, may cause *hypokalemia,* or loss of plasma potassium. Hypokalemia may lead to electrolyte abnormalities; cardiac irregularity; disturbed kidney and neuromuscular function; and in rare case muscle tissue breakdown, known as rhabdomyolysis. In a case study, Mayr and others reported hypokalemic paralysis in a professional bodybuilder who used furosemide, a potent diuretic, prior to a competition. Although this patient responded favorably to gradual potassium replacement over 7 hours, dehydration strategies that alter electrolyte balance can be fatal. In their review, Cadwallader and colleagues note a 200 percent increase in positive tests for diuretic use by World Anti-Doping Agency laboratories from 2005 to 2009.

Weight-Loss Drugs Lifestyle interventions such as increased physical activity and healthy nutrition have not been completely effective in controlling obesity and its co-morbidities. Therefore, various drugs have been developed to stimulate weight loss and generally are prescribed for the obese, not for those individuals who want to lose a few pounds. Nevertheless, it appears that individuals across the weight spectrum, including physically active individuals and athletes, are using drugs for weight-control purposes. Some drugs are available without prescription, whereas others should be used only under medical supervision.

Anti-obesity drugs may help reduce body weight by either enhancing the production or activity of serotonin and norepinephrine in the hypothalamus or suppressing neuropeptide Y (NPY) to curb the appetite. Other medications interfere with the action of gastric and intestinal lipases, thus blocking intestinal absorption of dietary fat and decreasing caloric intake. Other drugs may be used to increase energy expenditure (thermogenesis) in the peripheral tissues. Of particular interest is the development of drugs that might stimulate adrenergic receptors in brown fat and abdominal adipose tissue, and possibly muscle tissue, to increase resting energy expenditure (REE).

Silbutramine (Meridia®), a serotonin and norepinephrine re-uptake inhibitor in the brain, reduced hunger, stimulated thermogenesis, and was considered effective for long-term weight loss. However, it was linked to an increased risk for heart attack and removed from the marketplace in 2010. Currently, there are four prescription anti-obesity drugs approved for long-term use in the USA. The oldest, orlistat (Xenical®), is a lipase inhibitor that blocks fat absorption. Reported side effects include diarrhea, fatty stools, and flatulence. Chaput and others noted that orlistat is able to induce significant weight loss, with important co-morbidity reduction, with maintenance of reduced body weight for at least 1–2 years. Orlistat is also available as over-the-counter drug called *alli*, which is half the dose of Xenical and has been reported to be effective. In 2012, Phentermine-topiramate (Qsymia®) and lorcaserin (Belviq®) were approved by the FDA. Phentermine is a sympathomimetic amine that suppresses the appetite. Lorcaserin is a serotonin receptor agonist that improves control of eating. According to a review by Hainer and Aldhoon-Hainerová, phentermine-topiramate and lorcaserin are effective in promoting weight loss and reducing cardio-metabolic risk. Both agents have modest side effects (e.g., dizziness, nausea, constipation, and dry mouth) that tend to diminish over time. In September 2014, a naltrexone HCl/bupropion HCl combination obesity drug marketed under the trade name Contrave® received FDA approval. Contrave® is indicated for the treatment of overweight/obesity and components of the metabolic syndrome. Bupropion and naltrexone have been shown to stimulate receptors that suppress food intake and increase energy expenditure. In essence, Contrave® modulates CNS reward pathways. In clinical trials, Apovian and colleagues reported significantly greater weight loss with Contrave® at 32 weeks (6.5 percent) and 56 weeks (6.4 percent) compared to placebo along with improvements in waist circumference, blood lipids, fasting insulin levels, and control of eating. Rimonabant, previously marketed in Europe under the trade name Accomplia, enhances cannabinoid receptor activity in the nervous system and has been shown to be effective. However, it was never approved for use in the United States and was removed from the European market in 2009 amid concerns about psychological side effects.

Although research shows that weight-loss drugs may be effective, the lost weight is regained upon cessation of use of the drug if lifestyle is not changed. The Food and Drug Administration (FDA) recommends that weight-control drugs be used only on a short-term basis in conjunction with an education program stressing proper diet, exercise, and behavior modification. Several studies by Wadden and his associates reported twice as much weight loss when use of a weight-loss drug was combined with such an educational program, as compared to use of the drug alone. They concluded that the results underscore the importance of prescribing weight-loss medications in combination with, rather than in lieu of, lifestyle modification.

Some scientists contend that obesity is an incurable disease, somewhat comparable to type 1 diabetes. Type 1 diabetics need to take insulin daily to control their disease. It is hoped that continued research into the neural mechanisms underlying the etiology of obesity will eventually provide the database for pharmaceutical companies to develop more effective and safe drugs to prevent and treat obesity. For example, a new hormone, obestatin, has been discovered in some animals. Obestatin is derived from the same prohormone as ghrelin but has the opposite effects; obestatin actually depresses the appetite and thus may serve as the basis for developing an effective and safe weight-loss drug, which, as Halford and others note, is a major focus of pharmaceutical companies.

Very Low-Calorie Diets Starvation-type diets may involve either complete fasting or **very low-Calorie diets (VLCD)** (<800 Calories/day), often referred to as modified fasts. These diet plans are most often used with inpatient programs in hospitals. According to Jensen and others, guidelines by the American Heart Association, the American College of Cardiology, and The Obesity Society state that VLCD, under proper medical supervision, are generally regarded as safe and have been effective in inducing rapid weight loss in very obese patients. In their meta-analysis of 20 studies comparing post-VLCD interventions on weight-loss maintenance, Johansson and others reported a mean weight loss during the VLCD or low-Calorie diet (<1,200 Calories/day) of 12.3 kg (27 lbs) over a median period of 8 weeks. In their guidelines, Jenson and others state that VLCD result in 14 to 21 kg (31 to 46 lbs) over 11 to 14 weeks. The efficacy and safety of VLCD may depend on the duration.

Apparently little or no harm is caused by a 1- or 2-day fast, and some authorities have reported that a healthy man or woman can fast completely for 2 weeks with no permanent ill effects. Although VLCD may be safe and effective for promoting short-term weight loss, evidence of successful post-VLCD long-term weight maintenance is scant. Compared to control groups, Johansson and others reported greater post-VLCD weight maintenance with meal replacement, anti-obesity drugs, and high-protein diets. Exercise and other dietary supplements did not improve post-VLCD weight-loss maintenance compared to controls.

VLCDs should only be used after a medical exam and under medical supervision. Contraindications, as described by Atkinson, include fatigue, weakness, headaches, nausea, constipation, loss of libido, kidney stones, gallbladder disease, decreased HDL-cholesterol, impaired phagocytic function of the white blood cells, inflammation of the intestines and pancreas, decreases in blood volume, decreases in heart muscle tissue, low blood pressure, cardiac arrhythmias, and even death. Jenssen and Johansson and others describe the low long-term success of VLCD alone in weight maintenance. Therefore, the VLCD approach should be considered as the first step of a life-long weight-management program and is successful only when it is followed by a maintenance program consisting of lifestyle interventions involving behavior modification, dietary changes, and increased physical activity.

Weight Cycling **Weight cycling** (yo-yo syndrome) is a controversial practice of intermittent weight loss followed by weight gain with unknown long-term consequences. Experts have speculated that the practice may ultimately be counterproductive because of a net weight gain consisting of increased fat mass and loss of lean body mass. During the VLCD phase, the neural circuitry regulating energy balance may respond to caloric deprivation by decreasing both diet-induced thermogenesis and resting energy expenditure (REE), as well as enhancing food storage efficiency. Severe caloric deprivation may also result in catabolism of muscle protein to generate amino acids for conversion into glucose by the liver for central nervous system metabolism. When normal (or greater) caloric intake resumes, energy-conservation mechanisms may continue to function for some time, with storage of the extra calories as fat instead of being used to replace the lost tissue protein. Moreover, resumption of normal dietary habits may lead to binge eating due to alterations in neural pathways controlling eating. A meta-analysis by the National Task Force on the Prevention and Treatment of Obesity revealed that weight cycling does not exert any adverse effect on body composition, metabolism, risk factors for cardiovascular disease, or the effectiveness of future efforts to lose weight. The Task Force noted that although the evidence currently available indicates that weight cycling does not affect morbidity and mortality, conclusive data regarding its long-term health effects are lacking.

In more recent research partially supporting the previously described mechanisms, Bosy-Westphal and colleagues subjected obese subjects to a weight cycle (13-week low-Calorie diet with 6 months' follow-up) and divided the subjects into weight-regain and weight-stable groups. Woman had a higher regain of fat in the extremities, whereas men had a lower regain in both extremity and visceral fat. Regain of extremity skeletal muscle tissue was greater than that of the trunk. A lower REE was observed in the weight-regain group after weight loss. In their review, Bosy-Westphal and Müller describe several methodological obstacles to assessing the impact of weight cycling on body composition. One of these challenges, discussed earlier in this chapter, is the lack of valid and reliable techniques for *in vivo* body composition assessment in measuring different components contributing to small regains in weight.

Another potential health-related consequence of weight cycling is chronic inflammation, a known pathology of cardiovascular disease and type 2 diabetes. In their review, Strohaker and McFarlin comment that weight cycling may alter adipose tissue to increase secretion of pro-inflammatory cytokines. Barbosa-da-Silva and others fed mice weight-cycle diets consisting of standard chow (SC)/high-fat chow (HF) in different orders over durations of 2, 4, or 6 weeks. Greater pro-inflammatory cytokine levels were observed following the HF phase. The HF phase length was directly proportional to the time for inflammatory changes to return to baseline.

Some investigators believe the issue of weight cycling and health is still open for debate. Brownell and Rodin have suggested that although there has been no consistent demonstration that, as was first thought, weight cycling makes subsequent weight loss more difficult or regain more rapid, it is possible that this does occur under some conditions or in particular individuals. Although the mechanisms are not clear at present, they also note stronger and more consistent links between body-weight variability and negative health outcomes. In a large study, Field and others reported that weight cycling was associated with a higher prevalence of binge eating, lower levels of physical activity, and greater weight gain. It is generally agreed that any perceived risks of weight cycling should not deter an obese individual from attempts to lose weight, but the best strategy is a lifelong commitment to healthy behavior, diet, and exercise. There is a clear need for further research on the effects of weight cycling on behavior, metabolism, and health.

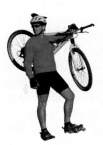

Young Athletes One of the major medical concerns is the effect that severe weight restriction over a longer period may have on children who are still in the growth and development stages of life. Young athletes are at a critical age as far as nutritional needs are concerned, but the importance of making weight for certain sports may outweigh consideration of a balanced diet, adequate fluid intake, and a minimum caloric requirement. As a result, young athletes may receive inadequate intakes of protein, zinc, iron, calcium, and other nutrients, described in earlier chapters, as essential for normal growth and development. Although numerous studies have revealed nutrient deficiencies and pathogenic weight-control behaviors in young athletes such as wrestlers and ballet dancers, there are very few data on the long-range effects of such practices. In a comparison of highly and moderately trained competitive female gymnasts, Daly and others indicated that in athletes who have long-term, clinically delayed maturation, catch-up growth may be incomplete and reported a high frequency of reduced growth velocity in some, but not all, female gymnasts. Theintz and others theorized that lower growth rates observed in gymnasts compared to swimmers over 2 to 3 years might be explained by heavy training ($\geq$18 hours/week), possibly combined with the metabolic effects of dieting, leading to impaired hypothalamus-pituitary-gonadal axis activity with resultant suppression of proper sexual development. In an extensive review in 2013, Malina and others concluded that gymnasts, while of shorter average stature, are still within a normal range, with no evidence of impairment of attained adult stature. There were insufficient data upon which to base any association between training behaviors and altered hormonal function. The short stature associated with successful, persistent gymnasts may be the result of self-selection or simply being selected by coaches based on stature. The American College of Sports Medicine also concluded that participation in high school wrestling, which normally involves weight cycling, does not adversely affect normal growth patterns. Nevertheless, there has been increasing concern over the development of chronic dieting problems, that is, eating disorders in children, adolescents, and young adults, which could have serious adverse health consequences.

What are the major eating disorders?

Eating behaviors vary among individuals and may be influenced by a number of factors, including ethnicity, religion, economics, environmentalism, and others. Some eating behaviors may be regarded as abnormal, and two such behaviors have been designated as *disordered eating* and *eating disorders*. The following discussion uses the criteria for such eating behaviors as presented in the fifth edition of *Diagnostic and Statistical Manual of Mental Disorders* (*DSM-V*) published by the American Psychiatric Association (APA) in 2013.

Disordered eating reflects atypical eating behaviors such as restrictive dieting, the use of diet pills or laxatives, bingeing, and purging. Disordered eating patterns may occur in response to a stressful event, an illness, personal appearance, or in preparation for athletic competition. In general, these behaviors occur less frequently or are less severe than those required to meet the full criteria for the diagnosis of an eating disorder as described in *DSM-V*. Nevertheless, medical professionals consider disordered eating behaviors to be suggestive of a potential unhealthy relationship with food and body image. For example, a condition called purging disorder, identified by Keel and others, is similar to bulimia but does not involve binge eating, only purging, usually by self-induced vomiting.

The APA defines **eating disorders** as illnesses in which the victims suffer severe disturbances in their eating behaviors and related thoughts and emotions. According to a national survey, Hudson and others estimate the lifetime prevalence of individual eating disorders as 0.6 to 4.5 percent. Currently, the APA recognizes four clinical eating disorders in *DSM-V*:

- Anorexia nervosa (AN)
- Bulimia nervosa (BN)
- Binge eating disorder (BED)
- Other specified feeding or eating disorder (OSFED)

Anorexia nervosa (AN) is a complex disorder that is not completely understood but is thought to be a sign of other psychological problems. Rask-Andersen and others report that AN is a complex, multifactorial disease with high heritability, including genetic influences on mental disorders, hunger regulatory systems, reward systems, and systems regulating energy metabolism and sex hormones. Research has suggested that AN cases possess characteristics that underlie compulsive personality disorders, and the prevalence of AN is greatest in groups that abuse psychoactive substances. The diagnostic criteria for AN, as developed by the APA, are summarized as follows:

1. Refusal to maintain the body weight over a minimal normal weight for age and height. A weight loss leading to maintenance of body weight less than 85 percent of that expected, including the expected weight gain during the period of growth.
2. An intense fear of gaining weight or becoming fat, even though underweight.
3. A disturbance in the way one's body weight or shape is perceived.

Individuals with AN may be the binge eating/purging type, engaging in binge eating or purging behavior, such as self-induced vomiting or the misuse of laxatives, diuretics, and enemas. The restricting type does not engage in such behaviors.

According to Hudson and others, the lifetime prevalence of anorexia nervosa for females and males in the general population is 0.9 and 0.3 percent, respectively. Young females, usually under the age of 25, account for about 85 to 90 percent of AN cases. As noted earlier, there appears to be a strong genetic predisposition to AN. Bulik and others found that AN was more prevalent between identical twins as compared to fraternal twins, and they indicated that about 56 percent of AN causality is associated with genetics. Sodersen and others suggest that brain mechanisms for reward may be critical; they may be stimulated when food intake is reduced, thus sustaining disordered eating behaviors.

Multiple factors underlie the development of AN. Perfectionist tendencies, low-esteem with poor body image, and self-criticism are personality traits that appear to be associated with AN. Upper-middle socioeconomic status, an overprotective home environment, and a culture that idealizes thinness are also associated with AN. Susceptible individuals desire to have control over something in their lives. Individuals with AN are more likely to be depressed, to be anxious, and to suffer obsessive-compulsive disorders. One review noted that up to 80 percent of anorexia nervosa patients engage in excessive exercise to lose weight. Although most anorexics are female, male anorexics possess similar characteristics.

Treatment of AN, as well as other eating disorders, involves an interdisciplinary team consisting of professionals from medical, nursing, nutritional, and mental health disciplines. In its 2011 position stand on treatment of eating disorders, the Academy of Nutrition and Dietetics (formerly the American Dietetic Association) emphasized a team approach, including nutritional counseling by a registered dietitian. Psychotherapeutic techniques, such as cognitive behavioral therapy, are designed to foster body acceptance. Intervention programs may use self-help or group approaches and may be prolonged for several years. Medical consequences of AN can be very serious, including hormonal imbalances, anemia, decreased heart muscle mass, heartbeat arrhythmias attributed to electrolyte imbalances, and even death. Amenorrhea, the absence of three consecutive menstrual cycles, is also common in females with AN. However, amenorrhea is also observed in other conditions, including the female athletic triad, discussed later in this chapter, and has been dropped as a diagnostic criterion for AN in *DSM-V*.

Success in treating AN is limited. The dropout rate from AN treatment programs is high. In their review, Bailey and others found that relapse prevention strategies such as cognitive behavioral therapy, psycho-education, and use of selective serotonin re-uptake inhibitors were addressed in only six of 64 AN treatment trials. More research is needed to identify effective strategies to prevent AN relapse. Mayer and others found that women with a lower percent body fat experienced a poorer long-term outcome. Attila states that AN is associated with significant morbidity and a mortality rate as high as that seen in any psychiatric illness. Crow and colleagues followed 177 diagnosed AN cases from 1979 to 1997 and cross-referenced this list with deaths from 1997 to 2004 using the National Death Index compiled by the National Center for Health Statistics. They reported a crude mortality rate of 4.0 percent, a standardized mortality rate (SMR) of 1.7 percent, and a suicide-specific SMR of 4.68 percent in AN cases.

The term **bulimia nervosa (BN)** means *morbid hunger,* and the disorder involves a loss of control over the impulse to binge. The bulimic individual repeatedly ingests large quantities of food within a discrete period of time, such as 2 hours but follows this by self-induced vomiting and other measures to avoid weight gain. This is known as the binge-purge syndrome. Bulimics may use other techniques, such as fasting or excessive exercise, to compensate for the binge. The APA *DSM-V* criteria for bulimia nervosa include the following:

1. Recurrent episodes of binge eating, at least one per week for 3 months
2. Lack of control over eating during the binge
3. Regular use of self-induced vomiting, laxatives, diuretics, fasting, or excessive exercise to control body weight
4. Persistent concern with body weight and body shape

BN is more common than anorexia nervosa. According to Hudson and others, lifetime prevalence rates for BN are 1.5 and 0.5 percent for females and males, respectively. However, the prevalence of BN among college students may be much higher. As with AN, certain characteristics may underlie the development of BN, including the desire for thinness and chronic low self-esteem.

According to the Mayo Clinic, dehydration, irregularity in heart rhythm, tooth decay, erosion of dental enamel, gum disease, amenorrhea, digestive problems, and substance abuse are associated with BN. Many of these complications are the result of self-induced purging or vomiting. Anxiety and depression are also associated with BN. As with anorexics, bulimics are in need of psychological counseling by qualified medical professionals. Prozac (fluoxetine), an antidepressant drug that helps increase serotonin levels, has been approved for medically supervised use in treating BN. Shapiro and others report that Prozac helps decrease the core symptoms of BN and associated psychological factors, at least on a short-term. Behavioral treatment may also be effective.

Although treatment of BN appears to produce better results than treatments available for AN, the outcome is still unsatisfactory for many patients. Crow and colleagues reported a crude mortality rate of 3.9 percent, a standardized mortality ratio (SMR) of 1.57 percent, and a suicide-specific SMR of 6.51 percent in BN deaths from 1997 to 2004.

Beginning with *DSM-V,* **binge eating disorder (BED)** is a third category of eating disorder. Previously, BED was described under a "catch-all" category entitled "eating disorders not otherwise specified" (EDNOS). Individuals with BED often eat an unusually large amount of food and feel out of control during the binge, which may include the following behaviors:

1. At least one episode/week over 3 months of consuming a large amount of food in a short time
2. Eating until uncomfortably full
3. Eating when not hungry
4. Eating alone because of embarrassment
5. Feeling disgusted, depressed, or guilty after eating

These behaviors are also common to BN, but the individual with BED does not purge. The causes of BED are similar to those of BN. Health consequences include weight gain and obesity, along with increases in CHD risk factors, cancer, and other health problems previously discussed. Crow and others reported a crude mortality rate of 5.2 percent, a standardized mortality ratio (SMR) of 1.81 percent, and a suicide-specific SMR of 3.91 percent in 802 diagnosed eating disorders or otherwise specified (EDNOS) cases. Prior to *DSM-V,* the EDNOS diagnosis included BED. Although EDNOS was considered a somewhat "less severe" eating disorder under earlier diagnostic criteria, Crow and others conclude it is associated with mortality and suicide rates similar to those of AN and BN. Treatment of BED is comparable to that for BN, which may involve medication such as antidepressants; treatment for obesity may also be involved.

The prevalence of full-blown clinical eating disorders in the general population is only about 1–3 percent. However, as noted previously, many more individuals exhibit signs of disordered eating. Research suggests that disordered eating may be more prevalent in certain professions or personal pursuits, one in particular being sports.

www.womenshealth.gov This is the U.S. Department of Health and Human Services Website for women's health. Type eating disorders, or the specific eating disorder, in the Search box to access numerous reputable Websites providing information on causes, symptoms, health risks, prevention, and treatment.

What eating problems are associated with sports?

Depending on the nature of the sport, the loss of excess body weight may enable an athlete to compete in a lower weight class or improve appearance and/or biomechanics and enhance the potential for success. Thus, some athletes may use weight loss as an ergogenic aid. Examples of such sports include wrestling, gymnastics, ballet, cheerleading, bodybuilding, figure skating, diving, lightweight football, lightweight rowing, and distance running. To lose weight, athletes in these sports, particularly athletes with perfectionistic tendencies, may exhibit some, but not all, of the characteristics associated with clinical eating disorders, thus meeting the criteria for Other Specified Feeding or Eating Disorders (OSFED).

The APA uses OSFED for individuals who do not meet the criteria for AN, BN, or BED. Included in this category is anorexia athletica. In recent years, the term **anorexia athletica (AA)** has been applied to those athletes who become overly concerned with their weight and exhibit some of the diagnostic criteria associated with AN or BN. According to Sundgot-Borgen, individuals must meet the following criteria for AA:

1. Excessive fear of becoming obese
2. Restriction of caloric intake
3. Weight loss
4. No medical disorder to explain leanness
5. Gastrointestinal complaints

In addition, they must meet one or more of these related criteria:

1. Disturbance in body image
2. Compulsive exercising
3. Binge eating
4. Use of purging methods
5. Delayed puberty
6. Menstrual dysfunction

Additional characteristics related to AA discussed by Sudi and colleagues include dieting and excessive overtraining, resulting in a lean physique; a motivation to lose weight based on performance; voluntary initiation of dieting and excessive training either by the athlete or at the coach's encouragement; and a pattern of weight cycling.

Although male athletes, particularly those in bodybuilding, distance running, and wrestling, may be at risk for disordered eating, most studies have focused on female athletes in weight-control aesthetic sports such as gymnastics and dance, as well as female distance runners. Bratland-Sandra and Sundgot-Borgen report prevalence rates of disordered eating and eating disorders in the literature of 0 to 19 percent in male and 6 to 45 percent in female athletes. In a meta-analysis of 34 studies, Smolak and others found that elite athletes in sports emphasizing thinness are particularly at risk. Studies by Torstveit and Sundgot-Borgen and Hoch also report a significant proportion of nonathletes were at risk for behaviors associated with the female athlete triad, a condition characterized by disordered eating, menstrual irregularity, and loss of bone mineral content.

According to a review by Knapp and others, subclinical eating disorder prevalence estimates in female athletes are much higher than in the general population, as high as 50 percent at the high school level and ranging from 20 to 62 percent at the collegiate level. In a cross-sectional survey of Norwegian athletes, Sundgot-Borgen and Torstveit reported significantly higher eating disorder prevalence rates in athletes (13.5 percent) compared to control subjects (4.6 percent), with a 42 percent prevalence rate in female aesthetic athletes. Currie and Morse reported that eating behaviors improve when the athletic season is completed and the athlete resumes normal dietary habits. Sudi reports that, in general, symptoms of AA diminish or disappear at the end of the athlete's career. However, short-term behaviors meant to control weight for training and athletic competition may develop into long-term medical problems.

Female Athlete Triad   In 2008, Bonci and others in the National Athletic Trainers' Association developed an excellent position statement with 50 recommendations for detecting, preventing, and managing disordered eating in athletes, including predisposing risk factors, clinical features and behavioral warning signs, screening methods, therapeutic interventions, special considerations for adolescent athletes, and prevention strategies. Athletic trainers, team physicians, sports nutritionists, and others involved in the health care of athletes should be aware of these recommendations.

The **female athlete triad**—disordered eating, amenorrhea, and osteoporosis—was introduced in chapter 8, with a focus on calcium balance. The triad may have serious health consequences, particularly premature osteoporosis, which is one of the reasons the American College of Sports Medicine (ACSM) revised its original 1997 position stand on the female athlete triad in 2007. In their 2014 consensus statement following international conferences in 2012 and 2013, De Souza and colleagues noted that the three components of the female athletic triad are interrelated and have adverse effects on health and performance. The following discussion highlights the key points of the ACSM position stand, along with other research findings.

www.acsm-msse.org   To view the American College of Sports Medicine position stand on the female athlete triad, click on ACSM Position Stands and Joint Position Statements, and then the PDF for the female athlete triad.

Disordered eating   Triad experts such as Loucks, Manore, De Souza, Javed, and others contend that disordered eating, either decreased energy intake and poor food selection or excessive exercise energy expenditure that is not balanced by energy intake, may be contributing factors to the triad. The ACSM stresses that the key factor in the triad is low energy availability. Inadequate caloric intake may be inadvertent, intentional, or psychopathological. Whatever the reason, the ACSM notes that most adverse effects of the triad appear to occur when energy intake availability is below 30 Calories per kilogram of fat-free mass per day, which may lead to impaired reproductive and skeletal health. Manore notes, however, that there appears to be wide individual variability in the response of athletes to factors that may influence low energy availability.

Amenorrhea   *Amenorrhea* is the absence of a menstrual period. Primary amenorrhea represents a delay in the onset of puberty and the menarche (first menstrual period), whereas secondary amenorrhea represents an interruption of the normal menstrual cycle, with an interval of 3–6 months or more between periods. Both types of amenorrhea may occur in athletes due to low energy availability, which may be associated with a number of factors, such as exercise intensity and training practices, body weight and composition, disordered eating behaviors, and physical and emotional stress. Collectively, the interaction of low-energy availability and other factors may disturb the hypothalamic-pituitary-gonadal (HPG) axis. The HPG axis is an endocrine feedback loop in which gonadotropin-releasing hormone (GnRH) secreted by the hypothalamus stimulates the subsequent release of follicle-stimulating hormone (FSH) and luteinizing hormone (LH) by the anterior pituitary, which in turn regulates the secretion of estrogen and progesterone by the ovaries. Interruption of the normal HPG axis may interfere with the reproductive cycle and contribute to cessation of menstruation. The ACSM indicates that amenorrhea may be related to infertility and other health problems.

Although eating disorders and low-energy availability may also occur in males, Loucks indicates that the consensus is that reproductive dysfunction is uncommon in male athletes and that the long-term physiological consequences of the suppression of the HPG axis in male athletes probably have little clinical significance.

Osteoporosis   Premature osteoporosis is one of the most serious consequences of the female athlete triad. One of the major consequences in disruption of the normal HPG axis may be decreased amounts of estrogen from the ovaries. In addition, hormones released by the adrenal glands may be converted by fat tissue into one form of estrogen; with lower levels of body fat, less estrogen may be produced. As noted in chapter 8, estrogen helps regulate bone metabolism and increase bone mass. Additionally, dietary restrictions will reduce the intake of nutrients important for bone health, such as calcium and protein. Thus, disordered eating predisposes the athlete to osteoporosis. The ACSM notes that bone mineral density decreases as the number of menstrual cycles missed increases. Stress fractures occur more commonly in females with low bone mineral density, and the relative risk for stress fractures is two to four times greater in amenorrheic than eumenorrheic athletes. Moreover, the loss of bone mineral density in young athletes may not be reversible. In separate reviews, Javeb and De Souza and colleagues commented that suppressed estrogen secretion may also decrease nitric oxide production, which could impair endothelial function and increase cardiovascular disease risk.

Prevention   Prevention of eating disorders in young athletes should receive more attention. Several investigators have suggested that special attention should be devoted to young female athletes, particularly those involved in sports such as gymnastics and ballet, because they may meet the age, gender, and socioeconomic status criteria that may predispose them to AN. The ACSM indicates that for prevention and early intervention, education of athletes, parents, coaches, trainers, judges, and administrators is a priority. Athletes should be assessed for the triad at the preparticipation physical and/or annual health screening exam, and whenever an athlete presents with any of the triad's clinical conditions. Coaches and others should look for the following:

- Unexplained weight losses
- Frequent weight fluctuations
- Sudden increases in training volume
- Obsession with exercise
- Excessive concern with body weight
- Appearance, as well as evidence of bizarre eating practices

The NCAA may provide brochures and other materials to help develop awareness among athletes of the potential health risks associated with these disorders. A summary of some possible warning signs developed by the NCAA is presented in table 10.4. The ACSM further notes that sport administrators should also consider rule changes to discourage unhealthy weight-loss practices, similar to what has been done with males in the sport of wrestling at both the high school and college levels.

In this regard, coaches and others should be aware of the limitations associated with body composition measurement. Unfortunately, imprecise measurement of body composition may be a predisposing factor to the development of eating disorders in athletes. As noted previously, prediction of body fat may vary considerably, so an athlete who may predict to be 10 percent by one method or prediction equation may predict to be 15–20 percent by others. If, for some reason, a coach believes that an athlete should achieve a set body-fat percentage (e.g., 8 percent), it would be wise to use a variety of techniques to predict body-fat percentages and use the lowest value predicted. This might be the safest approach to help prevent an excessive target loss of body fat that might lead to disordered eating.

Elliot and colleagues at Oregon Health and Science University have reported on the efficacy of a preventive and health promotion program called ATHENA (Athletes Targeting Healthy Exercise & Nutrition Alternatives) in reducing risky dietary practices and promoting healthy body weight in female high school athletes. Research reports for ATHENA can be accessed at the following Website. A link to an online calculator from the Female Athletic Triad International Coalition is also provided below.

www.athenaprogram.com   Access this Website for the school-based program ATHENA, or Athletes Targeting Healthy Exercise & Nutrition Alternatives, to promote a healthy body weight in physically active girls. The program includes eight sessions and is peer led and coach facilitated.

www.femaleathletetriad.org/calculators   The Female Athletic Triad International Coalition online calculators for estimated dietary energy, exercise energy expenditure, and body-fat percentage.

Treatment   The ACSM indicates that the first aim of treatment for any triad component is to increase energy availability by increasing energy intake and/or reducing exercise energy expenditure. A multidisciplinary treatment team should include a physician or other health-care professional and a registered dietitian. Nutrition counseling and monitoring may be sufficient for many athletes. Simply decreasing the amount of weekly exercise by about 10 percent or gaining several pounds may help. Dietary changes should include additional Calories and increased amounts of dietary protein. However, the ACSM notes that for athletes with eating disorders, a mental health practitioner may be needed, as the treatment may warrant psychotherapy. Local dietitians and psychologists are excellent contacts if assistance is needed in dealing with eating disorders. Many hospitals have eating disorder programs that also may be able to provide assistance.

As discussed Chapter 8, a controversial International Olympic Committee consensus statement by Mountjoy and colleagues has proposed replacing the term "female athletic triad" with "relative energy deficiency in sport (RED-S)." The group defends the rationale that RED-S is a more comprehensive term for a constellation of health problems in both females and males with low energy intake and/or excessive energy expenditure as the root cause. This proposed change has been refuted by De Souza and others based on more than 30 years of research on the female athletic triad.

TABLE 10.4	National Collegiate Athletic Association warning signs for anorexia nervosa and bulimia nervosa
Warning Signs for Anorexia Nervosa	
Dramatic loss in weight	
A preoccupation with food, Calories, and weight	
Wearing baggy or layered clothing	
Relentless, excessive exercise	
Mood swings	
Avoiding food-related social activities	
Warning Signs for Bulimia Nervosa	
A noticeable weight loss or gain	
Excessive concern about weight	
Bathroom visits after meals	
Depressive moods	
Strict dieting followed by eating binges	
Increasing criticism of one's body	

National Collegiate Athletic Association.

Body Composition and Physical Performance

Modifying body weight and composition is considered by some to be an ergogenic aid. Over the years athletes have used a variety of techniques, including surgery such as liposuction and body sculpting and drugs such as anabolic steroids and human growth hormone (discussed in chapter 13), but most have used diet and specific exercise programs. Healthy diet and exercise programs to lose excess body fat or gain muscle mass are presented in chapters 11 and 12, respectively, but let us look at some examples as to how body weight change may affect sports performance.

What effect does excess body weight have on physical performance?

Although extra body weight might increase stability in contact sports such as football, ice hockey, and sumo wrestling, this advantage may be neutralized if the individual loses a corresponding amount of speed. In rare instances, such as long-distance swimming in cold water, extra body fat may be helpful for its insulation and buoyancy effects. In a cross-sectional study of high school and college football players, Steffes and others observed the greatest risk for metabolic syndrome in offensive and defensive linemen, (players with the highest fat mass) and the lowest risk in other positions. As a general rule, increases in body weight for sports competition should maximize muscle mass and minimize body-fat gains.

In contrast, there are many sports in which excess body weight may be disadvantageous. Whenever the body has to be moved rapidly or efficiently, excess weight in the form of body fat serves only as a burden. Body-fat percentage is extremely low in sprinters, jumpers, distance runners, dancers and gymnasts.

According to basic principles of physics, body fat in excess of the amount necessary for optimal functioning will impair physical performance. Body fat increases the mass, or inertia, of the

individual but does not contribute directly to energy production, so excess fat will detract from performance in events in which the body must be moved. According to the laws of physics and all other factors, including force production, remaining the same, a high jumper who gains 5 pounds of fat would clear a lower height due to the resulting smaller displacement of her center of gravity. Similarly, extra mass on a distance runner could add a considerable energy cost. Adding body fat would slow the running pace. In essence, the body becomes a less efficient machine when it must transport extra weight that has no useful purpose. Losing excess fat will not influence the total VO_{2max}, but will increase VO_{2max} when expressed in milliliters of oxygen per kilogram body weight. A 70 kg male runner with 15 percent fat and a total body VO_{2max} of 4.9 liters/min has a weight-relative VO_{2max} of 70 ml/kg/min. A decrease in body fat to 10 percent would reduce his body weight to 66.1 kg (based on a two-compartment model) and increase his weight-relative VO_{2max} to 74 ml/kg/min. Amby Burfoot, editor-at-large for *Runner's World* magazine, wrote a science-based article on the ideal weight for runners. Based on changes in VO_{2max} expressed in milliliters/kilogram body weight, he calculated that for every pound you lose, you will save about 2 seconds per mile run. For example, if you lose 5 pounds, you will save about 31 seconds in a 5-kilometer (3.1-mile) race, and more than 4 minutes in a marathon; if you lose 20 pounds of excess fat, corresponding savings would be 2:04 and 17:28 in the 5K and marathon, respectively. These beneficial effects are most relevant for those runners who have excess body fat to lose, and may not be applicable to runners who are already at their optimal body weight. Losing too much weight may also adversely affect running performance.

For a number of reasons, it is difficult to predict with certainty a precise percentage of body fat for a given athlete that will result in optimal performance. Nevertheless, studies with elite athletes have given us some general guidelines. Male sprinters, long-distance runners, wrestlers, gymnasts, basketball players, soccer players, swimmers, bodybuilders, and football backs have functioned effectively with 5–10 percent body fat. Other male athletes such as baseball players, football linemen, tennis players, weight lifters, and weight men in track and field may average 11–15 percent, or just below the average for the nonathletic individual. Several authorities have suggested that female athletes should carry no more than 20 percent fat, whereas others note that it should be below 15 percent. Female gymnasts and distance runners have been recorded well below 15 percent; some gymnasts were even below 10 percent. Most other female athletes range between 15 and 20 percent, with some of the strength-type athletes, such as discus throwers, recording values of 25 percent or greater. Although these are some general guidelines, it should be noted that body-fat percentage is only one of many factors that may influence physical performance, and athletes may perform very well even though their body fat is above these levels. However, everything else being equal, excess body fat is a disadvantage when energy efficiency of body movement in sport is an important consideration.

Excess body fat may also increase injury risk and be related to cognitive impairment. Wilder and Cicchetti indicated that a high BMI is associated with an increased risk for musculoskeletal injuries. Yard and Comstock noted that compared with normal-weight athletes, obese athletes sustained a larger proportion of knee injuries. It is possible that the increased body mass created more torque on the knee and exceeded the injury threshold of ligaments and tendons. In separate studies, Fedor and Willeumier reported significant associations between high BMI and cognitive impairment.

Coaches and practitioners should exercise caution in advising athletes to lose body weight to achieve an arbitrary predetermined goal for the following reasons. As discussed earlier, estimation of body fat percentage will have a 2–4 percent or higher standard error of measurement depending on the assessment technique. The athlete's current body fat percentage may already be near or at the arbitrarily low goal level. Finally, as suggested by Benardot and Thompson, excessive weight losses may actually lead to a decrease in physical performance, just the opposite of the desired goal.

Does excessive weight loss impair physical performance?

In 1998, the National Collegiate Athletic Association adopted a rule mandating testing to establish a minimum wrestling weight for each wrestler. Oppliger and others reported that the NCAA weight-management program appears effective in reducing unhealthy weight-cutting behaviors, such as rapid weight losses and gains associated with competition, and promoting competitive equity. However, some studies found that a significant percent of the high school, college, and international-style wrestlers still used potentially harmful weight-loss methods.

Weight-reduction programs used by wrestlers and other athletes have been condemned by sports medicine groups, not only for health reasons but also because these practices may impair physical performance. In its position stand on weight loss in wrestlers, the American College of Sports Medicine noted that the practice of weight cutting involving food restriction, fluid deprivation, and dehydration could not only affect physical health and growth and development but also impair competitive performance. This impairment in performance may be attributed to decreased blood volume, decreased testosterone levels, impaired cardiovascular function, decreased ability to regulate body temperature, hypoglycemia, or depletion of muscle and liver glycogen stores. However, the ultimate effect on performance may be dependent on the technique used—dehydration or starvation—and the time over which the weight is lost.

The effect of rapid weight loss by voluntary dehydration on physical performance was covered in chapter 9. In general, events characterized by power, strength, and speed may not be adversely affected by short-term dehydration, whereas performance in aerobic and anaerobic endurance events is likely to deteriorate, particularly if exercising under warm environmental conditions.

Starvation and semistarvation studies have been conducted over periods ranging from 1 day to 1 year. Short-term starvation, involving rapid weight loss, may impair physical performance if blood glucose and muscle glycogen levels are lowered substantially. Although strength and VO_{2max} generally are not affected by acute starvation, studies using a 24-hour fast have shown that anaerobic and aerobic endurance performance will suffer if

dependent on muscle glycogen or normal blood glucose levels. Long-term semistarvation may lead to significant losses of lean muscle tissue and decreased performance in almost all fitness components. For example, Roemmich and Sinning compared body composition and strength measures of adolescent wrestlers with controls over the course of a wrestling season and found that the wrestlers decreased body weight, body fat, and various measures of strength and power from pre-season to late-season. The wrestlers failed to gain lean tissue during this time frame, which the authors associated with the decrease in strength and power. However, body weight, strength, and power returned to normal during the post-season. Garthe and others reported a slow weekly rate of weight loss (0.7 percent; ~1 pound) increased lean body mass by 2.1 percent compared to no change in a fast weekly rate of weight loss (1.4 percent; ~2 pounds). The athlete who avoids the loss of lean body mass would be less likely to experience a decline in performance during weight loss. Overall, although research findings regarding the effects of rapid weight loss on physical performance are somewhat mixed, as evidenced in the study by Koral and Dosseville, numerous studies involving wrestlers, boxers, and judo athletes have indicated that rapid weight loss over the course of several days to a week may impair physical performance, particularly prolonged, sport-specific anaerobic performance.

Gradual weight loss and a diet with adequate carbohydrate and protein appear to be the keys to maintaining optimal physical performance during weight loss. In some semistarvation studies in which fewer than 1,000 Calories were consumed daily, vigorous exercise programs were maintained even though the subjects were losing substantial amounts of body weight. In general, the authors noted that the key point was to prevent hypoglycemia, dehydration, and excessive loss of lean muscle mass. If these goals could be achieved, physical performance need not deteriorate on weight-loss programs. For example, Zachwieja and others reported that 2 weeks of moderate dietary energy restriction (750 Calories less per day) induced a weight loss of about 3 pounds in physically fit young men and women but had no effect on muscle strength and endurance, anaerobic capacity as evaluated by the Wingate test, or aerobic endurance as measured by a 5-mile run.

It is difficult to predict the specific body weight at which physical performance will begin to deteriorate for a given individual. For those athletes who are on a weight-loss program, it may be wise to monitor performance through certain standardized tests appropriate for their sport. Some examples include basic fitness tests with measures of strength, local muscular endurance, and cardiovascular endurance. A decrease in performance may be indicative that the weight loss is excessive. Personality changes, excessive tiredness, weakness, and lack of enthusiasm may also be telltale clues.

Weight losses have the potential to either improve or diminish performance. The interested reader is referred to the recent International Olympic Committee review and position statement by Sundgot-Borgen and others on minimizing health risks in weight-sensitive sports. The key is to lose weight properly, primarily body fat. The basic guidelines for the development of such a weight–control program to improve physical performance, or health, are presented in chapter 11.

Key Concepts

▶ Although the average body-fat percentages for young men and women are, respectively, 15–20 percent and 23–30 percent, those involved in certain types of athletic competition may be advised to reduce those levels.

▶ Excessive loss of body weight may impair sports performance. For athletes in sports where weight loss may enhance performance, basic specific fitness tests may be used periodically to ascertain that performance is maintained or improved.

APPLICATION EXERCISE

Case Study	Current Body Mass	Estimated Percent Fat	Fat Mass	Lean-Body Mass	Body Mass at 7 percent fat (see appendix C)
A wrestling coach would like his 152-pounder to make the 145-pound weight class for the upcoming season, scheduled to begin in 1 month, and seeks your professional advice as a sports nutritionist on the feasibility of this plan. The high school league mandates minimum wrestling weight determination based on a minimum 7 percent fat. The table includes body composition assessment data (estimated fat percentages) using four different methods.					
Skinfold measurements		9	13.7	138.3	148.7
Bioelectrical impedance	152	8	12.2	139.8	150.4
Air displacement plethysmography		10	15.2	136.8	147.1
Hydrostatic weighing		11	16.7	135.3	145.5

Discuss with the coach and athlete issues affecting the feasibility of this plan. Include in this discussion the potential effects of pre-season conditioning and restriction of caloric intake on LBM and the standard errors of measurement of the various body composition assessment methodologies.

Review Questions—Multiple Choice

1. Which of the following best describes the role of leptin in the human body?

   a. It is secreted by the hypothalamus and stimulates lipolysis in adipose cells.

   b. It is secreted by the liver and inhibits the digestion of fats.

   c. It is secreted by the adipose cells and inhibits hunger.

   d. It is secreted by the stomach and stimulates appetite.

   e. It is secreted by the intestines and stimulates appetite.

2. Which of the following statements regarding android/gynoid obesity is false?
   a. Gynoid obesity is associated with a higher incidence of certain diseases, such as hypertension.
   b. Android obesity is characterized by excess accumulation of fat deposits in the abdominal area.
   c. Android obesity is seen more often in men, while gynoid obesity is more prevalent in women.
   d. Gynoid-type fat deposits are more resistant to weight loss compared to android obesity.
   e. Development of both types of obesity is influenced by heredity.

3. If a skinfold technique for body composition has a standard error of estimate of 3 percent, you can have 70 percent confidence that for a person who has a predicted body fat of 18 percent, the actual value is within a range of
   a. 6–18 percent
   b. 18–21 percent
   c. 12–24 percent
   d. 15–21 percent
   e. 18–30 percent

4. Which of the following ranges of the body mass index (BMI) is indicative of a normal height-to-weight relationship?
   a. 5–8
   b. 10–12
   c. 15–17
   d. 20–22
   e. 27–28

5. In which sports might the condition of anorexia athletica appear to be more prevalent?
   a. football and basketball
   b. swimming and baseball
   c. wrestling and field hockey
   d. ballet and gymnastics
   e. tennis and golf

6. The set-point theory of weight control is based upon a feedback system, suggesting that the individual is programmed to be a certain body weight and that the body will always attempt to maintain that weight by regulating hunger and metabolism. What part of the body is believed to be the regulatory center for the control of the various feedback mechanisms?
   a. liver receptors
   b. stomach receptors
   c. blood receptors in the kidney
   d. receptors in the hypothalamus in the brain
   e. receptors in the small intestine where absorption takes place

7. The disorder of bulimia, which is often characterized by the binge-purge syndrome, is found
   a. only in those with anorexia nervosa.
   b. only in extremely underweight individuals.
   c. only in normal-weight individuals.
   d. only in moderately or morbidly obese individuals.
   e. in individuals across the body-weight spectrum.

8. Which of the following is mainly an environmental rather than a possible hereditary factor in the multicausal etiology of obesity?
   a. sedentary lifestyle
   b. hormonal imbalance
   c. disorder in the brain's hunger and satiety centers
   d. lower basal metabolic rate
   e. higher set point

9. Obesity has been associated as a potential risk factor in all the following diseases or health problems except which one?
   a. coronary heart disease
   b. anemia
   c. hyperlidemia
   d. diabetes
   e. hypertension

10. Protein consumed during a starvation-type diet most likely will be
   a. used to rebuild muscle tissue.
   b. used to replace worn-out cells.
   c. converted to glucose for energy.
   d. used to stabilize fluid balance.
   e. stored as fat.

Answers to multiple-choice questions: 1. c; 2. a; 3. d; 4. d; 5. d; 6. d; 7. e; 8. a; 9. b; 10. c

Review Questions—Essay

1. List and describe five different techniques used to evaluate body composition, and highlight at least one value of each.
2. Discuss the set-point theory of body-weight control and relate it to body-fat levels, leptin, and neuropeptide Y.
3. List the various genetic and environmental factors that may be involved in the etiology of obesity. Highlight two of each and explain their possible role.
4. Explain the metabolic syndrome and associated health risks.
5. List the three components of the female athlete triad. Discuss the underlying theories regarding its etiology, the potential effects on hormonal status, and subsequent serious health problems.

References

Books

American Psychiatric Association. 2013. *Diagnostic and statistical manual of mental disorders* (5th ed.). Washington, DC: American Psychiatric Association.

Heyward, V., and Wagner, D. 2004. *Applied Body Composition Assessment.* Champaign, IL: Human Kinetics.

National Academy of Sciences. 2002. *Dietary Reference Intakes for Energy, Carbohydrates, Fiber, Fat, Protein and Amino Acids (Macronutrients).* Washington, DC: National Academies Press.

National Research Council. 1989. *Diet and Health: Implications for Reducing Chronic Disease Risk.* Washington, DC: National Academies Press.

Shils, M., et al., eds. 2006. *Modern Nutrition in Health and Disease.* Philadelphia: Lippincott Williams & Wilkins.

U.S. Department of Health and Human Services Public Health Service. 2010. *Healthy People 2020.* Washington, DC: U.S. Government Printing Office.

World Cancer Research Fund/American Institute for Cancer Research. *Food, Nutrition, Physical Activity, and the Prevention of Cancer: a Global Perspective.* Washington DC: AICR, 2007.

Reviews and Specific Studies

Abizaid, A. 2009. Ghrelin and dopamine: New insights on the peripheral regulation of appetite. *Journal of Neuroendocrinology* 21:787–93.

Ackland, T. R., et al. 2012. Current status of body composition assessment in sport: Review and position statement on behalf of the *ad hoc* research working group on body composition health and performance, under the auspices of the I.O.C. Medical Commission. *Sports Medicine* 42 (3):227–49.

Alberti, K. G. M. M., et al. 2009. Harmonizing the metabolic syndrome. A joint interim statement of the International Diabetes Federation Task Force on Epidemiology and Prevention; National Heart, Lung, and Blood Institute; American Heart Association; World Heart Federation; International Atherosclerosis Society; and International Association for the Study of Obesity. *Circulation* 120:1640–45.

American College of Sports Medicine. 1996. American College of Sports Medicine position stand: Weight loss in wrestlers. *Medicine & Science in Sports & Exercise* 28 (6):ix–xii.

American College of Sports Medicine. 2007. The female athlete triad: Position stand. *Medicine & Science in Sports & Exercise* 39:1867–82.

American College of Sports Medicine. 2009. ACSM position stand on the appropriate intervention strategies for weight loss and prevention of weight regain for adults. *Medicine & Science in Sports & Exercise* 41:459–71.

American Dietetic Association, Dietitians of Canada, American College of Sports Medicine, and Rodriguez, N., et al. 2009. American College of Sports Medicine position stand: Nutrition and athletic performance. *Medicine & Science in Sports & Exercise* 41:709–31.

American Dietetic Association. 2011. Position of the American Dietetic Association: Nutrition intervention in the treatment of anorexia nervosa, bulimia nervosa, and eating disorders not otherwise specified (EDNOS). *Journal of the American Dietetic Association* 111:1236–41.

Andersen, R., et al. 1998. Relationship of physical activity and television watching with body weight and level of fatness among children. *Journal of the American Medical Association* 279:938–42.

Apovian, C. M., et al. 2013. A randomized, phase 3 trial of naltrexone SR/bupropion SR on weight and obesity-related risk factors (COR-II). *Obesity* 21 (3):935–43.

Arena, R., et al. 2014. The role of worksite health screening: A policy statement from the American Heart Association. *Circulation* 130:719–34.

Astrup, A. 2001. The role of dietary fat in the prevention and treatment of obesity. Efficacy and safety of low-fat diets. *International Journal of Obesity and Related Metabolic Disorders* 25:S46–S50.

Astrup, A., and Rossner, S. 2000. Lessons from obesity management programmes: Greater initial weight loss improves long-term maintenance. *Obesity Reviews* 1:17–19.

Atkinson, R. 1989. Low and very low calorie diets. *Medical Clinics of North America* 73:203–16.

Attila, E. 2010. Anorexia nervosa: Current status and future directions. *Annual Review of Medicine* 61:425–35.

Aubin, H. J., et al. 2012. Weight gain in smokers after quitting cigarettes: Meta-analysis. *British Journal of Medicine* 345:e4439. doi: 10.1136/bmj.e4439.

Aucott, L. 2008. Influences of weight loss on long-term diabetes outcomes. *Proceeding of the Nutrition Society* 67:54–59.

Aune, D., et al. 2014. Maternal body mass index and the risk of fetal death, stillbirth, and infant death: A systematic review and meta-analysis. *Journal of the American Medical Association* 311(15):1536–46.

Avram, M., et al. 2007. Subcutaneous fat in normal and diseased states 3. Adipogenesis: From stem cell to fat cell. *Journal of the American Academy of Dermatology* 56:472–92.

Baile, C. 2000. Regulation of metabolism and body mass by leptin. *Annual Reviews in Nutrition* 20:105–27.

Bailey, A. P., et al. 2014. Mapping the evidence for the prevention and treatment of eating disorders in young people. *Journal of Eating Disorders* 2:5. doi:10.1186/2050-2974-2-5.

Ball, S., and Altena, T. 2004. Comparison of the Bod Pod and dual energy x-ray absorptiometry in men. *Physiological Measurement* 25:671–78.

Bar-Or, O. 2000. Juvenile obesity, physical activity, and lifestyle changes. *Physician and Sportsmedicine* 28 (11):51–58.

Barbosa-da-Silva, S., et al. 2012. Weight cycling enhances adipose tissue inflammatory responses in male mice. *Public Library of Science One* 7 (7):e39837.

Barry, V. W., et al. 2014. Fitness vs. fatness on all-cause mortality: A meta-analysis. *Progress in Cardiovascular Diseases* 56:382–90.

Bays, H. E., et al. 2013. Obesity, adiposity, and dyslipidemia: A consensus statement from the National Lipid Association. *Journal of Clinical Lipidology* 7 (4):304–83.

Bellisle, F., and Drewnowski, A. 2007. Intense sweeteners, energy intake and the control of body weight. *European Journal of Clinical Nutrition* 61:691–700.

Beltrán-Sánchez, H., et al. 2013. Prevalence and trends of metabolic syndrome in the adult U.S. population, 1999–2010. *Journal of the American College of Cardiology* 62 (8):697–703.

Benardot, D., and Thompson, W. R. 1999. Energy from food for physical activity: Enough and on time. *ACSM's Health & Fitness Journal* 3 (4):14–18.

Berger, N. A. 2014. Obesity and cancer pathogenesis. *Annals of the New York Academy of Sciences* 1311:57–76. doi: 10.1111/nyas.12416.

Blüher, M. 2014. Are metabolically healthy obese individuals really healthy? *European Journal of Endocrinology* pii: EJE-14-0540.

Bonci, C., et al. 2008. National Athletic Trainers' Association position statement: Preventing, detecting, and managing disordered eating in athletes. *Journal of Athletic Training* 43:80–108.

Bosy-Westphal, A., and Müller, M. J. 2014. Measuring the impact of weight cycling on body composition: A methodological challenge. *Current Opinion in Clinical and Metabolic Care* 17 (5):396–400.

Bosy-Westphal, A., et al. 2013. Effect of weight loss and regain on adipose tissue distribution, composition of lean mass and resting energy expenditure in young overweight and obese adults. *International Journal of Obesity* 37 (10):1371–77.

Bouchard, C., et al. 1990. The response to long-term overfeeding in identical twins. *New England Journal of Medicine* 322:1477–82.

Bowman, S., et al. 2004. Effects of fast-food consumption on energy intake and diet quality among children in a national household survey. *Pediatrics* 113:112–18.

Bray, G. 2004. How do we get fat? An epidemiologic and metabolic approach. *Clinics in Dermatology* 22:281–88.

Bray, G. 2004. Medical consequences of obesity. *Journal of Clinical Endocrinology and Metabolism* 89:2583–89.

Brownell, K., and Liebman, B. 2010. In your face: How the food industry drives us to eat. *Nutrition Action Health Letter* 37 (4):1–6.

Brownell, K., and Rodin, J. 1994. Medical, metabolic, and psychological effects of weight cycling. *Archives of Internal Medicine* 154:1325–29.

Brożek, J., et al. 1963. Densitometric analysis of body composition: Revision of some quantitative assumptions. *Annals of the New York Academy of Sciences* 110:113–40.

Brunstrom, J. M. 2014. Mind over platter: Pre-meal planning and the control of meal size in humans. *International Journal of Obesity* 38:S9–S12.

Budd, G. 2007. Disordered eating: Young women's search for control and connection. *Journal of Child and Adolescent Psychiatric Nursing* 20:96–106.

Bulik, C., et al. 2006. Prevalence, heritability, and prospective risk factors for anorexia nervosa. *Archives of General Psychiatry* 63:305–12.

Bulik, C., et al. 2007. Anorexia nervosa treatment: A systematic review of randomized controlled trials. *International Journal of Eating Disorders* 40:310–20.

Buresh, R. 2014. Exercise and glucose control. *Journal of Sports Medicine and Physical Fitness* 54(4):373–82.

Burfoot, A. 2007. What's your ideal weight? *Runner's World* 42 (7):67–69.

Busetto, L. 2001. Visceral obesity and the metabolic syndrome: Effects of weight loss. *Nutrition, Metabolism and Cardiovascular Disease* 11:195–204.

Butterick, T. A., et al. 2013. Orexin: Pathways to obesity resistance? *Reviews in Endocrine and Metabolic Disorders* 14 (4):357–64.

Cadwallader, A. B., et al. 2010. The abuse of diuretics as performance-enhancing drugs and masking agents in sports doping: Pharmacology, toxicology and analysis. *British Journal of Pharmacology* 161:1–16.

Calle, E., et al. 2003. Overweight, obesity, and mortality from cancer in a prospectively studied cohort of U.S. adults. *New England Journal of Medicine* 348:1625–38.

Carmichael, A., and Bates, T. 2004. Obesity and breast cancer: A review of the literature. *Breast* 13:85–92.

Carroll, S., and Dudfield, M. 2004. What is the relationship between exercise and metabolic abnormalities? A review of the metabolic syndrome. *Sports Medicine* 34:371–78.

Carvalho, R., et al. 2008. Clinical profile of the overweight child in the new millennium. *Clinical Pediatrics* 47 (5):476–82.

Catenacci, V., et al. 2009. The obesity epidemic. *Clinics in Chest Medicine* 30:415–44.

Cawley, J., and Meyerhoefer, C. 2010. The medical care costs of obesity: An instrumental variables approach. National Bureau of Economics Research. Working paper 16467. www.nber.org/papers/w16467.

Chaput, J., et al. 2007. Currently available drugs for the treatment of obesity: Sibutramine and orlistat. *Mini Reviews in Medicinal Chemistry* 7:3–10.

Chaput, J. P., et al. 2014. Findings from the Quebec Family Study on the etiology of obesity: Genetics and environmental highlights. *Current Obesity Reports* 3:54–66.

Christakis, N. A., and Fowler, J. H. 2013. Social contagion theory: Examining dynamic social networks and human behavior. *Statistics in Medicine* 32 (4):556–77.

Christakis, N., and Fowler, J. 2007. The spread of obesity in a large social network over 32 years. *New England Journal of Medicine* 357:404–7.

Clark, A. L., et al. 2014. Obesity and the obesity paradox in heart failure. *Progress in Cardiovascular Diseases* 56 (4):409–14.

Clark, R., et al. 2002. Cross-validation of the NCAA method to predict body fat for minimum weight in collegiate wrestlers. *Clinical Journal of Sport Medicine* 12:285–90.

Clark, R., et al. 2004. Minimum weight prediction methods cross-validated by the four-component model. *Medicine & Science in Sports & Exercise* 36:639–47.

Claussnitzer, M. et al. 2015. FTO obesity variant circuitry and adipocyte browning in humans. *New England Journal of Medicine* doi: 10.1056/NEJMoa1502214.

Cohen, D., and Farley, T. 2008. Eating as an automatic behavior. *Preventing Chronic Disease* 5:A23.

Consumers Union. 2004. Outwitting your appetite. *Consumer Reports on Health* 16 (9):8–10.

Crow, S. J., et al. 2009. Increased mortality in bulimia nervosa and other eating disorders. *American Journal of Psychiatry* 166:1342–46.

Currie, A., and Morse, E. 2005. Eating disorders in athletes: Managing the risks. *Clinics in Sports Medicine* 24:871–83.

Dallman, M., et al. 2004. Minireview: Glucocorticoids—Food intake, abdominal obesity, and wealthy nations in 2004. *Endocrinology* 145:2633–38.

Daly, R., et al. 2005. Growth of highly versus moderately trained competitive female artistic gymnasts. *Medicine & Science in Sports & Exercise* 37:1053–60.

Dattilo, A. 1992. Dietary fat and its relationship to body weight. *Nutrition Today* 27 (January/February):13–19.

De Coster, S., and van Larabeke, N. 2012. Endocrine-disrupting chemicals: Associated disorders and mechanisms of action. *Journal of Environmental and Public Health* Article ID 713696. doi: 10.1155/2012/713696.

de Groot, L., and van Staveren, W. 1995. Reduced physical activity and its association with obesity. *Nutrition Reviews* 53:11–12.

De Souza, M. J., et al. 2014. 2014 female athletic triad coalition consensus statement on treatment and return to play of the female athletic triad. *British Journal of Sports Medicine* 48:289–308.

De Souza, M. J., et al. 2014. Misunderstanding the female athletic triad: Refuting the IOC consensus statement on relative energy deficiency in sport (RED-S). *British Journal of Sports Medicine* 48 (20). doi:10.1136/bjsports-2014-093502.

De Vadder, F., et al. 2013. Satiety and the role of mu-opoid receptors in the portal vein. *Current Opinion in Pharmacology* 13:959–63.

Dham, S., and Banerji, M. 2006. The brain-gut axis in regulation of appetite and obesity. *Pediatric Endocrinology Reviews* 3 (Supplement 4):544–54.

Dixon, J. B. 2010. The effect of obesity on health outcomes. *Molecular and Cellular Endocrinology* 316:104–8.

Ebbeling, C., et al. 2006. Effects of decreasing sugar-sweetened beverage consumption on body weight in adolescents: A randomized, controlled pilot study. *Pediatrics* 117:673–80.

Eckel, R., and Krauss, R. 1998. American Heart Association call to action: Obesity as a major risk factor for coronary heart disease. *Circulation* 97:2099–100.

Egecioglu, E., et al. 2011. Hedonic and incentive signals for body weight control. *Reviews in Endocrine and Metabolic Disorders* 12:141–51.

Ekelund, U., et al. 2006. TV viewing and physical activity are independently associated with metabolic risk in children. *Public Library of Science Medicine* 3 (12):e448. doi:1-.1371/journal.pmed.0030488.

Elliot, D. L., et al. 2008. Long-term outcomes of the ATHENA (Athletes Targeting Healthy Exercise & Nutrition Alternatives) program for female high school athletes. *Journal of Alcohol and Drug Education* 52 (2):73–92.

Ervin, R. B. 2009. *Prevalence of Metabolic Syndrome among Adults 20 Years of Age and over, by Sex, Age, Race and Ethnicity, and Body Mass Index: United States, 2003–2006.* National Health Statistics reports, no 13. Hyattsville, MD: National Center for Health Statistics.

Esposito, S., et al. 2013. Adenovirus 36 infection and obesity. *Journal of Clinical Virology* 55 (2):95–100.

Fallon, E. A., et al. 2014. Prevalence of body dissatisfaction among a United States adult sample. *Eating Behaviors* 15:151–58.

Fantuzzi, G., and Mazzone, T. 2007. Adipose tissue and atherosclerosis: Exploring the connection. *Arteriosclerosis, Thrombosis, and Vascular Biology* 27:996–1003.

Farrell, S., et al. 2010. Cardiorespiratory fitness, adiposity, and all-cause mortality in women. *Medicine & Science in Sports & Exercise* 42:2006–12.

Fawcett, K., and Barroso, I. 2010. The genetics of obesity: FTO leads the way. *Trends in Genetics* 26:266–74.

Federal Trade Commission. 2014. FTC testifies before Senate commerce subcommittee on agency efforts to combat fraudulent and deceptive claims for weight-loss products. www.ftc.gov/news-events/press-release/2014/06.

Fedor, A., and Gunstad, J. 2013. Higher BMI is associated with reduced cognitive performance in Division I athletes. *Obesity Facts* 6:185–92.

Fehm, H., et al. 2006. The selfish brain: Competition for energy resources. *Progress in Brain Research* 153:129–40.

Field, A., et al. 2004. Association of weight change, weight control practices, and weight cycling among women in the Nurses' Health Study II. *International*

Journal of Obesity and Related Metabolic Disorders 28:1134–42.

Fields, D., et al. 2002. Body-composition assessment via air-displacement plethysmography in adults and children: A review. *American Journal of Clinical Nutrition* 75:453–67.

Flegal, K. M., et al. 2013. Association of all-cause mortality with overweight and obesity using standard body mass index categories: A systematic review and meta-analysis. *Journal of the American Medical Association* 309 (1):71–82.

Flood, J., et al. 2006. The effect of increased beverage portion size on energy intake at a meal. *Journal of the American Dietetic Association* 106:1984–90.

Fosbøl, M. Ø., and Zerahn, B. 2014. Contemporary methods of body composition measurement. *Critical Physiology and Functional Imaging* (April 15). doi: 10.1111/cpf.12152. [Epub ahead of print]

Garthe, I., et al. 2011. Effect of two different weight-loss rates on body composition and strength and power-related performance in elite athletes. *International Journal of Sports Nutrition and Exercise Metabolism* 21 (2):97–104.

Geier, A., et al. 2006. Unit bias. A new heuristic that helps explain the effect of portion size on food intake. *Psychological Science* 17:421–25.

Gerson, L., and Braun, B. 2006. Effect of high cardiorespiratory fitness and high body fat on insulin resistance. *Medicine & Science in Sports & Exercise* 38:1709–15.

Gibbs, W. 1996. Gaining on fat. *Scientific American* 275 (August):88–94.

Going, S., et al. 2014. Top 10 research questions related to body composition. *Research Quarterly for Exercise and Sport* 85 (1):38–48.

Green, S., and Blundell, J. 1996. Effect of fat- and sucrose-containing foods on the size of eating episodes and energy intake in lean dietary restrained and unrestrained females: Potential for causing overconsumption. *European Journal of Clinical Nutrition* 50:625–35.

Grundy, S. 1999. Hypertriglyceridemia, insulin resistance, and the metabolic syndrome. *American Journal of Cardiology* 83:25F–29F.

Grundy, S. 2007. Metabolic syndrome: A multiplex cardiovascular risk factor. *Journal of Clinical Endocrinology and Metabolism* 92:399–404.

Hainer, V., and Aldhoon-Hainerová, I. 2014. Tolerability and safety of the new anti-obesity medications. *Drug Safety* 37 (9):693–702.

Halford, J., et al. 2010. Pharmacological management of appetite expression in obesity. *Nature Reviews Endocrinology* 6:255–69.

Hansen, J., et al. 2010. Is thermogenesis a significant causal factor in preventing the "globesity" epidemic? *Medical Hypotheses* 75:250–6.

Harrington, M., et al. 2009. A review and meta-analysis of the effect of weight loss on all-cause mortality risk. *Nutrition Research Reviews* 22 (1):93–108.

Hetherington, M., and Cecil, J. 2010. Gene-environment interactions in obesity. *Forum on Nutrition* 63:195–203.

Heyward, V. H. 1998. Practical body composition for children, adults, and older adults. *International Journal of Sports Nutrition* 8:285–307.

Hills, A., et al. 2007. The contribution of physical activity and sedentary behaviours to the growth and development of children and adolescents: Implications for overweight and obesity. *Sports Medicine* 37:533–45.

Hirsch, J., and Leibel, R. 1998. The genetics of obesity. *Hospital Practice (Office Edition)* 33:55–70.

Hoch, A., et al. 2009. Prevalence of the female athlete triad in high school athletes and sedentary students. *Clinical Journal of Sport Medicine* 19:421–8.

Hubert, H. B., et al. 1983. Obesity as an independent risk factor for cardiovascular disease: A 26-year follow-up of participants in the Framingham Heart Study. *Circulation* 67 (5):968–77.

Hudson, J. I., et al. 2007. The prevalence and correlates of eating disorders in the National Co-Morbidity Survey Replication. *Biological Psychiatry* 61:348–58.

Hur, S. J., et al. 2013. Effect of adenovirus and influenza virus infection on obesity. *Life Sciences* 93 (16):531–35.

Inadera, H. 2013. Developmental origins of obesity and type 2 diabetes: Molecular aspects and role of chemicals. *Environmental Health and Preventive Medicine* 18:185–97.

Institute of Medicine. 2013. *Challenges and Opportunities for Change in Food Marketing to Children and Youth: Workshop Summary.* Washington, DC: National Academies Press.

Jackson, A., and Pollock, M. 1978. Generalized equations for predicting body density of men. *British Journal of Nutrition* 40:497–504.

Jackson, A., et al. 1980. Generalized equations for predicting body density of women. *Medicine & Science in Sports & Exercise* 12:175–82.

Jacobs, E., et al. 2010. Waist circumference and all-cause mortality in a large US cohort. *Archives of Internal Medicine* 170:1293–301.

Jaffrin, M. 2009. Body composition determination by bioimpedance: An update. *Current Opinion in Clinical Nutrition & Metabolic Care* 12:482–6.

James, W., 2008. WHO recognition of the global obesity epidemic. *International Journal of Obesity* 32 (Supplement 7):S120–6.

Javed, A., et al. 2013. Female athletic triad and its components: Toward improved screening and management. *Mayo Clinic Proceedings* 88 (9):996–1009.

Jensen, M. D., et al. 2014. American Heart Association/American College of Cardiology/The Obesity Society: Guidelines for the management of overweight and obesity in adults. *Circulation* 129:S102–38.

Johansson, K., et al. 2014. Effects of anti-obesity drugs, diet, and exercise on weight loss maintenance after a very-low-calorie diet or low-calorie diet: A systematic review and meta-analysis of randomized controlled trials. *American Journal of Clinical Nutrition* 99:14–23.

Johnson, R., et al. 2009. Dietary sugars intake and cardiovascular health: A scientific statement from the American Heart Association. *Circulation* 120:1011–20.

Keel, P., et al. 2007. Clinical features and physiological response to a test meal in purging disorder and bulimia nervosa. *Archives of General Psychiatry* 64:1058–66.

Keesey, R., and Hirvonen, M. 1997. Body weight set-points: Determination and adjustment. *Journal of Nutrition* 127:1875S–83S.

Kenchaiah, S., et al. 2009. Body mass index and vigorous physical activity and the risk of heart failure among men. *Circulation* 119:44–52.

Kessler, D., and Liebman, B. 2009. Why we overeat. *Nutrition Action Health Letter* 16 (6):1–6.

Kiliaan, A. J., et al. 2014. Adipokines: A link between obesity and dementia? *The Lancet Neurology* 13 (9):913–23. doi: 10.1016/S1474-4422(14)70085-7.

Kim, Y., and Park, H. 2013. Does regular exercise without weight loss reduce insulin resistance in children and adolescents? *International Journal of Endocrinology* 2013:402592. doi: 10.1155/2013/402592.

King, B. 2006. The rise, fall, and resurrection of the ventromedial hypothalamus in the regulation of feeding behavior and body weight. *Physiology & Behavior* 87:221–44.

King, P. 2005. The hypothalamus and obesity. *Current Drug Targets* 6:225–40.

Klok, M., et al. 2007. The role of leptin and ghrelin in the regulation of food intake and body weight in humans: A review. *Obesity Reviews* 8:21–34.

Knapp, J., et al. 2014. Eating disorders in female athletes: Use of screening tools. *Current Sports Medicine Reports* 13 (4):214–18.

Kojima, M., and Kangawa, K. 2005. Ghrelin: Structure and function. *Physiological Reviews* 85:495–522.

Koral, J., and Dosseville, F. 2009. Combination of gradual and rapid weight loss: Effects on physical performance and psychological state of elite judo athletes. *Journal of Sports Sciences* 27:115–20.

Kotz C. M., et al. 2007. Neuroregulation of nonexercise activity thermogenesis and obesity resistance. *American Journal of Physiology Regulatory and Integrative Physiology* 294 (3):R699–R710.

Kral, T., and Rauh, E. 2010. Eating behaviors of children in the context of their family environment. *Physiology & Behavior* 100:567–73.

Kramer, C. K., et al. 2013. Are metabolically healthy overweight and obesity benign conditions? A systematic review and meta-analysis. *Annals of Internal Medicine* 159 (11):758–69.

Lachat, C. 2012. Eating out of home and its association with dietary intake: A systematic review of the evidence. *Obesity Research* 13 (4):329–46.

Lafontan, M. 2005. Fat cells: Afferent and efferent messages define new approaches to treat obesity. *Annual Review of Pharmacology and Toxicology* 45:119–46.

Lara, J. et al. 2014. Accuracy of aggregate 2- and 3-component models of body composition relative to 4-component for the measurement of changes in fat mass during weight loss in overweight and obese subjects. *Applied Physiology Nutrition and Metabolism* 39 (8):871–79.

Lee, M. J., et al. 2013. Adipose tissue heterogeneity: Implications of depot differences in adipose tissue for obesity complications. *Molecular Aspects of Medicine* 34 (1):1–11.

Lee, R. E. et al. 2014. Obesogenic and youth oriented restaurant marketing in public housing neighborhoods. *American Journal of Health Behavior* 38(2):218–24.

Lee, Y. 2009. The role of genes in the current obesity epidemic. *Annals Academy of Medicine Singapore* 38:45–3.

Levin, B. 2000. Metabolic imprinting on genetically predisposed neural circuits perpetuates obesity. *Nutrition* 16:909–15.

Levin, B. 2002. Metabolic sensors: Viewing glucosensing neurons from a broader perspective. *Physiology & Behavior* 76:387–401.

Levin, B. 2006. Metabolic sensing neurons and the control of energy homeostasis. *Physiology & Behavior* 89:486–89.

Levine, J. 2004. Non-exercise activity thermogenesis. *Nutrition Reviews* 62:S82–S97.

Levine, J., et al. 2006. Non-exercise activity thermogenesis: The crouching tiger hidden dragon of societal weight gain. *Arteriosclerosis, Thrombosis, and Vascular Biology* 26:729–36.

Liu, C., et al. 2013. FTO gene variant and risk of overweight and obesity among children and adolescents: A systematic review and meta-analysis. *Public Library of Science One* 8 (11):e82133. doi: 10,1371/journal.pone.0082133.

Loef, M., and Walach, H. 2013. Midlife obesity and dementia: Meta-analysis and adjusted forecast of dementia prevalence in the United States and China. *Obesity* 21 (1):E51-E55. doi: 10.1002/oby.2037.

Loenneke, J. P., et al. 2011. Validity of the current NCAA minimum weight protocol: A brief review. *Annals of Nutrition and Metabolism* 58:245–49.

Lohman, T., and Going, S. 2006. Body composition assessment for development of an international growth standard for preadolescent and adolescent children. *Food and Nutrition Bulletin* 27:S314–25.

Lohman, T., et al. 1997. Body fat measurement goes high-tech: Not all are created equal. *ACSM's Health & Fitness Journal* 1 (1):30–35.

Loucks, A. 2003. Energy availability, not body fatness, regulates reproductive function in women. *Exercise and Sports Sciences Reviews* 31:144–48.

Loucks, A. 2004. Energy balance and body composition in sports and exercise. *Journal of Sports Sciences* 22:1–14.

Loucks, A. 2006. The endocrine system: Integrated influences on metabolism, growth, and reproduction. In ACSM's *Advanced Exercise Physiology,* ed. C. M. Tipton. Philadelphia: Lippincott Williams & Wilkins.

Loyd, C., and Obici, S. 2014. Brown fat fuel use and regulation of energy homeostasis.

Current Opinion in Clinical Nutrition and Metabolic Care 17:368–72.

Lucassen, E., and Cizza, G. 2012. The hypothalamic-pituitary-adrenal axis, obesity, and chronic stress exposure: Sleep and the HPA axis in obesity. Current Obesity Reports (4):208–15.

Lutter, M., and Nestler, E. 2009. Homeostatic and hedonic signals interact in the regulation of food intake. Journal of Nutrition 139:629–32.

Major, G., et al. 2007. Clinical significance of adaptive thermogenesis. International Journal of Obesity 31:204–12.

Malik, V. S., et al. 2013. Sugar-sweetened beverages and weight gain in children and adults: A systematic review and meta-analysis. American Journal of Clinical Nutrition 98:1084–102.

Malina, R. M., et al. 2013. Role of intensive training in the growth and maturation of artistic gymnasts. Sports Medicine 43:783–802.

Malis, C., et al. 2005. Total and regional fat distribution is strongly influenced by genetic factors in young and elderly twins. Obesity Research 13 (12):2139–45.

Manore, M. 2002. Dietary recommendations and athletic menstrual dysfunction. Sports Medicine 32:887–901.

Marra, M., et al. 2007. BMR variability in women of different weight. Clinical Nutrition 26 (5):567–72.

Marshall, S., et al. 2004. Relationships between media use, body fatness and physical activity in children and youth: A meta-analysis. International Journal of Obesity and Related Metabolic Disorders 28:1238–46.

Mattson, M. 2010. Perspective: Does brown fat protect against diseases of aging? Ageing Research Reviews 9:69–76.

Mayer, L., et al. 2007. Does percent body fat predict outcome in anorexia nervosa? American Journal of Psychiatry 164:970–2.

Mayr, F. B., et al. 2012. Case report. Hypokalemic paralysis in a professional bodybuilder. American Journal of Emergency Medicine 30:1324.e5–1324.e8.

McNeil, J., et al. 2013. Inadequate sleep as a contributor to obesity and type 2 diabetes. Canadian Journal of Diabetes 37 (2):103–8.

Melby, C., et al. 1998. Exercise, macronutrient balance, and weight control. In Exercise, Nutrition, and Weight Control, ed. D. Lamb and R. Murray. Carmel, IN: Cooper.

Mendoza, J., et al. 2007. Dietary energy density is associated with obesity and the metabolic syndrome in U.S. adults. Diabetes Care 30:974–79.

Miller, Y., and Dunstan, D. 2004. The effectiveness of physical activity interventions for the treatment of overweight and obesity and type 2 diabetes. Journal of Science and Medicine in Sport 7:52–59.

Mitra, A., and Clarke, K. 2010. Viral obesity: Fact or fiction? Obesity Reviews 11:289–96.

Moon, J. R., et al. 2007. Percent body fat estimations in college women using field and laboratory methods: A three-compartment model approach. Dynamic Medicine 7:7. doi: 10.1186/1476-5918-7-7.

Moon, J. R., et al. 2007. Percent body fat estimations in college women using field and laboratory methods: A three-compartment model approach. Journal of the International Society of Sports Nutrition 7:4–16.

Moon, J. R. 2013. Body composition in athletes and sports nutrition: and examination of the bioimpedance analysis technique. European Journal of Clinical Nutrition 67:554–59.

Moran, T. 2006. Gut peptide signaling in the control of food intake. Obesity 14:250S–53S.

Moreno, L., and Rodríguez, G. 2007. Dietary risk factors for development of childhood obesity. Current Opinion in Clinical Nutrition and Metabolic Care 10:336–41.

Moreno, L. A. et al. 2010. Trends of dietary habits in adolescents. Critical Reviews in Food Science and Nutrition 50(2):106–112.

Mottillo, S., et al. 2010. The metabolic syndrome and cardiovascular risk a systematic review and meta-analysis. Journal of the American College of Cardiology 56:1113–32.

Mountjoy, M., et al. 2014. The IOC consensus statement: Beyond the female athletic triad-relative energy deficiency in sport (RED-S). British Journal of Sports Medicine 48:491–97.

Nader, P., et al. 2006. Identifying risk for obesity in early childhood. Pediatrics 118:594–601.

Nago, E. S., et al. 2014. Association of out-of-home eating with anthropometric changes: A systematic review of prospective studies. Critical Reviews in Food Science and Nutrition 54 (9):1103–16.

National Center for Health Statistics. 2013. Health, United States, 2013: With Special Feature on Prescription Drugs. Hyattsville, MD:

National Institutes of Health. NHLBI. North American Association for the Study of Obesity. 2000. The Practical Guide: Identification, Evaluation, and Treatment of Overweight and Obesity in Adults. NIH Publication Number 00–4084.

National Task Force on the Prevention and Treatment of Obesity. 1994. Weight cycling. Journal of the American Medical Association 272:1196–202.

Naukkarinen, J., et al. 2012. Causes and consequences of obesity: The contribution of recent twin studies. International Journal of Obesity 36:1017–24.

Newbold, R. 2010. Impact of environmental endocrine disrupting chemicals on the development of obesity. Hormones 9:206–17.

Ng, M., et al. 2014. Global, regional, and national prevalence of overweight and obesity in children and adults during 1980–2013: A systematic analysis for the Global Burden of Disease Study 2013. Lancet (May 28). pii: S0140-6736(14)60460-8. doi: 10.1016/S0140-6736(14)60460-8. [Epub ahead of print]

Niemeier, B. S., et al. 2012. Parent participation in weight-related health interventions for children and adolescents: A systematic review and meta-analysis. Preventive Medicine 55:3–13.

Nihiser, A. J., et al. 2009. BMI measurement in schools. Pediatrics 124:S89. doi: 10.1542/peds.2008–3586L.

Noreen, E., and Lemon, P. 2006. Reliability of air displacement plethysmography in a large, heterogeneous sample. Medicine & Science in Sports & Exercise 38:1505–9.

O'Brien, M., et al. 2007. The ecology of childhood overweight: A 12-year longitudinal analysis. International Journal of Obesity 31:1469–78.

O'Connor, D., et al. 2010. Generalized equations for estimating DXA percent body fat of diverse young women and men: The TIGER study. Medicine & Science in Sports & Exercise 42:1959–65.

Ode, J., et al. 2007. Body mass index as a predictor of percent fat in college athletes and nonathletes. Medicine & Science in Sports & Exercise 39:403–9.

Ogden, C. L., et al. 2010. Obesity and socio-economic status in adults: United States, 2005–2008. United States Department of Health and Human Services. Data Brief 50.

Ogden, C. L., et al. 2014. Prevalence of childhood and adult obesity in the United States, 2011–2012. Journal of the American Medical Association 311 (8):806–14.

Oppliger, R., et al. 2006. NCAA rule change improves weight loss among National

Championship wrestlers. *Medicine & Science in Sports & Exercise* 38:963–70.

Orphanidou, C., et al. 1994. Accuracy of subcutaneous fat measurement: Comparison of skinfold calipers, ultrasound, and computed tomography. *Journal of the American Dietetic Association* 94:855–58.

Owen, C. G., et al. 2009. Is body mass index before middle age related to coronary heart disease risk in later life? Evidence from observational studies. *International Journal of Obesity* 33 (8):866–77.

Owen, N., et al. 2010. Too much sitting: The population health science of sedentary behavior. *Exercise and Sport Sciences Reviews* 38:105–13.

Pate, R. R., et al. 2013. Factors associated with development of excessive fatness in children and adolescents: A review of prospective studies. *Obesity Reviews* 14 (8):645–58.

Pereira, M., et al. 2005. Fast-food habits, weight gain, and insulin resistance (the CARDIA study): 15-year prospective analysis. *The Lancet* 365:36–42.

Peters, J. 2006. Obesity prevention and social change: What will it take? *Exercise and Sport Sciences Reviews* 34:4–9.

Peters, J., et al. 2002. From instinct to intellect: The challenge of maintaining healthy weight in the modern world. *Obesity Reviews* 3:69–74.

Pi-Sunyer, F. 2002. The medical risks of obesity. *Obesity Surgery* 12:6S–11S.

Pi-Sunyer, F. 2006. The relation of adipose tissue to cardiometabolic risk. *Clinical Cornerstone* 8 (Supplement 4):S14–23.

Pi-Sunyer, F. 2007. How effective are lifestyle changes in the prevention of type 2 diabetes mellitus? *Nutrition Reviews* 65:101–10.

Pichard, C., et al. 1997. Body composition by x-ray absorptiometry and bioelectrical impedance in female runners. *Medicine & Science in Sports & Exercise* 29:1527–34.

Pourhassan, M., et al. 2013. Impact of body-composition methodology on the composition of weight loss and weight gain. *European Journal of Clinical Nutrition* 67:446–54.

Pulgarón, E. R. 2013. Childhood obesity: A review of increased risk for physical and psychological co-morbidities. *Clinical Therapies* 35 (1):A18–A32.

Rankinen, T., et al. 2006. The human obesity gene map: The 2005 update. *Obesity* 14:529–644.

Rask-Andersen, M., et al. 2010. Molecular mechanisms underlying anorexia nervosa: Focus on human gene association studies and systems controlling food intake. *Brain Research Reviews* 62:147–64.

Reaven, G. 2006. Metabolic syndrome: Definition, relationship to insulin resistance, and clinical utility. In *Modern Nutrition in Health and Disease,* ed. M. Shils et al. Philadelphia: Lippincott Williams & Wilkins.

Reaven, G. 2006. The metabolic syndrome: Is this diagnosis necessary? *American Journal of Clinical Nutrition* 83:1237–47.

Renehan, A. G., et al. 2010. Interpreting the epidemiological evidence linking obesity and cancer: A framework for population-attributable risk estimations in Europe. *European Journal of Cancer* 46:2581–92.

Renehan, A., et al. 2008. Body-mass index and incidence of cancer: A systematic review and meta-analysis of prospective observational studies. *The Lancet* 371:569–78.

Riondino, S., et al. 2014. Obesity and colorectal cancer: Role of adipokines in tumor initiation and progression. *World Journal of Gastroenterology* 20 (18):5177–90.

Riu, L. 2013. Brain regulation of energy balance and body weight. *Reviews in Endocrine and Metabolic Disorders* 14:387–407.

Rodriguez-Sanchez, N., and Galloway, S. D. R. 2014. Errors in dual energy x-ray absorptiometry of body composition induced by hypohydration. *International Journal of Sports Nutrition and Exercise Metabolism* (July 14). doi: 10.1123/ijsnem.2014.0067. [Epub ahead of print]

Roemmich, J., and Sinning, W. 1996. Sport-seasonal changes in body composition, growth, power and strength of adolescent wrestlers. *International Journal of Sports Medicine* 17:92–99.

Romero-Corral, A., et al. 2010. Modest visceral fat gain causes endothelial dysfunction in healthy humans. *Journal of the American College of Cardiology* 56:662–6.

Rossi, A. M., and Katz, B. E. 2014. A modern approach to the treatment of cellulite. *Clinics in Dermatology* 32 (1):51–59.

Rowland, T. 1998. The biological basis of physical activity. *Medicine & Science in Sports & Exercise* 30:392–99.

Sallis, J. F., et al. 2012. Role of built environments in physical activity, obesity, and cardiovascular disease. *Circulation* 125:729–37.

Salvy, S. J., et al. 2011. Influence of parents and friends on children's and adolescents' food intake and food selection. *American Journal of Clinical Nutrition* 93 (1):87–92.

Salvy, S. J., et al. 2012. Influence of peers and friends on overweight/obese youths' physical activity. *Exercise and Sport Science Reviews* 40 (3):127–32.

Salvy, S., et al. 2009. The presence of friends increases food intake in youth. *American Journal of Clinical Nutrition* 90:282–7.

Sarafrazi, N., et al. 2014. *Perception of Weight Status in US Children and Adolescents Aged 8-15 Years,* 2005–2012. NCHS data brief, no. 158. Hyattsville, MD: National Center for Health Statistics.

Sarjeant, K., and Stephens, J. M. 2012. Adipogenesis. *Cold Spring Harbor Perspectives in Biology* 4:a008417.

Saunders, T. J., et al. 2014. Sedentary behaviours as an emerging risk factor for cardiometabolic doseases in children and youth. *Canadian Journal of Diabetes* 38:53–61.

Schnirring, L. 2005. NFHS finalizes weight cutting rules for wrestlers. *Physician and Sportsmedicine* 33 (7):9–12.

Schulz, T. J., and Tseng, Y. H. 2013. Brown adipose tissue: Development, metabolism and beyond. *Biochemical Journal* 453 (2):167–78.

Sclafani, A., and Ackroff, K. 2012. Role of gut nutrient sensing in stimulating appetite and conditioning food preferences. *American Journal of Physiology Regulatory and Integrative Physiology* 302 (10):R1119–33.

Shah, M., and Garg, A. 1996. High-fat and high-carbohydrate diets and energy balance. *Diabetes Care* 19:1142–52.

Shapiro, J., et al. 2007. Bulimia nervosa treatment: A systematic review of randomized controlled trials. *International Journal of Eating Disorders* 40:321–36.

Shetty, P. S., and James, W. P. T. 1994. Body mass index—A measure of chronic energy deficiency in adults. Food and Agriculture Organization of the United Nations.

Siri, W. E. 1961. Body composition from fluid space and density. In *Techniques for Measuring Body Composition,* ed. J. Brożek and A. Hanschel. Washington, DC: National Academy of Science.

Small, K., et al. 2011. Identification of an imprinted master trans regulator at the KLF14 locus related to multiple metabolic phenotypes. *Nature Genetics* 43:561–4.

Smolak, L., et al. 2000. Female athletes and eating problems: A meta-analysis. *International Journal of Eating Disorders* 27:371–80.

Sodersen, P., et al. 2006. Understanding eating disorders. *Hormones and Behavior* 50:572–78.

Speakman, J. R., et al. 2011. Set points, settling points and some alternative models: Theoretical options to understand how genes and environments combine to regulate body adiposity. *Disease Models and Mechanisms* 4:733–45.

Steffes, G. D., et al. 2013. Prevalence of metabolic syndrome risk factors in high school and NCAA Division I football players. *Journal of Strength and Conditioning Research* 27 (7):1749–57.

Stein, D., et al. 2014. Psychosocial perspectives and the issue of prevention in childhood obesity. *Frontiers in Public Health* 2:104. doi: 10.3389/fpubh.2014.00104.

Stobbe, M. 2010. Obesity's impact on costs bigger than thought. *Associated Press,* October 17.

Stock, M. 1989. Thermogenesis and brown fat: Relevance to human obesity. *Infusiontherapie* 16:282–84.

Stout, J., et al. 1995. Validity of skinfold equations for estimating body density in youth wrestlers. *Medicine & Science in Sports & Exercise* 27:1321–25.

Strecker, L. 2010. School nutrition and childhood obesity. *Update Plus* (September/October):4–5.

Strohaker, K., and McFarlin, B. K. 2010. Influence of obesity, physical inactivity, and weight cycling on chronic inflammation. *Frontiers in Bioscience* (Elite Edition) 2:98–104.

Stubbs, R. 1999. Peripheral signals affecting food intake. *Nutrition* 15:614–25.

Stunkard, A., et al. 1990. The body-mass index of twins who have been reared apart. *New England Journal of Medicine* 322:1483–87.

Sturm, R., and Hattori, A. 2013. Morbid obesity rates continue to rise rapidly in the US. *International Journal of Obesity* 37 (6):889–91.

Sudi, K., et al. 2004. Anorexia athletics. *Nutrition* 20:657–61.

Sui, X., et al. 2007. Cardiorespiratory fitness and adiposity as mortality predictors in older adults. *Journal of the American Medical Association* 298:2507–16.

Sullivan, E., et al. 2011. Perinatal exposure to high-fat diet programs energy balance, metabolism and behavior in adulthood. *Neuroendocrinology* 93:1–8.

Sundgot-Borgen, J. 2000. Eating disorders in athletes. In *Nutrition in Sport,* ed. R. J. Maughan. Oxford: Blackwell Science.

Sundgot-Borgen, J., and Torstveit, M. K. 2004. Prevalence of eating disorders in elite athletes is higher than in the general population. *Clinical Journal of Sports Medicine* 14:25–32.

Sundgot-Borgen, J., et al. 2013. How to minimize the health risks to athletes who compete in weight-sensitive sports review and position statement on behalf of the ad hoc research working group on body composition, health and performance, under the auspices of the IOC Medical Commission. *British Journal of Sports Medicine* 47:1012–22.

Swinburn, B., and Shelly, A. 2008. Effects of TV time and other sedentary pursuits. *International Journal of Obesity* 32 (Supplement 7):S132–6.

Swinburn, B., and Shelly, A. 2008. Effects of TV time and other sedentary pursuits. *International Journal of Obesity* 32:S132–36.

Tang, L., et al. 2014. Meta-analysis between 18 candidate genetic markers for overweight/obesity. *Diagnostic Pathology* 9:56.

Teske, J. A., et al. 2008. Neuropeptidergic mediators of spontaneous physical activity and non-exercise activity thermogenesis. *Neuroendocrinology* 87 (2):71–90.

Thaiss, C. A., et al. 2014. Transkingdom control of microbiota diurnal oscillations promotes metabolic homeostasis. *Cell* 159 (3):514–29.

Theintz, G., et al. 1993. Evidence for a reduction of growth potential in adolescent female gymnasts. *Journal of Pediatrics* 122:306–13.

Torstveit, M., and Sundgot-Borgen, J. 2005. The female athlete triad exists in both elite athletes and controls. *Medicine & Science in Sports & Exercise* 37:1449–59.

Torstveit, M., and Sundgot-Borgen, J. 2005. Participation in leanness sports but not training volume is associated with menstrual dysfunction: A national survey of 1276 elite athletes and controls. *British Journal of Sports Medicine* 39:141–47.

Townsend, K. L., and Tseng, Y. H. 2013. Brown fat fuel utilization and thermogenesis. *Trends in Endocrinology and Metabolism* 25 (4):168–77.

Tremblay, A., et al. 1995. Alcohol and a high-fat diet: A combination favoring overfeeding. *American Journal of Clinical Nutrition* 62:639–44.

Tremblay, M. S., et al. 2011. Systematic review of sedentary behaviour and health indicators in school-aged children and youth. *International Journal of Behavioral Nutrition and Physical Activity* 8:98. doi: 10.1186/1479-5868-8-98.

Tsai, A. G., et al. 2011. Direct medical cost of overweight and obesity in the USA: A quantitative systematic review. *Obesity Reviews* 12 (1):50–61.

Tsai, A., and Wadden, T. 2006. The evolution of very-low-calorie diets: An update and meta-analysis. *Obesity* 14:1283–93.

Tso, P., and Liu, M. 2004. Ingested fat and satiety. *Physiology & Behavior* 81:275–87.

Utter, A., and Hager, M. 2008. Evaluation of ultrasound in assessing body composition of high school wrestlers. *Medicine & Science in Sports & Exercise* 40:943–49.

Vangipuram, S. D., et al. 2007. Adipogenic human adenovirus-36 reduces leptin expression and secretion and increases glucose uptake by fat cells. *International Journal of Obesity* 31:87–96.

Vartanian, L. R., et al. 2013. Disgust, contempt, and anger and the stereotypes of obese people. *Eating and Weight Disorders* 18 (4):377–82.

Vella-Zarb, R., and Elgar, F. 2009. The "freshman 5": a meta-analysis of weight gain in the freshman year of college. *Journal of the American College of Health* 58:161–6.

Ventura, A. K., and Worobey, J. 2013. Early influences on the development of food preferences. *Current Biology* 23 (9):R401–8.

Wadden, T., et al. 2005. Randomized trial of lifestyle modification and pharmacotherapy for obesity. *New England Journal of Medicine* 353:2111–20.

Wadden, T., et al. 2006. Obesity: Management. In *Modern Nutrition in Health and Disease,* ed. M. Shils et al. Philadephia: Lippincott Williams & Wilkins.

Wagner, D., and Heyward, V. 1999. Techniques of body composition assessment: A review of laboratory and field methods. *Research Quarterly for Exercise and Sport* 70:135–49.

Wagner, D., et al. 2000. Validation of air displacement plethysmography for assessing body composition. *Medicine & Science in Sports & Exercise* 32:1339–44.

Walker, T. B., et al. 2014. Lessons from the war on dietary fat. *Journal of the American College of Nutrition* 33 (4):347–51.

Wang, L., et al. 1992. The five-level model: A new approach to organizing body-composition research. *American Journal of Clinical Nutrition* 56:19–28.

Wang, Y., and Lim, H. 2012. The global childhood obesity epidemic and the association between socio-economic status and childhood obesity. *International Review of Psychiatry* 24 (3):176–88.

Wang, Y., et al. 2005. Comparison of abdominal adiposity and overall obesity in predicting risk of type 2 diabetes among men. *American Journal of Clinical Nutrition* 81:555–63.

Wang, Z., et al. 1998. Six-compartment body composition model: Inter-method comparisons of total body fat measurement. *International Journal of Obesity and Related Metabolic Disorders* 22:329–37.

Waterland, R. 2014. Epigenetic mechanisms of energy balance: Many questions, few answers. *Annual Review of Nutrition* 34:337–55.

Webster, B., and Barr, S. 1993. Body composition analysis of female adolescent athletes: Comparing six regression equations. *Medicine & Science in Sports & Exercise* 25:648–53.

Weinsier, R., et al. 2000. Do adaptive changes in metabolic rate favor weight regain in weight-reduced individuals? An examination of the set-point theory. *American Journal of Clinical Nutrition* 73:1088–94.

Weinstein, A., et al. 2008. The joint effects of physical activity and body mass index on coronary heart disease risk in women. *Archives of Internal Medicine* 168:884–90.

Wells, J. 2006. The evolution of human fatness and susceptibility to obesity: An ethological approach. *Biological Reviews of the Cambridge Philosophical Society* 81:183–205.

Welsh, J. A., et al. 2011. Consumption of added sugars is decreasing in the United States. *American Journal of Clinical Nutrition* 94:726–34.

Welsh, J. A., et al. 2013. The sugar-sweetened beverage wars: Public health and the role of the beverage industry. *Current Opinion in Endocrinology, Diabetes, and Obesity* 20 (5):401–6.

Wiecha, J., et al. 2006. When children eat what they watch: Impact of television viewing on dietary intake in youth. *Archives of Pediatrics & Adolescent Medicine* 160:436–42.

Wilder, R., and Cicchetti, M. 2009. Common injuries in athletes with obesity and diabetes. *Clinics in Sports Medicine* 28:441–53.

Wildman, R. 2009. Healthy obesity. *Current Opinion in Clinical Nutrition & Metabolic Care* 12:438–43.

Willeumeier, K., et al. 2012. Elevated body mass in National Football League players linked to cognitive impairment and decreased prefrontal cortex and temporal lobe activity. *Translational Psychiatry* 2:e68. doi:10.1038/tp.2011.67.

Williams, P. 1990. Weight set-point theory and the high-density lipoprotein concentrations of long-distance runners. *Metabolism* 39:460–67.

Wolin, K., et al. 2010. Obesity and cancer. *Oncologist* 15:556–65.

Woods, S. 2007. The endocannabinoid system: Mechanisms behind metabolic homeostasis and imbalance. *American Journal of Medicine* 120 (Supplement 1):S9–S17.

Woods, S. C. 2013. Metabolic signals and food intake. Forty years of progress. *Appetite* 71:440–44.

World Cancer Research Fund/American Institute for Cancer Research. 2007. *Food, Nutrition, Physical Activity, and the Prevention of Cancer: A Global Perspective*. Washington, DC: AICR.

Yard, E., and Comstock, D. 2011. Injury patterns by body mass index in US high school athletes. *Journal of Physical Activity and Health* 8:182–91.

Yeo, G. S. H. 2014. The role of the FTO (fat mass and obesity related) locus in regulating body size and composition. *Molecular and Cellular Endocrinology*. doi: 10.1016/j.mce.2014.09.012.

Yusuf, S., et al. 2005. Obesity and the risk of myocardial infarction in 27,000 participants from 52 countries: A case-control study. *Lancet* 366:1640–49.

Zachwieja, J., et al. 2001. Short-term dietary energy restriction reduces lean body mass but not performance in physically active men and women. *International Journal of Sports Medicine* 22:310–16.

Zeller, M., et al. 2008. Relation between body mass index, waist circumference, and death after acute myocardial infarction. *Circulation* 118:482–90.

Zhang, C., et al. 2008. Abdominal obesity and the risk of all-cause, cardiovascular, and cancer mortality: Sixteen years of follow-up in US women. *Circulation* 117:1658–67.

Zhang, J., et al. 2005. Obestatin, a peptide encoded by the ghrelin gene, opposes effects on food intake. *Science* 310:996–99.

Zimberg, I. Z., et al. 2012. Short sleep duration and obesity: Mechanisms and future perspectives. *Cell Biochemistry and Function* 30 (6):524–29.

Weight Maintenance and Loss through Proper Nutrition and Exercise

CHAPTER ELEVEN

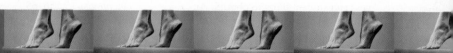

LEARNING OBJECTIVES

After studying this chapter, you should be able to:

1. Determine how many Calories per day are needed to maintain one's current body weight with either a sedentary or physically active lifestyle.

2. Calculate the amount of weight loss needed to attain a healthier BMI or body-fat percentage.

3. Identify behavior modification techniques that are appropriate to incorporate into a recommended weight-loss program.

4. Determine the number of daily Calories needed to lose body fat by diet alone, or with a combination diet-exercise program.

5. State the key principles underlying a weight-control diet designed to maintain a healthy body weight for a lifetime.

6. Use the Food Exchange System to plan a healthy, balanced diet containing sufficient Calories to meet one's daily energy needs for weight loss or weight maintenance.

7. Describe the value of exercise, including type, intensity, duration, and frequency, in a comprehensive weight-loss or weight-maintenance program.

8. Use heart rate responses as a guide to appropriate aerobic exercise intensity.

9. Design a progressive exercise program that will increase caloric expenditure to 300–500 Calories per day as part of a comprehensive weight-loss or weight-maintenance program.

10. Understand how diet and exercise complement each other to help lose or maintain body weight, citing the benefits of each that help compensate for the possible deficiencies of the other.

According to Ogden and colleagues, 34.8 percent of American adults (78.6 million) were obese in 2011–2012. Many millions more were overweight. The desire of so many individuals to lose weight has led to a weight-loss industry with a 2013 economic value of $60.5 billion http://www .marketdataenterprises.com/studies/#FS45. Weight-loss centers and health and fitness spas cater to this obsession by promising lean bodies just in time for the swimsuit season. Pharmaceutical companies produce prescription and over-the-counter drugs designed to promote fat loss the easy way. Food manufacturers market convenient, low-Calorie, prepackaged—but expensive—meals. Exercise equipment manufacturers advertise devices that burn twice as many Calories as a treadmill. Advertisements in the print and TV media include "before" and "after" pictures of successful customers with promises to "Lose weight while you sleep" or "Lose 30 pounds in just 30 days." Each year at least one diet book on the best-seller list is advertised as the last diet one will ever need.

A variety of techniques, some useful and some not, are used in attempts to stimulate weight loss. Dietary supplements are marketed to depress the appetite or increase metabolism. Creams are applied to specific body parts to shrink local fat deposits. Surgical techniques include intestinal bypasses, removal of or stapling part of the stomach, excision or suction removal of subcutaneous fat tissue, and wiring the jaw shut. Weight-loss diets involve almost every possible manipulation, including the high-fat diet, the high-protein diet, the chocolate diet, the grapefruit diet, the starvation diet, and even the "no diet" diet. Advertisements claim that specially designed clothing worn during exercise can help you lose inches of fat in hours. Psychological techniques such as hypnosis or behavior modification are designed to change your eating habits.

The National Academy of Sciences Institute of Medicine's Committee to Develop Criteria for Evaluating the Outcomes of Approaches to Prevent and Treat Obesity identified three types of programs and approaches to treat obesity or overweight: clinical programs, nonclinical programs, and do-it-yourself programs. No matter which program an individual selects to lose weight, the Committee recommended consultation with one's primary health-care provider before engaging in a weight-loss program.

In severe cases of clinical obesity, treatment usually is administered in a *clinical program* under medical supervision and may involve a combination of many techniques, including surgery, hormone therapy, drugs, and very low-calorie diets. An individualized, medically supervised weight-control program is very important for the clinically obese because so many health risks are related to obesity. Surgery may be effective, and various techniques may be used, including gastric bypass surgery and insertion of a small, flexible gastric band around the top part of the stomach. Government regulations indicate that individuals who have a BMI greater than 40, or a lower BMI with a serious health condition, such as diabetes, may benefit from weight-loss surgery. In a 24-month follow-up study of almost 74,000 bariatric surgery patients, Benoit and others reported significantly greater reductions in BMI and weight loss following gastric bypass and sleeve gastrectomy compared to the adjustable gastric band procedure.

Gastric electrical stimulation devices, or stomach pacemakers, were originally developed to treat delayed gastric emptying of a solid meal. These devices may also be used to combat obesity through decreasing caloric intake by neural/hormonal effects on energy intake centers in the brain and/or by stomach muscle stimulation. The devices are available in the European Union and were approved in 2015 by the Food and Drug Administration for use in the United States.

Unfortunately, however, clinical obesity is very resistant to other forms of treatment, particularly dieting: More than 95 percent of those individuals who lose weight regain it within 1–5 years, and they may do this repeatedly. As noted in chapter 10, these fluctuations in body weight are known as weight cycling. Although some uncertainty remains about the long-term effects of weight cycling on health and metabolism, there is insufficient evidence to deter an obese individual from attempts to lose weight. The National Institutes of Health notes that other groups may need medically supervised weight-loss programs, including children, pregnant women, persons over the age of 65, and individuals with medical conditions that could be exacerbated by weight loss.

Nonclinical programs for the treatment of obesity are primarily commercial franchises, using packaged materials provided by counselors who usually are not professional health-care providers. These programs may or may not be managed or advised by appropriate health-care professionals. In general, there is little scientific research on the effectiveness of nonclinical programs.

Do-it-yourself programs include any effort by the individual to lose weight by himself or herself; through use of popular diet books, dietary aids, or counseling/support groups; or through community-based and work-site programs. These treatment programs may be well suited for individuals who have accumulated excess body fat through environmental conditions, such as excessive eating and decreased physical activity. Such programs may be beneficial to the typical adult, for substantial amounts of body fat appear to accumulate between the ages of 25 and 35. The prevalence of overweight individuals, as measured by the body mass index (BMI), in the United States has increased in the past quarter-century in both children and adults, and this weight gain has been associated with an increased incidence of health complications. However, a 2013 expert panel by the National Heart, Lung, and Blood Institute reported evidence that even small (2 to 5 percent) decreases in weight or BMI may decrease the risk and symptoms of diabetes, improve lipids and blood pressure, and decrease mortality from cardiovascular diseases and all causes.

Because the majority of obese people who lose weight put it back on, most weight-control experts indicate that the focus should be on prevention and maintenance. Prevention of excess weight gain is more effective than treatment. Prevention should be a lifelong lifestyle, beginning in childhood and continuing through adulthood. Preventive techniques

may be especially helpful during the first 2 years of college, when young females typically gain weight. In their review of discordant (obese and non-obese) twin studies, Naukkarinen and others noted the non-obese twin offers strong evidence for the role of healthy lifestyle choices to counteract genetic and environmental tendencies toward obesity. Many overweight individuals often note that the hard part is not losing weight, it's keeping it off, but that may not necessarily be so. Maintenance of a healthy body weight is a simple form of prevention; preventing weight regain is comparable to preventing weight gain in the first place.

This chapter centers on some basic questions relative to the construction, implementation, and maintenance of a sound weight-control program using the *do-it-yourself* approach. The principles and suggestions advanced here apply to the overweight individual who wants to lose excess body fat, as well as to the person with normal body weight who wants to maintain that weight level or even lose additional poundage in order to improve physical performance. Individuals who are already lean should consult with qualified health professionals before attempting to lose weight. Fontana and Klein note that caloric restriction for weight change may be beneficial in many adults, but it may be detrimental in extremely lean individuals and other patient populations. One potential problem is the development of an eating disorder, as discussed in chapter 10. For individuals interested in participating in *nonclinical* or *clinical programs,* some guidelines are offered later in this chapter.

A comprehensive weight-control program involves three components: (1) a dietary regimen stressing balanced nutrition but with reduced caloric intake; (2) an aerobic and resistance exercise program to increase caloric expenditure

and maintain lean body mass; and (3) a behavior modification program to facilitate the implementation of the first two components. These components are emphasized in this chapter.

Although proper dieting and exercise are the two keys to weight control, the same diet and exercise plan may not be appropriate for all individuals. Genetic mutations related to obesity were discussed in chapter 10. Adamo and Tesson comment that the large interindividual variability in weight-loss success is also a function of environmental, genetic, and epigenetic influences.

Weight loss is difficult, but it can be done. Haruki Murakami, in his book *What I Talk About When I Talk About Running,* cited a sign he saw in a Tokyo gym that read "Muscles are hard to get and easy to lose, fat is easy to get and hard to lose." There is a lot of truth in that statement, as many individuals find it very difficult to lose body fat and maintain that loss. Kraschnewski and colleagues reported that only 17.3 percent of overweight and obese U.S. adults who lose at least 10 percent of their weight are successful at maintaining their weight loss for at least 1 year. However, Thomas and others report that 87 percent of 2,886 participants in the National Weight Control Registry (NWCR) have successfully maintained at least a 10 percent weight loss for up to 10 years. The diet and exercise strategies of the NWCR will be presented throughout this chapter.

However one does it, creating a negative energy balance in the body will lead to weight loss. As we shall see, a wide variety of diet and exercise programs may satisfy the criteria for a healthy weight-loss program and most individuals can find a program to meet their individual needs. The best diet and exercise strategy for weight loss is the one that works for you.

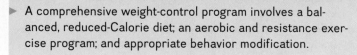

Key Concept

▶ A comprehensive weight-control program involves a balanced, reduced-Calorie diet; an aerobic and resistance exercise program; and appropriate behavior modification.

Basics of Weight Control

How many Calories are in a pound of body fat?

One pound is equivalent to 454 grams. Because we know that 1 gram of fat is equal to 9 Calories, it would appear that a pound of body fat would equal about 4,086 Calories (9 × 454).

However, the fat stored in adipose tissue contains small amounts of protein, minerals, and water, which reduces the caloric content of 1 pound of body fat to approximately 3,500 Calories.

Is the caloric concept of weight control valid?

The caloric concept of weight control is relatively simple. As illustrated in figure 11.1, if you take in more Calories than you expend, you will gain weight, a positive energy balance. If you expend more than you take in, you lose weight, a negative energy balance. To maintain your body weight, caloric input and output must be equal. As far as we know, human energy systems are governed by the same laws of physics that rule all energy transformations. The First Law of Thermodynamics is as pertinent to us in the conservation and expenditure of our energy sources as it is to any other machine. Because a Calorie is a unit of energy, and because energy can neither be created nor destroyed, those Calories that we eat must either be expended in some way or conserved in the body. No substantial evidence is available to disprove the caloric theory. It is still the physical basis for body-weight control. In a recent survey, Meerman and Brown observed that some family physicians, dietitians, and personal trainers lack a complete understanding of thermodynamics and fat catabolism.

Keep in mind that the total body weight is made up of different components, those notable in weight-control programs being body water, protein in the fat-free mass, small amounts of carbohydrate, and fat stores. Changes in these components may bring about daily body-weight fluctuations of 3–5 pounds that would appear to be contrary to the caloric concept because protein and carbohydrate contain only 4 Calories per gram and water contains no Calories. You may gain water weight by consuming a high-salt diet for a day, or by menstrual cycle changes. You may lose 5 pounds in an hour, but it will be mostly water weight lost through sweating. Starvation techniques may lead to rapid weight losses, but some of the weight loss will be in glycogen stores, body-protein stores such as muscle mass, and the water associated with glycogen and protein stores. In programs to lose body weight, we usually desire to lose excess body fat, and certain dietary and exercise techniques may help to maximize fat losses while minimizing protein losses. The results of safe weight-loss programs are observed over weeks to months, not hours or days.

The metabolism of human energy sources is complex, and although the caloric theory is valid relative to body-weight control, one must be aware that weight changes will not always be exactly in line with caloric input and output, and that weight losses may not be due to body-fat loss alone. Also keep in mind one of the concepts advanced in the last chapter relative to individual variability in metabolic rates; two individuals with the same body weight may consume the same amount of Calories, yet one may gain while the other may maintain or even lose weight. It is also important to remember that genetics may affect the rate of weight loss, as discussed by Adamo and Tesson. Other than differences in metabolism, this possibility also may be related to the type of Calories in the diet; research has suggested that the body may store dietary fat Calories in the adipose tissue more efficiently than carbohydrate or protein Calories. In essence, compared to dietary fat, it may take more energy to convert dietary carbohydrate and protein into body fat. These concepts are explored further in this chapter.

How many Calories do I need per day to maintain my body weight?

This depends on a number of factors, notably age, body weight, gender, resting energy expenditure (REE), the thermic effect of food (TEF), and physical activity levels.

Age   The caloric requirement per kilogram of body weight (Calories/kg) is very high during the early years of life when a child is developing and adding large amounts of body tissue. The Calorie/kg requirement decreases throughout the years from birth to old age, with exceptions during pregnancy and lactation.

Body Weight   Body weight influences the total amount of daily Calories you need, but not the Calorie/kg of body weight. The

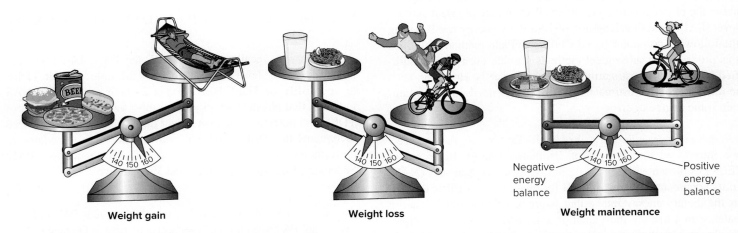

FIGURE 11.1 Weight control is based on energy balance and governed by the Laws of Thermodynamics. Too much food input or too little exercise output can result in a positive energy balance or weight gain, which can adversely affect health. Decreased food intake or increased physical activity can result in a negative caloric balance or weight loss, which can also adversely affect health. Attaining true energy balance to maintain a healthy body weight is the focus of this chapter.

large individual simply needs more total Calories to maintain body weight. Body weight is the most significant factor determining daily caloric intake necessary to maintain weight, although body composition also may be important.

Gender Up to the age of 11 or 12, the caloric needs of boys and girls are similar in terms of Calories/kg body weight. After puberty, however, males need slightly more Calories/kg, probably because of their greater percentage of muscle tissue in comparison to females.

REE Individual variations in REE may either increase or decrease daily caloric needs, depending on whether the REE is above or below normal. Individual variations may deviate 10–20 percent from normal. An extended discussion of the REE was presented in chapter 3.

TEF The TEF effect may also vary among individuals. The TEF is also covered in more detail in chapter 3.

Physical Activity Physical activity levels above resting may have a very significant impact on caloric needs. Some activities, like bowling, may increase energy needs only slightly, whereas others, such as running for an hour or more, may add 1,000–1,500 or more Calories to the daily energy requirement. You may wish to review chapter 3 regarding the caloric cost of exercise.

All of these factors make it difficult to make an exact recommendation relative to daily caloric needs. As noted in chapter 3, the doubly labeled water (DLW) technique may provide a fairly accurate measure of total daily energy expenditure (TDEE). However, it is rather expensive and not readily available to most individuals.

The following methods are available to help you determine the amount of Calories you need to consume daily to maintain a stable body weight. Some are more detailed than others. Calculating your daily energy needs by the Estimated Energy Requirement (EER) technique will provide you with an in-depth understanding of the role physical activity may play in daily caloric expenditure. It is a labor-intensive protocol but provides you with more details about the physical activity quotient (PA) and the physical activity level (PAL) used in calculation of your daily energy needs. Using the following computer-based ChooseMyPlate method simplifies this process, and subsequent methods provide even more simplified approaches to estimating daily energy needs. However, keep in mind that all are estimates of daily energy needs and may contain some degree of error.

Estimated Energy Requirement (EER) Technique In chapter 3 we introduced the concept of Estimated Energy Requirement (EER) as presented by the National Academy of Sciences (NAS) in its document focusing on DRI for energy. The EER is defined as the dietary energy intake that is predicted to maintain energy balance in a healthy individual of a defined age, gender, weight, height, and level of physical activity consistent with good health. As you may recall, total daily energy expenditure (TDEE) includes resting energy expenditure (REE), the thermic effect of food (TEF), and the thermic effect of exercise (TEE). The EER

TABLE 11.1 Estimated Energy Requirement (EER) formulas

Females age 19 and over:

EER = 354 − (6.91 × Age) + [PA × (9.361 × Weight + 726 × Height)]

Males age 19 and over:

EER = 662 − (9.53 × Age) + [PA × (15.91 × Weight + 539.6 × Height)]

Females age 9–18:

EER = 135.3 − (30.8 × Age) + [PA × (10.0 × Weight + 934 × Height)] + 25 (Calories/day for energy deposition)

Males age 9–18:

EER = 88.5 − (61.9 × Age) + [PA × (26.7 × Weight + 903 × Height)] + 25 (Calories/day for energy deposition)

Age: In years
Weight: In kilograms (kg). To convert weight in pounds to kilograms, multiply by 0.454.
Height: In meters (m). To convert height in inches to meters, multiply by 0.0254.

Adapted from National Academy of Sciences. 2002. *Dietary Reference Intakes for Energy, Carbohydrates, Fiber, Fat, Protein and Amino Acids (Macronutrients).* Washington, DC: National Academies Press.

equations for gender and different age categories are presented in table 11.1. As noted, the equations require age, height, weight, and physical activity coefficient (PA). You can easily determine the first three criteria, which is all you need to obtain an estimate of your energy requirements if you are sedentary, but determination of your PA requires some effort.

To calculate your EER, you should first determine your energy needs for a sedentary lifestyle. Select the appropriate formula for your gender and age category from table 11.1 and use the value of 1.0 as the PA. For example, a 20-year-old sedentary male weighing 175 pounds (80 kilograms) who is 71 inches (1.8 meters) tall would have a daily EER of 2,715 Calories.

EER = 662 − (9.53 × 20) + [1.0 × (15.91 × 80 + 539.6 × 1.8)] = 2,715

As you may recall from chapter 3, the PA is based on your physical activity level (PAL), which is the ratio of your TDEE to your BEE, or TDEE:BEE, over a 24-hour period. The NAS indicates that physical activity is the most variable component of TDEE and notes that the assessment of physical activity–induced increments in TDEE is fraught with considerable uncertainties. Nevertheless, the NAS has developed four categories of PAL: Sedentary, Low Active, Active, and Very Active.

www.nap.edu If you would like to calculate your PAL and resultant PA based on the NAS protocol, type in Dietary Reference Intakes for Energy in the Search box, click on the book title, and then peruse chapters 5 and 12 for details of the procedure.

EER can be calculated using a modified method based on a daily record of physical activities and metabolic equivalents (METS) of activities found in the Compendium of Physical Activities (https://sites.google.com/site/compendiumofphysicalactivities/). METS are exercise intensities expressed in multiples of the resting metabolic cost (~3.5 mL oxygen/kg/min).

The NAS bases the PAL on the amount of daily physical activity that is the equivalent of walking at a rate of 3–4 miles per hour. In the Compendium, "walking, 2.8 to 3.2 mph, level, moderate pace, firm surface" (activity code 17190) requires 3.5 METS, whereas "jogging, general" (activity code 12020) requires 7.0 METs. To reach a specific PAL category, one must expend the energy equivalent of walking a set number of miles. Although the NAS bases the PAL on an energy equivalent of walking, a multitude of physical activities of similar intensities may be used to reach the energy equivalent for a PAL category. Use the Compendium to find other activities requiring a similar intensity in METS. A MET value can be converted to C/kg/min. Total calories required for an activity can then be calculated by multiplying C/kg/min by body weight in kilograms and the total time of the activity in minutes. The agreement between the NAS procedure and the use of the Compendium to estimate exercise caloric expenditure is not exact because different calculations are used. However, both provide reasonable values for the energy cost of daily physical activity.

The following is a brief summary of the amount of physical activity needed for each PAL category. Table 11.2 complements this discussion and provides estimated exercise calories for an 80-kg individual at selected durations of walking and jogging. Some guidelines based on the energy expenditure equivalents of walking (~3 mph) or jogging are presented.

Sedentary category The energy expenditure of individuals in the Sedentary category represents their REE, including the TEF, plus various physical activities associated with independent living. Examples are activities found in "Inactivity," "Self-Care," and "Miscellaneous" Compendium categories such as dressing, grooming, light household tasks, and other forms of very light activity. The PAL will range from 1.00 to 1.39 for no daily physical activity, but the PA coefficient in the NAS EER formula is set at a baseline of 1.0. Individuals who walk less than 30 minutes daily generally fall in this category.

Low active category In addition to the normal daily activities of independent living, the energy equivalent of walking about 2.2 miles/day is required to be in the Low Active category. The PAL for this category will range from 1.40 to 1.59, but the NAS PA coefficient for the formula is set at 1.11–1.16 depending on gender and stage of life. Individuals who walk 45–50 minutes, or jog 20–25 minutes, daily generally fit this category.

Active category In addition to the normal daily activities of independent living, the energy equivalent of walking about 7 miles/day is required be in the Active category. The PAL for this category will range from 1.60 to 1.89, but the PA coefficient for the EER formula is set at 1.25–1.31 depending on gender and stage of life. Individuals who walk 115–120 min, or jog 55–60 minutes, daily generally fall in this category.

Very active category In addition to the normal daily activities of independent living, the energy equivalent of walking about 17 miles/day is required to be in the Very Active category. The PAL for this category will range from 1.90 to 2.50, but the PA coefficient for the formula is set at 1.42–1.56 depending on gender and stage of life. Individuals who walk 3.75–4 hours, or jog 1.75 hours, daily generally fit this category.

The following calculations on the 20-year-old 80-kg male provide EER values based on PA coefficients of 1.11, 1.25, and 1.48 for the Low Active, Active, and Very Active categories, respectively.

Low Active:
$$EER = 662 - (9.53 \times 20) + [1.11 \times (15.91 \times 80 + 539.6 \times 1.8)]$$
$$= 2,962 \text{ Calories}$$

Active:
$$EER = 662 - (9.53 \times 20) + [1.25 \times (15.91 \times 80 + 539.6 \times 1.8)]$$
$$= 3,276 \text{ Calories}$$

Very Active:
$$EER = 662 - (9.53 \times 20) + [1.48 \times (15.91 \times 80 + 539.6 \times 1.8)]$$
$$= 3,793 \text{ Calories}$$

As his EER for the Sedentary category is 2,715 Calories, he would need to expend about 247,561, or 1,078 Calories through physical activity to attain, respectively, the Low Active, Active, and Very Active PAL categories.

The Compendium of Physical Activity (https://sites.google.com/site/compendiumofphysicalactivities/) was introduced in chapter 3 with an explanation of how it may be used to estimate caloric expenditure through physical activity. You may wish to review that discussion. Appendix B provides estimated total (resting + exercise) Calories/minute as a function of MET value and body mass. For example, the estimated rate of total caloric expenditure for a 176-lb (80-kg) individual exercising at an intensity of 10 METS is 14.0 Calories/min. The total caloric cost of an activity can be calculated using METS, body weight in kg, and minutes of activity, as described in table 11.2. The following weekly physical activity log for an 80-kg male uses MET intensities from the Compendium of Physical Activities and the duration of the activities to calculate total weekly and average daily caloric expenditure. Thus, with an average daily energy expenditure through physical activity totaling 640 Calories, he is in the Active PAL category and can use that formula to calculate his EER. Alternatively, he may simply add the 640 Calories to his Sedentary EER to determine the number of Calories needed to maintain his body weight if it has been stable. Using the formula for the Active category, his EER as noted would total 3,276 Calories. Adding the 640 Calories to his Sedentary category EER of 2,715 would total 3,355 Calories. The difference between the two estimates is negligible in this case but may vary some in other cases.

Using this same procedure, you may calculate your EER to maintain your normal body weight. Use the formula in table 11.1 that is appropriate for your gender and age and, using the appropriate PA values from table 11.2, calculate your EER for each of the four PAL categories. Next, as per the previous example, record the type and amount of time devoted to various physical activities

Day	PA	Compendium Code	METS	Weight	Calories/minute	Duration	Total Calories*
Mon	Tennis, singles	15690	8.0	80	11.2	40	448
	Walking, 3 mph	17190	3.5	80	4.9	20	98
Tues	Running, 7 mph	12070	11.0	80	15.4	40	616
Wed	Tennis, singles	15690	8.0	80	11.2	40	448
	Walking, 3 mph	17190	3.5	80	4.9	20	98
Thurs	Running, 8 mph	12090	11.8	80	16.52	30	496
Fri	Tennis, singles	15690	8.0	80	11.2	40	448
	Bowling	15090	3.0	80	4.2	30	126
Sat	Golf, carrying clubs	15365	4.3	80	6.02	180	1,084
Sun	Running, 7 mph	12070	11.0	80	15.4	40	616
Total weekly Calories *(= Exercise Calories + Resting Calories)							4,477
Average daily Calories *(= Total weekly Calories ÷ 7 days)							640

TABLE 11.2 Physical Activity Level (PAL) Categories with conversion of MET values for two walking and jogging activities to Total Calories based on weight and duration of activity

PAL Category	PAL	Activity Description*	METS*	Weight (kg)	Minutes	Total Calories[†]	Physical Activity Coefficient			
							Males	Females	Boys	Girls
Sedentary	≥1.0 to <1.4	Only Activities of Daily Living with walking <30 minutes/day					1.00	1.00	1.00	1.00
Low Active	≥1.4 to <1.6	Walking, 2.8–3.2 mph	3.5	80	50	245	1.11	1.12	1.13	1.16
		Jogging, general	7.0	80	25	245				
Active	≥1.6 to <1.9	Walking, 2.8–3.2 mph	3.5	80	115	563.5	1.25	1.27	1.26	1.31
		Jogging, general	7.0	80	57.5	563.5				
Very Active	≥1.9 to <2.5	Walking, 2.8–3.2 mph	3.5	80	220	1078	1.48	1.45	1.42	1.56
		Jogging, general	7.0	80	110	1078				

*From the Compendium of Physical Activties, https://sites.google.com/site/compendiumofphysicalactivities/.
Click on the Activity Categories tab, such as walking or running.
[†]Total Calories = METS × 3.5 ml/kg/min × body weight (kg)÷1,000 mL/liter O_2 × 5 Cal/liter O_2 × minutes of activity.
Total Calories = Exercise Calories + Resting Calories

over the course of a week and calculate your average daily physical activity energy expenditure; you may then either add this amount to your Sedentary EER or use the appropriate formula to estimate your total daily EER.

Estimated Energy Requirement (EER) ChooseMyPlate Technique You may more easily calculate your EER by using the SuperTracker program available in the *ChooseMyPlate* Website. When you join, you enter your age, height, and weight, which are used as part of the basis to calculate your EER and can be updated as needed. There are two options available. In step #1

of creating a profile, you may select one of the following three options of moderate-intensity physical activity: <30 min/day, 30–60 min/day, or 60+ min/day. This option may not generate results that are as accurate as option 4, where one may enter specific activities for a day or a week such as in the table above. You may also create an account and save your profile. For option 4, you must enter all activities you performed in the past 24 hours, including sleeping, eating, sitting while reading or watching television, personal hygiene, housework, transportation, employment, leisure, and exercise. The total duration of these activities should add up to 1,440 minutes (24 hours).

An accurate description of your physical activity over a typical week will provide a good estimate of your EER. Using Physical Activity Tracker, type one of your activities in the search window and click "Go." Under activity details, provide the duration (minutes/session) and designate the days/week you participated in this activity. For convenience, you can designate activities as "Favorite Activities" and also copy activities on multiple days. For example, jogging (selected activity = Jogging, general) for 45 minutes four days per week totals 180 minutes per week, or an average of 26 minutes daily. Physical activity data linked to a created profile will provide estimated calories burned. For example, the 45 minutes of jogging by a 71" tall (1.8 m) 59 year old male weighing 145 pounds (65.9 kg) will burn an estimated 456 exercise Calories/session which is 1824 exercise Calories/week or 261 (=1824/7) exercise Calories/day. Calculate a daily average for other activities as well. Once you input the data, you can generate and save a physical activity report by selecting the "My Report" option at the top of the page.

Mayo Clinic Calorie Calculator   The prestigious Mayo Clinic provides a computerized estimate of daily energy needs based on age, gender, height, weight, and level of physical activity ranging from sedentary to very active. The estimated daily energy needs may be found at the Mayo Clinic Website, www.mayoclinic.org/calorie-calculator/itt-20084939.

Calorie Counting Technique   If your body weight has been stable, keeping track of the Calories you eat for 3–7 days may provide you with a good estimate of your daily energy requirement. Eat your normal diet, but record everything you consume. Some guidelines for measuring, recording, and calculating your daily caloric intake are presented later in this chapter. Computerized dietary analysis programs are available to facilitate this task. For example, the MyTracker program also has a dietary analysis program to assess your daily caloric intake.

How much weight can I lose safely per week?

If you decide to lose weight without medical supervision, keep in mind that the recommended maximal weight loss is 2 pounds per week. Because there are 3,500 Calories in a pound of body fat, this would necessitate a deficit of 7,000 Calories for the week, or 1,000 Calories per day. For growing children who carry excess fat, the general recommendation is about 1 pound per week, or a daily 500-Calorie deficit. Keep in mind that these are *maximal* recommended weight-loss values for medically unsupervised programs. Lower weight-loss goals, such as 1 pound per week for adults and 1/2 pound per week for children and adolescents, may be more appropriate, realizable goals. These recommendations are in line with the American College of Sports Medicine position stand on weight loss by Donnelly and others.

As we shall see later in this chapter, weight losses may not parallel the caloric deficit we incur during early stages of a weight-reduction program, and the 2-pound limit may be adjusted during this time period. In addition, as mentioned previously, we want our weight loss to be body-fat tissue, not lean body mass. A loss of 10 pounds of body weight may help improve physical performance, but if 5 pounds is muscle tissue, then performance could deteriorate. Thus, you should monitor your weight loss not only with a scale but also with skinfolds and girth measures, or other body-composition procedures, discussed in chapter 10, to help ensure that you are losing body fat, and in the right places.

How can I determine the amount of body weight I need to lose?

As noted in chapter 10, individuals desire to lose weight for one of three reasons—to improve appearance, health, or physical performance. As for your appearance, you are the judge, but consult with your physician or other health professional. You do not want your weight-loss program to induce an eating disorder. Losing excess body fat for health is a good reason. Check with your physician, who can also monitor increases in blood pressure, serum lipids, blood glucose, and visceral adiposity that are associated with excess body weight. A loss of 5–10 percent body weight or 2–4 inches off the waist, easily achieved in 3–4 months, may help reduce several health risk factors. Losing weight in attempts to enhance physical performance should involve interactions between the athlete, coach, and team physician; in the case of young athletes, parents should also be involved. The National Athletic Trainers' Association Position Stand, authored by Turocy and colleagues, recommends the most scientific assessment for body composition for athletes in order to identify competitive weights for sports requirements while allowing for appropriate energy and nutritional intake.

In their review, Lowe and Timko commented that dieting safety and effectiveness depend on who is attempting to lose weight as well as the motives and strategies for losing weight. The same reasoning applies for appearance and physical performance standards. They note that pursuit of an unrealistic ideal may lead to various health problems.

Several procedures may be used to estimate desired weight loss. Using the body mass index (BMI) as a guide, you will need to calculate your current BMI and determine your target BMI. Calculation of the BMI was presented in chapter 10 and a healthy BMI range is approximately 18.5–25. The formula to calculate your desired body weight in kilograms is

$$\text{Target body weight (kg)} = \text{Target BMI} \times \text{Height in meters}^2$$

As an example, if you are 5′7″ (1.70 meters) tall and weigh 170 pounds (77.2 kilograms), then you have a BMI of 26.7 ($77.2/1.70^2$). If you want to achieve a healthier BMI of 24, simply multiply 24 by 1.70^2 to determine your body-weight goal; 24 times 2.89 equals 69.4 kilograms, or 153 pounds. The desired weight loss would be 17 pounds (170–153), which represents a 10 percent reduction in total body weight ($17/170 = 0.10$; $0.10 \times 100\% = 10\%$).

If you want to use body-fat percentage as the guide to weight loss, you will need to measure your current body-fat percentage and determine your target goal. Methods of determining body-fat percentage are presented in appendix C. If you are an athlete with 20 percent body fat who desires to get down to 15 percent, you may use the following formula:

$$\text{Target body weight} = \frac{\text{Lean body mass in pounds}}{1.00 - \text{Desired body-fat percentage}}$$

As an example, an athlete who weighs 150 pounds and is 20 percent body fat has 30 pounds of body fat, and the remaining 120 pounds (150–30) is lean body mass. Substituting in the formula provides the following data:

$$\frac{120}{1.00-0.15} = \frac{120}{0.85} = 141 \text{ pounds}$$

Thus, this athlete would need to lose 9 pounds of body fat (150–141) to achieve a 15 percent body-fat percentage. If proper methods of weight loss are used, as discussed later in this chapter, the losses will be in body fat, not lean body mass.

Key Concepts

▶ One pound of body fat contains about 3,500 Calories.

▶ The caloric deficit, which represents caloric intake minus caloric expenditure, may be useful as a means to predict body-weight losses on a long-term basis, because 3,500 Calories equal approximately 1 pound of body fat.

▶ Various procedures are available to estimate daily energy requirements. Although all are estimates, calculating the Estimated Energy Requirement from 24-hour records of activity will provide the best estimate. A program on ChooseMyPlate provides a computerized analysis of estimated daily energy requirements.

▶ For the overweight adult who desires to lose weight without the guidance of a health professional, the recommended maximal weight loss is 2 pounds per week. Losing 1 pound a week is a more reasonable goal. Weight loss in children and adolescents should be about half the recommendations for adults.

Check for Yourself

▶ Based on your age, gender, height, and weight, calculate your Estimated Energy Expenditure (EER) for a sedentary lifestyle based on the formula in table 11.1. Use a PA value of 1.0. Compare this value to your REE determined in chapter 3. Using the guidelines presented in the text, you may also wish to calculate your EER based on your daily physical activity level.

▶ If you want to lose weight, use the text information to determine an appropriate total weight loss and recommended weight loss per week.

Behavior Modification

What is behavior modification?

In his book *Mindless Eating: Why We Eat More Than We Think,* Wansink indicates that we make numerous food-related decisions every day. Most of these decisions are made at the subconscious level, many triggered by cues in the food environment that modify our behavior and encourage us to eat more.

One of the key components of a successful weight-control program is the need to identify and modify those behaviors that contribute to the weight problem. The subject of human behavior development and change is very complex, but psychologists note that three factors are generally involved: the physical environment, the social environment, and the personal environment. For the person with a weight problem, a refrigerator brimming with food (physical environment), a family that consumes high-Calorie snack foods around the house (social environment), and an acquired taste for high-fat or sweet foods (personal environment) may trigger behaviors that make it very difficult to maintain a proper body weight.

A model often used to explain the development or modification of health behaviors, such as a proper diet and exercise program for weight control, involves three steps: knowledge, values, and behavior. First, proper knowledge is essential. A considerable amount of misinformation relative to the roles of nutrition and exercise in weight control exists, so you need to possess accurate information. Second, the health implications of this knowledge may help you develop a set of personal values, or attitudes, toward a specific health behavior. If you perceive excess body fat as a threat to your personal physical or psychological health, you are more likely to initiate behavioral changes. Third, your health behavior should then reflect the knowledge you acquired and the values you developed.

Behavior modification is a technique often used in psychological therapy to elicit desirable behavioral changes. The rationale underlying behavior modification is that many behavioral patterns are learned via stimulus-response conditioning; for example, a stimulus in your environment such as a commercial break in a television program elicits a response of a mad dash to the refrigerator. Because such responses are learned, they also may be unlearned. For a discussion of a comprehensive program conducted by a behavioral psychologist, the reader is referred to the review by Brownell and Kramer.

Relative to a self-designed program of weight control, behavior modification is used primarily to reduce or eliminate physical or social stimuli that may lead to excessive caloric intake or decreased physical activity. In his book, Bray noted that the most important component of any weight-control program is the associated behavior modification through which the individual learns new ways to deal with old problems. In a study stressing the importance of behavior modification, Haus and others recommended that potential weight-program participants learn and practice the weight-maintenance behavior of reduced dietary fat and regular exercise, independent of and before any weight-reduction attempts. The Consumers Union notes that exercising more and switching to a leaner, healthier diet will yield innumerable health benefits even if you don't lose a single pound.

How do I apply behavior-modification techniques in my weight-control program?

Willpower and self-discipline are keys to changing any habit. The individual is ultimately responsible for achieving goals associated with behavioral change. The overweight person must *want* to lose weight, *understand* the adverse effects of overweight and inactivity on health, and *take responsibility* for achieving the goal of weight loss. The individual must *value* the effect of weight loss on enhancement of life, establish weight loss as a high-priority goal, *adopt behaviors* that are consistent with goal attainment, and be willing to tolerate some discomfort in initiating change. According to Thomas and colleagues, the majority of National Weight Control Registry participants are successful in maintaining the majority of weight loss of 10 percent weight loss over 10 years through sustained behavioral change. Ultimately, the desire to lose weight must be greater than the desire to overeat or remain sedentary. Your cerebrum, the higher cognitive control center of the brain, must learn to control the hypothalamus, the subconscious appetite center.

Both long-range and short-range realistic goals should be established. Several experts in weight control, such as Tremblay and Wadden, indicated that for overweight individuals, a 10–15 percent weight loss is a reasonable goal over 4–6 months. For example, a 300-pound individual may want to lose 30 pounds (10 percent) over 6 months, whereas a short-range goal would be to lose about 1–2 pounds per week. Losing 30 pounds may seem like a daunting task, but setting small goals, a few pounds at a time, is one of the keys to success indicated by the National Weight Control Registry. A long-range goal may also include a large number of behavioral changes to achieve the 30-pound weight loss, but the number of changes would be phased in gradually on a short-term basis. As illustrated in figure 11.2, it will take time and patience to implement all behavioral changes and accomplish all goals.

As the saying goes, nothing breeds success like success, so it is extremely important to set short-term goals that may be attainable in a reasonable length of time so that you experience multiple successes in pursuit of your long-term goal. When you achieve your first short-term goal, a new short-term goal should be established as you progress toward your long-term goal. It is also important to remember that no initial short-term goal is too small, nor is any new short-term goal too small in the progress toward your long-term goal.

https://goramsey.co.ramsey.mn.us/Documents/adult_fitness_ideas.pdf This Website contains 171 small steps to a healthier diet and increased physical activity. As you achieve each short-term goal, you should reward yourself with something appropriate to the occasion in order to provide positive feedback for your commitment to your weight-loss program. One example might be to purchase a new pair of designer jeans with your lower waist measurement to encourage you to continue with your program.

One of the first steps in a behavior-modification program is to identify physical and social environmental factors that may lead to problem behaviors. Keeping a diary of your daily activities in your daily planner for a week or two may help you identify some behavioral patterns that may contribute to overeating, inactivity

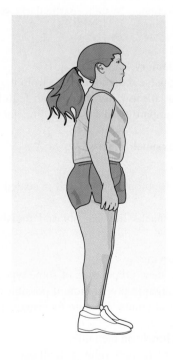 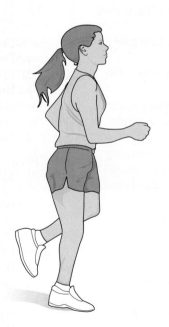 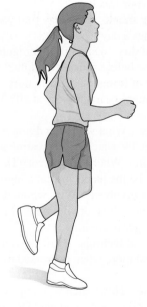

Time	Baseline	1 month (short-term)	6 months (long-term)
Weight	150	144	120
Weight loss		6	30
Activity goal		Run 1 mile nonstop	Run 5 miles nonstop

FIGURE 11.2 Goal setting is an important factor in an exercise program.

Record of 24-hour diet and physical activity

Time of day	Activity	Total minutes	Meal or snack	Degree of hunger*	Activity while eating	Place of eating	Food and quantity	Others present	Reason for choice

Note: Record time, activity such as sleeping, sitting, watching TV, and exercise, and minutes of activity. For meals, fill in the other columns. You may also use these columns for comments regarding activities other than eating. You can expand this table to incorporate a 24-hour period of time. Entering the data into a computer, such as in a Microsoft Excel format, may be helpful.
*Degree of hunger: 0 = none; 1 = little; 2 = moderate; 3 = high.

Self-discipline, self-control, and advanced planning:

1. Establish realistic weight-loss goals. A loss of 10 percent can produce significant health benefits.
2. Establish weight loss as a high priority; commit to permanent lifestyle changes.
3. Think about this priority before eating.
4. Take small helpings deliberately as a means to control your weight.
5. Plan for a modest daily energy deficit, about 300–500 Calories, which will result in a gradual weight loss.
6. Check your body weight and shape on a regular basis, either daily or two or three times a week. Use this as a motivational tool.

and extra body weight. The following are some of the factors that might be recorded each time you eat, along with a brief explanation of their possible importance. You should also record your daily physical activity. You may use the record of 24-hour activity form as a guide, which also may help in the calculation of your EER in the MyTracker program.

Type of food and amount   This may be related to the other factors. For example, do you eat a high-Calorie food during your snacks?

Meal or snack   You may find yourself snacking four or five times a day.

Time of day   Do you eat at regular hours or have a full meal just before retiring at night?

Degree of hunger   How hungry were you when you ate—very hungry or not hungry at all? You may be snacking when not hungry.

Activity   What were you doing while eating? You may find that TV watching and eating snack foods are related.

Location   Where do you eat? The office or school cafeteria may be the place you eat a high-Calorie meal.

Persons involved   With whom do you eat? Do you eat more when alone or with others? Being with certain people may trigger overeating.

Emotional feelings   How do you feel when eating? You might eat more when depressed than when happy, or vice versa.

Exercise   How much walking, stair climbing, or regular aerobic exercise do you get? Do you ride when you could walk? How much time do you just sit?

Recording this information may make you more aware of the physical and social circumstances under which you tend to overeat or be physically inactive. This awareness may be useful to help implement behavioral changes that may make weight control easier. The following suggestions are often helpful:

Foods to eat:
1. Use low-Calorie, healthful foods for snacks.
2. Plan low-Calorie, high-nutrient meals.
3. Plan your food intake for the entire day.
4. Eat only foods that have had minimal or no processing.
5. Allow yourself very small amounts of high-Calorie foods that you like, but stay within daily caloric limitations.
6. Know the Food Exchange System, particularly serving size and high-fat foods.

Food purchasing:
1. Do not shop when hungry.
2. Prepare a shopping list and do not deviate from it.
3. Buy only foods that are low in Calories and high in nutrient value. Read and compare food labels to limit fat and sugar content.
4. Buy natural foods as much as possible.

Food storage:
1. Keep high-Calorie food out of sight and in sealed containers or cupboards.
2. Have low-Calorie snacks like carrots and radishes readily available.

Food preparation and serving:
1. Buy only foods that need preparation of some type.
2. Do not add fats or sugar in preparation, if possible.
3. Prepare only small amounts. Be able to visualize 1 serving size for any given food.
4. Do not use serving bowls on the table.
5. Put the food on the plate, preferably a small one.

Location:
1. Eat in only one place, such as the kitchen or dining area.
2. Avoid food areas such as the kitchen or snack table at a party.
3. Avoid restaurants where you are most likely to buy high-Calorie items.

Restaurant eating:

1. When eating out, select the low-Calorie items.
2. Request that your meals be prepared without fat.
3. Have condiments like butter, mayonnaise, and salad dressing served on the side; use sparingly.
4. Order water, not a high-Calorie beverage.
5. Be wary of portion sizes, as most restaurant servings contain 2–3 normal servings. Ask for a take-home box before you eat, and put half of your meal in the box.

Methods of eating:

1. Eat slowly; chew food thoroughly or drink water between bites.
2. Eat with someone, for conversation can slow down the eating process.
3. Cut food into small pieces.
4. Do not do anything else while eating, such as watching TV.
5. Relax and enjoy the meal.
6. Eat only at specified times.
7. Eat only until pleasantly satisfied, not stuffed.
8. Spread your Calories over the day, eating small amounts more often.

Activity:

1. Decrease the amount of time spent in sedentary activities. Increase the amount of nonexercise activity thermogenesis (NEAT) by moving more and sitting less.
2. Walk more. Park the car or get off the bus some distance from work. Briskly walk the dog.
3. Use the stairs instead of the elevator when possible.
4. Do *exercise snacks*. Take a brisk 10-minute walk instead of a coffee-donut break. Do this several times a day.
5. Get involved in activities with other people, preferably physical activities that will burn Calories.
6. Avoid sedentary night routines.
7. Start a regular exercise program, including both aerobic and resistance exercises.
8. Schedule exercise as an appointment in your daily planner.

Sleep and stress reduction:

1. Try to get 7 to 8 hours of sleep each night.
2. Reduce emotional stress; try yoga or other stress-reduction techniques.

Mental attitude:

1. Recognize that you are not perfect and lapses may occur.
2. Deal positively with your lapse; put it behind you and get back on your program.
3. Put reminders on the refrigerator door at home or on your telephone at work.
4. Reward yourself for sticking to your plans.

For the interested reader, the books by Dusek and Miller provide an in-depth coverage of behavior modification for weight-control purposes. Many of the commercial, medically oriented weight-loss centers, as well as organizations such as Weight Watchers International, also may be sources of information. Self-taught, self-administered weight-loss programs may also be very effective, as indicated in the study by Miller and his associates.

Stress-reduction techniques may also be important in a weight-control program. Dallman comments that emotional stress can adversely affect weight control by increasing cortisol release, which conserves fat and increases hunger, and by degrading executive function whereby thoughtful responses are replaced by formed habits such as overeating. Exercise in itself may help reduce emotional stress, as may various relaxation techniques such as meditation and yoga.

Lack of adequate sleep may contribute to weight gain. In a study with more than a thousand subjects, Taheri and others concluded that getting less than 7 to 8 hours of sleep per night, such as only 4 to 5 hours, may decrease serum leptin and increase serum ghrelin levels, leading to an increased appetite and possible weight gain. In their meta-analysis of 45 studies conducted worldwide on almost 640,000 children and adults, Cappuccio and colleagues reported significant associations between short sleep duration and obesity. More research is needed to identify potential mechanisms and confounders to an association between sleep duration and weight gain.

Individuals with clinical obesity may need professional assistance from health counselors to implement a behavior-modification program for weight control. However, others with less severe weight problems may be able to initiate their own program if they have adequate accurate information.

Research has shown that most individuals initiating a weight-loss program do use acceptable strategies, such as exercising and eating a low-fat, low-Calorie diet, but use of these strategies becomes inconsistent in subsequent years, resulting in weight regain.

The 2009 Academy of Nutrition and Dietetics (formerly the American Dietetic Association) position statement on weight management by Seagle and colleagues commented that successful weight management requires a lifelong commitment to healthful, enjoyable, and sustainable eating behaviors and daily physical activity. The remainder of this chapter focuses on the development of a proper lifelong diet and exercise program for losing weight safely and keeping it off. What usually happens is that individuals suffer a lapse in the weight-loss program, such as an injury that prevents participation in their normal exercise program. If they do not have an alternative exercise program, some weight gain may occur until they can resume exercising. Brownell, in the LEARN (Lifestyle, Exercise, Attitudes, Relationships, Nutrition) program for weight control, indicates that one of the keys in weight control is to prevent a lapse from becoming a relapse, or a resumption of old behaviors and total weight regain. When a lapse occurs, Brownell recommends that you stay calm, analyze the lapse, and renew your diet and exercise commitment. By analyzing your lapse, you should be able to find a solution to help you get back on track. If unable to do so, seek some assistance from a qualified health professional.

Key Concepts

▶ Keeping a record of your daily eating habits will help you identify behavioral patterns relative to overeating and may be used as a basis for the elimination of cues that trigger eating.

▶ Behavior modification is a very important part of a weight-control program. For weight control to be effective over a lifetime, you may need to adjust dietary and exercise behaviors to curtail caloric intake and increase energy expenditure.

Check for Yourself

▶ Using information presented in the text, keep a record of your dietary and physical activity behaviors for a period of 3–7 days. Compare your findings to the text discussion regarding dietary and physical activity behaviors that may help you maintain a healthy body weight.

Dietary Modifications

Numerous weight-loss dietary plans are available and each is based on some combination of macronutrient—carbohydrate, fat, protein—content. To achieve weight loss, the key to each diet plan is to consume fewer Calories than expended. Most diet plans do so. The Consumers Union rated 15 different diet books and plans varying in macronutrient content. The daily range was 1,340 to 1,910 Calories and most averaged about 1,500 Calories, an energy intake that would lead to weight loss in most individuals.

As we shall see, there are high-carbohydrate, high-fat, and high-protein diets, and supporters for each. In a recent interview, Taubes, author of *Good Calories, Bad Calories,* indicates that the key to weight loss is to eat fewer carbohydrates. He recommends the original Atkins diet, which is basically a high-fat diet. In contrast, Dean Ornish, in his book *Eat More, Weigh Less,* recommends a diet containing 70 percent or more carbohydrate with no more than 10 percent fat. Barry Sears, who developed the Zone diet, stresses the importance of a high-protein diet.

A key concept of weight-loss diets supported by numerous studies is to consume fewer Calories than are expended. Moreover, as far as Calories are concerned, the macronutrient content of the diet is irrelevant. For example, in one study, Sacks and others assigned more than 800 subjects to one of four diets with an equal amount of Calories but varying percentages derived from carbohydrate (35 to 65 percent), fat (20 to 40 percent), and protein (15 to 25 percent). They reported that all diets resulted in meaningful weight loss, with no differences among them. To stress this point, Albers cites a case study of a professor of human nutrition who ate what was referred to as the Twinkie diet. Sixty percent of his caloric intake consisted of such items as cookies, chips, sugar cereal, snack cakes, and other sugary, processed foods, while the remaining 40 percent was healthier, such as vegetable snacks. However, total daily intake was limited to 1,600 Calories, much less than his total daily energy expenditure, and he lost 27 pounds in 10 weeks. Although not a recommended healthy diet for weight loss, it does support the point that it does not matter what you eat as long as your caloric intake is less than your daily caloric expenditure.

However, Foreyt and others note that although this "*a Calorie is a Calorie*" concept of weight control is valid as a metabolic unit,

its interpretation may be much more complex in the free-living situation. They note that the different diet-related factors that condition energy balance, including total energy intake, satiety and hunger sensory triggers, and palatability, must be considered when assessing the efficacy of weight-reducing diets of different macronutrient composition. These points are discussed later.

Sufficient evidence is available to provide prudent dietary guidelines for not only weight loss and maintenance but also health promotion. For example, Ma and others compared the dietary quality of popular weight-loss plans for their capacity to prevent cardiovascular disease, and we discussed the concepts of healthful sources of carbohydrate, fat, and protein in the DASH and OmniHeart diets in chapter 9. In general, healthful weight-control diets are based on selecting *good* carbohydrates, *good* fats, and *good* proteins. You can use the *ChooseMyPlate* food guide as a means to plan a healthful diet to achieve your desired body weight goal. In addition, the Academy of Nutrition and Dietetics Website provides sound advice on a number of weight-control topics.

www.ChooseMyPlate.gov Click Weight Management and Calories for guidance on what you *currently* eat and drink, what you *should* eat and drink, how to make better dietary choices, and how to increase activity.
www.eatright.org For weight control, click on *Public,* then *Healthy Weight.*

How can I determine the number of Calories needed in a diet to lose weight?

To answer this question you need to provide two figures. First, you need an estimate of how many Calories to consume daily to maintain your current body weight. As previously described, several techniques are available, so you should select one to provide an estimate of the number of Calories you may need to consume daily to maintain your current body weight. Second, you need an estimate of the amount of weight that you want to lose, as discussed on page 483, and then determine how much you want to lose per week. One pound is the preferable goal, but you may lose up to 2 pounds safely. Some computerized dietary analysis programs will calculate your estimated energy intake needed to lose about 1–2 pounds per week.

http://caloriecount.about.com/tools/calories-goal Consult this Website to provide a calculation of your daily caloric intake needed to achieve a given weight loss over a specified amount of time.
www.health24.com/Diet-and-nutrition/Tools/Am-I-eating-correctly-to-lose-weight-20130227 Take this quiz to check the health of your weight-loss diet.

For our purposes, we will use the value of 3,500 Calories to represent 1 pound of body-fat, or body-weight, loss. To lose 1 pound of body fat, you must create a 3,500-Calorie deficit. To lose 1 pound per week, your daily caloric deficit should be 500 (3,500/7). To lose 2 pounds per week, the recommended maximum unless under medical supervision, the daily caloric deficit should be 1,000 (7,000/7).

Once you calculate your daily energy needs to maintain your current body weight, simply subtract your daily caloric deficit from it; the result will be your recommended daily caloric intake. An example is presented below:

Example: 35-year-old female with low physical activity (PA = 1.12) who weighs 140 lbs (63.6 kg) and is 62.5 inches tall (1.59 m) desires to lose 1 pound per week

1. From tables 11.1 and 11.2—predicted number of Calories needed to maintain 140 pounds of body weight:

$$EER = 354 - (6.91 \times 30) + [1.12 \times (9.361 \times 63.6 \text{ kg} + 726 \times 1.59 \text{ m})] = 2{,}106 \text{ Calories}$$

2. Recommended daily caloric deficit = 500 Calories/day
3. Recommended daily caloric intake = 2,106 − 500 = 1,606

However, it is important to note that most health professionals do not recommend weight-loss diets lower than 1,000 Calories unless medically supervised.

How can I predict my body-weight loss through dieting alone?

As mentioned in chapter 10, the human body is composed of different components, most commonly compartmentalized into body fat and lean body mass; lean body mass is about 70 percent water. On a dietary program, weight loss may reflect decreases in body fat, body water, or muscle mass, all of which present different caloric values. For example, 1 pound of body fat equals about 3,500 Calories, whereas an equivalent weight of water contains no Calories. Because of this fact, it is difficult to predict exactly how much body weight one will lose on any given diet, but an approximate value of the time it will take to lose excess body fat may be obtained.

The key point is the caloric deficit. The number of days it takes for this daily deficit to reach 3,500 is how long it will take you to lose 1 pound.

Table 11.3 illustrates the importance of the caloric deficit in determining the rapidity of weight loss by dieting. This table is based upon the value of 3,500 Calories for a pound of body fat. The higher the deficit, the faster you lose weight. However, rapid weight-loss programs are not usually desirable, and the dieter should realize that a moderate caloric deficit, say 500 Calories/day, may effectively reduce weight in time and yet provide a satisfying diet. As noted later, however, as body weight is lost the caloric intake must be reduced slightly if one wants to maintain a standard daily caloric deficit.

Although these prediction methods are good for the long run, daily body-weight changes may not coincide with daily caloric deficits.

It is very important to note that although we are discussing dieting alone to create a daily caloric deficit, exercise also may be used to increase this deficit. When starting a weight-loss program,

the National Institutes of Health recommends that most of the 500–1,000 daily Calorie deficit be achieved by eating less food. However, 100–200 Calories of this deficit is achievable through daily exercise, such as walking for 30 minutes or so. Using exercise to contribute to your daily caloric deficit means your food caloric deficit may be reduced accordingly.

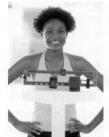

Why does a person usually lose the most weight during the first week on a reducing diet?

The principal objective of a diet is to lose body fat, not just body weight. If you start a diet with a significant caloric deficit, say 1,000 Calories/day, it would normally take you about 3.5 days to lose 1 pound of body fat. However, body-weight loss would be more rapid than this during the first several days, possibly totaling as much as 3–4 pounds. A large percentage of this weight loss would be due to a decrease in body carbohydrate and associated water stores. When you restrict your food intake, the body will use its reserves to meet its energy needs. These reserves consist of both fat and carbohydrate stores, but much of the carbohydrate, stored as liver and muscle glycogen, could be used up in several days, particularly with low carbohydrate intake, such as the Atkins diet. The use of stored glycogen for energy during a caloric deficit could result in significant early weight loss because 1 gram of glycogen is stored with about 3 grams of water. For example, 300 grams of glycogen, along with 900 grams of water stored with it, would account for a loss of

TABLE 11.3	Approximate number of days required to lose weight for a given caloric deficit				
Daily caloric deficit	To lose 5 pounds	To lose 10 pounds	To lose 15 pounds	To lose 20 pounds	To lose 25 pounds
100	175	350	525	700	875
200	87	175	262	350	438
300	58	116	175	232	292
400	44	88	131	176	219
500	35	70	105	140	175
600	29	58	87	116	146
700	25	50	75	100	125
800	22	44	66	88	109
900	19	39	58	78	97
1,000	17	35	52	70	88
1,250*	14	28	42	56	70
1,500*	12	23	35	46	58

See text for explanation.

*Note: Weight loss more than 2 pounds per week generally not recommended.

1,200 grams, or 1.2 kilograms; this would equal more than 2.5 pounds alone. About 70 percent of the weight loss during the first few days of a reduced-Calorie diet may be due to body-water losses. About 25 percent comes from body-fat stores and 5 percent from protein tissue. As body protein is used for energy, the excess nitrogen has to be excreted, and this increases water output, about 4–5 grams of water per gram of protein. As noted later, very low-Calorie diets may lead to greater protein losses, but slower weight losses, such as with a daily 500-Calorie deficit, will help conserve body protein.

If you desired to lose a maximal amount of weight during a 2- to 3-day period, water restriction would cause an even greater weight loss. However, this practice is not recommended, as you would only be decreasing body-water levels. As discussed in chapter 9, normal hydration is important for many physiological functions, including regulation of core temperature. Body water levels would return to normal when you returned to normal water intake. There is one additional point relative to body water. At the conclusion of your diet, if you return to a normal caloric diet to maintain your new body weight, you may experience a rapid weight gain of 2 or 3 pounds. This may represent a replenishment of your body glycogen stores with the accompanying water weight. It is important to keep in mind that rather large fluctuations in daily body weight, say in the order of 2 to 3 pounds, are not due to rapid changes in body fat or lean body mass. Instead, these fluctuations are due primarily to body-water changes accompanying carbohydrate and protein losses.

Why does it become more difficult to lose weight after several weeks or months on a diet program?

Weight loss may be rapid during the first few days on a diet, primarily because of water loss. Because water contains no Calories, caloric loss does not have to total 3,500 to lose 1 pound of weight. We may lose 1 pound of body weight with a deficit of only about 1,200 Calories, because 70 percent of the weight loss is water. The 1,200 Calories are mostly from fat with a small amount of protein. However, by the end of the second week of dieting, water loss may account for only about 20 percent of body-weight loss; 1 pound of weight loss will now cost us approximately 2,800 Calories. At the end of the 3 week, water losses are minimal. The energy deficit to lose 1 pound of body weight now approximates 3,500 Calories. In essence, as you continue your diet, weight losses cost you more Calories because less body water is being lost. At the end of 3 weeks, you still can be losing weight, but at a much slower rate than during the early stages.

Another factor also slows down the rate of weight loss. As you lose weight, you need fewer Calories to maintain your new body weight. As an example, a 200-pound (90.9 kg), 72.25-inch (1.84-m), active (PA = 1.25) male recreational athlete desires to decrease his weight to 180 pounds in 10 weeks. Using the information in tables 11.1 and 11.2, he would need approximately 3,501 Calories to maintain 200 pounds and a 1,000-Calorie/day deficit (2,501 dietary Calories/day) to lose 20 lbs in 10 weeks.

$$EER = 662 - (9.53 \times 22) + (1.25 \times (15.91 \times 90.9 + 539.6 \times 1.84))$$
$$= 3,501 \text{ Calories}$$

Daily caloric intake = 3,501 − 1,000 = 2,501 Calories

After 10 weeks, his new EER would be 3,320 Calories based on the lower body weight of 180 pounds, a difference of 181 calories.

$$EER = 662 - (9.53 \times 22) + (1.25 \times (15.91 \times 81.8 + 539.6 \times 1.84))$$
$$= 3,320 \text{ Calories}$$

Difference between 200-pound EER and 180-pound
EER = 3,501 − 3,320 = 181 Calories

If the athlete wanted to continue losing weight at a rate of 2 pounds/week, he would need to continue a 1,000-Calorie/day deficit based on the new EER of 3,320 Calories to maintain 180 lbs.

New daily caloric intake = 3,320 − 1,000 = 2,320 Calories

If he did not adjust his diet from 3,320 Calories, then the daily deficit would only be 819 Calories/day (3,320 − 2,501), not the standard 1,000 he wanted. Weight loss would continue, but at a slower rate.

You should realize that the rate of weight loss will slow as a natural consequence of your diet, but the weight you are losing at that point is primarily body fat. Depending on how much weight you want to lose, maintaining a standard caloric deficit may require additional reductions in caloric intake as you progress on your diet. Knowledge of these factors may help you through the latter stages of a diet designed to attain a set weight goal. Other factors associated with very low-Calorie diets and exercise, discussed later, may also influence the magnitude of the caloric intake necessary to sustain a given rate of weight loss.

What are the major characteristics of a sound diet for weight control?

Many different diet plans are available to help you lose weight. Diet books frequently appear on the *New York Times* Bestseller List. These diet plans are recycled over the years as variations of the same themes. Although some of these plans satisfy the criteria for safe and effective weight loss and can be highly recommended, others may be nutritionally deficient or even potentially hazardous to health. Fad diets should be avoided. Diets that restrict or eliminate various foods, including one-food diets such as the rice diet or the bananas-and-milk diet, may be deficient in certain key nutrients. Miracle diets that claim to contain a special weight-reducing formula or fat-burning enzymes should be also avoided, for such compounds simply do not exist or are not effective. You should avoid diets that promise fast and easy weight losses because there *is* no fast and easy dietary method to lose excess body fat. In their meta-analysis, Johnston and others noted significant and similar weight losses with low-carbohydrate and low-fat diets. In their study of metabolic syndrome patients, Ma and colleagues reported that meaningful weight loss occurred following a simple diet emphasizing only increased intake of fiber and may be preferred to a more complicated diet. These two studies underscore the potential effectiveness of any diet to which a given individual will adhere, provided the diet has reduced total energy content and appropriate nutrient density.

Carbohydrate, fat, and protein, and alcohol for those who drink, are the only dietary sources of Calories. Alcohol is not an essential nutrient but as noted later may play a significant role in weight gain. The majority of our dietary Calories come from carbohydrate and fat, with smaller amounts from protein. As you may recall, the National Academy of Sciences has published an Acceptable Macronutrient Distribution Range (AMDR) for carbohydrate, fat, and protein, which represents the percent of dietary Calories that should be derived from each.

- Carbohydrate AMDR: 45–65 percent
- Fat AMDR: 20–35 percent.
- Protein AMDR: 10–35 percent

Most popular weight-control diets have focused on limiting intake of either fat or carbohydrate, although some have stressed increased protein intake. Data comparing the caloric and macronutrient content of some popular diets are presented in table 11.4. The key point is that each diet is relatively low in Calories.

Riley has placed popular self-help weight-loss diets on a continuum of themes ranging from antifat to anticarbohydrate. The benefits and drawbacks of both the high-carbohydrate, low-fat (antifat) and low-carbohydrate, high-fat (anticarbohydrate) diets, along with diets somewhere between the two extremes, have been the subject of detailed reviews. In general, these reviews indicate that weight loss can be achieved with a variety of diet interventions, and that it is unlikely that one diet is optimal for all overweight or obese persons. Both low-fat and low-carbohydrate diets have been shown to induce weight loss and reduce obesity-related comorbidities. Reducing caloric intake is the key to the success of any diet. In a meta-analysis of 12 randomized clinical trials with a follow-up period of at least 12 months, Atallah and colleagues concluded that modest, long-term weight loss occurred with Atkins, Weight Watchers, and Zone diets and that no one diet could be viewed as more effective than other. All reduced-Calorie diets appear to be modestly successful in inducing modest weight loss. As noted previously, most studies indicate no significant differences in weight loss with diets of varying macronutrient content, provided caloric intake is similar. The interested reader is referred to the reviews by Brehm and D'Alessio and Nordmann.

Low-Fat, High-Carbohydrate Weight-Loss Diets   At the antifat end of Riley's continuum are diets such as those proposed by Dean Ornish and Nathan Pritikin, recommending that only 10–15 percent of dietary Calories be derived from fat, which is lower than the AMDR.

Reducing fat in the diet is a sound strategy to lose weight. The American College of Sports Medicine notes that a 10 percent reduction in fat intake can have a significant impact on energy balance and body weight over the long term. In a meta-analysis of 43 studies, Hooper and colleagues reported evidence for small but clinically meaningful reductions in weight and BMI 6 months to 8 years after low-fat intake compared to normal fat intake in children and adults. A 1 percent decrease in dietary fat intake was associated with a 0.19-kg (0.42-lb) decrease in weight.

Not all carbohydrates may be equal when it comes to weight loss, and some diets have focused on the glycemic index as the key to carbohydrate intake, as highlighted in such books as *The GI Diet* and *Good Carbs, Bad Carbs*. In his review on how to maintain a healthy body weight, Astrup indicated that the role of the glycemic index diet plan for body-weight control is controversial. Roberts indicates that consumption of high-glycemic-index (GI) carbohydrates may increase hunger and promote overeating compared to lower GI foods, but Das and others found that Calorie-restricted diets differing substantially in glycemic load (GL) can result in similar long-term weight loss. In their review, Esfahani and others found greater weight loss with low GI/GL diets or insignificant trends favoring low GI/GL diets in promoting weight loss. Thomas and others examined the outcomes of six studies and reported greater weight loss and improved lipid profiles following low GI/GL diets compared to higher GI/GL diets. Pittas and Roberts suggest the importance of individualized diet plans based on insulin sensitivity and other metabolic factors. Ebbeling and others note that reducing glycemic load may be especially important to achieve weight loss among individuals with high insulin secretion. According to Olsen and Heitmann, there is consistent evidence for a strong association between sugar-sweetened beverage (SSB) intake and weight gain. Avery and others report that educational and fluid replacement interventions may reduce consumption of SSB and subsequent weight gain in children. Added sugar accounts for about 16 percent of the daily caloric intake of average Americans. The U.S. Food and Drug Administration is proposing the inclusion of "added sugars" on food labels.

Proposed changes to the Nutrition Facts Label.   Go to www.fda.gov/; then click "Food," then "Guidance & Regulation," then "Guidance Documents Regulatory Information," then "Labeling and Nutrition," then "Proposed Changes to the Nutrition Facts Label."

As noted in chapter 4, *good* carbohydrates are rich in dietary fiber, which may play an important role in weight-loss diets. Howarth and others reported strong relationships between BMI and intake of fiber and fat, especially in women. A six-fold increase in overweight or obesity was observed in women consuming a low-fiber, high-fat diet compared to those consuming a high-fiber, low-fat diet. In 26 studies of normal-weight and overweight populations, Pol and colleagues reported a small effect of

TABLE 11.4   Calorie and macronutrient content of popular diets

Diet plan	Average daily calories	% carbohydrates	% fat	% protein
Weight Watchers	1,450	56	24	20
Atkins	1,520	11	60	29
South Beach	1,340	38	39	23
Volumetrics	1,500	55	23	22
Jenny Craig	1,520	62	18	20
Zone	1,660	40	30	30
Ornish	1,520	77	6	17

Adapted from Consumers Union. 2005. Rating the diets. *Consumer Reports* 70 (6):21.

whole-grain intake in reducing body fat, but not weight. In their meta-analysis, Ramage and others found increased fiber intake was the third most successful diet-related weight-loss strategy behind reduced energy and fat. Increasing fiber from 15 to the recommended 25–38 grams/day may be an effective component of weight loss. According to Ford and Frost, the action of gut bacteria on fermentable fiber found in a low GI diet may stimulate hormonal secretions to suppress appetite. Fiber also increases the volume of the food you eat, which can suppress hunger.

A fiber-rich diet is the principle underlying popular diet books such as *The Volumetrics Eating Plan* and *Eat More, Weigh Less.*

In a comparison of National Weight Control Registry groups who are weight-stable or struggling with weight, Ogden and others reported that weight-stable groups consumed approximately 1,400 Calories/day, with carbohydrate, fat, and protein intakes of 53–54, 26–27, and 18 percent, respectively. They also ate breakfast at least 6 days/week, engaged in regular physical activity, and reported less difficulty maintaining weight. A low-fat or moderate-fat, high-carbohydrate weight-loss diet may be effective, but selection of nutrient-dense carbohydrates is the key. Although some have suggested that low-fat diets may induce weight gain because of the increased carbohydrate in the diet, Howard and others found that such was not the case over the course of 7 years if vegetables, fruits, and whole grains replaced the dietary fat. As will be noted, the choice of the fat and protein content in a high-carbohydrate diet is also important.

Low-Carbohydrate, High-Fat Weight-Loss Diets

On Riley's anticarbohydrate end of the continuum are diets such as *Dr. Atkins' New Diet Revolution.* The Atkins diet has various phases, starting off as low as 20 grams of carbohydrate a day, mainly from nutrient-dense foods such as leafy green salads. The heart of the diet contains foods high in fat and protein, such as poultry, fish, red meat, and eggs, but gradually progresses to other stages with increasing amounts of carbohydrates, but much lower than AMDR levels. Such diets are also referred to as low-carbohydrate, high-fat, and high-protein weight-loss diets. The South Beach diet, by Agatston, limits saturated fats and focuses on healthier carbohydrates, which health professionals indicated appears to be a healthier version of the Atkins diet.

Research suggests that such diets may be effective. Liebman indicated that the Atkins diet may work because it virtually eliminates a whole category of food (carbohydrates), whereas a Tufts University report indicates that individuals who adopt the Atkins diet generally cut an average of 1,000 Calories per day from their diet, which is most likely the reason underlying its success. Correspondingly, Bravata and others reviewed 109 studies involving the use of low-carbohydrate diets and concluded that participant weight loss was principally associated with decreased caloric intake.

One of the criticisms of the Atkins diet was the possible adverse effects on the serum lipid profile and predisposition to cardiovascular disease. However, in their meta-analysis of 17 clinical studies, Santos and colleagues reported low-carbohydrate diets decreased weight, BMI, and waist circumference while improving blood pressure, insulin response, blood glucose, and triglycerides in 1,141 obese subjects. Bueno and others reported that studies of very low-carbohydrate ketogenic diets (VLCKD, <50 grams) resulted in greater weight loss and lower triglycerides and diastolic blood pressure at 12 months or more of follow-up than studies of low-fat (<30 percent of Calories) diets. They concluded that VLCKD may be effective in combating obesity. The Consumers Union notes that individuals with healthy lipid profiles will likely suffer no harm from adopting the Atkins diet plan for a short time.

Low-carbohydrate diets such as the Atkins diet may be successful. There is insufficient evidence to make recommendations against their use. However, Phelan and others reported that low-carbohydrate dieters represented only 10.8 percent of National Weight Control Registry participants who lost and maintained a weight loss of at least 30 pounds for at least 1 year.

Moderation in dietary fat intake may be the key. As noted, individuals in the National Weight Control Registry consume about 30 percent of daily energy from fat, which is considered moderate. In a 14-month study, Azadbakht and others reported significantly greater reductions in body weight, waist circumference, and cardiovascular risk factors in subjects consuming a moderate-fat (30 percent) versus a low-fat (20 percent) diet. The authors suggested that better dietary adherence with the moderate-fat diet may be the reason for its successful effects. Shai and others also suggested that the Mediterranean diet, which is a moderate-fat diet, may be an effective alternative to low-fat diets.

High-Protein Weight-Loss Diets

Some diets, such as the Zone diet, recommend that protein should account for 30 percent or more of energy and are marketed as high-protein diets. Although this recommendation falls within the AMDR for protein (10–35 percent), it is generally regarded as high because it may be twice the typical protein intake of 12–15 percent. However, other diets such as Atkins and South Beach also may be regarded as somewhat high in protein.

High-protein weight-loss diets have been recommended for several reasons. Westerterp-Plantenga, Wycherley, and Leidy, along with their associates, cited several possible benefits from increased protein intake.

- Increased satiety—increased oxidation of excess amino acids and decrease in ghrelin may help suppress the appetite.
- Increased thermogenesis—increased body temperature suppresses appetite.
- Decreased energy efficiency—more energy is used to process protein, such as in gluconeogenesis.
- Maintenance of lean body mass—muscle is the main protein reservoir in the body.

Some recommend that weight-loss diets contain 20–30 percent of energy content from protein. In a study with normal-weight individuals who were not on a weight-loss diet, Weigle and others found that increasing dietary protein content from 15 to 30 percent of energy intake, while keeping carbohydrate content constant, produced a sustained decrease in caloric intake. In another study involving high-protein diets (30 percent), Leidy and others reported improved perceptions of satiety and pleasure during dietary energy restriction, and the diet helped women preserve lean body mass. Mettler and others also reported that a high-protein (35 percent) diet, as compared to normal protein (15 percent) intake, was significantly superior for maintenance of lean body mass during a short-term weight-loss program.

In their meta-analysis, Schwingshackl and Hoffmann reported evidence of greater insulin sensitivity following a low-fat, high-protein diet compared to a low-fat, low-protein diet but no differences in weight loss, fat mass, lipids, blood pressure, or blood glucose. However, Hu concluded that short-term, high-protein diets induce weight loss and improve blood lipids. Layman and others indicated that high-protein, low-carbohydrate diets have been found to have some positive health effects, such as reducing serum triglycerides and blood pressure, increasing HDL-cholesterol, and improving glycemic control, factors that could reduce risk for heart disease and diabetes. Partial replacement of refined carbohydrates in the diet with protein sources that are low in fat may explain these changes.

In a position statement from the American Heart Association's Nutrition Committee, St. Jeor and others concluded that while high-protein diets may not be harmful to most healthy individuals in the short term, such diets are not recommended as substitutes for other diets that better meet nutritional needs. Animal sources of protein may be high in saturated fat and cholesterol. The observed changes in weight following high-protein diets may be attributed to fluid loss from low carbohydrate intake and from caloric deficit instead of high protein content *per se*. In their meta-analysis, Santesso and colleagues caution that small improvements in body fat, blood pressure, and lipids following high-protein diets must be considered against potential risks. Noto and others reported an increase in relative risk for all-cause mortality in four observational studies of over 143,000 subjects following low-carbohydrate, high-protein diets. Kappagoda and colleagues have expressed concern about high-protein diets followed by those with metabolic syndrome and at high risk for cardiovascular disease. Hu notes there are no long-term scientific studies to support the overall efficacy and safety of high-protein diets.

However, Westerterp-Plantenga and others comment that high-protein diets appear to present no risk to individuals with normal kidney function, but those at risk for chronic kidney disease should be screened for serum creatinine and proteinuria before starting such a diet. Although high intakes of protein may increase calcium loss, Calvez and others reported no adverse effects of such diets on calcium balance. Although diets containing 25–30 percent protein may be marketed as high-protein, such diets are actually within the AMDR of 10–35 percent of energy from protein. Nevertheless, individuals who have any health concerns should check with their health professionals before initiating such dietary changes.

Balanced Weight-Loss Diets   In the middle of Riley's continuum of popular weight-loss diets are mainly those recommended by most professional health organizations, such as the American Heart Association, Academy of Nutrition and Dietetics (formerly the American Dietetic Association) and American Diabetes Association. The Food Exchange System diet, developed by the latter two associations, is the basis of the diet plan advocated in this text.

Highly recommended diets are based upon sound nutritional principles and are designed to satisfy the individual's personal food tastes. Research with dieters has shown that any weight-reduction diet, to be safe, effective, and realistic, should adhere to the following principles:

1. It should be reduced in Calories and yet supply all nutrients essential to normal body functions. It is important to stress the importance of dietary Calories. Dich and others purposely overfed normal young men, about 1,200 additional Calories per day, with either a carbohydrate-rich or a fat-rich diet for 21 days. They found that the increase in body weight and fat mass was no different between the two diets. Excess dietary Calories lead to weight gain and this study indicates that it does not matter if they come from carbohydrate or fat. As far as energy is concerned, a Calorie from a banana is the same as a Calorie from a brownie.

2. It should contain a wide variety of foods that appeal to your taste and help prevent hunger sensations between meals. Low-glycemic-index diets with dietary fiber and moderate amounts of protein and fat may help to suppress the appetite. With respect to weight control, Kris-Etherton and others suggest that a moderate-fat diet can be as effective as, or even more effective than, a lower-fat diet, because of advantages with long-term adherence and potentially favorable effects on lipids and lipoproteins. However, they also note that because fat is energy dense, moderation in fat intake is essential for weight control.

3. It should be suited to your current lifestyle and personal preferences, being easily obtainable whether you eat most of your meals at home or you dine out frequently.

4. It should provide for a slow rate of weight loss, about 1–2 pounds per week.

5. It should be a lifelong diet, one that will satisfy the first three principles once you attain your desired weight.

In any diet plan, foods should be selected that adhere to the principles of healthful eating. This information was summarized in chapter 2, and 20 guidelines you can use in the selection and preparation of foods to reduce caloric intake are presented later in this chapter. As proper knowledge is a key to behavior modification, learning the caloric and nutrient content of a wide variety of foods may be a very important strategy in a weight-control program.

Is it a good idea to count Calories when attempting to lose body weight?

There are both disadvantages and advantages to counting Calories. Counting Calories may not be practical for many who are too busy to plan a daily menu designed around a caloric limit. Challenges in counting Calories, especially when dining out, include estimating serving sizes, which may vary from one source to another, and calories added in different methods of food preparation. Although these problems are not difficult to solve, it does take some effort.

On the other hand, counting Calories may be very helpful during the early stages of a diet. The dieter who understands the Food Exchange Lists and how to use Nutrition Facts on food labels can substitute one low-Calorie food for another in the daily menu. Research suggests that recording everything at the beginning of a diet, including the caloric content, can help you stick with your weight-loss program. In their meta-analysis of behavioral techniques in successful weight management, Hartmann-Boyce and colleagues reported counting Calories is significantly associated with weight loss. As one becomes more familiar with the caloric content of food, it is easier to select low-Calorie, nutrient-dense food and avoid high-Calorie foods that are low in nutrients. It will require a little effort in the beginning phases of a diet to learn the Calories in a given quantity of a certain food, but once learned and incorporated into your lifestyle, this knowledge is a valuable asset, not only when trying to lose weight but also when maintaining a healthy weight over a lifetime. As you incorporate low-Calorie, high-nutrient foods into your diet, it will eventually become second nature to you, and you may eliminate the need to count Calories.

The key to keeping track of Calories is to keep track of dietary fat and sugar and portion sizes. With knowledge of the Food Exchange System and Nutrition Facts food labels, you should be able to determine the grams of fat that you consume daily. Less than 30 percent of your dietary Calories should be derived from fat. On a diet of 1,800 Calories per day, fewer than 540 Calories should come from fat (1,800 × 0.30), which is the equivalent of 60 grams of fat because 1 gram of fat contains 9 Calories (540/9). Diets containing only 20 percent fat Calories may also be recommended. Less than 10 percent of your dietary Calories should come from sugar. On this 1,800-Calorie diet, that would be fewer than 180 Calories (45 grams) from sugar. As noted later, reducing the amount of fat and sugar in the daily diet may be a very effective means to reduce daily energy intake and lose excess body fat.

How often should I weigh myself?

Once you have attained your desired weight, a good set of scales would be most helpful. Keeping track of your weight on a day-to-day or weekly basis will enable you to decrease your caloric intake for several days once you notice your weight beginning to increase again. According to Ogden and colleagues, regular self-monitoring of weight is associated with successful weight loss and maintenance in 85 percent of National Weight Control Registry participants, noting that it is easier to deal with a gain of a few pounds rather than 10 or 20. Short-term prevention is more effective than long-term treatment. The dietary habits you acquire during the Calorie-counting phase of your diet will help you during these short-term prevention periods.

What is the Food Exchange System?

At this time it is important to expand our discussion of the Food Exchange System, which was introduced in chapter 2. The Food Exchange System was developed by a group of health organizations, including the American Diabetes Association and the Academy of Nutrition and Dietetics, as a means of advising patients about healthy eating. In essence, six food groups were established, and foods were assigned to these groups on the basis of similar caloric content and nutritional value. For our purposes at this time, we will concentrate on the caloric value, but you may also want to refresh your memory on the grams of fat per food exchange.

The six Food Exchange Lists may be found in appendix D. You should study these lists and get an idea of the types and amounts of foods in each that constitute one exchange. Memorizing the caloric

value of each food exchange is instrumental in determining the number of Calories you consume daily and in planning a healthful, low-Calorie diet. In their study, Benezra and others found that the intake of most nutrients can remain at recommended levels when the Food Exchange System is used to plan a weight-loss program. The caloric content and grams of fat of 1 serving from each of the six exchanges are listed below and expressed in figure 11.3.

1 vegetable exchange	=	25 Calories; 0 g fat
1 fruit exchange	=	60 Calories; 0 g fat
1 fat exchange	=	45 Calories; 5 g fat
1 starch exchange	=	80 Calories; 0–1 g fat
1 meat exchange	=	35–100 Calories
Very lean	=	35 Calories; 0–1 g fat
Lean	=	55 Calories; 3 g fat
Medium fat	=	75 Calories; 5 g fat
High fat	=	100 Calories; 8 g fat
1 milk exchange	=	90–150 Calories
Skim	=	90 Calories; 0–3 g fat
Low fat	=	120 Calories; 5 g fat
Whole	=	150 Calories; 8 g fat

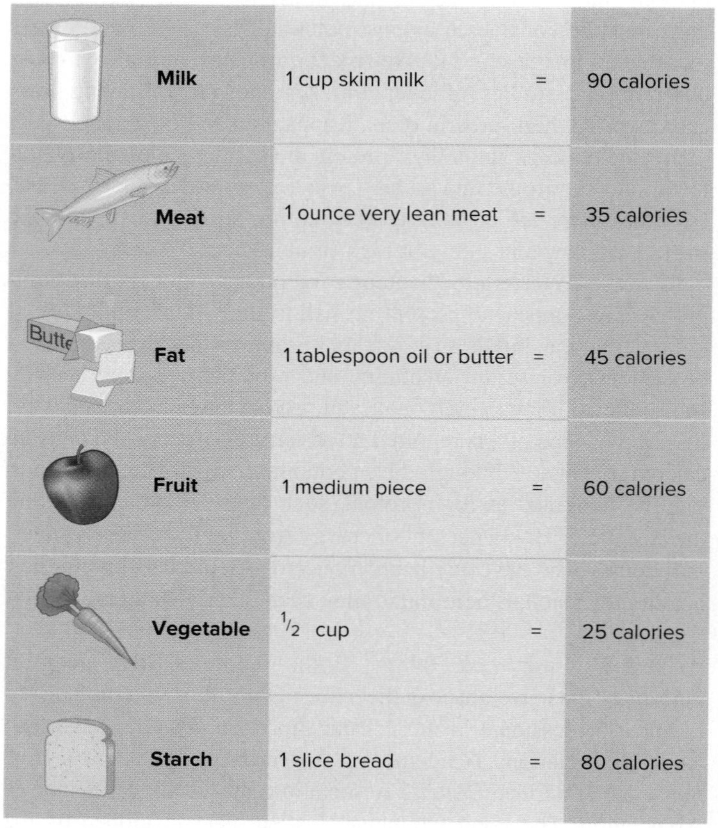

Milk	1 cup skim milk	=	90 calories
Meat	1 ounce very lean meat	=	35 calories
Fat	1 tablespoon oil or butter	=	45 calories
Fruit	1 medium piece	=	60 calories
Vegetable	1/2 cup	=	25 calories
Starch	1 slice bread	=	80 calories

FIGURE 11.3 Knowledge of the various food exchanges and their caloric values can be very helpful in planning a diet. With a little effort, you can learn to estimate the caloric value of most basic foods. See appendix D for other food examples and serving sizes.

TABLE 11.5 Carbohydrate, fat, protein, and Calories in the six food exchanges

Food exchange	Carbohydrate	Fat	Protein	Calories	Average serving size*
Vegetables	5	0	2	25	½ cup cooked; 1 cup raw
Fruits	15	0	0	60	½ cup fresh fruit or juice
Fat	0	5	0	45	1 teaspoon (5 grams)
Meat and meat substitutes					1 ounce
Very lean	0	0–1	7	35	
Lean	0	3	7	55	
Medium fat	0	5	7	75	
High fat	0	8	7	100	
Starch	15	0–1	3	80	⅓–½ cup cereal or pasta; 1 slice of bread
Milk					1 cup (8 fluid ounces)
Skim and very low fat	12	0–3	8	90–110	
Low fat	12	5	8	120	
Whole	12	8	8	150	

Carbohydrate, fat, and protein in grams
1g carbohydrate = 4 Calories
1g fat = 9 Calories
1g protein = 4 Calories

*See appendix D for specific foods.
Source: *Exchange Lists for Meal Planning,* American Diabetes Association and Academy of Nutrition and Dietetics, Chicago, ADA, 1995.

Table 11.5 presents a breakdown of the carbohydrate, fat, protein, and Calorie content of each food exchange.

How can I determine the number of Calories I eat daily?

You may use the guide presented earlier in this chapter to record your daily physical activity, including what you eat and drink. Carry a small notebook with you along with some reminder, such as a rubber band around your wrist, to record your activity and food intake in detail. One suggestion to document your food intake is to take a photo of what you eat with your cell phone, which provides you with a daily record. To calculate your caloric intake, you can use information provided by food labels or from the Food Exchange System in appendix D. Food intake should be recorded over a 3- to 7-day period, as a single day may give a biased value. Experiments have shown that this method may provide relatively accurate accounts of caloric intake if the amounts of food ingested are measured accurately. The main problem for most people is determining what and how much has been eaten. An 8-ounce glass of skim milk may be easy to record, and the caloric value from the food label or from appendix D is rather precise. However, the caloric value of a slice of pizza would likely vary from one restaurant to another because of differences in slice size; the kind and amount of toppings, sauce, and dough ingredients; and other factors. As a result, estimates of the caloric content of complex food combinations are much less precise. Nevertheless, some estimates are presented in appendix D in the section on combination foods. For example, one-quarter of a 10-inch cheese pizza with thin crust contains two starch, two medium-fat meat, and one fat exchange, or the equivalent of 355 Calories.

Although you may wish to use a ruler, a small measuring scale, and a measuring cup at home to accurately record the amount of food you eat, they are not practical for many dining situations. Young, in her book *The Portion Teller Plan: The No-Diet Reality Guide to Eating, Cheating and Losing Weight Permanently,* states that learning how to eyeball portion sizes accurately is an important skill. Some common objects in everyday life may serve as representative portion sizes for various foods, and some examples are presented in figure 11.4. The following may serve as guidelines for you to record the type and amount of food you eat:

1. In your notebook, record the foods you have eaten as soon as possible, noting the kind of food and the amount. Keep in mind that many servings today are supersized so that 1 of these "servings" may actually contain the Calories of 2–3 standard servings. Learn to visualize proper portion sizes and the associated Calorie content in various foods.

2. Check the labels of the foods you eat. Most commercial products have nutritional information listed, including the number of Calories per serving. Record these data when available.

3. Calories for most fluids are given in relation to ounces. For fluids, remember that 1 cup or regular glass is about 8 ounces, but many glasses now hold 12–16 ounces. Most regular

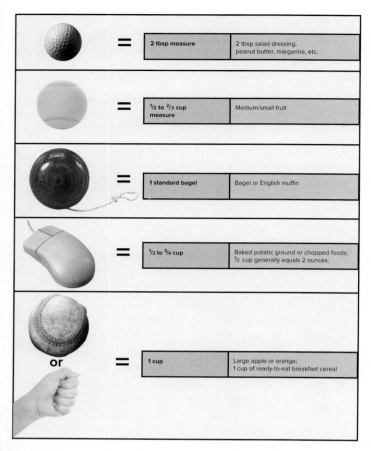

		2 tbsp measure	2 tbsp salad dressing, peanut butter, margarine, etc.
		½ to ⅔ cup measure	Medium/small fruit
		1 standard bagel	Bagel or English muffin
		½ to ¾ cup	Baked potato; ground or chopped foods; ½ cup generally equals 2 ounces.
or		1 cup	Large apple or orange; 1 cup of ready-to-eat breakfast cereal

FIGURE 11.4 A golf ball, tennis ball, large yo-yo, computer mouse, baseball, and fist make convenient guides to judge MyPyramid serving sizes. Additional handy guides include

thumb = 1 oz of cheese;
4 stacked dice = 1 oz cheese;
thumb tip to first joint = 1 tsp;
matchbox = 1 oz meat;
bar of soap or deck of cards = 3 oz meat;

palm of hand = 3 oz
1 ice cream scoop = ½ cup
handful = 1 or 2 oz of a
snack food; and
ping-pong ball = 2 tbsp;

canned drinks contain 12 ounces, although smaller and larger sizes are available; 20-ounce bottles are becoming increasingly popular.

4. Calories for meat, poultry, fish, and other related products are usually given by ounces. To get an idea of how many ounces are in these products, you could purchase a set weight of meat, say 16 ounces, and cut it into four equal pieces. Each would weigh approximately 4 ounces, or about the visual size of a deck of playing cards. For cheese, 1 ounce is about the size of a ping-pong ball. Get a mental picture of these sizes and use them as a guide to portion sizes.

5. For fruits and vegetables the caloric values are usually expressed relative to ½ cup or a small piece. At home, measure ½ cup of vegetables or fruit and place it in a bowl or on a plate. Again, make a mental picture of this serving size and use it as a reference. Compare the sizes of different fruits and notice the difference between a small, medium, and large piece.

A medium piece of fruit is about the size of a tennis ball, while a medium potato is about the size of a computer mouse.

6. For starch products, the Calories are most often expressed per serving, such as an average-size slice of bread or a dinner roll. In these cases it is relatively easy to determine quantity, but one slice of bread may contain 50 to 150 Calories or more, depending on its size and density. Depending on the type of cereal, pasta, grain, or starchy vegetable, the measure for one exchange is usually ⅓ or ½ cup, but some serving sizes are larger, such as those of puffed cereals. See appendix D. Use a measuring cup and the mental-picture concept again to estimate quantities. A cup of cold cereal is about the size of a large handful, whereas ½ cup of hot cereal is about the size of a tennis ball. A 2-ounce bagel is the size of a yo-yo.

7. For substances such as sugar, jams, jellies, nondairy creamers, and related products, make a mental picture of a teaspoon and tablespoon. These are common means whereby Calories are given. A teaspoon of butter or margarine is about the size of the tip of your thumb. One level teaspoon of sugar is about 20 Calories; jams and jellies contain similar amounts. Caloric values of other products may be obtained from nutrition labels.

8. Some combination foods, such as a homemade casserole, are included in appendix D. However, for combination foods not listed, you will need to list the ingredients separately to calculate the caloric content. Labels on most food products list caloric content per serving.

9. Caloric values for some national chain and fast-food restaurant items may be found at websites listed in appendix E. Most fast-food restaurants provide fact sheets detailing information on the nutrient content of their products. The FDA proposed that national restaurant chains, as well as other businesses, such as convenience stores that sell prepared food, be required to display Calorie counts for menu items so that the consumer may make an informed judgment when ordering. Some national chains are marketing low-Calorie (400–500 Calories) meals. If caloric values are not displayed, you may access them at various Websites. If nutrition fact sheets are not available when dining out in restaurants, you may obtain the caloric value of food items via e-mail.

http://caloriecount.about.com/ Type a food in the search window *or* scroll to the bottom to "Calories in Foods & Activities"; then browse nutrient value by "Food," "Brands" (including restaurant chains), or "Recipes" categories.

www.fastfoodnutrition.org/ Search fast-food items by chain.

www.calorieking.com/foods/calories-in-fast-food-chains-restaurants_c-Y2lkPTlx.html This is another link for caloric values of fast foods.

Working with the Food Exchange System helps you learn the portion size and caloric content of various foods. Through experience you should be able to readily identify, within a small error range, the quantities of food you eat. This is not only helpful for determining your caloric intake but may also serve as a motivational device to restrict portion sizes when you are on a weight-loss diet.

The following represents an example of how you might record one meal and calculate the caloric intake from appendix D or food labels.

Breakfast Food	Quantity	Calories
Milk, skim	1 glass, 8 ounces	90
Eggs	2, poached	150
Toast, whole wheat	2 slices	160
with butter	2 pats	90
with jelly	1 tablespoon	60
Orange juice	1 glass, 8 ounces	120
Coffee	1 cup, 8 ounces	0
with sugar	1 teaspoon	20
TOTAL		690

Reading food labels and consulting the Food Exchange System helps you learn the caloric and nutrient value of various foods and is recommended as a learning tool. You can then use computer programs to assess your diet on a daily basis. The ChooseMyPlate Website, discussed previously, gives you the opportunity to keep a detailed history of your caloric and nutrient intake, and you can use the *Energy Balance* option to plan a weight-control diet. Appropriate dietary analysis software is also provided with your purchase of this textbook.

https://www.supertracker.usda.gov/ Track your caloric intake using the supertracker software found at the ChooseMyPlate Website and described earlier in the chapter.

What are some general guidelines I can use in the selection and preparation of foods to promote weight loss or maintain a healthy body weight?

A 2013 *Consumer Reports* survey of more than 9,000 dieters found that more than 80 percent who successfully lost weight and kept it off did so without following a specific plan. Instead, they used sensible strategies such as cutting portion size and staying away from sweets and junk food. The following 20 guidelines for weight control and healthy eating are based on several reputable sources of information, including the Food Exchange System, the National Weight Control Registry, and the DASH and OmniHeart diets. In essence, the four key points are

- Eat fewer Calories from fat and sugar.
- Eat healthier carbohydrates.
- Eat healthier fats.
- Eat healthier proteins.

1. *Eat more nutrient-dense foods and fewer energy-dense foods.* You need to decrease the number of Calories you consume daily. The key principle is to select foods, in appropriate portion sizes, and with high-nutrient density from across the six food exchanges or the food groups in the MyPlate approach. Avoid energy-dense foods and drinks, such as bagels, soft pretzels, energy bars, smoothies, special coffees, and cocktails, all of which may be loaded with Calories. If you do buy convenience meals, select those that are low in Calories and fat. Check the label for total fat and total Calories from fat and sugar. This you can easily do by reading the label. Check figure 11.5.

2. *Eat foods that make you feel full.* Rolls based her excellent book, *The Volumetrics Eating Plan,* on this principle, as did Dean Ornish with his book *Eat More, Weigh Less.* Research from Rolls's laboratory reported that reducing dietary energy density is associated with weight loss in overweight individuals. High-volume, low-Calorie foods, such as salads, soups, vegetables, and whole grains, are rich in dietary fiber and water, and they help provide a sensation of fullness that curbs hunger.

3. *Restrict portion sizes.* Although the intake of high-volume, low-Calorie foods such as vegetables will help curtail hunger and promote weight loss, one of the major problems contributing to the increasing obesity in the United States is the consumption of large volumes of high-Calorie foods. Most fast-food eateries and convenience stores have increased portion sizes dramatically to give customers their *money's worth.* The "supersize" option is common today with *individual* soft-drink servings of 64 ounces replacing a 32-ounce *family* bottle of soda from years ago. Today's McDonald's meal of a hamburger, fries, and a soda may include 1,800 Calories, whereas decades ago the same menu items contained 600 Calories. Even manufacturers of "healthy" foods for dieters advertise "heartier" portions that weigh 50 percent more than the original version and contain more Calories. In contrast,

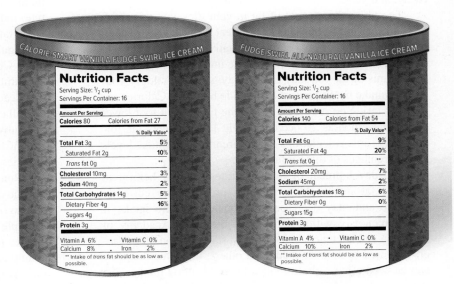

FIGURE 11.5 Reading labels helps you choose foods with less fat, sugar, and Calorie content.

some food manufacturers are now marketing 100-Calorie healthful snacks, such as almonds, and some restaurants are offering smaller portion sizes with reduced Calories and prices. Decreasing the volume of high-Calorie foods is one of the most important dietary means to reduced body fat.

4. *Eat less fat.* Although restricting dietary Calories is most important, and some experts such as Fogelholm and colleagues suggest the effect of macronutrient composition on weight gain is unclear, Hooper and colleagues report that reduced dietary fat is associated with meaningful weight reductions in adults and children. First, fat is rich in Calories—more than double the amount of Calories per gram as compared to carbohydrate and protein. In their study, Rolls and Bell found that when individuals were fed diets varying in caloric density (fat content) and could eat as much as they liked, they ate the same amount of food by weight, so the caloric intake varied directly with the caloric density of the food. Second, dietary fat does not appear to rapidly suppress the appetite. Increased dietary fat may contribute to an imbalance between "reward" brain centers and normal hypothalamic control on food intake as described by Egecioglu and colleagues. Third, dietary fat has a lower TEF, or higher metabolic efficiency, than carbohydrate and protein. Jéquier comments that dietary fat appears to be stored as fat more efficiently than either carbohydrate or protein, even if the caloric intake is similar. This is especially true in individuals who have lost weight and may be one of the most important reasons they regain weight so readily. Fourth, dietary fat may also be stored preferentially in the abdominal region, which may increase health risks. At 3 years into an 8-year study of over 48,000 postmenopausal women, Howard and others reported greater decreases in weight, BMI, and waist circumference in women consuming a low-fat diet. However, in a subsequent study of subsamples, Newhouser and colleagues reported increases in waist circumferences of 2.3 and 2.9 percent in low-fat and control groups, respectively, at 6 years.

To reduce the amount of fat in your diet, you may wish to count the total grams of fat you eat each day. A general recommendation is to keep your daily total fat intake to 30 percent or less of your total caloric intake. To calculate the total grams of fat you may eat per day, simply multiply your caloric intake by 30 percent and divide by 9 (the Calories per gram of fat). You may wish to get the fat content to a lower percentage, such as 20 percent. Table 11.6 presents the formula and some calculations for different caloric intake levels and percentages of dietary fat intake.

The development of fat substitutes may be helpful in reducing fat intake. Many fat-free products are currently available and may decrease total fat and caloric intake if used judiciously within a healthful diet. The Academy of Nutrition and Dietetics, in its position statement on fat replacers authored by Jonnalagadda and others, indicated that they can be used effectively to reduce fat and Calorie intake. The American Heart Association also noted that use of fat substitutes may be associated with reduced fat and Calorie intake compared with nonuse of any fat-modified products and

TABLE 11.6 Calculation of daily fat intake in grams

To use this table, determine the number of Calories per day in your diet and the percent of dietary Calories you want from fat, and then find the grams of fat you may consume daily. For example, if your diet contains 2,200 Calories and you desire to consume only 20 percent of your daily Calories as fat, then you could consume 49 grams of fat. The formula is % Fat × Daily Calories ÷ 9 Calories per fat gram = Daily fat grams [0.20 × 2,200 ÷ 9 = 49]

Daily caloric intake	30% fat Calories (maximal grams)	20% fat Calories (maximal grams)	10% fat Calories (maximal grams)
1,000	33	22	11
1,200	40	26	13
1,500	50	33	16
1,800	60	40	20
2,000	66	44	22
2,200	73	49	24
2,500	83	55	28

noted that when used appropriately, fat substitutes may provide some flexibility with diet planning. Miller and Groziak noted that some individuals using fat substitutes may compensate for reduced caloric intake from fat by increasing caloric intake, a speculation that was supported in a study by Shide and Rolls. However, in a recent review, Jandacek concluded there is no evidence in humans that use of olestra, a fat substitute, induces increased caloric intake. Manore indicated that some fat-free foods may have similar amounts of Calories as the regular-fat version, so you should always check the food label. Cotton and others suggest that you gradually blend fat substitutes into your diet. Making many changes at one time may lead to overconsumption of other foods, and hence your overall caloric intake may remain the same, or even increase. Fat substitutes can be part of an overall healthful diet for weight loss, provided you do not compensate for the saved Calories by ingesting other Calorie-rich foods.

Remember that you need some fat in your diet for essential fatty acids and fat-soluble vitamins, which you may be able to obtain in a diet containing 10 percent fat Calories. An example of grams of fat and Calories saved by using fat substitutes for a luncheon meal is presented in table 11.7. In this example, using fat substitutes reduced the energy density of the lunch by about 350 Calories.

Several modified fats have been proposed to facilitate weight loss. Diglycerides are components of a new cooking oil to replace the traditional triglycerides. Although the caloric

TABLE 11.7 Using foods with fat substitutes may help reduce Calories and fat from meals. In this example, the fat-substitute lunch contains about 350 fewer Calories and 40 fewer grams of fat.

Regular lunch	Calories/fat grams	Fat-substitute lunch	Calories/fat grams

Sandwich
  2 slices whole wheat bread
  2 oz bologna
	140/2
	180/16
		Sandwich
		  2 slices whole wheat bread
		  2 oz fat-free bologna
			140/2
			44/0.35

1 oz cheese	85/6.4	1 oz fat-free cheese	43/0
2 Tbsp mayonnaise	114/10	2 Tbsp fat-free mayonnaise	26/1.0
Banana, medium	105/0.4	Banana	105/0.4
1 cup ice cream	265/14	1 cup fat/sugar-free ice cream	182/0
Totals	889/43.8	Totals	540/3.75

content of the two fat compounds is the same, diglycerides are theorized to increase fat oxidation and not be stored as body fat as readily as triglycerides. Hibi and others reported evidence of enhanced fat metabolism in overweight women after consuming diglyceride compared to triglyceride oil. However, research data on diglycerides are limited, and the minor effects on weight loss do not justify its price. Health professionals recommend olive or canola oils, while limiting intake of other fats and oils.

Other suggestions for reducing dietary fat are included in the following guidelines, but you may wish to review chapter 5 for additional information. Once individuals adapt to a low-fat diet, they may prefer it because high-fat meals are digested more slowly, possibly leading to indigestion and some gastrointestinal distress.

5. *Eat fewer and smaller amounts of refined sugar.* This may be accomplished by restricting the amount of sugar added directly to foods and limiting the consumption of highly processed foods that may add substantial amounts of sweeteners, particularly sugar-sweetened beverages. A report in the Tufts University *Health & Nutrition Letter* indicated that Americans consume about 475 Calories daily from added sugars.

Artificial sweeteners may be helpful. For example, Raben and others found that overweight individuals who consumed large amounts of sucrose in their daily diets, mostly as beverages, had increased energy intake, body weight, and fat mass after 10 weeks, but these effects were not seen in a similar group that consumed artificial sweeteners. Early reviews by Pi-Sunyer and Drewnowskli noted that artificial sweeteners, such as aspartame, have been shown to reduce caloric intake without leading to an increased consumption of other foods and could increase weight loss. However, a more recent review by Shankar and others concluded there is insufficient evidence for or against the use of artificial sweeteners. More long-term research is recommended. Sugar substitutes, like fat substitutes, may be an effective part of a healthful

weight-loss diet, but individuals must be cautious not to compensate and eat more food later.

6. *Reduce the intake of both added fat and sugar.* In many cases, simply reducing the fat and sugar content in the diet will save substantial numbers of Calories and may be all that is needed. Fat and sugar together account for nearly 50 percent of the Calories in the average American diet. Many restaurant menu items are high in both fat and sugar. As examples, a large glass of sweet tea at McDonald's contains nearly 60 grams of sugar and 230 Calories, nearly 10 percent of your daily caloric requirement. A fried whole onion with dipping sauce contains about 2,100 Calories. Even supposedly healthy fast foods, such as salads, can contain as much fat and Calories as the burgers on the menu, mainly because large amounts of fat are added with the dressing. Table 11.8 provides some examples of how to save Calories via simple substitutions for comparable foods containing fat or sugar. As noted earlier, most national restaurant chains can provide you with the caloric content of their meal items.

7. *Eat more low-fat dairy products.* In separate reviews, Westerterp-Plantenga and Wycherley and their colleagues note that increased protein intake may help suppress the appetite more than equivalent amounts of carbohydrate or fat. In chapter 8, a dairy-rich diet was discussed as possibly promoting weight loss, but in general, research findings do not support this hypothesis. Nevertheless, milk exchange products are excellent sources of high-quality protein and other essential vitamins and minerals. Casein and whey dairy protein have long- and short-acting effects, respectively, on appetite suppression. Bendtsen and others reported no difference between casein and whey on hormonal response to suppress appetite. Select low-fat dairy products, such as skim milk and low-fat cottage cheese and yogurt, which are healthier-protein foods, instead of high-fat counterparts.

8. *Eat more low-fat meat and meat substitutes.* The meat and meat substitute exchange products also are sources of high-quality protein and many other nutrients but also may contain

TABLE 11.8 Simple food substitutions to save Calories

Instead of	Select	To save this many Calories by reducing sugar and fat
1 croissant	1 whole wheat bagel	80
1 whole egg	2 egg whites	50
1 ounce cheddar cheese	1 ounce mozzarella (skim)	30
1 ounce regular bacon	1 ounce Canadian bacon	100
3 ounces tuna in oil	3 ounces tuna in water	60
Cream of mushroom soup	Black bean soup	90
1 cup regular ice cream	1 cup fat-free frozen dessert	150
1 ounce turkey bologna	1 ounce turkey breast	50
1 McDonald's Big Mac	1 McDonald's grilled chicken	120
1 cup whole milk	1 cup skim milk	60
French fried potatoes	Baked potato	100
1 ounce potato chips	1 ounce pretzels	90
1 tablespoon mayonnaise	1 tablespoon fat-free mayonnaise	90
1 can regular cola	1 can diet cola	150

excessive fat Calories. To eat healthier proteins, select very lean and lean meat exchanges, including meat substitutes such as legumes. Very lean meat and meat substitutes contain only 35 Calories and less than 1 gram of fat per 1-ounce serving. Examples include the white meat of chicken and turkey, 99 percent fat-free ground turkey, tuna fresh or canned in water, shrimp, fat-free cheese, egg whites, and egg substitutes. See appendix D for other sources. If you enjoy beef and pork, use leaner cuts such as beef eye of round, flank steak, pork tenderloin, and 96 percent fat-free hamburger. Trim away excess fat; broil or bake your meats to let the fat drip away. If you eat in national chain and fast-food restaurants, select foods that are low in fat, such as grilled chicken, lean meats, and salads. Avoid the high-fat foods, which normally contain 40–60 percent fat Calories. Remember that serving sizes have increased dramatically in recent years. A large hamburger deluxe may have triple or more the Calories of a regular hamburger. Select legumes as an excellent meat substitute.

9. *Eat more whole, unprocessed carbohydrates.* The starch exchange contains healthy carbohydrates and is high in vitamins, minerals, and fiber. Eating a low-glycemic, high-fiber diet increases the gastric volume, which might help suppress appetite. Use whole-grain breads and cereals, brown rice, oatmeal, beans, bran products, and starchy vegetables for dietary fiber. Limit the use of processed grain products that add fat and sugar. Substitute products low in fat, such as standard-size whole wheat bagels, for those high in fat, like croissants.

10. *Eat more fruits.* Foods in the fruit exchange are high in vitamins and fiber. Select fresh, whole fruits or those canned or frozen in their own juices. Avoid those in heavy sugar syrups. Limit the intake of dried fruits, which are high in Calories. Eat at least one citrus fruit daily. Limit intake of fruit juices, which are rich in Calories.

11. *Eat more veggies.* The vegetable exchange foods are low in Calories yet high in vitamins, minerals, and fiber. Select dark-green leafy and yellow-orange vegetables daily. Low-Calorie items like carrots, radishes, and celery are highly nutritious snacks for munching. Many of these vegetables are listed as free exchanges in appendix D because they contain fewer than 20 Calories per serving. Fruits and vegetables may provide bulk to the diet and a sensation of fullness without excessive amounts of Calories.

12. *Consume fewer high-Calorie fat exchanges.* Use smaller amounts of high-Calorie fat exchanges. Many salad dressings, butter, margarine, and cooking oils are pure fat. If necessary, substitute low-Calorie or fat-free dietary versions instead. Fat-free mayonnaise tastes good and has 90 fewer Calories than a serving of regular mayonnaise. Do not prepare foods in fats, such as with frying. Use nonstick cooking utensils or nonfat cooking sprays.

13. *Reduce liquid Calories.* Individuals seeking to lose weight should consider limiting their intake of Calorie-containing beverages to milk and fruit juice. High-Calorie liquids, such as sodas and alcoholic beverages, may be especially harmful in weight-loss programs because they not only add Calories to the diet but also do not appear to suppress the appetite as well as similar amounts of Calories in solid foods. In a review of 32 high-quality studies, Malik and others found that the weight of epidemiological and experimental evidence indicates that a greater consumption of sugar-sweetened beverages is associated with weight gain and obesity in children and adults, and that sufficient evidence exists for public health strategies to discourage consumption of sugary drinks as part of a healthy lifestyle. Considerable controversy swirls around the health effects of the sweetener fructose, as evidenced in recent discordant reviews by Rippe and Bray. Popkin suggests that about half of the daily Calories that contribute to weight gain are consumed as sugary beverages. Other beverages may also contain excess Calories. For example, a 24-ounce Starbucks Vanilla Bean Frappuccino (whole milk with whipped cream) contains about as many Calories as a McDonald's Big Mac.

However, fluid intake should remain high, for it helps create a sensation of satiety during a meal. Concerned with the increase in obesity in the United States, Popkin and others assembled a Beverage Guidance Panel to provide guidance on the relative health and nutritional benefits and risks of various beverage categories. Plain drinking water was ranked as the preferred beverage to fulfill daily water needs, whereas calorically sweetened, nutrient-poor beverages were ranked as least preferred. The panel recommends that the consumption of beverages with no or few calories should take precedence over the consumption of beverages with more Calories.

14. *Limit your intake of alcohol.* It is high in Calories and devoid of nutrient value. One gram of alcohol contains 7 Calories, almost twice the value of protein and carbohydrate, but has no nutrient value. A 1.5-ounce shot of gin contains 100 Calories with no other nutrient value, whereas 2 ounces of grilled skinless chicken breast provides the same energy with nearly one-third of the protein RDA plus substantial amounts of iron, zinc, niacin, and other vitamins. Yeoman comments that instead of substituting for other Calories, alcohol actually increases the total caloric intake of the meal. Additionally, excess alcohol Calories are stored as body fat. If you desire alcohol, select light varieties of wine and beer. Substitution of a light beer for a regular beer will save about 50 Calories. A nonalcoholic wine or beer may contain even fewer Calories. Alcohol will be discussed in chapter 13.

15. *Limit salt intake.* Salt intake should be limited to that which occurs naturally in foods. Try to use dry herbs, spices, and other nonsalt seasonings as substitutes to flavor your food. Salt may increase the appetite or thirst for Calorie-containing beverages.

16. *Eat slowly.* Slowing down the process of eating, by taking time to smell the aromas from your food and chewing slowly, will provide time to help curb your appetite. In their meta-analysis, Robinson and others reported a significant association between eating rate and energy intake. Eat a salad or soup as an appetizer, which may help curb your appetite for the main course.

17. *Eat at least three meals a day.* In their review, Leidy and Campbell reported that eating fewer than three meals daily could negatively affect appetite control. They noted several studies that have found an increase in appetite and reduction in perceived satiety when a meal or two were eliminated from the daily diet. Individuals who want to graze, or eat five or six smaller meals a day instead of the traditional three meals, may find that it helps curb the appetite. In particular, low-Calorie but high-protein and moderate-fat snacks, such as a hard-boiled egg or a handful of nuts with a total of 100 Calories, may be rather satiating. Nevertheless, current research suggests that grazing may not be more effective than a traditional meal pattern if total daily caloric intake is the same.

18. *Eat breakfast.* According to Wyatt and others, 78 percent of National Weight Control Registry participants eat breakfast. It has been suggested that the appetite may be more easily suppressed in the morning than in the evening. Breakfast may therefore help curb hunger throughout the morning hours. Daily caloric intake may be less when more Calories are consumed in the morning compared to later in the day. A high-protein breakfast may be important. Leidy and colleagues reported that breakfast reduced daily hunger with greater evidence of satiety in overweight adolescent females following a high-protein breakfast. Daily caloric intake was no different following skipping breakfast versus eating a high-protein breakfast. Examples of high-protein breakfast items include egg substitutes (egg whites), whole-grain cereals with skim milk, and whole wheat toast with smoked salmon. Conversely, Giovannini and others suggested that breakfast skipping may lead to up-regulation of appetite throughout the day, possibly leading to weight gain over time. McCrory notes the need for longer-term experimental studies of the effect of breakfast on energy intake.

19. *Learn to cook!* Microwaves and electric grills make cooking easy. Microwave cooking needs no fat for preparation, and electric grilling helps remove fat from meats. Cook and serve small portions of food for meals. The temptation to overeat may be removed.

20. *Learn low-Calorie foods.* Learn what foods are low in Calories in each of the six food exchanges and incorporate those palatable to you in your diet. Learn to substitute low-Calorie foods for high-Calorie ones. The key to a lifelong weight-maintenance diet is your knowledge of sound nutritional principles and the application of this knowledge to the design of your personal diet. Knowledge, however, is not the total answer; your behavior should reflect your knowledge. You may know that whole milk contains about 60 more Calories per glass than skim milk, but if you cannot switch, then the advantage of your knowledge is lost in this instance. Sometimes making changes in small steps helps, such as first switching from whole to low-fat milk, and then to skim milk.

How can I plan a nutritionally balanced, low-Calorie diet?

The key to a sound diet for weight loss is nutrient density, or the selection of low-Calorie, high-nutrient foods. The 20 points addressed in the previous section represent important guidelines to implement such a diet. Table 11.9 presents a suggested meal pattern based on the Food Exchange System. The foods should be selected from the Food Exchange Lists found in appendix D. You may use the form shown in the next column as a guide.

The total caloric values are close approximations for a three-meal pattern. If you decide to include snacks in your diet, such as a fruit or vegetable, then remove each snack from one of the main meals. The salads should contain vegetables with negligible Calories, such as lettuce and radishes. Note that under the exchange system, starchy vegetables such as potatoes are included in the starch group because their caloric content is similar. The beverages, other than milk and fruit juice, should contain no Calories. Although you may drink as many noncaloric beverages as you wish over the course of the day, drinking at least one at each meal will help provide a feeling of satiation and may help suppress the appetite somewhat.

Calories: _____

Meal	Number of servings	Calories per serving	Total Calories	Foods selected
Breakfast				
Milk, skim		90		
Meat, very lean		35		
Fruit		60		
Vegetable		25		
Starch		80		
Fat		45		
Beverage		0		
Lunch				
Milk, skim		90		
Meat, very lean		35		
Fruit		60		
Vegetable		25		
Salad		20		
Starch		80		
Fat		45		
Beverage		0		
Dinner				
Milk, skim		90		
Meat, very lean		35		
Fruit		60		
Vegetable		25		
Salad		20		
Starch		80		
Fat		45		
Beverage		0		

Daily meal plan	1,500 Calories	
Milk exchange, skim	(2)	1 2
Meat exchange, very lean	(7)	1 2 3 4 5 6 7
Starch exchange	(6)	1 2 3 4 5 6 7
Vegetable exchange	(3)	1 2 3 4
Salads	(2)	1 2
Fruit exchange	(4)	1 2 3 4
Fat exchange	(2)	1 2 3
Beverages	(3)	1 2 3

Keep in mind that this is not a rigid diet plan. At a minimum you should have 2 skim milk exchanges, 5 very lean meat exchanges, 5 starch exchanges, 2–3 vegetable exchanges, and 2–3 fruit exchanges. Once you have guaranteed these minimum requirements, you may do some substitution between the various exchanges so long as you keep the total caloric content within range of your goals. For example, you may delete 2 starch exchanges (160 Calories) in the model and substitute 1 skim milk and 2 very lean meat exchanges (160 Calories). You may also shift a limited number of the exchanges from one meal to another. If you prefer a more substantial breakfast and a lighter lunch, simply shift some of the exchanges from lunch to breakfast.

It may be a good idea to take a little time and construct a diet for yourself, using the following guidelines for your calculations. Use the form on this page. Table 11.10 presents an example of a 1,500-Calorie diet based on the Food Exchange System.

1. Calculate the number of Calories you want per day. See pages 488–489 for guidelines.
2. Use table 11.9 to determine how many servings you need from each food exchange.
3. Multiply the number of servings by the Calories per serving to get the total Calories. Add the total Calories column to get total daily intake.
4. Select appropriate foods from the Exchange List in appendix D.

If your diet contains less than 1,600 Calories, it would be wise to take a daily vitamin/mineral supplement with the RDA for all essential vitamins and key minerals.

The purpose of creating your own diet plan is to familiarize yourself with the caloric and nutrient content of the majority of foods that constitute your diet. You can plan your diet manually, or with computer-based programs if preferred. For example, the ChooseMyPlate program permits you to develop a personalized diet; an example of a 2,000-Calorie diet is presented in appendix G. Other computerized diet plans are available, such as the following:

www.shapeup.org This program from Shape Up America provides you with a diet plan, labeled the Cyberkitchen (under the "Adults" menu), to balance your diet and physical activity to lose weight. Moreover, various diet plans are compatible for use with your cell phone. Simply Google the terms *diet plan cell phone* to review those applications (apps) available.

Although only seven levels of caloric intake are presented in table 11.9, you may adjust it according to your needs by simply adding or subtracting appropriate food exchanges. For example, if you wanted a 1,700-Calorie diet, you could subtract one starch exchange and one-half fat exchange (about 100 Calories) from the 1,800-Calorie diet.

After you have determined the number of Calories you need daily, select the appropriate diet plan from table 11.9. To help implement your diet plan and to keep day-to-day track of the food exchanges you eat, you should design a 3″ × 5″ card similar to the model below for the number of food exchanges in your daily diet. As you consume an exchange at each meal, simply cross it off on the card. Make a new card for each day. The example in table 11.10 is based on a 1,500 Calorie intake.

TABLE 11.9 Suggested daily meal pattern based on the Food Exchange System

	Approximate daily caloric intake						
	1,000	1,200	1,500	1,800	2,000	2,200	2,500
Breakfast							
Milk, skim	1	1	1	1	1	1	1
Meat, very lean	1	1	2	2	2	3	3
Starch	1	2	2	3	3	3	3
Fruit	1	1	1	1	2	2	2
Fat	0	0	1	1	1	2	2
Beverage	1	1	1	1	1	1	1
Lunch							
Milk, skim	1	1	1	1	1	1	2
Meat, very lean	2	2	2	3	3	3	4
Starch	2	2	2	2	2	3	3
Vegetable	1	1	2	2	2	2	2
Salad	1	1	1	1	1	1	1
Fruit	1	2	2	2	2	2	2
Fat	½	½	1	2	2	2	2
Beverage	1	1	1	1	1	1	1
Dinner							
Milk, skim	0	0	0	1	1	1	1
Meat, very lean	2	2	3	3	3	4	4
Starch	2	2	3	3	4	4	5
Vegetable	1	2	2	2	2	2	3
Salad	1	1	1	1	1	1	1
Fruit	0	0	1	2	2	2	3
Fat	½	1	1	1	1	2	2
Beverage	1	1	1	1	1	1	1
Totals							
Milk, skim	2	2	2	3	3	3	4
Meat, very lean	5	5	7	8	8	10	11
Starch	5	6	7	8	9	10	11
Vegetable	2	3	4	4	4	4	5
Salad	2	2	2	2	2	2	2
Fruit	2	3	4	5	6	6	7
Fat	1	2	3	4	5	6	6
Beverage	3	3	3	3	3	3	3

Key points
1. Caloric values:
    Milk exchange, skim = 90
    Meat exchange, very lean = 35
    Fruit exchange = 60
    Vegetable exchange = 25
    Starch exchange = 80
    Fat exchange = 45
    Beverage = 0
    Salad = 20
2. See appendix D for a listing of foods in each exchange. Note the following:
    a. Foods other than milk, such as yogurt, are included in the milk exchange.
    b. The meat list includes foods such as eggs, cheese, fish, and poultry; low-fat legumes, like beans and peas, may be considered as meat substitutes.
    c. Some starchy vegetables are included in the bread list.
3. Foods should not be fried or prepared in fat unless you count the added fat as a fat exchange. Broil or bake foods instead.
4. Low-Calorie vegetables like lettuce and radishes should be used in the salads. Use only small amounts of very low-Calorie salad dressing.
5. Beverages should contain no Calories.

TABLE 11.10 A 1,500-Calorie diet based on the Food Exchange System

Exchange	Number of servings	Calories per exchange	Total Calories	Foods selected
Breakfast				
Meat, very lean	2	35	70	1 ounce very lean ham and
Fat	1	45	45	1 ounce low-fat cheese melted on
Starch	2	80	160	2 pieces whole-grain toasted bread
Fruit	1	60	60	4 ounces orange juice
Beverage	1	0	0	1 cup coffee with noncaloric sweetener
Lunch				
Milk, low-fat	1	120	120	8 ounces plain, low-fat yogurt
Fruit	1	60	60	
Meat, very lean	2	35	70	2 ounces turkey breast on
Starch	2	80	160	whole-grain bun
Vegetable	1	25	25	1 carrot
Salad	1	20	20	lettuce with
Fat	1	45	45	low-Calorie dressing
Beverage	1	0	0	diet cola
Dinner				
Milk, skim	1	90	90	1/2 cup ice milk
Meat, very lean	3	35	105	3 ounces broiled fish
Starch	3	80	240	1 baked potato and 1 slice whole wheat
Vegetable	3	25	75	bread
Salad	1	20	20	1 1/2 cups steamed broccoli and
Fat	1	45	45	cauliflower
				cucumbers
				small amount of margarine for potato and
				low-Calorie dressing for salad
Fruit	2	60	120	1 banana cut up on ice milk
Beverage	1	0	0	iced tea
TOTAL			**1,530**	

Are very low-Calorie diets effective and desirable as a means to lose body weight?

As noted in chapter 10, very low-Calorie diets (VLCD) are defined technically as containing less than 800 Calories per day and are often referred to as modified fasts. In some medical institutions, total fasting programs are used. VLCD should only be administered under proper medical supervision and are described in guidelines authored by Jensen and others as safe and effective in inducing rapid weight losses in very obese patients. However, VLCD are not recommended for the individual who wants to lose 10–20 pounds or for the individual who is not under medical supervision, not only because of the possible adverse health consequences as noted in chapter 10 but also because VLCD may be counterproductive to the ultimate goal of long-term weight loss. They do not satisfy the criteria for a recommended weight-loss program for individuals who are not medically supervised and they often lead to weight cycling.

It is recommended that any individual contemplating the use of VLCD consult a physician and a dietitian.

Are weight-loss dietary supplements effective and safe?

Products classified as dietary supplements may enter the marketplace without the rigorous clinical testing to document efficacy that is required of drugs. As a result, numerous weight-loss dietary supplements are sold over-the-counter or on the Internet with dubious advertisements such as *Lose 30 Pounds in 30 Days without Dieting or Exercising* or *Lose Belly Fat and Gain Muscle While You Sleep*. Despite these claims, there is little research evidence for the efficacy of many weight-loss supplements.

Weight-loss dietary supplements are theorized to induce weight loss by several mechanisms, including inducing a sense of satiety to suppress the appetite, stimulating fat oxidation and thermogenesis, and blocking brain receptors. For example, yohimbine, an alpha adrenergic antagonist, is thought to suppress appetite by blocking receptors in the brain, whereas caffeine may stimulate thermogenesis through fat oxidation. The essential nutrients carnitine and chromium, discussed in chapters 5 and 8, have been purported to facilitate the loss of body fat or increase in muscle mass. Pekala and others reported no effect of l-carnitine on body weight or composition. Separate meta-analyses by Onakpoya and Tian and their colleagues revealed minimal and no efficacy, respectively, of chromium on body weight or composition. Metabolites, herbals, and extracts such as conjugated linoleic acid, caffeine, synephrine, green tea catechins, guarana, and others are also purported weight-loss dietary supplements. A meta-analysis by Onakpoya and colleagues reported little efficacy of conjugated linoleic acid supplementation in changing body composition.

Most research has focused on caffeine, herbals, or other supplements that promote thermogenesis. Caffeine, covered in detail in chapter 13, is a stimulant drug found in many popular beverages, particularly coffee and tea. Caffeine may stimulate metabolism and play a small beneficial role in weight control. Heckman and others reported a link between caffeine use and weight loss, with a consequent reduction of the overall risks for developing the metabolic syndrome. Caffeine is also present in many weight-loss dietary supplements and is found naturally in guarana and yerba mate, two herbals marketed for weight loss. Green tea contains caffeine and catechins, a combination marketed for weight control. Rains and others noted that green tea catechins, like caffeine, may influence the sympathetic nervous system, increasing energy expenditure and fat oxidation. Hursel and others reported in their meta-analysis increases of 5 percent in daily energy expenditure following catechin-caffeine and caffeine-only supplementation, while catechin-caffeine supplementation increased daily fat oxidation by 12 to 16 percent. However, in their meta-analysis, Phung and others concluded that although green tea catechins with caffeine did reduce body weight and waist circumference, the clinical significance of these reductions was modest at best. They also noted that the data do not suggest an independent effect of catechins. In general, research supports a modest effect of caffeine, either alone or combined with catechins, on weight loss, but additional research is warranted. According to Saito and Yoneshiro, capsaicin and capsinoids also induce thermogenesis by activating brown adipose tissue, which was discussed in chapter 10.

Other related herbal stimulants have been studied as a means to induce weight loss. Ma huang, or *Ephedra sinica,* contains ephedrine, a stimulant drug. Ephedrine, covered in detail in chapter 13, was marketed until 2006 as a weight-loss dietary supplement, at which time it was removed from the marketplace because its use was associated with serious health problems. Ephedrine-based products have since been replaced with synephrine, also known as *bitter orange,* which is chemically similar to ephedrine. However, as noted in chapter 13, research does not appear to support a beneficial effect of synephrine supplementation on weight loss. Synephrine may also be associated with health risks. Rossato and others reported that synephrine use has been linked to reports of adverse cardiac effects, including hypertension, angina, ventricular fibrillation, myocardial infarction, and sudden death. They note that the mechanisms involved in synephrine-induced cardiotoxicity are still unknown, because studies related to its safety are scarce. Kearney and others reported a substantial increase in the prevalence of adverse effects associated with herbal products containing yohimbine and questioned whether yohimbine should continue to be considered a safe dietary supplement.

Numerous other herbals and extracts, such as ginseng, yohimbine, and *Garcinia cambogia,* have been studied for their effect on weight loss, but research that evaluates their efficacy is very limited. Pawar and colleagues note the increasing use of herbal and botanical ingredients in so many products presents a challenge to develop analytical methods and techniques to ensure public safety. Egras and others, in a review of such dietary supplements used for weight loss, concluded that to date there is little clinical evidence to support their use and indicated that more data are necessary to determine the efficacy and safety of these supplements. The safety of weight-loss dietary supplements has been a concern. Although Heckman and others indicate that moderate caffeine consumption is considered safe and its use as a food ingredient has been approved, within certain limits, by numerous regulatory agencies around the world, its use may increase health risks for some, such as individuals with hypertension or women who are pregnant, as discussed in chapter 13.

Other stimulant supplements may pose significant health risks. The FDA removed Hydroxycut products—popular weight-loss dietary supplements—from the market in 2009 because their use was associated with serious liver damage. Contamination of dietary supplements may contribute to such health problems. As noted in chapter 2, dietary supplements are not subject to the same quality control as drugs and food. In their review, Judkins and Prock discussed the prevalence of supplements available on the Internet that are contaminated with steroids, stimulants, and other substances that are prohibited in most sports. Athletes who use weight-loss supplements in conjunction with their sport may consume products containing such contaminants and risk suspension from competition for a positive drug test.

www.fda.gov Type "Weight loss products" in the search box for updated information on dietary supplements for weight loss.

www.ods.od.nih.gov Click on *Dietary Supplement Fact Sheets* to get information on a specific dietary supplement.

Some organizations, such as U.S. Pharmacopeia (USP), may place a seal on the supplement label indicating that the product has been treated for purity and quality. However, the seal does not guarantee that the product will be effective as advertised.

Is it harmful to overeat occasionally?

Most of us occasionally overindulge in food, particularly on holidays and other festive occasions or when we dine at all-you-can-eat restaurants. Eating is a pleasurable activity, and the occasional overindulgence is not harmful as long as it does not become a habit. As noted in chapter 5, try to avoid high-fat meals if you are prone to cardiovascular disease, because such meals may increase the risk of heart attacks. After a very large meal, you may step on the scale the next day and find that you have gained 5 pounds or more. This should not be alarming, since most of that weight is water, which may be bound to the increased carbohydrate (glycogen stores) in your body. Additionally, if the meal was high in sodium, your extracellular water stores will also increase. Going back to your regular diet and exercise program will reduce these water stores in a day or so, and your body weight will return to normal.

It is important to recognize that occasional overeating may be a lapse in your diet and that you treat it as such. Renew your commitment to your weight-loss plan and prevent the occasional lapse from becoming a relapse.

Key Concepts

▶ Rapid loss of body weight, which may occur during the early stages of dieting, is due primarily to body-water changes. The rate at which weight loss occurs will slow down as your body weight decreases, for then body-fat stores are the prime source of weight loss and necessitate a greater caloric deficit.

▶ Numerous weight-loss diet plans are available, including low-fat diets, low-carbohydrate diets, and high-protein diets. All may be effective and safe if the daily caloric energy intake is less than the daily caloric energy expenditure. The DASH and Omni Heart diets may be highly recommended for weight control, as may a healthful Mediterranean diet.

▶ Counting Calories and grams of fat may be a useful technique during the early stages of a diet, for the more knowledge you have about the caloric and nutrient content of foods, the better equipped you are to make wise selections.

▶ The key principle of dieting is to select from among the six food exchanges low-Calorie, high-nutrient foods that appeal to your taste and are easily incorporated into your daily lifestyle.

▶ Very low-Calorie diets (VLCD) may be effective for weight loss under strict medical supervision but are not recommended for the average individual trying to lose some excess fat.

▶ In general, weight-loss dietary supplements do not appear to be effective, and their use may be associated with adverse health effects.

Check for Yourself

▶ Using the Food Exchange System, plan a balanced, healthy diet of 1,600 Calories for an individual who needs to consume this much to lose excess body fat.

▶ Go to a local health food store and ask the clerk for weight-loss products. Check those available and determine the active ingredient in each. How many contain various herbals or caffeine? Alternatively, ask only for those with herbals or herbals with caffeine (guarana), and inquire about the safety of each. Compare your findings to the text discussion.

Exercise Programs

In their review of interactions between genes and physical activity, Rankinen and Bouchard noted considerable research indicating that the level of physical activity plays a role in the risk of excessive weight gain, in weight-loss programs, and particularly in the prevention of weight regain. This section highlights the development of an exercise program to help prevent weight gain, promote weight loss, and maintain a healthy body weight. The following government Website provides information on exercise and weight loss for Americans.

www.cdc.gov/healthyweight/

What role does exercise play in weight reduction and weight maintenance?

Humans are meticulously designed for physical activity, and yet our modern mechanical age has eliminated many of the opportunities that our ancient ancestors had to incorporate moderate physical activity as a natural part of daily living. The regulation of our food intake has not adapted to the highly mechanized conditions in today's society. As discussed in chapter 10, physical inactivity may be one of the major contributing factors to the development and maintenance of obesity. For example, a sedentary lifestyle, principally TV watching, has been significantly associated with obesity in adolescents and adults. Indeed, the late Jean Mayer, an international authority on weight control, reported that no single factor is more frequently responsible for obesity than lack of physical exercise.

There are basically two ways you can become more physically active and increase your total daily energy expenditure. First, decrease the amount of time that you are physically inactive, particularly time watching television. In a review of 232 studies, Tremblay and others reported a significant reduction in children's BMI with decreased time spent in sedentary activities, including watching television. The same thinking applies to adults as well. In general, you want to increase your level of nonexercise activity themogenesis (NEAT). Keep moving throughout the day by walking rather than riding, standing instead of sitting, and fidgeting when you have to sit. Levine and others comment that obese individuals generally remain seated for about 2.5 more hours per day than their lean counterparts, which could result in 350 fewer Calories expended daily.

Second, start a planned exercise program. The Consumers Union noted that to slim down permanently, you need to make a lifelong commitment to regular exercise, including not only aerobic exercise to burn Calories but also strength (resistance) training to build or at least preserve muscle. According to Shaibi and others, regular exercise lowers cardio-metabolic risk of obese children by improving glucose tolerance, lipid status, and vascular health even in the absence of weight loss.

Resistance Exercise Training Resistance-training, or weight-training, programs are detailed in chapter 12 in relation to gaining body weight as muscle mass, but such programs may also be very helpful during weight-loss programs. One possibility, as suggested by the American College of Sports Medicine, is that increased strength through resistance training may lead to a more active lifestyle in sedentary overweight and obese individuals, thus leading to health benefits that may include weight loss and prevention of weight regain. Another possibility is maintenance of REE during weight loss. According to Hansen and colleagues, the more significant role of resistance training on body composition during weight loss is in maintaining or increasing fat-free mass rather than through energy expenditure leading to loss of fat mass. Recall that protein tissue, primarily muscle, may be lost along with body fat during a weight-reduction program. However, resistance training may stimulate muscular development and help prevent significant decreases in lean body mass. Such an effect may also help prevent decreases in the REE. Additionally, as is noted in chapter 12, the typical resistance-training workout does not burn many Calories, mainly because of frequent recovery periods; however, dynamic circuit-type resistance-training programs may also be used to burn additional Calories.

Aerobic Exercise Exercise burns Calories (figure 11.6). The primary function of aerobic exercise in a weight-control program is simply to increase the level of energy expenditure and help tip the caloric equation so that energy output is greater than energy input. As mentioned in chapter 3, the metabolic rate may be increased tremendously during aerobic exercise. For example, while the average person may expend only 60–70 Calories per hour during rest, this value may approach 1,000 Calories per hour during a sustained, high-level activity such as rapid walking, running, swimming, or bicycling. Athletes involved in extreme endurance bicycling and running events have been reported to consume between 6,000 and 13,000 Calories per day.

If you are overweight, the same amount of aerobic weight-bearing exercise will cost you more Calories than your leaner counterpart. Because you have more weight to move, you will expend more energy and lose more body fat in the long run. For example, the energy cost of jogging 1 mile would be about 70 Calories for

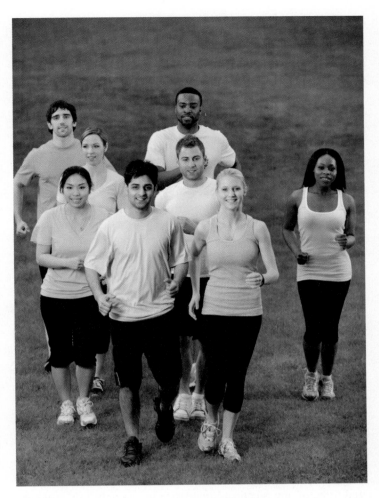

FIGURE 11.6 Exercise can be an effective means of increasing energy expenditure and losing excess Calories.

the 100-pound individual and about 140 Calories for someone twice that weight. Figure 11.7 depicts this concept graphically for one type of exercise—walking.

Many individuals may be discouraged to learn that 1 pound of fat contains about 3,500 Calories. Since approximately 100 Calories are expended in walking or running 1 mile, one must walk or jog 35 miles to lose that pound of fat. As a result, they hesitate to become physically active because they mistakenly believe exercise expends few Calories. However, individuals must consider the **long-haul concept** of weight control. The extra weight did not appear overnight, nor will it disappear overnight. Walking or jogging 2 miles a day will increase caloric expenditure by 6,000 Calories a month (about 1.7 pounds lost), provided the individual does not compensate by consuming more Calories. At this rate, you may lose 10 pounds in 6 months.

In addition to the direct effect of increased energy output during exercise, exercise has been theorized to facilitate weight loss by other means. As noted in chapter 3, aerobic exercise may increase the REE during the period immediately following the exercise bout and may increase the thermic effect of food (TEF) if you exercise after eating a meal. Unfortunately, the magnitude

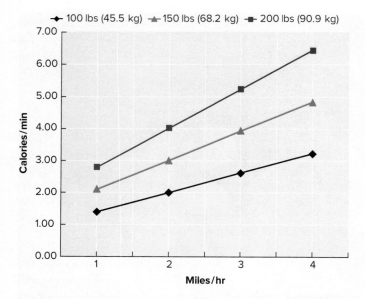

FIGURE 11.7 Effect of speed (mph) and gross body weight (lbs) on energy expenditure (Calories/minute) of walking. The heavier the individual, the greater the expenditure of Calories for any given speed of walking. The same would be true for running and other physical activities in which the body must be moved by foot. Data points in Figure 11.7 are calculated using the ACSM metabolic equations for steady-state walking exercise.

Source of equation: American College of Sports Medicine. 2014. *ACSM's Guidelines for Exercise Testing and Prescription*, 9th ed. Baltimore: Lippincott Williams & Wilkins.

of this increased REE or TEF is relatively minor and not considered to be of any practical importance in a weight-loss program. Related to the TEF, it does not matter if you exercise before or after a light meal, although as noted in the following text, exercise before a meal may help curb the appetite.

However, like resistance exercise, aerobic exercise may have a beneficial effect on the REE, but to a lesser degree. Although aerobic exercise will not totally prevent the decrease in the REE normally seen with weight loss, particularly with large weight losses, some studies suggest that it may help minimize the decrease, thereby helping maintain energy expenditure near normal levels during rest. However, not all research supports this finding. The interested reader is referred to the review by Schwartz and others.

Moreover, during aerobic exercise, the body mobilizes its fat cells to supply energy to the muscle cells. Hence, body-fat stores are reduced. In the long run, this change in body composition may actually favor a slight increase in the REE because muscle tissue is more active metabolically than fat tissue. Recall that in dieting alone, some lean muscle mass may be lost. According to Stiegler and Cunliffe, exercise combined with dietary restrictions is better at sustaining fat-free mass while decreasing fat mass than either exercise or diet alone.

Some research suggests that aerobic exercise may decrease the REE in individuals who are already lean, indicating that the body is attempting to preserve its energy reserves. This may be particularly true among elite endurance athletes, as noted by Sjodin and

others. Although this does not appear to be of any concern to overweight individuals who desire to lose weight, it may pose a problem to the lean athlete who is attempting to shed a few additional pounds for competition.

In addition to the physiological effects on energy expenditure, exercise may also confer significant psychological and medical benefits, even without any weight loss. As the fitness level and body composition improve, the individual may experience improvements in mood, energy levels, body image, and self-esteem. In a meta-analysis of 57 studies, Campbell and Hausenblas reported an improved body image following an exercise program. Exercise may also be the psychological catalyst that helps individuals to improve their nutritional habits and other health-related behaviors.

Aerobic exercise may yield other significant health benefits. For example, as documented in the *Surgeon General's Report on Physical Activity and Health,* exercise, as a form of physical activity, is becoming increasingly important as a means to help prevent, and even treat, many chronic diseases, such as cardiovascular disease, diabetes, and osteoporosis. Separate reviews by Vissers and others and Kay and Fiatarone Singh conclude that physical activity significantly reduces abdominal and visceral fat in overweight and obese males and females, which may reduce symptoms of the metabolic syndrome. Many of the health benefits of exercise related to weight loss were discussed in chapters 1 and 10.

For individuals with normal body weight, exercise is highly recommended for its preventive role, not only to prevent weight gain in the first place but also to prevent weight regain in those who have lost weight and are on a weight-maintenance program. It is generally recognized that prevention of obesity or excess body weight is more effective than treatment. Clark noted that organized exercise programs that elicit a physiological response are more effective in combating childhood obesity than general physical activity. Most people do not become overweight overnight but rather accumulate an extra 75–150 Calories per day, which over time will lead to excessive fat tissue. A daily exercise program could easily counteract the effect of these additional Calories and is a key component of a weight-maintenance program. Jakicic and Gallagher noted that although exercise may have a modest impact on initial short-term weight loss, it may have its greatest effect on long-term weight loss and prevention of weight regain. Catenacci and Wyatt also emphasize the essential role of physical activity in weight-loss maintenance. For those who like to eat but not gain weight, exercise is the intelligent alternative.

Does exercise affect the appetite?

Short-Term Effects On a short-term basis, exercise appears to depress the appetite. Schubert and others examined the results of 20 studies and concluded that acute exercise decreases ghrelin levels, which are known to stimulate appetite, and increases other gut hormones known to decrease food intake. In their review, Elder and Roberts concluded that the loss of body fat associated with exercise may be mediated by the spontaneous reduction in hunger associated with the exercise task.

The intensity of the exercise may be an important consideration. Intense exercise may be used to curb the appetite on a short-term basis at an appropriate time. In their review of 20 studies, Horner and colleagues reported that higher exercise intensities slowed the rate of gastric emptying. Research has related the appetite-suppressing effect of exercise to increased body temperature. The close anatomical relationship of the temperature and hunger centers in the hypothalamus may provide a rationale for the inhibition of the hunger center. Both exercise and the TEF will increase the core temperature of the body, so the body simply may be attempting to protect itself against an excessive rise in core temperature by suppressing the appetite to avoid the TEF. Exercise also will stimulate the secretion of several hormones in the body, notably epinephrine, which may also depress the appetite by affecting the hypothalamus or by increasing serum levels of both glucose and free fatty acids.

If you exercise before a meal, your food intake may be reduced considerably. If you have the facilities available, a half-hour of intense exercise may be an effective substitute for a large lunch. You may lose Calories two ways, expending them through exercise and replacing the large lunch with a low-Calorie, nutritious snack. However, King and others noted that although intense exercise may be an effective means of suppressing the appetite, the effects are brief. Thus, while intense exercise may help to curb your appetite at lunch, unless you are cautious you may increase your caloric intake above normal at dinner. Laan and others reported that although aerobic exercise decreased the appetite at 30 minutes postexercise, caloric intake increased by 14 percent at the next meal.

Long-Term Effects   On a long-term basis, increased energy expenditure through physical activity is generally counterbalanced by an increased food intake. The body compensates for the increased energy expenditure by consuming more energy. This is one of the major mechanisms whereby normal body weight is controlled in the average individual. Melanson and others indicated that there may be substantial individual variability in responses to exercise as a means to weight control and discuss compensatory behaviors such as increased caloric intake and/or decreased activity that counterbalance expected weight loss. In contrast, some individuals may not increase food intake and thus will experience weight loss. Donnelly and Smith reported that women generally lose less weight than men in response to exercise, suggesting as a reason that women may be more likely to exhibit a compensatory increase in energy intake in response to exercise. Since there is considerable inter-individual variability in behavioral and metabolic compensatory responses, exercise prescriptions might be more effective if tailored to suit individuals.

An important concern for the athletic individual is the fact that the appetite may not normally decrease with a decreased activity level, as recently reported by Stubbs. If you are physically active, but then must curtail your activity because of an injury or some other reason, your appetite may remain elevated above what you need to maintain body weight at your reduced energy levels. Hence, if you decrease your level of physical activity, you must reduce your food intake to balance the caloric equation to avoid weight gain.

Does exercise affect the set point?

As you may recall from chapter 10, the set-point theory suggests each individual possesses an inborn mechanism that attempts to maintain a certain level of energy balance, or body weight, by modifying energy intake or energy expenditure. In simple terms, the settling-point theory, another theory, suggests that the set point can be adjusted to a new level. Physical activity may have a significant impact on the settling point, or the body weight and body fatness at which a new steady state is reached. Hill and Commerford suggested that physical activity will increase total energy expenditure and fat oxidation, which can lead to an overall energy imbalance if there is not complete compensation in terms of increased energy intake and fat intake, and possibly decreased spontaneous daily activities. Increased physical activity can help individuals reach fat and energy balances at lower levels of body fatness than would have been achieved with lower levels of physical activity. Body weight and fat should decrease until a new steady state is achieved. However, there may be a limit to lowering the set point. Foster-Schubert and others reported that exercise-induced weight loss over 1 year resulted in an increase in plasma ghrelin, which stimulates the appetite. Unless the hypothalamus becomes less sensitive to ghrelin, the appetite will be stimulated to help deter additional weight loss.

What types of exercise programs are most effective for losing body fat?

There are a number of available exercise programs designed to reduce body weight. There are numerous media advertisements for various weight reduction programs, many of which use sophisticated equipment and claim to be the best or fastest way to lose body fat. The truth is that you do not need any special apparatus or any specially designed program. You can design your own program once you know a few basic principles about exercise and energy expenditure. However, a personal fitness trainer may be helpful in getting you on the right track during the early stages of an exercise program and may provide psychological support to help you maintain or increase your exercise program.

Although resistance exercise may play an important role in weight control, as discussed in chapter 12, the best type of exercise program for losing body fat involves aerobic exercises, those that utilize the oxygen energy system (figure 11.8). This type of exercise program is also the one that conveys the most significant health benefits. The key points of an aerobic exercise program are as follows.

Mode of Exercise   The mode of exercise must involve large muscle groups. The muscles of the legs constitute a good portion of the total body mass, as do the muscles of the arms. The major

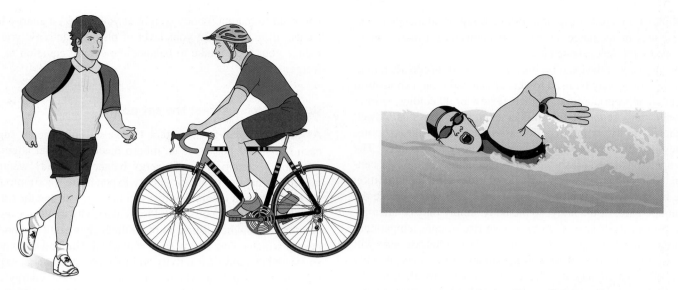

FIGURE 11.8 Aerobic-mode exercises—such as running, bicycling, or swimming—must involve large muscle groups.

muscles in the chest and back are also attached to the upper arm and are actively involved in almost all arm movements. Walking, jogging, hiking, stair climbing, running, in-line skating, and bicycling primarily involve the legs, whereas swimming primarily stresses the arms. The use of hand-held weights in walking incorporates arm action with the legs. Cross-country skiing, rowing, and rope jumping use both the arms and legs, as does an aerobic dance routine. These are good large-muscle activities, although there are a host of others.

Intensity of Exercise   The second factor is the intensity level. The higher the **exercise intensity**, the more Calories you expend per unit of time, and so the less time you need to burn a given amount of Calories. However, it is important to note that individuals beginning an exercise program should *not* engage in high-intensity training. Low- to moderate-intensity exercise training is preferred for beginners, who may increase the exercise intensity as they increase their fitness level. Normal walking uses fewer Calories than easy jogging, which uses fewer Calories than fast running. Simply put, it costs you more energy to move your body weight at a faster pace.

However, there is an optimal intensity level for each person depending on how long the exercise will last. You can run at a very high intensity for 50 yards, but you certainly could not maintain that same fast pace for 2 miles. Intensity and duration are interrelated, but for burning the most total Calories, duration becomes more important, and the intensity must be adapted for the amount of time you plan to exercise.

To get an idea of exercises with high intensity, check the Compendium of Physical Activities (https://sites.google.com/site/compendiumofphysicalactivities/) for the metabolic cost of many sporting, recreational, leisure-time, occupational, household, daily, and other activities. The Compendium values are in METs or multiples of resting metabolic cost (1 MET = 3.5 mL oxygen/kg/min).

Higher MET values represent more intense activity. When using the Compendium, keep these points in mind:

1. The figures are approximate and include the resting metabolic rate. Values for body weight and exercise time are needed to convert METS to Calories expended. The total cost of the exercise includes not only the Calories expended by the exercise itself but also the resting Calories you would have used anyway during the same period. As an example, a 154-pound (70-kg) person bicycles for 1 hour at a speed of 13 miles/hr. Go to the Compendium Website, click the "Activity Category" tab; then click "Bicycling." The bicycling activity described as "bicycling, 12–13.9 mph, leisure, moderate effort" (Compendium code 01030) has a total intensity of 8 METS, with 1 MET representing the resting metabolic cost. The actual (or net) intensity of the bicycling activity is 7.0 METS. As illustrated in the following table, the calculated energy cost is approximately 588 Calories. The bicyclist would have expended approximately 74 Calories at rest, so the net cost of the 1 hour bicycle ride is approximately 514 Calories.

2. The figures in the table are only for the time you are performing the activity. For example, in an hour of basketball, you may exercise strenuously only for 35–40 minutes, as you may take time-outs and may rest during foul shots. In general, record only the amount of time that you are actually moving during the activity.

3. The figures may give you some guidelines to total energy expenditure, but actual caloric costs might vary somewhat according to such factors as skill level, environmental factors (running against the wind or up hills), and so forth.

4. There may be small differences between men and women, but not enough to make a marked difference in the total caloric value for most exercises.

Activity: Bicycling, 12–13.9 miles/hr, leisure, moderate effort (Compendium code 01030)	Total Calories	Resting Calories	Net Calories
METS	8.0*	1.0	7.0
mL O$_2$/kg/min (= METS × 3.5 mL O$_2$/kg/min)	28.0	3.5	24.5
Body weight (154 pounds = 70 kg)[†]	70	70	70
mL O$_2$/min (= mL O$_2$/kg/min × kg)	1960	245	1715
Liters O$_2$/min (= mL O$_2$/min ÷ 1000)	1.96	0.245	1.715
Calories/min (= liters O$_2$/min × 5 Calories/liter O$_2$)	9.8	1.225	8.575
[‡]Minutes of activity	60	60	60
Total Calories (= Calories/min × minutes of activity)	588	74	514

Example of calculations to convert exercise intensity in METS to total calories, resting calories, and net calories.
*From the Compendium;
[†]subject's body weight in kilograms;
[‡]duration of the activity in minutes.

The Table of Caloric Expenditure based on the Compendium of Physical Activities, appendix B, or table 3.6 on page 112 may be useful to determine which types of activities may be of the appropriate intensity for your weight-control program. Listing those activities with higher caloric expenditure per minute may suggest several that you could blend into your lifestyle. Several Websites can provide you with an estimate of caloric expenditure in a wide variety of physical activities.

www.primusweb.com/fitnesspartner Enter your body weight and the amount of time you exercise and this program will provide you with your caloric expenditure for more than 200 physical activities.

http://ergo.human.cornell.edu/cutools.html Click the "METS to Calories Calculator" link under "Other Useful Tools" at the bottom of the screen.

http://lamb.cc/calories-burned-calculator These two sites calculate gross caloric expenditure from body weight, exercise time, and the intensity in METS (from the Compendium).

https://sites.google.com/site/compendiumofphysicalactivities/ The Compendium of Physical Activities, revised by Barbara Ainsworth and her associates in 2011, provides energy expenditure for more than 800 physical activities. The intensity of the activity is provided in MET values, and you may recall that 1 MET is your resting energy expenditure. You may review chapter 3 to convert METS to caloric expenditure.

Duration of Exercise Probably the most important factor in total energy expenditure is the duration of the exercise. In swimming, bicycling, running, or walking, distance is the key. For example, running a mile will cost the average-sized individual about 100 Calories. Five miles would approximate 500 Calories. An individual running 1 mile a day would take more than 1 month to expend the caloric equivalent of 1 pound of fat, whereas running 5 miles a day would shorten the time span to about 1 week. Thus, if the purpose of the exercise program is to lose weight, the individual should stress the **duration concept**. In their review, Catenacci and Wyatt reported that subjects lost substantially more weight in studies that prescribed greater amounts of exercise. For example, Tate and others found that over the course of 18 months, subjects who were encouraged to expend 2,500 Calories or more weekly lost significantly more weight than those who were encouraged to expend the standard 1,000 Calories weekly. At the end of 30 months, subjects who continued to expend 2,500 Calories or more weekly lost approximately 25 more pounds than those who exercised less.

A key point about the duration concept is the importance of constant movement rather than total time. For example, although tennis and running are both excellent physical activities, running will expend considerably more Calories in an hour than tennis. Running is a continuous activity, while tennis is an intermittent activity with a number of rest periods, during which the energy expenditure is lower. Consequently, two to three times more Calories may be expended in an hour of running compared to tennis. A similar differentiation can be made between runners and walkers with a greater accrued distance in an hour of running compared to walking.

In a survey of racially and ethnically diverse women, lack of time was reported by King and others to be a common barrier to regular physical activity. Shorter, more frequent bouts of exercise, or *exercise snacks,* may fit more conveniently into a busy schedule than the more traditional larger (30- to 40-min) blocks of time. In separate studies, Murphy and Macfarlane and their colleagues reported several short-duration bouts of exercise to be as effective as a single longer 30- to 40-minute bout in producing weight loss and improving cardiovascular fitness, respectively. Brisk walks before work, during work and lunch breaks, and before or after dinner may increase adherence to your exercise program and improve study or work productivity by providing a psychological boost during the day.

A major reason many adults do not use exercise as a weight-loss mechanism is that their level of physical fitness is so low they cannot sustain a moderate level of exercise intensity for very long.

However, keep in mind that as you continue to train, your body will begin to adapt so that in time you will be able to exercise for longer and longer periods.

Additionally, intensity and duration are interrelated and, if balanced, will result in equal weight losses. Melanson and others found that compared to a sedentary day, expending 400 Calories during exercise intensities of 40 and 70 percent of VO_2 max increased 24-hour energy expenditure, but there was no difference attributed to exercise intensity. Grediagin and others also found no significant difference in body-fat losses when women engaged in either high-intensity or low-intensity exercise, provided the total caloric expenditure per exercise session was the same. In both cases, it simply took the low-intensity exercise group longer to expend the same amount of Calories. However, in a study controlling total exercise energy expenditure in both exercise tasks, Irving and others reported that high-intensity exercise was more effective than low-intensity exercise as a means to reduce total abdominal fat. Hunter recommends incorporating some higher-intensity exercise in your program as your fitness level improves, not only because it burns Calories more rapidly but also because it will make your moderate-intensity workouts seem much easier. Additionally, as noted in chapter 1 and later in this chapter, additional health benefits may be associated with higher-intensity exercise.

Frequency of Exercise **Exercise frequency** complements duration and intensity. Frequency of exercise is how often each week you participate. As would appear obvious, the more often you exercise, the greater the total weekly caloric expenditure. In general, three to four times per week would be satisfactory, provided duration and intensity were adequate, but six to seven times would just about double your caloric output. A daily exercise program is recommended if weight control is the primary goal.

http://streaming.cdc.gov/vod.php?id=e6e0389dc5b6ce243 8443ae0c848c2a320111024101650742 This Centers for Disease Control and Prevention video is a good introduction to light-, moderate-, and vigorous-intensity aerobic exercise.

Enjoyment of Exercise An important factor is enjoyment of the exercise. For an activity to be effective in the long run, it should be one that you enjoy, yet one that will help expend Calories because it has a recommended intensity level, can be performed for a long time, or both. For example, you may not enjoy jogging or running, so other activities may be substituted. Fast walking with vigorous arm action, golf (pulling a cart), swimming, bicycling, tennis, handball, racquetball, aerobic dancing, and a variety of other activities may produce a greater feeling of enjoyment and still burn a considerable number of Calories. Even leisure activities and home chores done vigorously, such as gardening, yard work, washing the car, and home repairs, may be useful in burning Calories and developing fitness. Exercise need not be unpleasant. Enjoy your exercise. Try to make it a lifelong habit by viewing it as play. Next time you vacuum the house or mow the lawn, try to think about it as a good workout rather than work.

Practicality of Exercise Practicality is another important factor. You may enjoy swimming, tennis, racquetball, soccer, and a variety of other sports, but lack of facilities, poor weather conditions, no playing partners, or high costs may limit your ability to participate. For the active person who travels, this may be a major concern. Although there are many excellent activities that burn calories, the authors are admittedly biased toward walking and running because these activities are simple, are practical, and satisfy all of the previously mentioned criteria for maintaining body weight. All you need is a good pair of shoes and proper clothes for the weather, so nothing short of an injury should deter you from your daily exercise routine. Walking, jogging, or running can be very practical substitutes on those days when you cannot participate in your regular physical activity. Wood indicated that brisk walking is perhaps the best single exercise in regard to energy expenditure, feasibility, and acceptability to a large proportion of the population. It is probably the best activity for those who are unfit, overweight, or elderly. Some guidelines to an effective walking program are presented later.

Indoor exercise equipment is also very practical for a number of reasons. It can be used while watching children, avoiding inclement weather, or doing two things at one time, such as reading or watching television news. This is a highly recommended way to watch television. Numerous types of aerobic indoor exercise equipment are available, such as bicycling apparatus, cross-country skiing simulators, rowing machines, stair-steppers, and treadmills. Computerized fitness programs, such as Wii Fit, can provide a strenuous indoor workout. Zeni and others reported that treadmill exercise expended more Calories at a set rating of perceived exertion compared to other modes of indoor aerobic exercise. Low-intensity active office stations are becoming more prevalent in the workplace as a way to offset the sedentary nature of office work. In their review, Tudor-Locke and others comment that treadmill work stations significantly increase energy expenditure compared to traditional seated office work. Resistance- or strength-training indoor equipment, which may help preserve fat-free tissue, is also available. Resistance training will be discussed in detail in chapter 12. *Consumer Reports* magazine offers periodic analyses of various types of indoor exercise equipment. Although indoor exercise equipment can be expensive, there are inexpensive options such as elastic bands, dumbbells, an exercise mat, a stability ball, and DVDs with various aerobic exercise routines.

Versatility of Exercise Versatility is also an important factor. Learn and engage in a variety of physical activities, such as running, cycling, swimming, rowing on stationary machines, stair climbing, striding on elliptical trainers, aerobic dancing, and aerobic walking. By cross-training, such as running 3 days per week, cycling 2 days, and swimming 2 days, you are less likely to become bored with exercise or to sustain overuse injuries. Also, if you plan to exercise for an hour daily, 1/2 hour each of running and cycling, or some other combination of exercises, is also an effective way to cross-train. Moreover, if you become injured and cannot do your favorite type of exercise, you may be able to expend Calories and maintain fitness by using alternative exercises until you heal. For example, if weight-bearing activities such as jogging bother you, do nonweight-bearing activities such as cycling or swimming, or water-jogging wearing a buoyancy vest.

If I am inactive now, should I see a physician before I initiate an exercise program?

Various medical groups, such as the American College of Sports Medicine and the American Heart Association, have developed guidelines to determine who should receive a medical exam prior to initiating an exercise program. A thorough review of these guidelines is not presented here because they are extensive and beyond the scope of this text. However, the following points represent a synthesis of these guidelines.

1. Before initiating any exercise program, you should be aware of any personal medical problems that could be aggravated. If you have concern about any facet of your health, check with your physician before starting an exercise program. This is especially important in weight-reduction exercise programs where the main stress is placed on the heart and blood vessels, the cardiovascular system.
2. No matter what your age, if you have any of the coronary heart disease risk factors noted in table 11.11, you should have a medical examination. You may also wish to assess your cardiac risk profile at the American Heart Association's Website.

3. If you are young (twenties or early thirties), are healthy, and have no risk factors, it is probably safe to initiate an exercise program.
4. The older you are, the better the idea to get a medical examination. In fact, it is prudent for those over 40 to have an examination.

https://www.heart.org/gglRisk/main_en_US.html Use this American Heart Association website to estimate your risk of coronary heart disease. This is only a screening tool and does not replace a examination by a physician. A high risk individual should discuss the results with a physician prior to beginning an exercise program.

What other precautions would be advisable before I start an exercise program?

Your initial level of physical fitness is an important determinant of the intensity of exercise during the early stages of the program. If you are completely unconditioned, you should start at a lower intensity level—walk before you jog, for example. Keep in mind that it took time for you to gain weight and become unconditioned, so it will also take time to reverse the process. A gradual progression is the key point. Examples are presented later.

Other general precautions involve safety factors, timing of meals, environmental hazards, and equipment. The individual should adhere to safety principles for the activity selected, particularly swimming, bicycling, and pedestrian safety. Strenuous exercise should not be undertaken within 2 or 3 hours of a

TABLE 11.11 Major risk factors and symptoms of coronary artery disease

Risk Factors	1	Age: male >45 years, female >55 years
	2	Family history of heart disease in immediate family: <55 yr in father/brother, <65 yr in mother/sister
	3	Cigarette smoking: any within 6 months or exposure to significant secondhand smoke
	4	Sedentary lifestyle: <30 min moderate-intensity physical activity, 3 times/wk for the past 3 months
	5	Obesity: BMI >30 kg/m², or waist >102 cm [40 inches] (males); 88 cm [35 inches] (females)
	6	Hypertension: systolic >140 mmHg and/or diastolic > 90 mmHg, *or taking antihypertensive medication*
	7	Dyslipidemia: total cholesterol >200 mg/dL, low-density lipoprotein cholesterol (LDL-C) >130 mg/dL, or high-density lipoprotein cholesterol (HDL-C) <40 mg/dL, *or taking lipid-lowering medications. Note: high HDL (>60 mg/dL) is a protective factor.*
	8	Prediabetes: fasting glucose levels >100 mg/dL but <126 mg/dL or impaired 2-hr oral glucose tolerance test >140 mg/dL but ≤199 mg/dL
Important signs and symptoms	1	Chest discomfort—range of feelings from pain to "heavy feeling"
	2	Shortness of breath, rest or mild exertion
	3	Dizziness
	4	Severe shortness of breath at night
	5	Swelling in the ankles
	6	Irregular heartbeat or heart rhythm
	7	Cramping or fatigue in the legs
	8	Heart murmur
	9	Unusual fatigue with common activities

Source: *American College of Sports Medicine's Guidelines for Exercise Testing and Prescription, 9th ed.* 2014. Baltimore: Lippincott Williams & Wilkins.

heavy meal but may be done earlier with a light meal or just liquids. As noted in chapter 9, a hot environment poses the most serious threat to the person in training. Be aware of signs of heat stress such as dizziness, nausea, and weakness. If these occur, stop exercising and find a means to help cool your body. Proper equipment should be selected for the chosen activity. For example, of critical importance to the jogger or walker is a well-designed pair of shoes. They may help prevent certain medical problems, such as tendinitis and shin splints, which may occur during the early stages of training. Bicycling with a helmet is a must.

What is the general design of exercise programs for weight reduction?

Both resistance- and aerobic-exercise training are recommended components of a weight-loss program. Resistance training is covered in chapter 12. The basic principles of exercise training were discussed in chapter 1.

In essence, aerobic-exercise programs to reduce body fat or to help maintain an optimal weight are based on the same principles that underlie exercise programs to improve the efficiency of the cardiovascular system. The total exercise program is based on a balance of exercise intensity, duration, and frequency. However, each daily exercise bout is usually subdivided into three phases—warm-up, stimulus, and cool-down, in that order (figure 11.9). A proper warm-up and cool-down are important components of the aerobic-exercise prescription. Both may help prevent excessive strain on the heart and may be helpful in the prevention of muscular soreness or injuries.

The **warm-up** precedes the stimulus period and may be done in several ways. It may be general in nature, such as calisthenics, or specific to the type of exercise you plan to do, such as initially exercising at a lower level of intensity of the actual mode of exercise. Some gentle static stretching exercises are also helpful in the warm-up period.

For most aerobic-type exercise, it is probably better to warm up the specific muscles to be used. For example, if you plan to use jogging as your mode of aerobic exercise, you should stretch your leg muscles gently at first and then jog at a slower than normal pace for several minutes. Breaking into a sweat is a good external sign that you have sufficiently elevated your body temperature; by using a specific type of warm-up, the temperature of your exercising muscles will also be increased.

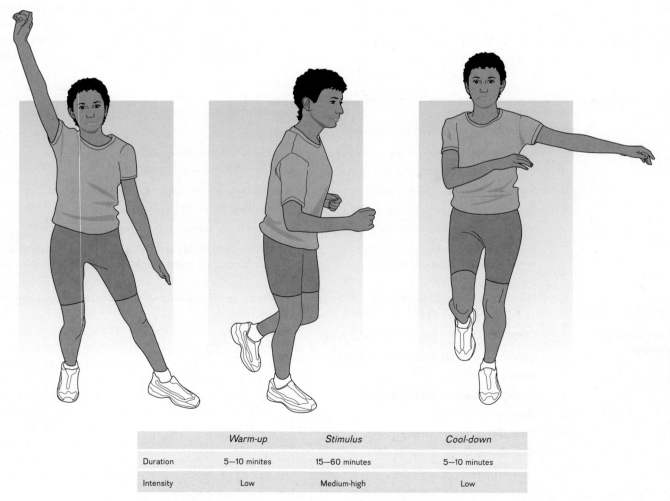

	Warm-up	Stimulus	Cool-down
Duration	5—10 minites	15—60 minutes	5—10 minutes
Intensity	Low	Medium-high	Low

FIGURE 11.9 The exercise prescription. The exercise prescription is divided into three phases: warm-up period, stimulus period, and cool-down period. The stimulus period is the key to burning Calories.

The **cool-down** phase follows the stimulus period and is designed primarily to help restore the cardiovascular system to normal. The abrupt cessation of exercise may provoke a number of undesirable outcomes. Blood may pool in the lower extremities, resulting in an increase in heart rate as a compensatory mechanism to maintain blood flow and pressure. There may be an increase in blood levels of certain hormones known to possibly cause an abnormal heart rhythm. These factors increase stress on the heart, which may induce a heart attack in individuals at risk. Decreased blood flow to the brain may cause dizziness and *exercise-associated collapse,* which was discussed in chapter 9. When the cool-down occurs gradually after strenuous exercise— by walking or jogging after a strenuous run, for example—the muscles help massage the blood through the veins back to the heart. These points emphasize the importance of a gradual cool-down. Complete your cool-down by stretching. Because the muscles are now warm from the exercise they are easier to stretch, which may help prevent muscle stiffness.

The warm-up and cool-down are important components of the daily exercise bout, but most of the Calories are expended during the stimulus period.

What is the stimulus period of exercise?

The **stimulus period** is the most important phase of the daily exercise bout. By modifying the intensity and duration of the exercise, the individual achieves the level of stimulus necessary to elicit a conditioning effect. As illustrated in figure 11.10, several important physiological and psychological measures increase in proportion to the exercise intensity.

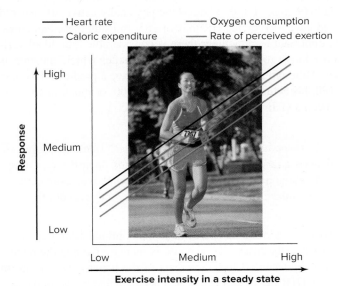

FIGURE 11.10 The relationship among various measures of energy expenditure. Heart rate (HR), oxygen consumption, caloric expenditure, and rate of perceived exertion (RPE) are, in general, directly related to the intensity of the exercise under steady-state conditions, that is, when the oxygen supply is adequate for the energy cost of the exercise. HR and RPE are practical methods to assess exercise intensity.

The two major components of the stimulus period are intensity and duration of exercise. In any exercise session, these two components are usually inversely related. In other words, if intensity is high, duration is short; if intensity is low, duration is long. Frequency (the number of exercise sessions per week) is also an important part of the exercise prescription. As discussed in detail in chapter 1, two joint reports from the American College of Sports Medicine and the American Heart Association, authored by Haskell and Nelson and their colleagues, provided recommendations on exercise for adults (age 18–65) and older adults (over age 65) as a means to help prevent chronic diseases. More recently, the American College of Sports Medicine, under the guidance of Donnelly and others, revised its position stand on appropriate physical activity intervention strategies for weight loss and prevention of weight regain for adults, and this position stand will be used as the basis for developing the aerobic exercise program here. However, some of the ACSM/AHA guidelines will be incorporated as deemed appropriate.

1. Intensity of training: For aerobic exercise, the ACSM position stand recommends moderate-intensity exercise, whereas the ACSM/AHA recommends both moderate- and vigorous-intensity exercise. Several techniques, such as heart rate measurement, to determine exercise intensity are discussed below. Intensity levels are based on the fitness level of the individual.
2. Duration of training: The ACSM position stand recommends a minimum of 150 minutes weekly, but 250 minutes or more may be recommended for specific weight-loss outcomes. For cardiovascular health, the ACSM/AHA guidelines recommend a minimum of 30 minutes daily for moderate-intensity exercise, or 20 minutes daily of vigorous-intensity exercise.
3. Frequency of training: The ACSM position stand recommends exercising about 5 days a week. The ACSM/AHA guidelines also recommend exercising 5 days weekly, but only 3 days may be needed if the exercise is vigorous.

Keep in mind that there are differences between these two sets of recommendations. The ACSM/AHA guidelines recommend exercise intensity, duration, and frequency for cardiovascular fitness and health, whereas the ACSM position stand focuses on exercise for weight loss and maintenance.

What is an appropriate level of exercise intensity?

The intensity of exercise is a very important component of the stimulus period; to receive the optimal benefits from the exercise program, you must attain a certain **threshold stimulus**, the minimal stimulus intensity that will produce a training effect. The intensity of exercise can be expressed in a number of different ways, such as percentage of VO_2 max and Calories/minute, but these techniques are not suitable for everyday exercise. However, other easily measured variables may provide you with a good estimate of your exercise intensity, including your heart rate, your perception of how strenuous the exercise is, and your ability to carry on a conversation.

Heart Rate As noted in figure 11.10, the heart rate is linearly related to oxygen consumption, which is the major measure of energy expenditure. Because the heart rate is easily obtained, it is usually used to determine the threshold level of exercise intensity.

To obtain the heart rate, press lightly with the index and middle fingers on the carotid artery, located just under the jawbone and beside the Adam's apple. Do not use the thumb, as it also has a pulse, and do not press hard on the carotid artery, for it may cause a reflex slowing of the beat in some persons. The radial artery pulse is obtained by placing your fingers on the inside of the wrist on the thumb side. These are the two most common locations for monitoring pulse rate, but other locations (the temple, inside the upper arm, and directly over the heart) may be used (see figure 11.11).

To obtain the heart rate per minute, simply count the pulse rate for 6 seconds and add a zero. Resting and recovery heart rates are easily obtainable, as they may be taken while you are motionless, but it is difficult to manually monitor the heart rate while exercising. Research has shown that the exercise heart rate correlates very highly with the heart rate during the early stages of recovery. Hence, to monitor exercise heart rate, secure the pulse *immediately* upon cessation of exercise and count the beats for 6 seconds. This provides a reliable measure of exercise heart rate, although it may be slightly lower due to the beginning of the recovery effect. If it is difficult for you to monitor your heart rate for 6 seconds, then use a 10-second period and multiply the count by six to obtain

your heart rate per minute. You probably should use 30 seconds to determine your resting heart rate; multiply your results by two. It may also be better to measure your resting pulse early in the morning, just after rising. Additionally, for the calculations to follow, you should take your resting heart rate in the position in which you will exercise—for example, lying down if you swim, seated if you cycle, or standing if you walk or run.

If you become serious about heart rate monitoring as the basis for your exercise training, you may want to invest in a device that monitors your heart rate while you exercise. Such devices usually use a comfortable chest band that transmits your heart rate to a wrist band so that you can easily see your heart rate response during any phase of exercise (see figure 11.11c).

One of the most prevalent techniques to determine the threshold stimulus for exercise is based upon the **maximal heart rate reserve (HR max reserve)**, the difference between the resting heart rate and the maximum heart rate. You may determine your resting heart rate shortly after you arise in the morning. You should not engage in strenuous physical activity to determine your maximal heart rate (HR max) if you have not been physically active in some time. If you have cardiovascular disease, more than one of the risk factors or any of the symptoms listed in table 11.11, you should discuss your exercise plans with your physician. There are various equations to predict HR max based on your age. The most commonly used and traditional equation in women and untrained men is 220 minus the person's age. As shown in table 11.12, other equations may be more relevant depending on gender, level of fitness, and body-composition status.

Using the traditional method, an untrained 40-year-old male would have a predicted HR max of 180 with a similar value using the Gellish method. The obese 40-year-old would also have a predicted HR max of 180, whereas the physically active 40-year-old would have a predicted HR max of 185. In using these equations, it is important to remember there is considerable individual variation relative to predicted HR max no matter which equation is used. Although a 40-year-old male may have a predicted HR max of 180, his actual HR max may be 200, 160, or much lower if he has been a victim of coronary heart disease.

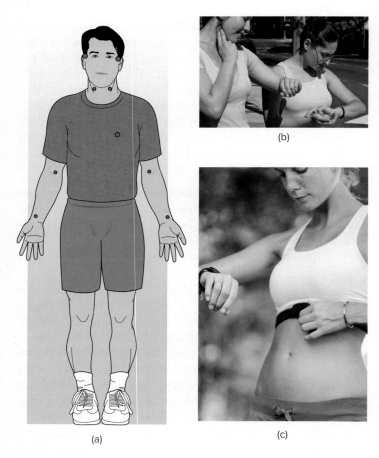

FIGURE 11.11 Palpation of heart rate. (a) Location of various palpation sites. (b) Carotid (left) and radial (right) pulse palpation are the two most commonly used to monitor the intensity of exercise. (c) Subject wearing a heart rate monitor.

www.stevenscreek.com/goodies/hr.shtml Use this link to calculate a target training heart rate based on entered resting heart rate and either actual maximal heart rate or predicted maximal heart rate based on age, gender, and level of fitness.

There is widespread agreement that optimal training effects occur when the heart rate response is increased above the resting level by between 50 and 85 percent of the **heart rate maximum reserve (HR max reserve)**, which is calculated as the maximum HR (HR max) minus the resting HR (RHR). Research has revealed that lower levels, 40–45 percent, may also be effective, particularly in individuals with poor levels of physical fitness.

Continuing with our example of the 40-year-old man, we can calculate the heart rate range needed to elicit a training effect. This is called the **target heart rate range**, or **target HR**. To complete the calculations, we need to know the age-predicted HR max

TABLE 11.12 Selected equations to predict maximum heart rate (HR max) in various populations

Equation	Authors	Comments	Age 10	20	30	40	50	60	70
220–age		Traditional	210	200	190	**180**	170	160	150
207–(0.7 × age)	Gellish	Avoids overestimating for those <40 and underestimating for those >40	NA	193	186	**179**	172	165	158
205–(0.5 × age)	Stevens Creek Software	Physically trained	NA	195	190	**185**	180	175	170
200–(0.5 × age)	Miller	Obese	NA	190	185	**180**	175	170	165
208–(0.7 × age)	Machado, Tanaka	Children and adolescents; healthy adults	201	194	187	**180**	173	166	159

and the resting heart rate (RHR); the latter should be determined under relaxed circumstances. If we assume a RHR of 70 and an a HR max of 180, the following formula, known as the **Karvonen equation**, would give us the target range:

$$\text{Target HR} = X\% \ (\text{HR max} - \text{RHR}) + \text{RHR}$$

For the 50 percent threshold level, the target heart rate for our example would be calculated as follows:

$$0.5 \ (180 - 70) + 70 =$$
$$0.5(110) + 70 = 55 + 70 = 125$$

For the 85 percent level, the target heart rate would be

$$0.85(180 - 70) + 70 =$$
$$0.85(110) + 70 = 93 + 70 = 163$$

Thus, to achieve a training effect, our 40-year-old man needs to train within a target HR range of 125–163.

If you wish to bypass the calculations, table 11.13 presents the target HR ranges for various age groups with RHR between 45 and 90 beats/minute. Simply find your age group and RHR in the headings and locate your target HR range. The table is based on a predicted HR max of 220 – age. If you prefer to use one of the other formulas to predict HR max, you may calculate your target HR range using the formula presented in table 11.12.

In general, table 11.13 is a useful guide to the threshold heart rate and target HR range. However, there is considerable variability in HR max among individuals, particularly in the older age groups. If your true HR max is below the predicted value (220 – age), the target HR range in the table would be higher than the recommended level. If your true HR max is higher than the predicted value, the target HR range in the table is lower than the recommended level. Although the target HR range might vary by a few beats, if your actual HR max is slightly higher or lower than the predicted value, you will still receive a good training effect—assuming you are in the middle of the range.

Once you have been training for a month or so, you may desire to determine your HR max in the specific activity you do. You may use the procedures described below, that is, running on a track at different speeds until you reach your maximal level, modifying the test dependent upon your aerobic exercise. For example, research has revealed that HR max is lower in swimming, possibly as much as 10 to 15 beats per minute, so the target heart rate may be slightly lower if this mode of exercise is used. One recommendation states that use of the formula 205 minus age may be appropriate to predict maximal heart rate while swimming.

As you can see, the range for the target heart rate may span about 30–50 beats. For example, a 36-year-old individual with a resting heart rate of 72 beats per minute has a target heart rate range of 127–167, or a span of 40 beats per minute. Exercising at the lower end of this range, about 127–147 beats per minute, may be considered moderate-intensity exercise, while exercising at about 148–167 beats may be considered vigorous-intensity exercise. However, for an untrained individual just starting a fitness program, a heart rate of 127–147 may appear to be vigorous at first, but as she continues to exercise and improves her physical fitness this same heart rate response may become less taxing and be perceived as moderate intensity. Moreover, as her fitness improves, her resting heart rate may decrease over time, possibly by 10 or more beats per minute, which will necessitate recalculation of the target heart rate range.

Rating of Perceived Exertion (RPE) Although the target heart rate approach is a sound means for monitoring exercise intensity, you may also wish to use other methods. One popular method, the **rating of perceived exertion (RPE)**, also known as the **Borg Scale**, is basically your perception of how hard you feel your body is working during exercise. The scale was originally designed to reflect heart rate responses by adding a zero to the rating. You simply rate the perceived difficulty or strenuousness of the exercise task according to the column A scale in table 11.14. If you are running, how do your legs feel? Do they feel light and easy to move, or are they heavy or possibly beginning to ache or burn? How is your breathing? Are you breathing easily and able to carry on a conversation, or are your sentences shortened to a few words? In general, how does your total body feel? Is the exercise too easy, or are you working too hard?

TABLE 11.13 Target heart rate zones

RHR	Age											
	15–19	20–24	25–29	30–34	35–39	40–44	45–49	50–54	55–59	60–64	65–69	70–74
45–49	125–180	123–175	120–171	118–167	115–163	113–158	110–154	108–150	105–146	103–141	100–137	98–133
50–54	127–181	125–176	122–172	120–168	117–164	115–159	112–155	110–151	107–147	105–142	102–138	100–134
55–59	130–181	128–176	125–172	123–168	120–164	118–159	115–155	113–151	110–147	108–142	105–138	103–134
60–64	132–182	130–177	127–173	125–169	122–165	120–160	117–156	115–152	112–148	110–143	107–139	105–135
65–69	135–183	133–178	130–174	128–170	125–166	123–161	120–157	118–153	115–149	113–144	110–140	107–136
70–74	137–184	135–179	132–175	130–171	127–167	125–162	122–158	120–154	117–150	115–145	112–141	110–137
75–79	140–184	138–180	135–176	133–172	130–168	128–163	125–159	123–155	120–151	118–146	115–142	113–138
80–84	142–185	140–181	137–177	135–173	132–169	130–164	127–160	125–156	122–152	120–147	117–143	115–139
85–89	145–186	143–181	140–177	138–173	135–169	133–164	130–160	128–156	125–152	123–147	120–143	118–139

The target zone (50–85 percent threshold) is based upon the median figure for each age range and resting heart rate range.

Borg also developed an abbreviated RPE scale with 0–10 points, which is depicted in column B in table 11.14. The OMNI-RPE scale uses a 0–10 pictorial version of exercisers displaying varying degrees of exertion. In separate studies, Utter and others validated its use in walking, running, and cycling exercise as comparable to the Borg RPE Scale. It has also been validated in children and older adults and for other activities such as bench stepping and elastic band exercise, as well as elliptical ergometry.

When you determine your exercise heart rate, it is a good idea to associate an appropriate RPE value with it so that you individualize the RPE to your specific exercise program. For example, at an exercise heart rate of 150 you might make a mental note of the exercise difficulty and assign a value of 15, or hard, to that level of exercise intensity. Research has shown that the RPE can be an effective means to measure exercise intensity in healthy individuals, particularly at heart rates above 150 beats/minute.

Talk Test   Another way to monitor your exercise effort, validated by Quinn and Coons and recently reviewed by Reed and Pipe, is associated with breathing and is often referred to as the *talk test*. If you are breathing harder but still able to carry on a conversation in complete sentences, you are probably exercising at a moderate intensity. However, if it is difficult for you to speak in complete sentences, you are probably exercising at a vigorous intensity. Another general rule of thumb is if you cannot maintain a conversation while exercising, you are probably exercising too hard, unless you are training for sports competition.

High-Intensity Interval Training   According to the American College of Sports Medicine, high-intensity interval training (HIIT) was the number one fitness trend for 2014. In contrast to a traditional continuous stimulus period, HIIT consists of repeated sets of high-intensity exercise followed by either rest or lower-intensity recovery intervals. For example, a person may alternate 1 minute at 90 percent

of HR reserve with 1 minute of exercise at 45 percent of HR reserve for a work: recovery ratio of 1:1. Advantages to HIIT include improvements in aerobic and anaerobic fitness, lipid profiles, insulin sensitivity, and blood pressure. HIIT may also reduce the weekly time commitment for exercise due to higher caloric expenditure at

TABLE 11.14 The RPE scales

A	B
6 Sitting, relaxing	0 Extremely easy
7 Very, very light	1
8	2 Easy
9 Very light	3
10	4 Somewhat easy
11 Light	5
12	6 Somewhat hard
13 Somewhat hard	7
14	8 Hard
15 Hard	9
16	10 Extremely hard
17 Very hard	
18	
19 Very, very hard	
20 Maximal effort	

the higher intensities of exercise. Some, but not all, research suggests HIIT may be an effective program for reducing abdominal and total fat while maintaining fat-free mass. In two studies comparing isocaloric HIIT and continuous aerobic exercise training, Sijie and others reported greater improvements in body composition with HIIT, whereas Keating and others found a significant reduction in android fat following continuous aerobic exercise but not HIIT. In his review, De Feo recommended continuous exercise over HIIT for obese subjects who generally have a low tolerance for high-intensity exercise. As previously discussed, the best weight-loss strategy is to exercise at the highest intensity that is safe and appropriate for age and health at a duration optimizing caloric expenditure.

> *www.acsm.org/docs/brochures/high-intensity-interval-training.pdf* This brochure, prepared by the American College of Sports Medicine, provides information on high-intensity interval training.

How can I determine the exercise intensity needed to achieve my target HR range?

To determine the exercise intensity necessary to reach your target HR range, all you need is a stopwatch. You may record your heart rate manually as explained previously, but use of a heart rate monitor would facilitate this task and probably increase the accuracy. Where distances are involved, such as with running, swimming, or cycling, an accurate measure is needed. An ideal situation for walking or running would be a quarter-mile (400 meters) high school or college track.

A steady-state HR response may be obtained in 3 to 5 minutes of evenly paced activity. A sound method for walking, jogging, or running follows, but this system may be adapted easily to other activities such as swimming, cycling, calisthenics, and aerobic dance.

Mark a 1/2-mile mile course. Two laps on a 1/4-mile track would be ideal, but you can pace out a quarter-mile on the sidewalks near your home. Measure your resting HR. Walk until you have an even pace and then time yourself for the 1/2 mile. Immediately record your HR at the conclusion of the exercise. During your walk, mentally record the RPE. Did you reach the target HR? Was your RPE related to your HR? If the HR response was in the target range or the RPE was not too strenuous, you are at a level to begin your training program. If the HR response was not in the target range, rest until your HR returns close to normal and then take the test at a faster pace. Repeat this procedure until you have a plot of the HR, RPE, and time for the 1/2 mile. Keep a record of this, as it will be useful in evaluating the effects of your conditioning program.

For example, suppose you recorded the following data on the 1/2-mile test on four trials (figure 11.12).

Test	Time	RPE	HR	Minutes/mile
1	8:00	11	108	16:00
2	7:10	13	132	14:20
3	6:30	15	156	13:00
4	6:00	18	180	12:00

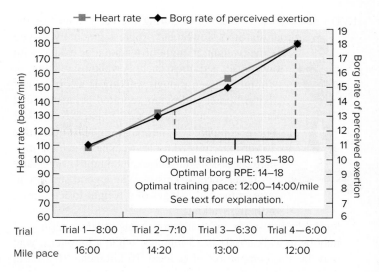

FIGURE 11.12 Plot of heart rate and RPE following a ½-mile walk in determination of the threshold heart rate.

As your speed increases, both RPE and HR naturally increase. If your predicted HR max is 200, and your resting HR is 70, the 50–85 percent target range approximates 135–180. Test 1 does not provide adequate stimulus intensity, Test 2 is just below the minimum target HR, Test 3 is in the middle of the range, while Test 4 is at your upper limit. Thus, your training intensity should be between 12 and 14 minutes per mile. The RPE may offer a means of judging the intensity of the exercise when you do not have a set distance and watch.

To determine your speed for these tests, simply double the time for the 1/2-mile and you have the time per mile. The last trial was 12 minutes per mile. The total caloric expenditure (resting + exercise) could be calculated from the intensity of exercise in METS found in the Compendium of Physical Activities (https://sites.google.com/site/compendiumofphysicalactivities/), your weight in kilograms (= pounds ÷ 2.2), and the minutes of exercise using either the following calculation

$$\text{Total calories} = \text{Exercise intensity in METS} \times 3.5 \text{ mL O}_2/\text{kg/min} \times \text{body weight in kg} \div 1,000 \text{ mL/liter O}_2 \times 5 \text{ Calories/liter} \times \text{minutes of exercise}$$

or one of these Websites: http://ergo.human.cornell.edu/cutools.html (click the "METS to Calories Calculator" link under "Other Useful Tools" at the bottom of the screen) or http://lamb.cc/calories-burned-calculator.

How can I design my own exercise program?

The exercise program that you design should not only be safe and effective but should also be one to which you will adhere for a lifetime. Unfortunately, in 2012 only 50 percent of U.S. adults met *HealthyPeople 2020* guidelines for physical activity (www.healthypeople.gov/2020/data-search/Search-the-Data). Many who begin an exercise program to lose excess body weight drop out within a short time. Research with successful exercisers has revealed several clues that increase the likelihood of staying with an exercise program.

1. Do not exceed your abilities during the early stages of the program. Start slowly and progress gradually. If you are overweight, it might be a good idea to start with low-impact activities, such as walking, cycling, or swimming. Even though walking is a low-impact activity, Lerner and others reported greater ground reaction forces to walking at 2.8 and 3.5 miles/hr in obese compared to normal-weight subjects due to lower-extremity muscle weakness, which may increase risk of musculoskeletal injury, especially at faster speeds. This may be a good strategy to use in the early stages of a weight-loss program utilizing walking.

2. Set both short-term and long-term goals. A short-term goal may be to walk a mile in 15 minutes, while a long-term goal may be the completion of a local 10-kilometer (6.2-mile) road race.

3. Keep a record of your exercise. This will allow you to evaluate your progress toward your goals. In a follow-up to two earlier reviews, Tudor-Locke and Lutes indicate that pedometers effectively promote physical activity and decrease body weight. It will help you document your daily physical activity in an objective way, evaluate your progress over time, and serve as a cue to remind you to be active that may motivate you to exercise more. According to Krenn and others, global positioning systems (GPS) are promising tools to track physical activity. Factors affecting the quality of GPS include patient adherence over longer monitoring periods, battery life, and receiver size. Garmin™ watches and the bodybugg™ system, can provide data on distance covered or Calories expended.

4. You must have time available to exercise. Most of us are busy with work, school, family, and friends, so finding the time to exercise is often difficult. Block out time in your daily schedule just as you do for other activities. Exercising before breakfast, at lunch, or immediately after work are some of the strategies used by busy individuals. As previously discussed, multiple *exercise snacks* during the day may substitute for a single, longer block of time. Multitasking, such as exercising while watching the television or using an active work station, are other possible strategies.

5. A place to exercise must be convenient. You are more likely to find an excuse not to exercise if you have to travel 5 miles in heavy traffic to a health club. Find a convenient location. A spare room or your garage could become a small gym.

6. Self-motivation is probably the most important determinant of adherence to an exercise program. In their review, Teixeira and others reported that women with the highest levels of autonomous motivation were more active 2 years after a 1-year intervention study compared to women with intermediate or low autonomous motivation. Enjoying your exercise program, being capable at the exercise task, and knowing that it will help you attain your goals will improve your motivation and make daily exercise a lifetime habit.

Although diverse modes of aerobic exercise may be used to lose body weight and to help condition the cardiovascular system, the major focus here will be on walk-jog-run programs. This is because they satisfy many of the criteria that may encourage adherence to an exercise program.

Former U.S. surgeon general C. Everett Koop indicated that walking for exercise should be elevated to a national priority. Walking may be the ideal exercise program for many individuals. Compared to jogging and running, there is less stress on the legs due to impact, because one foot is always on the ground supporting the body weight. However, leisurely walking usually will not provide an adequate stimulus to achieve the target HR, so the walking pace must be brisk. Walking at a faster-than-normal pace is often called **aerobic walking**, and if done properly can expend Calories at about the same rate as jogging or running. Vigorous arm action is needed, and the length of the stride as well as the step rate must be increased. Rowe and others suggested that 100 strides per minute is a good general recommendation for moderate-intensity walking but also suggested that height influences optimal stride rate. A 60-inch-tall person might have a stride rate of 113 per minute, whereas 90 strides per minute would be suitable for a 78-inch-tall person. Graves and others reported that adding 3-pound hand weights or ankle weights increased metabolic cost of brisk walking compared to no weights. Hand weights increased energy expenditure by about 1 Calorie per minute with no change in perceived exertion. Carrying the weights in the hands tends to increase the blood pressure more, so it may be helpful to use weights that strap around the wrist.

Another alternative is to wear a weighted vest. Puthoff and others reported that wearing weight vests adding 10, 15, and 20 percent to body weight increased energy expenditure, respectively, by 6.3, 9.4, and 11.5 percent while walking at 2 miles per hour, with even greater increases in energy expenditure at faster walking speeds. The authors also noted the added weight could provide an additional benefit by stimulating bone development but might be a detriment if it contributed to muscle injury or skeletal injury such as a stress fracture. Although hand weights and weighted vests may increase your energy expenditure at any given walking speed, you may expend similar amounts of Calories simply by walking faster or longer without added weight.

A wide variety of methods may be used to initiate an aerobic exercise program of walking, jogging, or running. The key is to begin slowly, gradually increasing the exercise intensity as you become better conditioned. Once you determine the intensity of exercise necessary to achieve the target HR, it becomes a relatively simple matter to individualize the exercise program. In the early weeks of training, you should attempt to exercise only at the 50–60 percent target HR range. However, if you find that the exercise intensity needed to achieve this level is too strenuous, reduce it to 40 percent of your calculated heart-rate reserve. As you become more fit, gradually increase your target HR to the 50–85 percent level. As recommended in the ACSM/AHA position stand, you may vary your exercise program by doing moderate-intensity exercise several days a week and vigorous-intensity exercise several other days.

Table 11.15 presents a sample aerobic walking program. It is designed to progress you gradually through 12 weeks to a point where the exercise intensity and duration may make a significant

TABLE 11.15 Sample aerobic walking program

	Warm-up	Target zone exercising	Cool-down	Total time
Week 1*	Walk slowly 5 minutes	Walk briskly 5 minutes	Walk slowly 5 minutes	15 minutes
Week 2	Walk slowly 5 minutes	Walk briskly 8 minutes	Walk slowly 5 minutes	18 minutes
Week 3	Walk slowly 5 minutes	Walk briskly 12 minutes	Walk slowly 5 minutes	22 minutes
Week 4	Walk slowly 5 minutes	Walk briskly 16 minutes	Walk slowly 5 minutes	26 minutes
Week 5	Walk slowly 5 minutes	Walk briskly 20 minutes	Walk slowly 5 minutes	30 minutes
Week 6	Walk slowly 5 minutes	Walk briskly 24 minutes	Walk slowly 5 minutes	34 minutes
Week 7	Walk slowly 5 minutes	Walk briskly 28 minutes	Walk slowly 5 minutes	38 minutes
Week 8	Walk slowly 5 minutes	Walk briskly 32 minutes	Walk slowly 5 minutes	42 minutes
Week 9	Walk slowly 5 minutes	Walk briskly 36 minutes	Walk slowly 5 minutes	46 minutes
Week 10	Walk slowly 5 minutes	Walk briskly 40 minutes	Walk slowly 5 minutes	50 minutes
Week 11	Walk slowly 5 minutes	Walk briskly 45 minutes	Walk slowly 5 minutes	55 minutes
Week 12	Walk slowly 5 minutes	Walk briskly 50 minutes	Walk slowly 5 minutes	60 minutes

From week 13 on, check your pulse periodically to see if you are exercising within your target heart rate range. As you become more fit, walk faster to increase your heart rate toward the upper levels of your target range. Follow the principle of progression. Note: If you find a particular week's pattern tiring, repeat it before going on to the next pattern. You do not have to complete the walking program in 12 weeks. Remember that your goal is to continue getting the benefits you are seeking—and to enjoy your activity. Listen to your body and progress less rapidly, if necessary.

*Program should include *at least* five, and preferably seven, sessions per week for weight loss.
Source: U.S. Department of Health and Human Services, modified to include recent American College of Sports Medicine guidelines for weight loss.

contribution to weight loss over time. If you feel fit, you may progress more rapidly than the table indicates, but stay within your target HR range and do not become unduly fatigued.

Table 11.16 presents an exercise program with a rapid progression to jogging, using an interval-training approach. **Interval training** alternates periods of rest and exercise. Again, the target HR method should be used during this exercise program. As compared to walking, jogging or running may expend two to three times the amount of Calories per unit of time. Thus, it may be worthwhile to interject short bouts of more intense exercise into a workout, such as jogging one block out of every three or four when walking. Kessler and others concluded that high-intensity interval exercise, discussed earlier in the chapter, may promote superior improvements in aerobic fitness with similar improvements in insulin sensitivity, blood pressure, and high-density lipoprotein cholesterol when compared to continuous aerobic exercise.

Whatever mode of exercise you select, the target HR should be maintained for 30 minutes or more. This may be continuous or intermittent. If 30 minutes is the allotted time, the target HR should be achieved for 30 continuous minutes or three 10-minute intervals of exercise with several minutes of rest in between.

The frequency of exercise should be daily or at least five times per week. During the early stages, however, it may be advisable to exercise daily in order to form sound habits. The exercise intensity at this time may not be too severe, such as walking, and hence daily exercise bouts may be undertaken without serious muscle soreness or related injury patterns. If you switch to jogging or running, decrease the frequency to three or four times per week to avoid overuse injuries. The frequency per week may be increased as you become better physically conditioned. To increase weekly energy expenditure and help prevent overuse injuries, engage in cross-training exercises on days you do not jog or run.

For weight-control purposes, duration and frequency of exercise are key elements. The longer and more often you exercise, the greater will be the total amount of energy expended. Aerobic walking for 5 miles on a daily basis is the equivalent of approximately 1 pound of body fat per week.

There are a number of other excellent conditioning programs available for the unconditioned individual. Probably the most popular is the aerobics program developed by Dr. Kenneth Cooper. Although dated, his programs may be found in *The Aerobics Program for Total Well Being,* a highly recommended paperback found in most bookstores. Books on initiating walking and other aerobic exercise programs are also available at your library or local bookstores, and various Websites provide very helpful information.

http://www.active.com/articles/america-on-the-move-small-steps-to-being-fit
www.walking.org These Websites provide detailed information on beginning and maintaining a fitness walking program and associated health benefits, including weight loss.

TABLE 11.16 Sample aerobic jogging program (interval training)

| Week | Warm-up | Stimulus | | Time (min) |
		Target zone exercise	Cool-down	
1	Stretch; limber up 5 min	Walk (non-stop) 10 min (×1)	Walk 3 min; stretch 2 min	20
2	Stretch; limber up 5 min	Walk (non-stop) 10 min (×1)	Walk 3 min; stretch 2 min	22
3	Stretch; limber up 5 min	Walk 5 min; jog 3 min (×2)	Walk 3 min; stretch 2 min	26
4	Stretch; limber up 5 min	Walk 5 min; jog 5 min (×2)	Walk 3 min; stretch 2 min	30
5	Stretch; limber up 5 min	Walk 4 min; jog 6 min (×2)	Walk 3 min; stretch 2 min	30
6	Stretch; limber up 5 min	Walk 4 min; jog 7 min (×2)	Walk 3 min; stretch 2 min	32
7	Stretch; limber up 5 min	Walk 4 min; jog 8 min (×2)	Walk 3 min; stretch 2 min	34
8	Stretch; limber up 5 min	Walk 4 min; jog 9 min (×2)	Walk 3 min; stretch 2 min	36
9	Stretch; limber up 5 min	Walk 4 min; jog 10 min (×2)	Walk 3 min; stretch 2 min	38
10	Stretch; limber up 5 min	Walk 4 min; jog 11 min (×2)	Walk 3 min; stretch 2 min	40
11	Stretch; limber up 5 min	Walk 4 min; jog 12 min (×2)	Walk 3 min; stretch 2 min	42
12	Stretch; limber up 5 min	Walk 4 min; jog 14 min (×2)	Walk 3 min; stretch 2 min	46
13	Stretch; limber up 5 min	Walk 2 min; jog slowly 2 min; jog 15 min (×2)	Walk 3 min; stretch 2 min	48
14	Stretch; limber up 5 min	Walk 1 min; jog slowly 3 min; jog 15 min (×2)	Walk 3 min; stretch 2 min	48
15	Stretch; limber up 5 min	Jog slowly 3 min; jog 17 min (×2)	Walk 3 min; stretch 2 min	50

www.10000steps.org.au This Australian Website provides advice on how to walk 10,000 steps daily, with a link on how to convert other activities into steps.

www.gmap-pedometer.com This program permits you to calculate distances of walking or jogging routes in your neighborhood or anywhere in the country.

www.health.gov/paguidelines/pdf/paguide.pdf This United States Department of Health and Human Services Website provides physical activity guidelines for Americans of all ages.

Numerous fitness applications are also available for cell phones. Google "fitness apps" to review recommended programs.

How much exercise is needed to lose weight?

Although a properly planned exercise program may produce significant health benefits even without weight loss, many individuals use exercise to decrease body fat. Weight loss depends on a balance between energy expenditure through exercise and energy intake through diet. Guidelines on recommended amounts of exercise for weight loss are available from professional and governmental health organizations.

The American College of Sports Medicine (ACSM)/American Heart Association (AHA) minimum recommendation (30 minutes of moderate-intensity exercise, 5 days per week) for cardiovascular health benefits totals 2.5 hours per week, which would approximate 1,000–1,200 Calories energy expenditure. However, the ACSM/AHA notes that *more exercise is better,* particularly for weight loss and maintenance. Increasing exercise duration and frequency is the key.

The ACSM, under the guidance of Donnelly and others, has revised its position stand on appropriate physical activity intervention strategies for weight loss and prevention of weight regain for adults. The following represent the key exercise recommendations emanating from this position stand, expressed in weekly minutes of moderate physical activity.

- 150–250 minutes
  - Prevent weight gain
  - Produce modest weight loss
  - Improve weight loss with moderate diet restriction
- 250 minutes or more
  - Produce clinically significant weight loss
  - Maintain weight after weight loss

The ACSM position stand recommends moderate-intensity exercise, which is appropriate for overweight individuals. Nybo and others found that moderate-intensity running was more effective than high-intensity exercise as a means to lose body fat, although the high-intensity exercise was more effective in promoting cardiorespiratory fitness. As weight loss increases, some vigorous exercise may be incorporated into the exercise regimen as a means to enhance cardiovascular fitness in addition to the weight loss.

Several other groups have also provided recommendations. Wing and Phelan noted that successful weight losers in the National Weight Control Registry exercised about 1 hour or more per day. Walking is their number one exercise, but they also engage in resistance training and other physical activities. Collectively, this amount of physical activity would approximate 1,500–2,000 Calories weekly. According to the National Academy of Sciences's Institute of Medicine, 30 minutes per day of regular activity is insufficient to maintain body weight within the recommended BMI range. Brooks and others state that moderate-intensity physical activity performed at least 60 minutes per day is required to maintain BMI in a healthy range and is recommended for children and adults. As an example, walking or jogging at 4–5 miles per hour for 6–7 days a week would approximate 2,000 Calories or more of energy expenditure. This corresponds to a physical activity level (PAL, discussed earlier in this chapter and in chapter 3) of 1.6 or greater.

Collectively, the optimal exercise energy-expenditure goal appears to be 1,500–2,000 Calories per week, or about 200–300 Calories per day. For walkers, this approximates 10,000 steps daily. According to Tudor-Locke and others, sedentary individuals walk no more than 5,000 steps a day and are more likely to be overweight or obese and have greater cardio-metabolic risk. Gradually adding about 5,000 or 6,000 steps of brisk walking per day to a sedentary routine would approximate 200–300 additional Calories expended, or about 1,500–2,000 per week. A pedometer can be used to record the number of steps taken each day and provide motivation to walk. The average person takes about 2,000 steps per mile. Walking 100 steps per minute (about 3 miles per hour) may be a moderate-intensity pace, whereas 130 steps per minute (about 4 miles per hour) is definitely a brisk pace and may be a recommended long-term goal. Walking even faster may approach the energy equivalency of jogging at the same pace. As noted by Rowe and others, the step rate may be modified based on the height of the individual, with shorter persons taking more steps per minute than taller persons.

Tudor-Locke and others have proposed daily walking guidelines for physical activity similar to the PAL categories presented earlier in this chapter and in chapter 3:

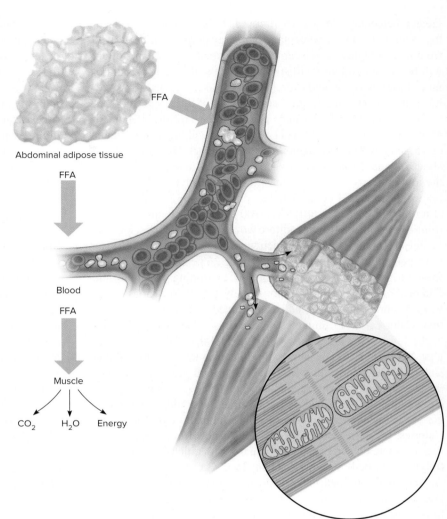

FIGURE 11.13 Exercise helps to release fat (free fatty acids) from the adipose tissue, particularly abdominal fat cells. The fat then travels by way of the bloodstream to the muscles, where the free fatty acids are oxidized to provide the energy for exercise. Thus, exercise is an effective means of reducing body fat.

Sedentary	<5,000 steps
Low active	5,000–7,499 steps
Somewhat active	7,500–9,999 steps
Active	10,000–12,499 steps
Highly active	>12,500 steps

From what parts of the body does the weight loss occur during an exercise weight-reduction program?

As mentioned previously, weight loss may come from any one of three body sources: body water, lean tissue such as muscle, and body-fat stores. A diet program, especially one very low in Calories, will cause a rapid weight loss due to decreases in body water and lean tissue. Body-fat losses are moderate at first but may increase in later stages of the diet. In contrast, weight lost through an exercise program alone is lost at a much slower rate.

Body-water levels remain relatively normal after replacement of water lost through exercise. The lean tissues, particularly muscle, might actually increase in amount from the stimulating effect of exercise on muscle development. Because a good proportion of the energy demand for exercise is met by the oxidation of fat, most of the body-weight reduction comes from the body-fat stores, particularly in the abdominal area (figure 11.13). As we learned previously, the caloric cost of 1 pound of fat is much higher than that of water or lean muscle tissue. Thus, loss of body fat through exercise takes time, highlighting the importance of the long-haul concept and long-term weight-loss goals.

Should I do low-intensity exercises to burn more fat?

The "fat burning myth," discussed in chapter 3, is based on the fact that a greater *percentage* of fat is used for energy during low-intensity exercise, whereas higher-intensity exercise uses a greater percentage of carbohydrate. This is somewhat misleading. Although a lower percentage of energy output will be derived from fat at a higher exercise intensity, the total energy expenditure will be greater and you will still burn almost the same amount of fat Calories as you would exercising at the lower intensity, providing you are exercising for the same amount of time.

For example, an 85-kg male could exercise to lose weight for 45 minutes at either 45 percent VO_2 max (walking 4 miles/hour) or 75 percent VO_2 max (running 5 miles/hour). He would derive about 60 and 26 percent, respectively, of his energy from fat at the low intensity and high intensities (figure 11.14a). At the low intensity, he would cover 3 miles, expending 332 total Calories at an energy cost of a little over 100 Calories per mile. The *net* (*total – resting*) caloric expenditure would be 268 Calories, approximately 160 (0.6 × 268), of which would be fat Calories. If he ran at 75 percent of VO_2 max, while deriving 26 percent of his energy from fat, he would cover 3.75 miles, expending 568 total and 502 net Calories, of which approximately 130 (0.26 × 502) would be fat Calories. However, he has expended 502 *net* Calories (568 total Calories) in 45 minutes compared to only 268 *net* Calories at the lower exercise intensity (figure 11.14b). This will lead to a greater weight loss or permit him to consume an additional 234 Calories in his daily diet. Moreover, the total grams of fat used during running are almost the same as he used during walking (figure 11.14c). If he had unlimited time, he could exercise longer at the lower exercise intensity and eventually burn more total Calories, including more fat Calories. As noted in chapter 3, you may estimate the energy it costs you to run 1 mile by simply multiplying your body weight in pounds by 0.73 Calorie.

Aerobically trained individuals are better able to burn fat and are able to oxidize fat at higher exercise intensities. According to Achten and Jeukendrup, the maximum rate of fat oxidation as a percent of VO_2 max occurs at 59 to 64 percent in endurance-trained individuals and 47 to 52 percent in normal subjects. If you want to burn 500 Calories per day by running 5 miles, it does not matter how fast you run. For weight-control purposes, the total distance covered, which translates into total Calories expended, is the key point. Most exercisers who want to achieve a healthy body weight and improve their fitness should exercise at the highest intensity appropriate for their age, health, motivation, and current fitness level. For optimal and safe weight loss, total energy expenditure is more important regardless of the fat or carbohydrates used during exercise. If you want to burn Calories to lose body fat, you should burn the greatest total Calories possible during the time you have to exercise.

Is spot reducing effective?

Spot reducing uses isolated exercises in an attempt to deplete local fat deposits in specific body areas. These techniques do not appear to be effective. Katch and others reported that 5,000 sit-ups performed over a 27-day period did not reduce abdominal adipose cell size as measured by biopsy. In another study, magnetic resonance imaging (MRI) was used to quantify the subcutaneous fat tissue in the upper arm. Kostek and others reported no changes in men and women engaged in resistance training of one arm for 12 weeks.

In their review, Caston and Dixon concluded that reduction of visceral fat is greater than subcutaneous fat with modest weight loss. However, greater weight loss diminished this difference. Fat reduction is most likely to occur in areas where fat deposits are the most conspicuous (usually the abdominal area), regardless of the weight-loss format, including exercise. However, some areas of the body are somewhat resistant to change, particularly the gynoid-type fat distribution around the hips and thighs. Although both large-muscle activities and local isolated-muscle exercises may help reduce fat stores, the former is recommended because the total caloric expenditure will be larger.

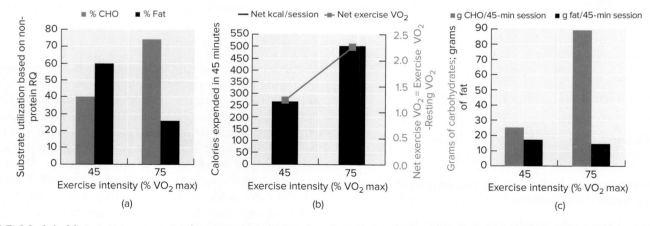

FIGURE 11.14 More intense exercise burns more calories. As a hypothetical example, an 187-pound (85-kg) man can exercise at either 45 percent (5.0 METS, walking 4 mi/hr) or 75 percent (8.6 METS, running 5 mi/hr) of VO_2 max for 45 minutes. (a) Fat provides 59.7 percent of the energy during low-intensity (45 percent VO_2 max) exercise, whereas carbohydrate provides 74.1 percent of the energy during high-intensity (75 percent VO_2 max) exercise. (b) The net (total – resting) Calories/session and VO_2 of high-intensity exercise is almost twice that of low-intensity exercise. (c) Compared to low-intensity exercise, 45 minutes of high-intensity exercise burns 250 percent more carbohydrate but only 16 percent less fat. Caloric expenditure is key to weight loss regardless of the contribution of fat vs. carbohydrate. See text for explanation.

Is it possible to exercise and still not lose body weight?

Many individuals are disappointed during the early stages of an exercise program because they do not lose weight very rapidly. Unless they understand what is happening in their bodies, the results on the scale may convince them that exercise is not an effective means of reducing weight, and they may quit exercising altogether. There are several reasons an individual may not lose weight during the early stages of a weight-reduction program, and why losing weight becomes more difficult after weight loss has occurred.

One reason may involve a compensation effect, such as increasing the amount of caloric intake or reducing the amount of other daily physical activities. For example, in a study involving the effects of exercise on weight loss, Manthou and others reported that nearly one-third of the subjects were responders, and lost body weight as expected. The remaining two-thirds were nonresponders, who did not lose and actually gained weight. Further analysis revealed that the nonresponders reduced their daily physical activities outside of their exercise sessions.

Another reason involves changes in body composition, but changes that are actually favorable to health. When a sedentary individual begins a daily exercise program, the body reacts to the exercise stress and changes so that it can more easily handle the demands of exercise (figure 11.15):

1. The muscles may increase in size because of hypertrophy of the muscle cells. The increased protein will hold water.
2. Mitochondria and other structures within the muscle cell that process oxygen, along with numerous enzymes involved in oxygen use, will increase in quantity.
3. Energy substances in the cell will increase, particularly glycogen, which binds water.
4. The connective tissue will toughen and thicken.
5. As discussed by Convertino, total blood volume may increase because of increased total body water and sodium retention. Plasma volume may increase by 500 milliliters, or about a pound, in the initial 1 to 2 weeks, after which both red cell and plasma volumes expand.

At the same time, however, body-fat stores will begin to diminish somewhat as fat is used as a source of energy for exercise. Overall, there may be an increase in body water and lean body mass, particularly the muscle tissues, and a decrease in body fat. These changes may counterbalance each other, and the individual may not lose any weight. However, although little or no weight is lost during those early phases, the body-composition changes are favorable. Body fat is being lost, particularly from the abdominal fat depots.

Once these adaptive changes have occurred, which may take about a month, body weight should decrease in relationship to the number of Calories lost through exercise. Keep in mind that

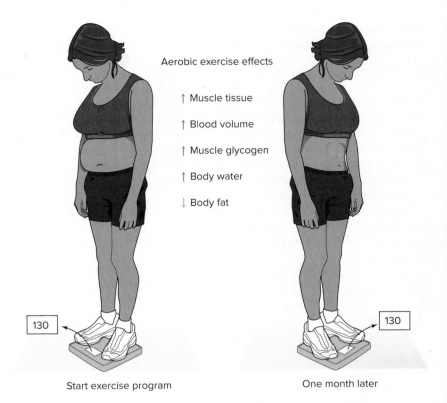

Aerobic exercise effects

↑ Muscle tissue

↑ Blood volume

↑ Muscle glycogen

↑ Body water

↓ Body fat

130

130

Start exercise program

One month later

FIGURE 11.15 Body weight may not change much during the beginning phases of an aerobic exercise program. However, body composition may change. The exercise stimulates an increase in muscle tissue, blood volume, and muscle glycogen stores, which tend to increase weight. Body fat is reduced, but the increases in the other components can balance out the fat losses with no net loss of body weight. Eventually, body weight, particularly abdominal fat, begins to drop as the exercise program is continued.

weight loss will be slow on an exercise program, but if you can build up to an exercise energy expenditure of about 300 Calories per day, then about 2.5 pounds per month will be exercised away, provided you do not compensate by eating more.

After several months you may begin to notice that your body weight has stabilized even though you continue to exercise and have not reached your weight goal. Part of the reason may be your lower body weight. The less you weigh, the fewer Calories you burn for any given exercise. If you have been doing the same amount of exercise all along, you may now be at the body weight where your energy output is matched by your energy input in food and your body weight has stabilized. In theory, you have reached your settling point. In addition, you may become more skilled, and hence more efficient, in your physical activity. Fewer Calories may then be expended for any given amount of time. However, this is usually true only of activities that involve a skill factor. It can be highly significant in swimming, but not as great in jogging.

In summary, your body weight may not change during the early stages of an exercise program; it may then begin to drop during a second stage, and then plateau at the third stage. If you are aware of these possible stages, your adherence to an exercise program may be enhanced. Also, during the third stage, if you desire to lose more weight by exercise, the amount of exercise will have to be increased.

What about the 5 or 6 pounds a person may lose during an hour of exercise?

A rapid weight loss may occur during exercise. Some individuals have lost as much as 10–12 pounds in an hour or so. As you probably suspect, this weight loss may be attributed to body-water losses. This is particularly evident while exercising in warm or hot weather. The weight loss is temporary, and under normal food and water intake the body-water content will return to normal. Each pound of weight lost this way is 1 pint of fluid, or 16 ounces. A 2.2-pound weight loss would be the equivalent of 1 liter.

In the heat of summer, you may occasionally see an individual training with heavy sweat clothes or a rubberized suit. The reason often given is to lose more body weight. The individual will lose more body weight, but again it will be body water, which will be regained as soon as he or she drinks fluids. This technique is worthless for weight loss, may excessively increase core temperature, and predisposes the individual to heat-related illness. Only sweat that actually evaporates will help reduce the heat stress on the body.

Any water lost through dehydration should be replaced before the next exercise session, especially when exercising in warm environments. The importance of rehydration and problems associated with exercise in the heat were covered in chapter 9.

Key Concepts

▶ Aerobic exercise can increase energy expenditure considerably, but in order to lose body fat through exercise one should think in terms of months, not days.

▶ To be aerobic, weight-reduction exercises must involve large muscle masses, such as the legs in jogging or bicycling or the arms and legs in swimming. Brisk walking is a highly recommended exercise program.

▶ The general design of the aerobic weight-reduction exercise programs involves three phases: warm-up, exercise stimulus, and cool-down.

▶ An effective means of monitoring aerobic exercise intensity is the exercise heart rate (HR). The exercise target HR varies depending upon age and level of conditioning. Ratings of perceived exertion (RPE) and the talk test may also be used to gauge exercise intensity.

▶ Walking is one of the recommended exercises for health and weight control. Here are a few historical quotes relative to the benefits of walking.

> Walking is our best medicine. *Hippocrates*
> Before supper take a little walk. After supper do the same. *Erasmus*
> I have two doctors, my left leg and my right leg. *Sir George Trevelyan*

▶ A slow, steady progression in exercise intensity is important in preventing excess stress and injuries.

▶ Duration and frequency of exercise are important considerations for weight loss. A weekly expenditure of

1,500–2,000 Calories from exercise appears to be a reasonable and effective means to induce and maintain weight loss.

▶ For several reasons, weight loss may not occur in the early stages of an exercise program; however, the body composition changes are favorable, that is, a decrease in body fat and increase in fat-free mass. A resistance-exercise program may be very helpful to maintain or increase fat-free mass.

▶ The rapid weight loss observed after a single bout of exercise is due to water loss through sweating.

Check for Yourself

▶ Using several different types of physical activity that you enjoy, use the Compendium of Physical Activities (https://sites.google.com/site/compendiumofphysicalactivities/) and appendix B and calculate how much time you would need to allocate to each in order to burn 500 Calories per day.

Comprehensive Weight Control Programs

Numerous well-designed studies with diet or diet-and-exercise interventions have reported significant weight loss. Unfortunately, most of these studies fail to document long-term success in maintenance of weight loss, with subjects regaining weight at a rate of 1–2 kg/year. Seagle and others, in the Academy of Nutrition and Dietetics (formerly American Dietetics Association) position statement on weight management, note that a lifetime commitment to change is fundamental to successful weight loss. Behavior modification incorporating properly designed diets and exercise programs, as detailed in this chapter, is the key to a comprehensive weight-control program not only to take off excess body fat but also to keep it off. A National Institutes of Health working group report by MacLean and others indicates that failure to maintain weight loss is due to poor adherence to behavioral changes and physiological adaptations that facilitate weight regain. The report calls for future weight-loss maintenance strategies to merge best behavioral strategies, better physiological understanding of energy balance, and new pharmacological interventions.

Which is more effective for weight control—dieting or exercise?

Dieting alone or exercise alone may be an effective means to reduce body fat, but each technique has certain advantages and disadvantages. However, the advantages of one approach help counterbalance the disadvantages of the other.

Dieting alone may be an effective means to lose excess body fat. Dieting will contribute to a negative caloric balance and may help bring about a rapid weight reduction early in the program. Redman and others found that dieting alone (25 percent reduction in caloric intake) induced similar total body fat and abdominal fat losses and changes in body composition in 6 months compared to subjects who created a similar energy deficit by both diet and aerobic exercise (12.5 percent reduction in caloric energy intake plus 12.5 percent increase in exercise energy expenditure). In their review, Stiegler and Cunliffe indicate that increasing the proportion of caloric intake from protein may also help maintain lean body mass on a weight-loss diet.

Aerobic exercise alone may also be an effective means to lose excess body fat. Stiegler and Cunliffe note that exercise training is associated with an increase in energy expenditure, thus promoting changes in body weight and composition, provided that dietary intake remains constant. Moreover, adding resistance exercise may provide additional benefits.

Contrary to the results of the study by Redman and others, Stiegler and Cunliffe also stated that research to date suggests that the addition of exercise programs to dietary restriction can promote more favorable changes in body composition than diet on its own. Miller and others note that adding exercise to a diet program significantly reduced decreases in lean body mass compared to energy restriction only, which could help maintain resting energy expenditure. Exercise may confer other benefits. Hansen and others contend that exercise may improve dietary compliance. Once the body-weight goal has been attained, expending 400–500 Calories daily through physical activity allows one to consume that many additional Calories. Instead of a 2,000-Calorie diet, one may consume 2,400 to 2,500 Calories. Hill notes that dieting alone to maintain weight is designed to fail in the long run. Although some can do it, they are few in number. Exercise enables one to eat more during the maintenance phase. Finally, Larson-Meyer and others note that despite similar effects of dieting or exercise on fat losses, combining caloric restriction with exercise increases aerobic fitness in parallel with improved insulin sensitivity, LDL-cholesterol, and diastolic blood pressure.

Some of the most meaningful data regarding long-term weight maintenance have been obtained by studying the habits of members of the National Weight Control Registry. (NWCR) Almost all NWCR participants modified food intake and increased activity to lose weight. According to Thomas and others, 87 percent participants have successfully maintained at least a 10 percent weight loss for 10 years. Some of their key behaviors include the following:

- Eat a low-Calorie diet, low in fat and high in carbohydrate.
- Eat breakfast; reduce hunger later in the day.
- Watch only a limited amount of television.
- Do about 60 minutes or more of physical activity daily; walking is the favorite exercise, but also engage in aerobic classes, resistance training, cycling, and swimming. They expend 2,000 or more Calories weekly through physical activity.
- Weigh oneself frequently (daily or several times a week) to help prevent a lapse from becoming a relapse.

Resistance training (covered in chapter 12) added to a weight-reduction program may also be very effective in helping to maintain lean body mass. Preferably, both aerobic and resistance exercise should be part of a comprehensive weight-control program. Kraemer and others reported that aerobic endurance training combined with resistance training exerted greater effects on body composition in overweight men compared to dieting alone. Sillanpää and colleagues found that 21 weeks of combined strength and endurance exercise optimized body composition in 40- to 65-year-old men compared to either exercise done separately. Combining aerobic and resistance exercise appears to provide the beneficial effects of both types of exercise.

Consider the following. A dietary reduction of 500 Calories per day, along with an exercise energy expenditure of 500 Calories per day, could lead to approximately 2 pounds of weight loss per week, about the maximal amount recommended unless under medical supervision. The removal of 500 Calories from the diet could be done immediately by simply reducing the amount of sugar and fat in the daily diet and using some of the behavior-modification techniques cited earlier. You should review those suggestions given earlier relative to the substitution of nutrient-dense foods for high-Caloric ones. Relative to exercise, it may take a month or more before you may be able to use 500 Calories daily, but by following the progressive plans outlined earlier in this chapter you should be able to reach that level safely. In the meantime, increase your level of NEAT by climbing stairs and walking more to add to your daily caloric expenditure.

A comprehensive weight-reduction program involving both a dietary and an exercise regimen, along with supportive behavior-modification techniques, is highly recommended by major health-related organizations such as the Academy of Nutrition and Dietetics and the American College of Sports Medicine. Three reviews and meta-analyses by Södlerlund, Brown, and Sweet, along with their associates, concluded that the most effective weight-loss programs included multiple components—diet, exercise, and behavior modification. The principles of developing such a program have been presented in the preceding three sections of this chapter.

If I want to lose weight through a national or local weight-loss program, what should I look for?

According to http://www.marketdataenterprises.com/studies/#FS45, the economic value of the U.S. weight-loss industry is $60.5 billion. National programs, such as NutriSystem, Weight Watchers, Jenny Craig, the South Beach diet, and the Atkins diet, may provide three flash-frozen meals daily, along with two snacks. Costs can range up to $10,000 per year, per person. The cost-effectiveness of several nonsurgical weight-loss strategies was recently estimated by Finkelstein and Kruger to range from $155 to $546 per kilogram of weight loss. Unfortunately, there is little governmental control over many of these programs, and although the national programs may be well designed, others may not provide appropriate programs for safe and effective long-term weight loss.

What do authorities recommend you should receive for your money if you want to enroll in a commercial weight-loss program? The following points are adapted and summarized from the report of a task force to establish weight-loss guidelines for the state of Michigan, and from other health professional sources, such as Partnership for Healthy Weight Management.

1. The staff should be well trained in their specialty, preferably having appropriate educational backgrounds, such as a physician, nurse, dietitian, or exercise physiologist.
2. You should receive a medical screening, verifying that you have no medical or psychological condition that might be exacerbated by weight loss through dieting or exercise.
3. A reasonable weight goal should be established, given your weight history.
4. The rate of weight loss, after the first 2 weeks, should not exceed 2 pounds per week.
5. You should receive an individualized treatment plan based on your weight-loss goal. You should also obtain an itemized list of costs.
6. The program should disclose in writing all health risks and benefits associated with the program, and you should have the opportunity to read them and sign an informed consent form.
7. The diet should be one that
   a. contains no less than 1,000–1,500 Calories per day.
   b. has at least 100 grams of carbohydrate per day.
   c. provides at least 100 percent of the RDA; supplements, if used, should not exceed 100 percent of the RDA.
   d. if under medical supervision, contains at least 600 Calories and 50 grams of carbohydrate per day.
8. The program should have a nutrition-education component that stresses permanent lifestyle changes in your eating habits.
9. Both aerobic and resistance exercise should be a component in the program. The focus should be on aerobic exercise, following the standards relative to mode, intensity, duration, and frequency discussed earlier in this chapter. It should be an exercise program you can live with for a lifetime. Guidelines for resistance exercise are presented in the next chapter.
10. Behavior-modification techniques should be individualized to help you incorporate sound dietary and exercise habits into your personal lifestyle.
11. There should be a weight-maintenance phase in the program once you have achieved your weight-loss goal. This should be a high priority to help you maintain your healthy body weight.
12. An effective, reputable weight-loss program should *not* have outrageous claims, small marketing print, dubious before-and-after photos, or any other marketing strategy that seems too good to be true.

http://win.niddk.nih.gov/publications/choosing.htm This U.S. Department of Health and Human Services publication provides information on effective weight-loss programs and questions a savvy consumer should ask in seeking a program.

http://health.usnews.com/best-diet U.S. News and World Reports best diet rankings for 2015.

The efficacy of commercial weight-loss programs has been evaluated in several reviews. Tsai and Wadden concluded that all programs can work to induce weight loss. Furlow and Anderson reported that individuals who completed supervised, commercial weight-loss programs involving meal replacement lost an average of about 1 kilogram per week over the course of about 18 weeks.

In a recent review of 45 studies, Gudzune and others reported that Jenny Craig® and Weight Watchers® resulted in significantly greater weight losses of 4.9 and 2.6 percent, respectively, at 12 months compared to control programs (education/counseling). They also concluded that more long-term studies are needed to examine the effectiveness of other programs such as Nutrisystem®. In 2015, *US News & World Report* rated Jenny Craig® and Weight Watchers® as the best commercial diet plans and easiest diets to follow. Regardless of the commercial program, compliance is the key to successful weight loss.

Guidelines similar to those just given should be used if you want to join a health or fitness club facility, particularly the qualifications of the staff and the availability of a variety of safe exercise equipment. Personal trainers should be certified by reputable professional organizations. The Consumers Union indicates that anyone can become a certified personal trainer, as there are no national standards for certification. Some Websites offer certification for minimal effort and several hundred dollars. The Consumers Union indicates that the best certification is provided by the following:

- The American College of Sports Medicine
- The American Council on Exercise
- The National Strength and Conditioning Association

Additionally, a Certified Specialist in Sports Dietetics (CSSD) would be a well-qualified contact for weight control, not only for the general population but also for athletes.

A personal trainer may help you plan an effective exercise program, including both aerobic and resistance exercise, to help you lose excess body weight. You can check with local fitness-oriented organizations, such as the YMCA, for a list of personal trainers, its certification, and its fees.

www.acsm.org
www.acefitness.org
www.nsca.com/membership/member-tools/find-a-trainer The Consumers Union indicates that the best certification programs for personal trainers are presented by the American Council on Exercise, the American College of Sports Medicine, and the National Strength and Conditioning Association. You can use the Website to obtain a list of certified trainers in your vicinity.
www.eatright.org The Academy of Nutrition and Dietetics Website provides a list of local registered dietitians (RD) with specialty in sports nutrition and weight control.

Although some individuals may need the structure of such programs, many successful individuals, including about half the members in the National Weight Control Registry, have lost excess body fat and kept it off with programs they designed by themselves.

www.nwcr.ws Access the National Weight Control Registry to review research findings as to how individuals lost weight and kept it off. Several success stories highlight methods used by individual members.

What type of weight-reduction program is advisable for young athletes?

The American Academy of Pediatrics notes that weight control is perceived to be advantageous for youths involved in sports such as bodybuilding, cheerleading, dancing, distance running, cross-country skiing, diving, figure skating, gymnastics, martial arts, rowing, swimming, weight-class football, and wrestling, which emphasize thinness, leanness, and/or competition at the lowest possible weight for aesthetic appeal or economy of movement. Such athletes may want to maintain or lose body weight, but weight lost should be fat, not muscle.

In general, athletes who desire to lose weight to enhance performance must rely primarily on dietary modifications because they are already exercising intensely. Excessive weight loss, especially in young athletes, is a major concern in sports.

As noted in chapter 10, use of improper weight-loss methods such as starvation, diuretics, laxatives, appetite-suppressing drugs, and dehydration may predispose young athletes to various health problems and impaired performance. Of particular concern are young female athletes in leanness sports who may develop long-term health problems associated with the female athlete triad, such as osteoporosis.

The American Academy of Pediatrics has recommended healthy weight-maintenance or weight-loss practices for young athletes. The following are some of its key points for young athletes:

- Start early to permit a gradual weight loss over a realistic time period.
- Eat enough to cover the energy costs of daily living, growth, building and repairing muscle tissue, and participating in sports.
- Lose excess fat without reducing lean muscle mass or causing dehydration, both of which can impair performance.
- Exceed no more than 1.5 percent of the total body weight, or 1 to 2 pounds per week.
- Lose excess weight by both diet and a safe amount of additional exercise.
- Obtain from the diet approximately 55–65 percent of energy from carbohydrate, 15–20 percent from protein, and 20–30 percent from fat.
- Maintain the desired body weight, once attained, rather than cycling up and down.
- Discuss any desired weight loss with a health-care professional and the family.

Other sports-related organizations, such as the National Collegiate Athletic Association and the National Federation of State High School Associations, have made regulations and recommendations specific to the sport of wrestling, including the following:

- Discourage rapid weight loss or weight gain with close monitoring of changes to no more than 1.5 percent per week.
- Prohibit dehydration techniques such as rubber suits, saunas, steam baths, hot rooms, laxatives, and diuretics.
- Weigh-in immediately prior to performance to discourage rapid dehydration and weight-gain techniques.

- Encourage methods to predict a minimum body-fat percentage or body weight, such as 7 and 12 percent for boys and girls, respectively.
- Encourage consumption of a nutritious diet.

Additionally, athletes on weight-loss programs should also increase the proportion of their energy intake from protein. Mettler and others reported that young athletes who consumed 35 percent of their energy intake as protein, as compared to others consuming 15 percent from protein, were better able to maintain lean body mass on a short-term weight-loss diet.

What is the importance of prevention in a weight-control program?

Health practices designed to prevent the development of chronic diseases currently are being promoted heavily by several major health organizations, and many have focused on the adverse health effects of obesity. For example, the Canadian Task Force on Preventive Health Care has recommended that obesity prevention be a high priority for health professionals. Changing your diet by reducing caloric intake, saturated fats, and cholesterol and eating more nutritious foods (quality Calories) as well as concurrently initiating and continuing a good aerobic- and resistance-type exercise program are considered to be two steps toward positive health and the prevention of obesity. James Hill, co-founder of the obesity-prevention program *America on the Move and the National Weight Control Registry,* indicated that walking an extra 2,000 steps a day and eating 100 fewer Calories will help prevent the average weight gain of 1–3 pounds per year. If you like to eat, additional exercise may help you burn these Calories and maintain your body weight (figure 11.16).

Although most of this chapter has focused on treatment programs for the reduction of excess body fat, the same guidelines may be applied to a prevention program. Obesity in our society is a serious medical problem of epidemic proportions. Although obesity treatment programs may be successful on a short-term basis, many ultimately regain lost weight. As noted by Levin, the formation of neural circuits in the brain that help perpetuate maintenance of excess body weight are not easily abolished. Strong prevention programs are needed, particularly early in life, because childhood and adolescence appear to be critical times in life for the development of chronic obesity.

Prevention of obesity on a large scale necessitates a multi-pronged effort involving various groups. Some examples are listed.

- Government can set standards for food advertisements to children.
- Food manufacturers could produce healthier products. One example was Fun Fruits, containing a variety of fruits and marketed specifically to kids.
- Communities could plan more bike paths, playgrounds, and recreation centers.
- Schools could schedule daily physical education classes and provide opportunities for students to participate in intramural sports and physical activity clubs after school. Schools could also provide healthier products in vending machines.

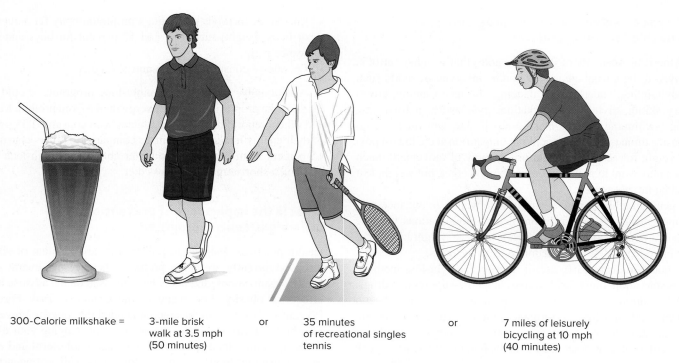

300-Calorie milkshake =   3-mile brisk   or   35 minutes   or   7 miles of leisurely
                           walk at 3.5 mph   of recreational singles   bicycling at 10 mph
                           (50 minutes)   tennis   (40 minutes)

FIGURE 11.16 It is very easy to consume 300 additional Calories per day, which can lead to an increase of about 2.5 pounds of body fat per month. However, increased physical activity may help to expend these Calories (170-pound individual).

- Parents could provide healthy foods and limit sedentary behaviors such as TV and computer time.

Various Websites to obtain helpful information relative to the prevention of obesity have been listed throughout this chapter, several of which have been recommended by the Consumers Union.

It is incumbent upon those involved with the food habits and physical activity of our youth, notably parents and health and physical educators, to instruct and motivate them toward sound health habits. According to the American Medical Association, prevention is the treatment of choice in dealing with obesity. The bottom line is *we need to eat less and move more.*

www.win.niddk.nih.gov An excellent source of information is the Weight-Control Information Network (WIN).

www.healthfinder.gov/prevention/ Free information and plans to help prevent excess weight gain in children. Click on *Nutrition and Physical Activity, then Physical Activity,* then *Help Your Child Stay at a Healthy Weight.*

Key Concepts

▶ Although diet and exercise may each be effective in losing body weight, a combination of the two would be even more beneficial, particularly when coupled with behavior-modification techniques.

▶ Prevention of obesity is more effective than treatment, and appropriate programs should be developed early for children and adolescents.

Albert's Weight Status

	Weight	Calorie intake	Maintenance calories
Current status			
Goal status			

Albert's Weight-Loss Plan

1. Desired weight loss per week:

2. Caloric energy intake reduction:

3. Caloric energy expenditure increase:

4. Total daily caloric deficit:

5. Maintenance Calories at goal weight:

Albert is overweight by 25 pounds and is very serious about reducing his body weight from 200 pounds down to 175 and a healthier BMI of 22. He is currently sedentary, is consuming an average 3,600 Calories per day, and is still gaining weight. You may assume that he needs 15 Calories per pound body weight to maintain his current weight. Using information presented in the text, develop a weight-loss program for Albert. Calculate an appropriate rate of weight loss per week. Based on your calculation, determine the daily caloric deficit needed to achieve his goal. The caloric deficit should incorporate reduced caloric energy intake and increased caloric energy expenditure through your recommended energy program. Once Albert is at his desired body weight and is involved in your exercise program, how many Calories may he consume daily to maintain that weight?

Review Questions—Multiple Choice

1. If you were to design an aerobic training program for a 30-year-old individual and wanted that person to maintain an exercise intensity of 60–80 percent of the predicted HR max (traditional method) as the target heart rate range, what exercise heart rate range would you recommend?
   a. 114–152
   b. 132–176
   c. 140–180
   d. 154–198
   e. 180–220

2. Which of the following statements relative to an exercise program for weight maintenance or loss is true?
   a. The mode of exercise should involve large muscle groups that are activated in rhythmic, continuous-type movement.
   b. The higher the intensity of aerobic exercise that the individual can sustain, the better because the greater the intensity, the greater the number of Calories burned per minute.
   c. The greater the duration of activity, the better.
   d. The more frequent the exercise during the week, the better.
   e. All statements are true.

3. Which of the following has the least amount of Calories per the Food Exchange System developed by the American Dietetic Association and the American Diabetes Association?
   a. 3 servings of skim milk
   b. 4 servings of lean meat such as turkey
   c. 5 servings of vegetables
   d. 4 servings of fruit
   e. 1 serving of whole milk

4. Aerobic-type exercise may be an effective part of a comprehensive weight-control program for all of the following reasons except which one?
   a. It increases the metabolic rate.
   b. It mobilizes and utilizes free fatty acids from the adipose tissues.
   c. It helps reduce body-water stores.
   d. It will increase the resting metabolic rate for 30 minutes or so after the exercise period.
   e. It may help to curb the appetite in some individuals if done prior to mealtime.

5. Suppose a young, sedentary woman wanted to lose 5 pounds of body fat in a period of 5 weeks. She now weighs 150 pounds and her activity level is so low that she needs only 13 Calories per pound of body weight to maintain her weight. Calculate the number of Calories she may consume daily in order to lose the 5 pounds by diet only.
   a. 800
   b. 1,250
   c. 1,450
   d. 1,750
   e. 1,950

6. In the exchange lists, high-fat foods are usually found in which two exchanges?
   a. fruit and vegetables
   b. starch/bread and lean meat
   c. whole milk and starch/bread
   d. fat and vegetable
   e. medium-meat and whole milk

7. Research with effective dieters has shown that to be successful, a diet should follow all the following principles except which?
   a. be low in Calories
   b. supply all essential nutrients
   c. contain bland foods to curb the intake of Calories
   d. be able to be accommodated within one's current lifestyle
   e. be a lifelong diet

8. The rate of weight loss on an appropriate low-Calorie diet may be rapid at first, but then may slow down. This decreased rate of weight loss is most likely due to
   a. an increased BMR and increased use of body-protein stores.
   b. a decrease in body weight and increased use of body-fat stores.
   c. an increased use of carbohydrate stores and retention of body water.
   d. a decreased BMR and an increased loss of body-water stores.
   e. an increased BMR and decreased use of body-fat stores.

9. Which of the following substitutes would not save Calories in a diet plan?
   a. skim milk in place of whole milk
   b. regular hard-stick margarine in place of butter
   c. plain yogurt in place of sour cream on a baked potato
   d. nonalcoholic beer in place of regular beer
   e. air-popped popcorn in place of potato chips

10. An example of a behavior-modification program for a weight-loss program is
    a. feel guilty after you overeat.

    b. eat fast so that there is no visible food to tempt you to eat more.
    c. keep a record of your eating habits so that you can see what situations cause you to overeat.
    d. always clean your plate when you eat.
    e. always wait until you are hungry to go food shopping.

Answers to multiple choice questions:
1. a; 2. e; 3. c; 4. c; 5. c; 6. e; 7. c; 8. b; 9. b; 10. c

Review Questions—Essay

1. Melinda wants to lose 30 pounds by summer, which is 20 weeks away. She currently weighs 150 pounds and is maintaining her body weight with an energy intake of 14 Calories per pound body weight. Based on dietary changes only, calculate her daily energy needs during the first week of the diet if she wants to lose weight at a steady level over the 20-week period.

2. Explain the concept of behavior modification in a weight-loss program, and describe some of the strategies one might employ to help change undesirable behaviors.

3. Discuss the potential positives and negatives of the high-carbohydrate, low-fat diet and the high-protein, high-fat, low-carbohydrate diet. What appears to be the key factor underlying the potential success of each on a short-term basis?

4. Discuss the importance of mode, intensity, duration, and frequency of exercise in a weight-loss program, and provide an example of an appropriate program incorporating each for a physically fit individual who wanted to lose 1 pound per week through exercise alone.

5. Both dieting and exercise may be helpful in a weight-loss program, but each may possess some drawbacks. Explain how the benefits of exercise may help counteract the possible drawbacks of dieting, and vice versa.

References

Books

Agatston, A. 2003. *The South Beach Diet*. Emmaus, PA: Rodale Press.

American College of Sports Medicine's Guidelines for Exercise Testing and Prescription. 2014. 9th ed. Baltimore: Lippincott Williams & Wilkins.

American Diabetes Association and American Dietetic Association. 1995. *Exchange Lists for Meal Planning*. Chicago: American Dietetic Association and American Diabetes Association.

Atkins, R. 1999. *Dr. Atkins' New Diet Revolution: Revised and Updated*. New York: M. Evans.

Brownell, K. 2004. *The LEARN Program for Weight Management*. Dallas: American Health.

Cooper, K. 1982. *The Aerobics Program for Total Well-Being*. New York: M. Evans.

Dusek, D. 1989. *Weight Management: The Fitness Way*. Boston: Jones and Bartlett.

Institute of Medicine. 1995. *Weighing the Options: Criteria for Evaluating Weight-Management Programs*. Committee to Develop Criteria for Evaluating the Outcomes of Approaches to Prevent and Treat Obesity.

Katzen, M., and Willett, W. 2006. *Eat, Drink, & Weigh Less*. New York: Hyperion.

Mayer, J. 1968. *Overweight: Causes, Cost and Control*. Englewood Cliffs, NJ: Prentice-Hall.

Miller, W. 1998. *Negotiated Peace: How to Win the War over Weight*. Boston: Allyn and Bacon.

Murakami, H. 2008. *What I Talk about When I Talk about Running*. London: Harvill Secker.

National Academy of Sciences. 2002. *Dietary Reference Intakes for Energy, Carbohydrates, Fiber, Fat, Protein and Amino Acids* (Macronutrients). Washington, DC: National Academies Press.

Ornish, D. 2001. *Eat More, Weigh Less: Dr. Dean Ornish's Life Choice Program for Losing Weight Safely While Eating Abundantly*. New York: HarperCollins.

Rolls, B. 2005. *The Volumetrics Eating Plan*. New York: HarperCollins.

Sears, B. 1995. *The Zone*. New York: Regan Books.

Taubes, G. 2007. *Good Calories, Bad Calories: Challenging the Conventional Wisdom on Diet, Weight Control, and Disease.* New York: Alfred A. Knopf.

Wansink, B. 2007. *Mindless Eating: Why We Eat More Than We Think.* New York: Bantam Books.

Young, L. 2006. *The Portion Teller Plan: The No-Diet Reality Guide to Eating, Cheating and Losing Weight Permanently.* New York: Morgan Road Books.

Reviews and Specific Studies

Achten, J., and Jeukendrup, A .E. 2004. Optimizing fat oxidation through exercise and diet. *Nutrition* 20(7–8):716–27.

Adamo, K., and Tesson, F. 2007. Genotype-specific weight loss treatment advice: How close are we? *Applied Physiology, Nutrition, and Metabolism* 32:351–66.

Ainsworth, B., et al. 2011. 2011 Compendium of physical activities: A second update of codes and MET values. *Medicine & Science in Sports & Exercise* 43:1575–81.

Albers, S. 2010. The Twinkie diet. www.psychologytoday.com. November 10.

American Academy of Pediatrics. 2005. Promotion of healthy weight-control practices in young athletes. *Pediatrics* 116:1557–64.

American Heart Association. 2006. Diet and lifestyle recommendations. *Circulation* 114:82–96.

Arciero, P., et al. 2006. Increased dietary protein and combined high intensity aerobic and resistance exercise improves body fat distribution and cardiovascular risk factors. *International Journal of Sport Nutrition and Exercise Metabolism* 16:373–92.

Astrup, A. 2006. How to maintain a healthy body weight. *International Journal for Vitamin and Nutrition Research* 76:208–15.

Atallah, R., et al. 2014. Long-term effects of 4 popular diets on weight loss and cardiovascular risk factors: A systematic review of randomized controlled trials. *Circulation. Cardiovascular Quality and Outcomes.* pii: CIRCOUTCOMES.113.000723.

Avery, A., et al. 2014. A systematic review investigating interventions that can help reduce consumption of sugar-sweetened beverages in children leading to changes in body fatness. *Journal of Human Nutrition and Dietetics.* 10.1111/jhn.12267.

Azadbakht, L., et al. 2007. Better dietary adherence and weight maintenance achieved by a long-term moderate-fat diet. *British Journal of Nutrition* 97:399–404.

Bendtsen, L. Q., et al. 2013. Effect of dietary proteins on appetite, energy expenditure, body weight, and composition: A review of the evidence from controlled clinical trials. *Advances in Nutrition* 4:418–38.

Benezra, L., et al. 2001. Intakes of most nutrients remain at acceptable levels during a weight management program using the food exchange system. *Journal of the American Dietetic Association* 101:554–61.

Benoit, S. C., et al. 2014. Use of bariatric outcomes longitudinal database (BOLD) to study variability in patient success after bariatric surgery. *Obesity Surgery* 24:936–43.

Borg, G. 1973. Perceived exertion: A note on "history" and methods. *Medicine & Science in Sports* 5:90–93.

Bravata, D., et al. 2003. Efficacy and safety of low-carbohydrate diets: A systematic review. *Journal of the American Medical Association* 289:1837–50.

Bray, G. 1990. Exercise and obesity. In *Exercise, Fitness and Health,* ed. C. Bouchard et al. Champaign, IL: Human Kinetics.

Bray, G. A. 2013. Energy and fructose from beverages sweetened with sugar or high-fructose corn syrup pose a health risk for some people. *Advances in Nutrition* 4 (2):220–25.

Brehm, B., and D'Alessio, D. 2008. Weight loss and metabolic benefits with diets of varying fat and carbohydrate content: Separating the wheat from the chaff. *Nature Clinical Practice. Endocrinology & Metabolism* 4:140–46.

Brooks, G. A., et al. 2004. Chronicle of the Institute of Medicine physical activity recommendation: How a physical activity recommendation came to be among dietary recommendations. *American Journal of Clinical Nutrition* 79:921S–30S.

Brown, T., et al. 2009. Systematic review of long-term lifestyle interventions to prevent weight gain and morbidity in adults. *Obesity Reviews* 10:627–38.

Brownell, K., and Kramer, F. 1989. Behavioral management of obesity. *Medical Clinics of North America* 73:185–202.

Brownell, K., and Rodin, J. 1994. The dieting maelstrom: Is it possible and advisable to lose weight? *American Psychologist* 49:781–91.

Bueno, N. B., et al. 2013. Very-low-carbohydrate ketogenic diet v. low-fat diet for long-term weight loss: A meta-analysis of randomized controlled trials. *British Journal of Nutrition* 110 (7):1178–87.

Calvez, J., et al. 2012. Protein intake, calcium balance and health consequences. *European Journal of Clinical Nutrition* 66 (3):281–95.

Campbell, A., and Hausenblas, H. 2009. Effects of exercise interventions on body image: A meta-analysis. *Journal of Health Psychology* 14:780–93.

Cappuccio, F. P., et al. 2008. Meta-analysis of short sleep duration and obesity in children and adults. *Sleep* 31 (5):619–26.

Catenacci, V., and Wyatt, H. 2007. The role of physical activity in producing and maintaining weight loss. *Nature Clinical Practice. Endocrinology & Metabolism* 3:518–29.

Chaston, T. B., and Dixon, J. B. 2008. Factors associated with percent change in visceral versus subcutaneous abdominal fat during weight loss: Findings from a systematic review. *International Journal of Obesity* 32 (4):619–28.

Clark, J. 2014. Does the type intervention method really matter for combating childhood obesity? A systematic review and meta-analysis. *Journal of Sports Medicine and Physical Fitness* (October 10).

Consumers Union. 2003. Eat more without gaining weight. *Consumer Reports on Health* 15 (6):8–9.

Consumers Union. 2005. Rating the diets. *Consumer Reports* 70 (6):1818–22.

Consumers Union. 2006. 10 ways to make exercise a lasting part of your life. *Consumer Reports on Health* 18 (5):1, 4–6.

Consumers Union. 2007. A truce in the diet wars. *Consumer Reports on Health* 19 (5):8–9.

Consumers Union. 2007. Gym traps—And solutions. *Consumer Reports on Health* 19 (2):7.

Consumers Union. 2007. New diet winners. *Consumer Reports* 72 (6):12–17.

Consumers Union. 2011. Pick your ideal diet. *Consumer Reports* 76 (6):14–16.

Consumers Union. 2013. Lose weight your way. *Consumer Reports* 78 (2): 26–29.

Convertino, V. A. 2007. Blood volume response to physical activity and inactivity. *American Journal of the Medical Sciences* 334 (1):72–79.

Cotton, J., et al. 1996. Replacement of dietary fat with sucrose polyester: Effects on energy intake and appetite control in non-obese males. *American Journal of Clinical Nutrition* 63:891–96.

Dallman, M. 2010. Stress-induced obesity and the emotional nervous system. *Trends in Endocrinology and Metabolism* 21:159–65.

Dansinger, M., et al. 2005. Comparison of the Atkins, Ornish, Watchers, and Zone diets for weight loss and heart disease risk reduction: A randomized trial. *Journal of the American Medical Association* 293:43–53.

Das, S., et al. 2007. Long-term effects of 2 energy-restricted diets differing in glycemic load on dietary adherence, body composition, and metabolism in CALERIE: A 1-y randomized controlled trial. *American Journal of Clinical Nutrition* 85:1023–30.

De Feo, P. 2013. Is high-intensity exercise better than moderate-intensity exercise for weight-loss? *Nutrition. Metabolism & Cardiovascular Diseases* 23:1037–1042.

Dich, J., et al. 2000. Effects of excessive isocaloric intake of either carbohydrate or fat on body composition, fat mass, de novo lipogenesis and energy expenditure in normal young men. *Ugeskrift for Laeger* 162:4794–99.

Donnelly, J., and Smith, B. 2005. Is exercise effective for weight loss with ad libitum diet? Energy balance, compensation, and gender differences. *Exercise and Sport Sciences Reviews* 33:169–74.

Donnelly, J., et al. 2009. American College of Sports Medicine position stand: Appropriate physical activity intervention strategies for weight loss and prevention of weight regain for adults. *Medicine & Science in Sports & Exercise* 41:459–71.

Drewnowski, A. 1995. Intense sweeteners and the control of appetite. *Nutrition Reviews* 53:1–7.

Ebbeling, C., et al. 2007. Effects of a low-glycemic load vs low-fat diet in obese young adults: A randomized trial. *Journal of the American Medical Association* 297:2092–102.

Egecioglu, E., et al. 2011. Hedonic and incentive signals for body weight control. *Reviews in Endocrine and Metabolic Disorders* 12:141–51.

Egras, A., et al. 2011. An evidence-based review of fat modifying supplemental weight loss products. *Journal of Obesity.* pii: 297315.

Elder, S., and Roberts, S. 2007. The effects of exercise on food intake and body fatness: A summary of published studies. *Nutrition Reviews* 65:1–19.

Finkelstein, E. A., and Kruger, E. 2014. Meta- and cost-effectiveness analysis of commercial weight loss strategies. *Obesity* 22 (9):1942–51.

Fogelholm, M., et al. 2012. Dietary macronutrients and food consumption as determinants of long-term weight change in adult populations. *Food and Nutrition Research* 56. doi: 10.3402/fnr.v56i0.19103.

Fontana, L., and Klein, S. 2007. Aging, adiposity, and calorie restriction. *Journal of the American Medical Association* 297:986–94.

Ford, H., and Frost, G. 2010. Glycaemic index, appetite and body weight. *Proceedings of the Nutrition Society* 69:199–203.

Foreyt, J., et al. 2009. Weight-reducing diets: Are there any differences? *Nutrition Reviews* 67 (Supplement 1):S99–101.

Foster-Schubert, K., et al. 2005. Human plasma ghrelin levels increase during a one-year exercise program. *Journal of Clinical Endocrinology and Metabolism* 90:820–25.

Furlow, E., and Anderson, J. 2009. A systematic review of targeted outcomes associated with a medically supervised commercial weight-loss program. *Journal of the American Dietetic Association* 109:1417–21.

Gellish, R., et al. 2006. Longitudinal modeling of the relationship between age and maximal heart rate. *Medicine & Science in Sports & Exercise* 38:822–29.

Giovannini, M., et al. 2010. Symposium overview: Do we all eat breakfast and is it important? *Critical Reviews in Food Science and Nutrition* 50:97–9.

Graves, J. E., et al. 1988. Physiological responses to walking with hand weights, wrist weights, and ankle weights. *Medicine and Science in Sports and Exercise* 20 (3):265–71.

Grediagin, M., et al. 1995. Exercise intensity does not effect body composition change in untrained, moderately overfat women. *Journal of the American Dietetic Association* 95:661–65.

Gudzune, K. A., et al. 2015. Efficacy of commercial weight-loss programs. An updated systematic review. *Annals of Internal Medicine* 162:501–12.

Hansen, D., et al. 2007. The effects of exercise training on fat-mass loss in obese patients during energy intake restriction. *Sports Medicine* 37 (1):31–46.

Hansen, D., et al. 2007. The effects of exercise training on fat-mass loss in obese patients during energy intake restriction. *Sports Medicine* 37:31–46.

Hartmann-Boyce, J., et al. 2014. Effect of behavioural techniques and delivery mode on effectiveness of weight management: Systematic review, meta-analysis and meta-regression. *Obesity Reviews* 15 (7):598–609.

Haskell, W., et al. 2007. Physical activity and public health: Updated recommendation for adults from the American College of Sports Medicine and the American Heart Association. *Medicine & Science in Sports & Exercise* 39:1423–34.

Haus, G., et al. 1994. Key modifiable factors in weight maintenance: Fat intake, exercise, and weight cycling. *Journal of the American Diebetic* Association 94:409–13.

Heckman, M., et al. 2010. Caffeine (1, 3, 7-trimethylxanthine) in foods: A comprehensive review on consumption, functionality, safety, and regulatory matters. *Journal of Food Science* 75:R77–87.

Hibi, M., et al. 2011. The short-term effect of diacylglycerol oil consumption on total and dietary fat utilization in overweight women. *Obesity* 19 (3):536–40.

Hill, J., and Commerford, R. 1996. Physical activity, fat balance, and energy balance. *International Journal of Sport Nutrition* 6:80–92.

Hooper, L., et al. 2012. Effect of reducing total fat intake on body weight: Systematic review and meta-analysis of randomized controlled trials and cohort studies. *British Medical Journal* 345:e-7666. doi 10.1136/bmj.e7666.trains

Horner, J. M., et al. 2014. Acute exercise and gastric emptying: A meta-analysis and implications for appetite control. *Sports Medicine* (November 15).

Howard, B., et al. 2006. Low-fat dietary pattern and weight change over 7 years: The Women's Health Initiative Dietary Modification Trial. *Journal of the American Medical Association* 295 (6):655–66.

Howarth, N. C., et al. 2005. Dietary fiber and fat are associated with excess weight in young and middle-aged US adults. *Journal of the American Dietetic Association* 105:1365–72.

Hu, F. 2005. Protein, body weight, and cardiovascular health. *American Journal of Clinical Nutrition* 82:242S–47S.

Hunter, G., et al. 1998. A role for high intensity exercise on energy balance and weight control. *International Journal of Obesity and Related Metabolic Disorders* 22:489–93.

Hursel, R., et al. 2011. The effects of catechin-rich teas and caffeine on energy expenditure and fat oxidation: A meta-analysis. *Obesity Reviews* 12:E-573-e581. doi: 10.1111/j.1467-789X.2011.00862.x.

Irving, B., et al. 2008. Effect of exercise training intensity on abdominal visceral fat and body composition. *Medicine & Science in Sports & Exercise* 40:1863–72.

Jakicic, J., and Gallagher, K. 2003. Exercise considerations for the sedentary, overweight adult. *Exercise and Sport Sciences Reviews* 31:91–95.

Jakicic, J., and Otto, A. 2006. Treatment and prevention of obesity: What is the role of exercise? *Nutrition Reviews* 64:S57–S61.

Jandacek, R. J. 2012. Review of the effects of dilution of dietary energy with olestra on energy intake. *Physiology and Behavior* 105(5):1124–31.

Jensen, M. D., et al. 2014. American Heart Association/American College of Cardiology/The Obesity Society: Guidelines for the management of overweight and obesity in adults. *Circulation* 129:S102–38.

Jequier, E. 2002. Pathways to obesity. *International Journal of Obesity and Related Metabolic Disorders* 26:S12–S17.

Johnston, B. C., et al. 2014. Comparison of weight loss among named diet programs in overweight and obese adults: A meta-analysis. *Journal of the American Medical Association* 312 (9):923–33.

Jonnalagadda, S. S., et al. 2005. Position of the American Dietetic Association: Fat replacers. *Journal of the American Dietetic Association* 105 (2):266–75.

Judkins, C., and Prock, P. 2012. Supplements and inadvertent doping—How big is the risk to athletes. *Medicine and Sport Science* 59:143–52.

Kappagoda, C. T., et al. 2004. Low-carbohydrate—high-protein diets. Is there a place for them in clinical cardiology? *Journal of the American College of Cardiology* 43 (5):725–30.

Karvonen, M. J., et al. 1957. The effects of training on heart rate; A longitudinal study. *Annales Medicinae Experimentalis et Biologicae Fenniae* 35 (3):307–15.

Katch, F. I., et al. 1984. Effects of sit-up exercise training on adipose cell size and adiposity. *Research Quarterly for Exercise and Sport* 55 (3):242–47.

Kay, S., and Fiatarone Singh, M. 2006. The influence of physical activity on abdominal fat: A systematic review of the literature. *Obesity Reviews* 7:183–200.

Kearney, T., et al. 2010. Adverse drug events associated with yohimbine-containing products: A retrospective review of the California Poison Control System reported cases. *Annals of Pharmacotherapy* 44:1022–9.

Keating, S. E., et al. 2014. Continuous exercise but not high intensity interval training improves fat distribution in overweight adults. *Journal of Obesity* 2014:834865. doi: 10.1155/2014/834865.

Kessler, H. S., et al. 2012. The potential for high-intensity interval training to reduce

cardiometabolic disease risk. *Sports Medicine* 42 (6):489–509.

King, A. C., et al. 2000. Personal and environmental factors associated with physical inactivity among different racial-ethnic groups of U.S. middle-aged and older-aged women. *Health Psychology* 19:354–64.

King, N., et al. 2007. Metabolic and behavioral compensatory responses to exercise interventions: Barriers to weight loss. *Obesity* 15:1373–83.

Kostek, M., et al. 2007. Subcutaneous fat alterations resulting from an upper-body resistance training program. *Medicine & Science in Sports & Exercise* 39:1177–85.

Kraemer, W., et al. 1999. Influence of exercise training on physiological and performance changes with weight loss in men. *Medicine & Science in Sports & Exercise* 31:1320–29.

Kraschnewski, J. L., et al. 2010. Long-term weight loss maintenance in the United State. *International Journal of Obesity* 34 (11):1644–54.

Krenn, P. J., et al. 2011. Use of global positioning systems to study physical activity and the environment: A systematic review. *American Journal of Preventive Medicine* 41 (5):508–15.

Kris-Etherton, P., et al. 2002. Dietary fat: Assessing the evidence in support of a moderate-fat diet; The benchmark based on lipoprotein metabolism. *Proceedings of the Nutrition Society* 61:287–98.

Laan, D., et al. 2010. Effects and reproducibility of aerobic and resistance exercise on appetite and energy intake in young, physically active adults. *Applied Physiology, Nutrition, and Metabolism* 35:842–7.

Larson-Meyer, D., et al. 2010. Caloric restriction with or without exercise: The fitness versus fatness debate. *Medicine & Science in Sports & Exercise* 42:152–9.

Layman, D., et al. 2005. Dietary protein and exercise have additive effects on body composition during weight loss in adult women. *Journal of Nutrition* 135:1903–10.

Layman, D., et al. 2008. Protein in optimal health: Heart disease and type 2 diabetes. *American Journal of Clinical Nutrition* 87:1571S–75S.

Leidy, H. J., et al. 2013. Beneficial effects of a higher-protein breakfast on the appetitive, hormonal, and neural signals controlling energy intake regulation in overweight/obese, "breakfast-skipping," late-adolescent girls. *American Journal of Clinical Nutrition* 97 (4):677–88.

Leidy, H., and Campbell, W. 2011. The effect of eating frequency on appetite control and food intake: Brief synopsis of controlled

feeding studies. *Journal of Nutrition* 141:154–7.

Leidy, H., et al. 2007. Effects of acute and chronic protein intake on metabolism, appetite, and ghrelin during weight loss. *Obesity* 15:1215–25.

Leidy, H., et al. 2007. Higher protein intake preserves lean mass and satiety with weight loss in pre-obese and obese women. *Obesity* 15:421–29.

Leidy, H., et al. 2011. The effects of consuming frequent, higher protein meals on appetite and satiety during weight loss in overweight/obese men. *Obesity* 19:818–24.

Lerner, Z. F., et al. 2014. Effects of obesity on lower extremity muscle function during walking at two speeds. *Gait and Posture* 39 (3):978–84.

Levin, B. 2002. Metabolic sensors: Viewing glucosensing neurons from a broader perspective. *Physiology & Behavior* 76:387–401.

Levine, J. A., et al. 2006. Non-exercise activity thermogenesis: The crouching tiger hidden dragon of societal weight gain. *Arteriosclerosis, Thrombosis, and Vascular Biology* 26 (4):729–36.

Liebman, B. 2004. Weighing the diet books. *Nutrition Action Health Letter* 31 (1):3–8.

Liebman, B. 2005. Bigger meals: Smaller waists. *Nutrition Action Health Letter* 32 (5):1–7.

Lowe, M. R., and Timko, C. A. 2004. Dieting: Really harmful, merely ineffective or actually helpful? *British Journal of Nutrition* 92 (Supplement 1):S19–S22.

Ma, Y., et al. 2007. A dietary quality comparison of popular weight-loss plans. *Journal of the American Dietetic Association* 107:1786–91.

Ma, Y., et al. 2015. Single-component verses multicomponent dietary goals for the metabolic syndrome: A randomized trial. *Annals of Internal Medicine* 162 (4):248–57.

Macfarlane, D. J., et al. 2006. Very short intermittent vs continuous bouts of activity in sedentary adults. *Preventive Medicine* 43:332–36.

Machado, F. A., et al. 2011. Validity of maximum heart rate prediction equations for children and adolescents. *Arquivos Brasileiros de Cardiologia* 97 (2):136–40.

MacLean, P. S., et al. 2015. NIH Working Group Report: Innovative research to improve maintenance of weight loss. *Obesity* 23 (1):7–15. doi: 10.1002/oby.20967.

Malik, V. S., et al. 2013. Sugar-sweetened beverages and weight gain in children and adults: A systematic review and meta-analysis. *American Journal of Clinical Nutrition* 98 (4):1084–102.

Manore, M. 1999. Low-fat foods and weight loss. *ACSM's Health & Fitness Journal* 3 (3):37–39.

Manthou, E., et al. 2010. Behavioral compensatory adjustments to exercise training in overweight women. *Medicine & Science in Sports & Exercise* 42:1221–8.

McCrory, M. A. 2014. Meal skipping and variables related to energy balance in adults: A brief review, with emphasis on the breakfast meal. *Physiology and Behavior* 134:51–54.

Meerman, R., and Brown, A. J. 2014. When somebody loses weight, where does the fat go? *British Medical Journal* 349:g7257. doi: 10.1136/bmj.g7257.

Melanson, E. L., et al. 2013. Resistance to exercise-induced weight loss: Compensatory behavioral adaptations. *Medicine and Science in Sport and Exercise* 45 (8):1600–9.

Melanson, E., et al. 2002. Effect of exercise intensity on 24-h energy expenditure and nutrient oxidation. *Journal of Applied Physiology* 92:1045–52.

Mettler, S., et al. 2010. Increased protein intake reduces lean body mass loss during weight loss in athletes. *Medicine & Science in Sports & Exercise* 42:326–37.

Miller, C.T., et al. 2013. The effects of exercise training in addition to energy restriction on functional capacities and body composition in obese adults during weight loss: A systematic review. *Public Library of Science One* 8(11):e81692. doi: 10.1371/journal.pone.0081692.

Miller, G., and Groziak, S. 1996. Impact of fat substitutes on fat intake. *Lipids* 31:S293–96.

Miller, W. C., et al. 1993. Predicting max HR and the HR-VO2 relationship for exercise prescription in obesity. *Medicine and Science in Sports and Exercise* 25 (9):1077–81.

Murphy, M., et al. 2002. Accumulating brisk walking for fitness, cardiovascular risk, and psychological health. *Medicine & Science in Sports & Exercise* 34:1468–74.

Murphy, M., et al. 2007. The effect of walking on fitness, fatness and resting blood pressure: A meta-analysis of randomized, controlled trials. *Preventive Medicine* 44:377–85.

National Heart, Lung, and Blood Institute. 2013. *Managing Overweight and Obesity in Adults. Systematic Evidence Review from the Obesity Expert Panel.* U.S. Department of Health and Human Services. National Institutes of Health.

Naukkarinen, J., et al. 2012. Causes and consequences of obesity: The contribution of recent twin studies. *International Journal of Obesity* 36:1017–24.

Nelson, M., et al. 2007. Physical activity and public health in older adults: Recommendation from the American College of Sports Medicine and the American Heart Association. *Medicine & Science in Sports & Exercise* 39:1435–45.

Newhouser, M. L., et al. 2012. A low-fat dietary pattern and risk for metabolic syndrome in post-menopausal women: The Women's Health Initiative. *Metabolism* 61 (11):1572–81.

Newman, B., et al. 1990. Nongenetic influences of obesity on other cardiovascular disease risk factors: An analysis of identical twins. *American Journal of Public Health* 80:675–78.

Nordmann, A., et al. 2006. Effects of low-carbohydrate vs low-fat diets on weight loss and cardiovascular risk factors: A meta-analysis of randomized controlled trials. *Archives of Internal Medicine* 166:285–93.

Noto, H., et al. 2013. Low-carbohydrate diets and all-cause mortality: A systematic review and meta-analysis of observational studies. *Public Library of Science ONE* 8(1):e55030. doi: 10.1371/journal. pone.0055030.

Nybo, L., et al. 2010. High-intensity training versus traditional exercise interventions for promoting health. *Medicine & Science in Sports & Exercise* 42:1951–58.

Ogden, C. L., et al. 2014. Prevalence of childhood and adult obesity in the United States, 2011–2012. *Journal of the American Medical Association* 311(8): 806–814.

Ogden, L. G., et al. 2012. Cluster analysis of the National Weight Control Registry to identify distinct subgroups maintaining successful weight loss. *Obesity* 20 (10):2039–47.

Olsen, N. J., and Heitman, B. L. 2009. Intake of calorically sweetened beverages and obesity. *Obesity Reviews* 10:68–75.

Onakpoya, I. J., et al. 2012. The efficacy of long-term conjugated linoleic acid (CLA) supplementation on body composition in overweight and obese individuals: A systematic review and meta-analysis of randomized clinical trials. *European Journal of Nutrition* 51 (2):127–34.

Onakpoya, I. J., et al. 2013. Chromium supplementation in overweight and obesity: A systematic review and meta-analysis of randomized clinical trials. *Obesity Reviews* 14(6):496–507.

Pawar, R. S., et al. 2013. Updates on chemical and biological research on botanical ingredients in dietary supplements. *Analytical and Bioanalytical Chemistry* 405 (13):4373–84.

Pawar, R.S., et al. 2013. Updates on chemical and biological research on botanical ingredients in dietary supplements. *Analytical and Bioanalytical Chemistry* 405(13):4373–4384.

Pekala, J., et al. 2011. L-carnitine-metabolic functions and meanings in human life. *Current Drug Metabolism* 12 (7):667–78.

Phelan, S., et al. 2007. Three-year weight change in successful weight losers who lost weight on a low-carbohydrate diet. *Obesity* 15 (10):2470–77.

Phung, O., et al. 2010. Effect of green tea catechins with or without caffeine on anthropometric measures: A systematic review and meta-analysis. *American Journal of Clinical Nutrition* 91:73–81.

Pi-Sunyer, F. 1990. Effect of the composition of the diet on energy intake. *Nutrition Reviews* 48:94–105.

Pittas, A., and Roberts, S. 2006. Dietary composition and weight loss: Can we individualize dietary prescriptions according to insulin sensitivity or secretion status? *Nutrition Reviews* 64:435–48.

Pol, K., et al. 2013. Whole grain and body weight changes in apparently healthy adults: A systematic review and meta-analysis of randomized controlled studies. *American Journal of Clinical Nutrition* 98:872–84.

Popkin, B., et al. 2006. A new proposed guidance system for beverage consumption in the United States. *American Journal of Clinical Nutrition* 83:529–42.

Puthoff, M., et al. 2006. The effect of weighted vest walking on metabolic responses and ground reaction forces. *Medicine & Science in Sports & Exercise* 38:746–52.

Quinn, T. J., and Coons, B. A. 2011. The talk test and its relationship with the ventilatory and lactate thresholds. *Journal of Sports Sciences* 29 (11):1175–82.

Raben, A., et al. 2002. Sucrose compared with artificial sweeteners: Different effects on ad libitum food intake and body weight after 10 wk of supplementation in overweight subjects. *American Journal of Clinical Nutrition* 76:721–29.

Rains, T., et al. 2011. Antiobesity effects of green tea catechins: A mechanistic review. *Journal of Nutritional Biochemistry* 22:1–7.

Ramage, S., et al. 2014. Healthy strategies for successful weight loss and weight maintenance: A systematic review. *Applied Physiology, Nutrition, and Metabolism* 39:1–20.

Rankinen, T., and Bouchard, C. 2008. Gene-physical activity interactions: Overview of human studies. *Obesity* 16 (Supplement 3) 3:S47–50.

Redman, L., et al. 2007. Effect of calorie restriction with or without exercise on body composition and fat distribution. *Journal of Clinical Endocrinology & Metabolism* 92:865–72.

Reed, J. L., and Pipe, A. L. 2014. The talk test: A useful tool for prescribing and monitoring exercise intensity. *Current Opinion in Cardiology* 29 (5):475–80.

Riley, R. 1999. Popular weight loss diets. *Clinics in Sports Medicine* 18:691–701.

Rippe, J. M. 2013. The metabolic and endocrine response and health implications of consuming sugar-sweetened beverages: Findings from recent randomized controlled trials. *Advances in Nutrition* 4 (6):677–86.

Roberts, S. 2000. High-glycemic index foods, hunger, and obesity: Is there a connection? *Nutrition Reviews* 58:163–69.

Robinson, E., et al. 2014. A systematic review and meta-analysis examining the effect of eating rate on energy intake and hunger. *American Journal of Clinical Nutrition* 100(1):123–51.

Rolls, B., and Bell, E. 1999. Intake of fat and carbohydrate: Role of energy density. *European Journal of Clinical Nutrition* 53:S166–73.

Rossato, L., et al. 2011. Synephrine: From trace concentrations to massive consumption in weight-loss. *Food and Chemical Toxicology* 49:8–16.

Rowe, D., et al. 2011. Stride rate recommendations for moderate-intensity walking. *Medicine & Science in Sports & Exercise* 43:312–18.

Sacks, F., et al. 2009. Comparison of weight-loss diets with different compositions of fat, protein, and carbohydrates. *New England Journal of Medicine* 360:859–73.

Saito, M., and Yoneshiro, T. 2013. Capsinoids and related food ingredients activating brown fat thermogenesis and reducing body fat in humans. *Current Opinions in Lipidology* 24 (1):71–77. doi: 10.1097/mol.0b013e32835a4f40.

Santesso, N., et al. 2012. Effects of higher-versus lower-protein diets on health outcomes: A systematic review and meta-analysis. *European Journal of Clinical Nutrition* 66:780–88.

Santos, F. L., et al. 2012. Systematic review and meta-analysis of clinical trials of the effects of low carbohydrate diets on cardiovascular risk factors. *Obesity Reviews* 13 (11):1048–66.

Schubert, M. M., et al. 2014. Acute exercise and hormones related to appetite regulation: A meta-analysis. *Sports Medicine* 44 (3):387–403.

Schwartz, A., et al. 2012. Greater than predicted decrease in resting energy expenditure and weight loss: Results from a systematic review. *Obesity* 20 (11):2307–10.

Schwingshackl, L., and Hoffman, H. 2013. Long-term effects of low-fat diets either low or high in protein on cardiovascular and metabolic risk factors: A systematic review and meta-analysis. *Nutrition Journal* 12:48. doi: 10.1186/1475-2891-12-48.

Seagle, H. M., et al. 2009. Position of the American Dietetic Association: Weight management. *Journal of the American Dietetic Association* 109 (2):330–46.

Shai, I., et al. 2008. Weight loss with a low-carbohydrate, Mediterranean, or low-fat diet. *New England Journal of Medicine* 359:229–41.

Shaibi, G. Q., et al. 2015. Exercise for obese youth: Refocusing attention from weight loss to health gains. *Exercise and Sport Sciences Reviews* 41 (1):41–47.

Shankar, P., et al. 2013. Non-nutritive sweeteners: Review and update. *Nutrition* 29 (11–12):1293–99.

Shide, D., and Rolls, B. 1995. Information about the fat content of preloads influences energy intake in healthy women. *Journal of the American Dietetic Association* 95:993–98.

Sijie, T., et al. 2012. High intensity interval exercise training in overweight young women. *Journal of Sports Medicine and Physical Fitness* 52 (3):255–62.

Sillanpää, E., et al. 2008. Body composition and fitness during strength and/or endurance training in older men. *Medicine & Science in Sports & Exercise* 40:950–58.

Sjodin, A., et al. 1996. The influence of physical activity on BMR. *Medicine & Science in Sports & Exercise* 28:85–91.

St. Jeor, S., et al. 2001. Dietary protein and weight reduction: A statement for health-care professionals from the Nutrition Committee of the Council on Nutrition, Physical Activity, and Metabolism of the American Heart Association. *Circulation* 104:1869–74.

Stiegler, P., and Cunliffe, A. 2006. The role of diet and exercise for the maintenance of fat-free mass and resting metabolic rate. *Sports Medicine* 36:239–62.

Stubbs, R., et al. 2004. A decrease in physical activity affects appetite, energy, and nutrient balance in lean men feeding ad libitum. *American Journal of Clinical Nutrition* 79:62–69.

Sweet, S., and Fortier, M. 2010. Improving physical activity and dietary behaviours with single or multiple health behaviour interventions: A synthesis of meta-analyses and reviews. *International Journal of Environmental Research and Public Health* 7:1720–43.

Södlerlund, A., et al. 2009. Physical activity, diet and behaviour modification in the treatment of overweight and obese adults: A systematic review. *Perspectives in Public Health* 129:132–42.

1996. *Surgeon General's Report on Physical Activity and Health*. 1996. U.S. Department of Health and Human Services, Public Health Service, Centers for Disease Control and Prevention, National Center for Chronic Disease Prevention and Health Promotion.

Taheri, S., et al. 2004. Short sleep duration is associated with reduced leptin, elevated ghrelin, and increased body mass index. *PLoS Medicine* 1 (3):e62.

Tanaka, H., et al. 2001. Age-predicted maximal heart rate revisited. *Journal of the American College of Cardiology* 37 (1):153–60.

Tate, D., et al. 2007. Long-term weight losses associated with prescription of higher physical activity goals. Are higher levels of physical activity protective against weight regain? *American Journal of Clinical Nutrition* 85:954–59.

Teixeira, P. J., et al. 2012. Exercise, physical activity, and self-determination theory: A systematic review. *International Journal of Behavioral Nutrition and Physical Activity* 9:78. doi: 10.1186/1479-5868-9-78.

Thomas, D. E., et al. 2007. Low glycaemic index or low glycaemic load diets for overweight and obesity. *Cochrane Database of Systematic Reviews* 18 (3):CD005105.

Thomas, J. G., et al. 2014. Weight-loss maintenance for 10 years in the National Weight Control Registry. *American Journal of Preventive Medicine* 46 (1):17–23.

Thompson, D., et al. 1988. Acute effects of exercise intensity on appetite in young men. *Medicine & Science in Sports & Exercise* 20:222–27.

Tian, H., et al. 2013. Chromium picolinate supplementation for overweight or obese adults. *Cochrane Database of Systematic Reviews* 11:CD010063. doi: 10.1002/14651858.CD010063.pub2.

Tremblay, A., and Doucet, E. 1999. Influence of intense physical activity on energy balance and body fatness. *Proceedings of the Nutrition Society* 58:99–105.

Tremblay, A., et al. 1999. Physical activity and weight maintenance. *International Journal of Obesity and Related Metabolic Disorders* 23 (Supplement 3):S50–S54.

Tremblay, M. S., et al. 2011. Systematic review of sedentary behaviour and health indicators in school-aged children and youth. *International Journal of Behavioral Nutrition and Physical Activity* 8:98. doi: 10.1186/1479-5868-8-98.

Tsai, A., and Wadden, T. 2005. Systematic review: An evaluation of major commercial weight loss programs in the United States. *Annals of Internal Medicine* 142:56–66.

Tudor-Locke, C., and Lutes, L. 2009. Why do pedometers work? A reflection upon the factors related to successfully increasing physical activity. *Sports Medicine* 39 (12):981–93.

Tudor-Locke, C., et al. 2008. Revisiting "How many steps are enough?" *Medicine & Science in Sports & Exercise* 40:S537–43.

Tudor-Locke, C., et al. 2013. A step-defined sedentary lifestyle index: <5000 steps/day. *Applied Physiology, Nutrition, and Metabolism* 38 (2):100–14.

Tudor-Locke, C., et al. 2014. Changing the way we work: Elevating energy expenditure with workstation alternatives. *International Journal of Obesity* 38 (6):755–65.

Tufts University. 2011. Extra sugar adds 475 calories a day. *Tufts University Health & Nutrition Letter* 28 (12):3.

Turocy, P., et al. 2011. National Athletic Trainers' Association position statement: Sage weight loss and maintenance practices in sport and exercise. *Journal of Athletic Training* 46 (3):322–36.

Utter, A. C., et al. 2004. Validation of the adult OMNI scale of perceived exertion for walking/running exercise. *Medicine and Science in Sport and Exercise* 36 (10):1776–80.

Utter, A., et al. 2006. Validation of Omni scale of perceived exertion during prolonged cycling. *Medicine & Science in Sport & Exercise* 38:780–86.

Vissers, D., et al. 2013. The effect of exercise on visceral adipose tissue in overweight adults: A systematic review and meta-analysis. *Public Library of Science One* 8 (2):e56415. doi: 10.1371/journal.pone.0056415.

Wadden, T., et al. 2004. Efficacy of lifestyle modification for long-term weight control. *Obesity Research* 12:151S–62S.

Weigle, D., et al. 2005. A high-protein diet induces sustained reductions in appetite, ad libitum caloric intake, and body weight despite compensatory changes in diurnal plasma leptin and ghrelin concentrations. *American Journal of Clinical Nutrition* 82:41–48.

Westerterp-Plantenga, M. S. et al., 2012. Dietary protein—Its role in satiety, energetics, weight loss and health. *British Journal of Nutrition* 108:S105–12.

Wing, R., and Phelan, S. 2005. Long-term weight maintenance. *American Journal of Clinical Nutrition* 82:222S–25S.

Wood, P. 1996. Clinical applications of diet and physical activity in weight loss. *Nutrition Reviews* 54:S131–35.

Wyatt, H. R., et al. 2002. Long-term weight loss and breakfast in subjects in the National Weight Control Registry. *Obesity Research* 10 (2):78–82.

Wycherley, T. P., et al. 2012. Effects of energy-restricted high-protein, low-fat compared to standard-protein, low-fat diets: A meta-analysis of randomized controlled trials. *American Journal of Clinical Nutrition* 96:1281–98.

Yeomans, M. R. 2010. Alcohol, appetite and energy balance: Is alcohol intake a risk factor for obesity? *Physiology and Behavior* 100 (1):82–89.

Zeni, A., et al. 1996. Energy expenditure with indoor exercise machines. *Journal of the American Medical Association* 275:1424–27.

Weight Gaining through Proper Nutrition and Exercise

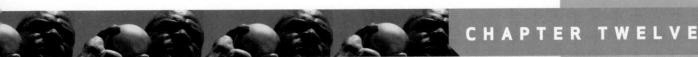

CHAPTER TWELVE

LEARNING OBJECTIVES

After studying this chapter, you should be able to:

1. Describe the steps an individual might take to gain body weight, mainly as muscle mass.

2. Plan a diet for an individual who desires to gain muscle mass in concert with a resistance-training program, focusing on recommended caloric intake and foods compatible with the Prudent Healthy Diet.

3. Identify dietary supplements used by physically active individuals to stimulate muscle building and body-fat loss, and list those, if any, that may be effective.

4. List and explain the principles of resistance training.

5. Understand the basic differences among resistance-training programs for muscular hypertrophy, muscular strength and power, and muscular endurance.

6. Design a total-body resistance-training program for an individual who desires to gain body weight as muscle mass.

7. Identify the potential health benefits of resistance exercise and compare them to the health benefits associated with aerobic endurance exercise, noting similarities and differences.

Introduction

As noted in chapter 11, there are basically three reasons individuals attempt to lose excess body weight—to improve appearance, health, or athletic performance. Some individuals may also wish to gain weight for the same three reasons and may use resistance training, also known as weight training or strength training, as a means to stimulate weight gain.

For those who wish to improve appearance, resistance training will increase muscularity, a desired physical attribute among many males. Resistance training is becoming increasingly popular. According to *Healthy People 2020* data (www.healthypeople.gov/2020), 23.9 percent of 18- to 64-year-old adults engaged in muscle-strengthening activities 2 or more days/week in 2012, including 28 percent of males and 19.9 percent of females. These percentages represent increases from 2008 of 8.9 and 8.7 percent for males and females, respectively, and are near the 2020 goal of 24.1 percent.

Gaining weight, particularly muscle mass stimulated by resistance training, may also be associated with some health benefits. An increased muscularity that improves physical appearance and body image may help elevate self-esteem, contributing to positive psychological health. Additionally, resistance training, done alone even without weight gain, is recommended for several other health benefits, such as increased bone mineral density. The American Heart Association and the American College of Sports Medicine, in their reports on physical activity and health, recommend resistance exercise as an effective means to promote overall good health. Resistance training is particularly recommended for older adults to help prevent the muscle wasting, and associated health problems, seen with aging, as documented by Nelson and Raymond and their respective colleagues. A popular book, *Dr. David Reuben's Quick Weight-Gain Program,* has been designed to provide sound medical advice for the 26 million Americans who need to gain weight for a variety of medical and cosmetic reasons.

Increased body weight, particularly increased muscle mass, may be associated with improvements in strength and power, two performance factors important for a wide variety of sports. Enhanced muscularity also may influence performance in judged aesthetic sports, such as diving and gymnastics. Most colleges and universities, as well as many high schools, have strength-training programs for their athletes, both males and females. At the elite level, sport-specific resistance-training programs are tailored to the individual athlete.

No matter what the reason for gaining body weight, you should be concerned about where the extra pounds will be stored. The energy-balance equation works as well for gaining weight as it does for losing weight, but excess body fat in general will not improve physical appearance, health, or athletic performance. On the contrary, it may detract from all three. To put on body weight, you have to concentrate on means to increase the fat-free mass, particularly muscle tissue, with little or no increase in body-fat stores.

Drummond and colleagues note that resistance exercise and nutritional provision are two independent and major stimuli of muscle protein synthesis and overall muscle growth, and numerous related approaches have been employed to increase muscle mass. Specialized exercise equipment or exercise techniques are advertised as the most effective methods available to build muscles. Protein supplements have been a favorite among weight lifters for years, but numerous dietary supplements currently on the market are advertised to produce an anabolic, or muscle-building, effect. Some athletes and nonathletes even

use drugs to gain weight for enhanced performance or appearance, a topic that is discussed in chapter 13. Although resistance training may confer significant health benefits, excessive weight lifting may be a symptom of a male-dominated psychological condition called muscle dysmorphia, also known as the Adonis complex. In their review, Suffolk and others commented that some very muscular individuals have a distorted body image, perceiving themselves as too thin or not sufficiently muscular. Murray and others noted that symptoms of muscle dysmorphia such as low self-esteem, body dissatisfaction, perfectionism, and obsessive-compulsive behavior are similar to those observed in females with eating disorders. McCreary and others suggest that muscle dysmorphia may lead to the use of anabolic-androgenic steroids to enhance muscularity. Skemp and others reported that competitive weight-training athletes scored higher than noncompetitive athletes in four of six muscle dysmorphia inventory subscales.

Like weight-loss programs, weight-gaining programs may be safe and effective or they can be potentially harmful to your health. Gaining weight, particularly as muscle mass, is difficult for some individuals. The purpose of this chapter is to present basic information on the type of diet and exercise program that is most likely to be effective as a means to put on weight without compromising your health.

Although some basic information regarding advanced resistance-training programs will be provided, detailed coverage of such programs is beyond the scope of this text. References to advanced resistance-training programs will be provided for the interested reader.

Basic Considerations

Why are some individuals underweight?

Being significantly under a healthy body weight may be due to several factors. Heredity may be an important factor, as genetic factors may predispose some individuals to leanness. For example, a lean body frame or high basal metabolic rate may have been acquired from your parents. Medical problems such as heartburn, infections, or cancer could adversely affect food intake and digestion, so a physician should be consulted to rule out nutritional problems caused by organic disease, hormonal imbalance, or inadequate absorption of nutrients. Social pressures, such as the strong desire of a teenage girl to have a slender body, could lead to undernutrition; an extreme example is anorexia nervosa, discussed in chapter 10. Emotional problems also may affect food intake. In many cases, food intake is increased during periods of emotional crisis, but the appetite may also be depressed in some individuals for long periods. Economic hardship may reduce food purchasing power, so some individuals simply may sacrifice food intake for other life necessities.

Being considerably underweight, such as a body mass index below 18.5, may be considered a symptom of malnutrition or undernutrition. It is important to determine the cause before prescribing a treatment. Our concern here is the individual who does not have any of these medical, psychological, social, or economic problems but who simply cannot create a positive energy balance because of excess energy expenditure or insufficient energy (Calorie) intake. Caloric intake has to be increased, and the output has to be modified somewhat.

What steps should I take if I want to gain weight?

The following guidelines may help you develop an effective program to maximize your gains in muscle mass and keep body-fat increases relatively low.

1. Have an acceptable purpose for the weight gain. The desire for an improved physical appearance and body image may be reason enough. For athletes, increased muscle mass may be important for a variety of sports, particularly if strength and power are improved. However, you do not want to gain weight at the expense of speed if speed is important to your sport.

2. Calculate your average energy needs daily, as discussed in chapter 11. For a weight-gain program, you may wish to use several techniques to estimate your daily energy needs and select the highest value.

3. Keep a 3- to 7-day record of what you normally eat. See pages 495–497 for guidelines to determine your average daily caloric intake. If the obtained value is less than your energy needs calculated under item 2 in this list, this may be a reason you are not gaining weight.

4. Check your living habits. Do you get enough rest and sleep? If not, you may be burning more energy than the estimate in item 2 of this list. Smoking increases your metabolic rate almost 10 percent and may account for approximately 200 Calories per day. Caffeine in coffee and soft drinks also increases the metabolic rate for several hours. Getting enough rest and sleep and eliminating smoking and caffeine will help decrease your energy output.

5. Set a reasonable goal within a certain time period. Weight gain may be rapid at first but then tapers off as you near your genetic potential. Lemon indicated that body mass may increase by as much as 20 percent in the first year of resistance training with subsequent yearly gains of only 1 to 3 percent. In general, about 0.5–1 pound per week is a sound approach for a novice, but weight gaining is difficult for some individuals and may occur at a slower rate. Specific goals may also include muscular hypertrophy in various parts of the body.

6. Increase your caloric and protein intake. A properly designed diet should include adequate Calories and protein and not violate the principles of healthful nutrition.

7. Start a resistance-training exercise program. This type of exercise program will serve as a stimulus to build muscle tissue. In a recent review, Phillips comments that resistance training plus the consumption of high-quality, rapidly digestible protein with high leucine content (0.25–0.30 gram/kg body mass/meal) can exert synergistic effects on muscle protein synthesis. Guidelines for developing a resistance-training program are presented later in this chapter.

8. Use a good cloth or steel tape to take body measurements before and during your weight-gaining program. Be sure you measure at the same points about once a week. Those body parts measured should include the neck, upper and lower arm, chest, abdomen, hips, thigh, and calf. This is to ensure that body-weight gains are proportionately distributed. You should look for good gains in the chest and limbs. The abdominal and hip girth increase should be kept low because that is where fat is more likely to be stored. If available, skinfold calipers may be used to measure subcutaneous fat skinfolds at multiple sites over the body. Fat skinfold thicknesses should remain the same or decrease to ensure that the weight gain is muscle rather than fat.

In summary, adequate rest; increased caloric intake; adequate intake of high-quality, highly digestible protein; and a proper resistance-training program may be very effective as a means to gain the right kind of body weight.

Key Concepts

▶ There may be a variety of reasons an individual is underweight, and the cause should be determined before a treatment is recommended.

▶ For those who want to gain weight, a weekly increase of 0.5–1.0 pound is a sound approach, but the desired weight gain should be muscle tissue and not body fat. In essence, adequate rest and sleep; increased caloric intake; adequate intake of high-quality, highly digestible protein; and a proper resistance-training program should be effective in helping to increase lean body mass.

Nutritional Considerations

In the last chapter, we discussed nutritional considerations for losing body weight, particularly body fat. In general, the recommendation consists of a healthy diet but with reduced caloric intake. In this chapter, we examine nutritional considerations for gaining body weight, particularly lean body mass as muscle. In this case, the recommendation still is to eat a healthy diet but with increased caloric intake.

Gaining weight as muscle mass may be difficult for some. Remember the quote from chapter 11: *Muscles are hard to get and easy to lose, fat is easy to get and hard to lose.* Resistance training, discussed later in this chapter, is important to help stimulate muscle growth so that extra Calories are used to develop muscle, not fat. As noted, gaining about 0.5–1.0 pound per week is a reasonable goal, although some may be able to gain more, while some may gain less.

How many Calories are needed to form 1 pound of muscle?

Muscle tissue consists of about 70 percent water and 22 percent protein, and the remainder is fat, carbohydrate, and minerals. Because the vast majority of muscle tissue is water, which has no caloric value, the total caloric value is only about 700–800 Calories per pound. However, extra energy is needed to help synthesize the muscle tissue.

It is not known exactly how many additional Calories are necessary to form 1 pound of muscle tissue in human beings, nor is it known in what form these Calories have to be consumed. The National Research Council notes that 5 Calories are needed to support the addition of 1 gram of tissue during growth. Because 1 pound equals 454 grams, a range of 2,300–3,500 additional Calories appears to be a reasonable amount. With a recommended weight gain of 1 pound per week, about 400–500 Calories above your daily needs would provide an amount in the suggested range, 2,800–3,500 Calories per week. Bartels and others reported that an additional 500 Calories per day resulted in nearly a 1-pound increase in lean body weight per week during a resistance-training program. For our purposes, we shall consider 3,500 Calories as the weekly excess energy intake necessary to support an increase in 1 pound of muscle tissue.

How can I determine the amount of Calories I need daily to gain 1 pound per week?

First, review the techniques presented in chapter 11 to determine the number of Calories needed simply to maintain your current body weight. Then add the Calories that you expend during exercise and the additional amount needed to synthesize the muscle tissue. Table 12.1 presents an example of a 154-pound, 18-year-old male who desires to gain a pound per week. You may modify the figures according to your own needs. You can use the ChooseMyPlate Website to plan a weight-gain diet as well as a weight-loss diet. Other methods presented in chapter 11, such as the Mayo Clinic Calorie Calculator, may also be used. Remember, a weight gain of 0.5–1.0 pound muscle mass per week is a reasonable goal during the early stages of resistance training. If you are maintaining your weight with your current dietary intake, adding 500 Calories per day may also be an acceptable approach.

TABLE 12.1 Caloric intake needed for a 154-pound, 18-year-old male to gain 1 pound per week

Energy expenditure	Daily Calories needed
Recommended caloric intake to maintain current weight 19 Calories/pound	2,468
Resistance training 200 Calories per session 4 sessions per week 800/7	115
Aerobic exercise 300 Calories per session 4 sessions per week 1,200/7	170
Muscle tissue synthesis 3,500 Calories per pound 3,500/7	500
Total daily caloric intake	3,253

Increased caloric intake is the key dietary principle, along with adequate protein intake, to gain mass during resistance training, as noted in a Gatorade Sports Science Institute review of weight-gain strategies in athletes by Butterfield, Kleiner, Lemon, and Stone.

Is protein supplementation necessary during a weight-gaining program?

One of the most researched areas in sports nutrition is the recommended protein intake for individuals who are attempting to increase muscle mass with resistance training. Topics of interest include amount, quality, timing, co-ingestion with carbohydrate, and cost.

Amount   From a mathematical viewpoint, adding a pound of muscle protein per week does not require a substantial increase in daily protein intake. Muscle tissue is about 22 percent protein and 70 percent water, with the remainder composed of carbohydrate and fat and trace amounts of vitamins and minerals. One pound of muscle is equal to 454 grams, but only about 100 grams (0.22 × 454 grams) is protein. If we divide 100 grams by 7 days, we would need approximately 14 grams of protein per day above our normal protein requirements to support the growth of 1 pound of muscle per week—if we are in protein balance. Incidentally, 14 grams of protein could be obtained in such small amounts of food as 2 glasses of milk; 2 ounces of meat, fish, or poultry; 2 eggs; or various combinations (see figure 12.1).

As you may recall, the Acceptable Macronutrient Distribution Range (AMDR) for protein is 10 to 35 percent of daily caloric intake. As noted in table 12.1, our 70-kilogram (154-pound) male needs a daily intake approximating 3,250 Calories to add a pound of muscle per week. If he consumed a diet containing 12 to 15 percent of energy from protein, his daily protein intake would approximate 98 (3,250 × 0.12 ÷ 4) to 122 (3,250 × 0.15 ÷ 4) grams, or 1.4 to 1.75 grams/kg body mass.

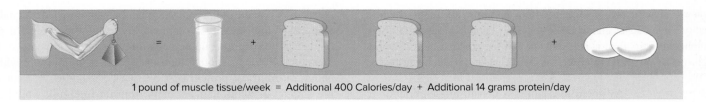

1 pound of muscle tissue/week = Additional 400 Calories/day + Additional 14 grams protein/day

FIGURE 12.1 To add a pound of muscle tissue per week, you need to consume approximately 400 additional Calories and 14 grams of additional protein per day. A weight-training program is an essential part of a muscle-building program. One glass of skim milk, three slices of whole wheat bread, and two hard-boiled egg whites provide the necessary Calories and about 23 grams of protein.

As noted in chapter 6, experts disagree on the necessity of protein over the RDA of 0.8 to 1.0 gram/kg for individuals seeking to gain muscle mass through resistance training. Some contend the RDA includes a safety factor providing adequate protein for muscle hypertrophy. In his 2012 review, Phillips notes the inconsistency in protein RDA and U.S./Canadian Dietetic Association recommendations of 1.2 to 1.7 grams/kg body mass for athletes. The RDA for our 70-kilogram male is 56 grams (0.8×70 kg) daily. An additional 14 grams totals 70 grams, which is less than would be consumed on a diet with 12–15 percent protein. If he consumed 1.6 grams/kg, as recommended by some, his daily protein intake would total 112 grams, still within the 12–15 percent range. Protein intake could be increased even more and still remain within the AMDR of 10–35 percent.

For individuals attempting to lose weight but maintain lean body mass, increasing the percentage of energy intake from protein may be recommended. In their meta-analysis of long-term effects of low-carbohydrate, high-protein diets on weight loss and maintenance, Clifton and colleagues reported that higher-protein diets (≥ 5 percent above baseline intake of protein at 12 months) exerted a three-fold greater reduction in fat mass compared to a normal (<5 percent over baseline) protein diet.

Timing Timing of protein intake is an important consideration. Hulmi and others indicated that protein intake close to a resistance exercise workout may alter messenger-RNA expression in a manner that may promote muscle hypertrophy. This may be the mechanism underlying the contention of Beelen and others that postexercise protein administration is warranted to stimulate muscle protein synthesis, inhibit protein breakdown, and allow net muscle protein accretion. In his review, Phillips concluded that evidence increasingly supports the efficacy of protein consumption in close temporal proximity to the performance of resistance exercise in promoting greater muscular hypertrophy.

Beelen and others quantified this recommendation, suggesting that the consumption of about 20 grams intact protein, or an equivalent of about 9 grams essential amino acids, has been reported to maximize muscle protein-synthesis rates during the first hours of postexercise recovery. They also suggested that ingestion of such small amounts of dietary protein five or six times daily (a total of about 100 to 120 grams) might support maximal muscle protein-synthesis rates throughout the day.

Although consuming protein within a short time of completing a resistance training workout appears to be beneficial to maximize muscle hypertrophy, and possibly strength and power, some have contended there would be little difference if the total amount of protein consumed throughout the day were similar, in essence hypothesizing that timing is not an important consideration. Several studies have tested this hypothesis. In general, the study protocol provided protein supplements to some subjects immediately before and/or after exercise, while other subjects consumed the supplements at different times of the day, either several hours after the workout or in the morning and evening. Both groups consumed the same total amount of protein daily.

Results from studies support both viewpoints. For example, Cribb and Hayes reported that consuming a protein/carbohydrate supplement, which also contained creatine, immediately before and after a resistance-training workout, as contrasted to consuming the same supplement in the morning and evening, resulted in greater increases in lean body mass and strength testing. In contrast, Hoffman and others conducted a similar study with resistance-trained men and concluded that the time of protein-supplement ingestion in resistance-trained athletes during a 10-week training program does not make any difference in strength, power, or body-composition changes. Studies with older subjects, men in their seventies, show a similar disparity. Esmarck and others concluded that oral protein supplement immediately after resistance training, as contrasted to 2 hours later, resulted in greater muscle hypertrophy in skeletal muscle of elderly men in response to resistance training. Conversely, Verdijk and others, in a similar 12-week study, concluded that timed protein supplementation immediately before and after exercise does not further augment the increase in skeletal muscle mass and strength after prolonged resistance-type exercise training in healthy elderly men who habitually consume adequate amounts of dietary protein.

In their review, Aragon and Schoenfeld comment that a postexercise protein intake for optimal muscle growth and repair may be less important if nutrient intake occurs within 1–2 hours of exercise. According to Bauer and colleagues, there is insufficient evidence for recommendations about the timing of protein intake in older individuals. Given the available research, consuming protein after resistance training appears to be prudent, as it may do some good and is unlikely to do any harm.

Quality Current research suggests that the quality of the ingested protein may also be an important consideration. In his most recent review on the science of muscle hypertrophy, Phillips indicated that certain types of proteins, particularly those that are digested rapidly and are high in leucine content, appear to be more efficient at stimulating muscle protein synthesis. In particular, Phillips notes that milk proteins, specifically whey and casein proteins, are of the highest quality. He indicates that whey protein is better able to support muscle protein synthesis than is soy protein, and the practice of consuming high-quality proteins after exercise should lead to greater hypertrophy.

Carbohydrate As noted in chapter 4, consuming carbohydrate after exercise is recommended to replace muscle glycogen, a key energy source for exercise. Phillips notes that carbohydrate alone is not sufficient for muscle protein synthesis but ingesting a protein and carbohydrate mixture immediately following resistance exercise or aerobic endurance exercise may be recommended. Both the carbohydrate and the protein will stimulate insulin secretion, which will help move glucose and amino acids into the muscle to facilitate recovery and support muscle protein synthesis.

Ivy and Portman recommend a tasty postworkout carbohydrate/protein drink, with a ratio of about 3–4 grams of carbohydrate for each gram of protein. As shown in figure 12.2, an 8-ounce glass of low-fat chocolate milk contains 32 grams of carbohydrate and 8 grams of protein (a 4:1 ratio) and is an affordable postexercise recovery beverage. In their review, Pritchett and Pritchett comment that ingestion of 1.0–1.5 grams/kg body weight immediately after and 2 hours after exercise may reduce muscle damage. Approximately 82 percent of cow's milk is casein protein and about 18 percent is whey protein. Some of the carbohydrate in chocolate milk is lactose, but most is glucose in the added chocolate syrup. Lactose-free chocolate milk is available for those with lactose intolerance. Several studies have shown that chocolate milk is an effective postexercise recovery fluid. Josse found that fat-free milk is also an effective drink to support favorable body-composition changes with resistance training.

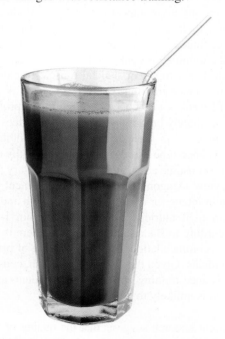

FIGURE 12.2 Chocolate milk may be an excellent source of nutrients before or after a resistance-training workout. One glass provides about 32 grams of carbohydrate and 8 grams of protein, a 4:1 ratio. Chocolate milk also provides important minerals and vitamins.

Cost As noted in table 6.8 on page 242 the cost for a standard amount of high-quality protein may vary considerably. In particular, protein sports supplements may be rather expensive. For example, Goldman noted that one popular product providing about 25 grams of protein cost $3 to $4 per bottle. A comparable amount of high-quality protein from fat-free milk would cost approximately 60 cents.

Are dietary supplements necessary during a weight-gaining program?

Dietary supplements appear to be very popular among athletes and others attempting to increase muscle mass and strength, if we can use advertisements as evidence to support this contention. For example, in a survey of only five magazines targeted to bodybuilding athletes, Grunewald and Bailey reported more than 800 performance claims made for 624 commercially available supplements. This survey was conducted over 20 years ago, but such marketing practices continue unabated. Numerous products are marketed not only to increase muscle mass, strength, and power but also to help prevent injuries during resistance training. According to Bloomer, nutritional supplements are aggressively marketed by the popular fitness media to athletes in order to attenuate strength training-related muscle injury with little scientific support for such claims.

Although there may be some truth underlying the alleged performance-enhancing mechanisms of these supplements, the effectiveness of most has not been evaluated by scientific research. In a review of nutritional supplements for strength-trained athletes, Williams indicated that there is little or no scientific evidence supporting positive effects on muscle growth, body-fat reduction, or strength enhancement in strength-trained athletes for most products. The effects of many of these supplements, such as specific individual amino acids, vitamins, minerals, and other individual nutrients, have been discussed in previous chapters and in general have not been found to be effective as performance-enhancing agents. Research has found that many are ineffective, whereas other supplements are inadequately researched.

Protein and creatine supplements may help increase muscle mass. Pasiakos and colleagues reported that protein may promote muscle hypertrophy and power with increased duration, frequency, and volume of resistance training. Phillips noted that whey and other high-quality proteins with high leucine content may increase muscle growth and repair. Creatine monohydrate, discussed in chapter 6, also appears to increase muscle mass. Numerous studies report increases in power and strength in high-intensity resistance exercise with short-term recovery. Early increases in muscle mass may be due to water retention, but increased resistance-training capacity may ultimately increase muscle mass. Creatine may help augment the anabolic effects of resistance training in the elderly, increasing muscle mass and strength, according to reviews by Candow and Rawson and Venezia. In their meta-analysis, Devries and Phillips reported that creatine and resistance training increased total mass and fat-free mass in adults over 60 years of age more than resistance training alone. The importance of resistance training to help prevent or reduce loss of muscle mass in the elderly will be covered in the next section.

Several other dietary supplements marketed to athletes are patterned after anabolic/androgenic steroids. Some herbal products are marketed for their supposed anabolic potential. In general, as noted in chapter 13, research indicates that such supplements do not increase muscle mass and may cause adverse health effects.

In a symposium sponsored by the Gatorade Sports Science Institute, five experts on muscle-building supplements provided this advice:

- Train hard.
- Follow a sound diet with adequate energy, protein, and carbohydrate.
- Don't rely on dietary supplements.

If you do use supplements, be sure to consult with an expert, such as a sports-oriented dietitan or physician, not the clerk at a health food store.

What is an example of a balanced diet that will help me gain weight?

As with losing weight, the Food Exchange System may serve as the basis for a sound weight-gaining diet. Foods must be selected for high nutrient value as well as additional Calories to support the weight gain.

The following suggestions may be helpful for those trying to gain weight as muscle. In general, the focus is on healthy dietary sources of carbohydrates, protein, and fats.

Milk exchange—Drink 1% or 2% milk instead of skim milk, which will add 15–30 Calories per glass. Chocolate milk provides both carbohydrate and high-quality protein. If you want to decrease caloric intake from fat, fat-free chocolate milk is available. Prepare milk shakes with dry milk powder and supplement with fruit. Add low-fat cheeses to sandwiches or snacks. Eat yogurt supplemented with fruit. The milk exchange is rich in high-quality protein.

Meat and meat substitute exchange—Increase your intake of lean meats, poultry, and fish, which are also sources of high-quality protein. Legumes such as beans and dried peas are high in protein, carbohydrate, and Calories and low in fat. Use nuts, seeds, and limited amounts of peanut butter for snacks. The meat exchange is also high in protein.

Starch exchange—Increase your consumption of whole-grain products. Pasta and rice are nutritious side dishes that provide adequate Calories. Starchy vegetables like potatoes are also nutritious sources of Calories. Breads and muffins can be supplemented with fruits and nuts. Whole-grain breakfast cereals can provide substantial Calories and even make a tasty dessert or snack with added fruit. The starch exchange is high in complex carbohydrates but also contains about 15 percent of its Calories as protein.

Fruit exchange—Add fruit to other food exchanges. Drink more fruit juices, which are high in both Calories and nutrients. Dried fruits such as apricots, pineapple, dates, and raisins are high in Calories and make excellent snacks.

Vegetable exchange—Use fresh vegetables like broccoli and cauliflower as snacks with melted low-fat cheese or a nutritious dip.

Fat exchange—Try to minimize the intake of saturated fats, using monounsaturated and polyunsaturated fats instead, particularly olive and canola oils. Nuts and seeds are good sources of monounsaturated fats. Salad dressings and soft margarine added to vegetables can increase their caloric content.

Beverages—Milk and juices are nutritious and high in Calories. Those who drink alcohol should obtain only limited amounts of Calories in this way. Some liquid supplements are available commercially and may contain 300–400 Calories with substantial amounts of protein. However, check the label for fat and sugar content.

Snacks—Eat three balanced meals per day supplemented with two or three snacks. Dried fruits, nuts, and seeds are excellent snacks. Some of the high-Calorie, high-protein, high-nutrient liquid meals, and sports bars on the market also make good snacks.

Table 12.2 presents an example of a high-Calorie diet plan based upon the Food Exchange System. It consists of three main meals and three snacks and totals about 4,000 Calories, with 160 grams of protein, which is 16 percent of the Calories. It is also high in carbohydrate, which may increase insulin release, facilitating amino acid transport into the muscle to help promote protein synthesis. Carbohydrate also spares the use of protein as an energy source. Alternative foods may be substituted from the food exchange list presented in appendix D. This suggested diet provides the necessary nutrients, Calories, and protein essential for increased development of muscle mass, and yet fewer than 30 percent of the Calories are derived from fat. The total number of Calories can be adjusted to meet individual needs. You may plan your weight-gain diet on the ChooseMyPlate Website.

Meal plans may be adjusted to the energy needs of individual athletes. For example, Lambert and others note that competitive bodybuilders should consume a diet that contains about 55–60 percent carbohydrate, 25–30 percent protein, and 15–20 percent fat for both the off-season and pre-contest phases. However, during the off-season, the diet should be slightly hyperenergetic (approximately 15 percent increase in energy intake) and during the pre-contest phase the diet should be hypoenergetic (approximately 15 percent decrease in energy intake). As noted previously, for 6–12 weeks prior to competition, bodybuilders attempt to retain muscle mass and reduce body fat to low levels, so they need to be in negative energy balance to facilitate oxidation of body fat. Lambert and others recommend that the diet contain 30 percent protein at this time to help prevent loss of muscle mass and possibly also provide a thermic effect to help burn fat.

For more detailed meal plans, the interested reader is referred to *Nutrient Timing* by Ivy and Portman.

Would such a high-Calorie diet be ill advised for some individuals?

As noted in chapter 5, one of the general recommendations for an improved diet is to reduce the consumption of fats, particularly saturated fats. Unfortunately, many high-Calorie diets are also high in fats. If there is a history of heart disease in the family

Exchange		Calories
TABLE 12.2 A high-Calorie diet based on the Food Exchange System		
Breakfast		
Milk	8 ounces 2% milk	120
Meat	1 poached egg	80
	2 ounces lean ham	110
Starch	2 slices whole wheat toast	160
Fruit	8 ounces orange juice	120
Other	1 tablespoon jelly	50
Midmorning snack		
Fruit	8 ounces apricot nectar	160
Starch	2 slices whole wheat bread	160
Meat	1 tablespoon peanut butter	100
Lunch		
Milk	8 ounces 2% milk	120
Meat	4 ounces lean sandwich meat	220
Starch	2 slices whole wheat bread	160
	2 granola cookies	100
Fruit	1 banana	120
Vegetable, starchy	1 order french fries	300
Afternoon snack		
Fruit	1/4 cup raisins	120
Dinner		
Milk	8 ounces 2% milk	120
Meat	5 ounces salmon	275
Starch	2 slices whole wheat bread	160
Fruit	1 piece apple pie	350
Vegetable, starchy	1 cup peas	160
	1 sweet potato, candied	300
Evening snack		
Fruit	1/2 cup dried peaches	210
Milk	8 ounces 2% milk with banana	240
Total		4,015

or if an individual is known to have high blood lipid levels, then high-fat diets may be contraindicated. Individuals with kidney problems also may have difficulty processing high-protein diets because of the increased need to excrete urea. Any person initiating such a weight-gaining program as advised here should consult with his or her physician.

Selection of food for a weight-gaining diet, if done wisely, can satisfy the criteria for healthful nutrition. Foods high in complex carbohydrates with moderate amounts of protein and a moderate fat content are able to provide substantial amounts of Calories and nutrients yet minimize health risks that have been associated with the typical American and Canadian diet. To gain weight wisely, you need to continue to eat healthful foods, but just more of them.

Key Concepts

▶ The individual attempting to gain body weight should obtain necessary high-quality protein for muscle synthesis through a well-balanced diet, rather than by consuming expensive protein supplements.

▶ Although creatine supplementation may help increase muscle mass during resistance training, most dietary supplements marketed to strength-trained individuals are not effective or have not been evaluated by scientific research.

▶ The Food Exchange System can serve as the basis for increasing caloric intake to gain body weight if the aspirant eats greater quantities of nutritious foods from each of the six lists, in three balanced meals plus several high-Calorie, high-nutrient snacks.

Check for Yourself

▶ Using the information presented in the text, calculate the additional number of Calories you would need in your daily diet to accumulate a weight gain of 0.5 pound per week. What foods could you add to your daily diet to provide these Calories?

Exercise Considerations

In chapter 11, we discussed the design of an aerobic exercise program for the loss of excess body fat but also mentioned that a resistance-training program could be helpful, for it might help prevent the loss of lean body mass and maintain normal resting-energy expenditure. In this chapter the focus is upon resistance training, sometimes called weight training or strength training, as a means to increase lean body mass and body weight. Before we discuss the principles underlying the design of a proper resistance-training program, let us introduce some basic terminology.

Repetition simply means the number of times you do a specific exercise. *Intensity* is determined by the weight, or resistance, that is lifted. A term used to describe the interrelationship between repetitions and intensity in weight training is **repetition maximum (RM)**. If you perform an exercise such as a bench press and lift 150 pounds once, but you cannot do a second repetition, you have done one repetition maximum, or 1RM. Individual workouts are generally based on a percentage of the RM, such as 80 percent of 1RM. For example, if your 1RM for the bench press is 150 pounds, 80 percent would be 120 pounds (0.8 × 150). If you bench press 120 pounds for five repetitions but cannot do a sixth, you have done five repetition maximum, or 5RM. A *set* is any particular number of repetitions, such as five or ten. The total volume of work you do in a single workout is the product of sets, repetitions, and resistance. For example, if you bench press three sets of five repetitions with a resistance of 100 pounds, your total volume of work is 1,500 pounds (3 × 5 × 100). The *recovery period* may represent the rest intervals between sets in a single workout or the rest interval between workouts during the week.

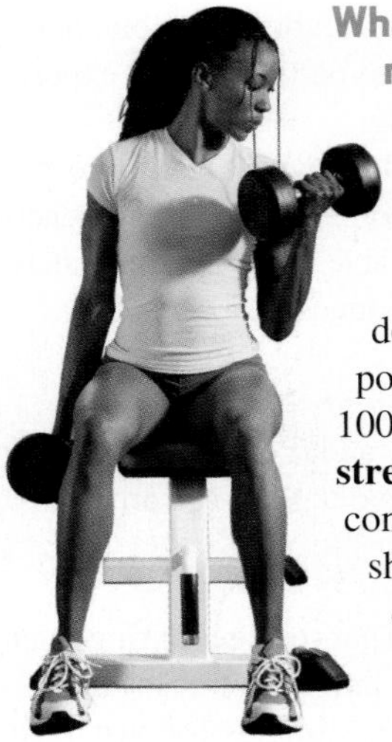

What are the primary purposes of resistance training?

As is probably obvious to you, there is an inverse relationship between the amount of weight you can lift and the number of repetitions you can do. If your 1RM in the bench press is 150 pounds, you can do more repetitions with 100 pounds than you can with 140. The **strength-endurance continuum** is a training concept that focuses upon the interrelationship between resistance and repetitions. As depicted in figure 12.3, to train for muscular strength you must combine high resistance with a low number of repetitions. Conversely, to train for muscular endurance, you must combine a low resistance with a high number of repetitions.

Resistance-training programs may be designed to train all three of the human energy systems. The ATP-PCr energy system predominates in strength and power activities, the lactic acid energy system is primarily involved in anaerobic endurance, and the oxygen system is involved in aerobic endurance activities. Thus, resistance-training programs may be developed for various purposes. One purpose may be to improve health, as discussed below. Another purpose may be to enhance sports performance, including improved strength and power for such sports as weightlifting and aesthetic appearance for sports such as bodybuilding.

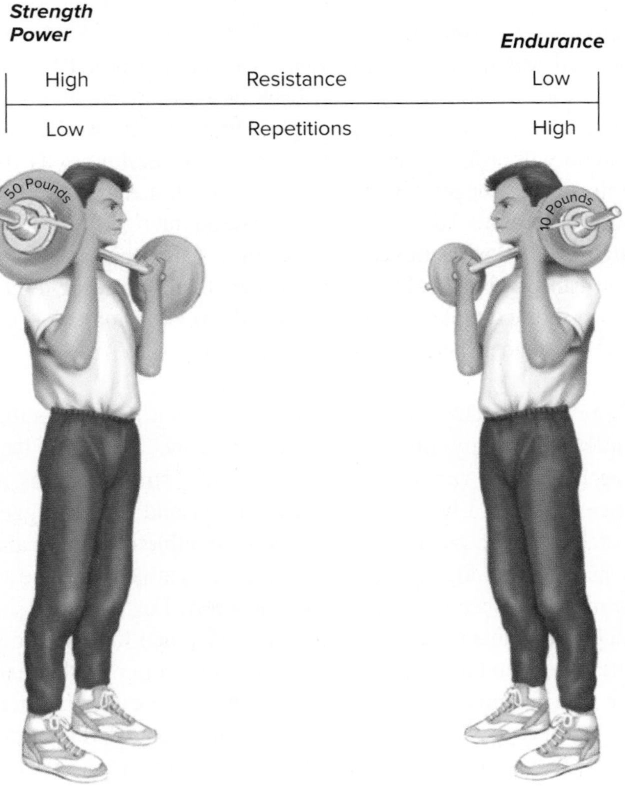

The American College of Sports Medicine (ACSM) and the American Heart Association (AHA), both separately and collectively, have provided recommendations for participation in resistance-training programs. The recommendations from the ACSM/AHA committee, chaired by Haskell, focus on resistance training as a component of an overall exercise program to improve muscular strength and endurance in healthy young adults, whereas those from the ACSM/AHA committee, chaired by Nelson, focus on programs for the elderly. The AHA scientific statement, developed by Williams and others, provides recommendations on resistance training for individuals with and without cardiovascular disease. The ACSM also developed a set of recommendations dealing with progression, or the gradual increase in overload placed on the body during training, and is more appropriate for the individual training to maximize muscular size and strength for bodybuilding or sports competition. Overall, these four sets of recommendations highlight the following purposes of resistance training, along with the recommended type of program.

Training for Muscular Hypertrophy Higher-volume, multiple-set programs are recommended for maximizing muscle hypertrophy. Emphasize a range of 6–12 RM per set.

Training for Strength and Power Multiple sets with fewer repetitions are recommended to maximize strength and power. Emphasize a range of 4–6 RM per set. Also, incorporate multiple sets of light loads (30–60 percent of 1 RM) at a fast contraction velocity.

Training for Local Muscular Endurance Multiple sets with more repetitions and light to moderate loads, such as 15 or more repetitions at 40–60 percent of 1 RM, are recommended. Use a short recovery period between sets.

Training for Health-Related Benefits Single sets are sufficient, approximating 8–12 RM. Include a variety of exercises that stress the major muscle groups of the body.

What are the basic principles of resistance training?

Given the different purposes for which individuals do resistance training, the design of the individual training program will vary accordingly. Athletes training to maximize muscle mass, strength, and power for their sport will engage in a more rigorous training program compared to someone doing resistance training for health benefits. Although the design of the resistance-training program may vary, the underlying principles are the same. The following discussion will highlight recommendations to gain muscle mass.

As noted in chapter 1, the following principles are not restricted to resistance training but apply to all forms of exercise training.

FIGURE 12.3 The strength-endurance continuum. To gain strength, you need to train on the strength end of the continuum; to gain endurance, you need to train on the endurance end of the continuum.

For example, intensity of exercise is simply another way of phrasing the overload principle.

Overload The *principle of overload* is the most important principle in all resistance-training programs. The use of weights places a greater than normal stress on the muscle cell. This overload stress stimulates the muscle to grow—to become stronger—in effect to overcome the increased resistance imposed by the weights (see figure 12.4).

To overload the muscle, you must increase the volume of work it must do. There are basically two ways to do this. One is to increase the amount of resistance or weight that you use; the other way is to increase the number of repetitions and sets you do.

A single set of eight to ten resistance exercises can increase muscle mass and strength gains in beginners. In their meta-analysis, Wolfe and others reported that single-set programs for an initial short training period in untrained individuals result in strength gains similar to those from multiple-set programs. A later meta-analysis by Fröhlich and colleagues confirmed the similar

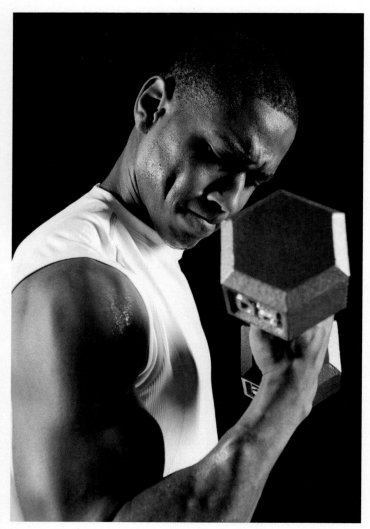

FIGURE 12.4 Lifting heavy weights illustrates the principle of overload in action with weight training. If improvement in strength is to continue, weights must be increased.

short-term efficacy of single and multiple sets but also concluded that multiple-set regimens elicit greater hypertrophy for experienced weightlifters over long-term training.

Using 60 to 80 percent of your 1 RM should provide a resistance that is approximately in the 8 to 10 RM range. For example, if your bench press 1 RM is 150 pounds, you should be able to do approximately 8 RM with 80 percent of that value, or 120 pounds (0.80 × 150).

> www.shapesense.com/fitness-exercise/calculators/1rm-calculator.aspx Use a resistance you can lift more than one but not more than ten times to estimate your 1 RM for any resistance exercise.

Progression As the muscle continues to get stronger during your training program, you must increase the amount of resistance—the overload—to continue to get the proper stimulus for sustained muscle growth. This is known as the *principle of progressive resistance exercise (PRE),* another basic principle of resistance training.

The ACSM provides guidelines on progression as the individual advances in weight lifting skill and strength, from novice to intermediate and advanced. As noted by Fröhlich and colleagues, multiple sets are more effective as progression occurs in order to elicit greater gains. Following a learning period, a recommended program for beginners is three to five sets using loads corresponding to 8–12 RM. The first step is to determine the maximum amount of weight that you can lift for 8 repetitions. If you can do more than 8 repetitions, the weight is too light and you need to add more poundage. As you get stronger during the succeeding weeks, you will be able to lift the original weight more easily. When you can perform 12 repetitions, add more weight to force you back down to 8 repetitions. This is the progressive resistance principle. Over several months' time, the weight will probably have to be increased several times as you continue to get stronger. Such a transition is illustrated in figure 12.5. The ACSM recommends that as you become an intermediate or advanced lifter, you should emphasize loads of 1–6 RM and progress when you can do about 1–2 more repetitions than the upper limit of the range. For example, if you are using the 6 RM protocol, you might add resistance when you can do 8 repetitions.

Specificity The *principle of specificity* is a broad training principle with many implications for resistance training, including specificity for various sports movements, strength gains, endurance gains, and body-weight gains. Frost and others suggest that to facilitate the greatest improvements to athletic performance, the resistance-training program employed by an athlete must be adapted to meet the specific demands of the sport. For example, a swimmer who wants to gain strength and endurance for a stroke should attempt to find a resistance weight-training program that exercises the specific muscles in a way as close as possible to the form used in that stroke. If you want to gain muscle mass in a certain part of the body, those muscles must be exercised. Strength coaches can help athletes develop resistance-training programs for specific sports.

Exercise Sequence Your exercise routine should be based upon the *principle of exercise sequence.* This means that if you have ten exercises in your routine, they should be arranged in

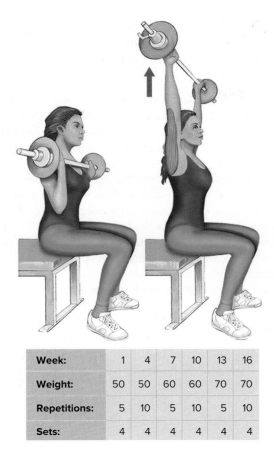

Week:	1	4	7	10	13	16
Weight:	50	50	60	60	70	70
Repetitions:	5	10	5	10	5	10
Sets:	4	4	4	4	4	4

FIGURE 12.5 The principle of progressive resistance exercise (PRE) states that as you get stronger, you need to progressively increase the resistance to continue to gain strength and muscle. In this example, the individual increases the resistance when she can complete ten repetitions with a given weight but then does only five repetitions with the increased weight.

logical order so that fatigue does not limit your lifting ability. For example, the first exercise in a sequence of ten might stress the biceps muscle, the second the abdominals, the third the quadriceps, and so forth. After you perform one full set of each of the ten exercises, you then do a complete second set, followed by the third set. This approach may be best for beginners and is the sequence for the eight exercises presented in this chapter.

Another popular option is to do three sets of the same exercise with a rest between sets; then do three sets of the second exercise, and so on. This approach may be a little more fatiguing because you are using the same muscle group in three successive sets, but it appears to be very effective. The time spent in recovery will also lengthen the total time for the workout. The ACSM also provides some guidelines on exercise sequence, recommending the following:

- Do multiple-joint exercises before single-joint exercises.
- Do large-muscle-group exercises before small-muscle-group exercises.
- Do higher-intensity exercises before lower-intensity exercises.

Recuperation Resistance training, if done properly to achieve the greatest gains, imposes a rather severe stress on the muscles,

requiring a period of recovery both during the workout and between workouts. Research has shown that high-intensity resistance exercise can lead to rapid depletion of ATP and PCr, the high-energy phosphates stored in the muscles; however, most of these high-energy compounds may be restored in about 2 to 3 minutes of recovery. This is the *principle of recuperation.* Thus, several minutes should intervene between sets if you are using the same exercise. Taking adequate rest between sets may help maintain the quality of the workout. In their review of 35 studies, de Salles and others concluded that rest intervals of 3 to 5 minutes resulted in a greater number of repetitions of resistances between 50 and 90 percent of 1 RM and produced greater training volumes, power production, and improvement in strength. Shorter (30- to 60-second) rest intervals may be more conducive to the development of both muscle hypertrophy and muscle endurance. If the goal is muscular endurance, the ACSM recommends that rest periods be shortened to less than 90 seconds.

Additionally, for beginners, resistance training should generally be done about 3 days per week, with a rest or recuperation day in between. This day of rest allows sufficient time for your muscle to repair itself and to synthesize new protein as it continues to grow, for research has shown that muscle protein synthesis occurs for up to 24 hours after a single bout of heavy resistance exercise. The ACSM indicates that advanced lifters could train 4–5 days per week. For health benefits, the ACSM and AHA recommended resistance exercise at least twice a week on nonconsecutive days.

Periodization **Periodization** is a training concept that divides training into time cycles of various durations determined by the individual. The volume and intensity of training vary within these cycles. A *microcycle* is a short period of time, typically 1 week, whereas a *macrocycle* may be a year or more. A *mesocycle* is an intermediate period, typically several months or more, and may include phases for tapering in preparation for competition. According to Selye's general adaptation theory, the body will adapt to exercise stress in ways beneficial to performance enhancement. However, as noted in chapter 3, excessive exercise may predispose athletes to overreaching and overtraining, which may contribute to impaired performance. Periodization is more applicable to competitive athletes than to beginning resistance exercisers. The classical linear periodization model includes successive mesocycles of increasing intensity and decreasing volume with variations in resistance, repetitions, and sets to emphasize endurance, hypertrophy, strength, and power. The undulating, or nonlinear, model includes greater variation in volume and intensity within a mesocycle. A more detailed discussion of periodization is beyond the scope of this text. The interested reader is referred to reviews by Harries and colleagues and Kraemer and Ratamess; texts by Bompa and Carrera and Stone and his colleagues; and the ACSM position statement on resistance-training progression models.

With the exception of periodization, these general principles should serve as guidelines during the beginning phase of your resistance-training program and should be used to guide your progress during the first 3 months of the basic resistance-training program described next. If you become serious about resistance training, additional reading is advised. Personal trainers may also be helpful.

What is an example of a resistance-training program that may help me to gain body weight as lean muscle mass?

If your goal is to gain significant amounts of muscle mass, you may wish to exercise on the strength end of the strength-endurance continuum, using six to ten different exercises that stress the major muscle groups of the body. About three to five sets of each exercise are done. In their review, Wernbom and others noted that increased muscle thickness has been reported following as little as one set of 8–12 repetitions. Although this may appeal to those with limited time, an optimal range of repetitions for hypertrophy is 30–60 repetitions per session. The repetition base can be 6–10, 8–12, or 10–12 repetitions per set. We will use the 8–12 model below and in the illustrations. The PRE concept is used, starting with resistance you can handle for eight repetitions and progressively increasing the repetitions to twelve. After you reach 12 repetitions, increase the resistance until you must come back to 8 repetitions.

Numerous resistance-training exercises are available to stress the major muscle groups in the body. The following exercises provide a sound basic resistance-training program for the adolescent and adult beginner.

1. Learn the proper technique for each exercise with a light weight, possibly only the bar itself, for 2 weeks. Do 8 to 12 repetitions of each exercise to develop form. Do not strain during this initial learning phase. Concentrate on lowering the weight slowly.
2. For each exercise, determine the maximum weight that you can lift for 8 repetitions after the 2-week learning phase.
3. A weekly record form, similar to the one presented in table 12.3, should be used to keep track of your progress.
4. Do one set of the 8 exercises shown in figures 12.6 to 12.13. The sequence of exercises should be
   a. Bench press: chest muscles
   b. Lat machine pulldown or bent-arm pullover: back muscles

TABLE 12.3 Weekly record for resistance-training program of eight exercises

Body Area		Chest	Back	Thigh	Shoulder	Calf	Front Arm	Back Arm	Abdomen
Resistance Exercise		Bench Press	Lat Pulldown	Half Squat	Lataral Raise	Heel Raise	Curls	Seated Press	Curlups
Date	Set	Wt/Reps	Wt/Reps	Wt/Reps	Wt/Reps	Wt/Reps	Wt/Reps	Wt/Reps	Wt/Reps
	1								
	2								
	3								
	4								
	5								
	1								
	2								
	3								
	4								
	5								
	1								
	2								
	3								
	4								
	5								
	1								
	2								
	3								
	4								
	5								

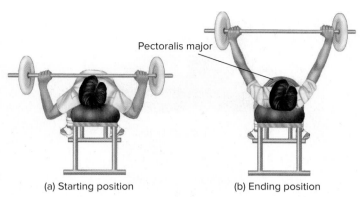

Pectoralis major

(a) Starting position   (b) Ending position

Chest	
Exercise	Bench press
Chest muscles	Pectoralls major
Other muscles	Deltoid, triceps
Sets	3–5
Repetitions	8–12, PRE concept
Safety	Have spotter stand behind bar to assist as fatigue sets in.
Equipment	Bench with support for weight, or two spotters to hand weight to you.
Description	Lie supine on bench. Use wide grip for chest development. Secure bar and lower *slowly* to chest. Press bar straight up to full extension. Do not arch back.

FIGURE 12.6 The bench press. The bench press primarily develops the pectoralis major muscle group in the chest; it also develops the deltoids in the shoulder and the triceps at the back of the arm.

Note: For safety reasons, a spotter should be present to assist in case of difficulty. The spotter is not depicted for purposes of illustration clarity.

    c. Half squat: thigh muscles
    d. Standing lateral raise: shoulder muscles
    e. Heel raise: calf muscles
    f. Standing curl: front upper arm muscles
    g. Seated overhead press: back upper arm muscles
    h. Curl-up: abdominal muscles

5. Because the exercise sequence is designed to stress different muscle groups in order, not much recuperation is necessary between exercises—possibly only 30 seconds or so.

6. Do three to five complete sets. You may wish to rest 2 to 3 minutes between sets.

7. Exercise 3 days per week; in each succeeding day try to do as many repetitions as possible for each exercise in each set. When you can do 12 repetitions each after a month or so, add more weight so you can do only 8 repetitions.

8. Repeat step 7 as you progressively increase your strength.

Because barbells and dumbbells appear to be the most common means of doing resistance training, this is the method utilized. However, other apparatus, such as the Nautilus, Hammer, and others, can also be used effectively to gain weight and strength. Most of the exercises described here using barbells or dumbbells have similar counterparts on other apparatus.

Note that muscles seldom operate alone, and that most resistance-training exercises stress more than one muscle group. Thus, keep in mind that although an exercise may be listed specifically for the chest muscles, it may also stress the arm and shoulder muscles. The exercises described in this section generally stress more than one body area, although their main effect is on the area noted.

It is important to note that your muscle contracts during both the up and down phase of weight lifting. As noted later, some training methods are based on this concept. When you lower a weight, your active muscle is actually contracting to help decrease the force of gravity. Lowering a weight slowly increases the time your muscle must contract. Raising the weight takes more force as you are working against gravity.

These eight exercises stress most of the major muscle groups in the body and thus provide an adequate stimulus for gaining body weight and strength through an increase in muscle mass. Literally hundreds of different resistance-training exercises and techniques to train are available; if you become interested in diversifying your program, consult a book specific to resistance training. Several may be found in the reference list at the end of this chapter. For example, nearly 30 different types of programs are presented in the classic text by Fleck and Kraemer, *Designing Resistance Training Programs*. Some professional organizations, such as the National Strength and Conditioning Association, also provide excellent resistance-training exercises.

Individuality in responses to resistance-training programs is an important consideration. According to Hayes and others, strength protocols elicit greater increases in the male anabolic hormone testosterone and greater gains in hypertrophy and strength in some individuals, whereas others respond preferentially to power or strength/endurance protocols. Other factors that may affect hypertrophy and strength gains between individuals include, but are not limited to, daily variations in testosterone and cortisol levels, which stimulate muscle synthesis and breakdown, respectively; the testosterone/cortisol ratio; and the time of day for resistance training. Testosterone will be discussed in chapter 13.

http://www.nsca.com/Videos For detailed illustrations of a wide variety of resistance-training exercises in video format, click on Exercise Techniques under Videos on the right of the page. The muscles involved in each exercise and safety tips are also provided.

www.nia.nih.gov/exercise Strength-training exercises for the elderly are presented using various types of equipment. Click on Chapter 4: Sample Exercises—Strength.

Are there any safety concerns associated with resistance training?

As noted later, several health problems may contradict participation in a strenuous resistance-training program. However, resistance training is generally regarded as a relatively safe sport, particularly if appropriate safety precautions are taken. The following guidelines should be incorporated into all resistance-training programs.

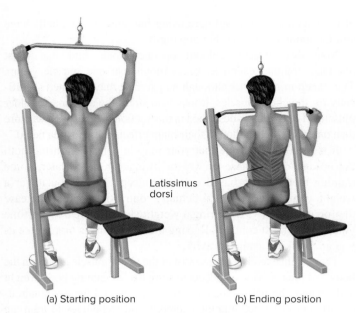

(a) Starting position   (b) Ending position

Latissimus dorsi

Back	
Exercise	Lat machine pulldown
Back muscles	Latissimus dorsi
Other muscles	Biceps, pectoralis major
Sets	3–5
Repetitions	8–12, PRE concept
Safety	A very safe exercise
Equipment	Lat machine
Description	From seated or kneeling position, take a wide grip at arm's length on the bar overhead. Pull bar down until it reaches your chest. Return slowly to starting position.

FIGURE 12.7A The lat machine pull down. The lat machine pull-down trains the latissimus dorsi in the back and side of the upper body, and it develops the biceps on the front of the upper arm and the pectoralis major in the chest.

Note: If a lat machine is not available, the bent-arm pullover may be substituted.

1. *Learn to breathe properly.* During the most strenuous part of the exercise, you are likely to hold your breath. This is a natural response to increase intrathoracic pressure, which stabilizes the spine and provides a stable base for muscle contraction. Usually, the breath hold is short and no problems occur. However, if prolonged, it may increase the chance of suffering a hernia if there is a weak area of the abdominal musculature.

Also associated with prolonged breath holding is a response known as the **Valsalva phenomenon** (Valsalva maneuver), which may lead to a blackout. As you reach a sticking point in your lift and strain to overcome it, you normally hold your breath. This causes your glottis to close over your windpipe and the pressure in your chest and abdominal area to rise rapidly. The pressure creates resistance to blood

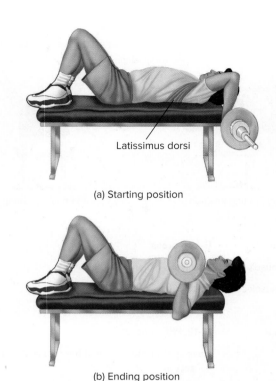

Latissimus dorsi

(a) Starting position

(b) Ending position

Back	
Alternate exercise	Bent-arm pullover
Back muscles	Latissimus dorsi
Other muscles	Pectoralis major
Sets	3–5
Repetitions	8–12, PRE concept
Safety	Do not arch back. Start with light weights when learning the technique.
Equipment	Bench
Description	Lie supine on bench, entire back in contact with the bench, feet on the bench, knees bent. Hold weight on chest with elbows bent. Swing weight over head, just brushing hair, and lower as far as possible without taking back off the bench. Keeping elbows in, return the weight to the chest.

FIGURE 12.7B The bent-arm pullover. The bent-arm pullover trains the latissimus dorsi and develops the pectoralis major.

Note: For safety reasons, a spotter should be present to assist in case of difficulty. The spotter is not depicted for purposes of illustration clarity.

flow, reducing the return of blood to the heart, and eventually leading to decreased blood flow to the brain and a possible blackout. Additionally, the Valsalva maneuver exaggerates the increase in blood pressure during resistance exercises, and although a brief Valsalva maneuver is unavoidable when doing near-maximal exercises, its effect may be minimized by proper breathing.

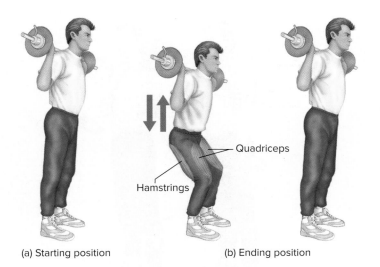

(a) Starting position (b) Ending position

Quadriceps

Hamstrings

Thigh	
Exercise	Half squat or parallel squat
Thigh muscles	Quadriceps (front), hamstrings (back)
Other muscles	Gluteus maximus
Sets	3–5
Repetitions	8–12, PRE concept
Safety	Have two spotters to assist if using free weights. Keep back straight. Drop weight behind you if you lose balance. Do not squat more than halfway down.
Equipment	Squat rack if available. Pad the bar with towels if necessary.
Description	In standing position, take bar from squat rack or spotters and rest on the shoulders behind the head. Squat until thighs are parallel to ground or until buttocks touch a chair at this parallel position. Do not squat beyond halfway. Keep back as straight as possible. Return to standing position, but do not lock your knees. This will maximize stress on your thighs.

FIGURE 12.8 The half squat or parallel squat. The half squat develops the quadriceps muscle group on the front of the thigh and the hamstrings on the back of the thigh.

Note: For safety reasons, spotters should be present to assist in case of difficulty. The spotters are not depicted for purposes of illustration clarity.

A recommended breathing pattern for beginning weightlifters that will help minimize these adverse effects is to breathe out while lifting the weight, especially through the sticking point, and breathe in while lowering it. You should breathe through both your mouth and nose while exercising. Practice proper breathing when you learn new resistance-training exercises.

2. *Use spotters.* When using free weights, use spotters when doing exercises that are potentially dangerous, such as the

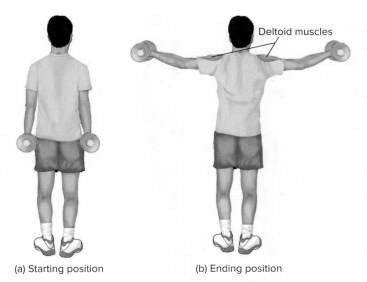

Deltoid muscles

(a) Starting position (b) Ending position

Shoulders	
Exercise	Standing lateral raise
Shoulder muscles	Deltoid
Other muscles	Trapezius
Sets	3–5
Repetitions	8–12, PRE concept
Safety	Do not arch back.
Equipment	Dumbbells
Description	Stand with dumbbells in hands at sides. With palms down, raise straight arms sideways to shoulder level. Bend elbows slightly. Return slowly to starting position.

FIGURE 12.9 Standing lateral raise. The standing lateral raise primarily develops the deltoid muscles in the shoulder. The trapezius in the upper back and neck area is also trained.

bench press. If you are doing a bench press alone and reach a sticking point in your lift, the Valsalva phenomenon may lead to serious consequences if you lose control of the weight directly above your head. The use of machines such as Nautilus helps eliminate the need for spotters.

3. *Use safety equipment.* If using free weights, place lock collars on the bar ends so that the plates do not fall off and cause injury to the feet. Again, the use of machines eliminates this safety hazard. However, do not attempt to change weight plates on machines while they are being used. Your fingers may get caught between the weights.

4. *Warm up.* Warm up with proper stretching exercises. Gently stretch the muscles to be used during exercise. Slow, static methods are recommended for cold muscles. Kokkonen and others reported that 10 weeks of static stretching for 40 minutes/day 3 days/week significantly improved knee extension

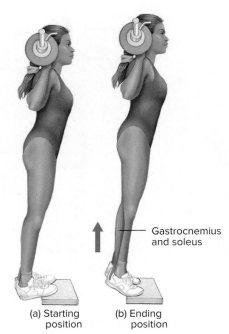

(a) Starting position   (b) Ending position

Calf

Exercise	Heel raise
Calf muscles	Gastrocnemius, soleus
Other muscles	Deep calf muscles
Sets	3–5
Repetitions	8–12, PRE concept
Safety	Have two spotters if you use free weights.
Equipment	Squat rack if available. Pad the bar with a towel if necessary.
Description	Place bar on back of shoulders as in squat exercise. Raise up on your toes as high as possible and then return to standing position. Place the toes on a board so heels can drop down lower than normal. Point toes in, out, and straight ahead during different sets to work the muscles from different angles.

FIGURE 12.10 Heel raise. The heel raise develops the two major calf muscles—the gastrocnemius and the soleus.

Note: For safety reasons spotters should be present to assist in case of difficulty. The spotters are not depicted for purposes of illustration clarity.

and flexion 1 RM. In a later study, Kokkonen and others reported that novice weight trainers assigned to static stretching and weight training significantly improved leg press and knee extension strength compared to only weight training. Stretching may facilitate a return to resistance training following injury as well as enhance early gains in strength.

5. *Use proper technique.* Use light weights to learn the proper technique of a given exercise so that you do not strain yourself if you do the exercise incorrectly. Learn to lift smoothly without jerking motions and using the full range of motion.

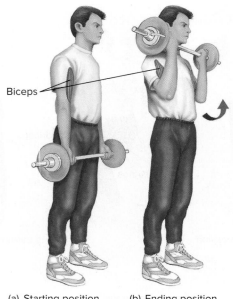

Biceps

(a) Starting position   (b) Ending position

Front of arm

Exercise	Standing curl
Arm muscle	Biceps
Other muscles	Several elbow flexors
Sets	3–5
Repetitions	8–12, PRE concept
Safety	Do not arch back. Place back against wall to control arching motion.
Equipment	Curl bar if available
Description	Stand with weight held in front of body, palms forward. Place back against wall. Bend the elbows and bring the weight to the chest. Lower it slowly.

FIGURE 12.11 The standing curl. The standing curl strengthens the biceps muscle in the front of the upper arm as well as several other muscles in the region that bend the elbow.

When the proper technique is mastered, the weights may be increased. Using proper technique ensures that the desired muscle group is being exercised.

6. *Protect your lower back.* Avoid exercises that may cause or aggravate low back problems. Try to prevent an excessive forward motion or stress in the lower back region. Figure 12.14 illustrates some positions that should be avoided.

7. *Lower weights slowly.* If you lower them rapidly, your muscles have to contract rapidly to slow the weights down as you reach the starting position. This necessitates the development of a large amount of force that may tear some muscle fibers or connective tissue and cause muscle soreness.

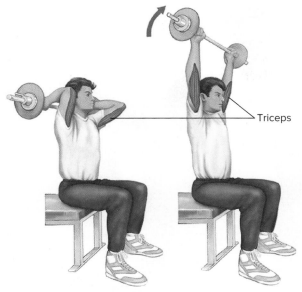

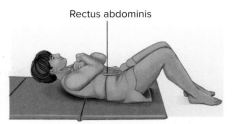

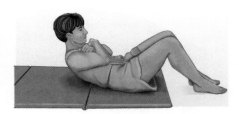

Triceps

(a) Starting position   (b) Ending position

Rectus abdominis

(a) Starting position

(b) Ending position

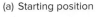

Back of arm	
Exercise	Seated overhead press (triceps extension)
Arm muscle	Triceps
Other muscles	Trapezius, deltoids
Sets	3–5
Repetitions	8–12, PRE concept
Safety	Do not arch back excessively. Have spotter available as fatigue sets in.
Equipment	Bench or chair
Description	Sit on bench with weight held behind the head near the neck. Hands should be close together, elbows bent. Keep elbows in. Straighten elbows and press weight over head to arm's length. Lower weight slowly to starting position.

FIGURE 12.12 The seated overhead press. The seated overhead press primarily develops the triceps muscle on the back of the upper arm; the exercise also trains the trapezius in the upper back and neck and the deltoids in the shoulder.

Note: For safety reasons spotters should be present to assist in case of difficulty. The spotters are not depicted for purposes of illustration clarity.

Abdominal area	
Exercise	Curl-up
Abdominal muscles	Rectus abdominis
Other muscles	Oblique abdominis muscles
Sets	3–5
Repetitions	8–12, PRE concept
Safety	Develop sufficient abdominal strength before using weights with this exercise. Do not arch back when exercising.
Equipment	Free-weight plates; incline sit-up bench if available
Description	Lie on back, knees bent with heels close to buttocks. Hands should hold weights on chest. Curl up about a third to halfway. Return to starting position slowly.

FIGURE 12.13 The curl-up. The curl-up trains the rectus abdominis and the oblique abdominis muscles.

Note: This exercise may be done without weights but with an increased number of repetitions.

How does the body gain weight with a resistance-training program?

Muscle hypertrophy simply means increased muscle size. Figure 12.15 depicts the microstructure of muscle tissue. Stimulation of DNA in skeletal muscle nuclei by resistance training increases RNA and results in protein synthesis. According to Zanou and Gailly, the activation of myogenic stem cells, also known as satellite cells, increases regulatory proteins controlling the formation of the contractile myofilament myosin

(see figure 12.15) as well as growth factors that play a key role in the repair of muscle damage. Chaillou and others describe the formation of new ribosomes, which translate mRNA into protein, as the result of signaling pathways, which also support muscle hypertrophy. Various hormones whose secretion is increased during exercise play important roles in stimulating muscle growth. In particular, Vingren and others state that testosterone is considered the major promoter of muscle growth and subsequent increase in muscle strength in response to resistance training in men. Human growth hormone and insulin-like growth factor are also involved. These hormones are discussed in more detail in chapter 13.

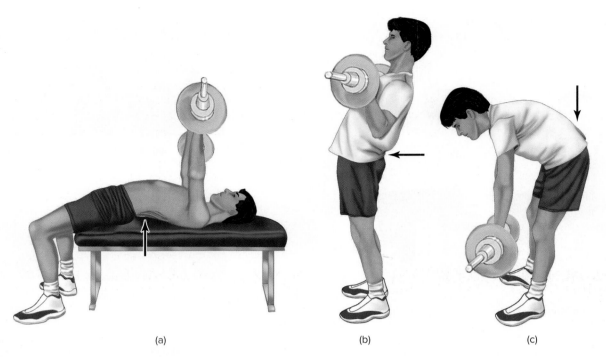

FIGURE 12.14 Avoid exercises or body positions that place excessive stress on the low-back region. Poor form in exercises like *(a)* the bench press and *(b)* the curl exaggerates the lumbar curve. Be sure to keep the lower back as flat as possible. Exercises similar to *(c)*, the bent-over row, place tremendous forces on the lower back because the weight or resistance is so far in front of the body.

Over time, the muscle cell tends to adapt to such stress by increasing its size. It may do so in several possible ways. First, the individual muscle cells and myofibrils may simply increase their size by incorporating more protein. Second, the myofibrils in each cell may multiply, which will increase the size of each muscle fiber. Third, the amount of connective tissue around each muscle fiber and around each bundle of muscle may increase and thicken, leading to an overall increase in the size of the total muscle. Fourth, the cell may increase its content of enzymes and energy storage, particularly ATP and glycogen. The increased muscle glycogen, along with increased muscle protein, binds additional water, which contributes to an increased body weight. Finally, the muscle fibers themselves may increase in number (hyperplasia), but current evidence suggests that this is much less likely to occur compared with the other four means to induce muscle hypertrophy. In their review, Folland and Williams noted that the primary factor contributing to increased overall muscle size is the increase in the size and number of the myofibrils. In addition to the effects on muscle, some but not all studies indicate that resistance-training may stimulate bone formation, possibly due to increased muscle tension on the bone. If so, this may account for a small increase in body weight. Whipple and others reported increases in urinary markers of bone formation 8 hours after a resistance exercise session.

Resistance training may be an effective means to increase muscle size and mass. Such increases help improve muscular strength and endurance and may be important components in weight-control programs. Traditionally, in research studies, females did not normally experience the same amount of hypertrophy that males did, although they did experience proportional gains in

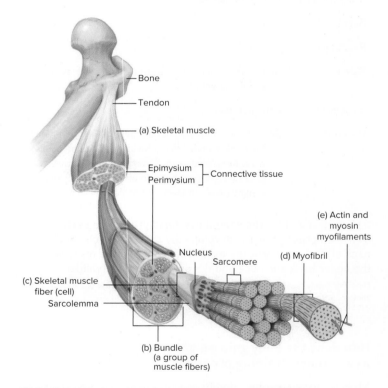

FIGURE 12.15 Muscle structure. The whole muscle is composed of separate bundles of individual muscle fibers. Each fiber is composed of numerous myofibrils, each of which contains thin protein filaments arranged so that they can slide by each other to cause muscle shortening or lengthening. Several layers of connective tissue surround the muscle fibers, bundles, and whole muscles, which eventually band together to form the tendon.

muscular strength and endurance. However, Staron and others revealed a significant increase in muscle cell size when women engaged in an intense, concentrated resistance-training program. Burd and others concluded that young males and females have similar relative changes in muscle hypertrophy following resistance training, but older subjects may have a diminished capacity for muscle hypertrophy. Vingren and others report decreased secretion of testosterone in older men and women during exercise. Burd and others reported that older women have a lower capacity for muscle protein synthesis and decreased hypertrophy in response to resistance training. However, in their meta-analysis, Peterson and others concluded that resistance training, particularly with higher-volume programs, is effective for gaining lean body mass in aging adults.

Is any one type of resistance-training program or equipment more effective than others for gaining body weight?

There are a variety of methods for resistance training. **Isometric methods** involve a muscle contraction against an immovable object, such as trying to pull a telephone pole out of the ground. However, if you succeed in moving the object, then you are doing an isotonic exercise. **Isotonic methods** are of two types. The **concentric method** means the muscle is shortening, as the biceps does in the up phase of a pull-up. The **eccentric method** means the muscle is lengthening even though it is trying to shorten. In the down phase of the pull-up, the biceps is now contracting eccentrically as it slows your rate of descent. Gravity is attempting to pull you down, but your bicep is resisting it. Finally, the **isokinetic method** uses machines or other devices to regulate the speed at which you can shorten your muscles. For example, you may try to move your arm as fast as possible, but you will be able to move only as fast as the setting on the isokinetic machine. Isokinetic exercise is also known as accommodating-resistance exercise because the resistance automatically adjusts to the force exerted, thus controlling the speed of movement.

Several different resistance-training products are available, such as Atlantis, Nautilus, Hammer, Cybex, Hydra-Gym, Soloflex, and other similar machines. Depending upon the model, they are designed to utilize one or more of the training methods cited previously.

A number of research studies have been conducted to determine which of these methods or machines is best, particularly in relation to strength and power gains. Research suggests that at present it is probably safe to say that the various training methods are comparable in their ability to produce gains in muscle size and strength. For example, in a comprehensive review comparing the effects of dynamic exercise (including free weights and weight machines), accommodating resistance (isokinetic and semi-isokinetic devices), and isometric resistance, Wernbom and others concluded that there is insufficient evidence for the superiority of any mode and/or type of muscle action over other modes and types of training.

In a study comparing the effects of concentric and eccentric muscle training in women, Nickols-Richardson and others reported no significant differences between the methods for improvements in muscular strength, fat-free body mass, or bone mineral content and density. However, Roig and others, in a meta-analysis of 20 studies, concluded that when eccentric exercise was performed at higher intensities compared with concentric training, total strength and eccentric strength increased more significantly. They suggested that the superiority of eccentric training to increase muscle strength and mass appears to be related to the higher loads developed during eccentric contractions. However, such training programs should be used with caution at least until the muscle adapts to a program of progression in intensity because high-intensity eccentric exercise may be more likely to cause muscle tissue damage and muscle soreness. Such programs would appear to be of interest primarily to highly trained athletes.

All methods may be effective in increasing body weight, provided the basic principles of resistance training, particularly the principle of overload, are followed. The ACSM recommends that your exercise program include both concentric and eccentric exercise, which are incorporated into most machines and free weights. If you use machines, be sure to exercise all major muscle groups. Free weights are relatively inexpensive and can be used for a wide variety of exercises. They also may be constructed at home, using pipe or solid broomstick handles for the bar and different-sized tin cans filled with cement for the weights.

There may be some specific training programs that are better suited for specific purposes, such as specific sports performance enhancement or injury rehabilitation. These topics are beyond the scope of this text, so the interested reader is referred to more detailed resources, such as the texts cited in the reference list at the end of this chapter.

If exercise burns Calories, won't I lose weight on a resistance-training program?

Although exercise does cost Calories, the amount expended during resistance training is relatively small compared to more active aerobic exercise. Resistance training can be a high-intensity exercise, but the time spent actually lifting during a typical workout is usually short, therefore limiting the number of Calories used. For example, in an hour workout, only about 15 minutes may be involved in actual exercise, the remaining time being recovery between each exercise. Based upon metabolic data collected in research studies, the average-sized male uses about 200 Calories in a typical workout, while the average-sized female uses about 150 (see figure 12.16). Resistance training appears to have a small effect on postexercise energy expenditure. In one study, Ormsbee and others reported that energy expenditure, mostly from fat, was increased following a 40- to 45-minute intense resistance-training workout. The increased caloric expenditure was only about 10 Calories over a 45-minute recovery period, not a very significant amount. However, Melanson and others indicated that circuit resistance training, as discussed later, may lead to a total daily energy expenditure comparable to aerobic cycling exercise.

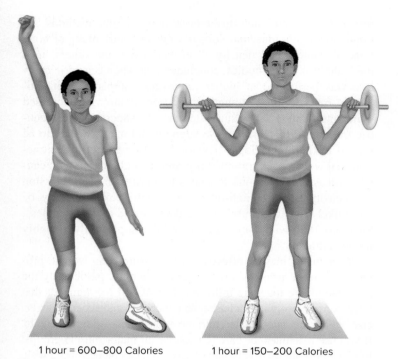

1 hour = 600–800 Calories   1 hour = 150–200 Calories

FIGURE 12.16 All models of exercise increase caloric expenditure. However, an hour of regular weight training expends only about one-third to one-fourth as many Calories as vigorous aerobic activity. Combining aerobic exercises with weight training (circuit aerobics) helps burn more Calories than weight training alone; it also provides cardiovascular health benefits while increasing muscular strength and endurance.

Are there any contraindications to resistance training?

Several health conditions may be aggravated by resistance training, primarily by the increased pressures that occur within the body when you strain to lift heavy weights and hold your breath at the same time. Because the blood pressure can increase rapidly and excessively during weight lifting, to 300 mmHg or higher, individuals with resting blood pressures of 140 mm Hg or higher (systolic) or 90 mm Hg or higher (diastolic) should refrain from heavy lifting, for they may be exposed to an increased risk of blood vessel rupture and a possible stroke. Lifting with the arms and straining exercises also increase the stress on the heart and thus should be avoided by individuals who have heart problems, such as arrhythmias. As previously noted, individuals with a hernia (a weakness in the musculature of the abdominal wall) also should refrain from strenuous weight lifting because the increased pressure may cause a rupture. Improper lifting technique may contribute to muscle strain, cause pain in the shoulder and other joints, and aggravate existing low back problems. Some individuals may suffer peripheral nerve injuries, such as carpal tunnel syndrome, involving weakness and numbness in the hand due to compressed nerves from improper lifting techniques. Individuals with these types of health problems should seek medical advice and be cleared by a physician before initiating or continuing with a resistance-training program.

There has been some concern about the advisability of prepubescent youth lifting weights. However, two recently updated policy and position statements, by the American Academy of Pediatrics (AAP) and by Faigenbaum and others for the National Strength and Conditioning Association (NSCA), provided an analysis of resistance-training programs for youngsters. The AAP and NSCA indicate the following benefits from participation in programs that are properly designed and supervised specifically for youth:

- They are safe.
- They can enhance muscular strength and power.
- They can help increase resistance to sports-related injuries.
- They may provide some health benefits, such as psychosocial well-being.
- They may promote the development of exercise habits.

The key to these benefits is a properly designed and supervised program. Gradual progression is important, as it is with adults. The AAP also recommends that both preadolescents and adolescents avoid power lifting, bodybuilding, and maximal lifts until they reach physical and skeletal maturity. Caution should be used with young athletes who have preexisting hypertension or other cardiovascular problems, as strength training may aggravate such conditions.

Are there any health benefits associated with resistance training?

Although resistance training has been recommended mainly as a means of gaining muscle mass, body weight, and strength, in the past its use normally was not associated with any health benefits. However, increasing research efforts focusing on the health implications of resistance training have suggested several favorable effects. Some of the health benefits are associated with increases in lean body mass and strength. Additionally, de Salles and others, in a review of 17 studies, concluded that resistance training could increase the secretion of beneficial cytokines, such as adiponectin, and decrease the secretion of harmful cytokines, such as tumor necrosis factor-alpha. Both an increase in muscle mass and beneficial cytokines could increase insulin sensitivity and protect against diabetes. Direct effects of resistance exercise on other body systems, such as the neuromuscular and skeletal systems, may produce health benefits. Various reviews, including those by the American College of Sports Medicine and American Diabetes Association, Deschenes and Kraemer, Phillips, Strasser and others, and Williams, have reported multiple health benefits associated with resistance training—benefits that, along with those cited in other reports, include the following:

1. Increased lean body mass to help prevent the development of **sarcopenia** (loss of muscle mass) as one ages, a major health benefit
2. Decreased risk of the metabolic syndrome and its co-morbities, such as high blood pressure

3. Increased strength and improved gait, to prevent falls and injury as one ages
4. Decreased pain in chronic low-back-pain patients to improve mobility
5. Increased bone mineral density to help prevent osteoporosis, particularly in females
6. Improved glucose metabolism and insulin sensitivity to help prevent diabetes or improve glucose control in diabetics
7. Improved serum lipid profiles, such as increased HDL-cholesterol and decreased LDL-cholesterol, to help prevent atherosclerosis and coronary heart disease
8. Improved ability to complete activities of daily living and enhance the quality of life in older individuals
9. Improved mood, body image, self-concept, and psychological health in children, adolescents, and adults
10. Improved rate of recovery from some types of surgery, such as hip replacement surgery

These findings are contrary to the belief that resistance training does not confer any health benefits comparable to aerobic exercise. It is also notable that many cardiac rehabilitation programs now incorporate resistance-training exercises.

Nevertheless, it still appears to be prudent health behavior to incorporate some aerobic exercise into your lifestyle, even when trying to gain body weight. Although the ACSM and AHA have incorporated resistance training into their recommended exercise program for healthy adults, it is designed to complement aerobic exercise, not to substitute for it. The American Academy of Pediatrics also noted that if long-term health benefits for children and adolescents are the goal, then strength training should be combined with an aerobic-training program. Aerobic exercise programs do consume more Calories, so you would have to balance the expenditure with increased food intake if you want to gain weight. However, the energy expenditure need not be excessive to provide a beneficial training effect. For example, running 2 to 3 miles about 4 days per week would provide you with an adequate aerobic-exercise training effect for your heart, but it would cost you only about 200–300 Calories a day. This 200- to 300-Calorie expenditure could be replaced easily by consuming two glasses of orange juice or similar small amounts of food.

Doing both resistance and aerobics exercise may provide additional health benefits. For example, Pitsavos and others, in a large study involving more than 3,000 subjects, suggested that combining aerobic and resistance-type activities may confer a better effect on lipoprotein profile in healthy individuals than aerobic activities alone.

Can I combine aerobic and resistance-training exercises into one program?

Although the principles underlying the development of an aerobic-training program and a resistance-training program are similar, the purposes of the two programs are rather different. An aerobic exercise program is designed to improve the efficiency of the cardiovascular system. The basic purpose of a resistance-training program is to increase muscle size, strength, and body weight.

One form of resistance training that has been used to provide some moderate benefits to the cardiovascular system is **circuit weight training**, a method in which the individual moves rapidly from one exercise to the next. Generally, this type of program uses lighter weights with greater numbers of repetitions, thus increasing the aerobic component of training. Research reported energy expenditure of approximately 10 Calories per minute for males and 7 Calories per minute for females. Circuit weight training can improve strength, but Harber and others indicated that strength gains are attributed more to neural adaptations because the relatively low resistance loads do not induce appreciable muscle hypertrophy.

A newer version of this method is **circuit aerobics**. Circuit aerobics may be done in a variety of ways, but basically it involves an integration of aerobic and resistance-training exercises. It is actually a form of interval aerobic training, but instead of resting or doing a lower level of aerobic activity during the recovery interval, you do resistance-training exercises. Circuit aerobics may offer multiple health and performance benefits, such as improved cardiovascular fitness, increased caloric expenditure for loss of body fat, improved muscular strength and endurance, and increased muscle tone in body areas not normally stressed by aerobic exercise alone. In their review, Romero-Arenas and colleagues concluded that circuit resistance training may improve cardiovascular fitness, muscle strength, body composition, bone mineral density, and risk factors for age-related diseases in elderly subjects. Curves, the largest fitness franchise in the world, have developed a 30-minute exercise program specifically for women using this concept.

However, if the main purpose of your resistance-training program is to gain body weight as muscle mass, then you need to train near the strength end of the strength-endurance continuum. For athletes who need to maximize gains in lean body mass, strength, and especially power, some sports scientists suggest that aerobic training should be markedly reduced if not eliminated. For example, Malisoux and others, reviewing studies involving single muscle fibers to help understand the effects of different forms of exercise training, reported that muscle fiber peak power is increased after resistance training but over time is decreased with endurance–training. Elliott and others indicate that cardiovascular endurance–training programs are detrimental for the performance of power athletes, suggesting contributing factors such as inappropriate neuromuscular adaptations, a catabolic hormonal profile, or ineffective motor learning environment. They note that there are unequivocal drawbacks to distance training in the power athlete.

http://growingstronger.nutrition.tufts.edu This Tufts University Website presents an evidence-based exercise program designed to increase muscle strength, maintain bone health, and improve balance, coordination, and mobility in older adults.

- A basic principle underlying all resistance-training programs is the overload principle, which simply means the muscle should be stressed beyond normal daily levels.
- Progressive resistance is also a basic principle of resistance training, for as you get stronger through use of the overload principle, you must progressively increase the resistance.
- To increase muscle mass and body weight, you should exercise near the strength end of the strength-endurance continuum.
- Your resistance-training program should exercise all major muscles groups in the body.
- A variety of methods and apparatuses are available for resistance training, but research suggests that they are equally effective as a means of gaining strength and muscle mass if the basic principles of resistance training are followed.

- Resistance training is generally regarded as a safe form of exercise, but it may be contraindicated in some individuals, for example, those with high blood pressure and hernias.
- Although resistance-training programs may confer some significant health benefits, it is also highly recommended that one add an aerobic exercise program to help condition the cardiovascular system.

Check for Yourself

- Do this after 2–3 weeks of resistance training. Using free weights or an appropriate weight-training machine, such as Nautilus, determine your one repetition maximum (1RM) for a given exercise, such as the bench press. Start out with a light weight that you know you can easily lift one time, and then gradually add on amounts until you reach your limit. You should need only three or four attempts. Record the weight of the last successful attempt.

APPLICATION EXERCISE

If you have time and are interested, start a resistance-training program, using the principles in the text. Record your 1 RM for an exercise (such as the bench press) initially and every 2 weeks for several months. Use a tape measure to determine body girth changes in the upper arm, chest, waist, and upper thigh. If you have access to skinfold calipers or other measures of body composition, keep similar records. Use a model comparable to those presented (adjusting the numbers in the vertical column to represent weight lifted for 1 RM, millimeters for skinfold measurement, and centimeters or inches for girth measurement), graph the results, and compare to the text discussion.

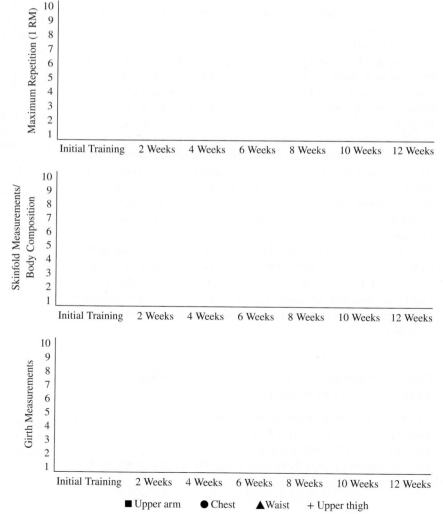

■ Upper arm   ● Chest   ▲ Waist   + Upper thigh

1. Which of the following would be least recommended for someone who wants to gain weight healthfully?
   a. stop smoking
   b. set a goal of about 0.5 pound per week
   c. get enough rest and sleep
   d. start a resistance-training program
   e. drink more caffeinated beverages

2. Which of the following is not one of the basic principles of resistance training?
   a. overload
   b. specificity
   c. progressive resistance
   d. aerobic
   e. sequence

3. The bench press exercise is designed to have the greatest effect on which group of muscles?
   a. calf
   b. thigh
   c. back
   d. chest
   e. abdominal

4. The standing lateral raise is designed to have the greatest effect on which group of muscles?
   a. shoulder
   b. thigh
   c. calf
   d. chest
   e. abdominal

5. Resistance training will stimulate muscle hypertrophy by a variety of mechanisms. Which of the following is considered to be least likely, according to the text discussion?
   a. Individual muscle cells and myofibrils increase in size.

   b. Myofibrils in each cell may multiply.
   c. Connective tissue in muscle may increase and thicken.
   d. Muscle cells will increase water content by binding to increased glycogen.
   e. Muscle fibers themselves increase rapidly in number.

6. For the purpose of gaining weight, which type of resistance-training equipment is best according to research findings, provided equal amounts of resistance work are done on each?
   a. isokinetic concentric machines
   b. isometric devices
   c. isotonic eccentric free weights
   d. isotonic concentric free weights
   e. No equipment is better than any other.

7. Which dietary supplement has the most research supporting its potential to help increase muscle mass and weight gain during a resistance-training program?
   a. HMB
   b. chromium
   c. creatine
   d. ginseng
   e. carnitine

8. Research suggests that proper resistance training may confer some significant health benefits. Which of the following is least likely?
   a. increased strength to prevent falls and injury as one ages
   b. increased bone mineral density to help prevent osteoporosis
   c. increased testosterone levels to help reduce serum HDL-cholesterol

   d. improved muscle mass and insulin sensitivity to help prevent type 2 diabetes
   e. improved body image and psychological health

9. Which of the following would be the least likely dietary recommendation for someone trying to gain weight in lean mass?
   a. Wait at least 4 hours after exercise before eating some protein and carbohydrate.
   b. Increase the intake of high-Calorie, high-nutrient foods.
   c. Keep the intake of saturated fats to a minimum.
   d. Eat three balanced meals a day supplemented with snacks.
   e. Supplement the diet with high-Calorie, high-nutrient liquids.

10. To gain 1 pound of muscle weight per week on a weight-training program, an individual might need an additional 14 grams of protein per day above the RDA, in addition to increased Calories. Which of the following would not supply that amount of protein daily?
    a. 2 glasses of skim milk
    b. 1 glass of orange juice and 2 eggs
    c. 1 slice of toast, 1 egg, and 1 ounce of ham
    d. 1 glass of orange juice, 2 slices of toast, and 1 banana
    e. 2 ounces of cheese

Answers to multiple choice questions:
1. e; 2. d; 3. d; 4. a; 5. e; 6. e; 7. c; 8. c; 9. a; 10. d

1. Explain the strength-endurance continuum as a training concept.
2. List the five basic principles of resistance training and provide an example of each.

3. Discuss the physiological means whereby resistance training leads to increases in muscle growth.
4. Describe at least five of the potential health benefits associated with resistance training.

5. Discuss the importance of protein in a weight-gaining diet and provide some recommendations for amounts of protein and types of protein-rich foods in the diet.

Books

Bompa, T., and Carrera, M. 2005. *Periodization Training for Sports.* Champaign, IL: Human Kinetics.

Fleck, S., and Kraemer, W. 2004. *Designing Resistance Training Programs.* Champaign, IL: Human Kinetics.

Ivy, J., and Portman, R. 2004. *Nutrient Timing: The Future of Sports Nutrition.* North Bergen, NJ: Basic Health Publications.

National Academy of Sciences. 2002. *Dietary Reference Intakes for Energy, Carbohydrate, Fiber, Fat, Protein and Amino Acids.* Washington, DC: National Academies Press.

Reuben, D. 1996. *Dr. David Reuben's Quick Weight-Gain Program.* New York: Crown.

Stone, M., et al. 2007. *Principles and Practices of Resistance Training.* Champaign, IL: Human Kinetics.

U.S. Department of Health and Human Services. 2010. *Healthy People 2020.* Washington, DC: U.S. Government Printing Office.

Reviews and Specific Studies

American Academy of Pediatrics Council on Sports Medicine and Fitness. 2008. Strength training by children and adolescents. *Pediatrics* 121:835–40.

American College of Sports Medicine, American Diabetes Association. 2010. American College of Sports Medicine and the American Diabetes Association joint position statement: Exercise and type 2 diabetes. *Medicine & Science in Sports & Exercise* 42:2282–303.

American College of Sports Medicine. 2009. American College of Sports Medicine position stand: Progression models in resistance training for healthy adults. *Medicine & Science in Sports & Exercise* 41:687–708.

Aragon, A. A., and Schoenfeld, B. J. 2013. Nutrient timing revisited: Is there a post-exercise anabolic window? *Journal of the International Society of Sports Nutrition* 10 (1):5. doi: 10.1186/1550-2783-10-5.

Bartels, R., et al. 1989. Effect of chronically increased consumption of energy and carbohydrate on anabolic adaptations to strenuous weight training. In *Report of the Ross Symposium on the Theory and Practice of Athletic Nutrition: Bridging the Gap,* ed. J. Storlie and A. Grandjean. Columbus, OH: Ross Laboratories.

Bauer, J., et al. 2013. Evidence-based recommendations for optimal dietary protein intake in older people: A position paper from the PROT-AGE study group. *Journal of the American Medical Directors Association* 14 (8):542–59.

Beelen, M., et al. 2010. Nutritional strategies to promote postexercise recovery. *International Journal of Sport Nutrition and Exercise Metabolism* 20:515–32.

Bloomer, R. 2007. The role of nutritional supplements in the prevention and treatment of resistance exercise-induced skeletal muscle injury. *Sports Medicine* 37:519–32.

Burd, N. A., et al. 2009. Exercise training and protein metabolism: Influences of contraction, protein intake, and sex-based differences. *Journal of Applied Physiology* 106(5):1692–701.

Candow, D. 2011. Sarcopenia: Current theories and the potential beneficial effect of creatine application strategies. *Biogerontology* 12:273–81.

Chaillou, T., et al. 2014. Ribosome biogenesis: Emerging evidence for a central role in the regulation of skeletal muscle mass. *Journal of Cellular Physiology* 229 (11):1584–94.

Clifton, P. M., et al. 2014. Long term weight maintenance after advice to consume low carbohydrate, higher protein diets—A systematic review and meta analysis. *Nutrition, Metabolism and Cardiovascular Diseases* 24 (3):224–35.

Cribb, P., and Hayes, A. 2006. Effect of supplement timing and resistance training on skeletal muscle hypertrophy. *Medicine & Science in Sports & Exercise* 38:1918–25.

de Salles, B. F., et al. 2009. Rest interval between sets in strength training. *Sports Medicine* 39 (9):765–77.

de Salles, B., et al. 2010. Effects of resistance training on cytokines. *International Journal of Sports Medicine* 31:441–50.

Deschenes, M., and Kraemer, W. 2002. Performance and physiologic adaptations to resistance training. *American Journal of Physical and Medical Rehabilitation* 81:S3–S16.

Devries, M. C,. and Phillips, S. M. 2014. Creatine supplementation during resistance training in older adults—A meta-analysis. *Medicine and Science in Sports and Exercise* 46 (6):1194–1203.

Drummond, M. J., et al. 2009. Nutritional and contractile regulation of human skeletal muscle protein synthesis and mTORC1 signaling. *Journal of Applied Physiology* 106 (4):1374–84.

Elliott, M., et al. 2007. Power athletes and distance training: Physiological and biomechanical rationale for change. *Sports Medicine* 37:47–57.

Esmarck, B., et al. 2001. Timing of postexercise protein intake is important for muscle hypertrophy with resistance training in elderly humans. *Journal of Physiology* 535:301–11.

Faigenbaum, A., et al. 2009. Youth resistance training: Updated position statement paper from the National Strength and Conditioning Association. *Journal of Strength and Conditioning Research* 23 (Supplement):S60–79.

Folland, J., and Williams, A. 2007. The adaptations to strength training: Morphological and neurological contributions to increased strength. *Sports Medicine* 37:145–68.

Frost, D., et al. 2010. A biomechanical evaluation of resistance: Fundamental concepts for training and sports performance. *Sports Medicine* 40:303–26.

Fröhlich, M., et al. 2010. Outcome effects of single-set versus multiple-set training—An advanced replication study. *Research in Sports Medicine* 18(3):157–75.

Gatorade Sports Science Institute. 1994. Methods of weight gain in athletes. *Sports Science Exchange Roundtable* 5 (1):1–4.

Goldman, M. 2011. Much ado about Muscle Milk. *University of California Berkeley Wellness Letter* 27 (4):2.

Grunewald, K., and Bailey, R. 1993. Commercially marketed supplements for bodybuilding athletes. *Sports Medicine* 15:90–103.

Harber, M., et al. 2004. Skeletal muscle and hormonal adaptations to circuit weight training in untrained men. *Scandinavian Journal of Medicine and Science in Sports* 14:176–85.

Harries, S. K., et al. 2015. Systematic review and meta-analysis of linear and undulating periodized resistance training programs on muscular strength. *Journal of Strength and Conditioning Research.* 29(4):1113–1125.

Haskell, W., et al. 2007. Physical activity and public health: Updated recommendation for adults from the American College of Sports Medicine and the American Heart Association. *Medicine & Science in Sports & Exercise* 39:1423–34.

Hayes, L., et al. 2010. Interactions of cortisol, testosterone, and resistance training: Influence of circadian rhythms. *Chronobiology International* 27:675–705.

Hoffman, J., et al. 2009. Effect of protein-supplement timing on strength, power, and body-composition changes in resistance-trained men. *International Journal of Sport Nutrition and Exercise Metabolism* 19:172–85.

Hulmi, J., et al. 2009. Acute and long-term effects of resistance exercise with or without protein ingestion on muscle hypertrophy and gene expression. *Amino Acids* 37:297–308.

Josse, A., et al. 2010. Body composition and strength changes in women with milk and resistance exercise. *Medicine & Science in Sports & Exercise* 42:1122–30.

Kokkonen, J., et al. 2007. Chronic static stretching improves exercise performance. *Medicine & Science in Sports & Exercise* 39:1825–31.

Kokkonen, J., et al. 2010. Early-phase resistance training strength gains in novice lifters are enhanced by doing static stretching. *Journal of Strength and Conditioning Research* 24 (2):502–6.

Kraemer, W., and Ratamess, N. 2005. Progression and resistance training. *President's Council on Physical Fitness and Sports Research Digest* 6 (3):1–8.

Kreider, R. 1999. Dietary supplements and the promotion of muscle growth with resistance exercise. *Sports Medicine* 27:97–110.

Lambert, C., et al. 2004. Macronutrient considerations for the sport of bodybuilding. *Sports Medicine* 34:317–27.

Lemon, P. 1996. Is increased dietary protein necessary or beneficial for individuals with a physically active lifestyle? *Nutrition Reviews* 54:S169–75.

Malisoux, L., et al. 2007. What do single-fiber studies tell us about exercise training? *Medicine & Science in Sports & Exercise* 39:1051–60.

McCreary, D. R., et al. 2007. A review of body image influences on men's fitness goals and supplement use. *American Journal of Men's Health* 1 (4):307–16.

Melanson, E., et al. 2002. Resistance and aerobic exercise have similar effects on 24-h nutrient oxidation. *Medicine & Science in Sports & Exercise* 34:1783–800.

Murray, S. B., et al. 2010. Muscle dysmorphia and the DSM-V conundrum: Where does it belong? A review paper. *International Journal of Eating Disorders* 43 (6):483–91.

Nelson, M., et al. 2007. Physical activity and public health in older adults: Recommendation from the American College of Sports Medicine and the American Heart Association. *Medicine & Science in Sports & Exercise* 39:1435–45.

Nickols-Richardson, S., et al. 2007. Concentric and eccentric isokinetic resistance training similarly increases muscular strength, fat-free soft tissue mass, and specific bone mineral measurements in young women. *Osteoporosis International* 18:789–96.

Ormsbee, M., et al. 2007. Fat metabolism and acute resistance exercise in trained men. *Journal of Applied Physiology* 102:1767–72.

Pasiakos, S. M., et al. 2015. The effects of protein supplements on muscle mass, strength, and aerobic and anaerobic power in healthy adults: A systematic review. *Sports Medicine* 45 (1):111–31.

Peterson, M., et al. 2011. Influence of resistance exercise on lean body mass in aging adults: A meta-analysis. *Medicine & Science in Sports & Exercise* 43:249–58.

Phillips, S. 2009. Physiologic and molecular bases of muscle hypertrophy and atrophy: Impact of resistance exercise on human skeletal muscle (protein and exercise dose effects). *Applied Physiology, Nutrition, and Metabolism* 34:403–10.

Phillips, S. M. 2012. Dietary protein requirements and adaptive advantages in athletes. *British Journal of Nutrition* 108:S158–67.

Phillips, S. M. 2014. A brief review of critical processes in exercise-induced muscular hypertrophy. *Sports Medicine* 44 (S1):S71–S77.

Pickett, T., et al. 2005. Men, muscles, and body image: Comparisons of competitive bodybuilders, weight trainers, and athletically active controls. *British Journal of Sports Medicine* 39:217–22.

Pitsavos, C., et al. 2009. Resistance exercise plus to aerobic activities is associated with better lipids' profile among healthy individuals: The ATTICA study. *Quarterly Journal of Medicine* 102:609–16.

Pritchett, K., and Pritchett, R. 2012. Chocolate milk: A post-exercise recovery beverage for endurance sports. *Medicine and Sports Science* 59:127–34.

Rawson, E., and Venezia, A. 2011. Use of creatine in the elderly and evidence for effects on cognitive function in young and old. *Amino Acids* 40:1349–62.

Raymond, M. J., et al. 2013. Systematic review of high-intensity progressive resistance strength training of the lower limb compared with other intensities of strength training in older adults. *Archives of Physical Medicine and Rehabilitation* 94:1458–72.

Roig, M., et al. 2009. The effects of eccentric versus concentric resistance training on muscle strength and mass in healthy adults: A systematic review with meta-analysis. *British Journal of Sports Medicine* 43:556–68.

Romero-Arenas, S., et al. 2013. Impact of resistance circuit training on neuromuscular, cardio-respiratory and body composition adaptations in the elderly. *Aging and Disease* 4 (5):256–63.

Skemp, K. M., et al. 2013. Muscle dysmorphia: Risk may be influenced by goals of the weightlifter. *Journal of Strength and Conditioning Research* 27 (9):2427–32.

Staron, R. S., et al. 1990. Muscle hypertrophy and fast fiber type conversions in heavy resistance-trained women. *European Journal of Applied Physiology and Occupational Physiology* 60 (1):71–79.

Strasser, B., et al. 2010. Resistance training in the treatment of the metabolic syndrome: A systematic review and meta-analysis of the effect of resistance training on metabolic clustering in patients with abnormal glucose metabolism. *Sports Medicine* 40:397–415.

Suffolk, M. T. 2013. Muscle dysmorphia: Methodological issues, implications for research. *Eating Disorders* 21(5):437–57.

Verdijk, L., et al. 2009. Protein supplementation before and after exercise does not further augment skeletal muscle hypertrophy after resistance training in elderly men. *American Journal of Clinical Nutrition* 89:608–16.

Vingren, J., et al. 2010. Testosterone physiology in resistance exercise and training: The up-stream regulatory elements. *Sports Medicine* 40:1037–53.

Wernbom, M., et al. 2007. The influence of frequency, intensity, volume and mode of strength training on whole muscle cross-sectional area in humans. *Sports Medicine* 37:225–64.

Whipple, T., et al. 2004. Acute effects of moderate intensity resistance exercise on bone cell activity. *International Journal of Sports Medicine* 25:496–501.

Williams, M. 1993. Nutritional supplements for strength trained athletes. *Sports Science Exchange* 6 (47):1–6.

Williams, M., et al. 2007. Resistance exercise in individuals with and without cardiovascular disease: 2007 update: A scientific statement from the American Heart Association Council on Clinical Cardiology and Council on Nutrition, Physical Activity, and Metabolism. *Circulation* 116:572–84.

Wolfe, B., et al. 2004. Quantitative analysis of single- versus multiple-set programs in resistance training. *Journal of Strength and Conditioning Research* 18:35–47.

Zanou, N., and Gailly, P. 2013. Skeletal muscle hypertrophy and regeneration: Interplay between the myogenic regulatory factors (MRFs) and insulin-like growth factors (IGFs) pathways. *Cellular and Molecular Life Sciences* 70 (21):4117–30.

Food Drugs and Related Supplements

CHAPTER THIRTEEN

LEARNING OBJECTIVES

After studying this chapter, you should be able to:

1. Explain the metabolic, physiological, and psychological effects of alcohol in the body, and evaluate its efficacy as an ergogenic acid.

2. Explain the possible beneficial and detrimental effects of alcohol consumption on health.

3. List and explain the several theories whereby caffeine supplementation is proposed to be an effective ergogenic aid, and summarize its effect on exercise performance.

4. Explain the possible beneficial and detrimental health-related effects of caffeine in the body, and cite current recommendations for coffee consumption.

5. Understand the potential health problems associated with dietary supplements containing stimulants such as ephedra.

6. Describe the theory underlying the use of sodium bicarbonate as an ergogenic aid, and understand the current research findings regarding its efficacy to enhance exercise performance.

7. Identify drugs and related dietary supplements used by physically active individuals to stimulate muscle building, and summarize the effects on exercise performance and potential health risks associated with their use.

8. Explain the theory as to how ginseng may enhance sports performance, and highlight the research findings regarding its ergogenic efficacy.

9. List those drugs or dietary supplements discussed in this chapter whose use is prohibited in sports.

10. Describe the four different recommendation levels for dietary supplements regarding their efficacy, safety, and permissibility as ergogenic aids for athletes, and cite examples of each.

Introduction

As noted in chapter 1, winning in sports is dependent not only on genetic endowment with physiological, psychological, and biomechanical attributes inherent to success in any given sport but also on optimal training of those attributes. However, over the years, athletes have attempted to go beyond training to gain a competitive edge on their opponents and have used a wide variety of ergogenic aids in the process.

The most historic and popular international sporting event is the Olympic Games. The first Olympics were held in Greece, starting in 776 BC and continuing for more than 1,000 years, being canceled in AD 393 because they were regarded as a pagan ritual. Similar to today, athletes who were successful in these ancient Olympics achieved fame and fortune.

Most elite Grecian athletes had personal trainers, called *paidotribes,* to plan their exercise program and their diet to prepare them for competition. In a sense, paidotribes were the first sports scientists and sports nutritionists. Several famous Greek scientists, including Galen and Pythagoras, were paidotribes who advocated specific, but different, diets for their athletes; Galen promoted beans as a staple of the athlete's diet, whereas Pythagoras prohibited them. During these early Olympic Games, various plants served as sources of ergogenic drugs. For example, certain mushrooms contained hallucinogens and *Strychnos nux vamica* was the source of strychnine; in small doses, both could serve as a stimulant. Athletes in the ancient Olympics were reported to consume such plants for their potential ergogenic effect.

The modern Olympic Games were resurrected in 1896 and continue today with competition among thousands of athletes in dozens of sports. As in the ancient Olympics, athletes in the modern Olympics have been reported to use drugs in attempts to obtain that competitive edge. As several of these drugs are found in some common foods or beverages that we may consume, they have been referred to as *food drugs.* Additionally, some plant extracts, or phytochemicals, may be marketed as dietary supplements designed to imitate ergogenic drugs. Others, particularly herbals, may be used for their pharmaceutical effects by practitioners of alternative medicine.

In this chapter, we will evaluate the effects of several food drugs and related dietary supplements on exercise performance and health. Two very common food drugs, alcohol and caffeine, have been studied for their ergogenic effects for more than 100 years and have been used by athletes as a means to enhance performance since the early 1900s. Each has also been studied extensively for possible health effects, both positive and negative.

The dietary supplement ma huang contains ephedra, or ephedrine, a stimulant theorized to enhance exercise performance, particularly when combined with caffeine. Ephedrine has also been studied for its potential health effects.

Sodium bicarbonate, or baking soda, is used in many food products and has been studied for 80 years as a means to enhance performance. It also has been marketed as part of a dietary supplement for athletes.

Several anabolic hormones, and related steroid drugs, are used to increase muscle mass and have been popular with strength/power athletes for more than 50 years. Because the use of such drugs has been controlled and illegal for sports competition for many years, companies have marketed prohormones, or precursors to these hormones, as dietary supplements to avoid drug regulations. However, now these prohormones have also been classified as controlled drugs and their use is illegal in sports. Use of these anabolic agents may also pose serious health risks.

Finally, several herbals and other phytochemicals, most notably ginseng, are used in alternative medicine for various purposes, one being enhancement of physical performance. Collectively, with the exception of alcohol and anabolic hormones, most of these performance-enhancing substances are marketed as dietary supplements, or sports supplements when targeted to athletes. The sports supplement industry has become a multibillion-dollar business. Some reports indicate that approximately 90 percent of elite athletes use sports supplements, while Greydanus and Patel note that the drive toward success in sport has driven many adolescents to use such products.

Some of the dietary supplements discussed in this chapter have been banned by the World Anti-Doping Agency (WADA) for use in sports competition, and others are being monitored by WADA. Specific details will be provided where warranted.

www.wada-ama.org The World Anti-Doping Agency (WADA) provides the complete list of drugs and doping techniques whose use is prohibited or monitored in sports competition. Click on *Prohibited List.* The list is updated annually.

Alcohol: Ergogenic Effects and Health Implications

The alcohol produced for human consumption is ethyl alcohol, or **ethanol**. Ethanol may be classified as a psychoactive drug, a toxin, or a nutrient.

The use of alcohol as a means to enhance exercise or sports performance has a long history. Ancient Greek athletes drank wine or brandy prior to competition, thinking that these alcoholic beverages enhanced performance. In more modern times, Olympic marathon runners in the Paris (1900) and London (1908) games drank brandy or cognac to enhance performance, while in the Paris Olympics in 1924 wine was served at fluid-replacement stations in the marathon. In 1939, Boje noted that in cases of extreme athletic exertion or in events of brief maximal effort, alcohol has been given to athletes to serve as a stimulant by releasing inhibitions and lessening the sense of fatigue. As of 2015, alcohol is banned by the WADA in archery, air, automobile, motorcycling, and power boating sports. A blood alcohol content of 0.10 g/l or higher is the doping threshold.

The use of alcohol as a social, psychoactive drug also has a long history, and its effects on human health have been studied extensively. Historically, most research has focused on the numerous adverse health effects of excessive alcohol consumption, but recent research has identified some potential health benefits of light to moderate alcohol consumption. According to Nova and colleagues, there is some evidence that moderate consumption is associated with improved insulin sensitivity and decreased CHD risk, but controversies remain based on insufficient research. Therefore, abstinence may be the best health-improvement strategy for some individuals.

What is the alcohol and nutrient content of typical alcoholic beverages?

Alcohol is a transparent, colorless liquid derived from the fermentation of sugars in fruits, vegetables, and grains. Although classified legally as a drug, alcohol is a component of many common beverages served throughout the world. In the United States, alcohol is consumed mainly as a natural ingredient of beer, wine, and liquors. As illustrated in figure 13.1, typical alcohol contents by volume are 4 to 5 percent for beer; 12 to 14 percent for wine; and 40 to 45 percent for distilled spirits such as whiskey, vodka, and rum. Based on these typical percentages, similar amounts of alcohol are found in a 4-oz glass of wine, a 12-oz bottle or can of beer, and a 1.25-oz shot of liquor. Other products containing alcohol are wine coolers and energy drinks, which contain 5 to 7 percent and 10 to 12 percent alcohol, respectively. Energy drinks will be discussed later in this chapter. The term **proof** is a measure of the alcohol content in a beverage and is double the percentage. It is very important to remember that the alcohol content can vary significantly among products within beer, wine, and liquor categories. As examples, certain craft and microbrews may contain 10 or more percent alcohol and some wines are fortified to 18 to 24 percent. An 86-proof bottle of whiskey contains 43 percent alcohol, but a 151-proof bottle of Caribbean rum contains over 75 percent alcohol.

Such beverages would provide significantly more alcohol per standard drink. Technically, alcohol may be classified as a nutrient because it provides energy, one of the major functions of food. Alcohol contains about 7 Calories per gram, almost twice the value of an equal amount of carbohydrate or protein. Beer and wine also contain some carbohydrate, a source of additional Calories. In general, a bottle of regular beer has about 150 Calories, while a 4-oz glass of wine or a shot glass of liquor contains about 100 Calories. Table 13.1 provides an approximate analysis of the caloric content of common alcoholic beverages and nonalcoholic beer.

In general, the alcohol Calories found in beer, wine, and liquor are empty Calories. Although wine and beer contain trace amounts of protein, vitamins, minerals, and phytochemicals, liquor is void of any nutrient value.

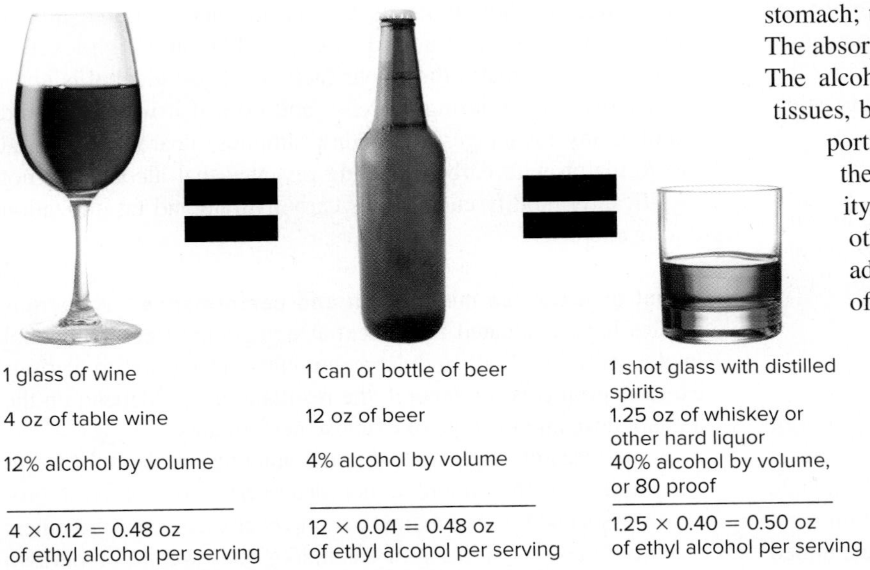

What is the metabolic fate of alcohol in the body?

About 20 percent of the alcohol ingested may be absorbed by the stomach; the remainder passes on to the intestine for absorption. The absorption is rapid, particularly if the digestive tract is empty. The alcohol enters the blood and is distributed to the various tissues, being diluted by the water content of the body. A small portion of the alcohol, about 3–10 percent, is excreted from the body through the breath, urine, or sweat, but the majority is metabolized by the liver, the organ that metabolizes other drugs. As the blood circulates, the liver of an average adult male will metabolize about 1/3 ounce (8–10 grams) of alcohol per hour, or somewhat less than the amount of alcohol in one drink.

Although alcohol is derived from the fermentation of carbohydrates, it is metabolized in the body as fat. The liver helps convert the metabolic by-products of alcohol into fatty acids, which may be stored in the liver or transported into the blood. Several other compounds, such as lactate, acetate, and acetaldehyde, may also be released into the blood. These products may eventually be utilized for energy and converted

1 glass of wine

4 oz of table wine

12% alcohol by volume

4 × 0.12 = 0.48 oz
of ethyl alcohol per serving

1 can or bottle of beer

12 oz of beer

4% alcohol by volume

12 × 0.04 = 0.48 oz
of ethyl alcohol per serving

1 shot glass with distilled spirits
1.25 oz of whiskey or other hard liquor
40% alcohol by volume, or 80 proof

1.25 × 0.40 = 0.50 oz
of ethyl alcohol per serving

FIGURE 13.1 Alcohol equivalencies in typical beverages.

TABLE 13.1   Caloric content of typical alcoholic beverages

| Beverage | Amount | Carbohydrate | | Alcohol | | Total |
		Grams	Calories	Grams	Calories	Calories
Beer, regular	12 ounces	13	52	13	91	150
Beer, light	12 ounces	7	28	11	77	109
Beer, nonalcoholic	12 ounces	12	48	1	7	55
Beer, alcohol-free	12 ounces	12	48	0	0	48
Wine, table	4 ounces	4	16	12	84	100
Liquor, 80-proof	1.25 ounces	0	0	14	98	100
Energy drink, alcoholic	12 ounces	32	128	15	105	233

The small discrepancies in the calculation of total Calories for beer and liquor may be attributed to a small protein content in beer and trace amounts of carbohydrate in liquor.

into carbon dioxide and water. A schematic of alcohol metabolism is presented in figure 13.2.

As noted, the liver of an average male can metabolize only about 1/3 ounce of alcohol, or less than one drink, per hour. The rate is lower in smaller individuals and higher in larger individuals. Thus, consumption of alcohol at a rate greater than one drink per hour will result in an accumulation of alcohol in the blood; this is measured as the **blood alcohol concentration (BAC)** in grams per 100 milliliters of blood. The ingested alcohol is diluted throughout the total body water, both inside and outside body cells, including the blood. For the average male, one drink will result in a BAC of about 0.025, or 0.025 gram (25 milligrams) per 100 milliliters of blood; four drinks in an hour would lead to a BAC of a little less than 0.10 because a small amount would be metabolized by the liver. However, BAC concentrations resulting from the same amount of drinks may vary widely among individuals, due to food intake, gender, differences in body weight and body fat, tolerance due to a history of alcohol consumption, genetics, and differences in activities of the enzymes in figure 13.2 that metabolize alcohol. The following Website may be used to calculate your BAC.

www.bloodalcoholcalculator.org Calculate your BAC based on your gender, body weight, number of drinks, and amount of time over which drinks were consumed.

Is alcohol an effective ergogenic aid?

For more than a century, athletes have consumed alcohol just prior to or during competition in attempts to improve performance. Potential ergogenic mechanisms attributed to alcohol include altered energy metabolism and improvements in physiological processes and psychological factors. These claims are examined in the following sections.

Use as an energy source Although alcohol contains a relatively large number of Calories and its metabolic pathways in the body are short, the available evidence suggests that it is not utilized to any significant extent during exercise. First, the major sources of energy for exercise are carbohydrates and fats, which are in ample supply in most individuals. Alcohol may help form fats, but there is no evidence that it can substitute for other fat sources in the body. Even if it could, this would be of no benefit because the body has more than enough fat to supply energy during prolonged exercise. Second, the by-products of alcohol metabolism that are released by the liver into the blood may enter the skeletal muscles but appear to be of little importance to exercising muscle. Third, even if the energy from alcohol could be used, it would represent an uneconomical source. The amount of oxygen needed to release the Calories from alcohol is greater than for an equivalent amount of carbohydrate and fat. And last, the rate at which the liver metabolizes alcohol limits its use as an energy source during exercise, particularly in an individual working at a high level of intensity. In summary, these four factors suggest alcohol is not a key energy source during exercise, and even if it were, it would not offer any advantages over natural supplies of carbohydrate and fat. Research with carbon labeling revealed that alcohol did not significantly modify endogenous carbohydrate and fat utilization during exercise.

Effect on exercise metabolism and performance Numerous studies have evaluated the potential ergogenic effect of alcohol intake, both in small and large amounts, just prior to various exercise protocols. In general, the resultant effects depend on the alcohol dose and the type of exercise performance.

Some research suggests that small amounts of alcohol (one to two drinks) neither improve nor deteriorate physiological processes associated with maximal aerobic exercise. Coiro and others recently reported that 0.5 g of alcohol/kg body weight (about two drinks) before a 15-minute exercise test to exhaustion had no effect

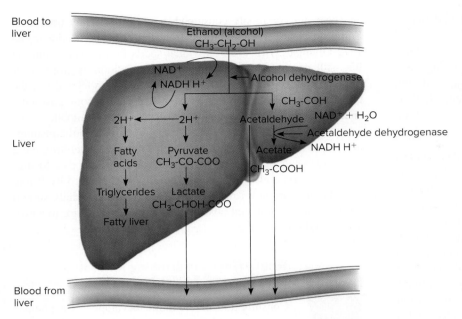

FIGURE 13.2 Simplified metabolic pathways of ethanol (alcohol) in the liver. Hydrogen ions are removed from ethanol as it is converted into acetaldehyde, which may be released into the blood for transport to other tissues. The excess hydrogen ions may combine with fatty acids to form triglycerides or with pyruvate to form lactate. Excessive accumulation of triglycerides may lead to the development of a fatty liver and eventually to cirrhosis.

on heart rate, blood pressure, ventilation, oxygen consumption, respiratory exchange ratio, cortisol, and growth hormone responses. However, hormonal response to exercise was decreased following a larger alcohol dose of 0.75 g/kg body weight. In an early study, Houmard and others reported no adverse effect of alcohol intake on 5-mile (8-km) treadmill run time, but they noted a trend for slower times with increased alcohol intake. In contrast, McNaughton and Preece reported greater detriments in 800- and 1,500-meter run performances with blood alcohol contents of 0.01 mg, 0.05 mg, and 0.10 mg/mL. Lecoultre and Schutz observed decreased power output, oxygen consumption, and glucose metabolism and increased heart rate and perceived exertion in trained male cyclists during a 60-min time-trial performance following alcohol (0.5 mL/kg fat-free mass) ingested with carbohydrate versus carbohydrate only.

Several studies have examined the effects of alcohol on high-intensity submaximal aerobic exercise performance. Kendrick and others reported nonsignificant increases in heart rate in four subjects at 30 minutes of a 60-min treadmill run at 80–85 percent VO_2 max following pre-exercise ingestion of 25 mL of alcohol compared to the placebo. However, the observed difference may have been significant with a larger sample. Furthermore, a second 25-mL dose of alcohol at 30 minutes resulted in a 24 percent decrease in blood glucose levels compared to placebo. Wang and others reported higher submaximal cycle exercise heart rate, blood pressure, oxygen consumption, and blood lactate response in women following alcohol ingestion (0.25 g/kg body weight) compared to a placebo treatment.

Anaerobic performance and sprint speed may be somewhat less affected by alcohol ingestion. McNaughton and Preece reported

declines in 200-m and 400-m sprint performance with increasing amounts of alcohol, but no effects on 100-m performance. Recent research suggests that alcohol may adversely affect neuromuscular function. Barnes reported that alcohol ingestion (1 g/kg) combined with exercise-induced muscle damage decreased maximal voluntary isometric force production of the quadriceps for up to 60 hours, possibly due to decreased neural activity. Haugvad and others observed that although alcohol did not delay post-resistance exercise muscle recovery, decreases in testosterone/cortisol ratios suggest the potential for adverse long-term effects on skeletal muscle repair. In their review, Bianco and others noted that alcohol may inhibit intracellular signaling pathways, which stimulate protein synthesis and hypertrophy.

Several metabolic effects of alcohol intake could impair endurance performance. Delgado and colleagues reported decreased left ventricular pumping action following low doses of alcohol. In their study, Burke and others observed that in some individuals, large amounts of postexercise alcohol may displace carbohydrate Calories that would otherwise facilitate glycogen synthesis. El Sayed and others noted studies suggesting that alcohol consumption decreases the use of glucose and amino acids by skeletal muscles, adversely affects energy supply, and impairs the metabolic process during exercise. Alcohol reduces gluconeogenesis by the liver and glucose uptake by the legs during the latter stages of exercise. In prolonged exercise, such as marathons, these effects could lead to an earlier onset of hypoglycemia or muscle glycogen depletion and a subsequent decrease in performance.

Alcohol intake during training could be counterproductive. Some studies have reported reduced absorption of thiamin (vitamin B_1) associated with moderate intakes of alcohol. Theoretically, this could impair physical performance of an endurance nature because vitamin B_1 is involved in the aerobic metabolism of carbohydrate.

The ACSM position stand on fluid replacement states that alcohol consumption increases urine output and delays full rehydration. Alcohol inhibits the release of antidiuretic hormone, which results in increased urine loss. Shirreffs and Maughan commented that higher alcohol content reduces the percent retention of ingested fluid. As a rehydration fluid after dehydration, drinks containing 4 percent alcohol or more, such as beer, tend to delay the restoration of blood and plasma volume. Consumption of a significant amount of alcohol in the dehydrated state is problematic for at least two reasons. First, increased urine output delays rehydration attempts, leading to impaired thermoregulation and performance in subsequent competition and training, especially in warm or hot weather. Second, Hobson and Maughan reported that the dehydrated individual will have a higher BAC for a given amount of ingested alcohol due to a lower total water volume. As noted later, a higher BAC could have adverse consequences. Alcohol consumed before cold-weather exercise has been reported by Graham to cause vasodilatation, to decrease core temperature, and to lower blood glucose levels. These changes could impair performance and possibly contribute to hypothermia.

Additional research is merited to document any adverse effects of alcohol on cardiovascular or metabolic processes during exercise, but at this time it appears that alcohol intake before or during aerobic and anaerobic endurance exercise is not ergogenic. In their recent review, Pesta and others described alcohol as an **ergolytic** agent that impairs athletic performance.

Effect on psychological processes   Because alcohol is a central nervous system depressant, one would not initially consider it to be a logical ergogenic aid. However, one of the effects of alcohol is a feeling of euphoria. In their review, Font and colleagues describe the involvement of alcohol and its metabolite, acetaldehyde (see figure 13.2), in the release of beta-endorphin, an analgesic (which dulls pain), and dopamine, a neurotransmitter associated with the pleasure center of the brain. The interaction of alcohol with beta-endorphin and dopamine may explain psychological effects sometime attributed to alcohol consumption such as suppression of inhibition, increased self-confidence, reduced anxiety, and a perceived decrease in sensitivity to pain, which may negate any depressant effects and benefit performance. Alcohol in small doses may exert a paradoxical stimulatory effect. Parts of the brain normally inhibiting behavior may be depressed by alcohol, leading to a transitory sensation of excitement.

Although these effects may occur, research does not support the use of alcohol in sports involving psychological processes such as perceptual-motor abilities. Perceptual-motor activities involve the perception of a stimulus, integration of this stimulus by the brain, and an appropriate motor response (movement). The evidence overwhelmingly supports the conclusion that alcohol adversely affects psychomotor performance skills, such as reaction time, balance, hand/eye coordination, and visual perception. These are important in events with rapidly changing stimuli, such as tennis.

Nevertheless, by reducing anxiety and related hand muscle tremor, alcohol could enhance performance in certain forms of athletic competition, such as riflery, pistol shooting, dart throwing, and archery. Although research generally is not supportive of improved performance, one study with archers revealed a tendency toward reduced tremor with low blood alcohol levels, resulting in a smoother release. However, no actual performance data were revealed. Throwing accuracy improved in darts at a BAC of 0.02 but was impaired at a BAC of 0.05. This area of study merits additional research.

Social drinking and sports   Based on limited research, there is general agreement that light social drinking will not impair performance the next day. Kruisselbrink and colleagues reported no change in grip strength, aerobic power, or levels of blood glucose and lactate in females the morning after consuming from zero to six bottles of beer. However, performance on a four-choice reaction-time test was adversely affected the morning following consumption of six beers compared to abstinence. Heavy drinking may impair some aspects of performance the next day due to hangover effects, involuntary eye movement, or dehydration.

Permissibility   The use of alcohol *in competition* by Olympic athletes had been banned previously by the IOC, but because wine and beer are commonly consumed as a part of many traditional European meals, it was removed from the banned list prior to the 1972 Olympics. However, individual sports federations within the IOC still may consider alcohol use in competition as grounds for disqualification. According to the 2015 WADA prohibited list, the use of alcohol in competition is banned by federations governing archery as well as air, automobile, motorcycle, and automobile sports.

In his review, Williams noted that although alcohol consumption is not prohibited for use by athletes *out of competition,* there are no data supporting an ergogenic effect, and some data to suggest an ergolytic effect. This viewpoint was supported by Burke and Maughan in their review. Athletes who drink socially should do so in moderation, and possibly abstain 24 hours prior to a prolonged endurance contest.

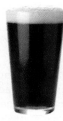

What effect can drinking alcohol have upon my health?

Consumption of alcoholic beverages is a popular pastime worldwide. People drink mainly for social reasons, but when and how much they drink may have a significant impact on their health and the health of others. As Klatsky noted, the basic disparity underlying all alcohol-health relations is between the effects of lighter and heavier drinking.

Alcohol consumption is associated with negative and positive health effects. Gunzerath and others described effects of moderate drinking (no more than one drink/day for females and no more than two drinks/day for males) in a 2003 report issued by the National Institute on Alcohol Abuse and Alcoholism (NIAAA). In its 2014 *Global Status Report on Alcohol and Health,* the World Health Organization (WHO) stated that alcohol abuse resulted in the death of 3.3 million people in 2012, accounting for 5.9 percent of all global deaths. The highest per capita alcohol consumption and rates of heavy, episodic alcohol consumption were observed in the European WHO region.

Although men and women of all ages may incur health problems with alcohol use, there are potential age- and gender-related differences in health risks. Women have less body water in which to dilute any ingested amount of alcohol and have lower levels of a form of alcohol dehydrogenase in the stomach that would decrease the rate of alcohol metabolism. These differences could result in a higher BAC for females, leading to increased short- and long-term health risk. Epstein and others noted these differences could place women at higher risk for negative physical, medical, and psychological consequences associated with at-risk and higher levels of alcohol consumption. In their review, Ferreira and Weems commented that more research is needed on the effects of alcohol use by the largest-growing U.S. age group, males and females over 65 years of age. Specific issues include interactions between alcohol and pharmacological agents commonly prescribed to older individuals and pathological changes associated with age-related diseases.

Negative Effects   Alcohol affects all cells in the body, and many of these effects may have significant health implications. According to the 2014 WHO *Global Status Report on Alcohol and*

Health, alcohol is causally related to more than 200 different medical conditions and is a major challenge to public health. Alcohol and its metabolite, acetaldehyde, can have direct toxic effects on cells, possibly damaging DNA. Alcohol may adversely affect functions of major body organs, particularly the liver and brain, and other metabolic functions important to good health.

Many of the adverse health effects of alcohol consumption are associated with heavy, or binge, drinking. Binge drinking in men is defined as consuming five or more drinks in one occasion, while the corresponding amount for women is four or more drinks.

Liver disease The liver is the only organ in the body that metabolizes alcohol, and alcohol may affect liver function in several ways. It may interfere with the metabolism of other drugs, increasing the effect of some and lessening the effects of others. Even with a balanced diet high in protein, consuming six drinks a day for less than a month has been shown to cause significant accumulation of fat in the liver. If continued for 5 years or more, the liver cells degenerate. Eventually, the damaged liver cells are replaced by nonfunctioning scar tissue, a condition known as **cirrhosis**. As liver function deteriorates, fat, carbohydrate, and protein metabolism are not regulated properly. This has possible pathological consequences for other body organs such as the kidney, pancreas, and heart.

In their meta-analysis to discern a threshold response of alcohol consumption for liver cirrhosis, Rehm and colleagues found no increase in *morbidity* between lifetime abstinence and up to two drinks per day in men and women. However, the risk of *mortality* was increased in women and men with only one and two drinks per day, respectively. Phospholipid extracts from soybean have been reported by Lieber to repair damaged liver cells and improve enzyme function. In a large prospective cohort study, Klatsky and others observed that four or more cups of coffee significantly decreased the risk of alcoholic cirrhosis and improved liver enzyme function. They concluded that coffee has an ingredient that protects against alcoholic cirrhosis. Resveratrol, an antioxidant in grape skin and red wine, has been reported by researchers such as Kasdallah-Grissa and colleagues to reduce oxidative stress in rat liver. As a result, some scientists theorize that wine may be the least damaging alcoholic beverage. However, liver damage is one of the most consistent adverse effects of excess alcohol intake, and Reuben noted that safe and effective therapies for alcoholic cirrhosis have yet to be discovered.

Psychological problems Many of the adverse health effects of alcohol consumption are associated with disturbed mental functions. As previously mentioned, a small amount of alcohol often provides pleasurable effects. However, alcohol generally acts as a depressant and its effects on the brain are dose-dependent. The effects occur in a hierarchical fashion related to the development of the brain. In general, alcohol first affects the higher brain centers. With increasing dosages, lower levels of brain function become depressed, with subsequent disturbance of normal functions. This hierarchy of brain functions, from higher levels to lower levels, and some of the functions affected by alcohol may be generalized as follows:

Thinking and reasoning—judgment
Perceptual-motor responses—reaction time
Fine motor coordination—muscles of speech
Gross motor coordination—Walking
Visual processes—double vision
Alertness—sleep, coma
Respiratory control—respiratory failure, death

As noted in table 13.2, a BAC of 0.06–0.09 may impair judgment, fine motor ability, and coordination—three factors that are extremely important in the safe operation of an automobile and other modes of transportation. A BAC of 0.08 or higher is the threshold for *driving under the influence (DUI)* in all 50 states. DUI has serious social and personal consequences, including death. In 2010, the economic cost of alcohol-impaired automobile accidents was $49.8 billion. These costs include but are not limited to lost productivity as well as medical and legal expenses. According to National Highway Traffic Safety Administration data, the number of alcohol-impaired driving fatalities has decreased by more than 50 percent since 1982, but 10,076 alcohol-related fatalities occurred in 2013. As the saying goes, "Don't drink and drive!"

www-nrd.nhtsa.dot.gov/Pubs/812102.pdf Use this link to access alcohol-impaired traffic safety facts for 2013. The information is from the National Highway Traffic Safety Administration's Fatality Analysis Reporting System, a repository of data on traffic safety.

TABLE 13.2 Typical effects of increasing blood alcohol content

Number of drinks consumed in 2 hours*	Blood alcohol content**	Typical effects
2–3	.02–.04	Reduced tension, relaxed feeling, relief from daily stress
4–5	.06–.09	Legally drunk (0.08) in all states; impaired judgment, a high feeling, impaired fine motor ability and coordination
6–8	.11–.16	Slurred speech, impaired gross motor coordination, staggering gait
9–12	.18–.25	Loss of control of voluntary activity, erratic behavior, impaired vision
13–18	.27–.39	Stupor, total loss of coordination
19 and above	>.40	Coma, depression of respiratory centers, death

*One drink = 12 ounces regular beer
    4 ounces wine
    1.25 ounces liquor
**BAC based on body weight of 160 pounds (72.6 kg). The BAC will increase proportionally for individuals weighing less (such as a 120-pound female) and will decrease proportionally for individuals weighing more (such as a 200-pound football player). For example, four to five drinks in 2 hours could lead to a BAC of 0.08–0.12 in a 120-pound individual.

In recent years, alcoholic energy drinks have become increasingly popular among the young. Some believe that the caffeine and other possible stimulants in these drinks may counteract the depressant effects of alcohol. Ulbrich and others found no evidence that alcohol consumed with either caffeine or an energy drink decreased subjective perception of alcohol intoxication. Furthermore, similar impairments in motor coordination, speech, and vision were observed compared to alcohol alone. Energy drinks are discussed in more detail in the next section, on caffeine.

An extensive body of literature supports a positive association between acute alcohol consumption and aggressive behaviors. In their review, Beck and Heinz note that alcohol is a contributing factor in half of the violent crimes and sexual assaults worldwide and is second only to depression in the the psychiatric diagnosis for suicide. The quantity of alcohol consumed also is related to aggression and fatal nontraffic outcomes. Smith and others reported intoxication (BAC $\geq$ 100mg/100mL) of 31.5, 31.0, and 22.7 percent in homicides, unintentional injury, and suicides, respectively. Galaif and others noted that suicide and alcohol use are related in young individuals. The suicide rate for those between 15 and 19 years of age is 9.7 per 100,000, while half of 12th graders have been intoxicated at least once. Monti and others reported that heavy drinking during the teenage years may cause permanent brain damage, which may be a related factor.

In their review, Attwood and Munafò comment that alcohol may disrupt signal processing between the frontal lobe and amygdala, brain centers involved in normal decision making and emotional reactions. Males are more prone to alcohol-related aggressive behavior than females. In susceptible individuals, such disruption may cue an increase in aggression and lead to learned aggressive behavior. Specific outcomes include disinhibition of suppressed behavior, heightened reaction to potentially aggressive situations, loss of empathy, and reduced recognition of submissive cues from others.

College students are known to engage in hazardous drinking. According to Karam and others, the prevalence of hazardous drinking among college students is similar in Australia, Europe, South America, and North America. Most of these adverse psychological effects are associated with excessive alcohol intake, particularly as practiced in binge drinking (5+ drinks for males; 4+ drinks for females). White and Hingson reported that 39 percent of full-time college students engaged in a binge drinking episode in 2011, a significant reduction from 2002–2010. Despite this encouraging reduction, the NIAAA notes that as many as 1,800 deaths, 599,000 injuries, 690,000 physical assaults, and 97,000 sexual assaults are related to alcohol use by college students. Even low drinking levels can cause problems. In their study, Gruenewald and others concluded that many problems among college students are associated with drinking relatively small amounts of alcohol (2 to 4 drinks). Poor academic performance related to alcohol use has been experienced by 25 percent of college students.

Many physically active individuals, including competitive athletes, consume alcohol on a regular basis. In a recent study of NCAA male athletes, Buckman and others noted that alcohol was the most widely used drug, with 82 percent of respondents reporting use within the last 12 months. El Sayed and others reported that alcohol continues to be the most frequently consumed drug among athletes and habitual exercisers and alcohol-related problems appear to be more common in these individuals. Ford commented that higher binge drinking among college athletes versus nonathletes may be related to differences in perceived social norms, peer influence, and athletes' "work hard, play hard" attitude. Sports participation may, in some way, be associated with increased alcohol use. In their study, the Wichstrøms found that sports participation in adolescence, and participation in team sports in particular, may increase the growth in alcohol intoxication during late adolescent and early adult years. Martens and others have developed and validated an Athlete Drinking Scale to explore the reasons athletes drink alcohol.

Cardiovascular disease   Heavy drinking may increase the risk of heart disease and stroke. O'Keefe and colleagues noted that heavier drinking may increase some of the possible risks to heart and vascular health, including the following:

- Alcoholic cardiomyopathy, or impaired heart function
- Hypertension (increased blood pressure)
- Increased risk of ischemic (lack of blood flow) and hemorrhagic (bleeding) stroke
- Increased risk of certain heart rate arrhythmias such as atrial fibrillation

As we shall see, drinking alcohol in moderation ($\leq$ 2 and $\leq$ 1 drinks/day for males and females, respectively) may help to prevent cardiovascular disease, but Cargiulo concludes that heavy drinking is associated with increased risk of coronary heart disease and stroke. According to Tonelo and others, heavy chronic or binge drinking may affect the heart's normal rhythm by increasing autonomic nervous activity, blood fatty acids, and/or acetaldehyde levels. The *holiday heart syndrome* is a rapid heart arrhythmia associated with heavy drinking around vacations and holidays. Although this syndrome is not normally dangerous, individuals with underlying heart problems may be at increased risk for a heart attack. George and Figueredo reported that numerous investigators have noted a causal relationship between alcohol and arrhythmias, as well as sudden cardiac death.

Cancer   Laboratory research has shown that, *in vitro* (that is, in a test tube), alcohol and acetaldehyde cause changes in DNA (the genetic material in body cells) comparable to changes elicited by carcinogens. This DNA damage may occur at an alcohol concentration equivalent to one to two drinks. Based on the carcinogenicity of acetaldehyde in animals, the Environmental Protective Agency has concluded that acetaldehyde is a probable human carcinogen.

In their comparative review of reports by the World Cancer Research Fund (WCRF)/American Institute of Cancer Research (AICR) and the International Agency for Research of Cancer (IARC) from 2007 and 2012, Roswall and Weiderpass noted that convincing links exist between alcohol use and cancers of the oral cavity, pharynx, larynx, and esophagus. These tissues directly contact ingested alcohol. Male colorectal and female breast cancers are also strongly linked to alcohol consumption.

The relationship between alcohol use and breast cancer is controversial. Although some positive health outcomes such as reduced cardiovascular disease risk have been associated with moderate alcohol use, the NIAAA states that even one drink/day increases the risk for breast cancer by 10 percent compared to women who do not drink. According to the WCRF/AICR report, there is an 8 percent increase in breast cancer risk for each 10 g/day increment in alcohol intake. Separate large epidemiological studies by Zhang and Allen and their associates have also reported associations between increased daily or cumulative intake of alcohol and breast cancer.

These findings are supported by several reviews. Michels and others reviewed the effects of 15 dietary variables on breast cancer and concluded that alcohol intake was one of the few whose association with breast cancer was consistent, strong, and statistically significant. Scoccianti and others noted that younger age at the start of drinking may also increase breast cancer risk by early and longer exposure of mammary tissue to the carcinogenic effects of acetaldehyde. In addition to potential DNA damage, alcohol ingestion may also increase estrogen levels, a factor that increases breast cancer risk. Alcohol also increases estrogen and progesterone receptor expression, which can in turn increase breast cancer risk. According to the NIAAA, women with significant family history for breast cancer or those on estrogen replacement therapy should discuss their alcohol intake with their health-care provider in order to weigh potential increases in breast cancer risk against potential decreases in cardiovascular disease risk.

Fetal alcohol spectrum disorders Women who drink should abstain during pregnancy because even moderate consumption of alcohol, or even a single drinking binge, may affect DNA in the embryo and fetus. Haycock indicates that ethanol is a classic teratogen capable of inducing a wide range of developmental abnormalities, particularly during peak periods of epigenetic reprogramming in the fetus. In their review, Burd and others reported that alcohol intake during pregnancy may have numerous adverse effects on the placenta, including placental dysfunction and decreased placental size. Given these effects, alcohol may cause health problems in the newborn, which Green identifies as *fetal alcohol spectrum disorder (FASD)*. FASD is the term used to describe birth anomalies associated with the mother's drinking alcohol while pregnant and refers to several conditions involving alcohol-related neurodevelopment disorders, birth defects, and other abnormalities in normal development.

Fetal alcohol syndrome (FAS) is the most severe of the FASD. The Centers for Disease Control and Prevention National Center on Birth Defects and Developmental Disabilities indicates that FAS is one of the leading known causes of mental retardation and birth defects. The incidence rate of FAS is very high in the United States, and FAS is currently the major cause of mental retardation in the Western world. The child may experience retardation in growth and mental development as well as facial birth defects (figure 13.3). In their meta-analysis, Lucas and others reported a significant association between prenatal alcohol exposure or FASD and impairment in gross motor skills such as balance, coordination, and ball-handling skills.

Fetal alcohol effects (FAE) may be observed in children when full-blown FAS is not present. Children with FAE are easily

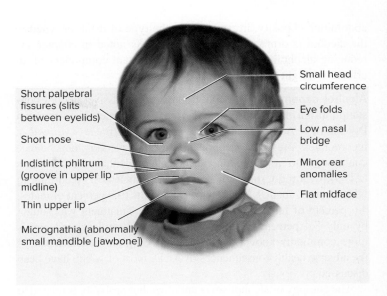

Short palpebral fissures (slits between eyelids)

Short nose

Indistinct philtrum (groove in upper lip midline)

Thin upper lip

Micrognathia (abnormally small mandible [jawbone])

Small head circumference

Eye folds

Low nasal bridge

Minor ear anomalies

Flat midface

FIGURE 13.3 Common facial characteristics of children with fetal alcohol syndrome (FAS).

distracted and have poor attention spans but do not have the facial features of FAS. Both FAS and FAE are associated with learning disorders in children. The Institute of Medicine has used more specific terms for FAE, including *alcohol-related neurodevelopmental disorder* and *alcohol-related birth defects*. Although Kelly and others reported that children of women who were classified as light drinkers (no more than one to two drinks a week) during pregnancy were not at increased risk for emotional or cognitive problems compared with children whose mothers did not drink while pregnant, abstinence still appears to be the safest approach. No "safe" amount of alcohol during pregnancy has been determined. Thus, the U.S. surgeon general indicated that the safest approach is abstinence.

Obesity Alcohol is a significant source of Calories, about 7 per gram, somewhat comparable to the caloric content of fat. Research has indicated that if small amounts of alcohol (5 percent of daily caloric intake) are interchanged for an equivalent caloric intake from carbohydrates, there is no effect on daily energy expenditure. In other words, alcohol Calories themselves will not increase body fat as long as total daily caloric intake matches daily caloric expenditure. In general, the NIAAA indicates that the relationship between moderate alcohol consumption and obesity remains inconclusive. In their study, Beulens and others reported that moderate alcohol consumption (40 grams daily for 4 weeks) was not associated with increased adiposity or increased weight circumference.

However, Yeomans noted that alcohol may increase energy intake in several ways. Alcohol stimulates the appetite, increasing food intake, and alcohol contains energy. In his review, Yeomans commented that alcohol Calories are generally additive to carbohydrate, fat, and protein Calories and can lead to obesity through overconsumption of energy. Suter noted that several metabolic studies have reported that alcohol decreases fat oxidation, leading to a positive fat balance. These points may underlie the conclusion of the study by Wannamethee and others, mainly that higher alcohol consumption is positively associated with both overall and abdominal adiposity, irrespective of the type of drink or whether the alcohol is drunk with meals or not. As noted in chapter 11, reducing alcoholic intake may be an important component of an effective weight-control program.

Alcohol dependence Alcohol abuse, or excessive alcohol consumption, is a major drug problem in the United States. The American Psychiatric Association's *Diagnostic Statistical Manual–V* incorporates previous alcohol abuse and alcohol dependence diagnoses into a single diagnosis called alcohol use disorders (AUD), with mild, moderate, and severe subclasses. According to NIAAA data, about 7.2 percent of U.S. adults (9.9 percent of males, 4.6 percent of females) had AUD in 2012. Treatment was sought by only 8.4 percent of those with AUD. Alcohol dependency is more commonly known as **alcoholism**. Cargiulo details many of the adverse health consequences of AUD, most of which have been discussed previously.

The etiology of alcoholism is unknown but probably is related to a variety of physiological, psychological, and sociological factors. Söderpalm and Ericson indicate that alcohol activates the dopamine system, an important part of the brain reward system, and the positive psychological effects may reinforce the desire to continue to consume alcohol. Morozova and others note that no single genetic locus explains alcohol dependence. Studies have reported many complex genetic and epigenetic factors that potentially influence an individual's susceptibility to alcohol dependence. According to the National Council on Alcoholism and Drug Dependence (NCADD), there is no single definition for alcoholism. It may be related to a variety of behaviors. A deficiency of B complex vitamins may contribute to many of the neuropsychiatric problems seen in alcoholism. The number of behaviors exhibited by the drinker may be related to various stages in the progression toward alcoholism.

> https://ncadd.org/get-help/take-the-test The NCAAD has developed an assessment of behaviors that may signal AUD. Access the questionnaire by clicking Take The Alcohol Test at the lower left of the page. A link to a teenager version can be accessed at the lower right link.
>
> www.testandcalc.com/etc/tests/audit.asp A shorter, online version known as the Alcohol Use Disorders Identification Test (AUDIT).

Positive Effects On the positive side, most recent epidemiological research and reviews have shown that light to moderate consumption of alcohol is associated with lessened mortality. For example, Ronksley and others noted a J-shaped relationship in their meta-analysis of 31 studies examining the association of alcohol use and all-cause mortality. Compared to nonusers, drinkers consuming 2.5–14.9 grams of alcohol/day had the lowest relative risk (0.83), but the risk significantly increased to 1.3 in heavy drinkers (>60 grams/day).

Alzheimer's disease, other dementia, and cognitive function
In their meta-analysis, Beydoun and others commented that 25 of 30 of studies reported evidence of improved cognitive function with moderate alcohol consumption. Proposed mechanisms include reduced cardiovascular risk, the reduced

platelet-aggregating effects of alcohol, and the memory-enhancing effects of acetylcholine on the hippocampus. Anstey and others found that drinkers, when compared with nondrinkers, had a reduced risk of Alzheimer's disease and any other dementia, but not cognitive decline. It is not clear whether the results reflected a protective effect of alcohol consumption throughout adulthood or a specific benefit of alcohol in late life. However, Piazza-Gardner and others observed that 9 of 19 studies reported no effect of alcohol on Alzheimer's disease. There were inconsistencies in measured alcohol consumption in 7 studies reporting moderate alcohol as protective against Alzheimer's disease. Given these discordant findings, additional research is merited to explore the links between cognitive function and alcohol consumption.

Cardiovascular Disease Most research on the possible health benefits of alcohol consumption has focused on heart health. Research suggests that light to moderate alcohol intake reduces risk of coronary heart disease and stroke, a major factor in reducing risk for all-cause mortality. For example, in their analysis of data from 52 countries, Leong and colleagues reported low alcohol consumption reduced myocardial infarction risk, while heavy drinking increased the risk. The mechanism is not known, but several have been proposed based on epidemiological and experimental studies.

One theory suggests small amounts of alcohol induce a relaxation effect, which may reduce emotional stress, a risk factor associated with CHD. Another theory suggests alcohol decreases platelet aggregability (clotting ability) by increasing the activity of a clot-dissolving enzyme in the blood. Still another theory involves an increased brain blood flow, which might help prevent certain forms of stroke. Other mechanisms, such as enhanced insulin sensitivity, may also play a role. Koppes and others reported a 30 percent lower risk for diabetes, a risk factor for CHD, in moderate drinkers compared to nonusers and heavy users.

The most prevalent theory involves the effect of alcohol to raise levels of HDL-cholesterol, the form of cholesterol that protects against the development of CHD (see discussion on pages 199–203). A significant number of studies have supported this effect. Brinton commented that moderate alcohol consumption (one to two drinks/day) generally increases smaller, dense, protein-rich HDL_3 levels by about 10 percent with decreased risk of CHD, while heavier consumption increases larger, less dense HDL_2 levels even more but with no additional decrease in CHD risk. Alcohol has been reported to positively affect certain steps in the transport by HDL of cholesterol from peripheral tissues to the liver and to favorably affect phospholipids of endothelial cells to improve vascular function. However, alcohol may increase the formation of ethyl fatty acid esters, which can promote liver damage. Although early research suggested that individuals with an alcohol dehydrogenase variant that metabolizes alcohol more slowly may have greater increases in HDL, more recent research has failed to confirm this genetic effect. The mechanisms of alcohol's effect on heart health are not fully understood.

Some investigators have theorized that the consumption of certain types of alcoholic beverages, most notably red wine, is responsible for the reported health benefits. In their review, Arranz and others concluded that polyphenols from moderate wine and beer consumption may protect against the atherosclerotic process. Resveratrol, a nonflavonoid, has received the most research attention. Specific mechanisms attributed to polyphenols include reductions in LDL oxidation, platelet aggregation, and biomarkers of inflammation as well as improved vasodilation, blood flow, and vascular function. There is less support for these effects in distilled spirits, which contain fewer polyphenols. They noted that individual differences in the absorptions of beneficial polyphenols would affect bioavailability and ultimately any protective effect. Rodrigo and others comment that alcohol increases polyphenol absorption. Compared to wine, beer contains more protein and B vitamins, is rich in flavonoids, and has an equivalent antioxidant content, but of different specific antioxidants derived from barley and hops. Mukamal and others found that men who consumed alcohol 3–4 days per week experienced a reduced risk of myocardial infarction, but the type of beverage consumed did not substantially alter this effect. Stackelberg and others reported a lower risk of abdominal aortic aneurysm with low to moderate consumption of either wine or beer, but not spirits, in Swedish men and women.

Although these factors may be important, Naimi and others contend that individuals who drink moderately may practice other lifestyle behaviors that reduce the risk for CHD. In their review, Piazza-Gardner and Barry reported a positive relationship between physical activity and alcohol consumption in studies of youth, college-aged students, and the general population. As noted in chapter 1, exercise itself may reduce the risk of CHD. However, Mukamal and others, reporting data from more than 50,000 males in the Health Professionals Follow-up Study over the course of 16 years, found that moderate alcohol intake, up to two drinks daily, is associated with lower risk of experiencing a heart attack even in men already at low risk for heart disease on the basis of body mass index, physical activity, smoking, and diet. However, using National Runners' Health Study data, Williams reported that men's blood pressure increases in association with the amount of alcohol intake, regardless of running level. Thus, it should be reemphasized that although there appear to be some positive health effects associated with light to moderate alcohol intake, or at least no detrimental effects, heavier drinking is another matter.

Others have challenged the health benefits of alcohol from another perspective. Although lifetime abstainers are the ideal comparison group for the health effects of alcohol use, nonusers in some studies have included individuals who decreased or stopped drinking due to illnesses. Such individuals have been classified as *sick quitters*. Fillmore and others suggested that sick quitters may represent a systematic error in studies supporting an association between moderate alcohol consumption and reduced CHD risk. Some alcohol abstainers who are ill and subsequently die may have decreased or stopped drinking because of their illness. In other words, their mortality was due to the underlying illness rather than lack of alcohol use. On the other hand, Mukamal and others reported heart benefits from moderate alcohol intake in only healthy men who exercised, ate a good diet, were not obese, and did not smoke. Rehm and others recommend using irregular, light lifetime drinkers with abstainers as the comparison group in future studies.

Holmes and colleagues recently reported that individuals with a genetic variant of alcohol dehydrogenase associated with no or low alcohol consumption have lower risk for cardiovascular disease. They concluded that reduction of alcohol consumption, even by moderate drinkers, can improve cardiovascular health. This finding calls into questions the cardio-protective effects of moderate alcohol consumption.

Because of the potential for abuse, addiction, and all types of injuries, abstinence from alcohol or prudent consumption is generally recommended by health authorities. *Low-risk drinking* is an emerging term to represent light to moderate alcohol intake. As noted previously, abstinence is the best policy for pregnant women or if you plan to operate a motor vehicle. Health professionals, however, generally support the view that low-risk drinking, along with a balanced diet, should not pose any health problem to the average, healthy individual. The definition of moderation varies, though. For example, in the United Kingdom and Denmark, sensible drinking limits are established at three drinks a day for men and two for women. In the United States, the NIAAA indicates that except for individuals at particular risk, consumption of two drinks a day for men and one for women is unlikely to increase health risks. As risks for some conditions and diseases do increase at higher levels of consumption, men should be cautioned not to exceed four drinks on any day and women not to exceed three on any day.

Nevertheless, although there are actually some possible health benefits associated with alcohol consumption in moderation, health authorities caution that these potential benefits are not sufficient cause to start drinking if you currently abstain. The NIAAA stipulates that *moderate alcohol use* should not be construed as *healthy alcohol use*, because numerous individual differences, such as age, genetics, and metabolic rate, may affect the response to alcohol. You should consult with your physician if you are considering drinking for its possible health benefits.

Key Concepts

▶ One drink of alcohol contains approximately 13–14 grams of alcohol, or about 1/2 ounce. One drink is typically the equivalent of 12 ounces of beer, 4 ounces of wine, or 1.25 ounces of 40-proof whiskey. However, the alcohol content in some beverages may be substantially greater.

▶ Alcohol is not an effective ergogenic aid; in fact, it may actually be ergolytic, that is, impair performance.

▶ Consumption of alcohol in moderation appears to cause no major health problems for the normal, healthy adult and may actually confer some health benefits. However, alcohol may be contraindicated for some, such as women during pregnancy. The effect of alcohol on breast cancer remains controversial. Heavy drinking is associated with numerous health problems.

Check Yourself

▶ Visit a local beer/wine store that carries a wide variety of products, including microbrews and fortified wines. Check the labels for percentage alcohol content, listing those from lowest to highest. Calculate how much alcohol would be in a standard drink from each.

www.niaaa.nih.gov This Website provides detailed information on a wide variety of alcohol-related topics. For example, if you want to decrease the amount of alcohol you drink, click on Publications and Multimedia, then Brochures and Fact Sheets, then Rethinking Drinking.

TABLE 13.3 Caffeine content in selected products

Product	Serving size	Caffeine (milligrams)
Coffee, brewed	8-ounce cup	80–135
Coffee, instant	8-ounce cup	65–100
Coffee, decaffeinated	8-ounce cup	3–4
Coffee, Starbucks	16-ounce cup	330
Tea, black or green	8-ounce cup	30–50
Hot cocoa	8-ounce cup	15
Sodas, cola	12-ounce can	35–45
Sodas, high caffeine	12-ounce can	55–70
POWERade Advance	16-ounce bottle	95
Energy drinks	8-ounce can	80–120
Performance candy	1 Buzz Bite	100
Stimulants	1 Vivarin tablet	200
Dietary supplements	5 grams guarana	250

Note: Check labels of over-the-counter stimulants and dietary supplements for caffeine content.

Caffeine: Ergogenic Effects and Health Implications

Coffee is one of the most widely consumed beverages throughout the world. The coffee bean, a plant product, contains caffeine, which has been theorized to enhance exercise performance. Indeed, Tunnicliffe and others noted that the majority of high-level Canadian athletes consume dietary caffeine, primarily in the form of coffee. Besides caffeine, coffee also contains numerous other biologically active phytonutrients, such as antioxidants, and has been studied for its possible beneficial or adverse effects on health.

What is caffeine, and in what food products is it found?

Caffeine is an odorless, bitter, white alkaloid that appears naturally in many plants. Technically, caffeine may be classified as a food ingredient, a dietary supplement, or a drug.

As a food ingredient, caffeine is found in many of the foods and beverages that we consume every day, not only coffee but tea, colas, caffeinated waters, juices, energy drinks, sports drinks and sports bars, and chocolate. Some approximate amounts in the beverages we consume are 80–135 mg in a cup of perked coffee, 40–60 mg in a cup of tea, 35–45 mg in a can of cola, and 80–120 mg or more in an 8-ounce serving of an energy drink. Mitchell and others indicate that 85 percent of Americans consume at least one caffeinated beverage per day, with coffee identified as the primary source. Caffeine is also found in various dietary supplements, such as kola nuts and guarana, and even in some over-the-counter stimulant supplements targeted to athletes; most recently, caffeine has been marketed as *performance candy*, such as Jolt Caffeine-Energy Gum and Buzz Bites, a chocolate chew candy. Such products may be construed to be sports supplements.

Caffeine is also legally classified as a drug and has some powerful physiological effects on the human body. A normal therapeutic dose of caffeine may range from 100 to 300 milligrams. As noted in table 13.3, some food products and supplements provide a therapeutic dose and meet the standards for classification as a drug. Indeed, caffeine has been identified as the most popular social drug in the United States (figure 13.4).

What effects does caffeine have on the body that may benefit exercise performance?

One of the primary effects of caffeine is to block the neurotransmitter adenosine, and thus influence a wide variety of metabolic processes throughout the body. Additionally, caffeine may stimulate the adrenal gland to release epinephrine (adrenaline) into the

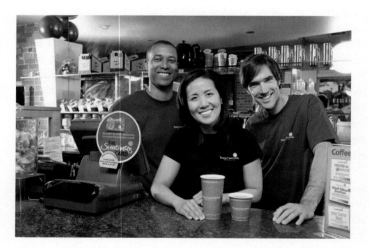

FIGURE 13.4 Caffeine is the most popular social drug in the United States. Up to 85 percent of all U.S. adults consume caffeine in one form or another, mainly as coffee.

circulation. Caffeine, in conjunction with epinephrine, stimulates a wide variety of tissues. Together, they stimulate the central nervous system, potentiate muscle contraction, raise the rate of muscle and liver glycogen breakdown, increase release of free fatty acids (FFAs) from adipose tissue, and increase use of muscle triglycerides. One of the most observed effects at rest is an increase in blood levels of FFAs.

Caffeine has been studied for its potential ergogenic effects for more than 100 years. Early research focused on improvements in strength, power, and psychomotor parameters such as reaction time. However, in the late 1970s, Costill and other researchers hypothesized caffeine could enhance performance of aerobic endurance athletes, such as marathoners, by increasing fat oxidation and sparing the use of muscle glycogen. Numerous investigators tested this hypothesis over the years. In his most recent review, Terry Graham, a noted caffeine researcher, and others concluded that there is very little evidence to support the hypothesis that caffeine has ergogenic effects as a result of enhanced fat oxidation and sparing of muscle glycogen use during prolonged aerobic endurance exercise.

> *www.caffeineinformer.com/* This Website contains an extensive database of drinks and foods containing caffeine, as well as a calculator to determine safe daily caffeine intake.

In his review of the potential ergogenic effects of caffeine, Tarnopolsky concluded that the ergogenic effect of caffeine on endurance exercise performance is multifactorial. For one, caffeine may stimulate the central nervous system, accelerating nerve cell activity in both the brain and spinal cord, and reduce the sensation of perceived effort (rating of perceived exertion, or RPE) during exercise. In a meta-analysis of 21 studies, Doherty and Smith concluded that in comparison to a placebo, caffeine reduced the RPE during exercise by 5.6 percent while improving exercise performance by 11.2 percent. The authors concluded that the effect of caffeine on the RPE could account for approximately 29 percent of the improvement in performance. The effect of caffeine to reduce the psychological effort of exercise appears to be an important factor underlying its ergogenic effect. Caffeine may increase the force of muscle contraction. In her review, Kalmar indicated that caffeine may influence muscle performance by stimulating the nervous system at various points along the motor pathway to the muscle. Caffeine may also increase the release of calcium from the sarcoplasmic reticulum in the muscle, possibly increasing the force of muscle contraction. Research by Tarnopolsky and Cupido, using electrical stimulation of the muscle, supports the hypothesis that some of the ergogenic effect of caffeine in endurance exercise performance occurs directly at the skeletal muscle level.

Overall, caffeine may influence central and peripheral metabolic processes, as well as psychological processes, to help delay the onset of fatigue and has been theorized to enhance performance in many types of exercise, including endurance, strength, speed, and power.

Does caffeine enhance exercise performance?

Hundreds of studies have been conducted to test the ergogenic effectiveness of caffeine. Considerable differences exist in the experimental designs of caffeine studies in such aspects as caffeine delivery system (caffeine in coffee or capsule form), caffeine dosage (3–15 mg per kg body weight), the type of exercise task (power, strength, reaction time, short-term endurance, prolonged endurance), the intensity of the exercise (submaximal exercise, maximal exercise), the training status of the subject (trained, untrained), the pre-exercise diet (high-carbohydrate, mixed), the subjects' caffeine status (user, abstainer), and individual variability (reactor, nonreactor). These differences complicate interpretation of the results. Additionally, some investigators have combined caffeine with other related stimulants, such as ephedrine.

Use by Athletes Caffeine appears to be a popular ergogenic aid among athletes. Using diet recall data from 270 elite Canadian athletes, Tunnicliffe and others reported that 67 percent consumed caffeine, mostly from chocolate or coffee. Desbrow and Leveritt noted that almost 90 percent of athletes competing in the 2005 World Championship Ironman Triathlon competition intended to use caffeine prior to or during the competition, while 75 percent believed that caffeine was ergogenic to their performance. Del Coso and others reported that caffeine was detected in 73.8 percent of almost 21,000 urine samples of elite Spanish athletes from 2004 to 2008 after caffeine was removed from the WADA prohibited list. Over 99 percent of these samples contained caffeine below the former threshold of 12 µg/mL. Overall, caffeine is one of the most popular sports supplements used worldwide by a wide variety of athletes.

Effect on Psychomotor Responses Caffeine may affect a number of psychomotor responses that may enhance performance in some sports. Caffeine can increase alertness, which may improve simple reaction time. Doses of 200 milligrams have been effective, particularly when subjects are mentally fatigued. Hogervorst and others have found that caffeine, as part of a carbohydrate-electrolyte solution or performance bar, improved cognitive function in trained athletes during and following an endurance cycling task. Maintaining cognitive function in many endurance activities may enhance performance. Stevenson and others theorized that a round of golf that lasts approximately 4 hours could be fatiguing from the prolonged walking and may result in impaired motor skill or cognitive performance. In their study with experienced golfers, they found that the consumption of a caffeinated sports drink prior to and during a round of golf improved putting performance and increased feelings of alertness. In its position statement on caffeine and exercise performance, the International Society of Sports Nutrition indicated that caffeine can enhance vigilance during bouts of extended exhaustive exercise, as well as periods of sustained sleep deprivation.

However, larger doses, above 400 milligrams, may increase nervousness and anxiousness in some individuals, and thus may adversely affect performance in events characterized by fine motor skills and control of hand steadiness, such as pistol shooting. Although caffeine may enhance visual attention, Hespel and others noted that in sports involving rapid visual stimuli, such as soccer, care must be taken not to overdose because visual information processing might be impaired.

Effect on Aerobic Endurance Performance Most research on the ergogenic effects of caffeine has focused on aerobic endurance

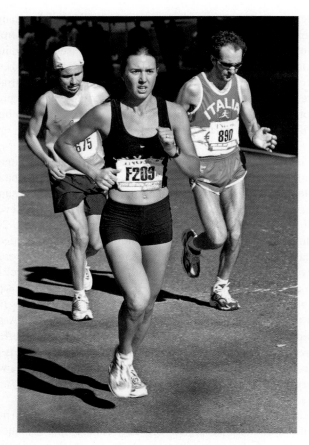

FIGURE 13.5 Caffeine may enhance performance in a wide variety of exercise endeavors, particularly events involving aerobic endurance.

performance, and numerous studies, reviews, meta-analyses, and position statements by sports-related associations support its efficacy as an ergogenic aid (figure 13.5).

Studies of rowing performance   Bruce and others reported that 6- and 9-mg/kg caffeine doses similarly decreased 2,000-meter rowing performance time by 1.2 percent and increased power by 2.7 percent compared to a placebo. However, Skinner and others found large interindividual differences in response to caffeine with no differences among placebo, 2-, 4-, and 6-mg/kg doses in rowing performance.

Studies of cycling performance   Foad and others observed that a 5-mg/kg dose resulted in a significant 3.5 percent increase in power during a 40-km cycling time trial. They also noted potentially meaningful 0.7 percent placebo and −1.9 percent *nocebo* (being correctly informed one did *not* receive caffeine) effects on power. Jenkins and others reported increased work performed in a maximal cycle ergometer task following 2- to 3-mg/kg caffeine doses.

Studies of running performance   In a field study, Bridge and Jones reported a 23.8-sec improvement in 8-kilometer run time following a 3-mg/kg caffeine dose, while Wiles and others found a 150- to 200-mg (~2- to 3-mg/kg) caffeine dose to improve 1,500-meter run performance in a laboratory setting. However, Candow

and others found no effect of a 2-mg/kg caffeine dose in a sugar-free energy drink compared to placebo on run time to exhaustion at 80 percent of VO_2 max. In their review, Schubert and Astorino identified an average improvement in running performance of 1.1 percent in seven studies of caffeine supplementation.

In their review, Ganio and others restricted their analysis to 21 studies that used only a time-trial endurance test, which has high reproducibility and is more applicable to sport. Although the amount of improvement varied among studies, the mean improvement in performance with caffeine ingestion was 3.2 percent. As previously noted, Doherty and Smith reported that caffeine improved exercise performance by 11.2 percent. In their review, Jeukendrup and Martin suggested that low doses of caffeine would improve 40-kilometer cycle performance time by 55–84 seconds. In his review, Spriet comments that low doses of caffeine (<3 mg/kg) ingested before and during exercise may be ergogenic in a variety of continuous and intermittent tasks, primarily due to improvement of vigilance, alertness, and cognitive function.

In its position stand on caffeine and exercise performance, the International Society of Sports Nutrition concluded that caffeine is ergogenic for sustained maximal endurance exercise and has been shown to be highly effective for time-trial performance, as noted earlier. The American College of Sports Medicine, in its position statement on fluid replacement during exercise, also noted that caffeine intake may help sustain performance. Although there are individual differences in response to caffeine, the available evidence supports its ergogenicity and popularity among endurance athletes.

Effect on High-Intensity Anaerobic Exercise   Davis and Green noted that the effect of caffeine on endurance performance is well founded, but comparatively less research has been conducted on the ergogenic potential of caffeine on anaerobic performance. For purposes of this discussion, high-intensity anaerobic exercise involves maximum exercise for 10–180 seconds, or intermittent high-intensity exercise in sports such as soccer, lacrosse, and field hockey.

In his 1991 review, Williams concluded that caffeine did not enhance performance in high-intensity anaerobic exercise tasks. However, Davis and Green noted that untrained subjects and flawed designs may account for nonsignificant findings in older studies and that more recent studies feature trained subjects and more appropriate sport-specific research designs. They concluded that caffeine is highly ergogenic for speed-endurance exercise ranging in duration from 60 to 180 seconds. Although traditional models examining anaerobic power and capacity such as the 30-second Wingate test have shown minimal effect of caffeine on performance, studies employing sport-specific (i.e., hockey, rugby, soccer), high-intensity, intermittent exercise of 4- to 6-second duration have reported an ergogenic effect of caffeine. For example, Glaister and others compared multiple 6-second cycle sprint performance in well-trained men following ingestion of 5 mg caffeine/kg or placebo. Caffeine increased maximal anaerobic power production and blood lactate levels in later sprints. In another review, Astorino and Roberson reported that 11 of 17 studies found significant improvements in team sports exercise and power-based sports with caffeine ingestion, but most commonly in elite athletes who do not regularly ingest caffeine. In its position stand on caffeine and exercise performance, the International Society of Sports Nutrition indicated that caffeine supplementation is beneficial for high-intensity exercise, including team sports such as soccer and rugby.

Caffeine appears to be an effective ergogenic for high-intensity, intermittent exercise, particularly within a period of prolonged duration, such as a soccer match.

Effect on Muscular Strength and Endurance

Research findings relative to the effect of caffeine supplementation on muscular strength and endurance are somewhat equivocal. Davis and Green note that research is somewhat limited regarding the effect of caffeine on resistance training and muscular strength and endurance. They also note recent studies showing that caffeine affects isometric maximal force and offers some evidence for enhanced muscle endurance for lower body musculature. However, the effects of caffeine on isokinetic peak torque, one-repetition maximum, and muscular endurance for upper body musculature are less clear. Astorino and Robinson indicate that 6 of 11 studies show that caffeine elicits significant benefits in resistance training. In their meta-analysis, Warren and others concluded that, overall, caffeine ingestion results in beneficial effect of about 7 percent on maximal voluntary contraction strength but primarily in the knee extensors and not in other muscle groups. They also reported that caffeine exerted a small beneficial effect on muscular endurance but only in some specific test protocols. However, Davis and Green conclude that because relatively few studies exist concerning caffeine and resistance training, a definite conclusion cannot be reached on the extent to which caffeine affects performance in this regard. The International Society of Sports Nutrition, in its position statement on caffeine and exercise performance, supports this viewpoint, concluding that the scientific literature is equivocal relative to the effects of caffeine supplementation on strength-power performance.

Effect of Dietary Carbohydrate

As noted in chapter 4, carbohydrate is the main energy source for aerobic endurance exercise, and sports scientists have studied both carbohydrates and caffeine to see if there could be a synergistic effect on performance. Yeo and others reported that consuming caffeine (5 mg/kg) with glucose during prolonged aerobic exercise increased both exogenous and total carbohydrate oxidation by 26 and 34 percent, respectively, compared to glucose alone. In a meta-analysis of 21 studies, Conger and others concluded that supplementation with carbohydrate and caffeine provides a small, but significant, effect to improve endurance exercise performance when compared to carbohydrate alone. Gant and others reported that when compared to a standard carbohydrate-electrolyte solution, a caffeinated version improved performance in a 90-minute intermittent shuttle-running trial designed to mimic a soccer match, suggesting that such a caffeine/carbohydrate combination also may be useful in prolonged intermittent, high-intensity sports.

Effect of Caffeine Status

Habituation to caffeine use has been identified as a possible factor influencing any ergogenic effect. Many studies reporting improved performance included a withdrawal period of 2–4 days in order to heighten a caffeine effect. This abstention period was based on some research reporting no effects of caffeine on epinephrine or free fatty acid levels if subjects abstained for less than 1 day. Bangsbo and others reported that 6 weeks of increased caffeine ingestion decreased caffeine sensitivity as reflected by decreased epinephrine levels during exercise. According to James and Rogers, caffeine's ergogenicity is largely due to the termination of adverse effects of caffeine withdrawal rather than a net effect. Ganio and others recommended abstaining from caffeine for at least 7 days before use to optimize an ergogenic effect.

However, Van Soeren and Graham reported no difference in exercise epinephrine levels in habitual users ingesting 6 mg/kg of caffeine following no withdrawal compared to 2 and 4 days of caffeine withdrawal. Similar results were reported by Irwin and others who observed that a 3-mg/kg caffeine dose significantly improves exercise performance irrespective of whether a 4-day withdrawal period is imposed on habitual caffeine users. Graham and Spriet suggested that caffeine withdrawal may have little effect on actual performance and that subjects may consume caffeine products up to the day of the event. As noted later, this issue may be related to the particular individual's sensitivity to caffeine.

Effect of Delivery System

Another factor influencing caffeine's effectiveness may be how it is consumed. Graham and others compared the effects of consuming the same dose of caffeine in coffee or as a capsule in water. In a well-designed, double-blind, repeated-measures study with 5 trials (3 caffeine and 2 placebo), they found that although the plasma epinephrine increased with the coffee, the increase was significantly greater with the caffeine capsule. Additionally, the caffeine capsule was the only treatment that improved exercise performance, a treadmill run to exhaustion at 85 percent VO_2 max. They suggested that some component or components in coffee may moderate the effect of caffeine. However, Liquori and others reported higher peak salivary caffeine levels and more rapid time to peak absorption in coffee or cola compared to capsule. Other studies have reported significant ergogenic effects when coffee was used to deliver caffeine. Nevertheless, in its position stand, the International Society of Sports Nutrition notes that caffeine exerts a greater ergogenic effect when consumed in an anhydrous, or pill, form as compared to coffee. For those who enjoy their coffee the morning of an event, McLellan and Bell reported that consuming coffee 30 minutes prior to taking capsulated caffeine did not negate its beneficial ergogenic effect on cycling endurance performance. Thus, drinking coffee would not seem to impair the potential ergogenic effect of caffeine tablets.

Effect of Exercise in the Heat

Caffeine has been classified as a diuretic and it stimulates metabolism. Theoretically, increased water losses and an elevated metabolism before competition could impair exercise performance under warm, humid environmental conditions, possibly because of retarded sweat losses and excessive increases in body temperature. However, research refutes any ergolytic effects of caffeine related to impairments in thermoregulation or fluid balance. Del Coso and others reported that caffeine, whether consumed alone or in combination with water or a sports drink, did not alter heat production, forearm skin blood flow, or sweat rate and did not impair heat dissipation when exercising for 120 minutes in a hot environment. Ganio and colleagues found that a 6-mg/kg caffeine dose increased performance under cool or warm conditions compared to a placebo, with no difference in rectal temperature.

These findings are supported by two recent meta-analyses. Armstrong and others concluded that in contrast to popular beliefs, caffeine consumption does not result in hypohydration, water-electrolyte imbalances, hyperthermia, or impaired exercise-heat tolerance. Zhang and colleagues concluded that although females were more susceptible to the diuretic effects of caffeine compared to males, increases in urine production following caffeine consumption are offset by the antidiuretic effect of exercise. Position statements of the ACSM and the ISSN conclude that moderate caffeine consumption will not markedly change urine output, induce dieresis during exercise, or harmfully change fluid balance leading to impaired performance.

Athletes will not incur detrimental fluid-electrolyte imbalances if they consume caffeinated beverages in moderation and eat a typical diet. Additionally, Armstrong and others reported that consuming caffeine, either 3 or 6 milligrams per kilogram body weight for 5 days, did not cause hypohydration, and they questioned the widely accepted notion that caffeine consumption acts chronically as a diuretic.

The Placebo Effect

As mentioned in chapter 1, subjects in a study may experience a placebo effect if they think they have received an effective ergogenic, such as caffeine. In a unique study, Beedie and others told subjects they would receive either a placebo, a moderate dose of caffeine, or high dose of caffeine before performing a 10-kilometer cycle time trial. Actually, in all trials, the subjects received only a placebo; no caffeine was provided. Afterward, the subjects were asked which treatment they received, and when they thought they had received caffeine, their performance was better, and even more so when they thought they received the high dose. Although this study clearly provides evidence of a placebo effect, Foad and others have shown there may also be clear pharmacological effects of caffeine on exercise performance. In a meticulous study with male competitive cyclists, six separate tests were used to establish a baseline for 40-kilometer cycling time-trial performance. The cyclists then performed eight more trials, two each under four experimental conditions (C-Y, P-Y, C-N, P-N) involving the interaction of caffeine (C) and placebo (P) and being informed they had (Y) or had not (N) received caffeine. They found that caffeine exerted a pharmacological ergogenic effect but also noted a possible beneficial psychological placebo effect, as the subjects performed somewhat better when informed they were given caffeine but were not. There was also a possible negative placebo (nocebo) effect when subjects were correctly informed they had received no caffeine. Their data support the ergogenic efficacy of caffeine but suggest that both positive and negative expectations may affect performance.

Effect of Dosage: Permissibility

Because caffeine is a stimulant drug, its use as an ergogenic in sports has been regulated by the International Olympic Committee and the WADA. The ISSN notes that caffeine is effective for enhancing sports performance in trained athletes when consumed in low to moderate dosages, about 3 to 6 mg/kg, and overall does not result in further enhancement in performance when consumed in higher dosages, such as greater than 9 mg/kg. However, the amount of caffeine Olympic and international-class athletes have been permitted to use has varied over the years. The International Olympic Committee (IOC) banned the use of caffeine as a drug prior to the 1972 Olympics, removed it from the doping list from 1972 to 1982, banned the use of large amounts (8–10 mg/kg) for the 1984 Olympics (possibly for its ergogenic effects), and under the recommendation of the WADA removed it from the banned list effective January 1, 2004. The WADA felt that the doping list should be adjusted to reflect changing times. The removal of caffeine from the prohibited list may be a reflection of the increased prevalence of caffeinated beverages, such as specialty coffees, fortified colas, energy drinks, and even sports drinks. These drinks, which may be larger and contain more caffeine, may be consumed in quantity by athletes. As noted earlier, caffeine is also found in a wide variety of other food products.

Currently, the WADA has caffeine in its monitoring list, meaning that caffeine levels in international-class athletes are tested and if caffeine abuse increases, it may be returned to the prohibited list. As previously discussed, Del Coso and others reported that many athletes use caffeine but only 0.6 percent had urine caffeine levels above the old limit of 12 μg/mL. Some athletic governing organizations, such as the National Collegiate Athletic Association (NCAA), may test urine samples for caffeine concentration, and a level of 15 micrograms/milliliter is considered to be evidence of doping. Research by Bruce and others found that subjects consuming about 9 mg/kg body weight exceeded this limit. However, athletes need not use such large doses, as they are no more effective than smaller ones. About 5 mg/kg body weight has been shown by multiple studies to be an effective dose.

Individuality

In general, studies have not reported a decrease in performance following caffeine ingestion. In separate studies, Jenkins and others reported a significant effect of caffeine on cycling performance, while Skinner and others found no effect on rowing performance. Both authors noted large interindividual responses to caffeine. In some subjects, adverse reactions to caffeine have resulted in impaired performance. Therefore, individual characteristics should be considered when administering caffeine for performance enhancement.

Caffeine appears to be an effective ergogenic aid in doses that are both safe and legal. However, some athletes believe that taking caffeine may be considered unethical because it is an artificial means of enhancing performance. Given its safety and legality, the decision to use caffeine as a performance enhancer rests with the ethical standards of the individual athlete. Although combining ephedrine with caffeine (as discussed in the next section) may increase the ergogenic effect of caffeine alone, ephedrine use may be illegal—so its use to increase sports performance is unethical.

Self-Experimentation If you are considering using caffeine as a potential ergogenic aid, it is wise to experiment with its use in training prior to use in competition. You might start by taking 200–400 milligrams of caffeine about an hour prior to some of your workouts. For example, if you are a distance runner, do your long runs periodically with and without the coffee or other caffeine source, and judge for yourself if it works for you. To make it a more valid case study, have someone randomly give you, blinded, a placebo (vitamin capsule) or a caffeine capsule before the runs, but without informing you which until you have done each several times. Try this procedure also after abstaining from caffeine for 4–5 days. Keep a record of your feelings and times after the runs so that you can compare differences.

Does drinking coffee, tea, or other caffeinated beverages provide any health benefits or pose any significant health risks?

The health effects of caffeine have been studied for nearly half a century. Early epidemiological research linked coffee or caffeine consumption with the development of a variety of health problems, including cancer, heart disease, osteoporosis, and birth defects. However, a recent Institute of Medicine workshop concluded that moderate consumption of products containing natural caffeine has no adverse effects and may actually benefit health. Concerns arise from the increased number of products with added caffeine and the use of such products by caffeine-naïve populations such as children and adolescents.

Current research involving the health effects of caffeine has used a variety of techniques, including epidemiological prospective cohort studies, randomized clinical trials, and animal models. Investigators have looked at a variety of factors, including different sources of caffeine, such as coffee versus tea, regular versus decaffeinated coffee, and even the method of preparing coffee, such as filtered versus boiled. Investigators suggest that some of the potential health benefits of coffee and tea may be attributed to substances other than the caffeine found in these beverages. For example, green tea contains caffeine and the catechin epigallocatechin-3-gallate (EGCG), which may reduce the risk of several chronic diseases such as the metabolic syndrome, as reviewed by Thielecke and Boschmann. Steinmann and others note its possible role in enhanced immune function.

The following sections highlight some of the key findings relative to the effect of caffeine on various health conditions. Most research involves the consumption of caffeinated beverages, but some involves caffeine in dietary supplements. A current hot topic involves the health effects of caffeinated energy drinks, particularly alcoholic energy drinks, and this is addressed separately from the other health conditions.

Energy Drinks Of special interest in recent years has been the increasing popularity of caffeinated energy drinks, particularly among youngsters and college-age adults. Temple noted that caffeine-containing drinks are marketed to and consumed regularly by young children. Red Bull, the first energy drink, appeared in Austria in 1987 and in the United States in 1997. Hundreds of energy drinks are currently available with caffeine contents ranging from 2.5 to 35.7 milligrams per fluid ounce, or about 50–500 milligrams per serving. According to Bloomberg Business, U.S. energy drink sales totaled almost $10 billion in 2013. Annual sales growth has recently slowed from double-digit rates amid FDA scrutiny over the caffeine content in these products.

Arria and O'Brien indicated that energy drinks are potentially harmful for various reasons, such as increased blood pressure in adolescents, and carry various risks for pregnant women, as discussed later. An American Academy of Pediatrics (AAP) committee report authored by Schneider and others comments on the role of excessive consumption of energy drinks in childhood obesity. The AAP report states that diets of children and adolescents should not include the caffeine and stimulants in energy drinks. Arria and O'Brien also note that the practice of mixing energy drinks with alcohol—a very common practice—has been consistently linked to drinking high volumes of alcohol per drinking session and subsequent serious, alcohol-related consequences, such as driving while intoxicated. As previously discussed, Ulbrich and others observed similar levels of impairment following consumption of alcohol alone compared to alcohol in an energy drink, with no "masking" of intoxication by caffeine in the energy drink. The inability to appraise the true level of impairment has been labeled "wide-awake drunkenness" and can lead to engaging in risky behavior.

Scientists indicate that additional research is needed to ascertain the potential health risks of energy-drink consumption but also suggest that the government should be proactive in protecting the public. For example, current FDA regulations limit the amount of caffeine in cola-type sodas to approximately 48 milligrams per 8-ounce serving, but a similar serving of one highly caffeinated energy drink may contain about 285 milligrams of caffeine. Some question why this FDA regulation does not apply to energy drinks. The FDA did undertake some action relative to energy drinks containing both caffeine and alcohol, announcing in November 2010 that caffeine is an unsafe food additive to alcoholic beverages. This action will prohibit the sale of caffeine/alcohol energy drinks in the United States.

Cardiovascular Disease and Associated Risk Factors Caffeine has been studied for its effect on various risk factors associated with cardiovascular disease. In their review, O'Keefe and others noted an association of two to three cups of coffee/day with reduced risk of coronary artery disease, diabetes, the metabolic syndrome, and all-cause mortality. Although the benefit of coffee is probably related to caffeine, they noted that decaffeinated coffee consumption may also benefit health, which suggests the existence of other potentially beneficial compounds. However, coffee, but not tea, may adversely affect lipid profiles based on the method of preparation. Compared to brewed and filtered coffee typically consumed in North America, boiled coffee, consumed in Europe, has higher levels of diterpenes, which are lipid-increasing compounds. Although research findings are inconsistent regarding the effects of coffee on the serum lipid profile, Reis and others observed no substantial association between coffee or caffeine intake and coronary and carotid atherosclerosis in a 20-year follow-up of 5,000 adults.

High blood pressure is another risk factor that may be affected by caffeine. Recall from chapter 9 that blood pressure is the product of blood flow and resistance to blood flow. Caffeine blocks receptors for adenosine, which is a potent vasodilator. In theory, caffeine may increase resistance to blood flow and increase blood pressure, especially in individuals who are caffeine sensitive and under stress. In a review, James concluded that blood pressure remains sensitive to the pressor effects of caffeine in the diet, with increases of 4 and 2 mmHg for systolic and diastolic blood pressures, respectively. These small increases could be related to increased premature deaths from heart disease and stroke. In a prospective study of almost 44,000 participants over almost 700,000 person-years, Liu and others reported positive associations between coffee consumption and cardiovascular and all-cause mortality. Astorino and others observed that caffeine (6 mg/kg) consumed 1 hour prior to resistance training elevated systolic blood pressure by 8–10 mmHg. An excessive increase in blood pressure during exercise could induce a heart attack or stroke.

However, Schardt cited one study that followed more than 150,000 women for 10 years that reported no difference in hypertension risk among non-coffee drinkers, regular-coffee drinkers, and decaffeinated-coffee drinkers. Steffen and others concluded there is no evidence linking caffeine or coffee consumption to hypertension. They also commented that the quality of the reviewed studies prevented making a recommendation. In their review, Guessous and others suggest that decreased sodium reabsorption by the kidney in individuals with a genotype for rapid caffeine metabolism may actually lead to lower blood pressure.

Some at-risk individuals should be cautious about caffeine use before exercise. Caffeine has also been found to cause a slight arrhythmia, or irregular heartbeat, in some caffeine-sensitive individuals, although in their review, Cheng and others concluded that caffeine consumption does not contribute to the most common type of serious arrhythmia, known as atrial fibrillation. However, individuals known to be caffeine sensitive, particularly those with high blood pressure, may be advised to use caution when exercising, as suggested in chapter 9. Although exercise is generally recommended in rehabilitation programs for those with coronary heart disease (CHD), caffeine consumption may pose a risk. In their review, Higgins and Baku noted an attenuation of the expected increase in coronary artery blood flow during exercise performed by normal subjects 1 hour after ingesting 200–300 mg of caffeine. Namdar and others reported this decreased flow occurs to a much greater degree in CHD patients.

Although caffeine may affect some of the risk factors associated with heart disease, Wu and others reported that their findings do not support the hypothesis that coffee consumption increases the long-term risk of CHD. Actually, habitual, moderate coffee drinking was associated with a lower risk of CHD in women.

Based on contemporary research, most health professional groups, such as the American Heart Association, recommend that moderate coffee consumption, about one to two cups daily, is safe and not associated with heart disease. However, the effects of consuming greater amounts of coffee are not as well known. James indicated that the effect of caffeine to increase blood pressure could account for premature deaths in the region of 14 percent for coronary heart disease and 20 percent for stroke and indicates that strategies for encouraging reduced dietary levels of caffeine deserve serious consideration. Heavy caffeine consumption has also been reported by Verhoef and others to increase levels of homocysteine, which is synthesized from the essential amino acid methionine and has been linked to vascular injury. Individuals who are hypertensive, who are under stress, or who may have other risk factors for heart disease should consult their physician regarding the use of caffeine.

Type 2 Diabetes   Over the past 15 years, several longitudinal studies and extensive reviews have indicated that consumption of caffeinated beverages, such as coffee and tea, was associated with a reduced risk of type 2 diabetes. In a recent meta-analysis of 28 studies, Ding and others found an inverse linear relationship between coffee consumption and reduced risk of type 2 diabetes. This dose-response relationship was observed for up to six cups/day of caffeinated or decaffeinated coffee. These findings suggest that other ingredients in coffee, and possibly tea, such as magnesium, chromium, lignans, and chlorogenic acid, may be involved. For example, chlorogenic acid can delay glucose absorption. Researchers recommend randomized clinical trials as a means to determine active ingredients, which may reveal a combination effect of multiple substances.

Cancer   The American Cancer Society, after reviewing the available scientific evidence, indicated that there is no known association between the consumption of coffee, tea, or other caffeinated beverages and the development of any type of cancer. In support of this viewpoint, Michels and others presented data from two large epidemiological studies involving men and women and reported that the consumption of caffeinated coffee, tea with caffeine, or caffeine was not associated with incidence of colon or rectal cancer. Schardt noted that a review of 66 studies of coffee and pancreatic cancer and 25 studies with kidney cancer concluded that coffee was unlikely to pose a substantial risk.

Lambert commented that tea shows promise in slowing the rate of cancer progression and modifying cancer biomarkers. More research is needed to better understand the cancer prevention mechanisms of action of caffeine and polyphenolic compounds in tea.

In their meta-analysis, Jiang and others reported no association between breast cancer and coffee or caffeine consumption. Among postmenopausal women, however, there was a significant decrease in breast cancer with caffeine consumption, which was even stronger in women with the *BRCA1* gene, which increases breast cancer risk.

Cognitive Functions   The extensive use of caffeine as a social drug is most likely attributable to its stimulating effect on cognitive functions. Lara stated that caffeine intake enhances mental energy; elevates mood; and increases alertness, attention, and cognitive function—effects that are more evident in longer or more difficult tasks or in situations of low arousal. Camfield and others concluded that L-theonine and caffeine in tea increase alertness and attention for up to 2 hours after ingestion. Moderate caffeine intake has been associated with lower risk of depression, cognitive failures, and suicide.

Caffeine intake may also be associated with less aging-related cognitive decline and lower risk for the onset of Alzheimer's disease (AD) and Parkinson's disease (PD). Blood–brain barrier (BBB) dysfunction is part of the pathology of AD and PD. Chen and others note that caffeine exerts protective effects against AD and PD by keeping the BBB intact. According to Cunha and Agostinho, caffeine alleviates AD and PD mental dysfunction in animal models. Research with humans also appears promising. Santos and others reported a trend toward a protective effect of caffeine but noted that the limited number of studies and different methodologies used preclude a more definitive statement. Petzer and Petzer note that caffeine is a promising PD agent not only as an adenosine antagonist but also by preventing the decline in dopamine-secreting neurons that often occurs during aging. Prediger concluded that caffeine is a promising therapeutic tool for the treatment of both motor and nonmotor symptoms in PD. Overall, research findings suggest habitual caffeine intake may be associated with less cognitive decline with aging. D'hooghe and others reported that coffee may provide some protection against relapsing onset multiple sclerosis. The protective effect of four to six cups of coffee/day on multiple sclerosis has recently been confirmed by results from large Swedish and U.S. cohort studies.

Asthma   According to Chapman and Mickleborough, one of the often overlooked effects of caffeine is its role as a very potent respiratory stimulant. Such an effect could be beneficial to individuals with various respiratory disorders. In their meta-analysis, Welsh and others concluded that caffeine, either as oral caffeine or coffee, appears to improve airway function modestly, for up to 4 hours, in people with asthma. Caffeine may help reduce exercise-induced asthma (EIA) symptoms. VanHaitsma and others reported similar protective EIA effects following 6 and 9 mg/kg of caffeine compared to albuterol, a common beta-2 agonist inhalant.

Osteoporosis   Factors underlying the development of osteoporosis are discussed in detail in chapter 8. Calcium loss may lead to osteoporosis. Caffeine tends to accelerate the loss of calcium from bones and lead to its excretion in the urine. However, only about 5 mg of calcium are lost per cup of coffee, which is replaced by 2 tablespoons of milk in the coffee. Barrett-Conner and others reported that one glass of milk/day offsets the decrease in bone mineral density associated with increased coffee consumption in postmenopausal women. In a 21-year prospective study of over 61,000 Swedish women, Hallström and others observed that high coffee consumption ($\geq$4 cups/day) was associated with a 2–4 percent decrease in bone density, but no increase in risk of fracture. The National Institutes of Health indicated that caffeine use does not cause significant losses of calcium. However, drinking milk or eating calcium-rich foods is highly recommended if you drink caffeinated beverages. Individuals with osteoporosis should consult with their physician about the use of calcium supplements.

Pregnancy-Related Health Problems   Animal research has suggested that very high doses of caffeine could cause various problems during pregnancy, including low birth weight, miscarriage, or birth defects, whereas consumption of moderate amounts did not produce such effects.

Similar findings are reported in research with humans. A large prospective study by the CARE Group found a significant association between low birth weight and caffeine consumption. Although Savitz and others found little indication of harmful effects of caffeine in 2,400 women who were light ($\leq$2 cups/day) coffee drinkers, Weng and others, in a prospective study of 1,000 women, reported that increased caffeine consumption, particularly over 200 mg/day, increased the risk of miscarriage. Browne reviewed studies of caffeine and birth defects and concluded that there is little evidence to support a teratogenic effect of caffeine in humans. Using data from the National Birth Defects Prevention Study, Browne and others did not find an association between caffeine intake and birth defects. However, Schardt states the data are not strong enough to conclude there is no increase in risk of birth defects with caffeine use. For example, in their meta-analysis of 60 studies, Greenwood and others found small but statistically significant associations between increased caffeine intake and spontaneous abortion, stillbirth, low birth weight, and small-for-gestational-age births. They concluded that associations between caffeine intake in the normal range and adverse birth outcomes are modest and recommend adherence to current intake limits but no further reduction in caffeine intake.

To be on the safe side, the Food and Drug Administration and the Academy of Nutrition and Dietetics recommend that pregnant women consider abstaining from caffeine use or, if they do drink caffeinated beverages, to do so in moderation. The American College of Obstetrics and Gynecology recommends a caffeine intake of no more than 200 mg/day during pregnancy. Caffeine consumed by the nursing mother gets into breast milk. Santos and others reported no association between maternal caffeine consumption and infant nighttime wakefulness.

Weight Control   Caffeine use may stimulate metabolism, increasing the resting metabolic rate about 10 percent for several hours, an effect that theoretically could facilitate weight loss. In an early review, Greenway noted that caffeine has a long history of safe, nonprescription use as a weight-loss supplement, and that the benefits of treating obesity appear to outweigh the small associated risk. Rudelle and others reported that a beverage containing caffeine, green tea catechins, and calcium increased 24-hour energy expenditure by 4.6 percent, but the contribution of the individual ingredients could not be distinguished. Although the increase in energy expenditure was modest, they concluded that such a beverage may prevent weight gain and provide benefits for weight control. Lopez-Garcia and others found that increased caffeine consumption was associated with decreased weight gain over the course of 12 years, but the differences were less than 1 pound. Regular consumption of coffee or caffeine would appear to make a very minor contribution to weight control, as contrasted to proper diet and exercise. More recently, Gurley and others caution that some weight-loss products may have different effects than traditional caffeine sources because of potential adverse interactions between caffeine and botanical extracts. Excessive amounts may cause adverse effects in some individuals using it for weight loss, especially when combined with ephedrine, as discussed in the following text. Proper weight-control procedures are discussed in chapters 10 and 11.

Sleeplessness   Caffeine use, particularly before retiring for the night, may delay the onset of sleep because of its stimulant effects. Inadequate sleep could be detrimental to cognitive functions the following day and, as noted in chapter 10, could be a contributing factor to weight gain. Individuals who want to improve the quality of their sleep may want to consider caffeine abstinence. Sin and others reported that abstaining from caffeine for a whole day improves sleep quality.

In contrast, preventing sleepiness may be beneficial in some situations. For example, decreased drowsiness and increased alertness may contribute to safer automobile operation under certain conditions. Philip and others found that drinking coffee with about 200 milligrams of caffeine helped improve the quality of nighttime driving. Mets and others reported that 80 mg of caffeine improved performance and reduced sleepiness during a monotonous driving task. These effects may help prevent vehicle accidents related to sleepiness.

Gastric Distress   Some individuals experience stomach irritation due to increased secretion of gastric acids following ingestion of caffeinated beverages. In such cases, individuals should consult their physician or avoid caffeine. In a large cross-sectional study of over 8,000 Japanese subjects, Shimamoto and others found no association between caffeine consumption and several gastric diseases.

Caffeine Naiveté   Abstainers or those who consume little caffeine may experience nervousness, irritability, headaches, or insomnia with moderate doses, although long-term consumption of coffee leads to the development of tolerance and reduction of these "coffee nerves" symptoms. Youngstedt and others reported that moderate aerobic exercise may reduce the anxiety sometimes associated with caffeine intake.

Caffeine Dependence   Although not classified as an addictive drug, some individuals may develop caffeine dependence, often referred to as *caffeinism.* Various health organizations differ on their classification of caffeine dependence. The World Health Organization recognizes caffeine dependence in its *Classification of Mental and Behavioral Disorders.* The American Psychiatric Association's *Diagnostic and Statistical Manual-V,* released in 2013, now lists caffeine withdrawal as a diagnosis under caffeine-related disorders. Juliano and Griffiths noted that caffeine-dependent individuals may experience various symptoms upon caffeine withdrawal, including headaches and nervousness, fatigue or drowsiness, depression, irritability, and difficulty concentrating. However, caffeine dependence is not considered a serious form of drug abuse.

Mortality   In their study of health professionals spanning about 20 years, Lopez-Garcia and others reported that regular coffee consumption was not associated with increased mortality rate in either men or women. However, Kerrigan and Lindsey indicated that in large doses, caffeine can be profoundly toxic, resulting in arrhythmia, tachycardia, vomiting, convulsions, coma, and death. Although rare, death may result from caffeine abuse, usually from overdoses of caffeine-containing diet or stimulant pills. Fatal caffeine overdoses in adults are typically in excess of 5 g. Individuals who take several different over-the-counter dietary supplements may be taking substantial amounts of caffeine along with other drugs. Such combinations, in excess, may be fatal.

Summary   In general, most professional health organizations note that caffeine is regarded as a safe drug. If you are healthy and are not on medications, several cups of coffee or caffeinated beverages should pose no health problems. A moderate dosage is the equivalent of about 200 to 300 milligrams of caffeine per day, or the amount in about two 6- to 8-ounce cups of coffee. One or more supersized 20-ounce cups from a convenience store or coffee house would easily exceed this moderate dose. Women who are pregnant may want to consider abstention, similar to the recommendations for alcohol intake during pregnancy. Moreover, keep in mind that individuals, based on their genetic variations, may respond differently to caffeine intake. Some may be more prone to its possible adverse effects as a potent stimulant.

Key Concepts

▶ Caffeine is a stimulant drug and can affect a variety of metabolic and psychological processes in the body that may affect exercise performance and health.

▶ Research suggests that caffeine may improve performance in a variety of athletic endeavors, particularly prolonged aerobic endurance exercise. An effective dose is approximately 5 milligrams per kilogram body weight.

▶ In general, caffeine is regarded as a safe drug, but physicians may recommend abstinence or use in moderation for some individuals. Various health professionals define moderation as the daily caffeine equivalent of one to two cups of coffee.

Check for Yourself

▶ Procure an automatic blood pressure monitor or have a colleague record your blood pressure. While resting, record your blood pressure several times over a course of 15–20 minutes. Drink a cup of coffee or two and then record your blood pressure again, about every 15 minutes over the course of an hour, again while resting. Plot the results. Does caffeine affect your blood pressure?

Ephedra (Ephedrine): Ergogenic Effects and Health Implications

What is ephedra (ephedrine)?

Ephedra sinica, a plant most commonly referred to as **ephedra**, contains a variety of naturally occurring alkaloids, including **ephedrine** and pseudoephedrine. The Chinese version of ephedra is known as **ma huang**. Ephedrine is considered the most active alkaloid, and its synthetic version is ephedrine hydrochloride. Pure ephedrine is regulated as a drug, and the FDA allows only very small amounts in over-the-counter drugs such as cold medications.

Like caffeine, ephedrine is a stimulant and, because it is derived from the plant ma huang, in the United States it had been classified as a dietary supplement. Ephedra or ephedrine-containing dietary supplements were marketed to promote weight loss, increase energy, and enhance sports performance, with such names as Xtreme Lean, Ultra Lean Extreme, and Ripped Force. These products were popular with some athletes. For example, Bents and Marsh found that almost half of the ice hockey players in one collegiate conference reported having used ephedra at least once in attempts to improve athletic performance.

In 2004, the FDA prohibited the sale of ephedra or ephedrine-containing dietary supplements, mainly because such products may pose some serious health threats, as noted later. Although banned by the FDA in the United States in 2004, several Internet sites still market ephedra. However, most of these products may be extracts from species of ephedra with little or no ephedrine, the active ingredient. It is legal to sell ephedra products that do not contain ephedrine. They are not believed to be harmful, but they also will not induce the pharmacological effects of ephedrine. Ephedra-free products are also marketed to physically active individuals, but they contain other stimulants, such as caffeine, discussed previously, and pseudoephedrine and synephrine, discussed later.

Does ephedrine enhance exercise performance?

In general, although a powerful stimulant, ephedrine by itself has not been shown to consistently enhance exercise performance. In their review, Rawson and Clarkson concluded that although there are few studies of the efficacy of ephedrine in improving exercise performance, these studies are consistent in their findings of no ergogenic effects. Shekelle and others, in a meta-analysis, supported this viewpoint, as did Magkos and Kavouras in their review, indicating that ephedrine and related alkaloids have not been shown, *as yet,* to result in any significant performance improvements. More recently, Jacobs and others reported increased local muscular endurance during the first set of traditional resistance-training exercise following ingestion of caffeine combined with ephedrine and ephedrine alone. They concluded that performance improvement was explained primarily by the effects of ephedrine with no additive effect of caffeine. However, Williams and others found differences in muscle strength or Wingate test performance among placebo, caffeine, and caffeine plus ephedrine.

Ephedrine with caffeine Graham indicated that the combination of ephedrine with caffeine has been suggested to be more potent than caffeine alone. Several studies by Bell and associates have shown that caffeine/ephedrine combinations may enhance exercise performance in various exercise performance tasks, many of a military nature. Using pharmaceutical-grade caffeine and ephedrine doses approximating 4–5 mg/kg and 0.8–1.0 mg/kg, respectively, they reported significant improvements in exercise tasks such as a 30-second Wingate test of anaerobic capacity, a maximal cycle ergometer performance about 12.5 minutes in duration, and a 3.2-kilometer run wearing combat gear weighing about 11 kilograms. In another study of 10-kilometer run performance wearing 11 kg of combat gear, they concluded that the ergogenic effect was due to ephedrine with no additive effect of caffeine. In their review, Magkos and Kavouras indicated that caffeine/ephedrine combinations have been reported in several instances to confer a greater ergogenic benefit than either drug by itself. Research appears to support an ergogenic effect of caffeine/ephedrine supplementation in a number of studies, several involving exercise tasks of a military nature that may be applicable to enhancement of sports performance.

Pseudoephedrine Herbal pseudoephedrine may be found in some dietary supplements but is most commonly found in over-the-counter cold medications. One Sudafed capsule contains 30 milligrams of pseudoephedrine.

Although research is limited, several studies have evaluated the ergogenic effect of pseudoephedrine supplementation and reported performance-enhancing effects on aerobic endurance. Hodges and others reported that pseudoephedrine (2.5 mg/kg), taken 90 minutes prior to a 1,500-meter run, improved performance by 2.1 percent, or about 6 seconds. There were no changes in measured blood parameters, so they assumed it was a central effect. Pritchard-Peschek and others, in a well-designed crossover study with well-trained athletes, reported that the ingestion of 180 milligrams of pseudoephedrine 60 minutes before a cycling time trial improved performance by 5.1 percent. They suggested that possible changes in metabolism or an increase in central nervous system stimulation is responsible for the observed ergogenic effect of pseudoephedrine. Although these two studies provide supportive evidence of an ergogenic effect of pseudoephedrine, a recent study by Pritchard-Peschek and others found no effect of a pseudoephedrine dose of 2.3 or 2.8 mg/kg on 30-minute cycle performance by trained cyclists compared to a placebo. Additional research is recommended.

Do dietary supplements containing ephedra pose any health risks?

Of all dietary supplements, the Consumers Union noted that the herbal supplement ephedra may be the most hazardous. Bent and others noted that ephedra use is associated with a greatly increased risk for adverse reactions compared with other herbs. They indicated that ephedra products accounted for 64 percent of all adverse reactions to herbs in the United States, even though these products represented less than 1 percent of herbal product sales.

Use of ephedra has been associated with numerous health problems. Maglione and others reported adverse psychiatric effects of ephedra use, including psychosis, severe depression, mania or agitation, hallucinations, sleep disturbance, and suicidal ideation. Andraws and others comment that ephedra alkaloids are associated with increased cardiovascular risks but have little health benefit. Even ephedra-free products may increase cardiovascular risk. Haller and others implicated ephedra in risk of seizures and noted that ephedra alone may be dangerous, but ephedra combined with caffeine exaggerates the potential adverse risks. A recent study by Cohen and others reported the presence of the amphetamine isomer β-methylphenylethylamine (BMPEA) in dietary supplements containing *Acacia rigidula,* a shrub found in Texas and Mexico. The researchers called for enforcement action by the U.S. Food and Drug Administration because the safety of BMPEA has not been studies in humans.

The Ephedra Education Council notes that 100 milligrams of ephedrine per day is safe and may be useful for individuals on a weight-loss program, mainly by increasing the resting metabolic rate. However, this dose may cause problems in individuals with existing disease, such as high blood pressure or heart disease, who are attempting to lose weight. Moreover, some individuals may exceed the recommended dosage. Indeed, Haller and Benowitz noted that ephedrine misuse may be associated with significant health risks.

In recent years, the deaths of several prominent collegiate and professional athletes made headlines when it was discovered they were using ephedra-containing supplements during training under warm environmental conditions. Ephedrine was linked to the 2001 heat-stroke death of Minnesota Vikings football player Korey Stringer. The risk-taking behavior associated with sports participants is well known, so athletes taking more than the recommended dose is one of the major problems. Additionally, the purity and amount of ephedra in a product are not well controlled, particularly in products marketed on the Internet. Given these possibilities, and given its physiological effects, ephedrine could be involved in such tragedies.

Synephrine   Ephedra-free dietary supplements have been marketed for weight loss (see figure 13.6). These products may contain synephrine, along with other stimulants such as caffeine. Synephrine is an extract from the Seville orange, or bitter, or sour orange. Neo-synephrine is also known as phenylephrine. Synephrine is a dietary supplement in the United States but classified as a drug in Europe. Synephrine is structurally similar to ephedrine and has been marketed as a safe alternative to ephedra.

There is little evidence to support weight loss with synephrine. Bent and others reported that synephrine was of no statistically significant benefit for weight loss. More recently, Astell and others also concluded that synephrine is not an effective agent to suppress appetite for weight loss.

The Consumers Union also indicates that there is little evidence showing that synephrine is safe, and experts suspect it could cause the same kinds of problems that ephedra does, particularly when it is combined with caffeine. Bui and others reported increases in systolic and diastolic blood pressure for 5 hours after ingesting a

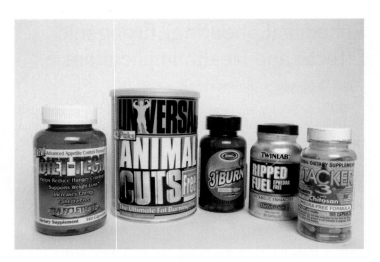

FIGURE 13.6 Ephedra-free dietary supplements are marketed for weight loss; many contain synephrine, a compound similar to ephedrine (see text for discussion).

900-mg dietary supplement containing 6 percent synephrine. Such supplements may increase risks for individuals with hypertension. Bouchard and others reported a case study indicating that synephrine may be associated with ischemic stroke. In their case report, Thomas and others describe a previously healthy 24-year-old male who presented with a myocardial infarction after taking a product containing synephrine.

For individuals interested in weight loss, safer approaches are available, as detailed in chapter 11.

Permissibility in Sports   The use of ephedrine, ephedra, and ma huang in competition is prohibited by the WADA and the IOC. Pseudoephedrine, which was previously on the WADA monitoring program, is now also prohibited in competition as of 2015. Urine limits for ephedrine and pseudoephedrine are 10 and 150 μg/mL, respectively. Synephrine was added to the 2015 monitoring program list. Since ephedra, ephedrine, and pseudoephedrine are banned in competition only, athletes may still use these agents in training. Magkos and Kavouras suggested that caffeine/ephedra mixtures may become one of the most popular ergogenic aids that athletes use in training. The use of pseudoephedrine in training may also increase. As previously mentioned, Gurley and others caution that caffeine/ephedra alkaloid combinations may have unpredictable side effects.

Key Concepts

▶ Ephedra, or ma huang, although classified as a dietary supplement, contains a potent stimulant drug, ephedrine.

▶ In general, research suggests that ephedra or ephedrine supplementation does not enhance exercise or sports performance. However, supplementation with caffeine/ephedrine compounds has been shown to enhance performance in various exercise tasks.

- Use of ephedra or ephedra-containing supplements has been associated with serious health problems, including psychiatric disorders, increased cardiovascular risk factors, and heat stroke in athletes that could be fatal. Ephedra, ephedrine, ma huang, and pseudoephedrine are banned for in-competition use by the WADA.

Check for Yourself

- Visit a local health food store that primarily sells dietary supplements, including sports supplements. Ask the clerk to show you products containing ephedra-related supplements for weight loss and enhanced sports performance; also ask if there are any health risks related to their use. Record the response for class discussion.

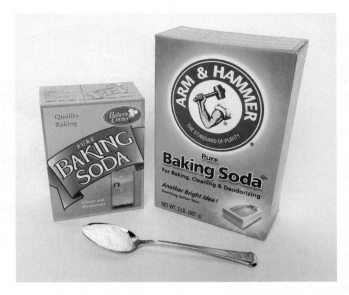

FIGURE 13.7 Baking soda is a commercial version of sodium bicarbonate.

Sodium Bicarbonate: Ergogenic Effects, Safety, and Legality

What is sodium bicarbonate?

Sodium bicarbonate is an alkaline salt found naturally in the human body. It is the major component of the alkaline reserve in the blood, whose major function is to help control excess acidity by buffering acids. Thus, sodium bicarbonate is also known as a buffer salt. Its action is comparable to that of medications you may take to control an upset stomach caused by gastric acidity. Sodium bicarbonate may be purchased in a supermarket as baking soda (see figure 13.7), and it has been marketed to athletes as part of a sports supplement.

Does sodium bicarbonate, or soda loading, enhance physical performance?

During high-intensity anaerobic exercise, sodium bicarbonate helps buffer the lactic acid that is produced when the lactic acid energy system is utilized. You may recall from chapter 3 that the accumulation of excess hydrogen ions from lactic acid in the muscle cell may interfere with the optimal functioning of various enzymes and thus lead to fatigue. The natural supply of sodium bicarbonate that you have in your blood can help delay the onset of fatigue during anaerobic exercise. It may facilitate the removal of the hydrogen ions associated with lactic acid from the muscle cell, thereby mitigating the adverse effects of the increased acidity (see figure 13.8). However, fatigue is inevitable if the rate of lactic acid production exceeds the capacity of your sodium bicarbonate supply to buffer it. Theoretically, an increase in the alkaline reserve could delay the onset of fatigue.

Alkaline salt supplementation has been studied for its ergogenic potential on all three human energy systems, but mainly the lactic acid energy system. Most studies have used a double-blind placebo design in which all subjects took all treatments. In the

popular literature, sodium bicarbonate supplementation has been referred to as *soda loading*, from baking soda, or *buffer boosting*, for increasing the natural blood buffer content.

Supplementation Protocol and Exercise Tasks A relatively standard supplementation protocol has been used, but variations also have been studied. As noted later, the lactic acid energy system has been studied extensively, but research has also studied the effect of sodium bicarbonate supplementation on the ATP-PCr and oxygen energy systems.

The usual experimental protocol has been to have subjects ingest the dose about 1–3 hours before the test. However, other protocols supplemented over the course of 5 days and up to 8 weeks. A typical dosage was 0.15–0.30 gram of sodium bicarbonate per kilogram body weight. Research by McNaughton has indicated that 0.30 gram per kilogram body weight appears to be the optimum dose, with higher dosages providing no additional benefits. This amount totals less than 1 ounce for the average adult. Some studies have used sodium citrate in similar dosages, because it has been shown to increase the alkaline reserve. The exercise task selected was normally one that stressed the lactic acid energy system, or about 1–3 minutes of maximal exercise. Often these exercise tasks were classified as supramaximal, because they used workloads greater than 100 percent VO_2 max. Repeated bouts of intense exercise interspersed with short rest periods have also been used, such as five 100-yard swims with a 2-minute rest between each.

Lactic Acid Energy System More than 70 years ago, German scientists reported that the ingestion of sodium bicarbonate and other alkaline salts could help improve anaerobic work capacity. Since then, many studies have failed to support this finding, but now a substantial number of well-controlled experiments by highly respected investigators in sports nutrition research have

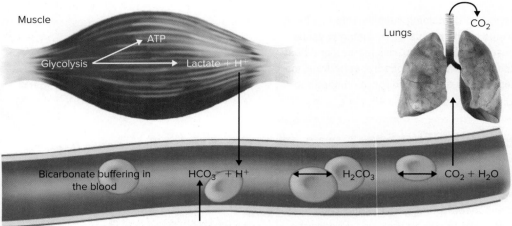

Muscle

Glycolysis → ATP → Lactate + H⁺

Lungs

CO_2

Bicarbonate buffering in the blood

$HCO_3^- + H^+$ ⟷ H_2CO_3 ⟷ $CO_2 + H_2O$

$NA^+HCO_3^-$ Sodium bicarbonate supplement (~300 mg/kg)

FIGURE 13.8 Alkaline salts, such as sodium bicarbonate, are theorized to reduce the acidity in the muscle cell by facilitating the efflux of hydrogen ions from the cell interior, promoting a more homeostatic environment for continued muscle contraction.

provided supportive data, not only for the underlying ergogenic mechanism but also for the performance-enhancing effects.

A study by Raymer and others, using magnetic resonance spectroscopy, provided support for the main theory underlying the ergogenic efficacy of sodium bicarbonate supplementation. They reported that sodium bicarbonate ingestion delayed the onset of intracellular acidification during incremental exercise, which would help maintain a more homeostatic cellular environment to delay the onset of fatigue.

Based on the available scientific evidence, sodium bicarbonate supplementation does appear to enhance performance in exercise tasks dependent upon the lactic acid energy system (see figure 13.9). A consistent finding is an increased serum pH following sodium bicarbonate supplementation, the desired effect to induce buffering of lactic acid. Regarding other factors that have been investigated, approximately half of the well-controlled laboratory studies suggest that ingestion of sodium bicarbonate will reduce acidosis in the muscle cell, decrease the psychological sensation of fatigue at a standardized level of exercise, and increase performance in high-intensity anaerobic exercise tasks to exhaustion.

Various field studies have reported significant improvements in events that primarily use the lactic acid energy system, such as 400 or 800 meters in highly trained track athletes, 100-meter swims in experienced swimmers, and 5-kilometer bicycle races in trained cyclists. In support of these field studies showing improved performance following sodium bicarbonate supplementation, a laboratory study by Van Montfoort and others, comparing different sodium mixtures, reported that sodium bicarbonate improved run time to exhaustion in a test designed to evaluate the lactic acid energy system;

the run to exhaustion approximated 77–82 seconds. Artioli and others reported a potential benefit of sodium bicarbonate supplementation in sports with multiple high-intensity bouts separated

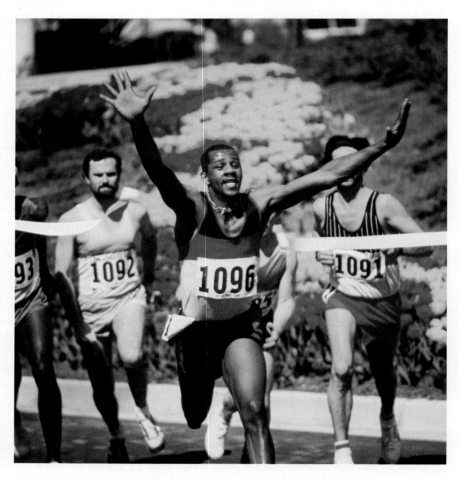

FIGURE 13.9 Sodium bicarbonate may enhance sports performance in a variety of events dependent primarily upon the lactic acid energy system (anaerobic glycolysis), such as the 400-meter sprint in track.

by brief periods of recovery. They reported that a standard bicarbonate-loading protocol (0.3 gram/kg 2 hours before testing) significantly improved performance in the latter phases of both a specific judo test and a Wingate test for anaerobic capacity of the upper arms. In a related study involving boxing, Siegler and Hirscher reported that sodium bicarbonate supplementation significantly increased the number of punches landed, or punch efficiency, during four 3-minute rounds, each separated by 1-minute seated recovery.

However, as with most research with nutritional ergogenic aids, not all studies find positive effects. For example, Kozak-Collins and her associates reported that sodium bicarbonate supplementation taken at moderate altitude did not improve the performance of competitive female cyclists on repeated 1-minute interval cycle tasks at 95 percent VO_2 max, nor did van Someren and others find any benefits on repeated 45-second high-intensity cycling bouts. More recently, Tan and others reported no effect of bicarbonate loading on sprint swim performance in female water polo players during a simulated match.

Although not all studies show ergogenic effects, separate reviews by Requena, McNaughton and others, and most recently Peart and others have all concluded that sodium bicarbonate is an effective ergogenic aid in events that depend primarily on the lactic acid energy system. In their meta-analysis of 40 studies generating 58 effect sizes, 27 of which were in tasks ≤ 2 minutes, Peart and others concluded that bicarbonate loading (200-400 mg/kg) was more effective in untrained compared to trained subjects and for single-bout compared to multiple-bout activities. Greater effects were observed in performance tasks measuring total work and time to exhaustion compared to performance time or power. The majority of the studies conducted subsequent to these reviews have indicated that sodium bicarbonate or sodium citrate supplementation was an effective ergogenic aid.

ATP-PCr Energy System Based on the available scientific data, alkaline salt supplementation does not appear to be an effective ergogenic aid for exercise tasks dependent primarily upon the ATP-PCr energy system. Most studies have reported no beneficial effects on performance in exercise bouts lasting less than 30 seconds or in resistive exercise tasks stressing strength, power, or short-term local muscle endurance. For example, McNaughton and Cedaro reported no ergogenic effect on maximal cycle ergometer performance in either 10-second or 30-second trials. This lack of an ergogenic effect is most likely because such exercise tasks do not maximally stress the normal alkaline reserve. However, Price and others reported that ingestion of sodium bicarbonate improved performance in multiple, intermittent 14-second maximal sprints (one sprint every 3 minutes) during a 30-minute cycle ergometer trial. Moreover, Bishop and Claudius reported that sodium bicarbonate ingestion can improve intermittent-sprint performance. The test protocol involved two 36-minute halves with sprints interspersed with lesser-intensity exercise tasks, and the investigators suggested that sodium bicarbonate may be a useful supplement for team-sport athletes. Performance in these multiple sprints may have been somewhat dependent on the lactic acid energy system.

Oxygen Energy System Although sodium bicarbonate has been studied mainly for its buffering effects, the sodium content could theoretically expand blood volume and benefit aerobic endurance performance, as suggested in chapter 9. The effect of alkaline salt supplementation on performance in events that depend increasingly on the oxygen energy system, such as events approximating 4 minutes or more in duration, are equivocal. Several early studies have shown ergogenic effects for sodium bicarbonate and sodium citrate. McNaughton and Cedaro reported greater cycle ergometer work output in a 4-minute trial as did Linossier and others in an exhausting exercise task at 120 percent of VO_2 peak lasting 4–5 minutes. Bicarbonate ingestion has also been reported by Bird and others to improve 1,500-meter run performance, while Shave and others found that sodium citrate improved performance in a 3,000-meter run by almost 11 seconds. Using well-trained male college runners as subjects, Ööpik and others found that sodium citrate supplementation improved performance in a simulated 5-kilometer treadmill run by 30 seconds. More recently, Egger and colleagues found 300 mg/kg of bicarbonate to increase time to exhaustion at 110 percent of anaerobic threshold in well-trained cyclists. Although primarily aerobic in nature, such exercise tasks may still depend somewhat on the lactic acid energy system. However, several studies have shown ergogenic effects of alkaline salt supplementation on exercise tasks that depend primarily on oxidative metabolism. Potteiger and others reported that sodium citrate supplementation significantly improved performance by 1.7 minutes in 30-kilometer cycling performance, and McNaughton and others reported that sodium bicarbonate supplementation, compared to the placebo trial, produced a 13 percent improvement in maximal cycle ergometer work over 60 minutes.

Conversely, other studies report no ergogenic effect of alkaline salt supplementation. Potteiger and others reported no beneficial effect of sodium bicarbonate supplementation to male runners on performance in a run to exhaustion at 110 percent of the lactate threshold following 30 minutes of running at the lactate threshold. Schabort and others also found no effect of varying doses of sodium citrate (0.2, 0.4, and 0.6 g/kg) on cycling endurance. The laboratory cycling protocol was designed to compare with an actual 40-kilometer road race, with ten sets of sprints within the 40-kilometer distance. Although the sodium citrate produced dose-dependent changes in blood alkalinity, there was no significant effect on total 40-kilometer time or on the various sprint performance times. Vaher and others reported that sodium citrate ingestion (500 mg/kg) increased water retention and plasma volume but did not decrease core temperature or improve 5-kilometer run time in a warm environment.

Stephens and others indicated that sodium bicarbonate ingestion has been shown to increase both muscle glycogenolysis and glycolysis during brief submaximal exercise, which could be detrimental to performance during more prolonged, exhaustive exercise. However, no studies have evaluated this potential ergolytic effect.

Is sodium bicarbonate supplementation safe and legal?

The dosage of sodium bicarbonate used in most of these studies, about 300 milligrams per kilogram body weight, appears to be effective yet medically safe. Relative to possible disadvantages, several investigators have noted that some subjects developed gastrointestinal distress, including nausea and diarrhea. Shave and others noted a high potential for gastrointestinal distress in their study that used 0.5 gram of sodium citrate per kilogram body weight, and suggested that this may limit the use of this strategy by athletes in competition. Excessive doses could lead to alkalosis, with symptoms of apathy, irritability, and possible muscle spasms. Some athletes experience gastrointestinal distress following an acute high dose of sodium bicarbonate. Driller and others compared an acute dose to the same dose spread serially over 3 days. They found no difference in 4-minute power output in well-trained cyclists and concluded that serial loading is as effective as an acute dose and may be more practical and convenient for some athletes.

Use of sodium bicarbonate currently is not prohibited by the WADA. As noted, sodium bicarbonate (baking soda) use by athletes has been dubbed *soda loading,* possibly to liken it to *carbohydrate loading.* As you may recall, the purpose of carbohydrate loading is to increase the storage of muscle and liver glycogen as a means to prevent fatigue in prolonged endurance events. Soda loading is viewed by some in a similar context, an attempt to increase the supply of a natural body ingredient helpful in delaying fatigue. However, because sodium bicarbonate may be regarded as a drug, it remains to be seen whether this technique will be deemed illegal. Tim Noakes, in the newest edition of his classic text *Lore of Running,* indicated that the use of sodium bicarbonate may be prohibited by the International Olympic Committee in the near future. Currently there is no test to detect its use, except for urinary pH, which can also be affected by some antacids, and at present sodium bicarbonate is considered to be legal for use in sports.

Key Concepts

▶ Sodium bicarbonate supplementation appears to be an effective ergogenic aid in exercise tasks that depend primarily upon the lactic acid energy system (anaerobic glycolysis), such as a 400-meter dash in track.

▶ Ingestion of sodium bicarbonate is generally regarded as safe but may cause acute gastrointestinal distress and diarrhea. Supplementation over a longer time frame may be effective and less likely to cause intestinal problems.

Anabolic Hormones and Dietary Supplements: Ergogenic Effects and Health Implications

Several natural hormones in the body may exert significant anabolic effects on body composition by stimulating protein synthesis, particularly human growth hormone (HGH), insulin, insulin-like growth factors (IGF-1), and testosterone. As noted in previous chapters, several nutrient supplements, such as specific amino acids, have been utilized in attempts to increase the secretion of these hormones for anabolic purposes. Two of these hormones, HGH and testosterone, as well as drugs patterned after testosterone, have been used directly to increase muscle mass. Additionally, several prohormones that may be converted into testosterone have been marketed as dietary supplements, and some herbal supplements are marketed for their potential to stimulate testosterone production.

It should be noted that the WADA prohibits the use of the anabolic hormones discussed in this section, including human growth hormone, anabolic/androgenic steroids, and anabolic prohormone dietary supplements.

Is human growth hormone (HGH) an effective, safe, and legal ergogenic aid?

HGH is a natural hormone, which is secreted by the anterior pituitary gland and then circulates via the bloodstream to affect most cells in the body. HGH increases insulin-like growth factor (IGF-1) secretion from the liver and within other tissues, such as muscle, which may function as an autocrine hormone and work directly in the muscle. IGF-1 mediates the various metabolic effects of HGH. Exercise stimulates release of HGH, which, according to Widdowson and others, may persist over 24 hours and potentially contribute to the physiological changes induced by exercise training.

HGH is an anabolic hormone that stimulates bone growth and the development of muscle tissue through its effects on protein, carbohydrate, and fat metabolism. A detailed discussion of the role of HGH is beyond the scope of this text. It is important to note, however, that extensive research into its effects began only when genetically engineered versions (recombinant HGH, or rHGH) of the natural body hormone became available in the early 1990s. rHGH was developed for medical applications, primarily for children and older adults with HGH deficiency. rHGH may optimize growth in young children and may confer some health benefits on aging adults. Available data suggest that in elderly men, who normally have reduced levels of HGH, injections of the hormone may help improve body composition and functional capacity. Meta-analyses and reviews, such as those by Rubeck and others, Widdowson and Gibney, and Widdowson and others, reported that rHGH therapy in individuals who suffered from HGH deficiency helped to improve body composition, such as decreases in body fat and increases in lean body mass, and increase aerobic exercise capacity, including VO_2max. However, these investigators noted that rHGH therapy failed to increase muscle strength, possibly because some studies have found that the increase in lean body mass was primarily water, not muscle tissue.

Whether or not rHGH injections enhance exercise performance is a subject of debate. In general, the available research does not support an anabolic or ergogenic effect of rHGH supplementation in younger individuals. For example, Yarasheski and others studied the effect of rHGH versus a placebo on adult males who weight-trained for 12 weeks. They reported significant increases in lean body mass in the group receiving rHGH, but there were no significant increases in skeletal muscle protein synthesis and size, as measured by magnetic resonance imaging, or in muscular strength, over the effects produced by weight training alone in the placebo group. Other studies have supported this general finding with resistance-trained athletes. In her review, Anne Loucks concluded that supraphysiological doses of rHGH have only increased total body water, lean body mass, and whole body protein synthesis in general without specifically increasing skeletal muscle protein synthesis or skeletal muscle mass, strength, or power in untrained young men or experienced young weight lifters. The review by Dean also concludes that there is no evidence of increased muscle strength with rHGH use in trained athletes.

However, a few studies have suggested that short-term rHGH use may benefit physical performance. For example, using recreationally trained young male and female athletes as subjects, Meinhardt and others found that rHGH injected subcutaneously (2 milligrams daily for 8 weeks) significantly reduced fat mass and significantly increased sprint capacity. However, the increase in sprint capacity was not maintained 6 weeks after discontinuation of the injections.

In a baseball scandal in the United States, some professional athletes admitted using rHGH to train harder and recover more rapidly, and anecdotal reports suggest that it may work for these intended purposes. In his review of rHGH as an ergogenic aid, Holt notes that although most scientific studies have not shown a performance-enhancing effect, athletes continue to use it. Based on his review, he believes the scientists are wrong. Time will tell.

Although athletes may continue to use rHGH, that may not be a wise idea based on its potential health risks and permissibility in sports. The potential adverse health effects of rHGH are substantial, including insulin resistance, high blood pressure, and increased risk of congestive heart failure. Liu and others indicated that because rHGH therapy is associated with increased rates of adverse events, it cannot be recommended as an antiaging therapy. Tentori and Graziani suggest that growth hormone or its mediator, IGF-1, has been associated with colon, breast, and prostate cancers. Most researchers caution that other long-term health risks of HGH administration are unknown. This is particularly distressing, as one report indicated that approximately 5 percent of high school students have used HGH.

Use of rHGH is prohibited by the WADA. Although Baumann noted that although detection of the application of rHGH is difficult, possibly because of its rapid half-life, some tests are available. They also note that as the tests for detection of rHGH doping become more sophisticated, athletes may turn to doping with recombinant rHIGF-1. Products identified as IGF-1 supplements are available on the Internet and the black market. Cox and Eichner reported that IGF-1 was detected in four of six commercial supplements marketed as all-natural and containing deer antler velvet. IGF-1 is also on the WADA prohibited list. According to Guha and others, progress is under way to develop an IGF-1 doping test.

Some dietary supplements are marketed as HGH products, such as HGH Surge™, but they contain only nutrients, such as amino acids and chromium, that are theorized to be ergogenic. However, as noted in previous chapters, such nutrients have not been shown to have anabolic effects and some may be contaminated with illegal drugs that may lead to a positive doping test.

Are testosterone and anabolic/androgenic steroids (AAS) effective, safe, and legal ergogenic aids?

Testosterone, the male steroid sex hormone produced by the testes, was one of the first anabolic agents used in attempts to enhance physical performance, possibly as early as the 1936 Berlin Olympic Games. As documented in the study by Bhasin and the review by Evans, testosterone is a very effective ergogenic aid, increasing lean muscle mass, decreasing body fat, and increasing strength even without resistance training; these anabolic effects were augmented in subjects who also trained. Rogerson and others reported that testosterone injection once per week to resistance-trained individuals increased muscular strength and 10-second cycle sprint performance in 3–6 weeks. Testosterone must be injected because ingested testosterone will be catabolized by digestive enzymes. Although injected testosterone use is still prevalent among various athletic groups, oral drug forms of testosterone have been developed, as noted here.

Testosterone therapy has been studied for its health potential as well. Bain cited a host of adverse symptoms such as fatigue, depression, irritability, decreased self-confidence, increased risk for the metabolic syndrome, type 2 diabetes, anemia, stroke, and coronary heart disease associated with decreasing testosterone levels in the aging male. In their meta-analysis of 29 randomized clinical trials, Isidori and others concluded that testosterone therapy in older males (mean = 64.5 years) decreased body fat, markers of bone resorption, and total cholesterol while increasing fat-free mass, leg/knee extension strength, and bone mineral density of the lumbar spine. Bain noted that testosterone therapy is controversial. For example, Basaria and others noted that a testosterone therapy study was terminated early because of a significantly higher rate of adverse cardiovascular events in the testosterone group than in the placebo group. However, a recent meta-analysis by Morgentaler and others suggests no increase in cardiovascular disease risk in older men receiving testosterone therapy. Furthermore, Grech and colleagues note no increased risk of prostate cancer, significant worsening of urinary symptoms, or sleep apnea. Bain suggests that short-term (4–6 months) testosterone therapy may be justified for some older men, particularly those at low risk for prostate cancer. In March 2015, the FDA required labels on testosterone replacement therapy products warning of increased risk for heart attacks and strokes.

Anabolic/androgenic steroids (AAS) represent a class of synthetic drugs designed to mimic the effects of testosterone. The chemical structure of testosterone may be modified in attempts to maximize the anabolic muscle-building effects and minimize the androgenic male secondary sex characteristics; both oral and injectable AAS have been developed.

In the United States, AAS are classified as Schedule III drugs under the Controlled Substances Act and may be used in testosterone therapy for aging adults, as noted earlier.

AAS are the drugs of choice for many strength athletes and bodybuilders to improve performance and appearance. AAS have been used by professional athletes for years. In recent years, Congress and the FBI have investigated anabolic steroid use among prominent baseball players.

Bahrke and others noted that AAS use is prevalent among adolescent athletes, particularly boys in strength-related sports. Yesalis and others commented that adolescent nonathletes and females also use AAS to enhance physical appearance and self-image, as well as to increase muscle mass. Pope and others note that lifetime AAS use by teenagers has been relatively stable since 1991. According to the Centers for Disease Control and Prevention's 2013 Youth Risk Behavior Survey, 2.2 percent of adolescent females and 4.0 percent of adolescent males have taken steroids at least one time.

Nyberg and Hallberg note that AAS influence opioid and dopamine secreting reward centers in the brain. An increased sensitivity of the AAS user to opioid narcotic and stimulant drugs may lead to addiction. In a cross-sectional survey, Ip and others reported that male AAS users were significantly more likely than nonusers to have used cocaine within the last 12 months and to meet the psychiatric diagnostic criteria for substance abuse disorder.

The effects of AAS on body composition and strength have been studied rather extensively. Although there may be some flaws in the experimental designs used, most reviewers agree that AAS use may increase muscle mass and strength and decrease total body fat, a judgment supported by reviews of laboratory studies that included meta-analysis as part of the evaluative criteria. In a cross-sectional comparison of strength-trained AAS users and nonusers, Nordström and others reported higher fat-free mass and lower gynoid fat in AAS users, but no difference between the groups in android fat. Schroeder and others found that AAS supplementation was also effective with healthy older men, significantly increasing muscle mass and strength after only 6 weeks. The increased muscle mass may be attributed to hypertrophy and the formation of new muscle fibers, in which key roles are played by the androgen receptors, as depicted in figure 13.10.

Baume and others note that although AAS are used mainly by strength athletes, endurance athletes have also used AAS because they are theorized to facilitate a better recovery and thus permit a higher training load. However, they found that compared to a placebo, two different anabolic steroids administered 12 times during a month of hard endurance training had no effect on standardized treadmill running performance test or blood markers for recovery from exercise. Research with AAS and endurance performance in young athletes is limited, but that which is available does not support an ergogenic effect. However, Sattler and others reported that supplemental testosterone and human growth hormone increased aerobic endurance in older men, which may have been associated with the accompanying significant reduction in body fat.

AAS use has been associated with a number of medical problems, listed in table 13.4, that are also discussed in reviews by Yesalis and Bahrke, Hartgens and Kuipers, and Talih and others, as well as in a recent Endocrine Society statement authored by Pope and others. Adverse cardiovascular effects include cardiomyopathy, myocardial infarction, stroke, clotting disorders, hypertension, decreased HDL-cholesterol, and polycythemia (abnormal increases in hematocrit and hemoglobin). Major mood disorders, aggressiveness, high-risk violent behavior, and psychosis may be observed with high AAS usage. AAS dependence, occurring in about 30 percent of AAS users, is related to muscle dysmorphia, which is discussed in chapter 12. Neurotoxic effects from long-term, high-dose use can cause permanent and irreversible cognitive impairments. AAS use can decrease endogenous testosterone production and lead to hypogonadism, decreased spermatogenesis, and male infertility. Intramuscular AAS injections can increase the risk of infections from unsterile needles. AAS use with high-volume weight lifting can increase the risk of rhabdomyolysis (abnormal muscle breakdown) and tendon rupture. Use of oral AAS can lead to liver damage, including elevated enzyme activity and peliosis hepatis (blood-filled cysts). AAS may cause premature cessation of bone growth in children and adolescents and may result in the appearance of several male secondary sex characteristics in females, some of which may be irreversible, such as deepening of the voice.

However, many of the adverse health effects of AAS use appear to be reversible. For example, Hartgens and others found that bodybuilders who cycled off AAS steroids for 3 months had similar lipoprotein profiles and liver enzymes as their non-drug-using counterparts. Moreover, earlier reviews noted that although the short-term health effects of AAS have been increasingly studied and reviewed, and while AAS use has been associated with adverse and even fatal effects, the incidence of serious effects thus far reported has been extremely low. In a review, van Amsterdam and others indicated that severe side effects of AAS use appear only following prolonged use at high doses, and their occurrence is limited. They conclude that, based on the scores for acute and chronic adverse health effects, the prevalence of use, social harm, and criminality, AAS were ranked a group of drugs with a relatively low harm. Nevertheless, Urhausen and others reported that several years after discontinuation of anabolic steroid abuse, strength athletes (bodybuilders and powerlifters) who used AAS showed a slight concentric left ventricular hypertrophy in comparison with AAS-free strength athletes. Left ventricular hypertrophy increases the risk of heart attack.

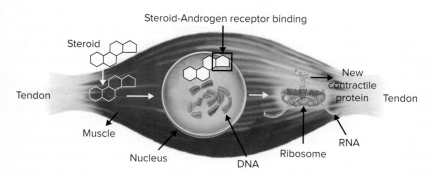

Steroid-Androgen receptor binding

Steroid

Tendon

New contractile protein

Tendon

Muscle

Nucleus

DNA

Ribosome

RNA

FIGURE 13.10 Anabolic steroids picked up by androgen receptors in the cell nucleus initiate the process of protein formation in cells such as muscle fibers, leading to muscle hypertrophy.

TABLE 13.4	Possible health risks associated with use of anabolic/androgenic steroids (AAS)

Cosmetic-related effects

Facial and body acne
Female-like breast enlargement in males (gynecomastia)
Premature baldness
Masculinization in females
Facial and body hair growth in females
Premature closure of growth centers in adolescents, leading to stunted growth
Deepening of the voice in females

Psychological effects

Increased aggressiveness and possible violent behavior

Reproductive effects

Reduction of testicular size
Reduction of sperm production
Decreased libido
Impotence in males
Enlargement of the prostate gland
Enlargement of the clitoris

Cardiovascular risk factors and diseases

Atherosclerotic serum lipid profile
  Decreased HDL-cholesterol
  Increased LDL-cholesterol
High blood pressure
Impaired glucose tolerance
Increased size of left ventricle
Stroke
Heart disease

Liver function

Jaundice
Peliosis hepatis (blood-filled cysts)
Liver tumors

Athletic injuries

Tendon rupture

One risk-reduction objective of *Healthy People 2020* is to decrease AAS use by middle and high school students. From 2009 to 2013, prevalence rates for AAS use decreased by 62, 49, and 33 percent, respectively, among 8th, 10th, and 12th graders. Moreover, the U.S. Congress has passed legislation to classify AAS as controlled substances, thus limiting their production and distribution by pharmaceutical companies. Penalties may be severe. According to Melnik and others, some AAS users obtain illegal prescriptions from physicians. However, many obtain these drugs illegally on the black market, where quality is not controlled, and chemical analysis has revealed some potentially hazardous constituents in these "homemade" drugs. As previously discussed, AAS users are known to use other illicit drugs as well,

each carrying independent health risks. The use of testosterone or AAS for the purpose of gaining body weight and strength is not recommended.

The WADA prohibits the use of AAS in training and competition. The American College of Sports Medicine (ACSM), the National Athletic Trainers' Association (NATA), and the National Strength and Conditioning Association (NSCA) have developed position stands regarding the use of AAS in sports. These groups condemn AAS use on the basis of ethics, the ideals of fair play in competition, and concerns for the athlete's health. The NSCA indicates that optimizing nutritional strategies for athletes is a key to preventing AAS use and abuse, and such strategies for strength/power athletes have been presented in chapter 12. Although an extensive discussion of AAS is beyond the scope of this text, the ACSM, NATA, and NSCA reports provide detailed reviews for the interested reader, as does the most recent review by Yesalis and Bahrke.

Are anabolic prohormone dietary supplements effective, safe, and legal ergogenic aids?

Several dietary supplements marketed to athletes as potent anabolic agents are of special interest, particularly dehydroepiandrosterone (DHEA), androstenedione, and related compounds. These supplements are classified as prohormones because they are precursors for testosterone and are thus theorized to increase muscle mass and decrease body fat. They may be derived from certain plants, such as wild yams. Although these prohormones have been marketed as dietary supplements, in 2005 the FDA classified them as controlled drugs, similar to anabolic steroids.

Dehydroepiandrosterone (DHEA) and its sulfated metabolite (DHEAS) are produced in the body by the adrenal and gonadal glands and may be converted into androstenedione with subsequent conversion to testosterone in peripheral tissues, including fat and muscle tissue. Body levels of DHEA are high in young adulthood and gradually decrease to low levels with aging. Although Abbasi and others reported a low, but significant, inverse relationship between natural DHEA levels and body fat in men age 60–80 years, Collomp and others noted that DHEA and DHEAS result in minimal increases in testosterone and that current research does not support an ergogenic effect. Studies by Wallace and Brown and their associates revealed no significant effects of DHEA supplementation (50–100 milligrams/day for 8–12 weeks) on serum testosterone levels, lean body mass, or muscular strength in either healthy middle-aged or young men involved in resistance training. In a 2-year study, Nair and others reported no effect on body composition, physical performance, insulin sensitivity, or quality of life in elderly men and women who received DHEA supplementation.

DHEA has also been marketed as an anti-aging agent to help prevent the development of chronic diseases, but Sirrs and Bebb noted that no good scientific data support this speculation. They caution against use of DHEA supplements, as high serum DHEA levels have been associated with several health risks, including several forms of cancer. Nevertheless, a study by Villareal and others provided some preliminary data supporting positive effects of DHEA supplementation on bone mineral density, body fat, and lean body mass in elderly subjects with very low levels of natural DHEA. Kenny and others reported that DHEA supplementation (50 milligrams daily for 6 months) improved muscle strength and physical function in frail older women who participated in 90-minute twice-weekly exercise sessions but had no effect on bone mineral density, even though calcium and vitamin D supplements were also provided. Although such effects may help prevent falls and fractures in the elderly, these research groups indicated that more defined and specific research is needed before DHEA supplementation may be recommended as a standard treatment.

These data with elderly subjects with very low DHEA levels do not support DHEA supplementation to young- or middle-aged individuals. Earnest reported that DHEA supplementation at relatively low doses (50–150 milligrams) does not enhance serum testosterone in young men. Acacio and others found that 6 months of supplementation with DHEA to young men age 18–42 elevated levels of a metabolite that raised concerns about the potential negative impact of DHEA supplementation on the prostate gland. The Consumers Union advised that individuals avoid DHEA supplementation, as there is not enough evidence concerning its effectiveness or safety.

Androstenedione and related compounds, such as androstenediol and norandrostenediol, are potent anabolic agents, one step removed from the formation of testosterone. Androstenedione received considerable notoriety during the 1998 baseball season when Mark McGwire, who established a home run record at that time, acknowledged using the dietary supplement. Subsequently, androstenedione-related products flooded the marketplace for resistance-trained individuals, even though no reputable research was available supporting beneficial effects.

Doses of androstenedione and related androgens used in studies varied, usually between 100 to 300 milligrams per day. Studies using the higher doses generally showed an increase in serum testosterone. Leder and others, although finding no significant effects of a 100-milligram dose, reported significant increases in serum testosterone in adult men following a 300-milligram dose, but no exercise performance was measured. Earnest and others also reported significant, but small, increases in total testosterone with a 200-milligram dose of androstenedione, but not androstenediol, supplementation. In a study with young women, Brown and others reported that androstenedione intake (100 or 300 milligrams) significantly increased serum testosterone concentrations.

In general, most studies that have evaluated the ergogenic effects of androstenedione supplementation have shown no beneficial effects. In a short-term study, Rasmussen and others found no effect of oral androstenedione supplementation (100 milligrams/day for 5 days) on serum testosterone or muscle protein anabolism in young men. In a more prolonged study, Wallace and others reported no significant effects of androstenedione supplementation (100 milligrams/day for 12 weeks) on serum testosterone levels, lean body mass, or muscular strength in resistance-trained middle-aged men. Using three individual 100-milligram androstenedione doses daily (total 300 milligrams/day), King and others reported no significant effects on serum testosterone, body fat, lean body

mass, muscle fiber diameter, or muscular strength in young men during 8 weeks of resistance training. Although androstenedione supplementation has been reported to increase testosterone in some studies, reviews by Earnest, Brown and others, and Ziegenfuss and Maughan have concluded there is no resulting increase in protein synthesis, muscle growth, muscle mass, or strength.

Use of androstenedione and related prohormones may be associated with increased health risks. Earnest indicated that androstenedione supplementation has been associated with impaired lipid metabolism, such as decreased HDL-cholesterol and increased LDL-cholesterol, which might increase risk for cardiovascular disease. Several studies have reported significant increases in estrogen hormones (estradiol or estrone), which could exert feminizing effects in males, such as gynecomastia (breast enlargement). Other adverse effects on gonadal hormones may be associated with testicular shrinkage and infertility. Leder also notes that women and children who use such supplements may be at risk. Unfortunately, given the recency of such supplements, no long-term safety data are available.

For athletes who may be tested for doping, the use of DHEA or androstenedione and related prohormones has been banned by the WADA and the International Olympic Committee; their use has also been banned by other sports organizations, including the National Collegiate Athletic Association and the National Football League. Although anabolic prohormones are currently banned for sale in the United States, a number of substitutes for these products are being marketed on the Internet. For example, Testosterone Factors™ is a blend of vitamins, amino acids, and herbal ingredients, none of which is banned. However, Maughan notes that some apparently legitimate dietary supplements on sale contain ingredients that are not declared on the label but that are prohibited by the doping regulations of the WADA and the International Olympic Committee. For example, Epstein and Dohrmann noted that in one study, 25 percent of 58 sports supplements tested contained steroids or stimulants. Geyer and others secured 634 nutritional supplements from 13 countries, and 14.8 percent contained anabolic/androgenic steroids not declared on the label. The administration of some of the supplements resulted in positive doping tests.

Key Concepts

▶ The use of anabolic drugs or hormones to increase body weight may be effective but may also lead to a variety of health problems. The WADA prohibits the use of anabolic hormones in sports training or competition.

▶ Research has shown that prohormone dietary supplements marketed as anabolic agents, such as androstenedione, do not effectively increase muscle mass or strength. Moreover, such prohormones have been classified as controlled anabolic steroids and their use is illegal and banned by the WADA.

Ginseng, Herbals, and Exercise and Sports Performance

Herbs contain various nutrients and phytonutrients, such as vitamins, minerals, and antioxidants, that may be part of a healthful diet. Herbal products have been used for centuries for their purported health benefits. For example, St. John's wort has been used to treat depression, kava kava to reduce stress and anxiety, echinacea to reduce symptoms of the common cold, and numerous herbals to promote weight loss. In some countries, many herbals are regulated as drugs, but in the United States, most are regulated as dietary supplements. A detailed discussion of the health effects of herbals is beyond the scope of this text. In general, however, well-controlled research with most herbal supplements and health outcomes is limited. Some may be effective and others not, and in many cases, the research findings are equivocal. For example, Shah and others, in a meta-analysis, found that echinacea decreased the odds of developing the common cold by 58 percent and the duration of a cold by 1.4 days and concluded that the published evidence supports echinacea's benefit in decreasing the incidence and duration of the common cold. In contrast, Karsch-Völk and others reported that the research results are inconsistent and that although the preventive effects of echinacea might exist, they have not been shown in rigorous randomized trials.

Numerous herbal supplements are marketed for weight control. For example, Hoodia gordonii is marketed for weight loss. In their review, Smith and Krygsman noted that decreased appetite and weight loss occur at high doses and may cause hypertension, loss of muscle mass, and gastrointestinal discomfort. Chitturi and Farrell noted that some herbal remedies marketed for weight reduction have been causally associated with significant liver injury. Moreover, the Consumers Union also notes that herbal supplements can interact dangerously with medications. For example, echinacea may interact with various drugs, including those for allergies, anxiety, asthma, diabetes, and high serum cholesterol. Individuals using herbal products for health purposes should consult with their physicians. As previously discussed, ephedra may be dangerous in and of itself.

Herbals have also been marketed as ergogenic aids for athletes. Unfortunately, with the exception of ginseng and related products, limited research has evaluated their ability to enhance exercise or sports performance.

Does ginseng or ciwujia enhance exercise or sports performance?

Ginseng and ciwujia are comparable herbs, and both have been studied for their potential effects on exercise or sports performance.

Ginseng Extracts derived from the plant family Araliaceae contain numerous chemicals that may influence human physiology, the most important being the glycosides, or ginsenosides. Collectively, these extracts are referred to as **ginseng**, and their physiological effects vary depending on the plant species, the part of the plant used, and the place of origin. The most common forms of ginseng include Chinese or Korean (*Panax ginseng*), American (*Panax quinquefolium*), Japanese (*Panax japonicum*), and Russian/Siberian (*Eleutherococcus senticosus*). *Eleutherococcus senticosus* is a totally different plant from Araliaceae, but it is recognized by some as a legitimate form of ginseng and its ginsenosides are also referred to as eleutherosides. The type and amount of ginsenosides present vary greatly among the different forms of ginseng.

Using such labels as Ginseng Energy, ginseng has been marketed in various forms as a means of enhancing health and physical performance (see figure 13.11). Although the underlying mechanisms are unknown, ginseng is believed to influence neural and hormonal activity in the body and has been theorized to enhance the immune system. The most prevalent theory suggests that ginseng may stimulate the hypothalamus, the neuroendocrine tissue in the brain that controls the pituitary gland. The pituitary gland in turn commands other endocrine glands in the body. For example, the hypothalamus secretes corticotropin-releasing hormone (CRH). This causes the anterior pituitary to secrete adrenocorticotropic hormone (ACTH), resulting in the release of cortisol by the adrenal gland in response to stress.

Much of the early ginseng research was conducted by Russians, who coined the term *adaptogens* to characterize ginseng's ability to

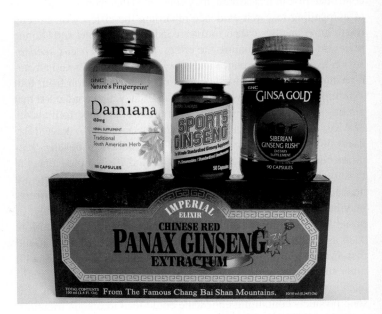

FIGURE 13.11 Various ginseng products are available as dietary supplements, some being marketed directly to athletes.

increase resistance to the catabolic effects of stress. They believed that ginseng helped develop resistance to the mental and physical stress associated with intense exercise training. Ginseng has been purported to influence physical performance in other ways as well, such as increased cardiac function, blood flow, and oxygen transport during exercise; increased oxygen utilization and decreased lactic acid levels during exercise; enhanced muscle glycogen synthesis after exercise; and a positive effect on nitrogen or protein balance. In essence, ginseng is theorized to enhance sports performance by allowing athletes to train more intensely and by inducing a physiological anti-fatiguing effect that increases stamina during competition. It should be noted that an underlying mechanism for this theorized ergogenic effect has not been determined.

Although numerous studies investigated the ergogenic possibilities of ginseng supplementation, few were well controlled. Research design flaws included no control or placebo group, no double-blind protocol, no randomization of order of treatment, and no statistical analysis.

More recent, well-designed studies using standardized ginseng abstracts and commercial products have reported no significant ergogenic effects. For example, Dowling and others reported no effect of *Eleutherococcus senticosus* on metabolic (oxygen uptake and lactic acid accumulation), physiological (heart rate and ventilation), or psychological (ratings of perceived exertion) responses to submaximal and maximal running. Using a similar research protocol but with cycling, Engels and Wirth reported no ergogenic effect of *Panax ginseng*. Other well-controlled studies by Engels and his associates have found no ergogenic effect of *Panax ginseng* on high-intensity, interval anaerobic exercise protocols. However, Ziemba and others reported that although *Panax ginseng* did not influence exercise capacity in soccer players, it did improve multiple choice reaction time before and during a cycling exercise task. Such an effect may be of benefit to athletes who must react quickly in sports. This finding merits additional research.

In their review, Bahrke and others noted that although more well-controlled research is needed, they concluded that there is an absence of compelling research evidence regarding the efficacy of ginseng use to improve physical performance in humans. Goulet and Dionne reviewed studies evaluating the effect of *Eleutherococcus senticosus* on exercise performance and concluded that it offers no advantage during exercise endurance tests ranging in duration from 6 to 120 minutes. In their review, Palisin and Stacy also concluded that ginseng cannot be recommended to improve athletic performance.

Most commercial ginseng preparations appear to have relatively low acute or chronic toxicity when taken in dosages recommended by the manufacturer. Coon and Ernst noted that the most commonly experienced adverse effects of *Panax ginseng* are headache and sleep and gastrointestinal disorders. These effects may be attributed to the postulated stimulant effect of ginseng, or possibly to additional substances in the commercial preparation, such as the stimulant ephedrine. In general, however, they found that *Panax ginseng,* when taken alone and not combined with other substances, is rarely associated with adverse effects. For athletes involved in sports that may use drug testing, the use of ginseng products containing ephedrine could lead to disqualification.

Some researchers theorize that long-term ginseng supplementation prevents some adverse effects of stress on the immune system,

which could help prevent illness or some of the symptoms of the overtraining syndrome during high-intensity training. However, Engels and others reported that *Panax ginseng* had no significant effect on immune functions during recovery from intense anaerobic exercise. Shergis and others concluded that *Panax ginseng* may boost cell-mediated immunity. Senchina and others noted that knowledge of the chemical characteristics of the botanical agents is essential to elucidate mechanisms of action for improved immune function.

Consumers should be aware of quality control problems with ginseng supplements. Cui and others reported that ginsenosides in 50 commercial preparations varied from 1.9 to 9.0 percent and that 12 percent contained no detectable ginsenosides. More recently, Harkey and others reported considerable product-to-product variability in the ginsenoside and eleutheroside content of 25 commercial ginseng products. Many ginseng products also contain alcohol.

Individuals who desire to experiment with long-term ginseng supplementation should consult with their physicians, because ginseng use may exacerbate various health problems, such as high blood pressure. Given the available scientific evidence, ginseng supplements cannot be recommended.

Ciwujias **Ciwujia**, a Chinese herb, is similar to ginseng. Cheuvront and others indicate that ciwujia is extracted from Araliaceae, the same plant family as *Panax ginseng*. Along with Plowman and others, they also note that it may be derived from the leaves of *Eleutherococcus senticosus*. Ciwujia was first marketed as the commercial sports supplement Endurox™. Currently it is marketed as Endurox Excel, whose advertisements suggest that it can increase fat oxidation (possibly sparing muscle glycogen), reduce lactate accumulation, raise the anaerobic threshold, lower the heart rate while maintaining the same level of workout intensity, and speed workout recovery. However, most of the claims for ciwujia are based on clinical trials with poor experimental designs. Plowman and others noted that none of the studies followed a randomized crossover or double-blind protocol, nor was the use of a placebo mentioned. None have been published in peer-reviewed journals.

Studies by Plowman, Cheuvront, and their associates, using double-blind, placebo-controlled, crossover experimental designs and published in peer-reviewed journals, reported that supplementation with Endurox™ (800 mg for 7–10 days) had no significant effect on heart rate, oxygen consumption, respiratory exchange ratio (a measure of fat oxidation), lactic acid accumulation, or ratings of perceived exertion during either cycle ergometer or stair-climbing exercise. The investigators indicated that their studies did not verify the claims made for Endurox™.

Based on the available evidence, products containing ciwujia do not appear to enhance exercise performance, and thus are not recommended for use by endurance athletes.

What herbals are effective ergogenic aids?

As noted earlier, caffeine may be derived from various herbals, such as guarana and the kola nut, whereas ephedra is a constituent of ma huang. Other than these and ginseng, athletes have experimented with a variety of other herbals, including cayenne for energy and gamma-oryzanol to increase muscle mass.

In her brief report, Kundrat indicated that double-blind, placebo-controlled human research on herb use by athletes is limited or nonexistent. One reason may be that, at least in the United States, herbs are regulated as dietary supplements and are not required to be standardized, so there is little consistency among brands. Moreover, herbal sports supplements may often contain several herbals and other substances in a commercial product, so it is difficult to isolate the potential ergogenic effect of a single ingredient. Studies conducted with such commercial herbal-based sports supplements, such as the study by Earnest and others, generally report no significant ergogenic effects.

Nevertheless, several reviews of herbal supplementation and exercise performance are available. In their review, Williams and Branch noted that much of what we know about the efficacy of herbal supplements as ergogenics is based on anecdotal data and poorly controlled studies. However, based on their analysis, they concluded that none of the following herbals have sufficient research support as a means of enhancing exercise or sports performance: bee pollen, capsicum, gamma-oryzanol, ginkgo biloba, kava kava, St. John's wort, *Tribulus terrestris,* and yohimbine. According to a recent review by Qureshi and others, there is little evidence that *Tribulus terristris* increases testosterone or its precursors, muscle mass, or strength. Some supplements such as kava kava and St. John's wort may induce adverse herbal/drug interactions by interfering with cytochrome P450 function in the liver. Ostojic reported that yohimbine (21 mg/day for 21 days) decreased fat mass but exerted no effect on body mass, muscle mass, or various and performance indicators in elite soccer players. However, the combination of certain herbals such as capsicum and yohimbine with other stimulants such as caffeine and ephedrine renders it difficult to isolate individual herbal effects and may cause adverse interaction effects.

Several other herbals have been studied for their purported ergogenic potential. The herb *Cordyceps sinensis* is a health tonic from China. Although it is rare, CordyMax Cs-4 is an available synthetic version. *Cordyceps sinensis* is theorized to have favorable effects on the heart and circulation to improve oxidative capacity and endurance performance. However, Parcell and others reported that 5 weeks of CordyMax Cs-4 supplementation had no effect on the aerobic capacity of endurance-trained male cyclists. In a study of a supplement containing *Cordyceps sinensis,* yohimbine, and other ingredients purported to increase ATP concentrations, Herda and others found no effect on vertical jump performance, isometric strength, or isokinetic endurance compared to a placebo.

Rhodiola rosea, like ginseng, is categorized as an adaptogen and has been theorized to enhance endurance performance through a stimulating effect and by increasing ATP turnover. However, Walker and others, using nuclear magnetic resonance spectroscopy, reported no significant effects of *Rhodiola rosea* supplementation on ATP turnover during a wrist flexion test to exhaustion. There were no differences between supplement and placebo conditions on perceived exertion (RPE) or time to exhaustion. De Bock and others found that an acute dose (200 milligrams) of *Rhodiola rosea* improved time to exhaustion by 3 percent on a cycle ergometer, but there was no effect on maximal strength or various measures of reaction time or movement time. In addition, there was no significant effect following supplementation with 200 milligrams daily for 4 weeks. Colson and others reported that a product containing *Cordyceps sinensis* and *Rhodiola rosea* had no effect on muscle-tissue oxygen saturation or on cycling time to exhaustion. Skarpanska-Stejnborn and others noted that 4 weeks of *Rhodiola rosea* supplementation increased plasma antioxidant levels in members of the Polish rowing team, but there was no effect on oxidative damage induced by exhaustive exercise. Overall, research findings do not support an ergogenic effect of *Rhodiola rosea* supplementation to trained athletes.

Epigallocatechin-3-gallate (EGCG) is an extract of green tea, a flavonol that functions as an antioxidant and has been theorized by some to enhance exercise performance by reducing oxidative stress. EGCG may also play a role in immune function, as previously discussed, in a review by Steinmann and others. Richards and others reported no effect on maximal heart rate, work rate, respiratory exchange ratio, or cardiac output following seven separate doses of EGCG (135 mg each) over 2 days. They did report a significant increase in VO$_2$ max, which may have been a chance finding. However, Dean and others reported no effect of 270 mg of EGCG/day for 6 days on a 40-km cycling time trial following 60 minutes of moderate-intensity cycling. In a similar study of green tea extract supplementation for 3 weeks, Eichenberger and others also reported no significant effect on a 30-minute cycling time trial following 2 hours of moderate-intensity cycling or on any markers of energy metabolism. In a comparison of 1 and 7 days of green tea extract ingestion, Randall and others reported increased lipolysis following 7 days but no evidence of increased fatty acid oxidation following either regimen. Overall, current research does not support an ergogenic effect of EGCG supplementation.

Cytoseira canariensis has been marketed as a new sports supplement designed to increase muscle mass and decrease body fat by inhibiting myostatin. Myostatin is a protein known as a growth and differentiation factor, and its role is to inhibit (not promote) the growth of muscles. Theoretically, by inhibiting the effects of myostatin, muscle growth may be increased. However, Willoughby reported that 1,200 milligrams/day of *Cystoseira canariensis* supplementation during 12 weeks of resistance training had no effect on serum myostatin levels, nor did it have any effect on muscle mass, muscle strength, or body fat.

As noted in chapter 8, increasing erythropoietin (EPO) levels by living at altitude may confer a beneficial effect on oxygen transport during exercise by increasing production of red blood cells. In one study, Whitehead and others found that subjects receiving 8,000 mg of echinacea daily for 28 days significantly increased their serum erythropoietin levels. However, there was no change in red blood cells or hemoglobin concentrations. This is an interesting finding, and more research is recommended to evaluate the ergogenicity of echinacea supplementation.

Kundrat indicated that athletes should be concerned about the safety of herbals, as there may be some side effects or herb-drug interactions. For athletes using herbals for weight loss, Pittler concluded that the potential health risks argue against such use due to an increased risk relative to benefit. Athletes contemplating using herbals should consult with their health-care professional.

Key Concepts

▶ Results from well-controlled research indicate that ginseng and related adaptogens, such as ciwujia, are not effective ergogenic aids.

▶ There is limited well-controlled research regarding the effect of herbals on exercise or sports performance, and that which is available suggests that herbal sports supplements are not effective ergogenic aids.

Sports Supplements: Efficacy, Safety, and Permissibility

What sports supplements are considered to be effective, safe, and permissible?

This text has addressed the effects of a wide variety of supplements on health and efficacy, safety, and permissibility as ergogenic aids in sports or exercise performance. Carbohydrate and fat metabolites, special proteins, numerous amino acids, vitamins, and minerals, as well as food drugs and herbal supplements, have all been studied for their health and ergogenic potential. In the joint position statement of the American College of Sports Medicine, the Academy of Nutrition and Dietetics (formerly the American Dietetic Association), and the Dietitians of Canada, Rodriguez and others conclude that performance and recovery from competition and training may be enhanced by research-based nutritional selections and strategies. This position statement has also classified nutritional supplements into four categories based on the supplements' legality and ability to enhance health, performance, or training when added to a healthful diet that already provides adequate Calories and essential nutrients. A similar classification system of the Australian Institute of Sport is presented in table 13.5. Group A supplements have research support for their efficacy and are permitted for use. Group B supplements require additional research but could be effective in certain circumstances. Group C includes supplements that are either not listed in Groups A and B or are abused Group A and B supplements. Group D supplements are banned and should not be used under any circumstances. The ergogenic effect of the supplement may also be limited to a specific type of athletic endeavor or characteristic. As examples, sodium bicarbonate may improve high-intensity, anaerobic exercise dependent primarily on anaerobic glycolysis. Females in weight-control sports may benefit from iron supplements to help prevent iron deficiency and anemia, as well as from calcium supplements to help maintain bone mass. Some supplements may be considered unsafe and not recommended if that is the research-based opinion of various health organizations. With few exceptions, research does not support the efficacy of most commercial sports supplements. Moreover, some supplements may be contaminated, intentionally or unintentionally, with substances that could lead to a positive doping test. In most cases athletes can meet their nutritional needs through consumption of a well-planned, healthful diet.

TABLE 13.5 Australian Institute of Sports classification system of nutritional supplements

Group	Evidence Level	Subcategory	Examples
A	Supported and permitted for use in specific situations	Sports foods	Carbohydrate/protein sports drinks/bars/gels; electrolyte replacements; whey protein
		Medical supplements	Iron, calcium, multi-vitamin/mineral, vitamin D
		Performance supplements	Caffeine, beta-alanine, sodium bicarbonate, beetroot juice, creatine
B	Deserving of additional research; permitted for use subject to clinical and/or research monitoring	Food polyphenols	Quercetin, montomorency, acai, gogi, curcumin
		Other	Vitamin C, Vitamin E, L-carnitine, hydroxymethylbutyrate, glutamine, eicosapentanoic acid, docosahexaenoic acid, glucosamine
C	Little proof of efficacy; not provided to athletes but may be permitted on an individual basis	Group A or B supplements not used according to approved protocols	
		Other supplements not listed in Groups A and B	Aspartate salts, bee pollen, boron, chromium, choline, condroitin, chromium, ciwujia, conjugated linoleic acids, coenzyme Q_{10}, *Cordyceps sinesis*, fat loading, gamma oryzanol, ginseng, hydroxycitrate, inosine, magnesium, medium-chain triacylglycerol, niacin, octacosanol, phosphate salts, pyruvate, *Rhodiola rosea*, ribose, selenium, tryptophan, vanadium, vitamin A, wheat germ oil, yohimbine, zinc
D	Banned by WADA or at high risk for contamination; should not be used by athletes	Stimulants	Ephedra/epidrine/ma huang, strychnine, sibutramine, methyhexanamine, others
		Prohormones	Dehydroeipandrosterone, androstenedione, 19-norandrostenedione, 19-norandrostenediol, *Tribulus terrestris*, maca root powder
		HGH releaser peptides	Glycine, ornithine, arginine, lysine
		Others	Glycerol, colostrum

Source: www.ausport.gov.au/ais/nutrition/supplements/classification.

If you or one of your colleagues is physically trained or an athlete, you might want to conduct a small case study with caffeine. Either of you should be physically trained to run a mile, swim 500 meters, or complete some comparable exercise task of 5–10 minutes of high-intensity exercise. Other exercise tasks of shorter duration may be selected. The activity is best done indoors to control environmental conditions. One of you can serve as the investigator and the other as the subject. A third colleague will administer the treatment on a double-blind basis. Randomly, over a 5-week period, the subject will participate in five trials, each involving maximal performance for the selected activity. Thirty minutes before the test, the subject should consume either two caffeine tablets, each containing 200 milligrams of caffeine (Vivarin or comparable over-the-counter tablet) or a comparable placebo (two multivitamin tablets) with some water. The subject's eyes should be closed while taking the tablets. Here is the weekly protocol.

Week 1—Learning protocol; no placebo or caffeine

Week 2—Placebo or caffeine

Week 3—Caffeine or placebo (opposite of week 2)

Week 4—Placebo or caffeine

Week 5—Caffeine or placebo (opposite of week 4)

Record the performance times (minutes: seconds) for each, average the two placebo and two caffeine trials, and compare the results for improvement, if any.

Caffeine Trial

	Week 1 (no placebo or caffeine)	Week 2 (placebo or caffeine)	Week 3 (opposite of week 2)	Week 4 (placebo or caffeine)	Week 5 (opposite of week 4)
Performance Time (minutes:seconds)	:	:	:	:	:

1. Of the drugs and supplements discussed in this chapter, which have the most research supporting their ability to enhance exercise or sports performance?
   (a) caffeine and androstenedione
   (b) ginseng and ephedrine
   (c) alcohol and DHEA
   (d) androstenedione and ephedrine
   (e) sodium bicarbonate and caffeine

2. About how many milligrams of caffeine are in a 6-ounce cup of perked coffee?
   (a) 25–30
   (b) 100–125
   (c) 300–400
   (d) 500–600
   (e) 1,000

3. Which of the following is not a physiological effect of caffeine?
   (a) decreases the metabolic rate
   (b) stimulates the central nervous system
   (c) increases the secretion of epinephrine
   (d) increases heart rate and force of contraction
   (e) increases force of skeletal muscle contractility

4. For an average-size male adult (150 pounds), the consumption of four drinks within a very short period of time would elevate the blood alcohol concentration (BAC) to about what level?
   (a) 0.01
   (b) 0.02
   (c) 0.05
   (d) 0.10
   (e) 0.15

5. As a potential ergogenic aid, sodium bicarbonate would be most likely suited to which type of athlete?
   (a) marathon runner (26.2 miles)
   (b) 100-meter sprinter (track)
   (c) 400-meter sprinter (track)
   (d) pole vaulter (field)
   (e) discus thrower (field)

6. Increasing research suggests that moderate alcohol consumption, or "low-risk" drinking, may reduce the risk of CHD and all-cause mortality. All but which of the following are hypothesized to contribute to this reduced risk?
   (a) a relaxation effect and reduced anxiety
   (b) decreased platelet aggregability (decreased possibility of blood clots)
   (c) increased blood flow to the brain
   (d) reduced caloric intake, induced weight loss, and prevented metabolic syndrome
   (e) an increase in HDL-cholesterol

7. Research generally supports the theory that caffeine may enhance performance in long-distance endurance events. Which of the following is the *least* likely hypothesis?
   (a) It may exert a psychologically stimulating effect.
   (b) It stimulates the release of epinephrine from the adrenal gland.
   (c) It decreases the use of both free fatty acids and muscle glycogen.
   (d) It may decrease the perception of effort during exercise.
   (e) It may exert a direct effect on the muscles to increase muscle contractile force.

8. Anabolic/androgenic steroids (AAS) are drugs popular with individuals with

muscle dysmorphia, or those who desire to increase muscle mass even though already very muscular. AAS are designed to mimic mainly the anabolic effects of which natural hormone in the body?

(a) insulin
(b) human growth hormone (HGH)
(c) testosterone
(d) androsterone
(e) estrogen

9. Which of the following dietary supplements marketed to strength-trained

individuals are precursors, or prohormones, for testosterone?

(a) creatine and conjugated linoleic acid
(b) gamma oryzanol and ginseng
(c) *Cordyceps sinensis* and *Cytoseira canariensis*
(d) HMB and *Tribulus terrestris*
(e) androstenedione and DHEA

10. Which of the following ergogenic aids are currently permitted for use by athletes in all sports competitions, according to the

doping list created by the World Anti-Doping Agency?

(a) caffeine and ephedrine
(b) sodium bicarbonate and caffeine
(c) caffeine and alcohol
(d) androstenedione and DHEA
(e) ginseng and ephedrine

Answers to multiple choice questions:
1. e; 2. b; 3. a; 4. d; 5. c; 6. d; 7. c;
8. c; 9. e; 10. b

Review Questions—Essay

1. Discuss both the potential beneficial and adverse health effects of consuming various amounts of alcohol.

2. Discuss the efficacy, safety, and legality of caffeine supplementation as an ergogenic aid for aerobic endurance athletes.

3. Discuss the efficacy, safety, and legality of sodium bicarbonate supplementation as an ergogenic aid. In which types of sports would it appear to be most effective?

4. Compare and contrast the effects of testosterone versus its congeners DHEA and androstenedione as ergogenic aids

for the development of muscle mass and strength. Discuss possible health risks associated with use of each.

5. What is ginseng, why is it purported to be an ergogenic aid, and does research support its efficacy as an ergogenic?

References

Books

American Psychiatric Association. 2013. *Diagnostic and Statistical Manual of Mental Disorders* (5th ed.). Washington, DC: APA.

Bahrke, M., and Yesalis, C. 2002. *Performance-Enhancing Substances in Sport and Exercise.* Champaign, IL: Human Kinetics.

Centers for Disease Control and Prevention. 2014. *Morbidity and Mortality Weekly Report.* Youth Risk Behavior Surveillance—United States, 2013. United States Department of Health and Human Services.

Institute of Medicine. 2014. *Caffeine in Food and Dietary Supplements: Examining Safety: Workshop Summary.* Washington, DC: National Academies Press.

Noakes, T. 2003. *Love of Running.* Champaign, IL: Human Kinetics. World Health Organization. 2014. *Global Status Report on Alcohol and Health.*

Reviews and Specific Studies

Abbasi, A., et al. 1998. Association of dehydroepiandrosterone sulfate, body composition, and physical fitness in independent community-dwelling older men and women. *Journal of the American Geriatric Society* 46:263–73.

Acacio, B., et al. 2004. Pharmacokinetics of dehydroepiandrosterone and its metabolites after long-term daily oral administration to healthy young men. *Fertility and Sterility* 81:595–604.

Allen, N., et al. 2009. Moderate alcohol intake and cancer incidence in women. *Journal of the National Cancer Institute* 101:296–305.

American College of Obstetrics and Gynecology. 2010. ACOG Committee opinion no. 462: Moderate caffeine consumption during pregnancy. *Obstetrics and Gynecology* 116 (2 Pt 1):467–68.

American College of Sports Medicine. 1987. American College of Sports Medicine

position stand on use of anabolic-androgenic steroids in sports. *Medicine & Science in Sports & Exercise* 19:534–39.

American College of Sports Medicine. 2007. Exercise and fluid replacement. *Medicine & Science in Sports & Exercise* 39:377–90.

Andraws, R., et al. 2005. Cardiovascular effects of ephedra alkaloids: A comprehensive review. *Progress in Cardiovascular Diseases* 47 (4):217–25.

Anstey, K., et al. 2009. Alcohol consumption as a risk factor for dementia and cognitive decline: Meta-analysis of prospective studies. *American Journal of Geriatric Psychiatry* 17:542–55.

Armstrong, L., et al. 2007. Caffeine, fluid-electrolyte balance, temperature regulation, and exercise-heat tolerance. *Exercise and Sport Sciences Reviews* 35:135–40.

Arranz, S., et al. 2012. Wine, beer, alcohol and polyphenols on cardiovascular disease and cancer. *Nutrients* 4:759–81.

Arria, M., and O'Brien, M. 2011. The "high" risk of energy drinks. *Journal of the American Medical Association* (January 25). doi:10.1001/jama.2011.109.

Artioli, G., et al. 2007. Does sodium-bicarbonate ingestion improve simulated judo performance? *International Journal of Sport Nutrition and Exercise Metabolism* 17:206–17.

Astell, K. J., et al. 2013. A review on botanical species and chemical compounds with appetite suppressing properties for body weight control. *Plant Foods for Human Nutrition* 68:213–21.

Astorino, T. A., et al. 2007. Caffeine-induced changes in cardiovascular function during resistance training. *International Journal of Sport Nutrition and Exercise Metabolism* 17 (5):468–77.

Astorino, T., and Roberson, D. 2010. Efficacy of acute caffeine ingestion for short-term high-intensity exercise performance: A systematic review. *Journal of Strength and Conditioning Research* 24:257–65.

Attwood, A., and Munafò. 2014. Effects of acute alcohol consumption and processing of emotion in faces: Implications for understanding alcohol-related aggression. *Journal of Psychopharmacology* 28(8):719–32.

Bahrke, M. S., et al. 1998. Anabolic-androgenic steroid abuse and performance-enhancing drugs among adolescents. *Child and Adolescent Psychiatric Clinics of North America* 7:821–38.

Bahrke, M., et al. 2009. Is ginseng an ergogenic aid? *International Journal of Sport Nutrition and Exercise Metabolism* 19:298–322.

Bain, J. 2010. Testosterone and the aging male: To treat or not to treat? *Maturitas* 66:16–22.

Bangsbo, J., et al. 1992. Acute and habitual caffeine ingestion and metabolic responses to steady-state exercise. *Journal of Applied Physiology* 72 (4):1297–303.

Barnes, M. J., et al. 2012. The effects of acute alcohol consumption and eccentric muscle damage on neuromuscular function. *Applied Physiology, Nutrition, and Metabolism* 37:63–71.

Barrett-Conner, E., et al. 1994. Coffee-associated osteoporosis offset by daily milk consumption. The Rancho Bernardo Study. *Journal of the American Medical Association* 271 (4):280–83.

Basaria, S., et al. 2010. Adverse events associated with testosterone administration. *New England Journal of Medicine* 363:109–22.

Baumann, G. P. 2012. Growth hormone doping in sports: A critical review of use and detection strategies. *Endocrine Reviews* 33 (2):155–86.

Baume, N., et al. 2006. Effect of multiple oral doses of androgenic anabolic steroids on endurance performance and serum indices of physical stress in healthy male subjects. *European Journal of Applied Physiology* 98:329–40.

Beck, A., and Heinz, A. 2013. Alcohol-related aggression—Social and neurobiological factors. *Deutsches Ärzteblatt International* 110 (42):711–15. doi: 10.3238/arztebl.2013.0711.

Beedie, C., et al. 2006. Placebo effects of caffeine on cycling performance. *Medicine & Science in Sports & Exercise* 38:2159–64.

Bell, D., and Jacobs, I. 1999. Combined caffeine and ephedrine ingestion improves run times of Canadian Forces Warrior Test. *Aviation and Space Environmental Medicine* 70:325–29.

Bell, D., et al. 2001. Effect of caffeine and ephedrine ingestion on anaerobic exercise performance. *Medicine & Science in Sports & Exercise* 33:1399–403.

Bell, D., et al. 2002. Effect of ingesting caffeine and ephendrine on 10-km run performance. *Medicine & Science in Sports & Exercise* 34:344–49.

Bent, S., et al. 2004. Safety and efficacy of citrus aurantium for weight loss. *American Journal of Cardiology* 94:1359–61.

Bents, R., and Marsh, E. 2006. Patterns of ephedra and other stimulant use in collegiate hockey athletes. *International Journal of Sport Nutrition and Exercise Metabolism* 16:636–43.

Beulens, J., et al. 2006. The effect of moderate alcohol consumption on fat distribution and adipocytokines. *Obesity* 14:60–66.

Beydoun, M. A., et al. 2014. Epidemiologic studies of modifiable factors associated with cognition and dementia: Systematic review and meta-analysis. *BioMed Central Public Health* 14:643.

Bhasin, S., et al. 1996. The effects of supraphysiologic doses of testosterone on muscle size and strength in normal men. *New England Journal of Medicine* 335:1–7.

Bianco, A., et al. 2014. Alcohol consumption and hormonal alterations related to muscle hypertrophy: A review. *Nutrition and Metabolism* 11:26. doi: 10.1186/1743-7075-11-26.

Bird, S., et al. 1995. The effect of sodium bicarbonate ingestion on 1500-m racing time. *Journal of Sports Sciences* 13:399–403.

Bishop, D., and Claudius, B. 2005. Effects of induced metabolic alkalosis on prolonged intermittent-sprint performance. *Medicine & Science in Sports & Exercise* 37:759–67.

Boje, O. 1939. Doping. *Bulletin of the Health Organization of the League of Nations* 8:439–69.

Bouchard, N., et al. 2005. Ischemic stroke associated with use of an ephedra-free dietary supplement containing synephrine. *Mayo Clinic Proceedings* 80:541–45.

Bridge, C. A., and Jones, M. A. 2006. The effect of caffeine ingestion on 8km run performance in a field setting. *Journal of Sports Sciences* 24(4):433–39.

Brinton, E. A. 2012. Effects of ethanol intake on lipoproteins. *Current Atherosclerosis Reports* 14(2):108–14.

Brown, G., et al. 1999. Effect of oral DHEA on serum testosterone and adaptations to resistance training in young men. *Journal of Applied Physiology* 87:2274–83.

Brown, G., et al. 2004. Changes in serum testosterone and estradiol concentrations following acute androstenedione ingestion in young women. *Hormone and Metabolic Research* 36:62–66.

Brown, G., et al. 2006. Testosterone prohormone supplements. *Medicine & Science in Sports & Exercise* 38:1451–61.

Browne, M. 2006. Maternal exposure to caffeine and risk of congenital anomalies: A systematic review. *Epidemiology* 17:324–31.

Browne, M. L., et al. 2011. Maternal caffeine intake and risk of selected birth defects in the National Birth Defects Prevention Study. *Birth Defects Research. Part A, Clinical Molecular Teratology* 91 (2):93–101.

Bruce, C., et al. 2000. Enhancement of 2000-m rowing performance after caffeine ingestion. *Medicine & Science in Sports & Exercise* 32:1958–63.

Buckman, J. F., et al. 2013. A national study of substance use behaviors among NCAA male athletes who use banned performance enhancing substances. *Drug and Alcohol Dependence* 131 (1-2):50–55.

Bui, L., et al. 2006. Blood pressure and heart rate effect following a single dose of bitter orange. *Annals of Pharmacotherapy* I40:53–57.

Burd, L., et al. 2007. Ethanol and the placenta: A review. *Journal of Maternal-Fetal & Neonatal Medicine* 20:361–75.

Burke, L. M. 2003. Effect of alcohol intake on muscle glycogen storage after prolonged exercise. *Journal of Applied Physiology* 95 (3):983–90.

Burke, L., and Maughan, R. 2000. Alcohol in sport. In *Nutrition in Sport,* ed. R. J. Maughan. Oxford: Blackwell Scientific.

Camfield, D. A., et al. 2014. Acute effects of tea constituents L-theanine, caffeine, and epigallocatechin gallate on cognitive function and mood: A systematic review and meta-analysis. *Nutrition Reviews* 72 (8):507–22.

Candow, D. G. 2009. Effect of sugar-free Red Bull energy drink on high-intensity run time-to-exhaustion in young adults. *Journal of Strength and Conditioning Research* 23 (4):1271–75.

CARE Study Group. 2008. Maternal caffeine intake during pregnancy and risk of fetal growth restriction: A large prospective observational study. *British Medical Journal* 337:a2332.

Cargiulo, T. 2007. Understanding the health impact of alcohol dependence. *American Journal of Health-Systems Pharmacy* 64:S5–S11.

Chapman, R., and Mickleborough, T. 2009. The effects of caffeine on ventilation and pulmonary function during exercise: An often-overlooked response. *Physician and Sportsmedicine* 37:97–103.

Chen, X., et al. 2010. Caffeine protects against disruptions of the blood-brain barrier in animal models of Alzheimer's and Parkinson's diseases. *Journal of Alzheimer's Disease* 20:S127–41.

Cheng, M., et al. 2014. Caffeine intake and atrial fibrillation incidence: Dose response meta-analysis of prospective cohort studies. *Canadian Journal of Cardiology* 30 (4):448–54.

Cheuvront, S., et al. 1999. Effect of ENDUROX™ on metabolic responses to submaximal exercise. *International Journal of Sport Nutrition* 9:434–42.

Chitturi, S., and Farrell, G. 2008. Hepatotoxic slimming aids and other herbal hepatotoxins. *Journal of Gastroenterology and Hepatology* 23:366–73.

Cohen, P. A., et al. 2015. An amphetamine isomer whose efficacy and safety in humans has never been studied, β-methylphenylethylamine (BMPEA), is found in multiple dietary supplements. *Drug Testing and Analysis.* doi: 10.1002/dta.1793.

Coiro, V., et al. 2007. Effects of moderate ethanol drinking on the GH and cortisol responses to physical exercise. *Neuro Endocrinology Letters* 28:145–8.

Collomp, K., et al. 2015. DHEA, physical exercise and doping. *Journal of Steroid Biochemistry and Molecular Biology* 145:206–12.

Colson, S., et al. 2005. Cordyceps sinensis- and Rhodiola rosea-based supplementation in male cyclists and its effect on muscle tissue saturation. *Journal of Strength and Conditioning Research* 19:358–63.

Conger, S., et al. 2011. Does caffeine added to carbohydrate provide additional ergogenic benefits for endurance? *International Journal of Sport Nutrition and Exercise Metabolism* 21:71–84.

Consumers Union. 2004. Ephedra: Heart dangers in disguise. *Consumer Reports* 69 (1):22–23.

Consumers Union. 2007. Risky herb-drug combos. *Consumer Reports on Health* 19 (1):10.

Consumers Union. 2008. Deflating the claims about DHEA. *Consumer Reports on Health* 20 (7):10.

Coon, J., and Ernst, E. 2002. Panax ginseng: A systematic review of adverse effects and drug interactions. *Drug Safety* 25:323–44.

Costill, D., et al. 1978. Effects of caffeine ingestion on metabolism and exercise performance. *Medicine & Science in Sports* 10:155–58.

Cox, H. D., and Eichner, D. 2013. Detection of human insulin-like growth factor-1 in deer antler velvet supplements. *Rapid Communication in Mass Spectrometry* 27 (19):2170–78.

Cui, J., et al. 1994. What do commercial ginseng preparations contain? *Lancet* 344 (8915):134.

Cunha, R., and Agostinho, P. 2010. Chronic caffeine consumption prevents memory disturbance in different animal models of memory decline. *Journal of Alzheimer's Disease* 20:S95–116.

Davis, J., and Green, J. 2009. Caffeine and anaerobic performance: Ergogenic value and mechanisms of action. *Sports Medicine* 39:813–32.

De Bock, K., et al. 2004. Acute Rhodiola rosea intake can improve endurance exercise performance. *International Journal of Sport Nutrition and Exercise Metabolism* 14:298–307.

Dean, H. 2002. Does exogenous growth hormone improve athletic performance? *Clinical Journal of Sport Medicine* 12:250–53.

Dean, S., et al. 2009. The effects of EGCG on fat oxidation and endurance performance in male cyclists. *International Journal of Sport Nutrition and Exercise Metabolism* 19:624–44.

Del Coso, J., et al. 2009. Caffeine during exercise in the heat: Thermoregulation and fluid-electrolyte balance. *Medicine & Science in Sports & Exercise* 41:164–73.

Del Coso, J., et al. 2011. Prevalence of caffeine use in elite athletes following its removal from the World Anti-Doping Agency list of banned substances. *Applied Physiology, Nutrition and Metabolism* 36:555–61.

Delgado, C. E., et al. 1975. Acute effects of low doses of alcohol on left ventricular function by echocardiography. *Circulation* 51 (3):535–40.

Desbrow, B., and Leveritt, M. 2006. Awareness and use of caffeine by athletes competing at the 2005 Ironman Triathlon World Championships. *International Journal of Sport Nutrition and Exercise Metabolism* 16:545–58.

Desbrow, B., and Leveritt, M. 2007. Well-trained endurance athletes' knowledge, insight, and experience of caffeine use. *International Journal of Sport Nutrition and Exercise Metabolism* 17:328–39.

Ding, M., et al. 2014. Caffeinated and decaffeinated coffee consumption and risk of type 2 diabetes: A systematic review and a dose-response meta-analysis. *Diabetes Care* 37 (2):569–86.

Doherty, M., and Smith, P. 2004. Effect of caffeine ingestion on exercise testing: A meta-analysis. *International Journal of Sport Nutrition and Exercise Metabolism* 14:626–46.

Doherty, M., and Smith, P. 2005. Effects of caffeine ingestion on rating of perceived exertion during and after exercise: A meta-analysis. *Scandinavian Journal of Medicine & Science in Sports* 15:69–78.

Dowling, E. et al. 1996. Effect of Eleutherococcus senticosus on submaximal and maximal exercise performance. *Medicine & Science in Sport & Exercise,* 28:482–89.

Driller, M. W., et al. 2012. The effects of serial and acute NaHCO₃ loading in well-trained cyclists. *Journal of Strength and Conditioning Research* 26 (10):2791–97.

D'hooghe, M. B., et al. 2012. Alcohol, coffee, fish, smoking and disease progression in multiple sclerosis. *European Journal of Neurology* 19:616–24.

Earnest, C. 2001. Dietary androgen supplements: Separating substance from hype. *Physician and Sportsmedicine* 29 (5): 63–79.

Earnest, C., et al. 2000. In vivo 4-androstene-3, 17-dione and 4-androstene-3 beta, 17 beta-diol supplementation in young men. *European Journal of Applied Physiology* 81:229–32.

Earnest, C., et al. 2004. Effects of a commercial herbal-based formula on exercise performance in cyclists. *Medicine & Science in Sports & Exercise* 36:504–9.

Egger, F., et al. 2014. Effects of sodium bicarbonate on high-intensity endurance performance in cyclists: A double-blind, randomized cross-over trial. *Public Library of Science One* 9 (12):e114729. doi: 10.1371/journal.pone.0114729.

Eichenberger, P., et al. 2010. No effects of three-week consumption of a green tea extract on time trial performance in endurance-trained men. *International Journal for Vitamin and Nutrition Research* 80:54–64.

El Sayed, M., et al. 2005. Interaction between alcohol and exercise: Physiological and haematological implications. *Sports Medicine* 35:257–69.

Engels, H., and Wirth, J. 1997. No ergogenic effect of ginseng (Panax ginseng C.A. Meyer) during graded maximal aerobic exercise. *Journal of the American Dietetic Association* 97:1110–15.

Engels, H., et al. 2001. Effects of ginseng supplementation on supramaximal exercise performance and short-term recovery. *Journal of Strength and Conditioning Research* 15:290–95.

Engels, H., et al. 2003. Effects of ginseng on secretory IgA, performance, and recovery from interval exercise. *Medicine & Science in Sports & Exercise* 35:690–96.

Epstein, D., and Dohrmann, G. 2009. What you don't know might kill you. *Sports Illustrated* 110 (30):54–63.

Epstein, E., et al. 2007. Women, aging, and alcohol use disorders. *Journal of Women & Aging* 19 (1–2):31–48.

Evans, N. 2004. Current concepts in anabolic-androgenic steroids. *American Journal of Sports Medicine* 32:534–42.

Ferreira, M. P., and Weems, M. K. 2008. Alcohol consumption by aging adults in the United States: Health benefits and detriments. *Journal of the American Dietetic Association* 108 (10):1668–76.

Fillmore, K., et al. 2007. Moderate alcohol use and reduced mortality risk: Systematic error in prospective studies and new hypotheses. *Annals of Epidemiology* 17:S16–S23.

Foad, A., et al. 2008. Pharmacological and psychological effects of caffeine ingestion in 40-km cycling performance. *Medicine & Science in Sport & Exercise* 40:158–65.

Font, L., et al. 2013. Involvement of the endogenous opioid system in the psychopharmacological actions of ethanol: The role of acetaldehyde. *Frontiers in Behavioral Neuroscience* 31 (7):93. doi: 10.3389/fnbeh.2013.00093.

Ford, J. A. 2007. Alcohol use among college students: A comparison of athletes and nonathletes. *Substance Use and Misuse* 42:1367–77.

Galaif, E., et al. 2007. Suicidality, depression, and alcohol use among adolescents: A review of empirical findings. *International Journal of Adolescent Medicine and Health* 19:27–35.

Ganio, M. S., et al. 2011. Effect of ambient temperature on caffeine ergogenicity during endurance exercise. *European Journal of Applied Physiology* 111:1135–46.

Ganio, M., et al. 2009. Effect of caffeine on sport-specific endurance performance: A systematic review. *Journal of Strength and Conditioning Research* 23:315–24.

Gant, N., et al. 2010. The influence of caffeine and carbohydrate coingestion on simulated soccer performance. *International Journal of Sport Nutrition and Exercise Metabolism* 20:191–7.

George, A., and Figueredo, V. 2010. Alcohol and arrhythmias: A comprehensive review. *Journal of Cardiovascular Medicine* 11:221–8.

Glaister, M., et al. 2014. Caffeine supplementation and peak anaerobic power output. *European Journal of Sport Science* 2:1–7.

Goulet, E., and Dionne, I. 2005. Assessment of the effects of Eleutherococcus senticosus on endurance performance. *International Journal of Sport Nutrition and Exercise Metabolism* 15:75–83.

Graham, T. 1981. Alcohol ingestion and man's ability to adapt to exercise in a cold environment. *Canadian Journal of Applied Sport Sciences* 6 (1):27–31.

Graham, T. 2001. Caffeine, coffee, and ephedrine: Impact on exercise performance and metabolism. *Canadian Journal of Applied Physiology* 26:S103–19.

Graham, T., and Spriet, L. 1996. Caffeine and exercise performance. *Sports Science Exchange* 9 (1):1–5.

Graham, T., et al. 1998. Metabolic and exercise endurance effects of coffee and caffeine ingestion. *Journal of Applied Physiology* 85:883–89.

Graham, T., et al. 2008. Does caffeine alter muscle carbohydrate and fat metabolism during exercise? *Applied Physiology, Nutrition, and Metabolism* 33:1311–8.

Graves, B., et al. 2010. International Society of Sports Nutrition position stand: Caffeine and performance. *Journal of the International Society of Nutrition* 7 (1):5.

Grech, A., et al. 2014. Adverse effects of testosterone replacement therapy: An update on the evidence and controversy. *Therapeutic Advances in Drug Safety* 5(5):190–200.

Green, J. 2007. Fetal alcohol spectrum disorders: Understanding the effects of prenatal alcohol exposure and supporting students. *Journal of School Health* 77:103–8.

Greenway, F. 2001. The safety and efficacy of pharmaceutical and herbal caffeine and ephedrine use as a weight loss agent. *Obesity Reviews* 2:199–211.

Greenwood, D. C., et al. 2014. Caffeine intake during pregnancy and adverse birth outcomes: A systematic review and dose-response meta-analysis. *European Journal of Epidemiology* 29 (10):725–34.

Greydanus, D., and Patel, D. 2010. Sports doping in the adolescent: The Faustian conundrum of Hors de Combat. *Pediatric Clinics of North America* 57:729–50.

Gruenewald, P., et al. 2010. A dose-response perspective on college drinking and related problems. *Addiction* 105:257–69.

Guessous, I., et al. 2014. Blood pressure in relation to coffee and caffeine consumption. *Current Hypertension Reports* 16 (9):468. doi: 10.1007/s11906-014-0468-2.

Guha, N., et al. 2013. Insulin-like growth factor-I (IGF-I) misuse in athletes and potential methods for detection. *Analytical and Bioanalytical Chemistry* 405 (30):9669–83.

Gunzerath, L. 2004. National Institute on Alcohol Abuse and Alcoholism report on moderate drinking. *Alcoholism, Clinical and Experimental Research* 28 (6):829–47.

Gurley, B. J., et al. 2014. Multi-ingredient, caffeine-containing dietary supplements: History, safety, and efficacy. *Clinical Therapeutics* (September 26). pii: S0149-2918(14)00550-5. doi: 10.1016/j.clinthera.2014.08.012. [Epub ahead of print]

Haller, C., and Benowitz, N. 2000. Adverse cardiovascular and central nervous system events associated with dietary supplements containing ephedra alkaloids. *New England Journal of Medicine* 343:1833–38.

Haller, C., et al. 2004. Enhanced stimulant and metabolic effects of combined ephedrine and caffeine. *Clinical Pharmacology and Therapeutics* 75:259–73.

Hallström, H., et al. 2013. Long-term coffee consumption in relation to fracture risk and bone mineral density in women. *American Journal of Epidemiology* 178 (6):898–909.

Harkey, M. R., et al. 2001. Variability on commercial ginseng products: An analysis of 25 preparations. *American Journal of Clinical Nutrition* 73:1101–6.

Hartgens, F., and Kuipers, H. 2004. Effects of androgenic-anabolic steroids in athletes. *Sports Medicine* 34:513–54.

Hartgens, F., et al. 1996. Body composition, cardiovascular risk factors and liver function in long term androgenic-anabolic steroids-using bodybuilders three months after drug withdrawal. *International Journal of Sports Medicine* 17:429–33.

Haugvad, A., et al. 2014. Ethanol does not delay muscle recovery but decreases testosterone/cortisol ratio. *Medicine and Science in Sport and Exercise* 46 (11):2175–83.

Haycock, P. 2009. Fetal alcohol spectrum disorders: The epigenetic perspective. *Biology of Reproduction* 81:607–17.

Herda, T. J., et al. 2008. Effects of a supplement designed to increase ATP levels on muscle strength, power output, and endurance. *Journal of the International Society of Sports Nutrition* 5:3. doi:10.1186/1550-2783-5-3.

Hespel, P., et al. 2006. Dietary supplements for football. *Journal of Sports Sciences* 24:749–61.

Higgins, J. P., and Baku, K. M. 2013. Caffeine reduces myocardial blood flow during exercise. *American Journal of Medicine* 126 (8):730.e1-8. doi: 10.1016/j.amjmed.2012.12.023.

Hobson, R., and Maughan, R. 2010. Hydration status and the diuretic action of a small dose of alcohol. *Alcohol and Alcoholism* 45:366–73.

Hodges, K., et al. 2006. Pseudoephedrine enhances performance in 1500-m runners. *Medicine & Science in Sports & Exercise* 38:329–33.

Hogervorst, E., et al. 1999. Caffeine improves cognitive performance after strenuous physical exercise. *International Journal of Sports Medicine* 20:354–61.

Hogervorst, E., et al. 2008. Caffeine improves physical and cognitive performance during exhaustive exercise. *Medicine & Science in Sports & Exercise* 40:1841–51.

Holmes, M. V., et al. 2014. Association between alcohol and cardiovascular disease: Mendelian randomization analysis based on individual participant data. *British Medical Journal* 349:g4164 doi: 10:1136/bmj.g4164.

Holt, R. 2009. Is human growth hormone an ergogenic aid? *Drug Testing and Analysis* 1:412–8.

Houmard, J. A., et al. 1987. Effects of the acute ingestion of small amounts of alcohol upon 5-mile run times. *Journal of Sports Medicine and Physical Fitness* 27 (2):253–57.

Irwin, C., et al. 2011. Caffeine withdrawal and high-intensity endurance cycling performance. *Journal of Sports Sciences* 29:509–15.

Isodori, A. M., et al. 2005. Effects of testosterone on body composition, bone metabolism and serum lipid profile in middle-aged men: A meta-analysis. *Clinical Endocrinology* 63 (3):280–93.

Jacobs, L., et al. 2004. Effects of ephedrine, caffeine, and their combination on muscular endurance. *Medicine & Science in Sports & Exercise* 35:987–94.

James, J. 2004. Critical review of dietary caffeine and blood pressure: A relationship that should be taken more seriously. *Psychosomatic Medicine* 66:63–71.

James, J. E., and Rogers, P. J. 2005. Effects of caffeine on performance and mood: Withdrawal reversal is the most plausible explanation. *Psychopharmacology* 182:1–8.

Jenkins, N., et al. 2008. Ergogenic effects of low doses of caffeine on cycling performance. *International Journal of Sport Nutrition and Exercise Metabolism* 18:328–42.

Jeukendrup, A., and Martin, J. 2001. Improving cycling performance: How should we spend our time and money? *Sports Medicine* 31:559–69.

Jiang, W., et al. 2013. Coffee and caffeine intake and breast cancer risk: An updated dose-response meta-analysis of 37 published studies. *Gynecologic Oncology* 129 (3):620–29.

Juliano, L., and Griffiths, R. 2004. A critical review of caffeine withdrawal: Empirical validation of symptoms and signs, incidence, severity, and associated features. *Psychopharmacology* 176:1–29.

Kalmar, J. 2005. The influence of caffeine on voluntary muscle activation. *Medicine & Science in Sports & Exercise* 37:2113–19.

Karam, E., et al. 2007. Alcohol use among college students: An international perspective. *Current Opinion in Psychiatry* 20:213–21.

Karsch-Völk, M., et al. 2014. Echinacea for preventing and treating the common cold. *Cochrane Database of Systematic Reviews* 2:CD000530. doi: 10.1002/14651858. CD000530.pub3.

Kasdallah-Grissa, A., et al. 2007. Resveratrol, a red wine polyphenol, attenuates ethanol-induced oxidative stress in rat liver. *Life Sciences* 80 (11):1033–39.

Kelly, Y., et al. 2010. Light drinking during pregnancy: Still no increased risk for socioemotional difficulties or cognitive deficits at 5 years of age? *Journal of Epidemiology and Community Health* (October 5).

Kendrick, Z., et al. 1993. Effect of ethanol on metabolic responses to treadmill running in well-trained men. *Journal of Clinical Pharmacology* 33:136–39.

Kenny, A., et al. 2010. Dehydroepiandrosterone combined with exercise improves muscle strength and physical function in frail older women. *Journal of the American Geriatric Society* 58:1707–14.

Kerrigan, S., and Lindsey, T. 2005. Fatal caffeine overdose: Two case reports. *Forensic Science International* 153:67–69.

Kersey, R. D., et al. 2012. National Athletic Trainers' Association position statement: Anabolic-androgenic steroids. *Journal of Athletic Training* 47 (5):567–88.

King, D., et al. 1999. Effect of oral androstenedione on serum testosterone and adaptations to resistance training in young men. *Journal of the American Medical Association* 281:2020–28.

Klatsky, A. 2007. Alcohol, cardiovascular diseases and diabetes mellitus. *Pharmacological Research* 55:237–47.

Klatsky, A., et al. 2006. Coffee, cirrhosis, and transaminase enzymes. *Archives of Internal Medicine* 166:1190–95.

Koppes, L., et al. 2005. Moderate alcohol consumption lowers the risk of type 2 diabetes: A meta-analysis of prospective observational studies. *Diabetes Care* 28:719–25.

Kozak-Collins, K., et al. 1994. Sodium bicarbonate ingestion does not improve performance in women cyclists. *Medicine & Science in Sports & Exercise* 26:1510–15.

Kruisselbrink, L. D., et al. 2006. Physical and psychomotor functioning of females the morning after consuming low to moderate quantities of beer. *Journal of Studies on Alcohol* 67 (3):416–20.

Kundrat, S. 2005. Herbs and athletes. *Sports Science Exchange* 18 (1):1–6.

Lambert, J. D. 2013. Does tea prevent cancer? Evidence from laboratory and human intervention studies. *American Journal of Clinical Nutrition* 98 (6S):1667S–75S.

Lara, D. 2010. Caffeine, mental health, and psychiatric disorders. *Journal of Alzheimer's Disease* 20:S239–48.

Lecoultre, V., and Schutz, Y. 2009. Effect of a small dose of alcohol on the endurance performance of trained cyclists. *Alcohol and Alcoholism* 44 (3):278–83.

Leder, B. et al. 2000. Oral androstenedione administration and serum testosterone concentrations in young men. *Journal of the American Medical Association* 283:779–82.

Leong, D. P., et al. 2014. Patterns of alcohol consumption and myocardial infarction risk: Observations from 52 countries in the INTERHEART case-control study. *Circulation* 130 (5):390–98.

Lieber, C. S. 2004. New concepts of the pathogenesis of alcoholic liver disease lead to novel treatments. *Current Gastroenterology Reports* 6(1):60–65.

Linossier, M. et al. 1997. Effect of sodium citrate on performance and metabolism of human skeletal muscle during supramaximal cycling exercise. *European Journal of Applied Physiology* 76:48–54.

Liquori, A., et al. 1997. Absorption and subjective effects of caffeine from coffee, cola, and capsules. *Pharmacology, Biochemistry, and Behavior* 58 (3):721–26.

Liu, H., et al. 2007. Systematic review: The safety and efficacy of growth hormone in the healthy elderly. *Annals of Internal Medicine* 146:104–15.

Lopez-Garcia, E., et al. 2006. Changes in caffeine intake and long-term weight change in men and women. *American Journal of Clinical Nutrition* 83:674–80.

Lopez-Garcia, E., et al. 2008. The relationship of coffee consumption with mortality. *Annals of Internal Medicine* 148:904–14.

Loucks, A. 2006. The endocrine system: Integrated influences on metabolism, growth, and reproduction. In ACSM's *Advanced Exercise Physiology,* ed. C. Tipton. Philadelphia: Lippincott Williams & Wilkins.

Lucas, B. R., et al. 2014. Gross motor deficits in children prenatally exposed to alcohol: A meta-analysis. *Pediatrics* 134 (1):e192–209.

Lui, J., et al. 2013. Association of coffee consumption with all-cause and cardiovascular disease mortality. *Mayo Clinic Proceedings* 88(10):1066–74.

Magkos, F., and Kavouras, S. 2004. Caffeine and ephedrine: Physiological, metabolic and performance-enhancing effects. *Sports Medicine* 34:971–89.

Maglione, M., et al. 2005. Psychiatric effects of ephedra use: An analysis of Food and Drug Administration reports of adverse events. *American Journal of Psychiatry* 162:189–91.

Martens, M. P., et al. 2008. Understanding sport-related drinking motives in college athletes: Psychometric analyses of the Athlete Drinking Scale. *Addictive Behaviors* 33:974–77.

Maughan, R. 2005. Contamination of dietary supplements and positive drug tests in sport. *Journal of Sports Sciences* 23:883–89.

Maughan, R., et al. 2004. Dietary supplements. *Journal of Sports Sciences* 22:95–113.

McLellan, T., and Bell, D. 2004. The impact of prior coffee consumption on the subsequent ergogenic effect of anhydrous caffeine. *International Journal of Sport Nutrition and Exercise Metabolism* 14:698–708.

McNaughton, L., and Cedaro, R. 1992. Sodium citrate ingestion and its effects on maximal anaerobic exercise of different durations. *European Journal of Applied Physiology* 64:36–41.

McNaughton, L., and Preece, D. 1986. Alcohol and its effects on sprint and middle distance running. *British Journal of Sports Medicine* 20(2):56–59.

McNaughton, L., et al. 1999. Sodium bicarbonate can be used as an ergogenic aid in high-intensity, competitive cycle ergometry of 1 h duration. *European Journal of Applied Physiology* 80:64–69.

McNaughton, L., et al. 2008. Ergogenic effects of sodium bicarbonate. *Current Sports Medicine Reports* 7:230–36.

Meinhardt, U., et al. 2010. The effects of growth hormone on body composition and physical performance in recreational athletes: A randomized trial. *Annals of Internal Medicine* 152:568–77.

Melnik, B., et al. 2007. Abuse of anabolic-androgenic steroids and bodybuilding acne: An underestimated health problem. *Journal der Deutschen Dermatologischen Gesellschaft* 5:110–7.

Mets, M. A. J., et al. 2012. Effects of coffee on driving performance during prolonged simulated highway driving. *Psychopharmacology* (2012) 222:337–42.

Michels, K., et al. 2005. Coffee, tea, and caffeine consumption and incident of colon and rectal cancer. *Journal of the National Cancer Institute* 97:282–92.

Michels, K., et al. 2007. Diet and breast cancer. A review of the prospective observational studies. *Cancer* 109 (Supplement 12):2712–49.

Mitchell, D. C., et al. 2014. Beverage caffeine intakes in the U.S. *Food and Chemical Toxicology* 63:136–42.

Monti, P., et al. 2005. Adolescence: Booze, brains, and behavior. *Alcoholism: Clinical & Experimental Research* 29:207–20.

Morgentaler, A., et al. 2015. Testosterone therapy and cardiovascular risk: Advances and controversies. *Mayo Clinic Proceedings* 90 (2):224–51.

Morozova, T. V., et al. 2014. Genetics and genomics of alcohol sensitivity. *Molecular Genetics and Genomics* 289 (3):253–69.

Mukamal, K., et al. 2003. Roles of drinking pattern and type of alcohol consumed in coronary heart disease in men. *New England Journal of Medicine* 348:109–18.

Mukamal, K., et al. 2006. Alcohol consumption and risk for coronary heart disease in men with healthy lifestyles. *Archives of Internal Medicine* 166:2145–50.

Naimi, T., et al. 2005. Cardiovascular risk factors and confounders among nondrinking and moderate-drinking U.S. adults. *American Journal of Preventive Medicine* 28:369–73.

Nair, K., et al. 2006. DHEA in elderly women and DHEA or testosterone in elderly men. *New England Journal of Medicine* 355:1647–59.

Namdar, M., et al. 2009. Caffeine impairs myocardial blood flow response to physical exercise in patients with coronary artery disease as well as in age-matched controls. *PLoS One* 4:e5665.

National Strength and Conditioning Association; Hoffman, J., et al. 2009. Position stand on androgen and human growth hormone use. *Journal of Strength and Conditioning Research* 23:S1–S59.

Nordström, A., et al. 2012. Higher muscle mass but lower gynoid fat mass in athletes using anabolic androgenic steroids. *Journal of Strength and Conditioning Research* 26 (1):246–50.

Nova, E., et al. 2012. Potential health benefits of moderate alcohol consumption: Current perspectives in research. *Proceedings of the Nutrition Society* 71:307–15.

Nyberg, F., and Hallberg, M. 2012. Interactions between opioids and anabolic androgenic steroids: Implications for the development of addictive behavior. *International Review of Neurobiology* 102:189–206.

O'Keefe, J. H., et al. 2013. Effects of habitual coffee consumption on cardiometabolic disease, cardiovascular health, and all-cause mortality. *Journal of the American College of Cardiology* 62 (12):1043–51.

O'Keefe, J. H., et al. 2014. Alcohol and cardiovascular health: The dose makes the poison or the remedy. *Mayo Clinic Proceedings* 89 (3):382–93.

Oopik, V., et al. 2003. Effects of sodium citrate ingestion before exercise on endurance performance in well-trained college runners. *British Journal of Sports Medicine* 37:485–89.

Ostojic, S. 2006. Yohimbine: The effects on body composition and exercise performance in soccer players. *Research in Sports Medicine* 14:289–99.

Palisin, T., and Stacy, J. 2006. Ginseng: Is it in the root? *Current Sports Medicine Reports* 5:210–14.

Parcell, A., et al. 2004. Cordyceps sinensis (CordyMax Cs-4) supplementation does not improve endurance exercise performance. *International Journal of Sport Nutrition and Exercise Metabolism* 14:236–42.

Peart, D. J., et al. 2012. Practical recommendations for coaches and athletes: A meta-analysis of sodium bicarbonate use for athletic performance. *Journal of Strength and Conditioning Research* 26 (7):1975–83.

Petzer, J. P., and Petzer, A. 2015. Caffeine as a lead compound for the design of therapeutic agents for the treatment of Parkinson's disease. *Current Medicinal Chemistry* 22 (8):975–88.

Philip, P., et al. 2006. The effects of coffee and napping on nighttime highway driving: A randomized trial. *Annals of Internal Medicine* 144:785–91.

Piazza-Gardner, A. K., and Barry, A. E. 2012. Examining physical activity levels and alcohol consumption: Are people who drink more active? *American Journal of Health Promotion* 26 (3):e95–e104.

Piazza-Gardner, A. K., et al. 2013. The impact of alcohol on Alzheimer's disease: A systematic review. *Aging and Mental Health* 17 (2):133–46.

Pittler, M., et al. 2005. Adverse events of herbal food supplements for body weight reduction: Systematic review. *Obesity Reviews* 6:93–111.

Plowman, S., et al. 1999. The effects of ENDUROX on the physiological responses to stair-stepping exercise. *Research Quarterly for Exercise and Sport* 70:385–88.

Pope, H. G., et al. 2014. Adverse health consequences of performance enhancing drugs: A Endocrine Society Scientific Statement. *Endocrine Reviews* 35 (3):341–74.

Pope, H. G., et al. 2014. The lifetime prevalence of anabolic-androgenic steroid use and dependence in Americans: Current best estimates. *American Journal on Addictions* 23:371–77.

Potteiger, J., et al. 1996. Sodium citrate ingestion enhances 30 km cycling performance. *International Journal of Sports Medicine* 17:7–11.

Potteiger, J., et al. 1996. The effects of buffer ingestion on metabolic factors related to

distance running performance. *European Journal of Applied Physiology* 72:365–71.

Prediger, R. 2010. Effects of caffeine in Parkinson's disease: From neuroprotection to the management of motor and non-motor symptoms. *Journal of Alzheimer's Disease* 20:S205–20.

Price, M., et al. 2003. Effects of sodium bicarbonate ingestion on prolonged intermittent exercise. *Medicine & Science in Sports & Exercise* 35:1303–8.

Pritchard-Peschek, K. R., et al. 2014. The dose-response relationship between pseudoephedrine ingestion and exercise performance. *Journal of Science and Medicine in Sport* 17 (5):531–34.

Pritchard-Peschek, K., et al. 2010. Pseudoephedrine ingestion and cycling time-trial performance. *International Journal of Sport Nutrition and Exercise Metabolism* 20:132–8.

Qureshi, A., et al. 2014. A systematic review of the herbal extract Tribulus terristris and the roots of its putative aphrodisiac and performance enhancing effect. Journal of Dietary Supplements 11 (1):64–69.

Randell, R. K., et al. 2013. No effect of 1 or 7 d of green tea extract ingestion on fat oxidation during exercise. *Medicine and Science in Sports and Exercise* 45 (5):883–91.

Rasmussen, B., et al. 2000. Androstenedione does not stimulate muscle protein anabolism in young healthy men. *Journal of Clinical Endocrinology and Metabolism* 85:55–59.

Rawson, E., and Clarkson, P. 2002. Ephedrine as an ergogenic aid. In *Performance-Enhancing Substances in Sport and Exercise,* ed. M. Bahrke and C. Yesalis. Champaign, IL: Human Kinetics.

Raymer, G., et al. 2004. Metabolic effects of induced alkalosis during progressive forearm exercise to fatigue. *Journal of Applied Physiology* 96:2050–56.

Rehm, J., et al. 2008. Are lifetime abstainers the best control group in alcohol epidemiology? On the stability and validity of reported lifetime abstention. *American Journal of Epidemiology* 168:866–71.

Rehm, J., et al. 2010. Alcohol as a risk factor for liver cirrhosis: A systematic review and meta-analysis. *Drug and Alcohol Review* 29:437–45.

Reis, J., et al. 2010. Coffee, decaffeinated coffee, caffeine, and tea consumption in young adulthood and atherosclerosis later in life: The CARDIA study. *Arteriosclerosis, Thrombosis, and Vascular Biology* 30:2059–66.

Requena, B., et al. 2005. Sodium bicarbonate and sodium citrate: Ergogenic aids. *Journal of Strength and Conditioning Research* 19:213–24.

Reuben, A. 2008. Alcohol and the liver. *Current Opinion in Gastroenterology* 24:328–38.

Richards, J., et al. 2010. Epigallocatechin-3-gallate increases maximal oxygen uptake in adult humans. *Medicine & Science in Sports & Exercise* 42:739–44.

Rodrigo, R., et al. 2011. Modulation of endogenous antioxidant system by wine polyphenols in human disease. *Clinica Chimica Acta* 412:410–424.

Rodriguez, N. R., et al. 2009. American College of Sports Medicine, American Dietetic Association, Dieticians of Canada joint position stand. Nutrition and athletic performance. *Medicine and Science in Sports and Exercise* 41 (3):709–31.

Rogerson, S., et al. 2007. The effect of short-term use of testosterone enanthate on muscular strength and power in healthy young men. *Journal of Strength and Conditioning Research* 21:354–61.

Ronksley, P. E., et al. 2011. Association of alcohol consumption with selected cardiovascular disease outcomes: A systematic review and meta-analysis. *British Medical Journal* 342:d671. doi: 10.1136/bmj.d671.

Roswall, N., and Weiderpass, E. 2015. Alcohol as a risk factor for cancer: Existing evidence in a global perspective. *Journal of Preventive Medicine and Public Health* 48:1–9.

Rubeck, K., et al. 2009. Impact of growth hormone (GH) substitution on exercise capacity and muscle strength in GH-deficient adults: A meta-analysis of blinded, placebo-controlled trials. *Clinical Endocrinology* 71:860–66.

Rudelle, S., et al. 2007. Effect of a thermogenic beverage on 24-hour energy metabolism in humans. *Obesity* 15:349–55.

Santos, C., et al. 2010. Caffeine intake and dementia: Systematic review and meta-analysis. *Journal of Alzheimer's Disease* 20:S187–204.

Santos, I. S., et al. 2012. Maternal caffeine consumption and infant nighttime waking: Prospective cohort study. *Pediatrics* 129 (5):860-868.

Sattler, F., et al. 2009. Testosterone and growth hormone improve body composition and muscle performance in older men. *Journal of Clinical Endocrinology and Metabolism* 94:1991–2001.

Savitz, D., et al. 2008. Caffeine and miscarriage risk. *Epidemiology* 19:55–62.

Schabort, E., et al. 2000. Dose-related elevations in venous pH with citrate ingestion do not alter 40-km cycling time-trial performance. *European Journal of Applied Physiology* 83:320–27.

Schardt, D. 2008. Caffeine: The good, the bad, and the maybe. *Nutrition Action Health Letter* 35 (2):1, 3–7.

Schneider, M. B., et al. 2011. Clinical report—Sports drinks and energy drinks for children and adolescents: Are they appropriate? *Pediatrics* 127:1182–89.

Schroeder, E., et al. 2005. Six-week improvements in muscle mass and strength during androgen therapy in older men. *Journals of Gerontology. Series A, Biological Sciences and Medical Sciences* 60:1586–92.

Schubert, M. M., and Astorino, T. A. 2013. Systematic review of the efficacy of ergogenic aids for improving running performance. *Journal of Strength and Conditioning Research* 27 (6):1699–1707.

Scoccianti, C., et al. 2014. Female breast cancer and alcohol consumption. A review of the literature. *American Journal of Preventive Medicine* 46 (W3S1):S16–S25.

Senchina, D. S., et al. 2009. Herbal supplements and athlete immune function—What's proven, disproven, and unproven? *Exercise Immunology Review* 15:66–106.

Shah, S., et al. 2007. Evaluation of echinacea for the prevention and treatment of the common cold: A meta-analysis. *The Lancet Infectious Diseases* 7:473–80.

Shave, R., et al. 2001. The effects of sodium citrate ingestion on 3,000-meter time-trial performance. *Journal of Strength and Conditioning Research* 15:230–34.

Shekelle, P., et al. 2003. Efficacy and safety of ephedra and ephedrine for weight loss and athletic performance: A meta-analysis. *JAMA* 289:1537–45.

Shergis, J.L., et al. 2013. Panax ginseng in randomised controlled trials: a systematic review. *Phytotherapy Research* 27(7):949–965.

Shimamoto, T., et al. 2013. No association of coffee consumption with gastric ulcer, duodenal ulcer, reflux esophagitis, and non-erosive reflux disease: A cross-sectional study of 8,013 healthy subjects in Japan. *Public Library of Science ONE* 8 (6):e65996. doi:10.1371/journal.pone.0065996.

Shirreffs, S.M. and Maughan, R.J. 2006. The effect of alcohol on athletic performance. *Current Sports Medicine Reports* 5:192–196.

Siegler, J., and Hirscher, K. 2010. Sodium bicarbonate ingestion and boxing performance. *Journal of Strength and Conditioning Research* 24:103–8.

Sin, C., et al. 2009. Systematic review on the effectiveness of caffeine abstinence on the quality of sleep. *Journal of Clinical Nursing* 18:13–21.

Sirrs, S., and Bebb, R. 1999. DHEA: Panacea or snake oil? *Canadian Family Physician* 45:1723–28.

Skarpanska-Stejnborn, A., et al. 2009. The influence of supplementation with Rhodiola rosea L. extract on selected redox parameters in professional rowers. *International Journal of Sport Nutrition and Exercise Metabolism* 19:186–99.

Skinner, T., et al. 2010. Dose response of caffeine on 2000-m rowing performance. *Medicine & Science in Sports & Exercise* 42:571–6.

Smith, C. and Krygsman, A. 2014. Hoodia gordonii: To eat, or not to eat. *Journal of Ethnopharmacology* 155 (2):987–91.

Smith, G., et al. 1999. Fatal nontraffic injuries involving alcohol: A meta-analysis. *Annals of Emergency Medicine* 33:699, 701.

Spriet, L. L. 2014. Exercise and sport performance with low doses of caffeine. *Sports Medicine* 44 (S2):S175–84.

Stackelberg, O., et al. 2014. Alcohol consumption, specific alcoholic beverages, and abdominal aortic aneurysm. *Circulation* 130 (8):646–52.

Steffen, M., et al. 2012.The effect of coffee consumption on blood pressure and the development of hypertension: A systematic review and meta-analysis. *Journal of Hypertension* 30 (12):2245–54.

Steinmann, J., et al. 2013. Anti-infective properties of epigallocatechin-3-gallate (EGCG), a component of green tea. *British Journal of Pharmacology* 168:1059–73.

Stephens, T., et al. 2002. Effect of sodium bicarbonate on muscle metabolism during intense endurance cycling. *Medicine & Science in Sports & Exercise* 34:614–21.

Stevenson, E., et al. 2009. The effect of a carbohydrate-caffeine sports drink on simulated golf performance. *Applied Physiology, Nutrition, and Metabolism* 34:681–8.

Suter, P. M. 2005. Is alcohol consumption a risk factor for weight gain and obesity? *Critical Reviews in Clinical Laboratory Sciences* 42(3):197–227.

Söderpalm, B., and Ericson, M. 2013. Neurocircuitry involved in the development of alcohol addiction: The dopamine system and its access points. *Current Topics in Behavioral Neurosciences* 13:127–61.

Talih, F., et al. 2007. Anabolic steroid abuse: Psychiatric and physical costs. *Cleveland Clinic Journal of Medicine* 74:341–4, 346, 349–52.

Tan, F., et al. 2010. Effects of induced alkalosis on simulated match performance in elite female water polo players. *International Journal of Sports Nutrition and Exercise Metabolism* 20 (3):198–205.

Tarnopolsky, M. 2008. Effect of caffeine on the neuromuscular system—Potential as an ergogenic aid. *Applied Physiology, Nutrition, and Metabolism* 33:1284–9.

Tarnopolsky, M., and Cupido, C. 2000. Caffeine potentiates low frequency skeletal muscle force in habitual and nonhabitual caffeine consumers. *Journal of Applied Physiology* 89:1719–24.

Temple, J. 2009. Caffeine use in children: What we know, what we have left to learn, and why we should worry. *Neuroscience and Biobehavioral Reviews* 33:793–806.

Tentori, L., and Graziani, G. 2007. Doping with growth hormone/IGF-1, anabolic steroids or erythropoietin: Is there a cancer risk? *Pharmacological Research* 55:359–69.

Thielecke, F., and Boschmann, M. 2009. The potential role of green tea catechins in the prevention of the metabolic syndrome—A review. *Phytochemistry* 70 (1):11–24.

Thomas, J. E., et al. 2009. STEMI in a 24-year-old man after use of a synephrine-containing dietary supplement. *Texas Heart Institute Journal* 36 (6):586–90.

Tonelo, D., et al. 2013. Holiday heart syndrome revisited after 34 years. *Arquivos Brasileiros de Cardiologica* 101(2):183–9.

Tunnicliffe, J., et al. 2008. Consumption of dietary caffeine and coffee in physically active populations: Physiological interactions. *Applied Physiology, Nutrition, and Metabolism* 33:1301–10.

Ulbrich, A., et al. 2013. Effects of alcohol mixed with energy drink and alcohol alone on subjective intoxication. *Amino Acids* 45:1385–93.

Urhausen, A., et al. 2004. Are the cardiac effects of anabolic steroid abuse in strength athletes reversible? *Heart* 90:496–501.

Vaher, I., et al. 2014. Impact of acute sodium citrate ingestion on endurance running performance in a warm environment. *European Journal of Applied Physiology.* doi: 10.1007/s00421-014-3068-6.

van Amsterdam, J., et al. 2010. Adverse health effects of anabolic-androgenic steroids. *Regulatory Toxicology and Pharmacology* 57:117–23.

Van Montfoort, M., et al. 2004. Effects of ingestion of bicarbonate, citrate, lactate, and chloride on sprint running. *Medicine & Science in Sports & Exercise* 36:1239–43.

van Soeren, M. H., and Graham, T. E. 1998. Effect of caffeine on metabolism, exercise endurance, and catecholamine responses after withdrawal. *Journal of Applied Physiology* 85(4):1493–501.

van Someren, K., et al. 1998. An investigation into the effects of sodium citrate ingestion on high-intensity exercise performance. *International Journal of Sport Nutrition* 8:356–63.

VanHaitsma, T. A., et al. 2010. Comparative effects of caffeine and albuterol on the bronchoconstrictor response to exercise in asthmatic athletes. *International Journal of Sports Medicine* 31 (4):231–36.

Verhoef, P., et al. 2002. Contribution of caffeine to the homocysteine-raising effect of coffee: A randomized controlled trial in humans. *American Journal of Clinical Nutrition* 76:1244–48.

Villareal, D., et al. 2000. Effects of DHEA replacement on bone mineral density and body composition in elderly women or men. *Clinical Endocrinology* 53:561–68.

Walker, T., et al. 2007. Failure of Rhodiola rosea to alter skeletal muscle phosphate kinetics in trained men. *Metabolism* 56:1111–17.

Wallace, M., et al. 1999. Effects of dehydroepiandrosterone vs androstenedione supplementation in men. *Medicine & Science in Sports & Exercise* 31:1788–92.

Wang, M. Q., et al. 1995. The acute effect of moderate alcohol consumption on cardiovascular responses in women. *Journal of Studies on Alcohol* 56 (1):16–20.

Wannamethee, S., et al. 2005. Alcohol and adiposity: Effects of quantity and type of drink and time relation with meals. *International Journal of Obesity* 29:1436–44.

Warren, G., et al. 2010. Effect of caffeine ingestion on muscular strength and endurance: A meta-analysis. *Medicine & Science in Sports & Exercise* 42:1375–87.

Welsh, E., et al. 2010. Caffeine for asthma. *Cochrane Database of Systematic Reviews* 20 (1):CD001112.

Weng, X., et al. 2008. Maternal caffeine consumption during pregnancy and the risk of miscarriage: A prospective cohort study. *American Journal of Obstetrics and Gynecology* (January 28).

White, A., and Hingson, R. 2013. The burden of alcohol use: Excessive alcohol consumption and related consequences among college students. Alcohol Research: *Current Reviews* 35 (2):201–18.

Whitehead, M., et al. 2007. The effect of 4 wk of oral echinacea supplementation on serum erythropoietin and indices of erythropoietic status. *International Journal of Sport Nutrition and Exercise Metabolism* 17:378–90.

Wichstrøm, T., and Wichstrøm, L. 2009. Does sports participation during adolescence prevent later alcohol, tobacco and cannabis use? *Addiction* 104:138–49.

Widdowson, W., and Gibney, J. 2010. The effect of growth hormone (GH) replacement on muscle strength in patients with GH-deficiency: A meta-analysis. *Clinical Endocrinology* 72:787–92.

Widdowson, W., et al. 2009. The physiology of growth hormone and sport. *Growth Hormone & IGF Research* 19:308–19.

Wiles, J., et al. 1992. Effect of caffeinated coffee on running speed, respiratory factors, blood lactate and perceived exertion during 1,500-meter treadmill running. *British Journal of Sports Medicine* 26:116–20.

Williams, A. D., et al. 2008. The effect of ephedra and caffeine on maximal strength and power in resistance-trained athletes. *Journal of Strength and Conditioning Research* 22 (2):464–70.

Williams, J. 1991. Caffeine, neuromuscular function and high-intensity exercise performance. *Journal of Sports Medicine and Physical Fitness* 31:481–89.

Williams, M. 2000. Smoking, alcohol, ergogenic aids, doping and the endurance performer. In *Endurance in Sport,* ed. R. Shephard and P. Astrand. Oxford: Blackwell Science.

Williams, M., and Branch, J. 2002. Herbals as ergogenic aids. In *Performance Enhancing Substances in Sports and Exercise,* ed. M. Bahrke and C. Yesalis. Champaign, IL: Human Kinetics.

Williams, P. 1997. Interactive effects of exercise, alcohol, and vegetarian diet on coronary artery disease risk factors in 9242 runners: The National Runners' Health Study. *American Journal of Clinical Nutrition* 66:1197–206.

Willoughby, D. 2004. Effects of an alleged myostatin-binding supplement and heavy resistance training on serum myostatin, muscle strength and mass, and body composition. *International Journal of Sport Nutrition and Exercise Metabolism* 14:461–72.

Wu, J., et al. 2009. Coffee consumption and risk of coronary heart diseases: A meta-analysis of 21 prospective cohort studies. *International Journal of Cardiology* 137:216–25.

Yarasheski, K., et al. 1993. Short-term growth hormone treatment does not increase muscle protein synthesis in experienced weight lifters. *Journal of Applied Physiology* 74:3073–76.

Yeo, S. E., et al. 2005. Caffeine increases exogenous carbohydrate oxidation during exercise. *Journal of Applied Physiology* 99 (3):844–50.

Yeomans, M. R. 2010. Alcohol, appetite and energy balance: Is alcohol intake a risk factor for obesity? *Physiology and Behavior* 100 (1):82–89.

Yesalis, C., and Bahrke, M. 2005. Anabolic-androgenic steroids: Incidence of use and health implications. *President's Council on Physical Fitness and Sports Research Digest* 5 (5):1–8.

Yesalis, C., et al. 1997. Trends in anabolic-androgenic steroid use among adolescents. *Archives of Pediatric and Adolescent Medicine* 151:1197–206.

Youngstedt, S., et al. 1998. Acute exercise reduces caffeine-induced anxiogenesis. *Medicine & Science in Sports & Exercise* 30:740–45.

Zhang, S., et al. 2007. Alcohol consumption and breast cancer risk in the Women's Health Study. *American Journal of Epidemiology* 165:667–76.

Zhang, Y., et al. 2014. Caffeine and dieresis during rest and exercise: A meta-analysis. *Journal of Science and Medicine in Sport* . doi: 10.1016/j. jsams.2014.07.017.

Ziegenfuss, T., et al. 2002. Effects of prohormones supplementation in humans: A review. *Canadian Journal of Applied Physiology* 27:628–46.

Ziemba, A., et al. 1999. Ginseng treatment improves psychomotor performance at rest and during graded exercise in young athletes. *International Journal of Sport Nutrition* 9:371–77.

Units of Measurement: English System— Metric System Equivalents

The Metric System and Equivalents

To measure ingredients, a standardized system known as the System Internationale (SI) has been established that is interpreted on an international basis. The SI is based on the metric system. However, in the United States, we also employ another set of measure and weight, the English system. In the field of dietetics, both systems are employed. The following tables give the quantities of the measures besides stating equivalents. With this information, it is possible to calculate in either system of measure and weight.

Household Measures (Approximations)

For easy computing purposes, the cubic centimeter (cc) is considered equivalent to 1 gram:

$$1 \text{ cc} = 1 \text{ gram} = 1 \text{ milliliter (mL)}$$

For easy computing purposes, 1 ounce equals 30 grams or 30 cubic centimeters.

1 quart	=	960 grams
1 pint	=	480 grams
1 cup	=	240 grams
1/2 cup	=	120 grams
1 glass (8 ounces)	=	240 grams
1/2 glass (4 ounces)	=	120 grams
1 orange juice glass	=	100–120 grams
1 tablespoon	=	15 grams
1 teaspoon	=	5 grams

Level Measures and Weights

1 teaspoon	=	5 cc or 5 mL 5 grams
3 teaspoons	=	1 tablespoon 15 cc 15 grams
2 tablespoons	=	30 cc 30 grams 1 ounce (fluid)
4 tablespoons	=	1/4 cup 60 cc 60 grams
8 tablespoons	=	1/2 cup 120 cc 120 grams
16 tablespoons	=	1 cup 240 grams 240 mL (fluid) 8 ounces (fluid) 1/2 pound
2 cups	=	1 pint 480 grams 480 mL (fluid) 16 ounces (fluid) 1 pound
4 cups	=	2 pints 1 quart 960 cc 960 mL (fluid) 2 pounds
4 quarts	=	1 gallon

Units of Weight

		Ounce	Pound	Gram	Kilogram
1 ounce	=	1.0	0.06	28.4	0.028
1 pound	=	16.0	1.0	454	0.454
1 gram	=	0.035	.002	1.0	0.001
1 kilogram	=	35.3	2.2	1,000	1.0

Units of Volume

		Ounce	Pint	Quart	Milliliter	Liter
1 ounce	=	1.0	0.062	0.031	29.57	0.029
1 pint	=	16.0	1.0	0.5	473	0.473
1 quart	=	32.0	2.0	1.0	946	0.946
1 milliliter	=	0.034	0.002	0.001	1.0	0.001
1 liter	=	33.8	2.112	1.056	1,000	1.0

Units of Length

		Millimeter	Centimeter	Inch	Foot	Yard	Meter
1 millimeter	=	1.0	0.1	0.0394	0.0033	0.0011	0.001
1 centimeter	=	10.0	1.0	0.394	0.033	0.011	0.01
1 inch	=	25.4	2.54	1.0	0.083	0.028	0.025
1 foot	=	304.8	30.48	12.0	1.0	0.333	0.305
1 yard	=	914.4	91.44	36.0	3.0	1.0	0.914
1 meter	=	1,000	100	39.37	3.28	1.094	1.0

1 kilometer	=	1,000 meters	= 0.6216 mile
1 mile	=	1,760 yards	= 1.61 kilometers

Units of mechanical, thermal, and chemical energy (approximate equivalents)

	Foot-pounds	Kilogram-meters	Kilojoules	Watts*	Kilocalories	Oxygen**
1 foot-pound	1	0.138	0.00136	0.0226	0.00032	0.000064
1 kilogram-meter	7.23	1	0.0098	0.163	0.0023	0.00046
1 kilojoule	737	102	1	16.66	0.239	0.047
1 watt*	44.27	6.12	0.06	1	0.0143	0.0028
1 kilocalorie	3,088	427	4.18	0.00024	1	0.198
1 liter oxygen**	15,585	2,154	21.1	351.9	5.047	1

Note: Read all tables across, such as 1 watt equals 44.27 foot-pounds per minute; 1 foot-pound equals 0.0226 watt.

* Watts are units of power expressed per minute.

** Equivalents are based upon 1 liter of oxygen metabolizing carbohydrate. Energy equivalents would be slightly less on a mixed diet of carbohydrate, fat, and protein. For example, 1 liter of oxygen would equal only 4.82 kilocalories on such a mixed diet.

Approximate Caloric Expenditure per Minute Based on the Metabolic Equivalents (METS) for Physical Activity

The caloric values presented in this appendix are based on the metabolic equivalents (METS) of various physical activities as presented in The Compendium of Physical Activities. You may find the MET value for a wide variety of physical activities, including common activities of daily living as well as physical activities and sports, on the following Website: https://sites.google.com/site/compendiumofphysicalactivities/. Consult the Website for activities you normally do and record the MET values for each. You may then consult this table in the column with your approximate body weight to find the caloric expenditure per minute for the given MET value. For example, if you weigh 154 pounds (70 kilograms) and engage in a physical activity that merits 10 METS, then you are expending 12.2 Calories per minute.

Please note that for some activities, such as walking, there are numerous choices from which to select, such as speed of walking, walking uphill, walking with a backpack, or walking with Nordic poles. Be sure to select the right activity.

					Body weight							
Kilograms	**45**	**48**	**50**	**52**	**55**	**57**	**59**	**61**	**64**	**66**	**68**	**70**
Pounds	**99**	**106**	**110**	**114**	**121**	**125**	**130**	**134**	**141**	**145**	**150**	**154**
METS												
1.0	0.8	0.8	0.9	0.9	1.0	1.0	1.0	1.1	1.1	1.2	1.2	1.2
1.5	1.2	1.3	1.3	1.4	1.4	1.5	1.5	1.6	1.7	1.7	1.8	1.8
2.0	1.6	1.7	1.8	1.8	1.9	2.0	2.1	2.1	2.2	2.3	2.4	2.5
2.5	2.0	2.1	2.2	2.3	2.4	2.5	2.6	2.7	2.8	2.9	3.0	3.1
3.0	2.4	2.5	2.6	2.7	2.9	3.0	3.1	3.2	3.4	3.5	3.6	3.7
3.5	2.8	2.9	3.0	3.2	3.4	3.5	3.6	3.7	3.9	4.0	4.2	4.3
4.0	3.2	3.4	3.5	3.6	3.9	4.0	4.1	4.3	4.5	4.6	4.8	4.9
4.5	3.5	3.8	3.9	4.1	4.3	4.5	4.6	4.8	5.1	5.2	5.4	5.5
5.0	3.9	4.2	4.4	4.6	4.8	5.0	5.2	5.3	5.6	5.8	6.0	6.1
5.5	4.3	4.8	4.8	5.1	5.3	5.5	5.7	5.9	6.2	6.4	6.5	6.7
6.0	4.7	5.0	5.3	5.5	5.8	6.0	6.2	6.4	6.7	6.9	7.1	7.4
6.5	5.1	5.4	5.7	5.9	6.3	6.5	6.7	7.0	7.3	7.5	7.7	8.0
7.0	5.5	5.8	6.1	6.4	6.7	7.0	7.2	7.5	7.8	8.1	8.3	8.6
7.5	5.9	6.2	6.6	6.8	7.2	7.5	7.7	8.0	8.4	8.7	8.9	9.2
8.0	6.3	6.7	7.0	7.3	7.7	8.0	8.3	8.5	9.0	9.2	9.5	9.8
8.5	6.7	7.1	7.4	7.7	8.2	8.5	8.8	9.1	9.6	9.8	10.1	10.4
9.0	7.1	7.5	7.9	8.2	8.7	9.0	9.3	9.6	10.1	10.4	10.7	11.0
9.5	7.5	8.0	8.3	8.6	9.1	9.5	9.8	10.1	10.6	11.0	11.3	11.6
10.0	7.9	8.4	8.8	9.1	9.6	10.0	10.3	10.7	11.2	11.5	11.9	12.2
10.5	8.3	8.8	9.2	9.6	10.1	10.5	10.8	11.2	11.8	12.1	12.5	12.8
11.0	8.7	9.2	9.6	10.0	10.6	11.0	11.4	11.7	12.3	12.7	13.1	13.4
11.5	9.1	9.6	10.1	10.5	11.1	11.5	11.9	12.3	12.9	13.3	13.7	14.0
12.0	9.5	10.0	10.5	10.9	11.6	12.0	12.4	12.8	13.4	13.9	14.3	14.6
12.5	9.8	10.5	10.9	11.4	12.0	12.5	12.9	13.3	14.0	14.4	14.9	15.2
13.0	10.2	10.9	11.4	11.8	12.5	13.0	13.4	13.9	14.6	15.0	15.5	15.8
13.5	10.6	11.3	11.8	12.3	13.0	13.5	13.9	14.4	15.1	15.6	16.1	16.4
14.0	11.0	11.7	12.2	12.7	13.5	14.0	14.5	14.9	15.7	16.2	16.7	17.0
14.5	11.4	12.1	12.7	13.2	14.0	14.5	15.0	15.5	16.2	16.7	17.3	17.6
15.0	11.8	12.6	13.1	13.7	14.4	15.0	15.5	16.0	16.8	17.3	17.9	18.4
15.5	12.2	13.0	13.6	14.1	14.9	15.5	16.0	16.5	17.4	17.9	18.4	19.0
16.0	12.6	13.4	14.0	14.6	15.4	16.0	16.5	17.1	17.9	18.5	19.0	19.6
16.5	13.0	13.8	14.4	15.0	15.9	16.5	17.0	17.6	18.5	19.1	19.6	20.2
17.0	13.4	14.2	14.9	15.5	16.4	17.0	17.6	18.1	19.0	19.6	20.2	20.8
17.5	13.8	14.7	15.3	15.9	16.8	17.5	18.1	18.7	19.6	20.2	20.8	21.4
18.0	14.2	15.1	15.8	16.4	17.3	18.0	18.6	19.2	19.8	20.8	21.4	22.0
18.5	14.6	15.5	16.2	16.8	17.8	18.5	19.1	19.7	20.7	21.4	22.0	22.6
19.0	15.0	16.0	16.6	17.3	18.3	19.0	19.6	20.3	21.2	21.9	22.6	23.2
19.5	15.4	16.4	17.1	17.7	18.8	19.5	20.1	20.8	21.8	22.5	23.2	23.9
20.0	15.8	16.8	17.5	18.2	19.3	20.0	20.6	21.3	22.4	23.1	23.8	24.5

APPENDIX B Approximate Caloric Expenditure per Minute Based on the Metabolic Equivalents (METS) for Physical Activity

73	75	77	80	82	84	86	89	91	93	95	98	100
161	165	169	176	180	185	189	196	200	205	209	216	220

METS

73	75	77	80	82	84	86	89	91	93	95	98	100
1.3	1.3	1.3	1.4	1.4	1.5	1.5	1.6	1.6	1.6	1.7	1.7	1.8
1.9	2.0	2.0	2.1	2.2	2.2	2.3	2.4	2.4	2.5	2.5	2.6	2.6
2.6	2.6	2.7	2.8	2.9	2.9	3.0	3.1	3.2	3.3	3.3	3.4	3.5
3.2	3.3	3.4	3.5	3.6	3.7	3.8	3.9	4.0	4.1	4.2	4.3	4.4
3.8	3.9	4.0	4.2	4.3	4.4	4.5	4.7	4.8	4.9	5.0	5.1	5.3
4.5	4.6	4.7	4.9	5.0	5.2	5.3	5.5	5.6	5.7	5.9	6.0	6.1
5.1	5.3	5.4	5.6	5.7	5.9	6.0	6.2	6.4	6.5	6.7	6.9	7.0
5.7	5.0	6.1	6.3	6.5	6.6	6.8	7.0	7.2	7.3	7.5	7.8	7.9
6.4	6.6	6.7	7.0	7.2	7.4	7.5	7.8	8.0	8.1	8.3	8.6	8.8
7.0	7.3	7.4	7.7	7.9	8.1	8.3	8.6	8.8	9.0	9.2	9.5	9.6
7.7	7.9	8.1	8.4	8.6	8.8	9.0	9.3	9.6	9.8	10.0	10.3	10.5
8.4	8.6	8.8	9.1	9.3	9,6	9.8	10.1	10.4	10.6	10.8	11.2	11.4
8.9	9.2	9.4	9.8	10.0	10.3	10.5	10.9	11.1	11.4	11.6	12.0	12.2
9.6	9.9	10.1	10.5	10.8	11.1	11.3	11.7	11.9	12.2	12/5	12.9	13.1
10.2	10.5	10.8	11.2	11.5	11.8	12.0	12.4	12.7	13.0	13.3	13.7	14.0
13.4	11.2	11.5	11.8	12.2	12.5	12.8	13.2	13.5	13.8	14/2	14.6	14.9
11.5	11.8	12.1	12.6	12.9	13.2	13.5	14.0	14.3	14.6	15.0	15.4	15.8
12.1	12.5	12.8	13.3	13.7	14.0	14.3	14.8	15.1	15.5	15.8	16.2	16.6
12.8	13.1	13.5	14.0	14.4	14.7	15.1	15.6	15.9	16.3	16.6	17.2	17.5
13.4	13.8	14.2	14.7	15.1	15.5	15.9	16.4	16.7	17.1	17.5	18.1	18.4
14.0	14.4	14.8	15.4	15.8	16.2	16.6	17.1	17.5	17.9	18.3	18.9	19.2
14.7	15.1	15.5	16.1	16.5	16.9	17.3	17.9	18.3	18.7	19.2	19.8	20.1
15.3	15.7	16.1	16.8	17.2	17.6	18.1	18.7	19.1	19.5	20.0	20.6	21.0
19.8	16.4	16.8	17.5	17.9	18.4	18.8	19.5	19.9	20.4	20.8	21.5	21.9
16.6	17.0	17.5	18.2	18.7	19.1	19.6	20.2	20.7	21.2	21.6	22.3	22.8
17.2	17.7	18.2	18.9	19.4	19.9	20,3	21.0	21.5	22/0	22/5	23.2	23.6
17.9	18.4	18.9	19.6	20.1	20.6	21.1	21.8	22.3	22.8	23.3	24.0	24.5
18.5	19.1	19.6	20.3	20.8	21.4	21.8	22.5	23.1	23.6	24.1	24.9	25.4
19.2	19.7	20.2	21.0	21.5	22.1	22.6	23.3	23.9	24.4	24.9	25.7	26.2
19.8	20.4	20.9	21.7	22.2	22.8	23.3	24.1	24/7	25.2	25.8	26.6	27.1
20.4	21.0	21.6	22.4	23.0	23.5	24.1	24.9	25.5	26.0	26.6	27.4	28.0
21.1	21.7	22.3	23.1	23.7	24.3	24.8	25.7	26.3	26.9	27.5	28.2	28.9
21.7	22.3	22.9	23.8	24.4	25.0	25.6	26.5	27.1	27.7	28.3	29.2	29.8
22.3	23.0	23.6	24.5	25.1	25.8	26.3	27.3	27.9	28.5	29.1	30.1	30.6
23.0	23.6	24.2	25.2	25.8	26.5	27.1	28.0	28.7	29.3	29.9	30.9	31.5
23.6	24.2	24.9	25.9	26.5	27.2	27.8	28.8	29.5	30.1	30.8	31.8	32.4
24.3	24.9	25.6	26.6	26.3	27.9	28.6	29.6	30.2	30.9	31.6	32.6	33.2
24.9	25.6	26.3	27.3	27.0	28.7	29.3	31.4	31.0	31.8	32.5	33.5	34.1
25.6	26.2	27.0	28.0	28.7	29.4	30.1	31.2	31.8	32.6	33.3	34.3	35.0

Determination of Healthy Body Weight

A number of different techniques are utilized to determine a healthy body weight. The following three methods offer you an estimate of an appropriate body weight. Method A is based on the body mass index (BMI). Method B is based on body-fat percentage. Method C, the waist circumference, does not determine a desirable body weight but provides an assessment of desirable body-fat distribution.

Method A

The BMI uses the metric system, so you need to determine your weight in kilograms and your height in meters. The formula is

$$\frac{\text{Body weight in kilograms}}{(\text{Height in meters})^2}$$

Dividing your body weight in pounds by 2.2 will give you your weight in kilograms. Multiplying your height in inches by 0.0254 will give you your height in meters.

$$\text{Your weight in kilograms} =$$
$$\frac{(\text{Your weight in pounds})}{2.2} = \underline{\quad}$$
$$\text{Your height in meters} =$$
$$(\text{Your height in inches}) \times 0.0254 = \underline{\quad}$$
$$\text{BMI} = \frac{\text{Body weight in kilograms}}{(\text{Height in meters})^2} = \underline{\quad}$$

Or you may use your weight in pounds and height in inches with the following formula:

$$\text{BMI} = \frac{\text{Body weight in pounds} \times 705}{(\text{Height in inches})^2}$$

A BMI range of 18.5 to 25 is considered to be normal, but a suggested desirable range for females is 21.3 to 22.1 and for males is 21.9 to 22.4. Individuals with BMI values between 25.0 and 29.9 are classified as overweight, those from 30.0 to 39.9 are classified as obese, and those 40 and above are classified as extremely obese. The higher the BMI, the greater the health risks faced by the individual, particularly diabetes, high blood pressure, and heart disease.

If you want to lower your body weight to a more desirable BMI, such as 22, use the following formula to determine what that weight should be; the weight is expressed in kilograms, so multiplying it by 2.2 will give you the desired weight in pounds.

$$\text{Kilograms body weight} =$$
$$\text{Desired BMI} \times (\text{Height in meters})^2$$

Here's a brief example for a woman who weighs 187 pounds and is 5′9″ tall; her BMI calculates to be 27.7, so her weight poses a health risk. If she wants to achieve a BMI of 23, she will need to reduce her weight to 155 pounds.

$$\text{Kilograms body weight} = 23 \times (1.753)^2 = 70.6$$

$$70.6 \text{ kg} \times 2.2 = 155 \text{ pounds}$$

To calculate your desired body weight:

$$\text{Kilograms body weight} =$$

$$(\text{Your desired BMI}) \times (\text{Your height in meters})^2$$

$$\text{Kilograms body weight} = \underline{\quad} \times \underline{\quad}$$

$$\underline{\quad} \text{ kg} \times 2.2 = \underline{\quad} \text{ pounds}$$

Keep in mind that the BMI does not discriminate between muscle mass and body fat, so a high BMI may reflect an increased muscle mass and body fat may actually be relatively low. Conversely, an individual with a low BMI may have a higher level of body fat if muscle mass is small. The BMI also does not account for regional fat distribution.

Method B

For this method, you will need to know your body-fat percentage as determined by the procedure described in table C.1 or another appropriate technique. You will also need to determine the body-fat percentage you desire to have. You may use table 10.2 as a guideline.

TABLE C.1 Generalized equations for predicting body fat

Measure the appropriate skinfolds for women (triceps, thigh, and suprailium sites) or men (chest, abdomen, and thigh sites) as illustrated in figures C.1–C.4. You may use either the appropriate formula or the appropriate table in appendix C to obtain the predicted body-fat percentage.

Women*	Men**
$BD = 1.0994921 - 0.0009929 (X_1) + 0.0000023 (X_1)^2 - 0.0001392 (X_2)$	$BD = 1.10938 - 0.0008267 (X_1) + 0.0000016 (X_1)^2 - 0.0002574 (X_2)$
BD = Body density	BD = Body density
X_1 = Sum of triceps, thigh, and suprailium skinfolds	X_1 = Sum of chest, abdomen, and thigh skinfolds
X_2 = Age	X_2 = Age

To calculate percent body fat, plug into Siri's equation.

$$\left(\frac{4.95}{BD} - 4.5 \right) \times 100$$

*From Jackson, A., Pollock, M., and Ward, A. 1980. Generalized equations for predicting body density of women. *Medicine & Science in Sports & Exercise* 12:175–82.
**Jackson, A., and Pollock, M. 1978. Generalized equations for predicting body density of men. *British Journal of Nutrition* 40:497–504.

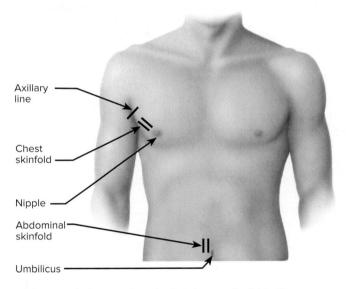

Axillary line

Chest skinfold

Nipple

Abdominal skinfold

Umbilicus

FIGURE C.1 The chest and abdomen skinfold. Chest—a diagonal fold is taken between the axilla and the nipple. Use a midway point. Abdomen—a vertical fold is taken about 2.5 centimeters (1 inch) to the side of the umbilicus.

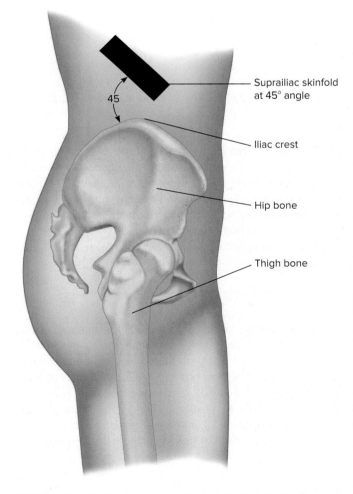

Suprailiac skinfold at 45° angle

Iliac crest

Hip bone

Thigh bone

45

FIGURE C.2 The suprailiac skinfold. A diagonal fold is taken at about a 45-degree angle just above the crest of the ilium.

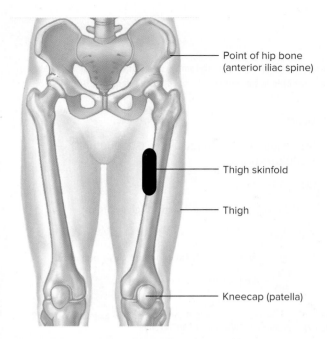

FIGURE C.3 The thigh skinfold. A vertical fold is taken on the front of the thigh midway between the anterior iliac spine and the patella.

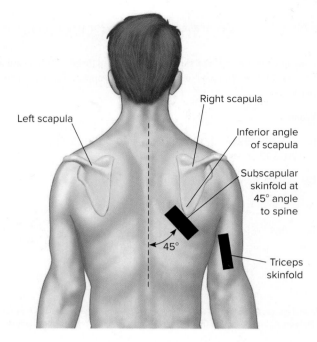

FIGURE C.4 The triceps and subscapular skinfolds. In the triceps skinfold, a vertical fold is taken over the triceps muscle one-half the distance from the acromion process to the olecranon process at the elbow. The subscapular skinfold is taken just below the lower angle of the scapula, at about a 45-degree angle to the spinal column.

You will need to do the following calculations for the formula:

1. Determine your current lean body weight (LBW). Multiply your current body weight in pounds by your current percent body fat expressed as a decimal (20 percent would be 0.20) to obtain your pounds of body fat. Subtract your pounds of body fat from your current weight to give you your lean body weight (LBW).
2. Determine your desired body-fat percentage and express it as a decimal.

$$\text{Desired body weight} = \frac{\text{LBW}}{1.00 - \text{Desired \% body fat}}$$

As an example, suppose we have a 200-pound male who is currently at 25 percent body fat but desires to get down to 20 percent as his first goal. Multiplying his current weight by his current percent body fat yields 50 pounds of body fat ($200 \times 0.25 = 50$); subtracting this from his current weight yields a LBW of 150 ($200 - 50$). If we plug his desired percent of 20 into the formula, he will need to reach a body weight of 187.5 to achieve this first goal.

$$\text{Desired body weight} = \frac{150}{1.00 - 0.20} = \frac{150}{0.8} = 187.5$$

Your current body weight _____
Your current percent body fat _____
Your pounds of body fat _____
Your LBW _____
Your desired percent body fat _____

$$\text{Desired body weight} \frac{\text{LBW}}{1.00 - ?} = \text{_____} = \text{_____}$$

Method C

The waist circumference is a measure of regional fat distribution. Using a flexible (preferably metal) tape, measure the narrowest section of the bare waist as seen from the front while standing. Wear tight clothing. Do not compress skin and fat with pressure from the tape. The waist measurement may be used as a simple screening technique for abdominal obesity. Females with a waist of 35 inches or over, and men with a waist of 40 inches or over may be at increased risk.

Waist girth _____

In the following table, use both your BMI and waist measurement to evaluate your risk of associated disease.

Risk of associated disease according to BMI and waist size

BMI		Waist less than or equal to 40 in. (men) or 35 in. (women)	Waist greater than 40 in. (men) or 35 in. (women)
18.5 or less	Underweight	—	N/A
18.5 – 24.9	Normal	—	N/A
25.0 – 29.9	Overweight	Increased	High
30.0 – 34.9	Obese	High	Very high
35.0 – 39.9	Obese	Very high	Very high
40 or greater	Extremely obese	Extremely high	Extremely high

Note: Recent research suggests that waist sizes greater than 37 inches in men and 31.5 inches in women may increase health risks when accompanied by other conditions, such as high blood pressure.
Source: www.consumer.gov/weightloss.bmi.htm

Percent fat estimate for men: sum of chest, abdomen, and thigh skinfolds

Sum of skinfolds (mm)	Age to last year								
	Under 22	23–27	28–32	33–37	38–42	43–47	48–52	53–57	Over 57
8–10	1.3	1.8	2.3	2.9	3.4	3.9	4.5	5.0	5.5
11–13	2.2	2.8	3.3	3.9	4.4	4.9	5.5	6.0	6.5
14–16	3.2	3.8	4.3	4.8	5.4	5.9	6.4	7.0	7.5
17–19	4.2	4.7	5.3	5.8	6.3	6.9	7.4	8.0	8.5
20–22	5.1	5.7	6.2	6.8	7.3	7.9	8.4	8.9	9.5
23–25	6.1	6.6	7.2	7.7	8.3	8.8	9.4	9.9	10.5
26–28	7.0	7.6	8.1	8.7	9.2	9.8	10.3	10.9	11.4
29–31	8.0	8.5	9.1	9.6	10.2	10.7	11.3	11.8	12.4
32–34	8.9	9.4	10.0	10.5	11.1	11.6	12.2	12.8	13.3
35–37	9.8	10.4	10.9	11.5	12.0	12.6	13.1	13.7	14.3
38–40	10.7	11.3	11.8	12.4	12.9	13.5	14.1	14.6	15.2
41–43	11.6	12.2	12.7	13.3	13.8	14.4	15.0	15.5	16.1
44–46	12.5	13.1	13.6	14.2	14.7	15.3	15.9	16.4	17.0
47–49	13.4	13.9	14.5	15.1	15.6	16.2	16.8	17.3	17.9
50–52	14.3	14.8	15.4	15.9	16.5	17.1	17.6	18.2	18.8
53–55	15.1	15.7	16.2	16.8	17.4	17.9	18.5	19.1	19.7
56–58	16.0	16.5	17.1	17.7	18.2	18.8	19.4	20.0	20.5
59–61	16.9	17.4	17.9	18.5	19.1	19.7	20.2	20.8	21.4
62–64	17.6	18.2	18.8	19.4	19.9	20.5	21.1	21.7	22.2
65–67	18.5	19.0	19.6	20.2	20.8	21.3	21.9	22.5	23.1
68–70	19.3	19.9	20.4	21.0	21.6	22.2	22.7	23.3	23.9
71–73	20.1	20.7	21.2	21.8	22.4	23.0	23.6	24.1	24.7
74–76	20.9	21.5	22.0	22.6	23.2	23.8	24.4	25.0	25.5
77–79	21.7	22.2	22.8	23.4	24.0	24.6	25.2	25.8	26.3
80–82	22.4	23.0	23.6	24.2	24.8	25.4	25.9	26.5	27.1
83–85	23.2	23.8	24.4	25.0	25.5	26.1	26.7	27.3	27.9
86–88	24.0	24.5	25.1	25.7	26.3	26.9	27.5	28.1	28.7
89–91	24.7	25.3	25.9	26.5	27.1	27.6	28.2	28.8	29.4
92–94	25.4	26.0	26.6	27.2	27.8	28.4	29.0	29.6	30.2
95–97	26.1	26.7	27.3	27.9	28.5	29.1	29.7	30.3	30.9
98–100	26.9	27.4	28.0	28.6	29.2	29.8	30.4	31.0	31.6
101–103	27.5	28.1	28.7	29.3	29.9	30.5	31.1	31.7	32.3
104–106	28.2	28.8	29.4	30.0	30.6	31.2	31.8	32.4	33.0
107–109	28.9	29.5	30.1	30.7	31.3	31.9	32.5	33.1	33.7
110–112	29.6	30.2	30.8	31.4	32.0	32.6	33.2	33.8	34.4
113–115	30.2	30.8	31.4	32.0	32.6	33.2	33.8	34.5	35.1
116–118	30.9	31.5	32.1	32.7	33.3	33.9	34.5	35.1	35.7
119–121	31.5	32.1	32.7	33.3	33.9	34.5	35.1	35.7	36.4
122–124	32.1	32.7	33.3	33.9	34.5	35.1	35.8	36.4	37.0
125–127	32.7	33.3	33.9	34.5	35.1	35.8	36.4	37.0	37.6

From A. S. Jackson and M. L. Pollock, "Practical Assessment of Body Composition," May 1985, in *Physician and Sportsmedicine*. Reprinted with permission of McGraw-Hill, Inc.

Percent fat estimate for women: sum of triceps, suprailium, and thigh skinfolds

Sum of skinfolds (mm)	Age to last year								
	Under 22	**23–27**	**28–32**	**33–37**	**38–42**	**43–47**	**48–52**	**53–57**	**Over 57**
23–25	9.7	9.9	10.2	10.4	10.7	10.9	11.2	11.4	11.7
26–28	11.0	11.2	11.5	11.7	12.0	12.3	12.5	12.7	13.0
29–31	12.3	12.5	12.8	13.0	13.3	13.5	13.8	14.0	14.3
32–34	13.6	13.8	14.0	14.3	14.5	14.8	15.0	15.3	15.5
35–37	14.8	15.0	15.3	15.5	15.8	16.0	16.3	16.5	16.8
38–40	16.0	16.3	16.5	16.7	17.0	17.2	17.5	17.7	18.0
41–43	17.2	17.4	17.7	17.9	18.2	18.4	18.7	18.9	19.2
44–46	18.3	18.6	18.8	19.1	19.3	19.6	19.8	20.1	20.3
47–49	19.5	19.7	20.0	20.2	20.5	20.7	21.0	21.2	21.5
50–52	20.6	20.8	21.1	21.3	21.6	21.8	22.1	22.3	22.6
53–55	21.7	21.9	22.1	22.4	22.6	22.9	23.1	23.4	23.6
56–58	22.7	23.0	23.2	23.4	23.7	23.9	24.2	24.4	24.7
59–61	23.7	24.0	24.2	24.5	24.7	25.0	25.2	25.5	25.7
62–64	24.7	25.0	25.2	25.5	25.7	26.0	26.2	26.4	26.7
65–67	25.7	25.9	26.2	26.4	26.7	26.9	27.2	27.4	27.7
68–70	26.6	26.9	27.1	27.4	27.6	27.9	28.1	28.4	28.6
71–73	27.5	27.8	28.0	28.3	28.5	28.8	29.0	29.3	29.5
74–76	28.4	28.7	28.9	29.2	29.4	29.7	29.9	30.2	30.4
77–79	29.3	29.5	29.8	30.0	30.3	30.5	30.8	31.0	31.3
80–82	30.1	30.4	30.6	30.9	31.1	31.4	31.6	31.9	32.1
83–85	30.9	31.2	31.4	31.7	31.9	32.2	32.4	32.7	32.9
86–88	31.7	32.0	32.2	32.5	32.7	32.9	33.2	33.4	33.7
89–91	32.5	32.7	33.0	33.2	33.5	33.7	33.9	34.2	34.4
92–94	33.2	33.4	33.7	33.9	34.2	34.4	34.7	34.9	35.2
95–97	33.9	34.1	34.4	34.6	34.9	35.1	35.4	35.6	35.9
98–100	34.6	34.8	35.1	35.3	35.5	35.8	36.0	36.3	36.5
101–103	35.3	35.4	35.7	35.9	36.2	36.4	36.7	36.9	37.2
104–106	35.8	36.1	36.3	36.6	36.8	37.1	37.3	37.5	37.8
107–109	36.4	36.7	36.9	37.1	37.4	37.6	37.9	38.1	38.4
110–112	37.0	37.2	37.5	37.7	38.0	38.2	38.5	38.7	38.9
113–115	37.5	37.8	38.0	38.2	38.5	38.7	39.0	39.2	39.5
116–118	38.0	38.3	38.5	38.8	39.0	39.3	39.5	39.7	40.0
119–121	38.5	38.7	39.0	39.2	39.5	39.7	40.0	40.2	40.5
122–124	39.0	39.2	39.4	39.7	39.9	40.2	40.4	40.7	40.9
125–127	39.4	39.6	39.9	40.1	40.4	40.6	40.9	41.1	41.4
128–130	39.8	40.0	40.3	40.5	40.8	41.0	41.3	41.5	41.8

From A. S. Jackson and M. L. Pollock, "Practical Assessment of Body Composition," May 1985, in *Physician and Sportsmedicine*. Reprinted with permission of McGraw-Hill, Inc.

Exchange Lists for Meal Planning*

What Are Exchange Lists?

Exchange Lists are foods listed together because they are alike. Each serving of a food has about the same amount of carbohydrate, protein, fat, and Calories as the other foods on that list. That is why any food on a list can be "exchanged," or traded, for any other food on the same list. For example, you can trade the slice of bread you might eat for breakfast for ½ cup of cooked cereal. Each of these foods equals one starch choice.

Exchange Lists

Foods are listed with their serving sizes, which are usually measured after cooking. When you begin, you should measure the size of each serving. This may help you learn to "eyeball" correct serving sizes.

The following chart shows the amount of nutrients in 1 serving from each list.

The Exchange Lists provide you with a lot of food choices (foods from the basic food groups, foods with added sugars,

Groups/lists	Carbohydrate (grams)	Protein (grams)	Fat (grams)	Calories
Carbohydrate group				
Starch	15	3	1 or less	80
Fruit	15	—	—	60
Milk				
Skim	12	8	0–3	90
Low-fat	12	8	5	120
Whole	12	8	8	150
Other carbohydrates	15	varies	varies	varies
Vegetables	5	2	—	25
Meat and meat substitutes group				
Very lean	—	7	0–1	35
Lean	—	7	3	55
Medium-fat	—	7	5	75
High-fat	—	7	8	100
Fat group	—	—	5	45

* The Exchange Lists are the basis of a meal planning system designed by a committee of the American Diabetes Association and the American Dietetic Association, now known as the Academy of Nutrition and Dietetics. While designed primarily for people with diabetes and others who must follow special diets, the Exchange Lists are based on principles of good nutrition that apply to everyone.
© 1995 American Diabetes Association, Inc., American Dietetic Association.

free foods, combination foods, and fast foods). This gives you variety in your meals. Several foods, such as dried beans and peas, bacon, and peanut butter, are on two lists. This gives you flexibility in putting your meals together. Whenever you choose new foods or vary your meal plan, monitor your blood glucose to see how these different foods affect your blood glucose level.

Most foods in the Carbohydrate group have about the same amount of carbohydrate per serving. You can exchange starch, fruit, or milk choices in your meal plan. Vegetables are in this group but contain only about 5 grams of carbohydrate.

A Word about Food Labels

Exchange information is based on foods found in grocery stores. However, food companies often change the ingredients in their products. That is why you need to check the Nutrition Facts panel of the food label.

The Nutrition Facts tell you the number of Calories and grams of carbohydrate, protein, and fat in 1 serving. Compare these numbers with the exchange information in this appendix to see how many exchanges you will be eating. In this way, food labels can help you add foods to your meal plans.

Ask your dietitian to help you use food label information to plan your meals, or read pages 63–69 for more tips on how to use food labels.

Getting Started!

See your dietitian regularly when you are first learning how to use your meal plan and the Exchange Lists. Your meal plan can be adjusted to fit changes in your lifestyle, such as work, school, vacation, or travel. Regular nutrition counseling can help you make positive changes in your eating habits.

Careful eating habits will help you feel better and be healthier, too. Best wishes and good eating with *Exchange Lists for Meal Planning*.

Starch List

Cereals, grains, pasta, breads, crackers, snacks, starchy vegetables, and cooked dried beans, peas, and lentils are starches. In general, one starch is

- ½ cup of cereal, grain, pasta, or starchy vegetable
- 1 ounce of a bread product, such as 1 slice of bread
- ¾ to 1 ounce of most snack foods (some snack foods may also have added fat)

Nutrition tips

1. Most starch choices are good sources of B vitamins.
2. Foods made from whole grains are good sources of fiber.
3. Dried beans and peas are a good source of protein and fiber.

Selection tips

1. Choose starches made with little fat as often as you can.
2. Starchy vegetables prepared with fat count as one starch and one fat.
3. Bagels or muffins can be 2, 3, or 4 ounces in size and can, therefore, count as 2, 3, or 4 starch choices. Check the size you eat.
4. Dried beans, peas, and lentils are also found on the Meat and Meat Substitutes list.
5. Regular potato chips and tortilla chips are found on the Other Carbohydrates list.
6. Most of the serving sizes are measured after cooking.
7. Always check Nutrition Facts on the food label.

One starch exchange equals
15 grams carbohydrate,
3 grams protein,
0–1 grams fat, and
80 Calories.

Bread

Bagel	½ (1 oz)
Bread, reduced-calorie	2 slices (1½ oz)
Bread, white, whole wheat, pumpernickel, rye	1 slice (1 oz)
Bread sticks, crisp, 4 in. long ×½ in	2 (⅔ oz)
English muffin	½
Hot dog or hamburger bun	½ (1 oz)
Pita, 6 in. across	½
Raisin bread, unfrosted	1 slice (1 oz)
Roll, plain, small	1 (1 oz)
Tortilla, corn, 6 in. across	1
Tortilla, flour, 7–8 in. across	1
Waffle, 4 ½ in. square, reduced-fat	1

Cereals and grains

Bran cereals	½ cup
Bulgur	½ cup
Cereals	½ cup
Cereals, unsweetened, ready-to-eat	¾ cup
Cornmeal (dry)	3 Tbsp
Couscous	⅓ cup
Flour (dry)	3 Tbsp
Granola, low-fat	¼ cup
Grape-Nuts	¼ cup
Grits	½ cup
Kasha	½ cup
Millet	¼ cup

Muesli	¼ cup
Oats	½ cup
Pasta	½ cup
Puffed cereal	1½ cups
Rice milk	½ cup
Rice, white or brown	⅓ cup
Shredded wheat	½ cup
Sugar-frosted cereal	½ cup
Wheat germ	3 Tbsp

Starchy vegetables

Baked beans	⅓ cup
Corn	½ cup
Corn on cob, medium	1 (5 oz)
Mixed vegetables with corn, peas, or pasta	1 cup
Peas, green	½ cup
Plantain	½ cup
Potato, baked or boiled	1 small (3 oz)
Potato, mashed	½ cup
Squash, winter (acorn, butternut)	1 cup
Yam, sweet potato, plain	½ cup

Crackers and snacks

Animal crackers	8
Graham crackers, 2 1/2 in. square	3
Matzoh	¾ oz
Melba toast	4 slices
Oyster crackers	24
Popcorn (popped, no fat added or low-fat microwave)	3 cups
Pretzels	¾ oz
Rice cakes, 4 in. across	2
Saltine-type crackers	6
Snack chips, fat-free (tortilla, potato)	15–20 (¾ oz)
Whole wheat crackers, no fat added	2–5 (¾ oz)

Dried beans, peas, and lentils (Count as 1 starch exchange, plus 1 very lean meat exchange.)

Beans and peas (garbanzo, pinto, kidney, white, split, black-eyed)	½ cup
Lentils	½ cup
Lima beans	⅔ cup
Miso ⚱	3 Tbsp

⚱ = 400 mg or more of sodium per serving.

Starchy foods prepared with fat (Count as 1 starch exchange, plus 1 fat exchange.)

Biscuit, 2 ½ in. across	1
Chow mein noodles	½ cup
Corn bread, 2 in. cube	1 (2 oz)
Crackers, round butter type	6
Croutons	1 cup
French-fried potatoes	16–25 (3 oz)
Granola	¼ cup
Muffin, small	1 (1 ½ oz)
Pancake, 4 in. across	2
Popcorn, microwave	3 cups
Sandwich crackers, cheese or peanut butter filling	3
Stuffing, bread (prepared)	⅓ cup
Taco shell, 6 in. across	2
Waffle, 4 ½ in. square	1
Whole wheat crackers, fat added	4–6 (1 oz)

Some food you buy uncooked will weigh less after you cook it. Starches often swell in cooking, so a small amount of uncooked starch will become a much larger amount of cooked food. The following table shows some of the changes.

Food (starch group)	Uncooked	Cooked
Oatmeal	3 Tbsp	½ cup
Cream of Wheat	2 Tbsp	½ cup
Grits	3 Tbsp	½ cup
Rice	2 Tbsp	⅓ cup
Spaghetti	¼ cup	½ cup
Noodles	⅓ cup	½ cup
Macaroni	¼ cup	½ cup
Dried beans	¼ cup	½ cup
Dried peas	¼ cup	½ cup
Lentils	3 Tbsp	½ cup
Common measurements		
3 tsp = 1 Tbsp	4 ounces = ½ cup	
4 Tbsp = ¼ cup	8 ounces = 1 cup	
5 ⅓ Tbsp = ⅓ cup	1 cup = ½ pint	

Fruit List

Fresh, frozen, canned, and dried fruits and fruit juices are on this list. In general, one fruit exchange is

- 1 small to medium fresh fruit
- 1/2 cup of canned or fresh fruit or fruit juice
- 1/4 cup of dried fruit

Nutrition tips

1. Fresh, frozen, and dried fruits have about 2 grams of fiber per choice. Fruit juices contain very little fiber.
2. Citrus fruits, berries, and melons are good sources of vitamin C.

Selection tips

1. Count 1/2 cup cranberries or rhubarb sweetened with sugar substitutes as free foods.
2. Read the Nutrition Facts on the food label. If 1 serving has more than 15 grams of carbohydrate, you will need to adjust the size of the serving you eat or drink.
3. Portion sizes for canned fruits are for the fruit and a small amount of juice.
4. Whole fruit is more filling than fruit juice and may be a better choice.
5. Food labels for fruits may contain the words "no sugar added" or "unsweetened." This means that no sucrose (table sugar) has been added.
6. Generally, fruit canned in extra light syrup has the same amount of carbohydrate per serving as the "no sugar added" or the juice pack. All canned fruits on the fruit list are based on one of these three types of pack.

One fruit exchange equals
15 grams carbohydrate and
60 Calories.
The weight includes skin, core, seeds, and rind.

Fruit

Apple, unpeeled, small	1 (4 oz)
Applesauce, unsweetened	½ cup
Apples, dried	4 rings
Apricots, canned	½ cup
Apricots, dried	8 halves
Apricots, fresh	4 whole (5½ oz)
Banana, small	1 (4 oz)
Blackberries	¾ cup
Blueberries	¾ cup
Cantaloupe, small	⅓ melon (11 oz) or 1 cup cubes
Cherries, sweet, fresh	12 (3 oz)
Cherries, sweet, canned	½ cup
Dates	3
Figs, dried	1½
Figs, fresh	1 ½ large or 2 medium (3 ½ oz)
Fruit cocktail	½ cup
Grapefruit, large	½ (11 oz)
Grapefruit sections, canned	¾ cup
Grapes, small	17 (3 oz)
Honeydew melon	1 slice (10 oz) or 1 cup cubes
Kiwi	1 (3 ½ oz)
Mandarin oranges, canned	¾ cup
Mango, small	½ fruit (5 ½ oz) or ½ cup
Nectarine, small	1 (5 oz)
Orange, small	1 (6 ½ oz)
Papaya	½ fruit (8 oz) or 1 cup cubes
Peach, medium, fresh	1 (6 oz)
Peaches, canned	½ cup
Pear, large, fresh	½ (4 oz)
Pears, canned	½ cup
Pineapple, canned	½ cup
Pineapple, fresh	¾ cup
Plums, canned	½ cup
Plums, small	2 (5 oz)
Prunes, dried	3
Raisins	2 Tbsp
Raspberries	1 cup
Strawberries	1¼ cup whole berries
Tangerines, small	2 (8 oz)
Watermelon	1 slice (13½ oz) or 1¼ cup cubes

Fruit juice

Apple juice/cider	½ cup
Cranberry juice cocktail	⅓ cup
Cranberry juice cocktail, reduced-calorie	1 cup
Fruit juice blends, 100% juice	⅓ cup
Grape juice	⅓ cup
Grapefruit juice	½ cup
Orange juice	½ cup
Pineapple juice	½ cup
Prune juice	⅓ cup

Milk List

Different types of milk and milk products are on this list. Cheeses are on the Meat list and cream and other dairy fats are on the Fat list. Based on the amount of fat they contain, milks are divided into skim/very low-fat milk, low-fat milk, and whole milk. One choice of these includes

	Carbohydrate (grams)	Protein (grams)	Fat (grams)	Calories
Skim/very low-fat	12	8	0–3	90
Low-fat	12	8	5	120
Whole	12	8	8	150

Nutrition tips

1. Milk and yogurt are good sources of calcium and protein. Check the food label.
2. The higher the fat content of milk and yogurt, the greater the amount of saturated fat and cholesterol. Choose lower-fat varieties.
3. For those who are lactose intolerant, look for lactose-reduced or lactose-free varieties of milk.

Selection tips

1. One cup equals 8 fluid ounces or 1/2 pint.
2. Look for chocolate milk, frozen yogurt, and ice cream on the Other Carbohydrates list.
3. Nondairy creamers are on the Free Foods list.
4. Look for rice milk on the Starch list.
5. Look for soy milk on the Medium-fat Meat list.

One milk exchange equals
12 grams carbohydrate and
8 grams protein.

Skim and very low-fat milk (0–3 grams fat per serving)

Skim milk	1 cup
½% milk	1 cup
1% milk	1 cup
Nonfat or low-fat buttermilk	1 cup
Evaporated skim milk	½ cup
Nonfat dry milk	⅓ cup dry

Low-fat (5 grams fat per serving)

2% milk	1 cup
Plain low-fat yogurt	¾ cup
Sweet acidophilus milk	1 cup
Plain nonfat yogurt	¾ cup
Nonfat or low-fat fruit-flavored yogurt sweetened with aspartame or with a nonnutritive sweetener	1 cup

Whole milk (8 grams fat per serving)

Whole milk	1 cup
Evaporated whole milk	½ cup
Goat's milk	1 cup
Kefir	1 cup

Other Carbohydrates List

You can substitute food choices from this list for a starch, fruit, or milk choice on your meal plan. Some choices will also count as one or more fat choices.

Food	Serving size	Exchanges per serving
Angel food cake, unfrosted	1/12th cake	2 carbohydrates
Brownie, small, unfrosted	2 in. square	1 carbohydrate, 1 fat
Cake, frosted	2 in. square	2 carbohydrates, 1 fat
Cake, unfrosted	2 in. square	1 carbohydrate, 1 fat
Cookie, fat-free	2 small	1 carbohydrate
Cookie or sandwich cookie with creme filling	2 small	1 carbohydrate, 1 fat
Cranberry sauce, jellied	1/4 cup	2 carbohydrates
Cupcake, frosted	1 small	2 carbohydrates, 1 fat
Doughnut, glazed	3 ¾ in. across (2 oz)	2 carbohydrates, 2 fats
Doughnut, plain cake	1 medium (1 ½ oz)	1 1/2 carbohydrates, 2 fats
Fruit juice bars, frozen, 100% juice	1 bar (3 oz)	1 carbohydrate
Fruit snacks, chewy (pureed fruit concentrate)	1 roll (¾ oz)	1 carbohydrate
Fruit spreads, 100% fruit	1 Tbsp	1 carbohydrate
Gelatin, regular	1/2 cup	1 carbohydrate
Gingersnaps	3	1 carbohydrate

Granola bar	1 bar	1 carbohydrate, 1 fat
Granola bar, fat-free	1 bar	2 carbohydrates
Hummus	⅓ cup	1 carbohydrate, 1 fat
Ice cream	½ cup	1 carbohydrate, 2 fats
Ice cream, light	½ cup	1 carbohydrate, 1 fat
Ice cream, fat-free, no sugar added	½ cup	1 carbohydrate
Jam or jelly, regular	1 Tbsp	1 carbohydrate
Milk, chocolate, whole	1 cup	2 carbohydrates, 1 fat
Pie, fruit, 2 crusts	⅙ pie	3 carbohydrates, 2 fats
Pie, pumpkin or custard	⅛ pie	1 carbohydrate, 2 fats
Potato chips	12–18 (1 oz)	1 carbohydrate, 2 fats
Pudding, regular (made with low-fat milk)	½ cup	2 carbohydrates
Pudding, sugar-free (made with low-fat milk)	½ cup	1 carbohydrate
Salad dressing, fat free ▲	¼ cup	1 carbohydrate
Sherbet, sorbet	½ cup	2 carbohydrates
Spaghetti or pasta sauce, canned ▲	½ cup	1 carbohydrate, 1 fat
Sweet roll or Danish	1 (2½ oz)	2 1/2 carbohydrates, 2 fats
Syrup, light	2 Tbsp	1 carbohydrate
Syrup, regular	1 Tbsp	1 carbohydrate
Syrup, regular	¼ cup	4 carbohydrates
Tortilla chips	6–12 (1 oz)	1 carbohydrate, 2 fats
Vanilla wafers	5	1 carbohydrate, 1 fat
Yogurt, frozen, fat-free, no sugar added	½ cup	1 carbohydrate
Yogurt, frozen, low-fat, fat-free	⅓ cup	1 carbohydrate, 0–1 fat
Yogurt, low-fat with fruit	1 cup	3 carbohydrates, 0–1 fat

▲ = 400 mg or more sodium per exchange.

Nutrition tips

1. These foods can be substituted in your meal plan, even though they contain added sugars or fat. However, they do not contain as many important vitamins and minerals as the choices on the Starch, Fruit, or Milk list.
2. When planning to include these foods in your meal, be sure to include foods from all the lists to eat a balanced meal.

Selection tips

1. Because many of these foods are concentrated sources of carbohydrate and fat, the portion sizes are often very small.
2. Always check Nutrition Facts on the food label. It will be your most accurate source of information.
3. Many fat-free or reduced-fat products made with fat replacers contain carbohydrate. When eaten in large amounts,

they may need to be counted. Talk with your dietitian to determine how to count these in your meal plan.
4. Look for fat-free salad dressings in smaller amounts on the Free Foods list.

One exchange equals
15 grams carbohydrate, or
1 starch, or 1 fruit, or 1 milk.

Vegetable List

Vegetables that contain small amounts of carbohydrates and Calories are on this list. Vegetables contain important nutrients. Try to eat at least 2 or 3 vegetable choices each day. In general, one vegetable exchange is

- ½ cup of cooked vegetables or vegetable juice
- 1 cup of raw vegetables

If you eat 1 to 2 vegetable choices at a meal or snack, you do not have to count the Calories or carbohydrates because they contain small amounts of these nutrients.

Nutrition tips

1. Fresh and frozen vegetables have less added salt than canned vegetables. Drain and rinse canned vegetables if you want to remove some salt.
2. Choose more dark green and dark yellow vegetables, such as spinach, broccoli, romaine, carrots, chilies, and peppers.
3. Broccoli, brussels sprouts, cauliflower, greens, peppers, spinach, and tomatoes are good sources of vitamin C.
4. Vegetables contain 1 to 4 grams of fiber per serving.

Selection tips

1. A 1-cup portion of broccoli is a portion about the size of a lightbulb.
2. Tomato sauce is different from spaghetti sauce, which is on the Other Carbohydrates list.
3. Canned vegetables and juices are available without added salt.
4. If you eat more than 4 cups of raw vegetables or 2 cups of cooked vegetables at one meal, count them as 1 carbohydrate choice.
5. Starchy vegetables such as corn, peas, winter squash, and potatoes that contain larger amounts of Calories and carbohydrates are on the Starch list.

One vegetable exchange equals
5 grams carbohydrate,
2 grams protein,
0 grams fat, and
25 Calories.

Artichoke
Artichoke hearts
Asparagus
Beans (green, wax, Italian)
Bean sprouts
Beets
Broccoli
Brussels sprouts
Cabbage
Carrots
Cauliflower
Celery
Cucumber
Eggplant
Green onions or scallions
Greens (collard, kale, mustard, turnip)
Kohlrabi
Leeks
Mixed vegetables (without corn, peas, or pasta)
Mushrooms

Okra
Onions
Pea pods
Peppers (all varieties)
Radishes
Salad greens (endive, escarole, lettuce, romaine, spinach)
Sauerkraut 🧂
Spinach
Summer squash
Tomato
Tomatoes, canned
Tomato sauce 🧂
Tomato/vegetable juice 🧂
Turnips
Water chestnuts
Watercress
Zucchini

🧂 = 400 mg or more sodium per exchange.

Meat and Meat Substitutes List

Meat and meat substitutes that contain both protein and fat are on this list. In general, one meat exchange is

- 1 oz meat, fish, poultry, or cheese
- ½ cup dried beans

Based on the amount of fat they contain, meats are divided into very lean, lean, medium-fat, and high-fat lists. This is done so you can see which ones contain the least amount of fat. One ounce (one exchange) of each of these includes

	Carbohydrate (grams)	Protein (grams)	Fat (grams)	Calories
Very lean	0	7	0–1	35
Lean	0	7	3	55
Medium-fat	0	7	5	75
High-fat	0	7	8	100

Nutrition tips

1. Choose very lean and lean meat choices whenever possible. Items from the high-fat group are high in saturated fat, cholesterol, and Calories and can raise blood cholesterol levels.
2. Meats do not have any fiber.
3. Dried beans, peas, and lentils are good sources of fiber.
4. Some processed meats, seafood, and soy products may contain carbohydrate when consumed in large amounts. Check the Nutrition Facts on the label to see if the amount is close to 15 grams. If so, count it as a carbohydrate choice as well as a meat choice.

Selection tips

1. Weigh meat after cooking and removing bones and fat. Four ounces of raw meat is equal to 3 ounces of cooked meat. Some examples of meat portions are

   - 1 ounce cheese = 1 meat choice and is about the size of a 1-inch cube
   - 2 ounces meat = 2 meat choices, such as
     1 small chicken leg or thigh
     ½ cup cottage cheese or tuna
   - 3 ounces meat = 3 meat choices and is about the size of a deck of cards, such as
     1 medium pork chop
     1 small hamburger
     ½ of a whole chicken breast
     1 unbreaded fish fillet

2. Limit your choices from the high-fat group to three times per week or less.
3. Most grocery stores stock Select and Choice grades of meat. Select grades of meat are the leanest meats.
4. Choice grades contain a moderate amount of fat, and Prime cuts of meat have the highest amount of fat. Restaurants usually serve Prime cuts of meat.
5. "Hamburger" may contain added seasoning and fat, but ground beef does not.
6. Read labels to find products that are low in fat and cholesterol (5 grams or less of fat per serving).
7. Dried beans, peas, and lentils are also found on the Starch list.
8. Peanut butter, in smaller amounts, is also found on the Fats list.
9. Bacon, in smaller amounts, is also found on the Fats list.

Meal planning tips

1. Bake, roast, broil, grill, poach, steam, or boil these foods rather than frying.
2. Place meat on a rack so the fat will drain off during cooking.
3. Use a nonstick spray and a nonstick pan to brown or fry foods.
4. Trim off visible fat before or after cooking.
5. If you add flour, bread crumbs, coating mixes, fat, or marinades when cooking, ask your dietitian how to count it in your meal plan.

Very lean meat and substitutes list (One exchange equals 0 grams carbohydrate, 7 grams protein, 0–1 grams fat, and 35 Calories.)

One very lean meat exchange is equal to any one of the following items.

Poultry: Chicken or turkey (white meat, no skin), Cornish hen (no skin) .... 1 oz

Fish: Fresh or frozen cod, flounder, haddock, halibut, trout; tuna fresh or canned in water .... 1 oz

Shellfish: Clams, crab, lobster, scallops, shrimp, imitation shellfish .... 1 oz

Game: Duck or pheasant (no skin), venison, buffalo, ostrich .... 1 oz

Cheese with 1 gram or less fat per ounce:

Nonfat or low-fat cottage cheese .... ¼ cup

Fat-free cheese .... 1 oz

Other: Processed sandwich meat with 1 gram or less fat per ounce, such as deli thin, shave meats, chipped beef 🜕, turkey ham .... 1 oz

Egg whites 2

Egg substitutes, plain .... ¼ cup

Hot dogs with 1 gram or less fat per ounce 🜕 .... 1 oz

Kidney (high in cholesterol) .... 1 oz

Sausage with 1 gram or less fat per ounce .... 1 oz

Count as one very lean meat and one starch exchange.

Dried beans, peas, lentils (cooked) .... ½ cup

🜕 = 400 mg or more sodium per exchange.

Lean meat and substitutes list (One exchange equals 0 grams carbohydrate, 7 grams protein, 3 grams fat, and 55 Calories.)

One lean meat exchange is equal to any one of the following items.

Beef: USDA Select or Choice grades of lean beef trimmed of fat, such as round, sirloin, and flank steak; tenderloin; roast (rib, chuck, rump); steak (T-bone, Porterhouse, cubed), ground round .... 1 oz

Pork: Lean pork, such as fresh ham; canned, cured, or boiled ham; Canadian bacon 🜕; tenderloin, center loin chop .... 1 oz

Lamb: Roast, chop, leg .... 1 oz

Veal: Lean chop, roast .... 1 oz

Poultry: Chicken, turkey (dark meat, no skin), chicken white meat (with skin), domestic duck or goose (well-drained of fat, no skin) .... 1 oz

Fish:

Herring (uncreamed or smoked) .... 1 oz

Oysters .... 6 medium

Salmon (fresh or canned), catfish .... 1 oz

Sardines (canned) .... 2 medium

Tuna (canned in oil, drained) .... 1 oz

Game: Goose (no skin), rabbit .... 1 oz

Cheese:

4.5%-fat cottage cheese .... ¼ cup

Grated Parmesan .... 2 Tbsp

Cheeses with 3 grams or less fat
per ounce .... 1 oz

Other:

Hot dogs with 3 grams or less fat per ounce .... 1½ oz

Processed sandwich meat with 3 grams or
less fat per ounce, such as turkey pastrami or
kielbasa .... 1 oz

Liver, heart (high in cholesterol) .... 1 oz

Medium-fat meat and substitutes list (One exchange equals 0 grams carbohydrate, 7 grams protein, 5 grams fat, and 75 Calories.)

One medium-fat meat exchange is equal to any one of the following items.

Beef: Most beef products fall into this category
(ground beef, meatloaf, corned beef, short
ribs, prime grades of meat trimmed of fat,
such as prime rib) .... 1 oz

Pork: Top loin, chop, Boston butt,
cutlet .... 1 oz

Lamb: Rib roast, ground .... 1 oz

Veal: Cutlet (ground or cubed,
unbreaded) .... 1 oz

Poultry: Chicken dark meat (with skin), ground
turkey or ground chicken, fried chicken
(with skin) .... 1 oz

Fish: Any fried fish product .... 1 oz

Cheese: With 5 grams or less fat per ounce

Feta .... 1 oz

Mozzarella .... 1 oz

Ricotta .... ¼ cup (2 oz)

Other:

Egg (high in cholesterol, limit to 3 per week) 1

Sausage with 5 grams or less fat
per ounce .... 1 oz

Soy milk .... 1 cup

Tempeh .... ¼ cup

Tofu .... 4 oz or ½ cup

High-fat meat and substitutes list (One exchange equals 0 grams carbohydrate, 7 grams protein, 8 grams fat, and 100 Calories.)

Remember these items are high in saturated fat, cholesterol, and Calories and may raise blood cholesterol levels if eaten on a regular basis. One high-fat meat exchange is equal to any one of the following items.

Pork: Spareribs, ground pork, pork
sausage .... 1 oz

Cheese: All regular cheeses, such as American, ▮
cheddar, Monterey Jack, Swiss .... 1 oz

Other: Processed sandwich meats with 8 grams or
less fat per ounce, such as bologna, pimento
loaf, salami .... 1 oz

Sausage, such as bratwurst, Italian, knockwurst,
Polish, smoked .... 1 oz

Hot dog (turkey or chicken) ▮ 1 (10/lb)

Bacon .... 3 slices (20 slices/lb)

Count as one high-fat meat plus one fat exchange.

Hot dog (beef, pork, or combination) ▮ 1 (10/lb)

Peanut butter (contains unsaturated fat) .... 2 Tbsp

▮ = 400 mg or more sodium per exchange.

Fat List

Fats are divided into three groups, based on the main type of fat they contain: monounsaturated, polyunsaturated, and saturated. Small amounts of monounsaturated and polyunsaturated fats in the foods we eat are linked with good health benefits. Saturated fats are linked with heart disease and cancer. In general, one fat exchange is

- 1 teaspoon of regular margarine or vegetable oil
- 1 tablespoon of regular salad dressing

Nutrition tips

1. All fats are high in Calories. Limit serving sizes for good nutrition and health.
2. Nuts and seeds contain small amounts of fiber, protein, and magnesium.
3. If blood pressure is a concern, choose fats in the unsalted form to help lower sodium intake, such as unsalted peanuts.

Selection tips

1. Check the Nutrition Facts on food labels for serving sizes. One fat exchange is based on a serving size containing 5 grams of fat.
2. When selecting regular margarine, choose those with liquid vegetable oil as the first ingredient. Soft margarines

are not as saturated as stick margarines. Soft margarines are healthier choices. Avoid those listing hydrogenated or partially hydrogenated fat as the first ingredient.

3. When selecting low-fat margarines, look for liquid vegetable oil as the second ingredient. Water is usually the first ingredient.

4. When used in smaller amounts, bacon and peanut butter are counted as fat choices. When used in larger amounts, they are counted as high-fat meat choices.

5. Fat-free salad dressings are on the Other Carbohydrates list and the Free Foods list.

6. See the Free Foods list for nondairy coffee creamers, whipped topping, and fat-free products, such as margarines, salad dressings, mayonnaise, sour cream, cream cheese, and nonstick cooking spray.

Monounsaturated fats list (One fat exchange equals 5 grams fat and 45 Calories.)

Avocado, medium	1/8 (1 oz)
Nuts	
almonds, cashews	6 nuts
mixed (50% peanuts)	6 nuts
peanuts	10 nuts
pecans	4 halves
Oil (canola, olive, peanut)	1 tsp
Olives: ripe (black)	8 large
green, stuffed 🛑	10 large
Peanut butter, smooth or crunchy	2 tsp
Sesame seeds	1 Tbsp
Tahini paste	2 tsp

Polyunsaturated fats list (One fat exchange equals 5 grams fat and 45 Calories.)

Margarine: stick, tub, or squeeze	1 tsp
lower-fat (30% to 50% vegetable oil)	1 Tbsp
Mayonnaise: regular	1 tsp
reduced-fat	1 Tbsp
Miracle Whip Salad Dressing®: regular	2 tsp
reduced-fat	1 Tbsp
Nuts, walnuts, English	4 halves
Oil (corn, safflower, soybean)	1 tsp
Salad dressing: regular	1 Tbsp
reduced-fat	2 Tbsp
Seeds: pumpkin, sunflower	1 Tbsp

🛑 = 400 mg or more sodium per exchange.

Saturated fats list* (One fat exchange equals 5 grams of fat and 45 Calories.)

Bacon, cooked	1 slice (20 slices/lb)
Bacon, grease	1 tsp

Butter: stick	1 tsp
reduced-fat	1 Tbsp
whipped	2 tsp
Chitterlings, boiled	2 Tbsp (1/2 oz)
Coconut, sweetened, shredded	2 Tbsp
Cream, half and half	2 Tbsp
Cream cheese: regular	1 Tbsp (1/2 oz)
reduced-fat	2 Tbsp (1 oz)
Fatback or salt pork, see below†	
Shortening or lard	1 tsp
Sour cream: regular	2 Tbsp
reduced-fat	3 Tbsp

*Saturated fats can raise blood cholesterol levels.
†Use a piece 1 in. × 1 in. × 1/4 in. if you plan to eat the fatback cooked with vegetables. Use a piece 2 in. × 1 in. × 1/2 in. when eating only the vegetables with the fatback removed.

Free Foods List

A *free food* is any food or drink that contains less than 20 Calories or less than 5 grams of carbohydrate per serving. Foods with a serving size listed should be limited to 3 servings per day. Be sure to spread them out throughout the day. If you eat all 3 servings at one time, it could affect your blood glucose level. Foods listed without a serving size can be eaten as often as you like.

Fat-free or reduced-fat foods

Cream cheese, fat-free	1 Tbsp
Creamers, nondairy, liquid	1 Tbsp
Creamers, nondairy, powdered	2 tsp
Margarine, fat-free	4 Tbsp
Margarine, reduced-fat	1 tsp
Mayonnaise, fat-free	1 Tbsp
Mayonnaise, reduced-fat	1 tsp
Miracle Whip®, nonfat	1 Tbsp
Miracle Whip®, reduced-fat	1 tsp
Nonstick cooking spray	
Salad dressing, fat-free	1 Tbsp
Salad dressing, fat-free, Italian	2 Tbsp
Salsa	¼ cup
Sour cream, fat-free, reduced-fat	1 Tbsp
Whipped topping, regular or light	2 Tbsp

Sugar-free or low-sugar foods

Candy, hard, sugar-free	1 candy
Gelatin dessert, sugar-free	
Gelatin, unflavored	
Gum, sugar-free	
Jam or jelly, low-sugar or light	2 tsp

Sugar substitutes[†]
Syrup, sugar-free .... 2 Tbsp

[†] Sugar substitutes, alternatives, or replacements that are approved by the Food and Drug Administration (FDA) are safe to use. Common brand names include
Equal® (aspartame)
Splenda® (sucralose)
Sprinkle Sweet® (saccharin)
Sugar Twin® (saccharin)
Sweet'n Low® (saccharin)
Sweet One® (acesulfame K)
Sweet-10® (saccharin)

Drinks

Bouillon, broth, consommé ♠
Bouillon or broth, low-sodium
Carbonated or mineral water
Club soda
Cocoa powder, unsweetened .... 1 Tbsp
Coffee
Diet soft drinks, sugar-free
Drink mixes, sugar-free
Tea
Tonic water, sugar-free

Condiments

Catsup .... 1 Tbsp
Horseradish
Lemon juice
Lime juice
Mustard

Pickles, dill ♠ .... 1 1/2 large
Soy sauce, regular or light ♠
Taco sauce .... 1 Tbsp
Vinegar

Seasonings

Be careful with seasonings that contain sodium or are salts, such as garlic or celery salt, and lemon pepper.

Flavoring extracts
Garlic
Herbs, fresh or dried
Pimento
Spices
Tabasco® or hot pepper sauce
Wine, used in cooking
Worcestershire sauce

♠ = 400 mg or more of sodium per choice.

Combination Foods List

Many of the foods we eat are mixed together in various combinations. These combination foods do not fit into any one Exchange List. Often it is hard to tell what is in a casserole dish or prepared food item. This is a list of exchanges for some typical combination foods. This list will help you fit these foods into your meal plan. Ask your dietitian for information about any other combination foods you would like to eat.

Food entrees	Serving size	Exchanges per serving
Chow mein (without noodles or rice)	2 cups (16 oz)	1 carbohydrate, 2 lean meats
Pizza, cheese, thin crust ♠	1/4 of 10 in. (5 oz)	2 carbohydrates, 2 medium-fat meats, 1 fat
Pizza, meat topping, thin crust ♠	1/4 of 10 in. (5 oz)	2 carbohydrates, 2 medium-fat meats, 2 fats
Pot pie ♠	1 (7 oz)	2 carbohydrates, 1 medium-fat meat, 4 fats
Tuna noodle casserole, lasagna, spaghetti with meatballs, chili with beans, macaroni and cheese ♠	1 cup (8 oz)	2 carbohydrates, 2 medium-fat meats

Frozen entrees	Serving size	Exchanges per serving
Entree with less than 300 calories ♠	1 (8 oz)	2 carbohydrates, 3 lean meats
Salisbury steak with gravy, mashed potato ♠	1 (11 oz)	2 carbohydrates, 3 medium-fat meats, 3–4 fats
Turkey with gravy, mashed potato, dressing ♠	1 (11 oz)	2 carbohydrates, 2 medium-fat meats, 2 fats

Soups	Serving size	Exchanges per serving
Bean ♠	1 cup	1 carbohydrate, 1 very lean meat
Cream (made with water) ♠	1 cup (8 oz)	1 carbohydrate, 1 fat
Split pea (made with water) ♠	1/2 cup (4 oz)	1 carbohydrate
Tomato (made with water) ♠	1 cup (8 oz)	1 carbohydrate
Vegetable beef, chicken noodle, or other broth-type ♠	1 cup (8 oz)	1 carbohydrate

♠ = 400 mg or more sodium per exchange.

Fast Foods*

Food entrees	Serving size	Exchanges per serving
Burritos with beef ⬛	2	4 carbohydrates, 2 medium-fat meats, 2 fats
Chicken breast and wing, breaded and fried ⬛	1 each	1 carbohydrate, 4 medium-fat meats, 2 fats
Chicken nuggets ⬛	6	1 carbohydrate, 2 medium-fat meats, 1 fat
Fish sandwich/tartar sauce ⬛	1	3 carbohydrates, 1 medium-fat meat, 3 fats
French fries, thin	20–25	2 carbohydrates, 2 fats
Hamburger, large ⬛	1	2 carbohydrates, 3 medium-fat meats, 1 fat
Hamburger, regular	1	2 carbohydrates, 2 medium-fat meats
Hot dog with a bun ⬛	1	1 carbohydrate, 1 high-fat meat, 1 fat
Individual pan pizza ⬛	1	5 carbohydrates, 3 medium-fat meats, 3 fats
Soft-serve cone ⬛	1 medium	2 carbohydrates, 1 fat
Submarine sandwich ⬛	1 sub (6 in.)	3 carbohydrates, 1 vegetable, 2 medium-fat meats, 1 fat
Taco, hard shell ⬛	1 (6 oz)	2 carbohydrates, 2 medium-fat meats, 2 fats
Taco, soft shell	1 (3 oz)	1 carbohydrate, 1 medium-fat meat, 1 fat

⬛ = 400 mg or more of sodium per serving.

*Ask at your fast-food restaurant for nutrition information about your favorite fast foods. Also, see appendix E.

Nutrient Content of Food Products from Selected Fast-Food Restaurants

Since the early 1950s, the number of fast-food restaurants has increased dramatically in the United States, as well as in many other countries throughout the world. Fast-food restaurants live up to their name, providing customers with various food selections in a short period of time. But such products are also usually inexpensive, another factor that attracts customers. However, such products may also contain substantial amounts of ingredients, such as sugar, refined grains, and fat, that may not be conducive to optimal health. Many fast-food restaurants now provide in-house menus, containing information on the nutrient content of their products.

Past editions of this book provided a list of about ten fast-food restaurants, along with the total Calories, percent fat Calories, cholesterol, sodium, and dietary fiber, for five or six of their most popular products. However, food offerings at fast-food restaurants may change rapidly, with modifications in the nutrient content, and thus the list would soon be outdated. Moreover, Restaurant Websites may provide options to select food products based on nutrient content to help you select a more healthful item.

This edition simply lists the major fast-food chains' Websites, where you can access the nutrient content of specific items in more detail. On each Website, look for terms such as *nutrient analysis,* which will provide you with details for each product the restaurant sells. Such information may include some or all of the following.

Calories	Cholesterol	Protein
Calories from fat	Sodium	Vitamin A
Fat, total	Total carbohydrate	Vitamin C
Saturated fat	Dietary fiber	Calcium
Trans fat	Sugars	Iron

Websites of Selected Fast-Food Restaurants

Arby's (www.arbys.com)
Click on the food item, then Nutritional Info on the bottom of the page.
Au Bon Pain (www.aubonpain.com) Click on Nutrition, then Nutrition Menu PDF.
Baja Fresh (www.bajafresh.com)
Click on Nutrition at the top, then the menu item, such as burritos.
Burger King (www.bk.com)
Scroll down to the bottom and click on Nutrition Information under BK cares.
Chipotle Mexican Grill (www.chipotle.com)
Click on Menu at the top of the page, then Nutrition Calculator on the pop-up list. Select a menu item, then ingredients and added extras.
Hardee's (www.hardees.com)
Click on Menu and Nutrition at the top of the page, then Nutrition Guide under Nutrition Downloads.
Jason's Deli (www.jasonsdeli.com)
Click on Interactive Nutrition Menu for prepared items, or click on Nutrition Calculator to prepare your own meal.
KFC (www.KFC.com)
Scroll to the bottom and under Nutrition click on Full Nutrition PDF.
Long John Silver's (www.longjohnsilvers.com)
Click on Menu and scroll to the bottom and click on Nutrition Information.
McDonald's (www.mcdonalds.com)
Click on Food, then Nutrition Choices, then Nutrition info for a PDF file.

Panera (www.panera.com) Click on Menu and Nutrition, then an item on the menu such as Panini. Click on a specific item and some nutrition information is provided, but click on Full Nutrition Details for more information.

Pizza Hut (www.pizzahut.com)

Scroll to the bottom and click on Nutrition Information.

Subway (www.subway.com)

At the top, click on Menu and Nutrition, then Nutrition Information on the pop-up screen.

Taco Bell (www.tacobell.com)

At the top of the page, click on Nutrition, then Full Nutrition Information.

Tropical Smoothie Café (www.tropicalsmoothie.com)

Scroll down and click on Nutritional Guide under Get the Facts.

Wendy's (www.wendys.com)

Scroll to the bottom and click on Nutrition Information under Quick Links, and then click on Nutrition and Ingredient Information. Choose a Menu Category such as cheeseburgers, and then click on a specific food item.

Energy Pathways of Carbohydrate, Fat, and Protein

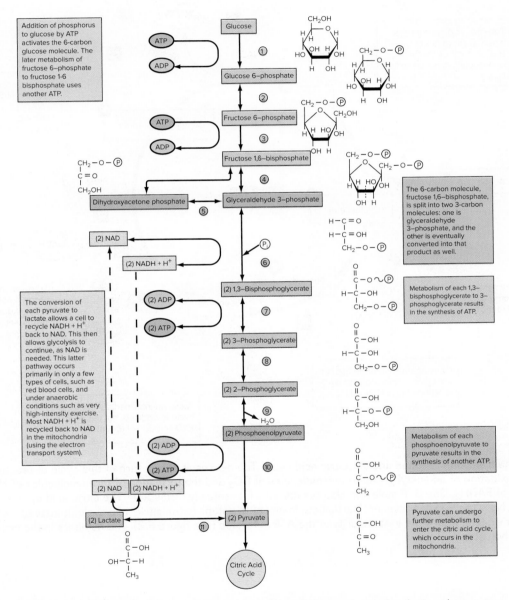

FIGURE F.1 Detailed depiction of the individual chemical reactions that constitute glycolysis—glucose to pyruvate. Glycolysis takes place in the cytosol of the cell. The enzymes in the cytosol that participate at the following steps are (1) hexokinase, (2) phosphohexose isomerase, (3) phosphofructokinase, (4) aldolase, (5) phosphotriose isomerase, (6) glyceraldehyde-3-phosphate dehydrogenase, (7) phosphoglycerate kinase, (8) phosphoglycerate mutase, (9) enolase, and (10) pyruvate kinase. Sometimes (11) lactate dehydrogenase is used to recycle NADH + H$^+$ back to NAD (anaerobic glycolysis). represents a phosphate group. Ⓟ represents a phosphate group.

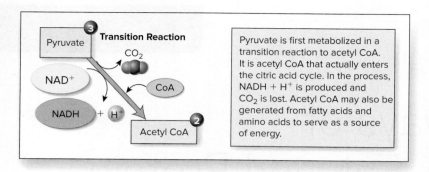

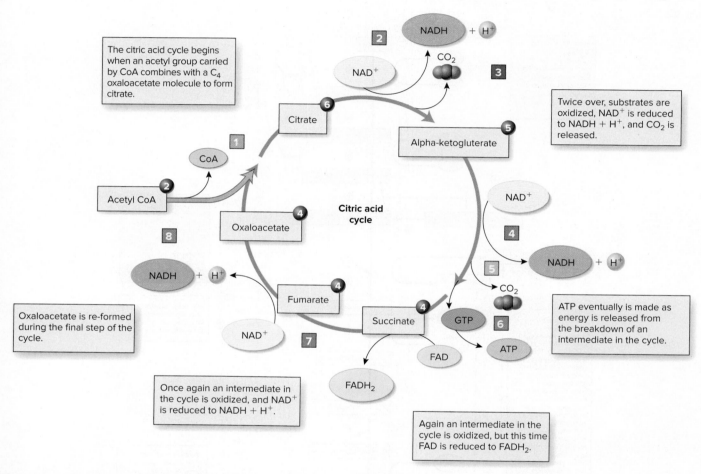

FIGURE F.2 The transition reaction and the citric acid cycle. The net result of one turn of this cycle of reactions (squares, steps 1–8) is the oxidation of an acetyl group to two molecules of CO_2 and the formation of three molecules of NADH + H$^+$ and one molecule of FADH$_2$. One GTP molecule also results, which eventually forms ATP. The citric acid cycle turns twice per glucose molecule. Note that oxygen does not participate in any of the steps in the citric acid cycle. It instead participates in the electron transport system, where the vast majority of the ATP is formed (see figure F.3). The numbers in the circles represent the number of carbon atoms.

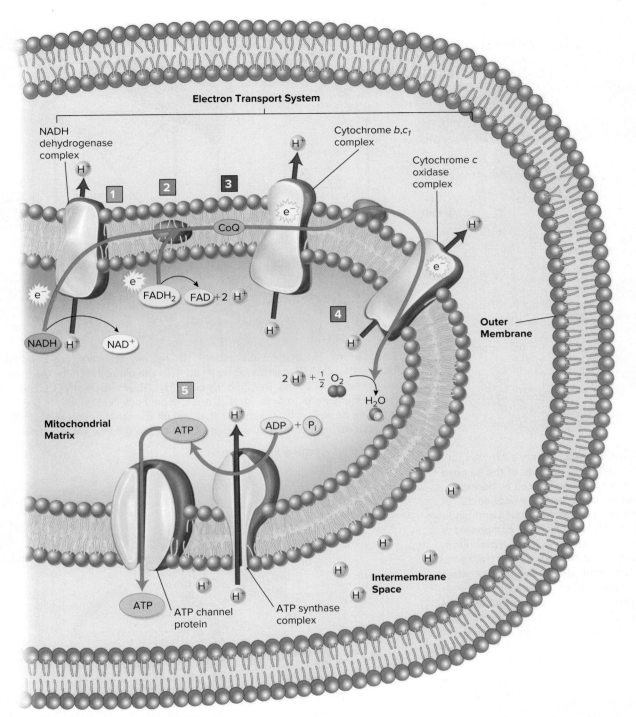

FIGURE F.3 Organization of the electron transport system. As electrons move from one molecular complex to the other, hydrogen ions (H$^+$) are pumped from the mitochondrial matrix into the intermembrane space (steps 1–4). (Note that each mitochondrion has an inner and outer membrane. Hydrogen ions flow down a concentration gradient from the intermembrane space into the mitochondrial matrix; ATP is then synthesized by the enzyme ATP synthase (step 5). ATP leaves the mitochondrial matrix by way of a channel protein.

Adipose Cells

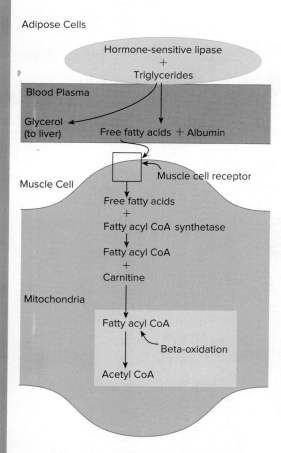

FIGURE F.4A Energy pathways for fatty acids. Triglycerides in the adipose tissue may be catabolized by hormone-sensitive lipase, with the fatty acids being released to the plasma and binding with albumin; the glycerol component is transported to the liver for metabolism. A receptor at the muscle cell transports the fatty acid into the muscle cell, where it is converted into fatty acyl CoA by an enzyme (fatty acyl CoA synthetase). The fatty acyl CoA is then transported into the mitochondria with carnitine (in an enzyme complex) as a carrier. The fatty acyl CoA, which is a combination of acetyl CoA units, then undergoes beta-oxidation, a process that splits off the acetyl CoA units for entrance into the Krebs cycle.

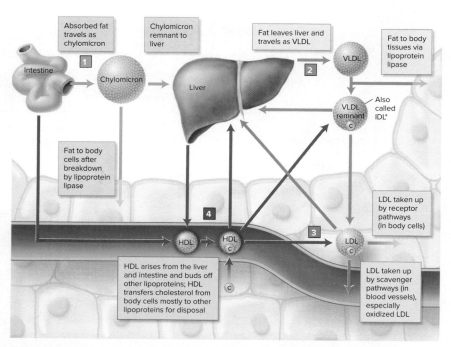

FIGURE F.4B Lipoprotein interactions. (1) Chylomicrons carry absorbed fat to body cells. (2) VLDL carries fat taken up from the bloodstream by the liver, as well as any fat made by the liver, to body cells. (3) LDL arises from VLDL and carries mostly cholesterol to cells. (4) HDL arises from body cells, mostly in the liver and intestine as well as from particles that bud off the other lipoproteins. HDL carries cholesterol from cells to other lipoproteins and to the liver for excretion.

*Intermediate-density lipoprotein.

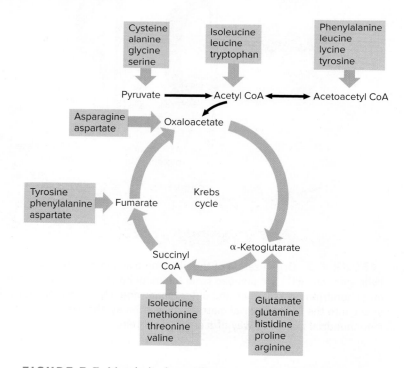

FIGURE F.5 Metabolic fates of various amino acids. Various amino acids, after deamination, may enter into energy pathways at different sites.

Sample Menu for a 2,000-Calorie Food Pattern

Sample menu for a 2,000-Calorie food pattern

Averaged over a week, this 7-day menu provides all of the recommended amounts of nutrients and food from each food group. (Italicized foods are part of the dish or food that precedes it.)

Sample Menu for a 2,000-Calorie Food Pattern

Use this 7-day menu as a motivational tool to help put a healthy eating pattern into practice and to identify creative new ideas for healthy meals. Averaged over a week, this menu provides the recommended amounts of key nutrients and foods from each food group. It features a large number of different foods to inspire ideas for adding variety to food choices. It is not intended to be followed day-by-day as a specific prescription for what to eat.

Spices and herbs can be used to taste. Try spices such as chili powder, cinnamon, cumin, curry powder, ginger, nutmeg, mustard, garlic powder, onion powder, or pepper. Try fresh or dried herbs such as basil, parsley, cilantro, chives, dill, mint, oregano, rosemary, thyme, or tarragon. Also try salt-free spice or herb blends.

While this 7-day menu provides the recommended amounts of foods and key nutrients, it does so at a moderate cost. Based on national average food costs, adjusted for inflation to March 2011 prices, the cost of this menu is less than the average amount spent for food, per person, in a four-person family.

DAY 1

BREAKFAST
Creamy oatmeal (cooked in milk):
  ½ cup uncooked oatmeal
  1 cup fat-free milk
  2 Tbsp raisins
  2 tsp brown sugar
Beverage: 1 cup orange juice

LUNCH
Taco salad:
  2 ounces tortilla chips
  2 ounces cooked ground turkey
  2 tsp corn/canola oil (to cook turkey)
  ¼ cup kidney beans*
  ½ ounce low-fat cheddar cheese
  ½ cup chopped lettuce
  ½ cup avocado
  1 tsp lime juice (on avocado)
  2 Tbsp salsa
Beverage:
1 cup water, coffee, or tea**

DINNER
Spinach lasagna roll-ups:
  1 cup lasagna noodles(2 oz dry)
  ½ cup cooked spinach
  ½ cup ricotta cheese
  1 ounce part-skim mozzarella cheese
  ½ cup tomato sauce*
1 ounce whole wheat roll
  1 tsp tub margarine
Beverage: 1 cup fat-free milk

SNACKS
2 Tbsp raisins
1 ounce unsalted almonds

DAY 2

BREAKFAST
Breakfast burrito:
  1 flour tortilla (8" diameter)
  1 scrambled egg
  ⅓ cup black beans*
  2 Tbsp salsa
½ large grapefruit
Beverage:
1 cup water, coffee, or tea**

LUNCH
Roast beef sandwich:
  1 small whole-grain hoagie bun
  2 ounces lean roast beef
  1 slice part-skim mozzarella cheese
  2 slices tomato
  ¼ cup mushrooms
  1 tsp corn/canola oil (to cook mushrooms)
  1 tsp mustard
Baked potato wedges:
  1 cup potato wedges
  1 tsp corn/canola oil (to cook potato)
  1 Tbsp ketchup
Beverage: 1 cup fat-free milk

DINNER
Baked salmon on beet greens:
  4 ounce salmon filet
  1 tsp olive oil
  2 tsp lemon juice
  ⅓ cup cooked beet greens (sauteed in 2 tsp corn/canola oil)
Quinoa with almonds:
  ½ cup quinoa
  ½ ounce slivered almonds
Beverage: 1 cup fat-free milk

SNACKS
1 cup cantaloupe balls

DAY 3

BREAKFAST
Cold cereal:
  1 cup ready-to-eat oat cereal
  1 medium banana
  ½ cup fat-free milk
1 slice whole wheat toast
  1 tsp tub margarine
Beverage: 1 cup prune juice

LUNCH
Tuna salad sandwich:
  2 slices rye bread
  2 ounces tuna
  1 Tbsp mayonnaise
  1 Tbsp chopped celery
  ½ cup shredded lettuce
1 medium peach
Beverage: 1 cup fat-free milk

DINNER
Roasted chicken:
  3 ounces cooked chicken breast
1 large sweet potato, roasted
½ cup succotash (limas & corn)
  1 tsp tub margarine
1 ounce whole wheat roll
  1 tsp tub margarine
Beverage:
1 cup water, coffee, or tea**

SNACKS
¼ cup dried apricots
1 cup flavored yogurt (chocolate)

Sample Menu for a 2,000-Calorie Food Pattern (cont'd)

DAY 4

BREAKFAST
1 whole wheat English muffin
1 Tbsp all-fruit preserves
1 hard-cooked egg
Beverage:
1 cup water, coffee, or tea**

LUNCH
White bean–vegetable soup:
1 ¼ cup chunky vegetable soup with pasta
*½ cup white beans**
6 saltine crackers*
½ cup celery sticks
Beverage: 1 cup fat-free milk

DINNER
Rigatoni with meat sauce:
1 cup rigatoni pasta (2 oz dry)
2 ounces cooked ground beef (95% lean)
2 tsp corn/canola oil (to cook beef)
*½ cup tomato sauce**
3 Tbsp grated parmesan cheese
Spinach salad:
1 cup raw spinach leaves
½ cup tangerine sections
½ ounce chopped walnuts
4 tsp oil and vinegar dressing
Beverage:
1 cup water, coffee, or tea**

SNACKS
1 cup nonfat fruit yogurt

DAY 5

BREAKFAST
Cold cereal:
1 cup shredded wheat
½ cup sliced banana
½ cup fat-free milk
1 slice whole wheat toast
2 tsp all-fruit preserves
Beverage:
1 cup fat-free chocolate milk

LUNCH
Turkey sandwich
1 whole wheat pita bread (2 oz)
3 ounces roasted turkey, sliced
2 slices tomato
¼ cup shredded lettuce
1 tsp mustard
1 Tbsp mayonnaise
½ cup grapes
Beverage: 1 cup tomato juice*

DINNER
Steak and potatoes:
4 ounces broiled beef steak
⅔ cup mashed potatoes made with milk and 2 tsp tub margarine
½ cup cooked green beans
1 tsp tub margarine
1 tsp honey
1 ounce whole wheat roll
1 tsp tub margarine
Frozen yogurt and berries:
½ cup frozen yogurt (chocolate)
¼ cup sliced strawberries
Beverage: 1 cup fat-free milk

SNACKS
1 cup frozen yogurt (chocolate)

DAY 6

BREAKFAST
French toast:
2 slices whole wheat bread
3 Tbsp fat-free milk and
⅔ egg (in French toast)
2 tsp tub margarine
1 Tbsp pancake syrup
½ large grapefruit
Beverage: 1 cup fat-free milk

LUNCH
3-bean vegetarian chili on baked potato:
¼ cup each cooked kidney beans, navy beans,* and black beans**
*½ cup tomato sauce**
½ cup chopped onion
2 Tbsp chopped jalapeno peppers
1 tsp corn/canola oil (to cook onion and peppers)
¼ cup cheese sauce
1 large baked potato
½ cup cantaloupe
Beverage:
1 cup water, coffee, or tea**

DINNER
Hawaiian pizza
2 slices cheese pizza, thin crust
1 ounce lean ham
¼ cup pineapple
¼ cup mushrooms
Green salad:
1 cup mixed salad greens
4 tsp oil and vinegar dressing
Beverage: 1 cup fat-free milk

SNACKS
3 Tbsp hummus
5 whole wheat crackers*

DAY 7

BREAKFAST
Buckwheat pancakes with berries:
2 large (7") pancakes
1 Tbsp pancake syrup
¼ cup sliced strawberries
Beverage: 1 cup orange juice

LUNCH
New England clam chowder:
3 ounces canned clams
½ small potato
2 Tbsp chopped onion
2 Tbsp chopped celery
6 Tbsp evaporated milk
¼ cup fat-free milk
1 slice bacon
1 Tbsp white flour
10 whole wheat crackers*
1 medium orange
Beverage: 1 cup fat-free milk

DINNER
Tofu–vegetable stir-fry:
4 ounces firm tofu
½ cup chopped Chinese cabbage
¼ cup sliced bamboo shoots
2 Tbsp chopped sweet red peppers
2 Tbsp chopped green peppers
1 Tbsp corn/canola oil (to cook stir-fry)
1 cup cooked brown rice (2 ounces raw)
Honeydew yogurt cup:
¾ cup honeydew melon
½ cup plain fat-free yogurt
Beverage:
1 cup water, coffee, or tea**

SNACKS
1 large banana spread with
*2 Tbsp peanut butter**
1 cup nonfat fruit yogurt

Notes

*Foods that are reduced sodium, low sodium, or no-salt added products. These foods can also be prepared from scratch with no added salt. All other foods are regular commercial products, which contain variable levels of sodium. Average sodium level of the 7-day menu assumes that no salt is added in cooking or at the table.

**Unless indicated, all beverages are unsweetened and without added cream or whitener.

Italicized foods are part of the dish or food that precedes it.

Source: www.choosemyplate.com.

Sample Menu for a 2,000-Calorie Food Pattern (cont'd)

Average amounts for weekly menu:

Food group	Daily average over 1 week
GRAINS	**6.2 oz eq**
Whole grains	3.8
Refined grains	2.4
VEGETABLES	**2.6 cups**
Vegetable subgroups (amount per week)	
Dark green	1.6 cups per week
Red/orange	5.6
Starchy	5.1
Beans and peas	1.6
Other vegetables	4.1
FRUITS	**2.1 cups**
DAIRY	**3.1 cups**
PROTEIN FOODS	**5.7 oz eq**
Seafood	8.8 oz per week
OILS	**29 grams**
CALORIES FROM ADDED FATS AND SUGARS	245 calories

Nutrient	Daily average over 1 week
Calories	1975
Protein	96 g
Protein	19% kcal
Carbohydrate	275 g
Carbohydrate	56% kcal
Total fat	59 g
Total fat	27% kcal
Saturated fat	13.2 g
Saturated fat	6.0% kcal
Monounsaturated fat	25 g
Polyunsaturated fat	16 g
Linoleic acid	13 g
Alpha-linolenic acid	1.8 g
Cholesterol	201 mg
Total dietary fiber	30 g
Potassium	4,701 mg
Sodium	1,810 mg
Calcium	1,436 mg
Magnesium	468 mg
Copper	2.0 mg
Iron	18 mg
Phosphorus	1,885 mg
Zinc	14 mg
Thiamin	1.6 mg
Riboflavin	2.5 mg
Niacin equivalents	24 mg
Vitamin B_6	2.4 mg
Vitamin B_{12}	12.3 mcg
Vitamin C	146 mg
Vitamin E	11.8 mg (AT)
Vitamin D	9.1 mcg
Vitamin A	1,090 mcg (RAE)
Dietary folate equivalents	530 mcg
Choline	386 mg

Glossary

A

accelerometer A small electronic device designed to monitor motion and is a component of various motion sensors marketed to measure daily physical activity. Some fitness devices contain triaxial accelerometers, which may measure motion in three planes.

Acceptable Daily Intake (ADI) The amount of a food additive an individual can consume without an adverse effect.

Acceptable Macronutrient Distribution Range (AMDR) A range of dietary intakes for carbohydrate, fat, and protein that is associated with reduced risk of chronic disease while providing adequate nutrients.

acclimatization The ability of the body to undergo physiological adaptations so that the stress of a given environment, such as high environmental temperature, is less severe.

acetaldehyde An intermediate breakdown product of alcohol.

acetic acid A naturally occurring saturated fatty acid; a precursor for the Krebs cycle when converted into acetyl CoA.

acetyl CoA The major fuel for the oxidative processes in the body, being derived from the breakdown of glucose and fatty acids.

acid-base balance A relative balance of acid and base products in the body so that an optimal pH is maintained in the tissues, particularly the blood.

acidosis A disturbance of the normal acid–base balance in which excess acids accumulate in the body. Lactic acid production during exercise may lead to acidosis.

acrylamide A cancer-causing agent that may be produced by prolonged, high-temperature cooking.

active couch potato An individual who is physically active yet spends many hours in seated, sedentary activity.

active transport A process requiring energy to transport substances across cell membranes.

activity-stat Center in the brain theorized to regulate daily physical activity.

acute exercise bout A single bout of exercise that will produce various physiological reactions dependent upon the nature of the exercise; a single workout.

adaptive thermogenesis The thermal effects of environmental, emotional, or pharmacological stimuli to increase metabolic rate above baseline levels.

added sugars Refined sugars added to foods during commercial food processing.

additives Substances added to food to improve flavor, color, texture, stability, or for similar purposes.

adenosine triphosphate *See* ATP.

Adequate Intake (AI) Recommended dietary intake comparable to the RDA but based on less scientific evidence.

adipokines Substances released from adipose (fat) cells that function as hormones in other parts of the body.

adiposopathy Pathological function of fat tissue that increases risk of the metabolic syndrome.

Adonis complex A disturbed body image in which muscular individuals consider themselves too thin or not sufficiently muscular; also known as muscle dysmorphia.

adrenaline A hormone secreted by the adrenal medulla; it is a stimulant and prepares the body for "fight or flight."

aerobic Relating to energy processes that occur in the presence of oxygen.

aerobic glycolysis Oxidative processes in the cell that liberate energy in the metabolism of the carbohydrate glycogen.

aerobic lipolysis Oxidative processes in the cell that liberate energy in the metabolism of fats.

aerobic walking Rapid walking designed to elevate the heart rate so that a training effect will occur; more strenuous than ordinary leisure walking.

air displacement plethysmography (ADP) A procedure to measure body composition via displacement of air in a special chamber; comparable to water displacement in underwater weighing techniques to evaluate body composition.

alanine A nonessential amino acid.

alcohol A colorless liquid with depressant effects; ethyl alcohol or ethanol is the alcohol designed for human consumption.

alcohol dehydrogenase An enzyme in the liver that initiates the breakdown of alcohol to acetaldehyde.

alcoholism A rather undefined term used to describe individuals who abuse the effect of alcohol; an addiction or habituation that may result in physical and/or psychological withdrawal effects.

aldosterone The main electrolyte-regulating hormone secreted by the adrenal cortex; primarily controls sodium and potassium balance.

allithiamine A derivative of thiamine.

alpha-ketoacid Specific acids associated with different amino acids and released upon deamination or transamination; for example, the breakdown of glutamate yields alpha-ketoglutarate.

alpha-linolenic acid An omega-3 fatty acid considered to be an essential nutrient.

alpha-tocopherol The most biologically active alcohol in vitamin E.

alpha-tocopherol equivalent The amount of other forms of tocopherol to equal the vitamin E activity of 1 milligram of alpha-tocopherol.

AMDR *See* Acceptable Macronutrient Distribution Range.

amenorrhea Absence or cessation of menstruation.

amino acids The chief structural material of protein, consisting of an amino group (NH_2) and an acid group (COOH) plus other components.

amino group The nitrogen-containing component of amino acids (NH_2).

aminostatic theory A theory suggesting that hunger is controlled by the presence or absence of amino acids in the blood acting upon a receptor in the hypothalamus.

ammonia A metabolic by-product of the oxidation of glutamine; it may be transformed into urea for excretion from the body.

amylopectin A branched-chain starch.

amylose A straight-chain starch that is more resistant to digestion compared to amylopectin.

anabolic/androgenic steroids (AAS) Drugs designed to mimic the actions of testosterone to build muscle tissue (anabolism) while minimizing the androgenic effects (masculinization).

anabolism Constructive metabolism, the process whereby simple body compounds are formed into more complex ones.

anaerobic Relating to energy processes that occur in the absence of oxygen.

anaerobic glycolysis Metabolic processes in the cell that liberate energy in the metabolism of the carbohydrate glycogen without the involvement of oxidation.

anaerobic threshold The intensity of exercise at which the individual begins to increase the proportion of energy derived from anaerobic means, principally the lactic acid system. *Also see* steady-state threshold and onset of blood lactic acid (OBLA).

android-type obesity Male-type obesity in which the body fat accumulates in the abdominal area and is a more significant risk factor for chronic disease than is gynoid-type obesity.

androstenedione An androgen produced in the body that is converted to testosterone; marketed as a dietary supplement.

anemia In general, subnormal levels of circulating RBCs and hemoglobin; there are many different types of anemia.

angina The pain experienced under the breastbone or in other areas of the upper body when the heart is deprived of oxygen.

anion A negatively charged ion, or electrolyte.

anorexia athletica (A'A) A form of anorexia nervosa observed in athletes involved in sports in which low percentages of body fat may enhance performance, such as gymnastics and ballet.

anorexia nervosa (AN) A serious nervous condition, particularly among teenage girls and young women, marked by a loss of appetite and leading to various degrees of emaciation.

anthropometry Use of body girths and diameters to evaluate body composition.

antibodies Protein substances developed in the body in reaction to the presence of a foreign substance, called an antigen; natural antibodies are also present in the blood. They are protective in nature.

antidiuretic hormone (ADH) Hormone secreted by the pituitary gland; its major action is to conserve body water by decreasing urine formation; also known as vasopressin.

antinutrients Substances in foods that can adversely affect nutrient status.

antioxidant A compound that may protect other compounds from the effects of oxygen. The antioxidant itself interferes with oxidative processes.

antipromoters Compounds that block the actions of *promoters,* agents associated with the development of certain diseases, such as cancer.

apolipoprotein A class of proteins associated with the formation of lipoproteins. A variety of apolipoproteins have been identified and are involved in the specific functions of the different lipoproteins.

appestat Term used for the neural center in the hypothalamus that helps control appetite by stimulating either hunger or satiety.

appetite A pleasant desire for food for the purpose of enjoyment that is developed through previous experience; believed to be controlled in humans by an appetite center, or appestat, in the hypothalamus.

arginine An essential amino acid.

arteriosclerosis Hardening of the arteries; *also see* atherosclerosis.

ascorbic acid Vitamin C.

aspartame An artificial sweetener made from amino acids.

aspartates Salts of aspartic acid, an amino acid.

atherosclerosis A specific form of arteriosclerosis characterized by the formation of plaque on the inner layers of the arterial wall.

athletic amenorrhea The cessation of menstruation in athletes, believed to be caused by factors associated with participation in strenuous physical activity.

ATP Adenosine triphosphate, a high-energy phosphate compound found in the body; one of the major forms of energy available for immediate use in the body.

ATPase The enzyme involved in the splitting of ATP and the release of energy.

ATP-PCr system The energy system for fast, powerful muscle contractions; uses ATP as the immediate energy source, the spent ATP being quickly regenerated by breakdown of the PCr. ATP and PCr are high-energy phosphates in the muscle cell.

B

BAT (brown adipose tissue) *See* brown fat.

baking soda A commercial form of sodium bicarbonate.

basal energy expenditure (BEE) The basal metabolic rate (BMR) total energy expenditure over 24 hours.

basal metabolic rate (BMR) The measurement of energy expenditure in the body under resting, postabsorptive conditions, indicative of the energy needed to maintain life under these basal conditions.

Basic Four Food Groups Grouping of foods into four categories that can be used as a means to educate individuals on how to obtain essential nutrients. The four groups are meat, milk, bread-cereal, and fruit-vegetable.

bee pollen A nutritional product containing minute amounts of protein and some vitamins that has been advertised to be possibly ergogenic for some athletes.

behavior modification Relative to weight-control methods, behavioral patterns, or the way one acts, may be modified to help achieve weight loss.

beriberi A deficiency disease attributed to lack of thiamin (vitamin B_1) in the diet.

beta-alanine A nonessential amino acid, also labeled as β-alanine, that is a part of the peptides carnosine and anserine; beta-alanine is purported to have ergogenic potential.

beta-carotene A precursor for vitamin A found in plants.

beta glucan Gummy form of water-soluble fiber useful in reducing serum cholesterol; oats are a good source.

beta-oxidation Process in the cells whereby 2-carbon units of acetic acid are removed from long-chain fatty acids for conversion to acetyl CoA and oxidation via the Krebs cycle.

bile A fluid secreted by the liver into the intestine that aids in the breakdown process of fats.

bile salts Active salts found in bile; cholesterol is part of their structure.

binge eating disorder Condition in which individuals demonstrate some of the same behaviors as those with bulimia nervosa, such as eating more quickly and until uncomfortably full, but do not purge.

binge-purge syndrome An eating behavior characterized by excessive hunger leading to gorging, followed by guilt and purging by vomiting. *Also see* bulimia nervosa.

bioavailability In relation to nutrients in food, the amount that may be absorbed into the body.

bioelectrical impedance analysis (BIA) A method to calculate percentage of body fat by measuring electrical resistance due to the water content of the body.

bioengineered foods Foods modified by genetic engineering to produce desirable traits.

biotin A component of the B complex.

bisphosphonates Drugs used to inhibit bone resorption, but not mineralization, to help prevent bone loss and increase bone mineral density; Fosamax is one brand.

blood alcohol concentration (BAC) The concentration of alcohol in the blood, usually expressed as milligram percent.

blood alcohol level *See* blood alcohol concentration.

blood glucose Blood sugar; the means by which carbohydrate is carried in the blood; normal range is 70–120 mg/mL.

blood pressure The pressure of the blood in the blood vessels; usually used to refer to arterial blood pressure. *Also see* systolic blood pressure and diastolic blood pressure.

BMI *See* body mass index.

BDNF *See* brain-derived neurotropic factor.

body image The image or impression the individual has of his or her body. A poor body image may lead to personality problems.

Body mass index (BMI) An index calculated by a ratio of height to weight, used as a measure of obesity.

body plethysmography A body composition technique using a special chamber to measure air displacement; similar to water displacement theory associated with underwater weighing.

brain-derived neurotropic factor (BDNF) Protein produced in the brain and other tissues that may promote growth and support of neurons.

branched-chain amino acids (BCAA) Three essential amino acids (leucine, isoleucine, and valine) that help form muscle tissue.

bread exchange One bread exchange in the Food Exchange System contains 15 grams of carbohydrate, 3 grams of protein, and 80 Calories.

brown fat Adipose tissue that is designed to produce heat; small amounts are found in humans in the area of vital organs such as the heart and lungs.

buffer boosting Term associated with use of sodium bicarbonate as an ergogenic aid to increase the acid-buffering capacity of the blood.

built environment environment built by humans for the comfort and convenience of humans. Some features of the built environment are proposed to contribute to obesity by increasing energy intake, decreasing energy expenditure, or both.

bulimia nervosa (BN) An eating disorder involving a loss of control over the impulse to binge; the binge-purge syndrome.

bulk-up method A method of weight training designed to increase muscle mass; uses high resistance and moderate volume with many different muscle groups.

C

CED *See* chronic energy deficiency.

caffeine A stimulant drug found in many food products such as coffee, tea, and cola drinks; stimulates the central nervous system.

calciferol A synthetic vitamin D.

calcitriol The hormone form of vitamin D.

calcium A silver-white metallic element essential to human nutrition.

caloric concept of weight control The concept that Calories are the basis of weight control. Excess Calories will add body weight while caloric deficiencies will contribute to weight loss.

caloric deficit A negative caloric balance whereby more Calories are expended than consumed; a weight loss will occur.

Calorie A measure of heat energy. A small calorie represents the amount of heat needed to raise 1 gram of water 1 degree Celsius. A large Calorie (kilocalorie, KC, or C) is 1,000 small calories.

calorimeter A device used to measure the caloric value of a given food, or heat production of animals or humans.

calorimetry The science of measuring heat production.

carbohydrate-electrolyte solutions (CES) Fluids containing water, various forms of carbohydrate such as glucose and fructose, and various electrolytes such as sodium, chloride, and potassium, in a solution designed to maintain optimal hydration and energy during exercise. *See also* sports drinks.

carbohydrate loading A dietary method used by endurance-type athletes to help increase the carbohydrate (glycogen) levels in their muscles and liver.

carbohydrates A group of compounds containing carbon, hydrogen, and oxygen. Glucose, glycogen, sugar, starches, fiber, cellulose, and the various saccharides are all carbohydrates.

carcinogenicity The potential of a substance to cause cancer.

carnitine A chemical that facilitates the transfer of fatty acids into the mitochondria for subsequent oxidation.

carnosine A peptide found in muscle tissue theorized to possess ergogenic potential via its buffering effect on lactic acid during high-intensity exercise; carnosine contains the nonessential amino acid beta-alanine.

catabolism Destructive metabolism whereby complex chemical compounds in the body are degraded to simpler ones.

catalase An enzyme that helps neutralize free radicals.

cation A positively charged ion or electrolyte.

cellulite Lumpy fat that often appears in the thigh and hip region of women. Cellulite is simply normal fat in small compartments formed by connective tissue but may contain other compounds that bind water.

cellulose The fibrous carbohydrate that provides the structural backbone for plants; plant fiber.

Celsius A thermometer scale that has a freezing point of 0° and a boiling point of 100°; also known as the centigrade scale.

central fatigue Fatigue caused by suboptimal functioning of neurotransmitters, most likely in the brain.

cerebrospinal fluid (CSF) The fluid found in the brain and spinal cord.

chloride A compound of chlorine present in a salt form carrying a negative charge; Cl^-, an anion.

cholecalciferol The product of irradiation of 7-dehydrocholesterol found in the skin. *Also see* vitamin D_3.

cholesterol A fat-like, pearly substance, an alcohol, found in all animal fat and oils; a main constituent of some body tissues and body compounds.

choline A substance associated with the B complex that is widely distributed in both plant and animal tissues; involved in carbohydrate, fat, and protein metabolism.

chondroitin Formed in the body from amino acids and involved in cartilage formation; marked as a dietary supplement.

ChooseMyPlate The program and Website designed by the United States Department of Agriculture to provide sound nutritional guidance to Americans as a means to promote optimal health.

chromium A whitish metal essential to human nutrition; it is involved in carbohydrate metabolism via its role with insulin.

chronic energy deficiency A long-term negative energy balance associated with abnormally low body mass index.

chronic fatigue syndrome Prolonged fatigue (over 6 months) of unknown cause characterized by mental depression and physical fatigue; may be observed in endurance athletes.

chronic training effect The structural and metabolic adaptations that occur in the body in response to exercise training over time; the adaptations are specific to the type of exercise, such as aerobic endurance training or resistance training.

chronic traumatic encephalopathy (CTE) Progressive degeneration of brain tissue caused by repeated brain concussions over the course of many years. CTE has been found in many athletes participating is sports associated with repetitive brain trauma, including boxing, American football, rugby, and ice hockey.

chylomicron A particle of emulsified fat found in the blood following the digestion and assimilation of fat.

circuit aerobics A combination of aerobic and weight-training exercises designed to elicit the specific benefits of each type of exercise.

circuit weight training A method of training in which exercises are arranged in a circuit or sequence. May be designed with weight training to help convey an aerobic training effect.

cirrhosis A degenerative disease of the liver, one cause being excessive consumption of alcohol.

cis **fatty acids** The chemical structure of unsaturated fatty acids in which the hydrogen ions are on the same side of the double bond.

citrulline An amino acid that may be converted in the body into arginine and hypothesized to possess ergogenic potential; citrulline is not needed to form any body tissues.

ciwujia A Chinese herb theorized to be ergogenic.

clinical obesity Obesity determined by a clinical procedure.

Clostridium A bacterium commonly involved in food poisoning.

cobalamin The cobalt-containing complex common to all members of the vitamin B_{12} group; often used to designate cyanocobalamin.

cobalt A gray, hard metal that is a component of vitamin B_{12}.

coenzyme An activator of an enzyme; many vitamins are coenzymes.

coenzyme Q10 *See* CoQ10.

colon The large intestine.

Compendium of Physical Activities A comprehensive list of the metabolic cost in METS (multiples of resting metabolic cost) of many recreational, leisure, and occupational activities as well as activities of daily living.

compensated heat stress A condition in which heat loss balances heat production, a set body temperature is maintained, and the individual can continue to exercise in warm environmental conditions.

complementary proteins Combining plant foods such as rice and beans so that essential amino acids deficient in one of the foods are provided by the other, in order to obtain a balanced intake of essential amino acids.

complete proteins Proteins that contain all nine essential amino acids in the proper proportions. Animal protein is complete protein.

complex carbohydrates Foods high in starch, such as bread, cereals, fruits, and vegetables, as contrasted to simple carbohydrates such as table sugar.

concentric method A method of weight training in which the muscle shortens.

conduction In relation to body temperature, the transfer of heat from one substance to another by direct contact.

conjugated linoleic acid (CLA) Isomers of linoleic acid, an essential fatty acid. CLA is found in the meat and milk of ruminants and is theorized to have health and exercise performance benefits, such as promotion of weight loss.

convection In relation to body temperature, the transfer of heat by way of currents in either air or water.

copper A reddish metallic element essential to human nutrition; it functions with iron in the formation of hemoglobin and the cytochromes.

CoQ10 A coenzyme involved in the electron transport system in the mitochondria.

core temperature The temperature of the deep tissues of the body, usually measured orally or rectally; *also see* shell temperature.

Cori cycle Cycle involving muscle breakdown of glucose to lactate, lactate transport via blood to the liver for reconversion to glucose, and glucose returning to the muscle.

coronary artery disease (CAD) Atherosclerosis in the coronary arteries.

coronary heart disease (CHD) A degenerative disease of the heart caused primarily by arteriosclerosis or atherosclerosis of the coronary vessels of the heart.

coronary occlusion Closure of coronary arteries that may precipitate a heart attack; occlusion may be partial or complete closure.

coronary risk factors Behaviors (smoking) or body properties (cholesterol levels) that may predispose an individual to coronary heart disease.

coronary thrombosis Occlusion (closure) of coronary arteries, usually by a blood clot.

cortisol A hormone secreted by the adrenal cortex with gluconeogenic potential, helping to convert amino acids into glucose.

creatine A nitrogen-containing compound found in the muscles, usually complexed with phosphate to form phosphocreatine.

crossover concept The concept that as exercise intensity increases, at some point carbohydrate rather than fat becomes the predominant fuel for muscle contraction.

cruciferous vegetables Vegetables in the cabbage family, such as broccoli, cauliflower, kale, and all cabbages.

CSSD Certification as a Specialist in Sports Dietetics; a certification program by the American Dietetic Association.

cyanocobalamin Vitamin B_{12}.

cysteine A breakdown product of cystine. It is also a sulfur-containing amino acid.

cystine A sulfur-containing amino acid.

cytochromes Any one of a class of pigment compounds that play an important role in cellular oxidative processes.

cytokine Small proteins or peptides produced in cells, such as adipokines by adipose tissue cells, that possess hormone-like functions on other cells in the body; the immune system secretes a number of different cytokines.

D

DSM-V (DSM-5) *See Diagnostic and Statistical Manual of Mental Disorders,* 5th edition.

Daily Reference Values (DRVs) Recommended daily intakes for the macronutrients (carbohydrate, fat, and protein) as well as cholesterol, sodium, and potassium. On a food label, the DRV is based on a 2,000-Calorie diet.

Daily Value (DV) A term used in food labeling; the DV is based on a daily energy intake of 2,000 Calories and for the food labeled presents the percentage of the RDI and the DRV recommended for healthy Americans. *See* RDI and DRV.

DASH diet The Dietary Approaches to Stop Hypertension diet plan that is designed to reduce or prevent an increase in blood pressure.

deamination Removal of an amine group, or nitrogen, from an amino acid.

dehydration A reduction of the body water to below the normal level of hydration; water output exceeds water intake.

dehydroepiandrosterone (DHEA) A natural steroid hormone produced endogenously by the adrenal gland. May be marketed as a nutritional sports ergogenic as derived from herbal precursors.

delayed onset of muscle soreness (DOMS) Soreness in muscles experienced a day or two after strenuous eccentric exercise, such as running downhill. Prolonged, excessive eccentric exercise may lead to small muscle tears, and the pain is believed to occur during the repair process when swelling activates pain receptors.

depressant Drug or agent that will depress or lower the level of bodily functions, particularly central nervous system functioning.

DHAP Dihydroxyacetone and pyruvate, the combination of two by-products of glycolysis.

DHEA *See* dehydroepiandrosterone.

diabesity Term coined to highlight the relationship between the development of diabetes following the onset of obesity.

diabetes mellitus A disorder of carbohydrate metabolism due to disturbances in production or utilization of insulin; results in high blood glucose levels and loss of sugar in the urine.

***Diagnostic and Statistical Manual of Mental Disorders,* 5th edition** The American Psychiatric Association's current diagnostic tool for psychiatric and psychological disorders. Published in 2013.

diarrhea Frequent passage of a watery fecal discharge due to a gastrointestinal disturbance.

diastolic blood pressure The blood pressure in the arteries when the heart is at rest between beats.

dietary fiber Nondigestible carbohydrates and lignin that are intrinsic and intact in plants.

dietary folate equivalents (DFE) Used in estimating folate requirements, adjusting for the greater degree of absorption of folic acid (free form) compared with folate naturally found in foods. One microgram food folate equals 0.5 to 0.6 microgram folic acid added to foods or as a supplement.

dietary-induced thermogenesis (DIT) The increase in the basal metabolic rate following ingestion of a meal. Heat production is increased.

Dietary Reference Intake (DRI) Standard for recommended dietary intake, consisting of various values. *See also* AI, EAR, RDA, AMDR, and UL.

dietary supplement A food product, added to the total diet, that contains either vitamins, minerals, herbs, botanicals, amino acids, metabolites, constituents, extracts, or combinations of these ingredients.

Dietary Supplement Health and Education Act (DSHEA) Act passed by the United States Congress defining a dietary supplement (*see* dietary supplement); legislation to control advertising and marketing.

2,3-diphosphoglyceride A by-product of carbohydrate metabolism in the red blood cell; helps the hemoglobin unload oxygen to the tissues.

disaccharide Any one of a class of sugars that yield two monosaccharides on hydrolysis; sucrose is the most common.

disordered eating Atypical eating behaviors such as restrictive dieting, using diet pills or laxatives, bingeing, and purging. In general, disordered eating behaviors occur less frequently or are less severe than those required to meet the full criteria for the diagnosis of an eating disorder.

dispensable amino acids *See* nonessential animo acids.

diuretics A class of agents that stimulate the formation of urine; used as a means to reduce body fluids.

diverticulosis Weak spots in the wall of the large intestine that may bulge out like a weak spot in a tire inner tube. May become infected, leading to diverticulitis.

DNA Deoxyribonucleic acid; a complex protein found in chromosomes that is the carrier of genetic information and the basis of heredity.

docasahexanoic acid (DHA) Docasahexanoic acid, an omega-3 fatty acid found in fatty fish.

dopamine A neurotransmitter secreted in the brain and involved in a number of functions, including sensations of pleasure. Decreased dopamine levels may be associated with Parkinson's disease.

doping Official term used by the WADA and the International Olympic Committee to depict the use of drugs in sports in attempts to enhance performance.

doubly labeled water technique A technique using labeled water to study energy metabolism.

dual energy X-ray absorptiometry (DEXA, DXA) A computerized X-ray technique at two energy levels to image body fat, lean tissues, and bone mineral content.

dual-intervention A theoretical model of weight gain that describes competition between physiological control factors which defend an upper point of weight or fat mass and environmental factors favoring either weight gain or loss.

dumping syndrome Movement of fluid from the blood to the intestines by osmosis. May occur when a concentrated sugar solution is consumed in large quantities, causing symptoms such as weakness and gastrointestinal distress.

duration concept One of the major concepts of aerobic exercise; refers to the amount of time spent exercising during each session.

E

EAH *See* exercise-associated hyponatremia.

eating disorders psychological disorders A psychological disorder centering on the avoidance, excessive consumption, or purging of food, such as anorexia nervosa and bulimia nervosa.

eccentric method A weight-training method in which the muscle undergoes a lengthening contraction.

eicosanoids Derivatives of fatty acid oxidation in the body, including prostaglandins, thromboxanes, and leukotrienes.

eicosapentaenoic acid (EPA) An omega-3 fatty acid found in fatty fish.

electrolyte A substance that, when in a solution, conducts an electrical current.

electrolytes solution A solution that contains ions and can conduct electricity; often the ions of salts such as sodium and chloride are called electrolytes; *also see* ions.

electron transfer system A highly structured array of chemical compounds in the cell that transport electrons and harness energy for later use.

element Relative to chemistry, a substance that cannot be subdivided into substances different from itself; many elements are essential to human life.

endocrine system The body system consisting of glands that secrete hormones, which have a wide variety of effects throughout the body.

energy The ability to do work; energy exists in various forms, notably mechanical, heat, and chemical in the human body.

English system A measurement system based upon the foot, pound, quart, and other nonmetric units; *also see* metric system.

enzymes Complex proteins in the body that serve as catalysts, facilitating reactions between various substances without being changed themselves.

ephedra *Ephedra sinica,* a source of ephedrine.

ephedrine A stimulant with somewhat weaker effects than amphetamine; found in some commercial dietary supplements; also known as ephedra.

epidemiological research A study of certain populations to determine the relationship of various risk factors to epidemic diseases or health problems.

epigenetics The study of various factors, including diet and exercise, that may influence gene expression without modifying the DNA, that influence gene expression. For example, exerkines produced during exercise may influence DNA activity, such as activating or deactivating genes, without changing the DNA sequence.

epigenome A structure located just outside the genome that may be influenced by various factors, such as nutrients in the foods eaten; activates or deactivates DNA and subsequent genetic and cellular activity that may have either positive or negative health effects.

epinephrine A hormone secreted by the adrenal medulla that stimulates numerous body processes to enhance energy production, particularly during intense exercise.

epithelial cells The layer of cells that covers the outside and inside surfaces of the body, including the skin and the lining of the gastrointestinal system.

ergogenic aids Work-enhancing agents that are used in attempts to increase athletic or physical performance capacity.

ergogenic effect The physiological or psychological effect that an ergogenic substance is designed to produce.

ergolytic An agent or substance that may lead to decreases in work productivity or physical performance. *See also* ergogenic effect.

ergometer A device, such as a cycle ergometer, to measure work output in watts or other measures of work.

Escherichia A bacterium commonly involved in food poisoning.

essential amino acids Amino acids that must be obtained in the diet and cannot be synthesized in the body. Also known as indispensable amino acids.

essential fat Fat in the body that is an essential part of the tissues, such as cell membrane structure, nerve coverings, and the brain; *also see* storage fat.

essential fatty acid Those unsaturated fatty acids that may not be synthesized in the body and must be obtained in the diet, e.g., linoleic fatty acid.

essential nutrients Those nutrients found to be essential to human life and optimal functioning.

ester Compound formed from the combination of an organic acid and an alcohol.

Estimated Average Requirement (EAR) Nutrient intake value estimated to meet the requirements of half the healthy individuals in a group.

Estimated Energy Requirement (EER) The daily dietary intake predicted to maintain energy balance for an individual of a defined age, gender, height, weight, and level of physical activity consistent with good health.

Estimated Minimal Requirement (EMR) Part of the RDA pertaining to the minimal daily requirement for sodium, chloride, and potassium.

Estimated Safe and Adequate Daily Dietary Intakes (ESADDI) Part of the previous RDA. Daily allowances for selected nutrients that are based upon available scientific evidence to be safe and adequate to meet human needs.

ethanol Alcohol; ethyl alcohol.

ethyl alcohol Alcohol; ethanol.

euhydration *See* normohydration.

evaporation The conversion of a liquid to a vapor, which consumes energy; evaporation of sweat cools the body by using body heat as the energy source.

exercise A form of structured physical activity generally designed to enhance physical fitness; usually refers to strenuous physical activity.

exercise-associated collapse Postexercise dizziness due to hypotension from venous pooling.

exercise-associated hyponatremia (EAH) Term associated with the decline in serum sodium levels during prolonged exercise with excessive fluid intake and/or sodium losses; *also see* water intoxication.

exercise frequency In an aerobic exercise program, the number of times per week that an individual exercises.

exercise intensity The tempo, speed, or resistance of an exercise. Intensity can be increased by working faster, doing more work in a given amount of time.

exercise metabolic rate (EMR) An increased metabolic rate due to the need for increased energy production; during exercise, the resting energy expenditure (REE) may be increased more than 20-fold.

exercisenomics General term regarding the effects of exercise on genetic expression and resultant metabolic adaptations.

exercise sequence *See* principle of exercise sequence.

exercise snacks The practice of shorter, more frequent bouts of exercise in place of fewer, but longer exercise sessions.

exercise stimulus The means whereby one elicits a physiological response; running, for example, can be the stimulus to increase the heart rate and other physiological functions.

exerkines Muscles may produce substances known as myokines, which are referred to as exerkines when produced during exercise. Exerkines may function like hormones and may influence cell activity throughout the body that may have multiple health benefits.

exertional heat stroke Heat stroke that is precipitated by exercise in a warm or hot environment.

experimental research Study that manipulates an independent variable (cause) to observe the outcome on a dependent variable (effect).

extracellular water Body water that is located outside the cells; often subdivided into the intravascular water and the intercellular, or interstitial, water.

F

facilitated diffusion Process whereby glucose combines with a special protein carrier molecule at the membrane surface, facilitating glucose transport into the cell; insulin promotes facilitated diffusion in some cells.

faddism Relative to nutrition, the use of dietary fads based upon theoretical principles that may or may not be valid; usually used in a negative sense, as in quackery.

fasting Starvation; abstinence from eating that may be partial or complete.

fast-twitch fibers Muscle fibers characterized by high contractile speed.

fat exchange A fat exchange in the Food Exchange System contains 5 grams of fat and 45 Calories.

fat-free mass The remaining mass of the human body following the extraction of all fat.

fatigue A generalized or specific feeling of tiredness that may have a multitude of causes; may be mental or physical.

fat loading Practices used to maximize the use of fats as an energy source during exercise, particularly a low-carbohydrate, high-fat diet.

fat patterning The deposition of fat in specific areas of the human body, such as the stomach, thighs, or hips. Genetics plays an important role in fat patterning.

fats Triglycerides; a combination, or ester, of three fatty acids and glycerol.

fat substitutes Various substances used as substitutes for fats in food products; two popular brands are Simplesse and Olestra.

fatty acids Aliphatic acids containing only carbon, oxygen, and hydrogen; they may be saturated or unsaturated.

feedback system The autoregulatory control of a physiological process in response to effects caused by the process. Feedback is important in physiological homeostasis and in endocrine control.

female athlete triad The triad of disordered eating, amenorrhea, and osteoporosis sometimes seen in female athletes involved in sports where excess body weight may be detrimental to performance.

female-type obesity *See* gynoid-type obesity.

ferritin The form in which iron is stored in the tissues.

fetal alcohol effects (FAE) Symptoms noted in children born to women who consumed alcohol during pregnancy; not as severe as fetal alcohol syndrome.

fetal alcohol spectrum disorders (FASD) Birth anomalies associated with drinking alcohol while pregnant; refers to several conditions involving alcohol-related neurodevelopment disorders, birth defects, and other abnormalities in normal development. *See also* fetal alcohol syndrome and fetal alcohol effects.

fetal alcohol syndrome (FAS) The cluster of physical and mental symptoms seen in the child of a mother who consumes excessive alcohol during pregnancy.

fiber In general, the indigestible carbohydrate in plants that forms the structural network; *also see* cellulose.

First Law of Thermodynamics The law that energy cannot be created or destroyed; energy can be converted from one form to another.

flatulence Gas or air in the gastrointestinal tract, particularly the intestines.

flexitarians Vegetarians who occasionally may eat meat, fish, or poultry. Flexitarians are also known as semivegetarians.

fluoride A salt of hydrofluoric acid; a compound of fluorine that may be helpful in the prevention of tooth decay.

folacin Collective term for various forms of folic acid.

folate Salt of folic acid; form found in foods.

folic acid A water-soluble vitamin that appears to be essential in preventing certain types of anemia.

food additive *See* additives.

food allergy An adverse immune response to an otherwise harmless food. *Also see* food hypersensitivity.

food cultism Treating a particular food as if it possesses special properties, such as prevention or treatment of disease or improvement of athletic performance, usually without scientific justification.

Food and Drug Administration (FDA) Federal agency tasked with the responsibilities to monitor safety of foods and drugs sold in the United States.

Food Exchange System The system developed by the American Dietetic Association and other health groups that categorizes foods by content of carbohydrate, fat, protein, and Calories; used as a basis for diet planning.

food hypersensitivity Term for some individuals who may develop clinical symptoms, such as migraine headaches, gastrointestinal distress, or hives and itching when certain foods are eaten.

food intolerance A general term for any adverse reaction to a food or food component not involving the immune system; an example is lactose intolerance.

food poisoning Foodborne illness caused by bacteria such as Salmonella, Escherichia, Staphylococcus, and Clostridium.

foot-pound A unit of work whereby the weight of 1 pound is moved through a distance of 1 foot.

Fosamax A commercial bisphosphonate product.

free fatty acids (FFA) Acids formed by the hydrolysis of triglycerides.

free radicals Atoms or compouds in which there is an unpaired electron; thought to cause cellular damage.

Freshman 15 An exaggerated reference to the typical weight gain in pounds by college freshmen. It is actually about 5 pounds.

fructose A monosaccharide known as levulose or fruit sugar; found in all sweet fruits.

fruitarian A type of vegetarian who subsists solely on fruits, fruit products, and nuts.

fruit exchange One fruit exchange in the Food Exchange System contains 15 grams of carbohydrate and 60 Calories.

fTRP:BCAA ratio The ratio of free tryptophan to branched-chain amino acids; a high ratio is theorized to elicit fatigue in prolonged endurance events.

functional fiber Isolated, nondigestible carbohydrate that has beneficial effects in humans.

functional foods Food products containing nutrients designed to provide health benefits beyond basic nutrition.

G

galactose A monosaccharide formed when lactose is hydrolyzed into glucose and galactose.

gastric emptying The rate at which substances, particularly fluids, empty from the stomach; high gastric emptying rates are advisable for sports drinks.

general model A theoretical model of weight gain that combined the set and settling point theories in describing regulation of intake as functions of social/environmental versus and genetics and feedback control factors.

genomics The study of the entire genome of an individual or organism; human genomics attempts to determine DNA sequence and gene mapping. Human genomic research may lead to genetic modifications to enhance health of individuals; genomics may also be involved in gene doping, or sports performance enhancement with gene manipulation.

ghrelin Hormone released by an empty stomach to stimulate the appetite.

ginseng A general term for a variety of natural chemical plant extracts derived from the family Araliaceae; extract contains ginsenosides and other chemicals that may influence human physiology.

Globesity A term referring to the worldwide increase in the prevalence rate of obesity and co-morbitities

glucagon A hormone secreted by the pancreas; basically it exerts actions just the opposite of insulin, i.e., it responds to hypoglycemia and helps to increase blood sugar levels.

glucarate A compound found in cruciferous vegetables that is thought to block the actions of cancer-causing agents.

glucogenic amino acids Amino acids that may undergo deamination and be converted into glucose through the process of gluconeogenesis.

gluconeogenesis The formation of carbohydrates from molecules that are not themselves carbohydrate, such as amino acids and the glycerol from fat.

glucosamine Formed in the body from amino acids and involved in cartilage formation; marketed as a dietary supplement.

glucose A monosaccharide; a thick, sweet, syrupy liquid.

glucose-alanine cycle The cycle in which alanine is released from the muscle and is converted to glucose in the liver.

glucose-electrolyte solutions Solutions designed to replace sweat losses; contain varying proportions of water, glucose, sodium, potassium, chloride, and other electrolytes.

glucose polymers Combinations A combination of several glucose molecules into more complex carbohydrates.

glucostatic theory The theory that hunger and satiety are controlled by the glucose level in the blood; the receptors that respond to the blood glucose level are in the hypothalamus.

GLUT-4 Receptors in cell membranes that transport glucose from the blood to the cell interior.

glutathione peroxidase An enzyme that helps neutralize free radicals.

gluten intolerance A sensitivity to gluten; the immune system recognizes gluten as a foreign substance but does not induce an allergic response.

glycemic index (GI) A ranking system relative to the effect that consumption of 50 grams of a particular carbohydrate food has upon the blood glucose response over the course of 2 hours. The normal baseline measure is 50 grams of glucose, and the resultant blood glucose response is scored as 100.

glycemic load (GL) A ranking system relative to the effect that eating a carbohydrate food has on the blood glucose level, but also includes the portion size. The formula is

$$GL = \frac{(GI) \times (\text{grams of nonfiber carbohydrate in 1 serving})}{100}$$

glycerate A commercial product containing glycerol; marketed to athletes.

glycerin *See* glycerol.

glycerol Glycerin, a clear, syrupy liquid; an alcohol that combines with fatty acids to form triglycerides.

glycogen A polysaccharide that is the chief storage form of carbohydrate in animals; it is stored primarily in the liver and muscles.

glycogen-sparing effect The theory that certain dietary techniques, such as the use of caffeine, may facilitate the oxidation of fatty acids for energy and thus spare the utilization of glycogen.

glycolysis The degradation of sugars into smaller compounds; the main quantitative anaerobic energy process in the muscle tissue.

gout The deposit of uric acid by-products in and about the joints contributing to inflammation and pain; usually occurs in the knee or foot.

gram calorie A small calorie; *see also* Calorie.

GRAS A classification for food additives indicating that they most likely are not harmful for human consumption.

green tea A Chinese beverage that contains caffeine and other constituents, such as epigallocatechin gallate (EGCG), which are theorized to possess numerous health benefits.

gums A form of water-soluble dietary fiber found in plants.

gynoid-type obesity Female-type obesity; body fat is deposited primarily about the hips and thighs. *Also see* android-type obesity.

H

HDL High-density lipoprotein; a protein-lipid complex in the blood that facilitates the transport of triglycerides, cholesterol, and phospholipids. *Also see* HDL-cholesterol.

HDL-cholesterol High-density lipoprotein cholesterol; one mechanism whereby cholesterol is transported in the blood. High HDL levels are thought to be somewhat protective against CHD.

HPA *See* hypothalamic-pituitary-adrenal axis.

HPG *See* hypothalamic-pituitary-gonadal axis.

health-related fitness Those components of physical fitness whose improvement have health benefits, such as cardiovascular fitness, body composition, flexibility, and muscular strength and endurance.

Healthy at Every Size (HAES®) an advocacy movement begun in the 1960s to promote weight-neutral promotion of healthy lifestyle choices and physical activity.

Healthy Eating Index (HEI) USDA computerized dietary analysis to assess personal diets to provide an overall rating as related to health.

heart rate maximum See HR max

healthy obese A proposed phenotype characterized by obesity without the typical co-morbidities of metabolic syndrome, diabetes, hypertension, and cardiovascular disease

heat-balance equation Heat balance is dependent on the interrelationships of metabolic heat production and loss or gain of heat by radiation, convection, conduction, and evaporation.

heat cramps Painful muscular cramps or tetany following prolonged exercise in the heat without water or salt replacement.

heat exhaustion Weakness or dizziness from overexertion in a hot environment.

heat index The apparent temperature determined by combining air temperature and relative humidity.

heat shock proteins Proteins released by the muscle, in response to increased temperature or exercise, that may (similar to the effect of cytokines) influence other body tissues and induce possible positive health effects.

heat stroke Elevated body temperature of 105.8°F or greater caused by exposure to excessive heat gains or production and diminished heat loss.

heat syncope Fainting caused by excessive heat exposure.

hematuria Blood or red blood cells in the urine.

heme iron The iron in the diet associated with hemoglobin in animal meats.

hemicellulose A form of dietary fiber found in plants. Differs from cellulose in that it may be hydrolyzed by dilute acids outside of the body. Not hydrolyzed in the body.

hemochromatosis Presence of excessive iron in the body, resulting in an enlarged liver and bronze pigmentation of the skin.

hemoglobin The protein-iron pigment in the red blood cells that transports oxygen.

hemolysis A rupturing of red blood cells with a release of hemoglobin into the plasma.

hepatitis An inflammatory condition of the liver.

hepcidin A hormone produced in the liver that helps regulate serum iron levels mainly by its effects on intestinal absorption. Elevated serum iron levels will stimulate hepcidin synthesis by the liver, which will inhibit iron absorption by the intestines. Conversely, decreased levels of serum iron will inhibit hepcidin synthesis and increase intestinal iron absorption.

heterocyclic amines (HCA) Carcinogens formed in foods that have been charred by excess grilling or broiling.

hidden fat In foods, the fat that is not readily apparent, such as the high fat content of cheese.

high blood pressure *See* hypertension.

high-density lipoprotein *See* HDL.

high-fructose corn syrup A common high-Calorie sweetener used as a food additive; derived from the partial hydrolysis of corn starch.

high-intensity interval training (HIIT) An exercise format involving short bouts of intense, near maximal, anaerobic exercise followed by a short recovery period. Exercise protocols are designed to provide health benefits comparable to more prolonged aerobic endurance exercise, but less overall time commitment.

histidine An essential amino acid.

HMB Beta-hydroxy-beta-methylbutyrate, a metabolic by-product of the amino acid leucine, alleged to retard the breakdown of muscle protein during strenuous exercise.

homeostasis A condition of normalcy in the internal body environment.

homocysteine A metabolic by-product of amino acid metabolism; elevated blood levels are associated with increased risk of vascular diseases.

hormone A chemical substance produced by specific body cells, secreted into the blood and then acting on specific target tissues.

hormone sensitive lipase (HSL) An enzyme that catalyzes triglycerides into free fatty acids and glycerol.

HR max The normal maximal heart rate of an individual during exercise.

HR reserve The mathematical difference, or reserve, between the resting HR and maximal HR. A percentage of this reserve may be added to the resting HR to determine exercise intensity.

human growth hormone (HGH) A hormone released by the pituitary gland that regulates growth; also involved in fatty acid metabolism; rHGH is a genetically engineered form.

hunger A basic physiological desire to eat that is normally caused by a lack of food; may be accompanied by stomach contractions.

hunger center A collection of nerve cells in the hypothalamus that is involved in the control of feeding reflexes.

hydrodensitometry Another term for the underwater weighing technique.

hydrogenated fats Fats to which hydrogen has been added, usually causing them to be saturated.

hydrolysis A mechanism for splitting substances into smaller compounds by the addition of water; enzyme action.

hydrostatic weighing An underwater weighing technique used to estimate body composition (body fat and lean body mass)

hypercholesteremia Elevated blood cholesterol levels.

hyperglycemia Elevated blood glucose levels.

hyperhydration The practice of increasing the body-water stores by fluid consumption prior to an athletic event; a state of increased water content in the body.

hyperkalemia An increased concentration of potassium in the blood.

hyperlipidemia Elevated blood lipid levels.

hyperplasia The formation of new body cells.

hypertension A condition with various causes whereby the blood pressure is higher than normal.

hyperthermia Unusually high body temperature; fever.

hypertonic Relative to osmotic pressure, a solution that has a greater concentration of solute or salts, hence higher osmotic pressure, in comparison to another solution.

hypertriglyceridemia Elevated blood levels of triglycerides.

hypertrophic cardiomyopathy An unusual thickening of the heart muscle, usually genetic in nature, that may elicit few, if any, symptoms in many people, but may cause abnormal heart rhythms and possible heart failure in some individuals.

hypertrophy Excessive growth of a cell or organ; in pathology, an abnormal growth.

hypervitaminosis A pathological condition due to an excessive vitamin intake, particularly the fat-soluble vitamins A and D.

hypoglycemia A low blood sugar level.

hypohydration A state of decreased water content in the body caused by dehydration.

hypokalemia A decreased concentration of potassium in the blood.

hyponatremia A decreased concentration of sodium in the blood.

hypothalamic-pituitary-adrenal axis The endocrine glands and hormones which regulate the response to psychological and physical stress.

hypothalamic-pituitary-gonadal axis The endocrine glands and hormones which regulate normal reproductive function in males and females.

hypothalamus A part of the brain involved in the control of involuntary activity in the body; contains many centers for neural control such as temperature, hunger, appetite, and thirst.

hypothermia Unusually low body temperature.

hypotonic Having an osmotic pressure lower than that of the solution to which it is compared.

I

IGF-1 *See* insulin-like growth factor.

incomplete proteins Protein foods that do not possess the proper amount of essential amino acids; characteristic of plant foods in general.

Index of Nutritional Quality (INQ) A mathematical means of determining the quality of any given food relative to its content of a specific nutrient.

indicator dilution method A technique for measuring water volume where a known amount of a substance known as a tracer is injected and equilibrates throughout the volume to be measured. Volume is calculated as tracer quantity divided by tracer concentration.

indicator nutrients The eight nutrients which, if provided in adequate supply through a varied diet, should provide adequate amounts of the other essential nutrients: protein, vitamin A, thiamin, riboflavin, niacin, vitamin C, calcium, and iron.

indispensable amino acids *See* essential amino acids.

indoles Phytochemicals believed to help prevent various diseases.

infrared interactance Use of infrared technology to estimate body composition.

initial fitness level The physical fitness level of an individual prior to the onset of a physical conditioning program.

in-line skating An exercise-skating technique with specially designed shoes for use on sidewalks and similar surfaces.

inosine A nucleoside of the purine family that serves as a base for the formation of a variety of compounds in the body; theorized to be ergogenic.

inositol A member of the B complex, although its role in human nutrition has not been established; not classified as a vitamin.

INQ *See* Index of Nutritional Quality.

insensible perspiration Perspiration on the skin not detectable by ordinary senses.

insoluble dietary fiber Dietary fiber that is not soluble in water, such as cellulose. *Also see* soluble dietary fiber.

insulin A hormone secreted by the pancreas, involved in carbohydrate metabolism.

insulin-like growth factor (IGF-1) A growth factor found in the blood that resembles insulin; produced in response to growth hormone release.

insulin response Blood insulin levels rise following the ingestion of sugar and the resultant hyperglycemia; the insulin causes the sugar to be taken up by the muscles and fat cells, possibly creating a reactive hypoglycemia.

intercellular water Body water found between the cells; also known as interstitial water.

intermittent high-intensity exercise Short-term bouts of high-intensity exercise interspersed with short periods of recovery.

International Unit (IU) A method of expressing the quantity of some substance, such as vitamins, which is an internationally developed and accepted standard.

International Unit System (SI) *Le Systeme International d'Unite,* or the International System of Units; a system of measurement based upon the metric system.

interstitial water *See* intercellular water.

interval training A method of physical training in which periods of activity are interspersed with periods of rest.

intestinal absorption The rate at which substances, particularly fluids and nutrients, are absorbed into the body; a fast rate of intestinal absorption is a desirable characteristic of sports drinks.

intracellular water Body water that is found within the cells.

intravascular water Body water found in the vascular system, or blood vessels.

involuntary dehydration Unintentional loss of body fluids during exercise under warm or hot environmental conditions.

IOC International Olympic Committee.

iodine A nonmetallic element that is necessary for the proper development and functioning of the thyroid gland.

ions Particles with an electrical charge; anions are negative and cations are positive.

iron A metallic element essential for the development of several chemical compounds in the body, notably hemoglobin.

iron-deficiency anemia Anemia caused by an inadequate intake or absorption of iron, resulting in impaired hemoglobin formation.

iron deficiency without anemia A condition in which the hemoglobin levels are normal but several indices of iron status in the body are below normal levels.

irradiation Process whereby foods are subjected to ionizing radiation to kill bacteria.

ischemia Lack of blood supply.

isoflavones Phytochemicals believed to help prevent various diseases.

isokinetic Literally meaning "same speed"; in weight training an isokinetic machine is used to control the speed of muscle contraction.

isoleucine An essential amino acid.

isometric Literally meaning "same length"; in weight training the resistance is set so that the muscle will not shorten.

isotonic Literally meaning "equal tension or pressure"; in weight training the resistance is set so there is supposed to be equal tension in the muscle through a range of motion, but this is rarely achieved owing to movement of body parts. Isotonic also means equal osmotic pressures between two solutions.

J

jogging A term used to designate slow running; although the distinction between running and jogging is relative to the individual involved, a common value used for jogging is a 9-minute mile or slower.

joule A measure of work in the metric system; a newton of force applied through a distance of 1 meter.

K

ketogenesis The formation of ketones in the body from other substances, such as fats and proteins.

ketogenic amino acids Amino acids that may be deaminated, converted into ketones, and eventually into fat.

ketones Organic compounds containing a carbonyl group; ketone acids in the body, such as acetone, are the end products of fat metabolism.

ketosis The accumulation of excess ketones in the blood; because ketones are acids, acidosis occurs.

key-nutrient concept The concept that if certain key nutrients are adequately supplied by the diet, the other essential nutrients will also be present in adequate amounts. *Also see* indicator nutrients.

kidney stones Compounds in the pelvis of the kidney formed from various salts such as carbonates, oxalates, and phosphates.

kilocalorie (KC) A large Calorie; *see also* Calorie.

kilogram A unit of mass in the metric system; 1 kilogram is the equivalent of 2.2 pounds.

kilogram-meter (KGM) A measure of work in the metric system whereby 1 kilogram of weight is moved through a distance of 1 meter; however, the joule is the recommended unit to express work.

kilojoule One thousand joules; 1 kilojoule (kJ) is approximately 0.25 kilocalorie.

Krebs cycle The main oxidative reaction sequence in the body that generates ATP; also known as the citric acid or tricarboxylic acid cycle.

L

lactic acid The anaerobic end product of glycolysis; it has been implicated as a causative factor in the etiology of fatigue.

lactic acid system The energy system that produces ATP anaerobically by the breakdown of glycogen to lactic acid; used primarily in events of maximal effort for 1 to 2 minutes.

lactose A white crystalline disaccharide that yields glucose and galactose upon hydrolysis; also known as milk sugar.

lactose intolerance Gastrointestinal disturbances due to an intolerance to lactose in milk; caused by deficiency of lactase, an enzyme that digests lactose.

lactovegetarians Vegetarians who include milk products in the diet as a form of high-quality protein.

LDL Low-density lipoprotein; a protein-lipid complex in the blood that facilitates the transport of triglycerides, cholesterol, and phospholipids. *Also see* LDL-cholesterol.

LDL-cholesterol Low-density lipoprotein cholesterol; a mechanism whereby cholesterol is transported in the blood. High blood levels are associated with increased incidence of CHD.

lean body mass The body weight minus the body fat, composed primarily of muscle, bone, and other nonfat tissue.

lecithin A fatty substance of a class known as phospholipids; said to have the therapeutic properties of phosphorus.

legumes The fruit or pods of vegetables, including soybeans, kidney beans, lima beans, garden peas, black-eyed peas, and lentils; high in protein.

leptin Regulatory hormone produced by fat cells; when released into the circulation, it influences the hypothalamus to control appetite.

leucine An essential amino acid.

leukotrienes Eicosanoids that possess hormone-like activity in numerous cells in the body.

levulose Fructose.

lignin A noncarbohydrate form of dietary fiber.

limiting amino acid An amino acid deficient in a specific plant food, making it an incomplete protein; methionine is a limiting amino acid in legumes, whereas lysine is deficient in grain products.

linoleic acid An essential fatty acid.

lipase An enzyme that catabolizes fats into fatty acids and glycerol.

lipids A class of fats or fat-like substances characterized by their insolubility in water and solubility in fat solvents; triglycerides, fatty acids, phospholipids, and cholesterol are important lipids in the body.

lipoic acid A coenzyme that functions in oxidative decarboxylation, or removal of carbon dioxide from a compound.

lipoprotein A combination of lipid and protein possessing the general properties of proteins. Practically all the lipids of the plasma are present in this form.

lipoprotein (a) Serum lipid factor very similar to the LDL, being in the upper LDL density range and containing apolipoprotein (a); high levels are associated with increased risk for CHD.

lipoprotein lipase An enzyme involved in the metabolism of lipoproteins.

lipostatic theory The theory that hunger and satiety are controlled by the lipid level in the blood.

liquid meals Food in a liquid form designed to provide a balanced intake of essential nutrients.

liquid-protein diets Protein in a liquid form; a common form consists of protein predigested into simple amino acids.

liver glycogen The major storage form of carbohydrate in the liver.

long-chain fatty acids (LCFAs) Fatty acids containing chains with 12 or more carbons.

long-haul concept Relative to weight control, the idea that weight loss via exercise should be gradual, and one should not expect to lose large amounts of weight in a short time.

L-tryptophan One form of tryptophan. L is for levo (left), or the direction in which polarized light is rotated when various organic compounds are analyzed.

lycopene A carotenoid that serves as an antioxidant.

lysine An essential amino acid.

M

macrominerals Those minerals essential to human nutrition with an RDA in excess of 100 mg/day: calcium, magnesium, phosphorous, sodium, potassium, chloride.

macronutrient Dietary nutrient needed by the body in daily amounts greater than a few grams, such as carbohydrate, fat, protein, and water.

magnesium A white metallic mineral element essential in human nutrition.

magnetic resonance imaging (MRI) Magnetic-field and radio-frequency waves used to image body tissues; useful for imaging visceral fat.

ma huang A Chinese plant extract theorized to be ergogenic; contains ephedrine, a stimulant.

major minerals *See* macrominerals.

male-type obesity *See* android-type obesity.

malnutrition Poor nutrition that may be due to inadequate amounts of essential nutrients. Too many Calories leading to obesity is also a form of malnutrition. *Also see* subclinical malnutrition.

maltodextrin A glucose polymer that exerts lesser osmotic effects compared with glucose; used in a variety of sports drinks as the source of carbohydrate.

maltose A white crystalline disaccharide that yields two molecules of glucose upon hydrolysis.

manganese A metallic element essential in human nutrition.

MAOD *See* maximal accumulated oxygen deficit.

maximal accumulated oxygen deficit An indirect marker for anaerobic contributions to energy expenditure during exercise obtained by measurement of oxygen consumption during recovery.

maximal heart rate *See* HR max.

maximal heart rate reserve The difference between the maximal HR and resting HR. A percentage of this reserve, usually 60–90 percent, is added to the resting HR to get the target HR for aerobics training programs.

maximal oxygen uptake *See* VO$_2$ max.

meat analogues Food products usually made from plant products and designed to have the flavor, texture, and appearance of meat products. Also known as imitation meat, mock meat, and meat substitute.

meat exchange One very lean meat exchange in the Food Exchange System contains 0–1 gram of fat, 7 grams of protein, and 35 Calories; a lean meat exchange contains 3 grams of fat, 7 grams of protein, and 55 Calories; a medium-fat meat exchange has an additional 2 grams of fat and totals 75 Calories; a high-fat exchange has 5 additional grams of fat and totals 100 Calories.

Mediterranean diet A diet associated with reduced risk of cardiovascular disease attributed to olive oil, the primary source of dietary fat. However, other elements of the Mediterranean diet, such as seafood and vegetables, may also be associated with reduced CHD risk.

Mediterranean Food Guide Pyramid A food group approach to healthful nutrition that includes basic food groups but also lists olive oil and wine as components of the diet.

medium-chain fatty acids (MCFAs) Fatty acids containing chains with 6–12 carbons.

medium-chain triglycerides (MCTs) Triglycerides containing fatty acids with carbon chain lengths of 6–12 carbons.

megadose An excessive amount of a substance in comparison to a normal dose of RDA; usually used to refer to vitamins.

menadione Vitamin K_3.

menoquinone The animal form of vitamin K.

meta-analysis A statistical technique to summarize the findings of numerous studies in an attempt to provide a quantitatively based conclusion.

metabolic aftereffects of exercise The theory that the aftereffects of exercise will cause the metabolic rate to be elevated for a time, thus expending Calories and contributing to weight loss.

metabolic rate The energy expended to maintain all physical and chemical changes occurring in the body.

metabolic syndrome The syndrome of symptoms often seen with android-type obesity, particularly hyperinsulinemia, hypertriglyceridemia, and hypertension.

metabolic water The water that is a by-product of the oxidation of carbohydrate, fat, and protein in the body.

metabolism The sum total of all physical and chemical processes occurring in the body.

metalloenzymes Enzymes that must have a mineral component, such as zinc, to function effectively.

methionine An essential amino acid.

methylmercury An industrial waste product dumped in the seas that may accumulate in large fish; may lead to subsequent nerve damage in children or pregnant females who eat contaminated fish.

metric system A method of measurement based upon units of ten.

METS A measurement unit of energy expenditure; 1 MET equals approximately 3.5 ml O_2/kg body weight/minute.

microgram One-millionth of a gram (μg).

micronutrient Dietary nutrient needed by the body in daily amounts less than a few grams, such as vitamins and minerals.

milk exchange One skim milk exchange in the Food Exchange System contains 12 grams of carbohydrate, 8 grams of protein, a trace of fat, and 90 Calories. A low-fat exchange contains 120 Calories, whereas whole milk has 150 Calories.

milligram One-thousandth of a gram.

millimole One-thousandth of a mole.

mineral An inorganic element occurring in nature.

mitochondria Structures within the cells that serve as the location for the aerobic production of ATP.

mole One mole is the gram molecular weight of a compound, which is the quantity of a substance that equals its molecular weight.

molybdenum A hard, heavy, silvery-white metallic element.

monosaccharides Simple sugars (glucose, fructose, and galactose) that cannot be broken down by hydrolysis.

monounsaturated fatty acids (MUFAs) Fatty acids that have a single double bond.

morbid obesity Severe obesity in which the incidence of life-threatening diseases is increased significantly.

MPF factor Muscle protein factor; an unknown property of meat, fish, and poultry that facilitates the absorption of nonheme iron found in plant foods.

muscle dysmorphia *See* Adonis complex.

muscle glycogen The form in which carbohydrate is stored in the muscle.

muscle hypertrophy An increase in the size of the muscle.

myocardial infarction Death of heart tissue following cessation of blood flow; may be caused by coronary occlusion.

myoglobin An iron-containing compound, similar to hemoglobin, found in the muscle tissues; it binds oxygen in the muscle cells.

myokines Cytokines secreted by muscle tissue.

MyPlate The graphic and program, introduced in 2011, representing the healthful food guidelines presented by the United States Department of Agriculture.

MyPyramid The former graphic and program representing the healthful food guidelines presented by the United States Department of Agriculture. It was replaced by the new model, MyPlate, in 2011.

N

narcotic Any agent that produces insensibility to pain.

National Weight Control Registry A registry of individuals who have lost at least 30 pounds and have kept it off for a year.

Nautilus A brand of exercise equipment designed for strength-training programs; uses a principle to help provide optimal resistance throughout the full range of motion.

NCAA National Collegiate Athletic Association.

negative caloric balance A condition whereby the caloric output exceeds the caloric intake, thus contributing to weight loss.

negative nitrogen balance A condition in which dietary protein is insufficient to meet the nitrogen needs of the body. More nitrogen is excreted than is retained in the body.

net protein utilization (NPU) A technique used to assess protein quality.

neural tube defects (NTD) Birth defects involving incomplete formation of the neural tube in the spinal column of newborn children; may lead to paralysis; may be prevented by adequate folate intake.

neuropeptide Y (NPY) Neuropeptide produced in the hypothalamus; a potent appetite stimulant.

neutron activation analysis A sophisticated, noninvasive method of analyzing body structure and function.

newton A unit of force that will accelerate 1 kilogram of mass 1 meter per second.

NIAAA National Institute on Alcohol Abuse and Alcoholism.

niacin Nicotinamide; nicotinic acid; part of the B complex and an important part of several coenzymes involved in aerobic energy processes in the cells.

niacin equivalents (NE) A unit of measure of niacin activity in a food related to both the amount of niacin present and that obtainable from tryptophan; about 60 mg tryptophan can be converted to 1 mg niacin.

nickel A silvery-white metallic element.

nicotinamide An amide of nicotinic acid; niacin.

nicotinic acid Niacin.

nitrogen A colorless, tasteless, odorless gas comprising about 80 percent of the atmospheric gas; an essential component of protein that is formed in plants during their developmental process.

nitrogen balance A dietary state in which the input and output of nitrogen is balanced so that the body neither gains nor loses protein tissue.

nonessential amino acids Amino acids that may be formed in the body and thus need not be obtained in the diet; also known as dispensable amino acids. *See also* essential amino acids.

nonessential nutrient A nutrient that may be formed in the body from excess amounts of other nutrients.

nonexercise activity thermogenesis (NEAT) Thermogenesis, or heat production by the body, that accompanies physical activity other than volitional exercise.

nonheme iron Iron that is found in plant foods; *see also* heme iron.

nonprotein nitrogen Nitrogen in the body and foods that is associated with nonprotein compounds.

non-shivering thermogenesis An increase in cellular metabolic rate and heat production induced by an increase in sympathetic nervous activity.

normohydration The state of normal hydration, or normal body-water levels, as compared with hypohydration and hyperhydration.

nutraceuticals Nutrients that may function as pharmaceuticals when taken in certain quantities.

nutrient Substance found in food that provides energy, promotes growth and repair of tissues, and regulates metabolism.

nutrient density A concept related to the degree of concentration of nutrients in a given food; *also see* the related concept INQ.

nutrigenomics General term regarding the effects of nutrition on genetic expression and resultant metabolic adaptions.

nutrition The study of foods and nutrients and their effect on health, growth, and development of the individual.

nutritional labeling A listing of selected key nutrients and Calories on the label of commercially prepared food products.

O

obesity An excessive accumulation of body fat; usually reserved for those individuals who are 20–30 percent or more above the average weight for their size.

obesogenic An environment that promotes the development of obesity.

octacosanol A solid white alcohol found in wheat germ oil.

odds ratio (OR) A probability estimate; OR of 1.0 is normal.

Olestra A commercially produced substitute for dietary fat.

oligomenorrhea Intermittent periods of amenorrhea.

omega-3 fatty acids Polyunsaturated fatty acids that have a double bond between the third and fourth carbon from the terminal, or omega, carbon. EPA and DHA found in fish oils are theorized to prevent coronary heart disease.

omega-6 fatty acids Polyunsaturated fatty acids that have a double bond between the sixth and seventh carbon from the terminal, or omega, carbon. Linoleic acid is an essential omega-6 fatty acid.

OmniHeart diet The Optimal MacroNutrient Intake diet, consisting of *healthy* carbohydrates, *healthy* fats, and *healthy* proteins designed to reduce risks of cardiovascular disease, particularly high blood pressure.

ONQI See Overall Nutritional Quality Index

onset of blood lactic acid (OBLA) The intensity level of exercise at which the blood lactate begins to accumulate rapidly.

oral contraceptives Birth control pills used to prevent conception.

oral rehydration therapy (ORT) Fluids balanced in nutrients that help restore normal hydration levels in the body and prevent excessive dehydration.

organic foods Foods that are stated to be grown without the use of manmade chemicals such as pesticides and artificial fertilizers.

orlistat A prescription drug for weight loss that blocks the digestion of dietary fat.

osmolality Osmotic concentration determined by the ionic concentration of the dissolved substance per unit of solvent.

osmoreceptors Receptors in the body that react to changes in the osmotic pressure of the blood.

osmotic pressure A pressure that produces a diffusion between solutions that have different concentrations.

osteomalacia A disease characterized by softening of the bones, leading to brittleness and increased deformity; caused by a deficiency of vitamin D.

osteoporosis Increased porosity or softening of the bone.

Other Specified Feeding or Eating Disorders (OSFED) A category of eating disorders described in *Diagnostic and Statistical Manual of Mental Disorders,* 5th edition (*DSM-V*) known in earlier *DSM* versions as Eating Disorders Not Otherwise Specified (EDNOS).

Overall Nutritional Quality Index Based on the Dietary Reference Intakes and the Dietary Guidelines of Americans, a measure designed to evaluate the nutritional quality of foods and beverages relative to the effects they may have on overall health.

overload principle *See* principle of overload.

overtraining syndrome Symptoms associated with excessive training, such as tiredness, sleeplessness, and elevated heart rate.

overweight Body weight greater than that which is considered normal; *also see* obesity.

ovolactovegetarians Vegetarians who also eggs and milk products as a source of high-quality animal protein.

ovovegetarians Vegetarians who include eggs in the diet to help obtain adequate amounts of protein.

oxalates Salts of oxalic acid, which are found in green leafy vegetables such as spinach and beet greens.

oxidized LDL An oxidized form of low-density lipoprotein that has increased atherogenic potential.

oxygen consumption The total amount of oxygen utilized in the body for the production of energy; it is directly related to the metabolic rate.

oxygen system The energy system that produces ATP via the oxidation of various foodstuffs, primarily fats and carbohydrates.

P

paidotribe Individual who served as a personal trainer in ancient Greece to advise athletes on proper diet and exercise training programs.

Paleolithic (Paleo) diet The diet plan based on what our ancient ancestors (cavemen) ate, often referred to as the hunter/gatherer or carnivore diet, consisting mainly of meat.

pangamic acid A term often associated with "vitamin B_{15}," the essentiality of which has not been established; often contains calcium gluconate and dimethylglycine.

pantothenic acid A vitamin of the B complex.

para-aminobenzoic acid (PABA) Although not a vitamin, often grouped with the B complex.

partially hydrogenated fats Polyunsaturated fats that are not fully saturated with hydrogen through a hydrogenation process; *also see trans* fatty acids.

peak bone mass The concept of maximizing the amount of bone mineral content during the formative years of childhood and young adulthood.

pectin A form of soluble dietary fiber found in some fruits.

pellagra A deficiency disease caused by inadequate amounts of niacin in the diet.

pentose A simple sugar containing five carbons instead of six as in glucose.

peptides Small compounds formed by the union of two or more amino acids; known also as dipeptides, tripeptides, and so on, depending on the number of amino acids combined.

perceptual-motor activities Physical activities characterized by the perception of a given stimulus and culminating in an appropriate motor, or movement, response.

periodization A technique applied to resistance training, as well as other forms of exercise training, that modifies the amount of exercise stress placed on the individual over the course of time. Various cycles, such as the microcycle, mesocycle, and macrocycle, are designed to allow the body to adapt to exercise stress in ways beneficial to performance enhancement.

peripheral vascular disease Atherosclerosis or blockage of the peripheral arteries.

pernicious anemia A severe, progressive form of anemia that may be fatal if not treated with vitamin B_{12}. Usually caused by inability to absorb B_{12}, not a dietary deficiency of B_{12}.

pescovegetarians Vegetarians who eat fish, but not poultry, or other animal meats.

pesticides Poisons used to destroy pests of various types, including plants and animals.

pH The abbreviation used to express the level of acidity of a solution; a low pH represents high acidity.

phenylalanine An essential amino acid.

phenylketonuria (PKU) Congenital lack of an enzyme to metabolize phenylalanine, an essential amino acid. May lead to mental retardation if not detected early in life.

phosphagens Compounds such as ATP and phosphocreatine that serve as a source of high energy in the body cells.

phosphates Salts of phosphoric acid, purported to possess ergogenic qualities.

phosphatidylserine Like phosphatidylcholine, a naturally occurring phospholipid found in cell membranes; as a dietary supplement, it is theorized to possess ergogenic potential.

phosphocreatine (PCr) A high-energy phosphate compound found in the body cells; part of the ATP-PCr energy system.

phospholipids Lipids containing phosphorus that in hydrolysis yield fatty acids, glycerol, and a nitrogenous compound. Lecithin is an example.

phosphorus A nonmetallic element essential to human nutrition.

phosphorus:calcium ratio The ratio of calcium to phosphorus intake in the diet; the normal ratio is 1:1.

photon absorptiometry An analytical, noninvasive technique designed to assess bone density.

phylloquinone Vitamin K; essential in the blood clotting process.

physical activity Any activity that involves human movement; in relation to health and physical fitness, physical activity is often classified as structured and unstructured.

physical activity level (PAL) Increase in energy expenditure through physical activity based on energy expended through daily walking mileage or equivalent activities; National Academy of Sciences lists four PAL categories: Sedentary, Low Active, Active, and Very Active.

Physical Activity Pyramid A guide to weekly physical activity, including aerobic endurance, muscular strength and endurance, and flexibility.

Physical Activity Quotient (PA) Coefficient used to calculate estimated energy requirement (EER) based on categories of physical activity level (PAL).

physical conditioning Methods used to increase the efficiency or capacity of a given body system so as to improve physical or athletic performance.

physical fitness A set of abilities individuals possess to perform specific types of physical activity. *Also see* health-related fitness and sports-related fitness.

phytates Salts of phytic acids; produced in the body during the digestion of certain grain products; can combine with some minerals such as iron and possibly decrease their absorption.

phytochemicals Chemical substances, other than nutrients, found in plants that are theorized to possess medicinal properties to help prevent various diseases.

phytoestrogens Phytochemicals that may compete with natural endogenous estrogens; believed to help prevent certain forms of cancer associated with excess estrogen activity in the body.

phytonutrients Substances found in plants, also known as phytochemicals, that help protect plants from threats, such as bugs. Although not essential nutrients, such as vitamins, Dome phytonutrients may elicit healthful effects in humans.

picolinate A natural derivative of tryptophan; commercially it is bound to chromium as a means of enhancing chromium absorption.

plaque The material that forms in the inner layer of the artery and contributes to atherosclerosis. It contains cholesterol, lipids, and other debris.

platelet aggregability Function of platelets to promote clumping together of red blood cells.

polypeptides A combination of a number of simple amino acids; *also see* peptides.

polysaccharide A carbohydrate that upon hydrolysis will yield more than ten monosaccharides.

polyunsaturated fatty acid Fat that contains two or more double bonds and thus is open to hydrogenation.

positive caloric balance A condition whereby caloric intake exceeds caloric output; the resultant effect is a weight gain.

Positive Health Lifestyle A lifestyle characterized by health behaviors designed to promote health and longevity by helping to prevent many of the chronic diseases afflicting modern society.

postabsorptive state The period after a meal has been absorbed from the gastrointestinal tract; in BMR tests it is usually a period of approximately 12 hours.

potassium A metallic element essential in human nutrition; it is the principal cation present in the intracellular fluids.

power Work divided by time; the ability to produce work in a given period of time.

power-endurance continuum In relation to strength training, the concept that power or strength is developed by high resistance and few repetitions, whereas endurance is developed by low resistance and many repetitions.

PRE See principle of progressive resistance exercise (PRE).

prediabetes A condition predisposing one to type 2 diabetes. Conditions include excess body weight, impaired fasting blood glucose, and glucose intolerance.

pre-event nutrition Dietary intake prior to athletic competition; may refer to a 2- to 3-day period prior to an event or the immediate pre-event meal.

premenstrual syndrome (PMS) A condition associated with a wide variety of symptoms during the time prior to menses.

principle of exercise sequence Relative to a weight-training workout, the lifting sequence is designed so that different muscle groups are utilized sequentially so as to be fresh for each exercise.

principle of overload The major concept of physical training whereby one imposes a stress greater than that normally imposed upon a particular body system.

principle of progressive resistance exercise (PRE) A training technique, primarily with weights, whereby resistance is increased as the individual develops increased strength levels.

principle of recuperation A principle of physical conditioning whereby adequate rest periods are taken for recuperation to occur so that exercise may be continued.

principle of specificity of training The principle that physical training should be designed to mimic the specific athletic event in which one competes. Specific human energy systems and neuromuscular skills should be stressed.

Pritikin program A dietary program developed by Nathan Pritikin, which severely restricts the intake of certain foods like fats and cholesterol and greatly increases the consumption of complex carbohydrates.

profile of mood states (POMS) An inventory to evaluate mood states such as anger, vigor, etc.

proline A nonessential amino acid.

promoters Substances or agents necessary to support or promote the development of a disease once it is initiated.

proof Relative to alcohol content, proof is twice the percentage of alcohol in a solution; 80-proof whiskey is 40 percent alcohol.

prostaglandins Eicosanoids that possess hormone-like activity in numerous cells in the body.

proteases Enzymes that catalyze proteins.

protein Any one of a group of complex organic compounds containing nitrogen; formed from various combinations of amino acids.

protein-Calorie insufficiency A major health problem in certain parts of the world where the population suffers from inadequate intake of protein and total Calories.

protein complementarity The practice among vegetarians of eating foods together from two or more different food groups, usually legumes, nuts, or beans with grain products, in order to ensure a balanced intake of essential amino acids.

Protein Digestibility Corrected Amino Acid Score (PDCAAS) A scientific measure used to assess the quality of protein in foods with values from 1.0 to 0.0, with 1.0 being the highest quality.

protein hydrolysate A high-protein dietary supplement containing a solution of amino acids and peptides prepared from protein by hydrolysis.

protein-sparing effect An adequate intake of energy Calories, as from carbohydrate, will decrease somewhat the rate of protein catabolism in the body and hence spare protein. This is the basis of the protein-sparing modified fast, or diet.

proteinuria The presence of proteins in the urine.

provitamin A Carotene, a substance in the diet from which the body may form vitamin A.

Prudent Healthy Diet A diet plan based upon healthful eating principles that is designed to help prevent or treat common chronic diseases in the United States, Canada, and Mexico, particularly cardiovascular disease and cancer.

psyllium A plant product that contains both water-soluble and insoluble dietary fiber.

purines The end products of nucleoprotein metabolism, which may be formed in the body; they are nonprotein nitrogen compounds that are eventually degraded to uric acid.

pyridoxal A component of the vitamin B group.

pyridoxamine A part of the vitamin B group; an analog of pyridoxine.

pyridoxine A component of the vitamin B complex, vitamin B_6.

pyruvate The end product of glycolysis. Under aerobic conditions it may be converted into acetyl CoA, whereas under anaerobic conditions it is converted into lactic acid.

PYY Peptide YY (PYY), a gut hormone fragment produced by the intestines; affects neurons in the hypothalamus to reduce appetite and food intake.

Q

quackery Misrepresentation of the facts to deceive the consumer.

quality Calories Calories in foods that are accompanied by substantial amounts of nutrients. Skim milk contains quality Calories, as it provides considerable amounts of protein, calcium, and other nutrients, whereas cola drinks provide similar Calories but no nutrients.

quercetin A dietary flavonol, part of polyphenolic compounds that functions as an antioxidant and may be an anti-inflammatory agent.

R

radiation Electromagnetic waves given off by an object; the body radiates heat to a cool environment.

radura International symbol of radiation; used on labels for irradiated foods.

rating of perceived exertion (RPE) (Borg Scale) A subjective rating, on a numerical scale, used to express the perceived difficulty of a given work task.

reactive hypoglycemia A decrease in blood glucose caused by an excessive insulin response to hyperglycemia associated with a substantial intake of high-glycemic-index foods.

Recommended Dietary Allowance(s) (RDA) The levels of intake of essential nutrients considered to be adequate to meet the known nutritional needs of practically all healthy persons.

recommended dietary goals Dietary goals for U.S. citizens that have been established by a U.S. Senate subcommittee on nutrition; goals stress dietary reduction of fat, cholesterol, salt, and sugar, and increase of complex carbohydrates.

recuperation principle *See* principle of recuperation.

Reference Daily Intakes (RDIs) Used in food labeling as the recommended daily intake for protein and selected vitamins and minerals. It replaces the old U.S. RDA (United States Recommended Daily Allowance).

regional fat distribution Deposition of fat in different regions of the body. *See also* android- and gynoid-type obesity.

relative energy deficiency in sport (RED-S) A controversial alternative reference to the condition known as the female athlete triad. Proponents claim RED-S is a more inclusive description for a group of symptoms directly related to restricted energy intake and/or excessive energy expenditure. *Also see* female athlete triad.

relative humidity The percentage of moisture in the air compared to the amount of moisture needed to cause saturation, which is taken as 100.

relative risk (RR) A probability estimate; RR of 1.0 is normal.

relative-weight method A method of determining obesity by comparing the weight of an individual to standardized height and weight tables.

repetition maximum (RM) In weight training, the amount of weight that can be lifted for a specific number of repetitions.

repetitions In relation to weight training or interval training, the number of times that an exercise is done.

resistin An adipokine secreted by adipose tissue that is thought to increase insulin resistance and may be the link between obesity and development of type 2 diabetes.

resting energy expenditure (REE) The energy required to drive all physiological processes while in a state of rest.

resting metabolic rate (RMR) *See* BMR and REE.

retinol Vitamin A.

retinol equivalents (RE) and **retinol activity equivalents (RAE)** Measures of vitamin A activity in food as measured by preformed vitamin A (retinol) or carotene (provitamin A). 1 RE or RAE equals 1 microgram of retinol or 3.3 IU.

rHGH *See* human growth hormone.

riboflavin Vitamin B_2, a member of the B complex.

ribose A five-carbon sugar found in several body compounds, such as riboflavin.

risk factor Associated factor that increases the risk for a given disease; for example, cigarette smoking and lung cancer.

RNA Ribonucleic acid; nuclear material involved in the formation of proteins in cells.

RRR-alpha-tocopherol One of the two major forms of vitamin E; serves as the basis for the RDA.

RRR-gamma-tocopherol One of the two major forms of vitamin E.

running Although the distinction between running and jogging is relative to the individual involved, a common value used for running is 7 mph or faster.

S

saccharide A series of carbohydrates ranging from simple sugars (monosaccharides) to complex carbohydrates (polysaccharides).

saccharine An artificial sweetener made from coal tar.

Salmonella A bacterium commonly involved in food poisoning.

sarcopenia Loss of muscle mass associated with the aging process.

satiety center A group of nerve cells in the hypothalamus that responds to certain stimuli in the blood and provides a sensation of satiety.

saturated fatty acid Fat that has all chemical bonds filled.

SCAN Sports and Cardiovascular Nutritionists, a practice group of the Academy of Nutrition and Dietetics focusing on applications of nutrition to sport and wellness.

scurvy A deficiency caused by a lack of vitamin C in the diet; symptoms include weakness, bleeding gums, and anemia.

SDA Specific dynamic action; often used to represent the increased energy cost observed during the metabolism of protein in the body. *Also see* dietary-induced thermogenesis and TEF.

seasonal affective disorder (SAD) Symptoms associated with various seasons of the year, e.g., depression in winter months.

secondary amenorrhea Cessation of menstruation after the onset of puberty; primary amenorrhea is the lack of menstruation prior to menarche.

Sedentary Death Syndrome (SeDS) Term associated with a sedentary lifestyle and related health problems that predispose to premature death.

selenium A nonmetallic element resembling sulfur; an essential nutrient.

selfish gene A genetic phenotype characterized by dominance of the dopamine-secreting reward-pleasure centers over the hypothalamus in regulating energy intake in favor of highly palatable foods with high energy density and low nutrient density.

semivegetarians Individuals who refrain from eating red meat but include white meat such as fish and chicken in a diet stressing vegetarian concepts.

serotonin A neurotransmitter in the brain; may induce a sense of relaxation and drowsiness, possibly associated with fatigue; may also depress the appetite.

serum lipid level The concentration of lipids in the blood serum.

set-point theory The weight-control theory that postulates that each individual has an established normal body weight. Any deviation from this set point will lead to changes in body metabolism to return the individual to the normal weight.

sets In weight training, a certain number of repetitions constitutes a set; for example, a lifter may do three sets of six repetitions per set.

settling-point theory Theory that the body weight set point may be increased or decreased through interactions of genetics and the environment; an environment rich in high-fat foods may lead to a higher set point so that the body settles in at a higher weight and fat content.

shell temperature The temperature of the skin; *also see* core temperature.

short-chain fatty acids (SCFAs) Fatty acids with chains containing fewer than six carbons.

sibutramine A prescription drug for weight loss that suppresses the appetite by affecting brain neurotransmitters.

sick fat *See* adiposopathy.

silicon A nonmetallic element.

simple carbohydrates Usually used to refer to table sugar, or sucrose, a disaccharide; also other disaccharides and the monosaccharides.

Simplesse A commercially produced fat substitute derived from protein.

skinfold technique A technique used to compute an individual's percentage of body fat; various skinfolds are measured and a regression formula is used to compute the body fat.

sling psychrometer A device that incorporates both a dry-bulb and wet-bulb thermometer, thus providing a heat-stress index incorporating both temperature and relative humidity.

slow-twitch fibers Red muscle fibers that have a slow contraction speed; designed for aerobic-type activity.

Smilax A commercial plant extract theorized to produce anabolic effects.

soda loading Term associated with use of baking soda (sodium bicarbonate) as an ergogenic aid.

sodium A soft metallic element; combines with chloride to form salt; the major extracellular cation in the human body.

sodium bicarbonate $NaHCO_3$; a sodium salt of carbonic acid that serves as a buffer of acids in the blood, often referred to as the alkaline reserve.

sodium citrate A white powder used as a blood buffer; *see also* sodium bicarbonate.

sodium loading Consumption of excess amounts of sodium; endurance athletes may use sodium loading in attempts to increase plasma volume, improve blood flow, and enhance aerobic endurance.

soluble dietary fiber Dietary fibers in plants such as gums and pectins that are soluble in water.

specific dynamic action *See* SDA.

specific heat The amount of energy or heat needed to raise the temperature of a unit of mass, such as 1 kilogram of body tissue, 1 degree Celsius.

specificity of training *See* principle of specificity of training.

sportomics The study of the metabolic response of the athlete in an actual sport environment, not in a laboratory.

sports anemia A temporary condition of low hemoglobin levels often observed in athletes during the early stages of training.

sports bars Commercial food products targeted to athletes and physically active individuals containing various concentrations of carbohydrate, fat, and protein; some products contain other nutrients, such as antioxidants.

sports drinks Popular term for various glucose-electrolyte fluid-replacement drinks.

sports gels Commercial food products targeted to athletes; consist primarily of carbohydrate in a gel form.

sports nutrition The application of nutritional principles to sport with the intent of maximizing performance.

sports-related fitness Components of physical fitness that, when improved, have implications for enhanced sports performance, such as agility and power.

sports supplements Dietary supplements marketed to athletes and physically active individuals.

spot reducing The theory that exercising a specific body part, such as the thighs, will facilitate the loss of body fat from that spot.

standard error of measurement or estimate A measure of variability about the mean. Sixty-eight percent of the population is within one standard error above and below the mean, while about 95 percent is within two standard errors.

standardized exercise An exercise task that conforms to a specific standardized protocol.

Staphylococcus A bacterium commonly involved in food poisoning.

steady state A level of metabolism, usually during exercise, when the oxygen consumption satisfies the energy expenditure and the individual is performing in an aerobic state.

steady-state threshold The intensity level of exercise above which the production of energy appears to shift rapidly to anaerobic mechanisms, such as when a rapid rise in blood lactic acid exists. The oxygen system will still supply a major portion of the energy, but the lactic acid system begins to contribute an increasing share.

sterols Substances similar to fats because of their solubility characteristics; the most commonly known sterol is cholesterol.

stimulus period In exercise programs, the time period over which the stimulus is applied, such as an HR of 150 for 15 minutes.

storage fat Fat that accumulates and is stored in the adipose tissue; *also see* essential fat.

strength-endurance continuum In relation to strength training, the concept that power or strength is developed by high resistance and few repetitions and that endurance is developed by low resistance and many repetitions.

structured physical activity A planned program of physical activities usually designed to enhance physical fitness; often referred to as exercise.

subclinical malnutrition A nutrient-deficiency state in which no clinical signs of the nutrient deficiency are observable, but other nonspecific symptoms such as fatigue may be present.

subcutaneous fat The body fat found immediately under the skin; evaluated by skinfold calipers.

sucrose Table sugar, a disaccharide; yields glucose and fructose upon hydrolysis.

sulfur A pale yellow, nonmetallic element essential in human nutrition; component of the sulfur-containing amino acids.

sumo wrestling A form of wrestling in Japan.

superoxide dismutase An enzyme in body cells that helps neutralize free radicals.

SuperTracker A free, online food and physical activity tracker developed by the U.S. Department of Agriculture, Center for Nutrition Policy and Promotion designed to help you plan, analyze, and track your diet and physical activity.

Syndrome X *See* metabolic syndrome.

synephrine A dietary supplement marketed for fat loss; synephrine is derived from a fruit plant known as bitter orange. Used as an alterative to ephedra, or ephedrine.

systolic blood pressure The blood pressure in the arteries when the heart is contracting and pumping blood.

T

target heart rate range (target HR) In an aerobic exercise program, the heart-rate level that will provide the stimulus for a beneficial training effect.

taurine A vitamin-like compound synthesized from amino acids, mainly methionine and cysteine.

teratogen Any substance that can interfere with the normal development of the embryo or fetus; may lead to various birth defects.

testosterone The male sex hormone responsible for male secondary sex characteristics at puberty; it has anabolic and androgenic effects.

thermic effect of exercise (TEE) Increased muscular contraction produces additional heat.

thermic effect of food (TEF) The increased body heat production associated with the digestion, assimilation, and metabolism of energy nutrients in a meal just consumed.

thermogenesis The production of heat; metabolic processes in the body generate heat constantly.

thiamin Vitamin B$_1$.

threonine An essential amino acid.

threshold stimulus The minimal level of exercise intensity needed to stimulate gains in physical fitness.

thrifty gene A genetic phenotype that increases the ability to store fat and energy in times of abundance. The thrifty gene served nomadic humankind well, but it is hypothesized to contribute to obesity and diabetes in contemporary humankind.

thromboxanes Eicosanoids that possess hormone-like activity in numerous cells in the body.

thyroxine A hormone secreted by the thyroid gland that is involved in control of the metabolic rate.

tin A white, metallic element.

tocopherol Generic name for an alcohol that has the activity of vitamin E.

Tolerable Upper Intake Level (UL) The highest level of daily nutrient intake likely to pose no adverse health risks.

tonicity Tension or pressure as related to fluids; fluids with high osmolality exhibit hypertonicity, whereas fluids with low osmolality exhibit hypotonicity.

total body electrical impedance A sophisticated method of measuring the resistance provided by water in the body as a means to predict body composition.

total body fat The sum total of the body's storage fat and essential fat stores.

total daily energy expenditure (TDEE) The total amount of energy expended during the day, including REE, TEF, and TEE.

total fiber Sum of dietary fiber and functional fiber.

trabecular bone The spongy bone structure found inside the bone, as contrasted with the more compact bone on the outside.

trace minerals Those minerals essential to human nutrition that have an RDA less than 100 mg.

trans **fatty acids** Unsaturated fatty acids in which the hydrogen ions are on opposite sides of the double bond.

triglycerides Fats formed by the union of glycerol and fatty acids.

triose A simple sugar having three carbon atoms.

tryptophan An essential amino acid.

Type I muscle fiber The slow-twitch red fiber that provides energy primarily by the oxygen system.

Type IIa muscle fiber The fast-twitch red fiber that provides energy by both the oxygen system and the lactic acid system.

Type IIb muscle fiber The fast-twitch white fiber that provides energy primarily by the lactic acid system.

tyrosine A nonessential amino acid.

U

ubiquinone *See* CoQ10.

uncompensated heat stress A condition in which heat loss is insufficient to offset heat production during exercise in the heat, the body temperature continues to rise, and exhaustion eventually occurs.

uncoupling protein (UPC) A protein believed to stimulate thermogenesis in fat tissues; uncouples thermogenesis with the production of ATP, so no ATP is generated in this process.

underwater weighing A technique for measuring the percentage of body fat in humans.

United States Recommended Daily Allowances *See* U.S. RDA.

Universal Gym A brand name for exercise equipment, particularly weights for strength development.

unsaturated fatty acids Fatty acids that contain double or triple bonds and hence can add hydrogen atoms.

unstructured physical activity Many of the normal, daily physical activities that are generally not planned as exercise, such as walking to work, climbing stairs, gardening, domestic activities, and games and other childhood pursuits.

urea The chief nitrogenous constituent of urine and the final product of the decomposition of proteins in the body.

uric acid A crystalline end product of purine metabolism; commonly involved in gout and the formation of kidney stones.

USDA United States Department of Agriculture.

USOC United States Olympic Committee.

U.S. RDA The United States Recommended Daily Allowances; the RDA figures used on labels, representing the percentage of the RDA for a given nutrient contained in a serving of the food. The U.S. RDA are now known as the Reference Daily Intake (RDI).

V

valine An essential amino acid.

Valsalva phenomenon A condition in which a forceful exhalation is attempted against a closed epiglottis and no air escapes; such a straining may cause the person to faint.

vanadium A light gray, metallic element.

vanadyl sulfate A salt form of vanadium; marketed for its anabolic potential.

vascular water The body water contained in the blood vessels; a part of the extracellular water.

vasodilation An increase in the size of the blood vessels, usually referring to the arterial system.

vasopressin *See* antidiuretic hormone (ADH).

vegan A vegetarian who eats no animal products.

vegetable exchange One vegetable exchange in the Food Exchange System contains 5 grams of carbohydrate, 2 grams of protein, and 25 Calories.

vegetarian One whose food is of vegetable or plant origin; *also see* lactovegetarian, ovovegetarian, ovolactovegetarian, pescovegetarian, semivegetarian, flexitarian, and vegan.

ventral tegmental area (VTA) One of the oldest parts of the brain; a group of neurons that integrates input from various neural centers and helps to control basic human needs by secreting neurotransmitters, such as dopamine, to other parts of the brain.

very low-Calorie diets (VLCD) Diets containing less than 800 Calories per day.

very low-density lipoprotein *See* VLDL.

visceral fat The deep fat found in the abdominal area; measurement of this fat requires special techniques, such as MRI.

vitamin, natural Often referred to as a vitamin derived from natural sources, i.e., food in nature, contrast with vitamin, synthetic.

vitamin, synthetic An artificial vitamin commercially produced from the separate components of the vitamin.

vitamin A Retinol, an unsaturated aliphatic alcohol; fat soluble.

vitamin B_1 Thiamin; the antineuritic vitamin.

vitamin B_2 Riboflavin.

vitamin B_6 Pyridoxine and related compounds.

vitamin B_{12} Cobalamin, Cyanocobalamin.

vitamin B_{15} Not a vitamin but marketed as one; usual composition is calcium gluconate and dimethylglycine (DMG).

vitamin C Ascorbic acid; the antiscorbutic vitamin.

vitamin D Any one of related sterols that have antirachitic properties; fat soluble.

vitamin D_3 The prohormone form of vitamin D, also known as cholecalciferol, formed in the skin by irradiation from the sun. Released into the blood and eventually converted by the kidney to the hormone form of vitamin D.

vitamin deficiency Subnormal body-vitamin levels due to inadequate intake or absorption; specific disorders are linked with deficiencies of specific vitamins.

vitamin E Various forms of tocotrienols and tocopherols; fat soluble.

vitamin K The antihemorrhagic, or clotting, vitamin; fat soluble.

vitamins A general term for a number of substances deemed essential for the normal metabolic functioning of the body.

VLDL Very low-density lipoproteins; a protein-lipid complex in the blood that transports triglycerides, cholesterol, and phospholipids; has a very low density. *Also see* HDL-cholesterol and LDL-cholesterol.

voluntary dehydration Intentional loss of body fluids in attempts to reduce body mass for sports competition; techniques include exercise, sauna, and diuretics.

VO$_2$ max Maximal oxygen uptake; measured during exercise, the maximal amount of oxygen consumed reflects the body's ability to utilize oxygen as an energy source; equals the cardiac output times the arteriovenous oxygen difference.

W

WADA The World Anti-Doping Agency, which develops and enforces regulations against the use of prohibited performance-enhancing substances by athletes in international sports competition.

waist circumference The circumference of the waist at its most narrow point as seen from the front; used as a measure of regional adeposity.

warm-up Low-level exercises used to increase the muscle temperature and/or stretch the muscles prior to a strenuous exercise bout.

water A tasteless, colorless, odorless fluid essential to life; composed of two parts hydrogen and one part oxygen (H_2O).

water intoxication Consumption of excessive amounts of water leading to dilution of body electrolytes. *See also* hyponatremia.

watt A unit of power in the SI; 1 watt equals about 6 kilogram-meters per minute.

WBGT index Wet-bulb globe thermometer index; a heat-stress index based upon four factors measured by the wet-bulb globe thermometer.

weight cycling Repetitive loss and regain of body weight; often called yo-yo dieting.

wet-bulb globe thermometer A device that takes into account the various factors determining heat stress: air temperature, air movement, radiation heat, and humidity.

wheat germ oil Oil extracted from the embryo of wheat, high in linoleic fatty acid, vitamin E, and octacosanol.

work Effort expended to accomplish something; in terms of physics, force times distance.

X

xerophthalmia Dryness of the conjunctiva and cornea of the eye, which may lead to blindness if untreated; caused by a deficiency of vitamin A.

xylitol A sugar alcohol that may be obtained from fruits.

Y

yohimbine A plant extract theorized to stimulate testosterone production and elicit anabolic effects.

Z

zinc A blue-white, crystalline, metallic element essential to human nutrition.

zone diet A high-protein diet plan; the 40-30-30 plan consisting of 40 percent Calories from carbohydrate and 30 percent each from protein and fat.

Photo Credits

Chapter 1

Opener and Intro: © Digital Vision/Getty Images RF; p. 2: © Author's Image/Glow Images RF; p. 3: © Image Source/Getty Images RF; 1.4: © moorboard/SuperStock RF; 1.8: © Corbis RF; p. 19: © McGraw-Hill Education; p. 20 (left): © SW Productions/Brand X Pictures/Getty Images RF; p. 20 (right): © Ingram Publishing RF; 1.11: © Mauro Femariello/Science Source

Chapter 2

Opener 2a&b and Intro: © Digital Vision/Getty Images RF; Table 2.2: © Oreste Gaspari/Getty Images RF; Fig 2.2 (All): © Greg Kidd and Joanne Scott; p. 43: © Pixtal/AGE Fotostock RF; 2.3: Courtesy U.S. Department of Agriculture, U.S. Department of Health and Human Services; Table 2.4 (top): © Verdina Anna/Getty Images RF; Table 2.4 (bottom): © D. Hurst/Alamy RF; 2.5: © Pixtal/AGE Fotostock RF; p. 49 (top): CMCD/Getty Images RF; p. 49 (bottom): © Photolink/Getty Images RF; 2.7: © Digital Vision/Getty Images RF; 2.8 (left): © McGraw-Hill Education/Mark Dierker, photographer; 2.7 (right): © Greg Kidd and Joanne Scott; 2.9: © McGraw-Hill Education/Mark Dierker, photographer; p. 62: © UpperCut Images/SuperStock RF; p. 63: © Sam Edwards/age fotostock RF; 2.11: © McGraw-Hill Education/Jill Braaten, photographer; 2.12: © Image Source, all rights Reserved RF; p. 79: © 2007 Getty Images RF; p. 80: © Iconotec/Alamy RF; p. 83 (trail mix): © Thomas Northcut/Getty Images RF; p. 83 (peanut butter): © McGraw-Hill Education/Jacques Cornell, photographer; p. 83 (tomatoes): © Adrian Burke/Getty Images RF; p. 83 (bagel): © Copyright © Foodcollection RF

Chapter 3

Opener and Intro: © Digital Vision/Getty Images RF; 3.3: © Samual Ashfield/SPL/Science Source; 3.4: © Delicious Delights/Corbis RF; 3.6: © People in Sports/Corbis RF; p. 102: © RubberBall Productions RF; Table 3.4 (top): © Stockbyte/Getty Images RF; Table 3.4 (bottom): © RubberBall Productions RF; 3.14: © Media for Medical/UIG via Getty Images; p. 109 (left): © RubberBall/Getty Images RF; 3.16: © Digital Vision/PunchStock RF; p. 110: © Purestock/SuperStock RF; p 111: © Hero/Corbis/Glow Images RF

Chapter 4

Opener and Intro: © Corbis/SuperStock RF; p. 138: © lynx/iconotec.com/Glowimages RF; p. 143: © Rubberball/Erik Isakson/Getty Images RF; p. 152: © Jupiterimages RF; p. 156: © lynx/iconotec.com/Glowimages RF; p. 159: © Steve Hambin/Alamy RF; p. 162: © McGraw-Hill Education/Jill Braaten, photographer; p. 166: © Image Source RF

Chapter 5

Opener and Intro: © Corbis/PunchStock RF; p. 189: © McGraw-Hill Education/Ken Karp, photographer; p. 196 and p. 198 (left): © Corbis RF; p. 198 (right): © Andresr/age fotostock RF; 5.17: © Ingram Publishing/SuperStock RF

Chapter 6

Opener and Intro: © Jules Frazier/Getty Images RF; 6.3: © McGraw-Hill Education/John Thoeming, photographer; p. 237: © RubberBall Selects/Alamy RF

Chapter 7

Opener and Intro: © Brand X Pictures/PunchStock RF; p. 284: © D. Hurst/Alamy RF; p. 292: © lynx/iconotec.com/Glow Images RF; p. 296: © Author's Image/Glow Images RF; p. 298: © Pixtal/AGE

Fotostock RF; p. 300 (left): © Ken Welsh/AGE Fotostock RF; p. 300 (right): © Image Source/Glow Images RF; p. 305: © PCN Photography/Alamy RF; p. 315: © Purestock/SuperStock RF

Chapter 8

Opener and Intro: © Digital Vision/Getty Images RF; 8.1: © Sam Edwards/AGE Fotostock RF; p. 336 and 342: © Royalty-Free/CORBIS; p. 352: © Photodisc/Alamy RF

Chapter 9

Opener and Intro: © Karl Weatherly/Getty Images RF; p. 372: © John Lund/Drew Kelly/Blend Images RF; p. 373 (left): © vm/Getty Images RF; p. 373 (faucet): © christopher gonata/SuperStock RF; p. 373 (right): © Purestock/SuperStock RF; p. 373 (faucet): © christopher gonata/SuperStock RF; p. 381: © McGraw-Hill Education; p. 391: © InsideOutPix/AGE Fotostock RF; 9.10 (intestine): © McGraw-Hill Education; p. 406: © BrandXPictures/PunchStock RF; 9.12: © Tony Duffy/Getty Images

Chapter 10

Opener and Intro: © Digital Vision/Getty Images RF; 10.2: © Rick O'Quinn/University of Georgia; 10.3: © Life Measurement Instruments; 10.4: © McGraw-Hill Education/Connie Mueller, photographer; 10.5: © Mauro Fermariello/Science Source; 10.6: © Mediscan/Corbis; p. 438: © Duncan Smith/Getty Images RF; 10.7 (scale): © iStock.com/jgroup RF; 10.7 (food): © John E. Kelly/Getty Images RF; 10.7 (bicyclist): © Chase Jarvis/Getty Images RF; 10.7 (stomach): © Purestock/SuperStock RF; p. 455 (left): © Image Source, all rights reserved RF; p. 455 (right): © Ryan McVay/Getty Images RF; p. 459: © Royalty Free/CORBIS

Chapter 11

Opener and Intro: © Digital Vision/Getty Images RF; p. 489: © JGI/Blend Images LLC; 11.4 (golf ball): © Royalty-Free/CORBIS; 11.4 (tennis ball): © Ron Chapple Stock/FotoSearch/Glow Images RF; 11.4 (yo-yo): © Lawrence Manning/Corbis RF; 11.4 (mouse): © PhotoDisc/Getty Images RF; 11.4 (baseball): © Ron Chapple Stock/FotoSearch/Glow Images RF; 11.4 (fist): © McGraw-Hill Education/Mark Dierker, photographer; 11.6: © Christopher Futcher/Getty Images RF; p. 508: © Trinette Reed/Blend Images LLC RF; 11.10: © Michael Krinkel/Getty Images RF; 11.11b: © McGraw-Hill Education/John Flournoy, photographer; 11.11c: © suedhang/Getty Images RF; p. 520: © Royalty Free/CORBIS

Chapter 12

Opener and Intro: © Digital Vision/Getty Images RF; 12.2: © Iconotec/Glowimages RF; p. 547: © Nice One Production/Corbis RF; 12.4: © Erik Isakson/Blend Images LLC RF

Chapter 13

Opener and Intro: © Lawrence M. Sawyer/Getty Images RF; p. 567 (left): © Planview/Getty Images RF; p. 567 (middle): © broken2/Getty Images RF; p. 567 (right): © gresei/Getty Images RF; p. 570: © Copyright © Foodcollection; 13.3 © Realistic Reflections; 13.4: © Image Source, all rights reserved RF; 13.5: © McGraw-Hill Education/Lars A. Niki, photographer; p. 581: © John A. Rizzo/Getty Images RF; 13.6 and 13.7: © McGraw-Hill Education/Jill Braaten, photographer; 13.8 (lungs): © SCIEPRO/Getty Images RF; 13.9: © Sports & Fitness CD/Corbis RF; 13.10 (oocyte) & (tRNA): © McGraw-Hill Education; 13.11: © McGraw-Hill Education/Jill Braaten, photographer

Glossary: © Digital Vision/Getty Images RF

Index

inosine, 260
protein/carbohydrate
preparations, 244–245
safety, 257–258
special protein
supplements, 241–242
summary, 261
taurine, 260
tyrosine, 259–260
whey and colostrum, 243
excessive protein intake
bone and joint health,
264–265
cardiovascular disease and
cancer, 263–264
heat illnesses, 265
liver and kidney function,
264
hydrolysate, 238
metabolism and function. *See*
Metabolism
plant and animal foods,
226–228
required, 226–227
supplementation
amount, 542–543
carbohydrate, 544
cost, 544
quality, 543–544
timing, 543
Protein and exercises
carbohydrate
protein hydrolysate, 238
protein intake after
exercise, 238–239
protein intake before
exercise, 238
daily energy intake, 237–238
energy intake
aerobic endurance
exercise, 232
leucine and the glucose-
alanine cycle, 233
mechanisms and
by-products, 232–233
protein use and
importance of
carbohydrate, 233
resistance training, 232
need for dietary protein
endurance-type activities,
236–237
strength-type activities,
236
protein losses
gastrointestinal losses,
234
sweat losses, 234
urinary losses, 234
prudent protein intakes,
240–241

recovery after exercise, 234
resistance-trained athletes,
237
before sleep protein intake,
240
supplementation
nutrient timing and
performance, 240
protein and carbohydrate
intake after exercise,
240
training, 234–235
Protein/carbohydrate
preparations, 244–245
Protein-sparing effect, 232
Proteinuria, 234
Prudent Healthy Diet, 14, 15
Purine, 260
Pyridoxine
deficiency, 294–295
DRI, 294
food sources, 294
functions, 294
recommendations, 295
supplementation, 295
Pyruvate, 159–160

Q

Quackery, nutritional
books, 26
cautions on using the
Internet, 27
consultants, 26–27
definition, 24–25
government, organizations,
and websites, 26
popular magazines, 26
prevalence in athletics, 25
recognition, 25–26
scientific journals, 26
Qualified health claims, 68
Quality Calories, 47
Quercetin, 307
Quetelet's Index, 430

R

Radiation, 382
Radura, 76
RAE. *See* Retinol activity
equivalents (RAE)
Rating of perceived exertion
(RPE), 517
RDA. *See* Recommended
Dietary Allowances (RDA)
Reactive hypoglycemia, 132
Reactive oxygen/nitrogen
species (RONS), 279
Reactive oxygen species (ROS),
279

Recommended Dietary
Allowances (RDA), 13, 40
Recommended dietary intakes,
40
REE. *See* Resting energy
expenditure (REE)
Refined sugars and starches
chronic diseases, 162
dental caries, 161–162
Regional fat distribution, 437
Relative energy deficiency in
sport (RED-S), 337
Repetition maximum (RM), 546
Research
creatine supplementation, 29
dietary recommendations,
basis for, 30–31
environmental nutrition, 30
epidemiological research
(observational research),
28
evidence-based medicine,
27–28
experimental research, 28–29
meta-analysis, 30
public understanding,
improving, 29–30
Resistance training
and aerobic exercise, 559
contraindications, 558
equipment, 557
exercises, 550
health benefits, 558–559
health-related benefits, 547
lean muscle mass, 550–551
muscle hypertrophy, 547,
555–558
muscular endurance, 547
primary purposes, 547
principles
exercise sequence,
548–549
overload, 548
periodization, 549
progression, 548
recuperation, 549
specificity, 548
safety concerns
bench press, 551
bent-arm pullover, 552
curl-up, 555
heel raise, 554
lower back protection,
554
machine pull-down, 552
proper breathing, 551–552
seated overhead press,
555
standing curl, 554
using proper technique,
554

using safety equipment,
553
using spotters, 553
warm up, 553–554
strength and power, 547
Resting energy expenditure
(REE), 102, 479–480
dieting and body
composition, 104
environmental factors, 104
estimating daily, 103
during exercise, 111–112
genetic factors, 103–104
Resting metabolic rate (RMR),
102
Retinol. *See* Vitamin A
Retinol activity equivalents
(RAE), 280
Retinol equivalents (RE), 283
Reverse cholesterol transport,
202
RHGH injections/therapy,
590–591
Rhodiola rosea, 597
Riboflavin
deficiency, 292–293
DRI, 292
food sources, 292
functions, 292
recommendations, 293
supplementation, 293
Ribose, 160–161
Risk factors
of coronary artery disease,
513
definition, 2
RM. *See* Repetition maximum
(RM)
RONS. *See* Reactive oxygen/
nitrogen species (RONS)
ROS. *See* Reactive oxygen
species (ROS)
RRR-alpha-tocopherol, 288
RRR-gamma-tocopherol, 288

S

Sarcopenia, 558
Satiety center, 440
Saturated fat
Calories, 179, 180
fatty acids, 177, 181–182
intake, 205–206
iron, 348–349
list, 628
Secondary amenorrhea, 337
Sedentary Death Syndrome
(SeDS), 6
Selenium (Se), 345
deficiency, 355
DRI, 354